SIDNEY HURWITZ, M.D.

Clinical Professor
Pediatrics and Dermatology
Yale University School of Medicine

SECOND EDITION

CLINICAL PEDIATRIC DERMATOLOGY

A Textbook of Skin Disorders of Childhood and Adolescence

W.B. SAUNDERS COMPANY
A Division of Harcourt Brace & Company
Philadelphia London Toronto Montreal Sydney Tokyo

W.B. SAUNDERS COMPANY
A Division of
Harcourt Brace & Company

The Curtis Center
Independence Square West
Philadelphia, Pennsylvania 19106

Library of Congress Cataloging-in-Publication Data

Hurwitz, Sidney
    Clinical pediatric dermatology / Sidney Hurwitz—2nd ed.
      p. cm.
    Includes bibliographical references and index.
    ISBN 0–7216–1515–5
    1. Pediatric dermatology. I. Title.
    [DNLM: 1. Skin Diseases—in adolescence. 2. Skin Diseases—in
infancy & childhood. WS 260 H967c]
    RJ511.H87   1993
    618.92′5—dc20
    DNLM/DLC   92-20398

CLINICAL PEDIATRIC DERMATOLOGY   ISBN 0–7216–1515–5

Printed in The United States of America

Last digit is the print number: 9   8   7   6   5   4   3   2   1

Dedicated to
my wife
TEDDY
and my daughters
WENDY, LAURIE, and ALISON
Without whose patience, encouragement, understanding and sacrifice
this book could not have come to fruition.

PREFACE

Although 20 to 30 per cent of children and adolescents seen by pediatricians, family practitioners, and internists present problems related directly or indirectly to the skin, primary care physicians are often inadequately prepared in the knowledge of pathogenesis, diagnosis, and therapy of cutaneous disorders found in this age group. Throughout my fifteen years of busy private pediatric practice, I came to recognize the ever present need for a wider understanding of the skin diseases that affect children and adolescents. Twenty years ago, my decision was to return to the Yale University School of Medicine to pursue a residency in dermatology, and subsequently to embark upon a career dedicated to the advancement of research, knowledge, and treatment of the skin in childhood and adolescence.

During the past two decades, there has been rapidly growing interest in the field of pediatric dermatology. Twelve years ago, the first edition of *Clinical Pediatric Dermatology* was published. This second edition is a major revision which includes six additional chapters, 700 clinical photographs in color, 97 tables, and more than 2100 updated annotated references.

The text is designed to provide the clinician with information that will enable him to deal effectively with skin problems of the young. The new and exciting disorders as well as the commonly known diseases have been included. Histopathology has been described in an effort to help non-dermatologists to understand the signs and symptoms of cutaneous disease and as an aid to proper diagnosis and appropriate therapy. Emphasis in terminology is placed upon the simple, preferred terms for each disease, with references to other terms of historical significance. Focus is upon diagnosis and treatment; presentation is comprehensive yet concise. Cutaneous lesions are described in detail and extensively illustrated; recent advances are stressed.

It is my feeling that in a textbook of this kind it is essential to reproduce skin disorders in color in an effort to portray variations in hue so valuable to accurate dermatological diagnosis. The cost of color reproduction is so great, however, that it is frequently impossible to utilize color plates and keep the price of the book within the range of practicality. In this book, the use of personal honoraria and the generosity of the following companies helped to underwrite the cost of reproduction of many color plates: Allergan Herbert Laboratories; Dermik Laboratories; Galderma/Owen Laboratories; Glaxo Dermatology; Janssen Pharmaceutica; Kimberly-Clark Corporation; Lever Brothers Company; Neutrogena Corporation; Ortho Pharmaceuticals; Proctor & Gamble; Roche Laboratories; Schering Corporation; Stiefel Laboratories; and Westwood-Squibb Pharmaceuticals.

Appreciation is expressed to my daughter, Dr. Wendy Hurwitz, for her invaluable help in the preparation of the text, and to Lynn Panza and Leslie Stein for their assistance in the typing of the manuscript.

By far the most important person concerned with the execution of this book has been my wife, Teddy. In the beginning, my wife was the only one who recognized my dream of a career in pediatric dermatology. Without her enthusiasm and constant encouragement to forge ahead despite all obstacles, without her sacrifices during my second residency and in the early days of my new venture, without her patience and devoted energy in reviewing my manuscripts, and without her support during my prolonged recovery from legionnaires' disease, my dream would never have become a reality.

In today's market, a single-authored textbook is a rarity, requiring personal sacrifice not only of the author but also of his loved ones. The writing of *Clinical Pediatric Dermatology* was done on "family time." The first edition took six years of nights, weekends, and holidays; the second edition took four years. I am deeply indebted to my wife, Teddy, and our three daughters, Wendy, Laurie, and Alison, who were forced to "wait in the wings" for both projects to be completed.

Without their sustained devotion and understanding, this textbook could never have come to fruition.

The research and writing of this text during a busy schedule of clinical practice, publishing, and lecturing have truly been a labor of love. My hope is that those who utilize this book will enjoy and benefit as much from the reading of it as I have from its research and writing.

SIDNEY HURWITZ, M.D.

CONTENTS

AN OVERVIEW OF DERMATOLOGIC DIAGNOSIS

Accurate diagnosis of cutaneous disease in infants and children is a systematic process that requires careful inspection, evaluation, and some knowledge of dermatologic terminology, morphology, and differential diagnosis. Disorders of the skin in infants and young children vary in many respects from occurrences of the same diseases in older children and adults. The diagnosis and treatment may be confused by more sensitive reaction patterns, a tendency toward vesicle and bulla formation, and therapeutic dosages and regimens that frequently differ from those of adults.

The same basic principles applied to the detection of disorders of any other organ of the body are applicable to the study of cutaneous disease. A thorough physical examination should be performed, an adequate history obtained, and, whenever possible, the clinical impression verified by appropriate laboratory studies. The easy visibility of skin lesions all too frequently results in cursory examination and hasty diagnosis. This tendency must be overcome. The entire skin should be examined routinely and carefully, including the hair, scalp, nails, oral mucosa, anogenital regions, palms, and soles, because findings often hold clues to the final diagnosis.

Examination should be conducted in a well-lighted room. Although natural daylight is the most effective type of illumination for an examination, fluorescent or incandescent lighting of adequate intensity may be satisfactory. A properly sequenced examination requires initial viewing of the patient at a distance in an effort to establish the overall status of the patient and his or her disorder. By this overall evaluation, distribution patterns and clues to the appropriate final diagnosis frequently can be recognized. This initial evaluation is followed by careful scrutiny of primary and subsequent secondary lesions in an effort to discern the characteristic feature of the disorder.

Although not always diagnostic, the morphology and configuration of cutaneous lesions are of considerable importance to the classification and diagnosis of cutaneous disease. Unfortunately, a lack of understanding of dermatologic terminology frequently poses a barrier to the description of cutaneous disorders by clinicians who are not dermatologists. Accordingly, a review of dermatologic terms is included.

GLOSSARY OF DERMATOLOGIC TERMS

Primary Lesions

The term *primary* refers to the most representative, but not necessarily the earliest, lesions; it does not refer to the cutaneous features brought about by secondary changes due to excoriation, eczematization, infection, or previous therapy.

Macules. Macules are flat, circumscribed changes of the skin. They may be of any size, may have no palpable manifestations, and are neither elevated nor depressed in reference to the surrounding skin. Macules may appear as areas of hyperpigmentation, hypopigmentation, or vascular abnormality. They are usually rounded, but may be oval or irregular, and they may be distinct or may fade into the surrounding area. Examples include freckles, lentigines, flat nevi, café au lait spots, tinea versicolor, areas of vitiligo or hypopigmentation, and flat vascular lesions such as telangiectases or capillary lesions of the salmon patch or port-wine type.

Papules, nodules, plaques, and tumors. *Papules* are circumscribed, nonvesicular or nonpustular, elevated lesions less than 0.5 to 1 cm in diameter. When viewed in profile they may be flat topped, or high or low domed, acuminate (tapering to a point), digitate (finger-like), smooth, eroded, or ulcerated; or they may be covered by scales, crusts, or a combination of secondary features. Examples include elevated nevi, verrucae, molluscum contagiosum, and individual lesions of lichen planus.

Nodules are circumscribed, elevated, usually solid lesions that measure 0.5 to 2 cm in diameter (some leeway in size is arbitrarily allowed here). They may be located only in the epidermis or may extend deeper into the dermis or subcutaneous tissue. Examples include fibromas, neurofibromas, xanthomas, intradermal or compound nevi, lesions of erythema nodosum, and various benign or malignant growths.

Plaques are broad, elevated, disk-shaped lesions that occupy a relatively large area. They are frequently formed by a confluence of papules and may be seen in psoriasis, lichen simplex chronicus (neurodermatitis), or lesions of lichen planus.

Tumors are larger and deeper circumscribed solid lesions of the skin or subcutaneous tissue. They may be benign or malignant processes and include lesions such as lipomas, strawberry or cavernous hemangiomas, and various neoplastic growths.

Wheals. *Wheals* are a distinctive type of solid elevation formed by local, superficial, transient edema. White to pink or pale red, compressible, and evanescent, they often disappear within a period of hours. They vary in size and shape and may be seen in dermographism, insect bites, and various forms of urticaria.

Vesicles and bullae. *Vesicles* are sharply circumscribed, elevated, fluid-containing lesions that measure 0.5 cm in diameter or less. Examples include lesions of herpes, dyshydrosis, pompholyx, varicella, and contact dermatitis.

Bullae are larger circumscribed, elevated fluid-containing lesions over 0.5 cm in diameter. They may be seen in burns, contact dermatitis, pemphigus, bullous impetigo, neonatal herpes simplex, and epidermolysis bullosa.

Pustules. *Pustules* are circumscribed elevations that contain a purulent exudate. They may be bacterial, as in pyoderma (impetigo), or may be sterile, as in pustular psoriasis, bromoderma, or smallpox.

Comedones. *Comedones* are plugged secretions of horny material retained within a pilosebaceous follicle. They may be flesh-colored, closed comedones (whiteheads), or slightly raised brown or black open comedones (blackheads). Closed comedones, in contrast to open comedones, may be difficult to visualize. They appear as pale, slightly elevated small papules without a clinically visible orifice. Since closed comedones are the precursors of the papules, pustules, cysts, or nodules of acne, they are of considerable clinical importance.

Burrows. *Burrows* are linear lesions produced by tunneling of an animal parasite in the stratum corneum. Burrows may be seen in scabies or cutaneous larva migrans (creeping eruption) and, when present, are highly characteristic and diagnostic of these disorders.

Telangiectasia. The term *telangiectasia* refers to a relatively permanent dilatation of superficial venules, capillaries, or arterioles of the skin. These dilatations may be seen in actinically damaged skin, rosacea, radiodermatitis, hereditary hemorrhagic telangiectasia (Osler-Weber-Rendu disease), essential telangiectasia, angiokeratomas, lesions of lupus erythematosus, lipomas, and basal cell epitheliomas; and when present in the cuticular region (cuticular telangiectasia) they are a pathognomic sign of connective tissue disease, such as lupus erythematosus, dermatomyositis, or scleroderma.

Secondary Lesions

Secondary lesions represent evolutionary changes that occur later on in the course of the cutaneous disorder. Although helpful in dermatologic diagnosis, they do not offer the same degree of diagnostic aid as that afforded by primary lesions of a cutaneous disorder.

Crusts and scales. *Crusts* are the result of dried remains of serum, blood, pus, or exudate overlying areas of lost or damaged epidermis. They may be seen in third-degree burns, in lesions of weeping eczematous dermatitis, or as dried honey-colored lesions of impetigo. Crusts are yellow when formed by dried serum, green or yellowish green when formed by purulent exudate, and dark red or brown when formed by bloody exudative serum.

Scales are formed by an accumulation of compact desquamation layers of stratum corneum. A result of abnormal keratinization and exfoliation of cornified keratinocytes, they may be greasy and yellowish (seborrheic dermatitis), silvery and mica-like (psoriasis), fine and barely visible (pityriasis alba or tinea versicolor), or large, adherent, and lamellar (in various forms of ichthyosis).

Fissures and erosions. A *fissure* is a dry or moist linear, often painful, cleavage in the cutaneous surface that results from marked drying and long-standing inflammation, thickening, and loss of elasticity of the integument. Fissures frequently appear in chronic dermatoses, calluses of the hands and feet, keratoderma of the palms and soles (tylosis), angular cheilitis, and perianal lesions such as perianal psoriasis and perianal streptococcal disease.

Erosions are moist, slightly depressed vesicular lesions in which part or all of the epidermis has been lost or denuded. Since erosions do not extend into the underlying dermis or subcutaneous tissue, healing occurs without subsequent scar formation.

Excoriations and ulcerations. The term *excoriation* refers to a traumatized or abraded (usually self-induced) superficial loss of skin caused by scratching, rubbing, or scrubbing of the cutaneous surface. Excoriations are seen in pruritic disorders such as atopic dermatitis, neurotic excoriations, contact dermatitis, fiberglass dermatitis, prurigo nodularis, icterus, varicella, papular urticaria, dermatitis herpetiformis, scabies, pediculosis, and acne excoriée.

Cutaneous ulcers are the result of necrosis of the epidermis and part or all of the dermis and/or the underlying subcutaneous tissue. Ulcers may occur as the result of bacterial, parasitic, or fungal infection, vasculitis, tissue infarction, halogenoderma, scleroderma, ecthyma, frostbite, sickle cell disease, and benign or neoplastic necrosis of tissue (as in decubitus ulcers, basal cell epithelioma, reticulum cell sarcoma, and proliferating tumors).

Atrophy. *Atrophy* refers to cutaneous changes that result in depression of the epidermis, dermis, or both. Epidermal atrophy is characterized by thin, almost translucent epidermis, a loss of the normal skin markings, and wrinkling when subjected to lateral pressure or pinching of the affected area. In dermal atrophy there is a depression of the skin without change in color or skin markings.

Scars (cicatrices) and keloids. *Scars* are permanent fibrotic skin changes that develop following damage to the dermis. Initially pink or violaceous, as the color fades they remain as permanent white, shiny, sclerotic areas. Although fresh scars often tend to be hypertrophic, with passage of time (frequently 6 months to 1 year) they usually contract and become less apparent.

Hypertrophic scars must be differentiated from keloids, which represent an exaggerated connective tissue response to skin injury. Keloids are pink, smooth, and rubbery and are often traversed by telangiectatic vessels. They tend to increase in size long after healing has taken place and can be differentiated from hypertrophic scars by the fact that the surface of keloidal scars tends to proliferate beyond the area of the original wound.

Configuration of Lesions

Annular, circinate, or ring-shaped lesions. A number of dermatologic entities assume annular shapes and are interpreted as "ringworm" or superficial fungal infections. Although tinea is indeed one of the common annular dermatoses of childhood, other disorders that must be included in the differential diagnosis of ringed lesions include pityriasis rosea, seborrheic dermatitis, nummular eczema, lupus erythematosus, granuloma annulare, psoriasis, erythema multiforme, erythema annulare centrifugum, erythema migrans, secondary syphilis, sarcoidosis, urticaria, pityriasis alba, tinea versicolor, lupus vulgaris, drug eruptions and cutaneous T-cell lymphoma (mycosis fungoides).

Arciform or arcuate lesions. The terms *arciform* and *arcuate* refer to lesions that assume arc-like configurations. Arciform lesions may be seen in erythema multiforme, urticaria, and pityriasis rosea.

Confluent lesions. Lesions that tend to join or run together are said to be confluent. Confluence of lesions is seen in childhood exanthems, *Rhus* dermatitis, erythema multiforme, and urticaria.

Dermatomal lesions. Lesions localized into a dermatome supplied by one or more dorsal ganglia are referred to as dermatomal. Prominent examples of this type of distribution include lesions of herpes zoster and segmental vitiligo.

Discoid lesions. *Discoid* is used to describe lesions that are solid, moderately raised, and disk shaped. Although the term is frequently used to differentiate cutaneous from systemic forms of lupus erythematosus, since one cannot determine from the clinical or histologic examination of a discoid lesion whether there is systemic involvement, a more appropriate term would be *cutaneous*.

Discrete lesions. Individual lesions that tend to remain separated and distinct are referred to as discrete. Discrete lesions appear in a variety of conditions; and although perhaps of descriptive value, this term is neither characteristic nor diagnostic of any specific disorder.

Eczematoid or eczematous disorders. *Eczematoid* and *eczematous* are adjectives relating to eczema and suggest inflammation with a tendency to thickening, oozing, vesiculation, or crusting.

Grouping or clustering. Grouping and clustering are characteristic of vesicles of herpes simplex or herpes zoster, insect bites, lymphangioma circumscriptum, contact dermatitis, and bullous dermatosis of childhood.

Guttate lesions. Guttate or drop-like lesions are characteristic of flares of psoriasis in children and adolescents that follow an acute upper respiratory tract infection that is usually, but not necessarily, streptococcal.

Gyrate lesions. *Gyrate* refers to twisted, coiled, or spiral-like lesions, such as may be seen in patients with urticaria and erythema annulare centrifugum.

Iris lesions. Iris or target-like lesions are concentric ringed lesions characteristic of erythema multiforme of both the regular and bullous (Stevens-Johnson) varieties.

Keratosis (keratotic). The term *keratosis* refers to circumscribed patches of horny thickening, as seen in seborrheic or actinic (solar) keratoses, keratosis pilaris, and keratosis follicularis (Darier's disease). *Keratotic* is an adjective pertaining or relating to keratosis and frequently refers to the horny thickening of the skin seen in chronic dermatitis and callus formation.

Koebner phenomenon (isomorphic response). The Koebner phenomenon refers to an isomorphic response with the appearance of lesions along the site of injury. This phenomenon may be seen with warts, molluscum contagiosum, *Rhus* dermatitis (poison ivy), psoriasis, lichen planus, lichen nitidus, pityriasis rubra pilaris, and keratosis follicularis (Darier's disease).

Linear disorders. Lesions in a linear or band-like configuration appear in the form of a line or stripe and may be seen in linear nevi (nevus unius lateris), Conradi's syndrome, linear morphea or scleroderma (the coup de sabre deformity or pansclerotic morphea), lichen striatus, striae, *Rhus* dermatitis, deep mycoses (sporotrichosis or coccidioidomycosis), incontinentia pigmenti, hypomelanosis of Ito, porokeratosis of Mibelli, or factitial dermatitis.

Moniliform lesions. The term *moniliform* refers to a banded or necklace-like appearance. This is seen in monilethrix, a hair deformity characterized by beaded nodularities along the hair shaft.

Multiform lesions. The term *multiform* refers to disorders in which more than one variety or shape of cutaneous lesions occurs. The most common manifestation of this configuration is typified by the varied lesions seen in patients with erythema multiforme, early Henoch-Schönlein purpura, and polymorphous light eruption.

Polycyclic. The term *polycyclic* refers to oval lesions containing more than one ring. This frequently is seen in patients with urticaria.

Reticular. A reticulated or net-like pattern may be seen in erythema ab igne, livedo reticularis, cutis marmorata, cutis marmorata telangiectatica congenita (congenital phlebectasia), and lesions of confluent and reticulated papillomatosis.

Serpiginous. The term *serpiginous* describes the shape or spread of lesions in a serpentine or snake-like configuration. This term is used to describe lesions of cutaneous larva migrans (creeping eruption) and elastosis perforans serpiginosa.

Umbilicated lesions. The terms *umbilication* and *umbilicated* refer to lesions that are depressed or shaped like an umbilicus or navel. Examples include lesions of molluscum contagiosum, varicella, vaccinia, variola, herpes zoster, and Kaposi's varicelliform eruption.

Universal (universalis). The terms *universal* and *universalis* imply widespread disorders affecting the entire skin (as in alopecia universalis).

Zosteriform. The term *zosteriform* is a descriptive term that implies a linear arrangement along a nerve. This configuration is typified by lesions of herpes zoster and linear forms of keratosis follicularis (zosteriform Darier's disease).

REGIONAL DISTRIBUTION AND MORPHOLOGIC PATTERNS

The regional distribution and morphologic configuration of cutaneous lesions are frequently helpful in dermatologic diagnosis.

Acneiform (acneform) or acne-like distribution patterns. Acneiform lesions are those appearing like or having the form of acne or lesions of acne. An acneiform distribution refers to lesions primarily seen on the face, neck, chest, upper arms, shoulders, and back.

Atopic dermatitis. Sites of predilection of atopic dermatitis include the face, trunk, and extremities in young children; the extremities (particularly the antecubital fossae and popliteal fossae) in older children and adults; and the face, neck, trunk, and antecubital fossae and popliteal fossae in adolescents and adults.

Erythema multiforme. Lesions of erythema multiforme may be widespread but have a distinct predilection for the hands and feet (particularly the palms and soles) and mucous membranes.

Herpes simplex. Lesions of herpes simplex may appear anywhere on the body but have a distinct predisposition for the areas about the lips, face, and genitalia. Herpes zoster generally has a dermatomal or nerve-like distribution and is usually but not necessarily unilateral. Over 75 per cent of cases occur between the second dorsal and second lumbar vertebrae, the fifth cranial nerve frequently is involved, and only rarely are lesions seen below the elbows or knees.

Lichen planus. Lesions of lichen planus frequently affect the limbs. Favorite sites include the lower extremities, the flexor surface of the wrists, the buccal mucosa, the trunk, and the genitalia.

Lupus erythematosus. The favorite locations include the bridge of the nose and the malar eminences, scalp, ears, buccal mucosa, arms, legs, hands, fingers, back, chest, or abdomen. The patches tend to spread at the border and clear in the center, with atrophy, scarring, and telangiectases. The malar or butterfly rash is neither specific for nor the most frequent sign of lupus erythematosus, and telangiectasia without the accompanying features of erythema, scaling, or atrophy is never a marker of this disorder.

Photodermatoses. Photodermatoses are cutaneous disorders caused or precipitated by exposure to light. Areas of predilection include the face, ears, anterior "V" of the neck, upper chest, the dorsal aspect of the forearms and hands, and exposed areas of the legs, with sparing of the shaded regions of the upper eyelids, subnasal, and submental regions. The major photosensitivity disorders are lupus erythematosus, dermatomyositis, polymorphous light eruption, drug photosensitization, and porphyria.

Photosensitive reactions cannot be distinguished on a clinical basis from lesions of photocontact allergic conditions, may reflect internal as well as external photoallergens, and may simulate contact dermatitis from airborne sensitizers. Lupus erythematosus can be differentiated by the presence of atrophy, scarring, hyperpigmentation, or hypopigmentation and the presence of cuticular telangiectases. Dermatomyositis with swelling and erythema of the cheeks and eyelids should be differentiated from allergic contact dermatitis by the heliotrope hue and other associated changes, particularly those of the fingers (telangiectases of the cuticles, Gottron's papules, and subungual hyperkeratosis) when present.

Pityriasis rosea. This benign, exceedingly common eruption is observed most frequently in children and young adults but also may appear in infants. In 70 to 80 per cent of cases the generalized eruption starts with a solitary round or oval lesion known as the herald patch followed, after an interval of 7 to 10 days, by a generalized symmetrical eruption that involves mainly the trunk and proximal limbs, with the long axis of oval lesions parallel to the lines of cleavage in what has been termed a *Christmas-tree pattern.*

Psoriasis. Classic lesions of psoriasis consist of round, erythematous, well-marginated patches with a rich red hue covered by a characteristic grayish or silvery white mica-like (micaceous) scale, which, on removal, may result in pinpoint bleeding (Auspitz's sign). Although exceptions occur, lesions generally are seen in a bilaterally symmetrical pattern with a predilection for the elbows, knees, scalp, and lumbosacral, perianal, and genital regions. Nail involvement, a valuable diagnostic sign, is characterized by pitting of the nail plate, discoloration, separation of the nail from the nail bed (onycholysis), and an accumulation of subungual scale (subungual hyperkeratosis). A characteristic feature of this disorder is the Koebner or isomorphic response in which new lesions appear at sites of local injury.

Scabies. The diagnosis of scabies is best made by a history of itching; a characteristic distribution of lesions on the wrists and hands (particularly the interdigital webs), forearms, genitalia, areolae, and buttocks; the recognition of primary lesions (particularly the pathognomonic burrow when present); and the presence of disease among the patient's family or associates. In infants and young children the diagnosis is often overlooked because of a lower index of suspicion; an atypical distribution that includes the head, neck, palms, and soles; and obliteration of demonstrable primary lesions due to vigorous hygienic measures, excoriation, crusting, eczematization, and secondary infection.

Seborrheic dermatitis. Seborrheic dermatitis is an erythematous, scaly or crusting eruption that characteristically occurs on the scalp, face, and postauricular, presternal, and intertriginous areas. The classic lesions are dull or pinkish yellow or salmon colored, with fairly sharp borders and overlying yellowish greasy scale. Morphologic and topographic variants occur in many combinations and with varying degrees of severity, from mild involvement of the scalp with occasional blepharitis to generalized and occasionally severe eczematous eruptions. The differential diagnosis includes atopic dermatitis, psoriasis, various forms of diaper dermatitis, Letterer-Siwe disease, scabies, pediculosis, tinea corporis or capitis, pityriasis rosea, pityriasis alba, contact dermatitis, Mucha-Habermann disease, Darier's disease, pityriasis rubra pilaris, and lupus erythematosus.

Warts. Warts are common viral cutaneous lesions characterized by the appearance of skin-colored small papules of several morphologic types. They may be elevated or flat lesions and tend to appear in areas of trauma, particularly the dorsal surface of the face, hands, periungual areas, elbows, knees, feet, and genital or perianal areas. Close examination may reveal capillaries appearing as punctate dots scattered over the surface.

Disorders associated with increased scaling. A large number of cutaneous diseases are associated with abnormalities of keratinization. These include the ichthyoses, keratosis pilaris, lichen spinulosus, palmar and plantar keratosis (keratoderma), pityriasis rubra pilaris, hypervitaminosis A (vitamin A intoxication), and keratosis follicularis (Darier's disease).

Variations in black skin and hair. The skin of black children varies in several ways from that of children of white and Asian backgrounds. Among the black population, (1) genetic background, (2) relatively poor socioeconomic status, and (3) mores and customs may at times alter the individual physician's therapeutic approach to cutaneous problems. Skin disorders more commonly seen are impetigo, papular urticaria, tinea capitis, sickle cell ulcers, sarcoidosis, sycosis barbae, acne keloidalis, and dissecting cellulitis of the scalp (perifolliculitis capitis abscedens et suffodiens). Tinea versicolor is very common in blacks because of a higher incidence in tropical climates and because of the easy visibility of lesions in marked contrast to uninvolved surrounding skin. Lichen nitidus is more apparent and possibly more common in black individuals; lichen planus is reported to be more severe; and keloids are seen more frequently.

Erythema in black skin is difficult to see and frequently has a purplish tinge that can be confusing to unwary observers. In atopic dermatitis there is often a variation in pigmentary change (areas of hypopigmentation or hyperpigmentation are more extensive and more obvious) and lesions frequently have a follicular quality. Secondary syphilis often has a follicular quality and is papular and annular. Psoriasis, dermatitis herpetiformis, pemphigus vulgaris, and pediculosis capitis are relatively uncommon, and lupus erythematosus is seen only half as frequently in black individuals as it is in white individuals.

Black skin tans on exposure to sunlight, and although slight erythema may develop after exposure to sun, sunburn and chronic sun-induced diseases such as actinic keratosis and actinically induced carcinomas of the skin (e.g., squamous cell carcinoma, keratoacanthoma, basal cell carcinoma, and malignant melanoma) have an extremely low incidence in blacks.

The hair of blacks varies from that of whites and Asians, as well. Black hair tends to tangle when dry and becomes matted when wet. As a result of its natural curly or spiral nature, pseudofolliculitis barbae is more common in blacks than whites. Frequent and liberal use of greasy lubricants and pomades produces a comedonal and papulopustular form of acne (pomade acne). Frequent use of picks for hair grooming, the use of hot pressing oils in hair-straightening techniques, and tight braiding of the hair are common causes of traumatic alopecia.

Disorders of pigmentation. Various disorders of hyperpigmentation and hypopigmentation may become manifest in infancy and childhood. Disorders of hyperpigmentation include postinflammatory hyperpigmentation, mongolian spots, various moles and nevi, café au lait spots, postinflammatory hyperpigmentation, incontinentia pigmenti, fixed drug eruption, photodermatitis, phytophotodermatitis, chloasma, Riehl's melanosis, argyria, acanthosis nigricans, and Addison's disease. Yellowish discoloration of the skin is common in infants. This condition generally is related to the presence of carotene derived from excessive ingestion of foods, particularly yellow vegetables containing carotenoid pigments.

Disorders of depigmentation or hypopigmentation may be seen as vitiligo, postinflammatory hypopigmentation, pityriasis alba, tinea versicolor, chemical depigmentation, halo nevi, achromic nevi, albinism and partial albinism (piebaldism), Waardenburg's syndrome, Vogt-Koyanagi syndrome, Tietz's syndrome, Chédiak-Higashi syndrome, tuberous sclerosis, incontinentia pigmenti achromians (hypomelanosis of Ito), and leprosy.

2

CUTANEOUS DISORDERS OF THE NEWBORN

NEONATAL SKIN

The skin of the infant differs from that of an adult in that it is thinner, is less hairy, has weaker intercellular attachments, and produces fewer sweat and sebaceous gland secretions (Table 2–1). Although much has been published on the various disorders and phenomena peculiar to the integument of infants, it is unfortunate that actually very little is known about the physiologic variations and reactivity of the skin in the neonatal age group. As a result, the skin of the newborn presents a broad area for research and investigation.

The concept that neonatal skin is more susceptible to external irritants remains controversial and requires further investigation. Percutaneous absorption is known to occur through two major pathways: through the cells of the stratum corneum and the epidermal malpighian layer (the transepidermal route) and through the hair follicle–sebaceous gland component (the transappendageal route). Although for years physicians have considered neonatal skin to be more susceptible to the percutaneous absorption of potentially toxic substances, current data reveal that although the skin of the premature infant is indeed more permeable, undamaged skin of normal full-term newborns (except for the scrotal area) is no more susceptible to percutaneous absorption than that of older children or adults.[1, 2] The problem of percutaneous permeability and absorption in infancy, therefore, is one of a greater relative skin surface to

Table 2–1. CHARACTERISTICS OF NEONATAL SKIN IN COMPARISON WITH ADULT SKIN

1. Thinner, less hairy, weaker intercellular attachments
2. Fewer eccrine and sebaceous gland secretions
3. Increased susceptibility to external irritants
4. Increased susceptibility to micrococcal infection
5. Depressed contact allergen reactivity
6. Percutaneous permeability increased only in premature infants or in damaged or scrotal skin

body volume ratio in infants and small children (as compared with that of older children and adults). This results in the risk of higher blood level accumulations of potentially toxic substances in this age group.

Skin Care of the Newborn. The skin of the newborn is covered with a grayish white greasy material termed *vernix caseosa.* The vernix represents a physiologic protective covering derived partially by secretion of the sebaceous glands and in part as a decomposition product of the infant's epidermis. Although its function is not completely understood, most studies suggest that it be left on as a protective coating for the newborn skin and that it be allowed to come off by itself with successive changes of clothing (generally within the first few weeks of life).

The skin acts as a protective organ. Any break in its integrity, therefore, affords an opportunity for initiation of infection. Skin care of the newborn is complicated by the fact that the infant does not have protective skin flora at birth, has at least one, and possibly two, open surgical wounds (the umbilicus and circumcision site), and is exposed to fomites and personnel that potentially harbor a variety of infectious agents.

Skin care should involve gentle cleansing with a nontoxic, nonabrasive neutral material. During the 1950s the use of hexachlorophene-containing compounds became routine for the skin care of newborns as prophylaxis against *Staphylococcus aureus* infection. In 1971 and 1972, however, the use of hexachlorophene preparations as skin cleansers for newborns was restricted because of studies demonstrating vacuolization in the central nervous system of infants and laboratory animals after prolonged application of these preparations. As a result, current recommendations for the management of skin care suggest gentle removal of blood from the face and head, and meconium from the perianal area, by careful water rinsing. The remainder of the skin is probably best left alone unless grossly soiled. Vernix caseosa should be removed from the face only, allowing that remaining on the rest of the body to come off by itself. For the remainder of the infant's stay in the hospital nursery, the buttocks and perianal regions should be cleansed with water and cotton. A mild soap with water rinsing may also be used at diaper changes if desired.

There is no single method of umbilical cord care that has been proven to limit colonization and dis-ease. Several methods include local application of alcohol, triple dye (an aqueous solution of brilliant green, proflavine, and crystal violet), and antimicrobial agents such as bacitracin (Neosporin, Polysporin) or silver sulfadiazine cream.

PHYSIOLOGIC DISORDERS OF THE NEWBORN

Neonatal dermatology, by definition, encompasses the spectrum of cutaneous disorders that arise during the first 4 weeks of life. Many such conditions are transient, appearing in the first few days to weeks of life, only to disappear shortly thereafter. The appreciation of normal phenomena and their differentiation from the more significant cutaneous disorders of the newborn is critical for the general physician, obstetrician, and pediatrician, as well as for the pediatric dermatologist.

At birth the skin of the full-term infant is normally soft, smooth, and velvety. Desquamation of neonatal skin generally takes place 24 to 36 hours after delivery and may not be complete until the third week of life. When seen at birth, this is an abnormal phenomenon and is indicative of postmaturity, intrauterine anoxia, or congenital ichthyosis.

The skin at birth has a purplish red color that is most pronounced over the extremities. Except for the hands, feet, and lips, where the transition is gradual, this quickly changes to a pink hue. In a great number of infants a purplish discoloration of the hands, feet, and lips occurs during periods of crying, breath holding, or chilling. This normal phenomenon, termed *acrocyanosis,* appears to be associated with an increased tone of peripheral arterioles, which in turn creates vasospasm, secondary dilatation, and pooling of blood in the venous plexuses, resulting in a cyanotic appearance to the involved areas of the skin. The intensity of cyanosis depends on the degree of oxygen loss and the depth, size, and fullness of the involved venous plexus. Acrocyanosis, a normal physiologic phenomenon, should not be confused with true cyanosis.

Cutis Marmorata

Cutis marmorata is a normal reticulated bluish mottling of the skin seen on the trunk and extremities of infants and young children (Fig. 2–1). This phenomenon, a physiologic response to chilling, with resultant dilatation of capillaries and small venules, usually disappears as the infant is rewarmed. Although a tendency to cutis marmorata may persist for several weeks or months, this disorder bears no medical significance and treatment generally is unnecessary. In some children cutis marmorata may tend to recur until early childhood, and in patients with Down's syndrome, trisomy 18, and the Cornelia de Lange syndrome, this reticu-

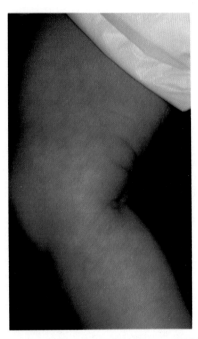

Figure 2-1. Cutis marmorata. A normal reticulated bluish pattern of the skin seen as a physiologic response to cool environmental temperatures in infants and, at times, young children.

Bronze Baby Syndrome

The *bronze baby syndrome* is a term used to describe infants who develop a grayish brown discoloration of the skin, serum, and urine while undergoing phototherapy for hyperbilirubinemia. Although the exact source of the pigment causing the discoloration is not clear, the syndrome usually begins 1 to 7 days after the initiation of phototherapy, resolves gradually over a period of several weeks after phototherapy is discontinued, and appears to be related to a combination of photoisomers of bilirubin or biliverdin or a photoproduct of copper–porphyrin metabolism.[4–6] The disorder should be differentiated from neonatal jaundice, cyanosis associated with neonatal pulmonary disorders or congenital heart disease, an unusual progressive hyperpigmentation (universal acquired melanosis, the "carbon baby" syndrome),[7] and chloramphenicol intoxication (the "gray baby" syndrome), which is a disorder in infants with immature liver function who are unable to conjugate chloramphenicol characterized by elevated serum chloramphenicol levels, progressive pallid cyanosis, abdominal distention, hypothermia, vomiting, irregular respiration, and vasomotor collapse.[8]

lated marbling pattern may be persistent. In some infants a white negative pattern of this phenomenon (*cutis marmorata alba*) may be created by a transient hypertonia of the deep vasculature. Cutis marmorata alba is also a transitory disorder and appears to have no clinical significance.

Harlequin Color Change

Harlequin color change, not to be confused with that of the harlequin fetus, is occasionally observed in full-term infants but usually occurs in premature infants. Seen in up to 10 per cent of infants, the harlequin color change occurs when the infant is lying on his or her side and consists of reddening of one half of the body with simultaneous blanching of the other half. Attacks develop suddenly and may persist for 30 seconds to 20 minutes. The side lying uppermost is paler, and a clear line of demarcation runs along the midline of the body. At times this line of demarcation may be incomplete; and when attacks are mild, areas of the face and genitalia may not be involved.

This phenomenon appears to be related to immaturity of hypothalamic centers that control the tone of peripheral blood vessels and has been observed in infants with severe intracranial injury as well as in infants who appear to be otherwise perfectly normal. Although the peak frequency of attacks of harlequin color change generally occurs between the second and fifth days of life, attacks may occur anywhere from the first few hours to as late as the second or the third week of life.[3]

COMPLICATIONS FROM FETAL AND NEONATAL DIAGNOSTIC PROCEDURES

Fetal complications associated with invasive prenatal diagnostic procedures include cutaneous puncture marks, scars or lacerations, exsanguination, ocular trauma, blindness, subdural hemorrhage, pneumothorax, cardiac tamponade, splenic laceration, porencephalic cysts, arteriovenous or ileocutaneous fistulas, digital loss (in 1.7 percent of newborns whose mothers had undergone chorionic villus sampling), musculoskeletal trauma, disruption of tendons or ligaments, and occasionally gangrene.[9] Cutaneous puncture marks, which occur in 1 to 3 per cent of newborns whose mothers had undergone amniocentesis, may be seen as single or multiple 1- to 6-mm pits or dimples on any cutaneous surface of the newborn (Fig. 2–2).[10, 11]

Fetal scalp monitoring can result in infection, bleeding, or fontanelle puncture, and prenatal vacuum extraction can produce a localized area of edema, ecchymosis, or localized alopecia. The incidence of scalp electrode infection varies from 0.3 to 5.0 per cent, and although local sterile abscesses account for the majority of adverse sequelae, *Staphylococcus aureus* or gram-negative rod infections, cellulitis, tissue necrosis, subgaleal abscess, osteomyelitis, necrotizing fasciitis, and neonatal herpes simplex infections may also occur as complications of this procedure (Fig. 2–3).[12–14]

Transcutaneous oxygen monitoring (application of heated electrodes to the skin thus allowing continuous detection of tissue oxygenation of adjacent areas) and pulse oximetry (a noninvasive oxygen-

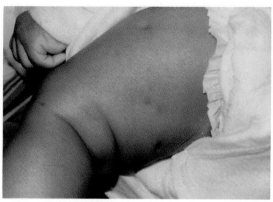

Figure 2–2. Multiple grouped depressed scars on the thigh of an infant born to a mother who had amniocentesis for diagnostic purposes during her pregnancy. (Courtesy of Lester Schwartz, M.D.)

monitoring technique for patients receiving general anesthesia) may also result in erythema, tissue necrosis, and first- or second-degree burns. Although lesions associated with transcutaneous oxygen monitoring generally resolve within 48 to 60 hours, persistent atrophic hyperpigmented craters may at times be seen as a complication. Frequent (2- to 4-hour) changing of electrode sites and reduction of the temperature of the electrodes to 43°C, however, can lessen the likelihood of this complication.[15, 16]

Calcinosis cutis may occur on the scalp or chest of infants or children at sites of electroencephalograph or electrocardiograph electrode placement, as a result of diagnostic heel sticks performed during the neonatal period, or following intramuscular or intravenous administration of calcium chloride or calcium gluconate for the treatment of neonatal hypocalcemia. Seen primarily in high-risk infants who receive repeated heel sticks for blood chemistry determinations, calcified nodules usually begin as small depressions on the heels. With time, generally after 4 to 12 months, tiny yellow or white papules appear, gradually enlarge to form nodular deposits, migrate to the cutaneous surface, extrude their contents, and generally disappear spontaneously by the time the child reaches 18 to 30 months of age. Although calcified heel nodules are usually asymptomatic, children may at times show signs of discomfort with standing or with the wearing of shoes. In such instances, gentle cryosurgery and curettage can be both diagnostic and therapeutic. Calcinosis cutis following electroencephalography or electrocardiography, which is more likely to be seen in infants and young children or individuals where the skin has been abraded and usually disappears spontaneously within 2 to 6 months, can be avoided by the use of an electrode paste that does not contain calcium chloride and, like calcified heel sticks, may be treated by gentle cryosurgery and curettage.[17, 18]

ABNORMALITIES OF SUBCUTANEOUS TISSUE

Skin turgor is generally normal during the first few hours of life. As normal physiologic dehydration occurs during the first 3 or 4 days of life (up to 10 per cent of birth weight), the skin generally becomes loose and wrinkled. Subcutaneous fat, normally quite adequate at birth, increases until about 9 months of age, thus accounting for the traditional chubby appearance of the healthy newborn. A decrease or absence of this normal panniculus is abnormal and suggests the possibility of prematurity, postmaturity, or placental insufficiency.

Sclerema neonatorum and subcutaneous fat necrosis appear to be clinical variants of the same disorder or closely allied abnormalities of subcutaneous tissue (Table 2–2). Although there is considerable confusion in the literature, evidence suggests that the biochemical abnormality in these two disorders may be identical.

Sclerema Neonatorum

Sclerema neonatorum is a diffuse, rapidly spreading, wax-like hardening of the skin and subcutaneous tissue that occurs in premature or debilitated infants during the first few weeks of life. The disorder, usually associated with a serious underlying condition such as sepsis or other infection, congenital heart disease, respiratory distress, diarrhea, or dehydration, is characterized by a diffuse nonpitting woody induration of the involved tissues. The process is symmetrical, usually starting on the legs and buttocks, and may progress to involve all areas except the palms, soles, and genitalia. As the disorder spreads, the skin becomes cold, yellowish white, mottled, stony hard, and cadaver-like. The limbs become immobile, and the face acquires a fixed mask-like expression. The infants become sluggish, feed poorly, show clinical signs of shock, and in a high percentage of cases

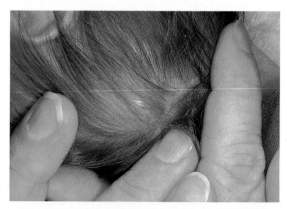

Figure 2–3. A staphylococcal abscess on the scalp of a 9-day-old infant as a complication of intrauterine fetal monitoring.

Table 2–2. CHARACTERISTIC DIFFERENCES BETWEEN SCLEREMA NEONATORUM
AND SUBCUTANEOUS FAT NECROSIS

Sclerema Neonatorum	Subcutaneous Fat Necrosis
1. Serious underlying disease (sepsis, congestive heart disease, respiratory distress, diarrhea, or dehydration)	1. Healthy newborns
2. Wax-like hardening of skin and subcutaneous tissue in premature or debilitated infants	2. Circumscribed indurated and nodular areas of fat necrosis
3. *Etiology:* hypothermia, peripheral chilling with vascular collapse, defect in fatty acid mobilization?	3. *Etiology:* pressure on bony prominences during delivery, asphyxia, hypothermia, or diabetes in mother
4. *Histopathology:* edema and thickening of connective tissue bands around fat lobules, needle-shaped clefts within fat cells	4. *Histopathology:* large fat lobules, inflammatory infiltrate in subcutaneous tissue, foreign body giant cells around crystals of fatty acid
5. *Management:* supportive care, heat, O₂, control of infection, intravenous fluids, systemic corticosteroids	5. *Management:* aspiration of fluctuant lesions as needed; most resolve spontaneously in 2 to 4 weeks.

often die. Although the etiology of this disorder is unknown, it appears to represent a nonspecific sign of grave prognostic significance rather than a primary disease. Infants with this disorder are characteristically small or premature, debilitated, weak, cyanotic, and lethargic. In 25 per cent of cases the mothers are ill at the time of delivery. Exposure to cold, hypothermia, peripheral chilling with vascular collapse, and an increase in the ratio of saturated to unsaturated fatty acids in the triglyceride fraction of the subcutaneous tissue (due to a defect in fatty acid mobilization) have been hypothesized, but lack confirmation, as possible causes for this disorder.[19, 20]

The histopathologic findings of sclerema neonatorum consist of edema and thickening of the connective tissue bands around the fat lobules. Although necrosis and crystallization of the subcutaneous tissue have been described, these findings are more characteristically seen in lesions of subcutaneous fat necrosis.

The prognosis of sclerema neonatorum is poor, and mortality occurs in 50 to 75 per cent of affected infants. Death, when it occurs, generally is due to inanition, debilitation, and the associated underlying pathologic disorder. In those infants who survive, the cutaneous findings resolve without residual sequelae. There is no specific therapy for sclerema neonatorum.

Supportive care with heat and administration of oxygen, control of infection, management of the underlying disorder, and intravenous therapy for correction of fluid and electrolyte imbalance are essential. Although indications for their use are unclear and controlled studies fail to confirm their efficacy, in view of the fact that these infants are critically ill and the mortality rate continues to be high, systemic corticosteroids in addition to antimicrobial agents have been advocated for infants with this disorder.[21, 22]

Subcutaneous Fat Necrosis

Subcutaneous fat necrosis is a benign self-limiting disease that affects apparently healthy full-term newborns and young infants. It is characterized by sharply circumscribed, indurated, and nodular areas of fat necrosis (Fig. 2–4). The etiology of this disorder remains unknown but appears to be related to trauma due to pressure on bony prominences during the time of delivery, asphyxia, hypothermia, and, in some instances, hypercalcemia.[23–27] Although the mechanism of hypercalcemia is not known, it has been attributed to aberrations in vitamin D or parathyroid homeostasis. The disorder has also been described in infants delivered by cesarean section and in infants born to diabetic mothers. The relationship between subcutaneous fat necrosis, maternal diabetes, and cesarean section, however, if any, is unclear.[28]

The onset of subcutaneous fat necrosis generally occurs during the first few days and weeks of life. Lesions appear as single or multiple localized, sharply circumscribed, usually painless areas of induration. At times, however, affected areas may be extremely tender and infants may be quite uncomfortable and may cry vigorously when they are handled. Lesions of subcutaneous fat necrosis vary from small nodules to large plaques and grow to several centimeters in diameter. Although lesions may occur in any cutaneous area, sites of predilection include the cheeks, back, buttocks, arms, and thighs. Involved tissues are nontender, of a reddish or violaceous hue, and of a nonpitting, stony consistency. Many lesions have an uneven lobulated surface with an elevated margin separating it from the surrounding normal tissue. Subcutaneous fat necrosis tends to have a good prognosis. Although lesions may develop extensive deposits of calcium, which may liquefy, drain, and heal with scarring, most areas undergo spontaneous resolution within several weeks.

Histologic examination of lesions of subcutaneous fat necrosis reveal larger than usual fat lobules and an extensive inflammatory infiltrate in the subcutaneous tissue consisting of lymphocytes, foreign body giant cells about crystals of fatty acid, and histiocytes. Although many authors consider necrosis and crystallization of the subcutaneous fat to be part of the histopathology of sclerema neonatorum, needle-shaped clefts within fat cells with necrosis and crystallization of the subcutaneous fat are more characteristic of sub-

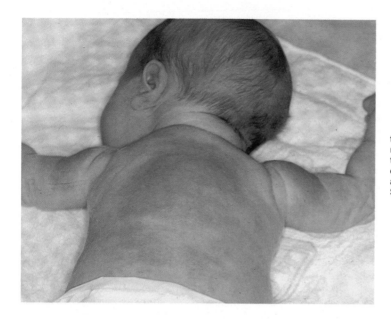

Figure 2–4. Subcutaneous fat necrosis of the newborn. Sharply circumscribed reddish to violaceous plaques or nodules on the cheeks, back, buttocks, arms, and thighs of otherwise apparently healthy newborns and young infants. (Courtesy of Richard Swint, M.D.)

cutaneous fat necrosis than sclerema of the newborn.

Most uncomplicated lesions of subcutaneous fat necrosis are self-limiting, resolve spontaneously within 2 to 4 weeks (usually without atrophy or scarring), and require no specific therapy. Fluctuant lesions, however, should be aspirated with a small-gauge needle in an effort to prevent rupture, thus diminishing the possibility of, or susceptibility to, subsequent scarring. Rarely infants with associated hypercalcemia may require low calcium intake, restriction of vitamin D, and systemic corticosteroid therapy.

MISCELLANEOUS CUTANEOUS DISORDERS

Miliaria

Differentiation of the epidermis and its appendages, particularly in the premature infant, is frequently incomplete at birth. As a result of this immaturity, a high incidence of sweat-retention phenomena may be seen in the newborn. Miliaria, a common neonatal dermatosis caused by sweat retention, is characterized by a vesicular eruption with subsequent maceration and obstruction of the eccrine ducts. The pathophysiologic events that lead to this disorder are keratinous plugging of eccrine ducts and the escape of eccrine sweat into the skin below the level of obstruction (see Chapter 6).

Virtually all infants develop miliaria under appropriate conditions. In infants there are two principal forms of this disorder: (1) miliaria crystallina (sudamina), which consists of clear superficial pinpoint vesicles without an inflammatory areola, and (2) miliaria rubra (prickly heat), which is character-

ized by small discrete erythematous papules, vesicles, or papulovesicles (Fig. 2–5). The incidence of miliaria is greatest in the first few weeks of life owing to the relative immaturity of the eccrine ducts, which favors poral closure and sweat retention.

Therapy for miliaria is directed toward avoidance of excessive heat and humidity. Lightweight clothing, cool baths, and air conditioning are invaluable in the management of this disorder. Resorcinol, 3 per cent (in Cetaphil lotion [Owen/Galderma]), is also helpful in instances in which more active therapeutic measures are desired.

Milia

Milia commonly occur on the face of the newborn. Seen in 40 to 50 per cent of infants, they result from retention of keratin and sebaceous ma-

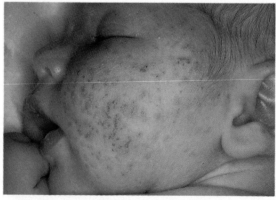

Figure 2–5. Miliaria rubra ("prickly heat"). Discrete erythematous papules, vesicles, and papulovesicles due to obstruction and rupture of epidermal sweat ducts.

terial within the pilosebaceous apparatus of the newborn. They appear as tiny 1- to 2-mm pearly white or yellow papules. Particularly prominent on the cheeks, nose, chin, and forehead, they may be few or numerous and are frequently grouped in the areas of involvement (see Figs. 6–22 and 8–47). Occasionally lesions may also be noted on the upper trunk, limbs, penis, or mucous membranes. Although milia of the newborn may persist into the second or third month, they usually disappear spontaneously during the first 3 or 4 weeks of life and, accordingly, require no therapy. Persistent milia in an unusual or widespread distribution, particularly when seen in association with other defects, may be seen as a manifestation of hereditary trichodysplasia (Marie-Unna hypotrichosis) or the oral-facial-digital syndrome type I.

Bohn's Nodules and Epstein's Pearls

Discrete, 2- to 3-mm round, pearly white or yellow, freely movable elevations at the gum margins or midline of the hard palate (termed *Bohn's nodules* and *Epstein's pearls*, respectively) are seen in up to 85 per cent of newborns. Clinically and histologically the counterpart of facial milia, they disappear spontaneously, usually within a few weeks of life, and require no therapy.

Sebaceous Gland Hyperplasia

Sebaceous gland hyperplasia represents a physiologic phenomenon of the newborn manifested by multiple, yellow to flesh-colored tiny papules that occur on the nose, cheeks, and upper lips of full-term infants. A manifestation of maternal androgen stimulation, these papules represent a temporary disorder that resolves spontaneously, generally within the first few weeks of life.

Acne Neonatorum

Occasionally infants develop an eruption that resembles acne vulgaris as seen in adolescents (see Fig. 6–21). Although the etiology of this disorder is not clearly defined, it appears to develop as a result of hormonal stimulation of sebaceous glands that have not yet involuted to their childhood state of immaturity. In mild cases of acne neonatorum, therapy is often unnecessary; daily cleansing with soap and water may be all that is required. Occasionally mild keratolytic agents may be helpful (see Chapter 6).

Erythema Toxicum Neonatorum

Toxic erythema of the newborn (erythema toxicum neonatorum) represents a characteristic, asymptomatic, benign self-limiting cutaneous eruption of the neonatal period of unknown etiology. Composed of erythematous macules, papules, pustules, or a combination of these lesions, lesions of toxic erythema may occur anywhere on the body, including at times the palms and soles, and may vary from a few (two or three) to several hundred (Fig. 2–6). The fact that these lesions frequently tend to spare the palms and soles may be explained by the absence of pilosebaceous follicles in these regions.

The eruption may first appear as a blotchy macular erythema that may develop into firm 1- to 3-mm, pale yellow or white papules, pustules, or a combination of these lesions on an erythematous base, the so-called flea-bitten rash of the newborn. The erythematous macules generally display an irregular or splotchy appearance, varying from a few millimeters to several centimeters in diameter. They may be seen in sharp contrast to the surrounding unaffected skin, may blend into a surrounding erythema, or may progress to present a confluent eruption.

Although erythema toxicum appears most frequently during the first 3 to 4 days of life, it has been seen at birth and may be noted as late as the 14th day of life.[29–31] Exacerbations and remissions may occur during the first 2 weeks of life. The duration of individual lesions varies from a few hours to 16 days (the average duration is approximately 2 days).

The etiology of erythema toxicum remains obscure. Its reported incidence is variable, owing to the fleeting nature of the disorder and the disparity among reported observations on the part of clinicians. Some authors report an incidence as low as

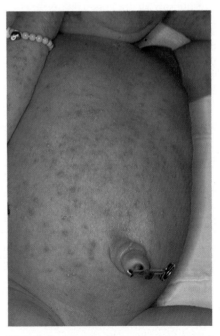

Figure 2–6. Toxic erythema of the newborn (erythema toxicum neonatorum) appears most frequently during the first 3 or 4 days of life. In this instance the disorder was present at birth.

4.5 per cent; others report incidences varying from 31 to 70 per cent of newborns.[31] No sexual or racial predisposition has been noted; discrepancies in racial incidence appear to be related to the difficulty of recognition of erythema on pigmented skin. The incidence does not differ significantly with respect to maternal history, condition at birth, or sex of the infant. It does, however, have a lower rate of incidence in premature as contrasted with full-term infants, with an increase in incidence (from 0 to 59 per cent) as the gestational age increases (from 30 weeks or less to 42 weeks or more).[32]

The histopathologic picture of a papule of erythema toxicum reveals a characteristic accumulation of eosinophils about the pilosebaceous apparatus just below the dermal-epidermal junction of the skin; pustular lesions are the result of a perifollicular accumulation of these cells in a subcorneal or intradermal location. Examination of the peripheral blood in affected infants has shown an eosinophilia in 7 to 15 per cent of cases. Although the eosinophilic response has led some observers to attribute the etiology of this disorder to a hypersensitivity reaction, specific allergens have never been implicated or confirmed. Studies of the acute inflammatory process in newborns reveal an eosinophilic response, suggesting that eosinophilia may be a normal neonatal response to the stimulus of injury.[33] At present, therefore, the etiology of erythema toxicum remains obscure. Perhaps it represents a transient reaction of neonatal skin to normal mechanical or thermal stimuli.[34]

Since erythema toxicum is a benign self-limiting asymptomatic disorder, no therapy is indicated. Occasionally, however, it may be confused with other eruptions of the neonatal period, namely, transient neonatal pustular melanosis, milia of the newborn, miliaria, congenital cutaneous candidiasis, herpes simplex, or impetigo neonatorum. Of these, herpes simplex neonatorum, congenital candidiasis, and impetigo are the most important because of the possibility of contagion or systemic involvement.

Toxic erythema can be rapidly differentiated by cytologic examination of the contents of a pustule. A smear of intralesional contents of erythema toxicum prepared with Wright's or Giemsa stain may reveal clusters of eosinophils and a relative absence of neutrophils. The presence of a predominance of neutrophils is suggestive of a bacterial infection; absence of bacteria on Gram staining and negative bacterial culture tend to rule out impetigo of the newborn. Congenital cutaneous candidiasis can be differentiated by potassium hydroxide or Gram-stained preparations of cutaneous scrapings and fungal culture.

Impetigo Neonatorum

Impetigo in newborns may occur as early as the second or third day or as late as the second week of life. It usually presents as a superficial vesicular, pustular, or bullous lesion on an erythematous base. Vesicles and bullae are easily denuded, leaving a round, red, raw, moist surface, usually without crust formation. Blisters are often wrinkled, contain some fluid, and are easily denuded without formation of crusts. Lesions tend to occur on moist or opposing surfaces of the skin, as in the diaper area, groin, axillae, and folds of the neck.

The term *pemphigus neonatorum* is an archaic misnomer occasionally applied to superficial bullous lesions of severe impetigo widely distributed over the surface of the body. The status of "pemphigus neonatorum" as a distinct nosologic entity is dubious. Fortunately, with improved neonatal care and appropriate antibiotic therapy, this severe form of neonatal pyoderma is rarely seen today.

Sucking Blisters

Sucking blisters, presumed to be induced by vigorous sucking on the affected part in utero, are seen in up to 0.5 per cent of normal newborns as 0.5- to 2.0-cm oval bullae or erosions on the dorsal aspect of the fingers, thumbs, wrists, lips, or radial aspect of the forearms. These lesions, which must be differentiated from bullous impetigo and the blisters of epidermolysis bullosa, epidermolytic hyperkeratosis, and herpes neonatorum, resolve rapidly without sequelae.

Transient Neonatal Pustular Melanosis

Transient neonatal pustular melanosis is a benign self-limiting disorder of unknown etiology characterized by superficial vesiculopustular lesions that rupture easily and evolve into evanescent hyperpigmented macules (Figs. 2–7 and 2–8). Seen in 0.2 to 4 per cent of newborns,[35–37] lesions are usually present at birth. They generally begin as superficial sterile vesiculopustular lesions that rupture easily during the first bathing and often leave a collarette of fine white scales around a pinhead-sized brown hyperpigmented macule that generally fades within several weeks to months (see Fig. 2–8). The lesions are most often seen in clusters under the chin and on the forehead, nape of the neck, lower back, and shins. Occasionally, lesions may also appear on the cheeks, trunk, and extremities. Rarely, blisters, which do not progress to pigmented macules, may be detected on the scalp, palms, and soles.

Lesions of transient neonatal pustular melanosis are sterile. Smears of vesicle fluid stained with Wright's stain, in contrast to lesions of erythema toxicum neonatorum, demonstrate variable numbers of neutrophils, few or no eosinophils, and cellular debris. Histopathologic examination of cutaneous biopsy specimens of vesiculopustular lesions are characterized by hyperkeratosis of the

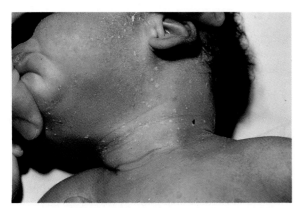

Figure 2–7. Transient neonatal pustular melanosis. Papulovesicles present at birth leave hyperpigmented macules surrounded by a collarette of fine scales. (Courtesy of Nancy B. Esterly, M.D.)

stratum corneum and intracorneal and subcorneal separation with polymorphonuclear infiltration. Histopathologic examination of pigmented macular lesions reveals basket-weave hyperkeratosis and areas of focal basilar hyperpigmentation.

Transient neonatal pustular melanosis is a benign disorder, appears to have no associated systemic manifestations, and requires no treatment. Lesions are distinguishable from those of erythema toxicum and must be differentiated from pustulovesicles of staphylococcal, candidal, or herpetic origin. Vesiculopustular lesions of transient neonatal pustular melanosis disappear in 24 to 48 hours, often leaving hyperpigmented macules, which in turn generally regress within 3 weeks to 3 months.

Congenital Erosive and Vesicular Dermatosis

Congenital erosive and vesicular dermatosis healing with reticulated supple scarring is an uncommon disorder characterized by erosive and bullous lesions that, as the name implies, are present at birth and heal with scarring. Although its cause is unknown, it appears to represent a nonhereditary intrauterine event, such as infection or amniotic adhesions, or perhaps an unusual healing defect of immature skin. The disorder generally occurs on the skin of the trunk, extremities, scalp, and at times the tongue, with sparing of the face, palms, and soles. Infants are often born prematurely and manifest extensive cutaneous ulcerations, reticulated crusts, and intact vesicles that heal during the first month of life. Generalized supple reticulated scars in which the elevated bands are of normal color to minimally hypopigmented result and the intervening depressed areas are of normal color or minimally hyperpigmented. Frequently involving as much as 75 per cent of the cutaneous surface, scars on the trunk and head,

which often have a cobblestone-like appearance, may be oriented along the cutaneous lines of cleavage; on the limbs they tend to follow the long axes of the extremities (Figs. 2–9 and 2–10).[38–40]

Although the eyebrows and cilia are usually normal, alopecia may be noted on the scalp, the nails may be absent or hypoplastic, and affected areas on the tongue may manifest areas of scarring and absence of papillae. Hyperthermia, especially in warm weather or after exertion, is common; and although sweating is absent in atrophic areas, compensatory hyperhidrosis in normal-appearing skin may be noted in response to warm weather or after physical exertion. Some patients affected with this disorder have also been found to have neurologic defects, such as mental and motor retardation, microcephaly, cerebral palsy, and seizures. Whether central nervous system features are part of the syndrome or merely coincidental features, however, remains unknown.

Histopathologic examination of affected areas reveals normal or nearly normal epidermis; and although the dermis may be normal, it may reveal a minimal increase in collagen (in a scarring pattern), a decrease in hair follicle density, and absence of eccrine glands.

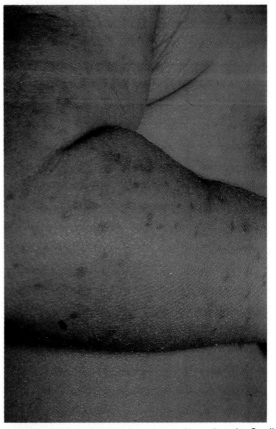

Figure 2–8. Transient neonatal pustular melanosis. Small brown hyperpigmented macules on the arm and forearm. (Courtesy of Nancy B. Esterly, M.D.)

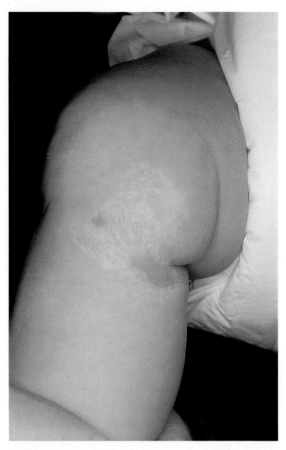

Figure 2–9. A hypopigmented scar on the knee of an infant with congenital erosive and vesicular dermatosis with reticulated scarring.

Seborrheic Dermatitis

Seborrheic dermatitis is a term that has been used to describe a self-limiting condition of the scalp, face, ears, trunk, and intertriginous areas characterized by greasy scaling associated with patchy redness, fissuring, and occasional weeping.

The cause of seborrheic dermatitis is not well understood. It appears to be an inflammatory disorder related to a dysfunction of the sebaceous glands and has a predilection for areas where the density of sebaceous glands is high. Ostensibly under hormonal influence, this disorder first appears during the first few months of infancy when transplacental hormone levels are elevated. It frequently improves between 8 and 12 months of age as these levels decline, is less common during childhood, and reappears with elevation of hormone levels during adolescence. Whether seborrheic dermatitis of adolescence and adulthood is related to that of infancy remains unknown. Studies suggest that *Pityrosporum ovale* (*Malassezia ovalis*), lipophilic yeast found in abundance on the human scalp, may be related to the pathogenesis of

this disorder. Whether this organism plays a primary or secondary etiologic role, however, is controversial.[41-44]

In newborns and infants seborrheic dermatitis often begins during the first 12 weeks of age, with a scaly dermatitis of the scalp termed *cradle cap* (Fig. 2–11). This disorder may spread over the face, including the forehead, ears, eyebrows, nose, and back of the head, and often clears spontaneously by 8 to 12 months of age (Fig. 2–12). Erythematous, greasy, salmon-colored, and sharply marginated oval scaly lesions may involve other parts of the body, particularly the intertriginous and flexural areas, the postauricular regions, the trunk, umbilicus, anogenital areas, and groin (Fig. 2–13). Infants with these lesions usually lack stigmata of atopy (itching, dry skin, follicular keratosis) and personal or family history of atopic disease.

The histologic picture of infantile seborrheic dermatitis is not specific and has features of both psoriasis and chronic dermatitis (see Chapter 3). Spongiosis, however, although seen in seborrheic dermatitis, is not present in psoriasis and is a helpful differentiating feature between these two disorders.

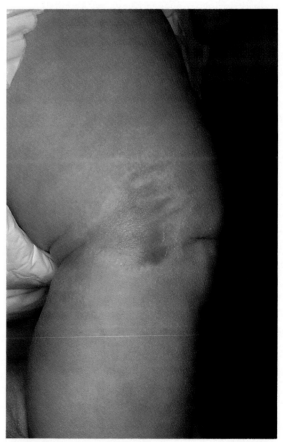

Figure 2–10. An atrophic scar on the knee of an infant with congenital erosive and vesicular dermatosis with reticulated scarring.

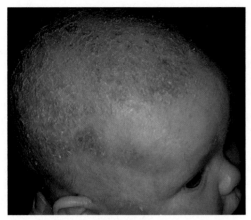

Figure 2–11. Seborrheic dermatitis of the scalp ("cradle cap").

The prognosis of infantile seborrheic dermatitis is good. In some patients the disorder clears within 3 to 4 weeks, even without treatment, and most cases clear spontaneously by 8 to 12 months of age. The diagnostic features include its early onset, the characteristic greasy nature of the eruption with its predilection for the scalp and intertriginous areas, and a general lack of associated pruritus. Occasionally seborrheic dermatitis may be followed by typical atopic dermatitis. Whether this represents a chance occurrence or perhaps a specific constitutional predisposition is still controversial.

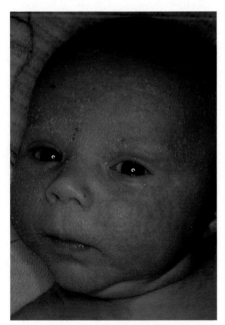

Figure 2–12. Seborrheic dermatitis on the face. Infantile seborrheic dermatitis may be differentiated from atopic dermatitis by its very early onset, a lack of pruritus and personal or family history of atopy, and the absence of vesiculation and lichenification.

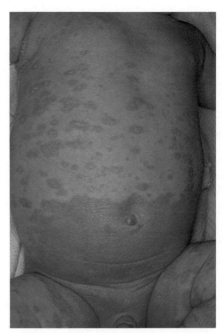

Figure 2–13. Greasy salmon-colored well-marginated scaly eruption of seborrheic dermatitis.

Infantile seborrheic dermatitis may be differentiated from atopic dermatitis by its early onset, a lack of pruritus and personal or family history of atopy, and the absence of vesiculation and lichenification. Although seborrheic dermatitis can at times be mistaken for Letterer-Siwe disease, the presence of discrete 1- to 3-mm yellowish to reddish brown infiltrated papules at the periphery of the eruption, purpuric lesions, hepatosplenomegaly, adenopathy, fever, anemia, thrombocytopenia, and skeletal tumors can help differentiate the latter disorder. When the diagnosis remains in doubt, a cutaneous punch biopsy may help differentiate the two conditions.

Treatment. Treatment of seborrheic dermatitis of the scalp is best managed by frequent shampooing, preferably with one of the commercially available antiseborrheic shampoos (those containing sulfur and salicylic acid are generally satisfactory). If the scales are thick and adherent, removal can be facilitated by the use of slightly warmed mineral oil or petrolatum. In stubborn or persistent cases, a phenol-saline solution (P & S liquid [Baker/ Cummins]) massaged into the scalp lesions at night and shampooed out the next morning will assist removal of thick scales and crusts.

When the scalp is shampooed, gentle scrubbing is safe and often necessary to facilitate removal of the thick adherent scales. Antiseborrheic agents should be left on for an appropriate period of time (long enough to soften and loosen the scales properly). Failure to allow the agent to stay on for the recommended period and inadequate scrubbing of the scales are common causes for failure of otherwise adequate antiseborrheic therapy. For stubborn or persistent lesions, a topical corticosteroid lotion, alone or in combination with 3 to 5 per cent sulfur precipitate or salicylic acid or both, is frequently effective. This preparation may be used three times a day initially and its frequency reduced or discontinued as the eruption improves.

Leiner's Disease

Leiner's disease is a disorder of infancy characterized by an intractable, generalized, seborrhea-like dermatitis; severe exfoliative erythroderma; severe diarrhea; marked wasting and dystrophy; and recurrent local and systemic infections, usually of gram-negative etiology. Described primarily in the preantibiotic era as an extensive form of seborrheic dermatitis of unknown etiology, Leiner's disease appears to represent the phenotype of a number of nutritional and immunologic disorders, such as acrodermatitis enteropathica, free fatty acid deficiency, biotin-responsive multiple carboxylase deficiency, C_3 or C_5 dysfunction, and other disorders of immunodeficiency that mimic each other in clinical features.[45] The disorder may occur during the first week of life but generally begins suddenly in infants between 2 and 4 months of age. Infants of both sexes appeared to be affected equally; and although the proportion of breast-fed infants was initially said to be high, this may have been a reflection of the feeding practice at the time the disorder was initially described.

The dermatosis is characterized by universal erythema and loosening of the epidermis with scale and crust formation (Fig. 2–14). Generally considered to be a severe exfoliative variant of seborrheic dermatitis, it commonly begins as a progressive increase in severity of seborrheic dermatitis of the scalp or flexures, or by the sudden development of intense erythema of the entire skin surface with profuse desquamation of fine, branny scales on the face; heavy crusting of the scalp and eyebrows; and a thick, profound exfoliation of the trunk and extremities. The scalp is often covered with thick, greasy, yellow crusts, as seen in severe seborrheic dermatitis, and a patchy or total alopecia may be noted. Severe protracted diarrhea, dehydration, fever, inanition, and death are frequent sequelae in patients with severe or untreated forms of this disorder.

Familial Leiner's Disease with C_5 Dysfunction. Familial cases of infants with severe forms of Leiner's disease (similar to those originally described by Leiner) have been reported in which affected infants have a defect in function of the fifth component of complement (C_5). This dysfunction of C_5 resulted in decreased phagocytosis (opsonic activity) of the patient's serum and in failure to thrive and recurrent sepsis with an ominous prognosis. In patients with Leiner disease's and C_5 dysfunction, vigorous antibiotic therapy combined with infusions of fresh frozen plasma or whole blood is helpful and may be lifesaving.[46, 47]

DEVELOPMENTAL ABNORMALITIES OF THE NEWBORN

Drug-Induced Fetal Malformations

In recent years there have been numerous reports of drugs, such as alcohol, hydantoin, trimethadione, paramethadione, valproic acid, warfarin, aminopterin, and retinoic acid, that when taken by pregnant women produce an adverse effect on the fetus and newborn. *Fetal alcohol syndrome,* the leading cause of mental retardation in the United States, occurs in approximately 1 in 500 to 1 in 1,000 live births. Other clinical features include prenatal and postnatal growth deficiency, facial abnormalities, microcephaly, hydrocephalus, hypotonia, poor fine motor coordination, hyperactivity, irregularly shaped teeth, clinodactyly, small distal phalanges with hypoplastic nails, hernias, meningomyelocele, limb abnormalities, cardiac defects, myopia, hearing disorders, renal malformation, the DiGeorge syndrome (an embryologic deficiency of

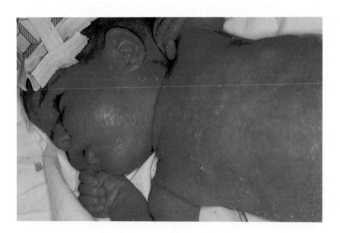

Figure 2–14. Leiner's disease. Generalized exfoliative seborrheic dermatitis with erythema, desquamation, and crusting.

the thymus and parathyroids associated with congenital defects of the heart and aortic arch), and lifelong mental and behavioral problems.[48, 49]

Clinical features of the *fetal hydantoin syndrome* (Fig. 2–15) include a pixy-like facies, short nose, broad or depressed nasal bridge, bowed upper lip, ocular hypertelorism, microcephaly, prenatal and postnatal growth deficiency, finger-like thumbs, hypoplasia of distal phalanges with small nails, longitudinal pigmentary streaks in the fingernails, and delays in mental performance.[50, 51] Infants born to mothers who take trimethadione or paramethadione during pregnancy (the *fetal trimethadione syndrome*) have intrauterine growth retardation, short stature, facial abnormalities, low-set ears with anteriorly folding helix, cleft lip and/or high arched palate, irregular teeth, microcephaly, ocular and cardiac abnormalities, and genital anomalies.[52] Fetal exposure to the anticonvulsant drug valproic acid (Depakene), the *fetal valproate syndrome*, is characterized by craniofacial and cardiovascular abnormalities, hyperconvex fingernails, long thin fingers and toes, meningomyelocele, triphalangeal thumbs, hernias, supernumerary nipples, hypospadias, and, at times, growth and mental deficiency.

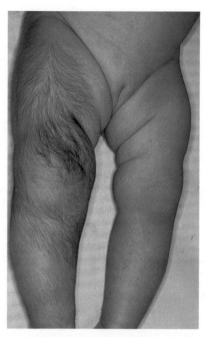

Figure 2–16. Congenital hemihypertrophy with hypertrichosis. (Hurwitz S, Klaus SN: Congenital hemihypertrophy with hypertrichosis. Arch. Dermatol. *103*:98–100, 1971.)

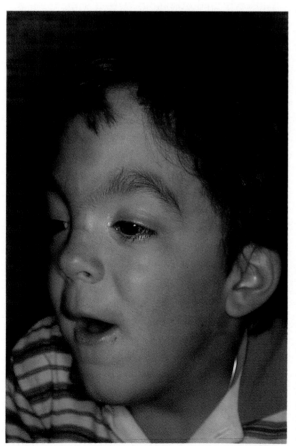

Figure 2–15. A 7-year-old boy with fetal hydantoin syndrome.

Retinoic acid embryopathy, the result of taking isotretinoin (13-*cis*-retinoic acid, Accutane) or etretinate (Tegison) during pregnancy, is characterized by microcephaly, macrocephaly, frontal bossing, microphthalmia, low-set malformed ears, occluded auditory canals, thymic defects, hepatic abnormalities, optic nerve and retinal disorders, and malformations of the cardiac and central nervous system.

Congenital Hemihypertrophy

Hemihypertrophy is a developmental defect in which one side of the body is larger than the other. Although differences in symmetry are often detectable during the newborn period, they usually become more striking with growth of the child. The cutaneous findings most often associated with hemihypertrophy are pigmentation, telangiectasia, abnormal nail growth, and hypertrichosis (Fig. 2–16). Body temperature and sweating differences have also been reported in patients with this disorder.[53]

Of particular significance is the fact that about 50 per cent of persons with hemihypertrophy have associated anomalies. Significant malformations include Wilms' tumor, aniridia, cataracts, ear deformities, internal hemangiomas, genitourinary tract anomalies, adrenocortical neoplasms, and brain tumors. Patients who exhibit congenital hemihypertrophy, therefore, should be evaluated

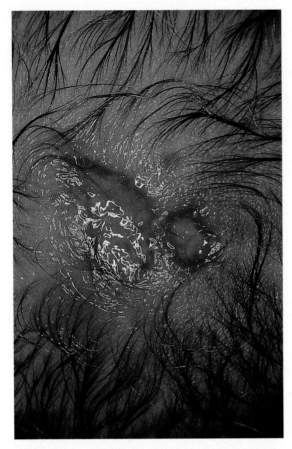

Figure 2–17. A sharply demarcated ulceration on the scalp of a newborn with aplasia cutis. (Courtesy of Suguru Imaeada, M.D.)

for the tumors and congenital malformations often associated with this disorder. During infancy and early childhood, these patients should be examined at regular intervals for possible development of liver, adrenocortical, or renal neoplasms.

Aplasia Cutis Congenita

Aplasia cutis congenita is a congenital defect of the integument characterized by localized absence of the epidermis, dermis, and, at times, subcutaneous tissues. The defect is present at birth; and although it generally occurs on the scalp, it may also involve the skin of the face, trunk, and extremities.[54, 55]

The disorder usually presents as solitary or multiple, sharply demarcated, weeping or granulating, oval, circular, elongated, stellate, or triangular defects ranging from 1 to 3 cm in diameter. In 70 per cent of cases the ulceration is singular, in 20 per cent it is double, and in 8 per cent of patients three or more cutaneous defects may be noted.[54] In 60 per cent of patients aplasia cutis congenita occurs on the scalp, usually near the sagittal suture of the

vertex or over adjacent parietal regions. In more than 50 per cent of reported cases the defect is located in the midline of the scalp, and in 30 per cent of patients it is seen in an area adjacent to this position. Although aplasia cutis congenita may also affect the occiput, the postauricular areas, and the face, involvement of these areas appears to be relatively rare.

At birth the cutaneous defect may vary from a denuded ulceration with a red weeping or granulating base to an area of erosion covered with a thin friable membrane (Fig. 2–17). Histologic examination reveals an absence of epidermis, absence or paucity of appendageal structures, a variable decrease in dermal elastic tissue, and, in deeper lesions, a complete deficit of all layers of the skin and subcutaneous tissues. As healing takes place the defect is replaced by smooth, gray, hairless, parchment-like scar tissue (Fig. 2–18). After the lesions heal, the total absence of epidermal appendages in the area of the defect and the presence of rudimentary or malformed appendages on histologic examination of the surrounding edge is highly characteristic.

Although most infants with aplasia cutis congenita have no other abnormalities, other developmental abnormalities reported in association with aplasia cutis congenita include cleft lip and palate, syndactyly, hydrocephalus, defects of the underlying skull, malformations of the brain, transverse defects at variable levels of the limbs manifested as hemimelia and aphalangia, colobomas, cranial stenosis, meningomyelocele, anencephaly, microphthalmus, congential heart disease, gastroschisis, omphalocele, congenital midline porencephaly, spastic paralysis, mental retardation, epidermolysis bullosa, nail dystrophy, clubbed hands and feet, tracheoesophageal fistula, and vascular anomalies.[56]

The etiology of aplasia cutis congenita remains unknown. Although most instances of this disorder are sporadic, familial cases are suggestive of autosomal dominant inheritance with reduced pene-

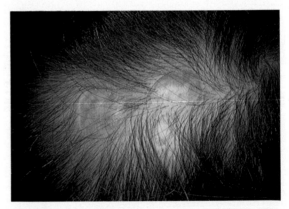

Figure 2–18. Parchment-like scars of the scalp (aplasia cutis congenita).

trance. Incomplete closure of the neural tube or an embryologic arrest of skin development has been suggested as an explanation of midline lesions. This hypothesis, however, fails to account for lesions of the trunk and limbs. In such instances, vascular abnormality of the placenta, with a degenerative rather than an aplastic or traumatic origin, has been postulated as the cause of the cutaneous defects.[57]

Recognition of aplasia cutis congenita and differentiation of it from forceps or other birth injury will help prevent possible medicolegal complications occasionally seen with this disorder. Except for residual scarring and defects that overlie the sagittal suture where fatal hemorrhage from the sagittal sinus has been reported, the prognosis of aplasia cutis generally is good. With conservative therapy designed to prevent further trauma and secondary infection, most small defects of the scalp heal well during the first few weeks to months of life. Defects of the lytic lesions of the skull generally heal spontaneously by 5 to 7 months. As the child matures, most scars become relatively inconspicuous and require no correction. Those that are large and obvious, however, generally respond to multiple punch graft transplants or surgical excision followed by plastic repair.

Setleis' Syndrome (Bitemporal Aplasia Cutis Congenita with Other Cutaneous Abnormalities). In 1963, Setleis and others described five children of three families, all of Puerto Rican ancestry, who presented with unique characteristic clinical defects confined to the face. Termed *congenital ectodermal dysplasia of the face*, features of the affected children were an aged leonine appearance; absent eyelashes from either eyelid or multiple rows of lashes on the upper lids with absence of those of the lower lids; eyebrows that slanted sharply upward and laterally; scar-like defects on each temple; puckered skin about the eyes; a scar-like median ridge of the chin; and a nose and chin that seemed rubbery when palpated (Fig. 2–19).[58]

Rudolph and co-workers subsequently described an 8-year-old Puerto Rican girl with a peculiar "old lady" facies with a prominent jaw; mild frontal bossing; flattened bridge of the nose; narrowed palpebral fissure; stenotic nares with shiny atrophic skin at the margins; low-set small and abnormally shaped ears; missing lateral eyebrows; flesh-colored hyperkeratotic papules on the arms, thighs, and back; bilaterally symmetrical, slightly hyperpigmented, depressed oval areas on the temples covered with smooth shiny skin with an apparent lack of underlying subcutaneous tissue; and small irregularities of the underlying skull.[59]

Although this entity was described as an example of "bitemporal aplasia cutis congenita with other cutaneous abnormalities," it appears that the patient had a defect similar to that described 14 years earlier by Setleis and associates as "congenital ectodermal dysplasia of the face." It appears that all six patients demonstrate a similar clinical

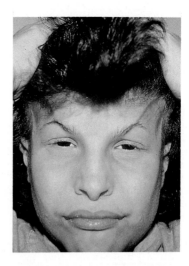

Figure 2–19. A young Puerto Rican woman with bilateral depressed oval areas overlying the temples, absence of lateral eyebrows, narrowed palpebral fissures, and stenotic nares (Setleis' syndrome). (Courtesy of Seth Orlow, M.D.)

syndrome, an autosomal recessive disorder with its origin near the towns of San Sebastian and Aguadilla in a rural part of the island of Puerto Rico.[60]

Other Developmental Defects

A *congenital dermal sinus* is a developmental epithelium-lined tract that extends inward from the surface of the skin. Since midline fusion of ectodermal and neuroectodermal tissue occurs at the cephalic and caudal ends of the neural tube, the majority of such defects are seen in the suboccipital and lumbosacral regions.

Dermal sinus openings may be difficult to visualize, particularly in the occipital region where they may be hidden by hair. A localized thickening of the scalp, hypertrichosis, dimpling, or vascular nevi in the midline of the neck or back should alert the physician to the possibility of such an anomaly. These sinuses are of clinical importance as portals for infections that may give rise to abscesses, osteomyelitis, or meningitis. Radiographs and/or magnetic resonance imaging (MRI) studies of suspicious areas should be obtained to rule out the possibility of associated spina bifida or other bony abnormality.

Most authorities agree that dermal sinuses occurring above the lumbosacral area can be excised during the newborn period; controversy, however, exists as to the management of congenital defects in the lumbosacral and coccygeal regions. Available evidence at this time suggests that asymptomatic infants with lumbosacral, sacral, or coccygeal sinuses can be followed for a 4- to 6-month period providing the parents have been instructed to contact a physician immediately if there is any evidence of inflammation, discharge of fluid, poor bladder or bowel control, or abnormality of the lower extremities. Sinography and probing are contraindicated because of the possibility of introducing infection. If infection develops, surgery should be undertaken as soon as the infection is brought under control. If abnormal neurologic signs develop or if after 4 to 6 months the bottom of a presumed sinus is not clearly visible, surgical exploration is advisable.[61]

Congenital fistulas of the lower lip (congenital lip pits) may be unilateral or bilateral and may be seen alone or in association with other anomalies of the face and extremities. They are characterized by single or paired, circular or slit-like depressions on either side of the midline of the lower lip at the edge of the vermilion border. Also known as labial fistulas or congenital pits of the lips, these depressions represent blind sinuses that extend inward through the orbicularis oris muscle to a depth of 0.5 cm or more. At times lip pits may also be seen to communicate with underlying salivary glands.

Congenital lip pits may be inherited as an autosomal dominant disorder with penetrance estimated at 80 per cent. They may be seen alone, or, in 70 per cent of patients, in association with cleft lip or cleft palate. Other associated anomalies include clubfoot, talipes equinovarus, syndactyly, and the popliteal pterygium syndrome (an autosomal dominant disorder with cleft lip with or without cleft palate, filiform adhesions between the eyelids, pterygium of the leg, limiting its mobility, anomalies of the genitourinary system, and congenital heart disease).[62]

Other than recognition of possible associated defects, most patients with congenital lip pits require no specific therapy. When communication with underlying mucous glands results in secretion of mucus onto the lip surface, surgical excision of the sinus tract and its glandular tissue, or transposition of the sinus tract onto a buccal surface, may be indicated.

Skin dimpling defects (depressions, deep pits, or creases) in the sacral area and over bony prominences may be seen in normal children and infants with diastematomyelia (a fissure or cleft of the spinal cord, usually in the lumbar area), the congenital rubella or congenital varicella-zoster syndromes, deletion of the long arm of chromosome 18, and Zellweger's (cerebrohepatorenal), Bloom's, and Freeman-Sheldon (craniocarpotarsal dysplasia, "whistling face") syndromes.

Amniotic constriction bands may produce congenital constriction deformities, and congenital amputation of one or more digits or extremities of otherwise normal infants may occur. The deformities are believed to result from intrauterine rupture of amnion with formation of fibrous bands that encircle fetal parts and produce permanent constriction of the underlying tissue.[63] *Pseudoainhum*, a term occasionally used to describe this disfigurement, should not be confused with *ainhum*, a

disorder of the toes, and sometimes the fingers, primarily seen in black men in Africa in which recurrent chronic fissuring, trauma, and infection are precipitating factors.

Preauricular pits and *sinus tracts* may develop as a result of imperfect fusion of the tubercles of the first two branchial arches. Unilateral or bilateral, these lesions may be seen in association with other anomalies of the ears and face and may become infected or result in chronic preauricular ulcerations, retention cysts, or both, often requiring surgical excision. *Accessory tragi* are multiple or single, unilateral or bilateral, soft or cartilaginous, sessile or pedunculated lesions that contain epidermal adnexal structures. Usually seen in the preauricular area, they may also occur on the neck (anterior to the sternocleidomastoid muscle) and, although generally seen as an isolated congenital defect, may be associated with other branchial arch syndromes. The most common error made in the treatment of accessory tragi is failure to consider the possibility of a more serious congenital anomaly and the fact that cartilaginous structures may be incorporated in these cutaneous projections.

Branchial cleft cysts and sinuses, formed along the course of the first and second branchial clefts as a result of improper closure during embryonic life and generally located along the lower third of the lateral aspect of the neck near the anterior border of the sternocleidomastoid muscle, may be unilateral or bilateral and may open onto the cutaneous surface or may drain into the pharynx. They are a common source of recurrent inflammation, and their treatment consists of complete surgical removal or marsupialization (exteriorization, resection of the anterior wall, and suturing of the cut edges of the remaining cyst to the adjacent edges of the skin). *Thyroglossal cysts and sinuses* are unilateral or bilateral defects located in or near the midline of the neck, which may open onto the cutaneous surface, extend to the base of the tongue, or drain into the pharynx. Although surgical excision is the treatment of choice, care must be exercised to preserve aberrant thyroid tissue occasionally seen in association with these disorders.

Congenital cartilaginous rests of the neck (also known as *wattles*, a term derived from the loose folds of skin hanging from the throat of certain birds, turkeys, cattle, or other mammals) may be seen as small fleshy appendages on the anterior neck or over or near the lower half of the sternocleidomastoid muscle. Treatment consists of surgical excision with recognition of the fact that these cutaneous appendages may contain cartilage and may at times communicate with deeper structures or congenital sinus tracts.[64] *Pterygium colli*, congenital folds of skin extending from the mastoid region to the acromion on the lateral aspect of the neck, not to be confused with the loose pendulous skin seen in persons with cutis laxa or congenital hypothyroidism, may be seen in individuals with the Turner, Noonan, Down, LEOPARD, or multiple pterygium syndromes, trisomy 18, short-limbed dwarfism, and combined immunodeficiency disease.

Supernumerary nipples (polythelia), present at times in males as well as females, are manifested as small brown or pink, concave, umbilicated or elevated papules along or slightly medial to the embryologic milk line. Usually seen on the chest or upper abdomen, below the normal position of the areola, they may at times also be seen in other locations, such as the face, neck, shoulder, back, vulva, or posterior thigh.[65] Although much has been written about a relatively high incidence of renal malformation in patients with supernumerary nipples, current studies suggest that this anomaly in an otherwise apparently normal individual does not appear to be a marker of urinary tract malformation.[66] Since supernumerary nipples may also contain breast tissue, however, they are subject, at least in women, to the same complications (fibroadenoma, papillary ademona, cysts, or carcinoma) as normally located breast tissue.

CONGENITAL INFECTIONS OF THE NEWBORN

Viral, bacterial, and parasitic infections during pregnancy are frequently associated with widespread systemic involvement, serious permanent sequelae, and, at times, a variety of cutaneous manifestations. Of these, congenital rubella, congenital varicella-zoster syndrome, neonatal varicella, herpes neonatorum, congenital syphilis, cytomegalic inclusion disease, maternally transmitted acquired immunodeficiency syndrome (AIDS), and congenital toxoplasmosis are the most significant.

Congenital Rubella

Ever since the work of Gregg in 1941, physicians have been aware of the teratogenic effects of rubella contracted during pregnancy. Congenital rubella occurs following maternal rubella infection during the first 20 weeks of pregnancy. At least 15 to 20 per cent of offspring of women who contract this disorder during the first trimester of pregnancy are afflicted with one or more serious congenital malformations. If infants are followed for a period of years, however, an additional 15 per cent may be added to this figure.

At present, the infection is primarily a result of underutilization of rubella vaccine, and not to waning immunity in immunized persons, and 10 to 20 per cent of young adults are susceptible to rubella. The earlier in pregnancy that maternal rubella occurs, the greater the risk to the fetus. Thus, 50 per cent or more of infants born to women who contract rubella during the first 4 weeks of pregnancy may have gross congenital anomalies; by the third or fourth month of gestation this incidence falls to 2 to 6 per cent; and by 18 to 20 weeks the risk is practically nil.[67, 68]

Clinical Manifestations. The clinical manifestations of congenital rubella are varied. Investigations of the consequences of the 1963–1965 rubella epidemic have shown that infants of mothers with rubella infection during early pregnancy may develop systemic involvement in addition to the classic triad of congenital cataracts, deafness, and congenital malformations of the heart. Infected infants are usually born at term, but with low birth weight. They may show only a few manifestations at birth or may be asymptomatic, with consequences of fetal rubella only apparent in subsequent months, or they may have a wide systemic involvement characterized by growth retardation, thrombocytopenic purpura, hyperbilirubinemia, hepatosplenomegaly, pneumonia, cardiac defects, eye disorders, deafness, osseous defects, and meningoencephalitis.

The most prominent cutaneous features of congenital rubella are thrombocytopenic purpura and bluish red infiltrated macules measuring 2 to 8 mm in diameter, the so-called *blueberry muffin* lesions (Fig. 2–20). Blueberry muffin lesions are usually noted at birth or within the first 24 hours. New lesions rarely appear after 2 days of age. Lesions may be few or numerous and generally appear on the head, neck, trunk, or extremities. Many of the larger lesions tend to be raised (1 to 2 mm above the surrounding skin surface). They are generally circular and vary from a dark blue to a purplish red (magenta) color. Smaller infiltrated macules are flat, oval, or circular and less violaceous, varying from dark red to pale grayish purple or copper brown. Blueberry muffin lesions usually disappear within 3 to 6 weeks (the larger lesions regressing more slowly than the smaller flat macules in this disorder).

Histologic studies of blueberry muffin lesions reveal discrete dermal aggregates of relatively large nucleated cells and nonnucleated erythrocytes. A result of dermal erythropoiesis (rather than true hemorrhage), these infiltrated lesions, characteristic of viral infection of the fetus, are not unique to infants with congenital rubella but may also be seen in patients with congenital toxoplasmosis, cytomegalic inclusion disease, neuroblastoma, congenital leukemia, erythroblastosis fetalis, and twin transfusion syndrome.[69]

Other cutaneous manifestations include a generalized maculopapular rash; reticulated erythema of the face and extremities; hyperpigmentation of the navel, forehead, cheeks, and sites of previous trauma; seborrhea of the cheeks, forehead, and body; eczema; and recurrent urticaria. Vasomotor instability, manifested by poor peripheral circulation, with generalized mottling of the face and acral areas, cyanosis of dependent extremities, and vivid flushing of the ears, cheeks, fingertips, and toes on elevation of the affected infant's surround-

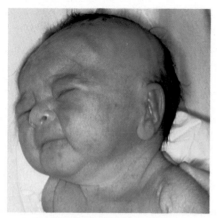

Figure 2–20. Congenital rubella syndrome with petechiae and blueberry muffin lesions. (Courtesy of Louis Gluck, M.D.)

ing environmental temperature, may also occur in association with this disorder.

Diagnosis. Congenital rubella syndrome should be suspected in infants with intrauterine growth retardation, congenital manifestations such as glaucoma, cataracts, deafess, thrombocytopenic purpura, blueberry muffin lesions, hepatosplenomegaly, cardiac defects, pneumonia, meningoencephalitis, or osseous defects. Bony abnormalities are seen in up to 80 per cent of affected infants at or near birth and include a large anterior fontanelle and characteristic small longitudinal areas of translucency in the metaphyses of long bones (especially the distal femur and proximal tibia) during the first 2 or 3 months of life. It must be noted, however, that these bony abnormalities also resemble those of other fetal viral infections such as cytomegalic inclusion disease and are not pathognomonic of the disorder.

The diagnosis of congenital rubella may be confirmed by isolation of rubella virus from respiratory secretions, urine, stool, cerebrospinal fluid, or tissues obtained at biopsy and identification of rubella IgM antibodies in the newborn, or by the persistence of rubella IgG antibodies in infants older than the age of 4 to 6 months. Although until recently the hemagglutination inhibition antibody test was the most frequently used method of screening for the presence of rubella antibodies, this test has generally been supplanted by a number of other equally or more sensitive assays, such as latex agglutination, fluorescence immunoassay, passive hemagglutination, hemolysis-in-gel, and enzyme immunoassay tests.

Management. Infants with neonatal rubella thrive poorly, and 20 to 30 per cent die within the first year of life. There is no specific treatment for the rubella-infected child apart from supportive therapy and recognition of potential disabilities. Because of the high incidence of ophthalmic complications, careful evaluation of eyes is important and ophthalmologic consultation should be ob-

tained for all affected infants. Although purpura and petechiae secondary to thrombocytopenia may be severe, true hemorrhagic difficulties do not appear to present a major problem, and corticosteroid therapy does not appear to be indicated for infants with this complication.

It must be remembered that over 80 per cent of infants with congenital rubella shed virus during the first month of life, some continue to shed virus for 6 to 9 months, and in severely affected infants (5 to 10 per cent) the virus may be detected for as long as 12 months. After 2 years the risk of viral shedding is extremely small. Affected infants should be isolated and handled only by personnel not considered at risk (those known to be seropositive for rubella with hemagglutinating antibody titers of 1 to 8 or greater). Following discharge from the hospital no special precautions are necessary other than prevention of potential risk to pregnant visitors.

With currently available live attenuated rubella vaccine and present recommendations for vaccination of all children between 1 year old and puberty, congenital rubella should be a preventable disease. It should be noted, however, that vaccination should not be administered to infants younger than 15 months of age, since the possible persistence of maternal antibody might interfere with an adequate immunologic response. Because infection with attenuated virus presents a potential risk to the fetus, rubella vaccine should not be administered to pregnant women or to those who might become pregnant within the next 2 months.

Because of the high risk of fetal damage, women known to have contracted maternal rubella during the early months of pregnancy may consider the option of therapeutic abortion. This decision, however, must be based on the age of the mother, the expectancy of other children, the gestational time of infection, and the patient's personal feeling regarding therapeutic abortion. Although limited data suggest that immune globulin, in dosages of 0.55 ml/kg, may prevent or modify infection if exposure can be documented to have taken place within 72 hours, this does not guarantee that fetal infection has been prevented. Thus, immune globulin administration to an exposed pregnant woman should be considered only if termination of the pregnancy is not an option.

Congenital Varicella-Zoster Syndrome

Although congenital varicella-zoster syndrome may on rare occasions be life threatening to the fetus, only about 40 cases have been reported in the world literature. Since 5 to 16 per cent of women of child-bearing age are susceptible to chickenpox, the fact that so few cases have been recognized may be related to the fact that not all women who develop varicella while pregnant are infected early (during the first 20 weeks of pregnancy), that some infants infected in fetal life may have infection without sequelae, and that the varicella-zoster virus does not cross the placenta as readily as other viruses. Although there are rare reports of fetal sequelae in infants born to mothers who develop herpes zoster infection during pregnancy, the vast majority of infants exposed to maternal herpes zoster infection appear to be normal, and reports of herpes zoster–related fetal abnormalities or deaths may have been related to other causes.[70–72] Manifestations of the congenital varicella-zoster syndrome include low birth weight for gestational age, eye defects (microphthalmia, cataracts, and chorioretinitis), encephalomyelitis (often with severe brain damage), hypoplastic limbs with flexion contractures, cutaneous cicatricial scars, micrognathia, pneumonitis, and increased susceptibility to infection.[73–76]

Because the risk of fetal malformation in an infant born to a mother exposed to varicella-zoster virus during pregnancy is so slight, therapeutic abortion is generally not recommended. Since there is a strong correlation between limb defects and brain damage, however, a possible exception would be a fetus found to have a limb abnormality by ultrasonography at 20 weeks of gestation or a fetus found to have varicella-zoster virus infection by prenatal viral testing. Since infants in utero exposed to neonatal herpes zoster are protected by transplacentally acquired antibody and the infection is not associated with viremia, herpes zoster infection during pregnancy does not appear to present a problem for newborns.[72]

Neonatal Varicella. Neonatal chickenpox is a varicella infection of the newborn that occurs when a pregnant woman develops chickenpox during the last 2 or 3 weeks of pregnancy or the first few days post partum. In such instances, the timing of the onset of disease in the mother and her newborn are critical. If the disease onset in the mother is 5 or more days before delivery or in the newborn during the first 4 days of life, the infection is mild. In contrast, however, if the onset in the mother is within 4 days prior to or within 48 hours after delivery, or in the newborn between 5 and 10 days of birth, the infant's infection is usually severe, disseminated, and fulminant, with pneumonia, hepatitis, or meningoencephalitis, and death occurs in approximately one third of the infants (Fig. 2–21).

In an effort to avoid the untoward effects of neonatal varicella infection, 125 to 250 units (1.25 or 2.5 ml) of zoster-immune globulin (ZIG) from convalescing zoster patients or varicella-zoster immune globulin (VZIG) from high-titered normal adults should be given intramuscularly as soon as possible after delivery to all infants in whom the mother has the onset of varicella within 5 days before, or within 48 hours after delivery. If zoster-immune or varicella-zoster immune globulin is not available, 0.1 to 0.3 ml/kg of regular immune serum globulin may be used.[76, 77] In addition, since vidarabine and acyclovir have been shown to be effective in the treatment of neonatal varicella, their use should be considered in severe

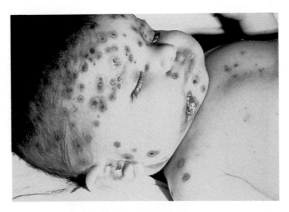

Figure 2–21. Neonatal varicella in an infant born to a mother who developed chickenpox several days prior to delivery.

neonatal varicella infection and when zoster immune globulin is not available or it is too late to use it effectively (preferably, if possible, within the first 48 hours after delivery). Of these agents, acyclovir currently appears to be the treatment of choice.

Herpes Neonatorum

Affecting 1,500 to 2,200 infants annually in the United States, herpes simplex virus infection in young infants may result in a broad spectrum of illness, ranging from death or recovery with severe central nervous system or ocular damage to mild or asymptomatic infection with apparent complete recovery. Most neonatal herpes simplex virus infections (approximately 80 per cent) are caused by type 2 (genital) *Herpesvirus hominis*, acquired either by ascending infection from the mother's genital area to the intrauterine infant, with or without premature rupture of membranes, or by spread to the infant during delivery through the birth canal of an infected mother. Infection of the newborn may also be acquired by intrauterine infection due to maternal viremia with transplacental spread (about 5 per cent of infants with the disease are infected in utero) or by postnatal hospital or household contact with other infants or persons with oral herpes simplex virus infection.[78–80]

Maternal genital herpes is estimated to occur in approximately one in 7,500 (one in 3,000 to 20,000) live births, and the risk of herpes simplex virus infection in an infant born vaginally to a mother with primary genital infection is high (40 to 50 per cent). The risk to an infant born to a mother with recurrent genital infection is much lower, probably less than 5 per cent. The lower rate of transmission when lesions are recurrent may reflect partial protection of the fetus by maternal herpes simplex virus antibodies. Although the risk of herpes neonatorum in infants born to mothers with asymptomatic herpes simplex virus infection is unknown, studies have indicated that at least 50 to 70 per cent

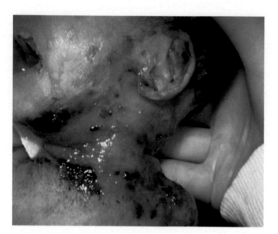

Figure 2–22. Neonatal herpes simplex with gangrenous lesions of face, head, and neck. (Courtesy of Louis Gluck, M.D.)

of infants with herpes neonatorum are born to mothers with asymptomatic shedding of the virus.[81, 82]

Neonatal herpetic infection may be categorized as disseminated, local, or asymptomatic. The relative frequency of the various forms of neonatal infection is still unknown. Similarly, the prognosis for each form is not completely elucidated. The disseminated form of neonatal herpes affects the visceral organs, chiefly the liver and adrenal glands; it may also involve the central nervous system and other organs and appears to be associated with the highest mortality. Of infants with neonatal herpes simplex virus infection, 72 per cent have skin lesions, and of these, 70 per cent if untreated will progress to systemic infection. Of further significance is the fact that untreated herpes simplex virus infection of the newborn has a fatality rate of 60 per cent and that at least one half of the survivors have significant ocular or neurologic sequelae. Any newborn, therefore, with vesicular, vesiculopustular, bullous, erosive, or ulcerated lesions should be considered as possibly having herpes simplex virus infection.

Intrauterine herpes virus infection may be termed *early* or *late*, depending on the time of infection. Early intrauterine infection with resulting disturbance of embryogenesis occurs during the first 8 weeks of gestation. Although evidence of early infection is limited, it may result in cutaneous scars, abortion, or severe congenital malformation (intrauterine growth retardation, diffuse brain damage, intracranial calcification, microcephaly, hydranencephaly, microphthalmia, chorioretinitis, retinal dysplasia, cardiac abnormalities, and short digits) with or without an associated vesicular cutaneous eruption. Late intrauterine infection produces effects that may range from congenital abnormalities (e.g., microcephaly, chorioretinitis, and intracranial calcification) to clinical disease similar to that seen in other neonatally acquired infection, ranging from fatal disease

with hepatoadrenal necrosis, pneumonia, fever, and associated cutaneous vesicular eruption, to recovery with neurologic and ophthalmologic sequelae and recurrent vesicular eruption, or recurrent vesicular lesions without evidence of associated sequelae.[79, 83, 84]

Clinical Manifestations. The clinical picture of herpes neonatorum is frequently that of an apparently previously well newborn who becomes ill on the fourth to eighth day of life, at which time vesicular lesions may be detected on the skin or buccal mucosa (Figs. 2–22 and 2-23). Although skin lesions may be present at birth, the incubation period of herpes neonatorum may vary from 2 to 21 days, with 6 days as the average age at onset. The eruption may vary from erythematous, flat, or depressed lesions to individual grouped vesicles or a widespread generalized vesicobullous eruption on the skin or buccal mucosa. The most common skin lesion is a vesicle, which usually measures 1 or 2 mm in diameter, has an erythematous halo around its base, becomes pustular after 24 to 48 hours, and eventually becomes crusted or ulcerated (Fig. 2–23). Other types of lesions include purpuric or petechial lesions, zosteriform lesions, erythematous macular lesions that eventually develop vesicular lesions within the macule, exanthems (without vesicles), pustules, erosions, and large bullae with skin denudation similar to those seen in epidermolysis bullosa.[85, 86]

Skin lesions occur most often on the scalp and face, the areas closest to and in longest contact with the cervical area from which the infection is transmitted under normal circumstances of childbirth. A zosteriform eruption has also been described in several patients with herpes simplex virus infection.[87] Occasionally, the presenting part of the in-

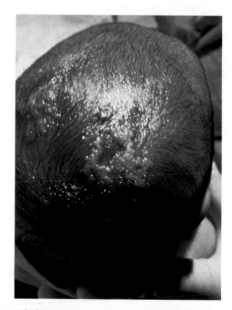

Figure 2–23. Herpes neonatorum on the scalp. (Courtesy of Louis Gluck, M.D.)

fant at time of delivery may be covered by a diffuse edematous swelling resembling that seen in association with caput succedaneum. Rather than resolving spontaneously during the first week of life (as normally occurs with caput succedaneum), the boggy swelling may become necrotic, with resultant draining sinus and eschar formation and tense, irregularly grouped herpetic vesicles in otherwise normal-appearing cutaneous tissue (see Fig. 2–23).

At times conjunctivitis and keratoconjunctivitis may be seen as the first presenting sign of this disorder. This is subsequently followed by lethargy, anorexia, fever or fluctuating temperature, icterus, hepatosplenomegaly, and widespread herpes simplex virus dissemination, with hepatitis, pneumonia, coagulopathy with severe bleeding diathesis, and, at times, disease of the central nervous system. Approximately 60 per cent of all infants with symptomatic infection will have prominent signs and symptoms of central nervous system involvement, such as irritability, bulging fontanelle, focal or generalized seizures, flaccid or spastic paralysis, opisthotonos, decerebrate rigidity, or coma. Since disseminated visceral herpes of the newborn, if untreated, will end fatally in 90 per cent of cases and antiviral therapy is most effective if started early in the course of the disease, treatment should be initiated as early as possible, preferably within 24 hours of presentation. Thus, when a newborn is suspected of having a herpes simplex virus infection, it is better to initiate antiviral therapy early rather than to withhold treatment until a definitive diagnosis is established.

Diagnosis. When cutaneous lesions are absent, disseminated neonatal herpes infection may be confused with sepsis, toxoplasmosis, or cytomegalic inclusion disease. The diagnosis of herpes simplex virus infection of the newborn may be aided by the Tzanck test, viral culture, or biopsy of cutaneous lesions. The characteristic histopathologic lesion of herpes simplex virus infection is an intraepidermal vesicle with balloon degeneration of the epidermal cells. Multinucleated giant cells containing intranuclear inclusions are of diagnostic significance when found in scrapings from the bases of lesions or undersides of blisters (the Tzanck test).

To perform the Tzanck test, the top of a vesicular lesion is removed with a scalpel and fluid contents are blotted away carefully to avoid disturbing the base of the lesion. The lesion is then pinched firmly to prevent bleeding and scraped gently with a sharp curet; the curettings are spread on a clean glass microscope slide. The specimen is air dried, fixed by a fixative spray or immersion for 1 minute in 95 per cent methyl alcohol, and stained with Giemsa's, Wright's, methylene blue, crystal violet, or Papanicolaou's stains or Sedi-stain. The finding of marginated multinucleated giant cells (balloon cells) on Tzanck smear indicates the presence of herpes simplex, herpes zoster, or varicella virus (Fig. 2–24), but without other clinical or laboratory

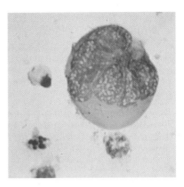

Figure 2–24. Tzanck smear with margination of nucleus and balloon cells. (Courtesy of Guinter Kahn, M.D.)

data it does not differentiate one from the other. Other diagnostic techniques such as direct fluorescent antibody staining of vesicle scrapings, enzyme-linked immunosorbent assay (ELISA), and DNA amplification tests using the polymerase chain reaction offer more rapid diagnosis.

Management. Several approaches to the prevention and treatment of herpes simplex virus infection of the newborn have been recommended. Instrumentation such as fetal monitoring should be avoided whenever possible for infants known to be at risk for herpes simplex virus infection (see Fig. 2–23), and until recently it was recommended that pregnant women with known genital herpes simplex virus infection be delivered by cesarean section if the membranes are intact or if they have been ruptured for no more than a 4-hour period. One must recognize, however, that although the risk of herpes simplex virus infection in an infant born vaginally to a mother with primary genital infection is approximately 50 per cent, the risk to an infant of a mother with recurrent herpes simplex virus infection is less than 5 percent; and over 70 per cent of infants with neonatal herpes infection are born to mothers who do not manifest any sign or symptom of genital infection at the time of delivery. Accordingly, the value of viral cultures and cytologic studies of mothers with suspected genital herpes simplex virus infection during the last few weeks before delivery and of routine prophylactic cesarean section, a procedure associated with appreciable maternal and neonatal morbidity, has led to careful scrutiny and reevaluation.[88]

If herpes simplex virus infection is suspected, the newborn should be isolated during evaluation, appropriate viral studies should be done, and baseline renal and hepatic studies should be performed to rule out the possibility of visceral involvement. In infants born to mothers with known genital herpes simplex virus infection, specimens from various sites (throat, stool, urine, peripheral blood buffy coat) should be obtained frequently for culture, and the infant should be carefully observed for signs of infection. Ophthalmologic examinations should be performed, and prophylactic topical ophthalmic preparations, such as iododeoxyuridine (Herplex, Stoxil), vidarabine (Vira-A Ophthalmic Ointment), or trifluridine (Viroptic Ophthalmic Solution), should be used for infants at risk (of these, the latter currently appears to be the therapeutic agent of choice).

Women with active congenital herpes simplex virus infection should be given a private room, and gown and glove precautions and thorough hand-washing techniques should be used to help avoid contact of the infant with lesions or infectious secretions. A mother with herpes labialis or stomatitis may handle and feed her infant, provided that she uses careful hand-washing techniques and wears a disposable surgical mask or dressing to cover her lesions until they have crusted and dried.[89] There is no unequivocal evidence that herpes simplex virus is transmitted by breast milk or that breast feeding by a mother with recurrent herpes simplex virus infection poses a risk to the infant. It therefore appears that if open lesions are covered and careful hand washing techniques and precautions are utilized, breast feeding by a mother with recurrent herpes simplex virus infection may be acceptable.[89] After discharge from the hospital, infants born to mothers with known genital herpes infection who appear to be clinically well should be examined every few days for at least 1 month.

Once a diagnosis of herpes neonatorum is established, intravenous vidarabine (Vira-A) or acyclovir (Zovirax) should be administered as soon as possible, preferably before central nervous system or other systemic complications occur. For reasons of lower toxicity and ease of administration, acyclovir (30 mg/kg/day in three divided doses) given intravenously for a minimum of 14 days is recommended.

Human Parvovirus Infection

Human parvovirus B19, the same virus that causes erythema infectiosum (fifth disease) has a special affinity for rapidly dividing cells, particularly erythroblasts, and therefore may at times result in hydrops fetalis and fetal death. Although the full extent of fetal loss to parvovirus infection is unknown, the risk of hydrops fetalis and fetal death to a pregnant women exposed to this infection appears to be less than 1 per cent, and current data suggest a 2 to 5 per cent risk following parvovirus infection during the first 20 weeks of pregnancy. Pregnant women exposed to this virus, therefore, should have this relatively low potential risk explained to them, and the option for having serologic tests (in an effort to determine previous immunity or the possibility of active infection) should be offered. For pregnant women with evidence of infection, maternal serum α-fetoprotein concentration may provide a marker of fetal aplastic crisis; if the α-fetoprotein concentration is increased, serial ultrasound examinations may be used to detect the possibility of fetal hydrops and fetal sampling may

indicate its severity. Since intrauterine infection tends to cause fetal hydrops and death, rather than abnormality, therapeutic abortion is not indicated, but in utero transfusion and early delivery and transfusion may at times be beneficial.[90, 91]

Neonatal Syphilis

As a result of advances in the detection and treatment of syphilis during the years following World War II, the incidence of neonatal syphilis dropped to relatively insignificant levels by the mid 1950s. Since 1959, however, the incidence of primary and secondary syphilis has increased, with a resultant resurgence in the incidence of congenital syphilis (a disorder that to a generation of physicians had been well documented but temporarily forgotten).[92, 93]

Congenital syphilis, more accurately termed *prenatal syphilis*, is a disorder in which the fetus becomes infected with organisms of the spirochete *Treponema pallidum* by way of the placenta usually, but not necessarily, sometime after the 16th week of pregnancy. For years it was believed that fetal infection did not occur earlier because the Langhans layer of the chorion allegedly functioned as a barrier to the passage of *T. pallidum* and did not begin to atrophy until after the 16th week of gestation. Although this concept was adhered to for generations, studies on early abortuses from syphilitic women refute it. Whatever the factors responsible for this attenuated virulence of early prenatal syphilis, they seem to have little to do with previous theories of mechanical barriers and perhaps are related to inability of the fetal immune system to marshal a plasma cell response, or perhaps to other unrecognized biochemical requirements of the spirochete in fetuses infected during the early weeks of pregnancy.[94]

The clinical manifestations of congenital syphilis can be divided into lesions of early congenital syphilis (those appearing before age 2) and late congenital syphilis (those occurring after age 2). The lesions of early congenital syphilis are generally infectious and, since there is no primary stage, may resemble those of acquired secondary syphilis. They differ from those of the second stage of syphilis in that the fetal lesions are generally more widely distributed, more severe, and of longer duration. The lesions of late congenital syphilis, conversely, may represent either a hypersensitivity reaction on the part of the host or scars and deformities that are direct consequences of the infection.

Clinical Manifestations

Early Congenital Syphilis. Fetal infection with *T. pallidum* results in multiple system involvement with considerable variation in clinical expression. Although infants with congenital syphilis frequently exhibit no external signs of disease at the time of birth, many present clinical manifestations in the first month. In a series of 206 infants, 31

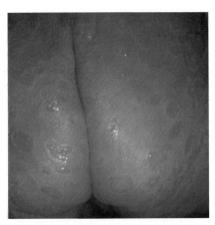

Figure 2–25. Eroded papular lesions of congenital syphilis. (Courtesy of Gabriela Lowy, M.D.)

per cent showed evidence of the disorder at birth (personal communication, Dr. Gabriela Lowy, Rio de Janeiro, Brazil). Those with florid manifestations at birth appear to be more severely infected, are often premature, and usually have a poor prognosis. The most common clinical manifestations are anemia, fever, wasting, hepatosplenomegaly, lymphadenopathy, rhinitis (usually known as "snuffles"), mucocutaneous eruptions, edema, desquamation, and pseudoparalysis.

Rhinitis or "Snuffles." Rhinitis (snuffles) is generally the first sign of congenital syphilis and is rarely absent in the infant with clinically manifest disease. It usually appears between the second and sixth weeks of life and is the result of an ulcerous lesion of the nasal mucosa. When ulceration is deep enough to involve the cartilage of the nasal bone, the normal architecture is destroyed, thus giving rise to the classic saddle-nose deformity characteristically seen in this disorder.

Cutaneous Manifestations. Cutaneous lesions of congenital syphilis may be seen in one third to one half of infants affected by this disorder. They may be quite varied, but most commonly appear as large round or oval maculopapular or papulosquamous lesions (Fig. 2–25) comparable to those seen in secondary syphilis of the adolescent or adult. The eruption may appear on any part of the body but usually is most pronounced on the face, the dorsal surface of the trunk and legs, the diaper area, and, at times, the palms and soles. The eruption generally develops slowly, is bright pink or red, and gradually fades to a coppery brown. It disappears spontaneously over 1 to 3 months, often leaving a residual area of hyperpigmentation or hypopigmentation. Vesiculobullous hemorrhagic lesions are relatively rare but, especially when seen on the palms and soles, are highly diagnostic of this disorder. The palms and soles may be fissured, erythematous, and, as a result of subcutaneous edema, indurated with a dull red, shiny, almost polished appearance. Concomitant with these changes, desquamation of the skin in large dry flakes may occur over the entire body. Even when not present elsewhere, this desquamation may still be detected around the nails of the fingers and toes of affected infants.

Mucous membrane patches, seen in approximately one third of infants, are among the most characteristic and most infectious of the early lesions seen in congenital syphilis. At mucocutaneous junctions they tend to weep and may cause fissures, which often extend out from the lips in a radiating fashion over the surrounding skin. When deep these may leave residual scars (rhagades) in the adjacent circumoral region (Fig. 2–26).

Raised, flat, moist wart-like lesions (condylomata lata) commonly appear in any of the moist areas of the body surface of infants with congenital syphilis. Also extremely infectious, they are most commonly seen in the anogenital regions, about the nares, and at the angles of the mouth.

Necrotizing funisitis, spiral zones of red and pale-blue umbilical cord discoloration interspersed with streaks of chalky white (hence the term *barber-pole umbilical cord*), has been described as a frequently overlooked, early diagnostic clinical feature of congenital syphilis. The external smooth surface of the umbilical cord without evidence of exudation apparently differentiates necrotizing funisitis from acute bacterial funisitis, an inflammation of the umbilical cord seen in newborns with acute bacterial infection.[95]

Visceral Involvement. Hepatomegaly may occur in 50 to 75 per cent of affected infants. It is frequently associated with icterus and, at times, ascites, splenomegaly, and generalized enlargement of the lymph nodes. Palpable epitrochlear nodes, although not pathognomonic, are highly suggestive of congenital syphilis. The jaundice, together with the anemia, edema, and cutaneous changes seen after the eruption has faded, produces a peculiar dirty, whitish brown (café au lait) appearance to the skin. Damage to the hemato-

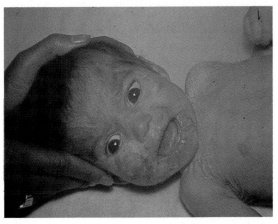

Figure 2–26. Congenital syphilis. Rhagades, infiltrated plaques, and café au lait color. (Courtesy of Gabriela Lowy, M.D.)

poietic system with hemolytic anemia, and at times thrombocytopenia, is an almost constant feature of early congenital syphilis. When seen with hepatosplenomegaly, jaundice, and large numbers of nucleated erythrocytes in the peripheral circulation, an erroneous diagnosis of erythroblastosis fetalis may be made.

Osseous Manifestations. Although only 15 per cent of infants with congenital syphilis show clinical signs of osteochondritis at birth, 90 per cent of infants will show radiologic evidence of osteochondritis and periostitis after the first month of life. Syphilitic osteochondritis may occur in any bone but is found most frequently in the long bones of the extremities. Radiographic findings consist of increased widening of the epiphyseal line with increased density of the shafts, spotty areas of translucency, and a resultant motheaten appearance. In most cases the bony lesions are asymptomatic. In some infants, however, severe involvement may lead to subepiphyseal fracture with epiphyseal dislocation and extremely painful pseudoparalysis of one or more extremity (the so-called pseudoparalysis of Parrot).

Dactylitis is a rare form of osteochondritis of the small bones of the hands and feet that usually appears between 6 months and 2 years of age. Commonly found in the metatarsals, metacarpals, and proximal phalanges of the hands, its presence can frequently be detected by a cylindrical swelling of the affected bone with reddening of the overlying skin and relatively little pain or discomfort of the involved area.

Periosteal lesions, unlike those of osteochondritis, are seldom present at birth. Periostitis of the frontal bones of the skull, when severe, is at least partially responsible for the flat overhanging forehead that persists as a stigma of children severely infected in infancy. The radiologic changes of periostitis are usually most pronounced during the second to sixth months of life and rarely persist beyond the age of 2 years. Lesions are usually diffuse (in contrast to the localized involvement characteristic of lesions of osteochondritis) and frequently extend the entire length of the involved bone. First seen as a thin, even line of calcification outside the cortex of the involved bone, the lesions progress and additional layers of opaque tissue are laid down, with the resulting "onion-peel" appearance of advanced periostitis. This eventually produces calcification and thickening of the cortex and, when severe, a permanent deformity. In the tibia, this results in an anterior bowing referred to as saber shins. In the skull it is seen (in 30 to 60 per cent of patients) as frontal or parietal bossing.

Central Nervous System Involvement. Even though clinical evidence of central nervous system involvement is a relatively uncommon finding, cerebrospinal fluid abnormalities may be detected in 40 to 50 per cent of infants with congenital syphilis. This is demonstrated by increased protein levels, by mononuclear pleocytosis of up to 200 or 300 cells/cubic millimeter (mm^3), or by positive results of a cerebrospinal fluid VDRL test. Clinical evidence of miningitis with bulging of the fontanelle, opisthotonos, and, at times, convulsions, generally portends a poor prognosis. Low-grade syphilitic meningitis may result in a mild degree of hydrocephalus, and children with central nervous system inolvement continuing beyond the period of infancy may go on to demonstrate marked residua with varying degrees of physical and mental retardation.

Late Congenital Syphilis

Late congenital syphilis is that form of congenital syphilis that persists beyond 2 years of age. It also includes varying signs and stigmata of congenital syphilis in individuals in whom the diagnosis was overlooked or in those patients who were inadequately treated early in the course of the disease. The stigmata most suggestive of congenital syphilis are interstitial keratitis (seen in 20 to 50 per cent of affected children), Hutchinson's incisors, mulberry (or Moon's) molars, and eighth nerve deafness.

Dental Changes. Perhaps the most pathognomonic signs of this disorder are the dental changes. Although the result of infection at an early age, their appearance at the time of eruption of the permanent teeth merits their inclusion among the manifestations of late congenital syphilis.

The deciduous teeth of children with early congenital syphilis are prone to caries but show no specific abnormalities characteristic of this disorder. The term *Hutchinson's incisors* is applied to deformities of the permanent upper central incisors characterized by central notching of the biting edges with tapering of the lateral side of the teeth toward the biting edge (so-called screwdriver teeth). The simultaneous appearance of interstitial keratitis, Hutchinson's incisors, and eighth nerve deafness is termed *Hutchinson's triad.* Although described as a time-honored sign of congenital syphilis, owing to the relative infrequency of eighth nerve deafness, this triad is actually extremely uncommon and rarely reported.

The *mulberry* or *Moon's molar* (named after the English surgeon who first described it) is a malformation of the lower first 6-year molars. The mulberry appearance is created by poorly developed cusps crowded together on the crown. Since these teeth are subject to rapid decay, mulberry molars are rarely seen past puberty. When present, however, they are pathognomonic of congenital syphilis. Carabelli's tubercle is the name given to an accessory cusp that develops on the inner aspect of the upper first molar. This deformity occurs with equal frequency in nonsyphilitic as well as congenital syphilitic patients. The presence of Carabelli's tubercle should not be regarded as a sign of congenital syphilis.

Gummas. Also occurring as a late manifestation of congenital syphilis and considered to be the result of a hypersensitivity phenomenon, gummas may appear in the bones of the skull (or in the tibias) where they may erode the bone and go on to involve the subcutaneous tissue and cutaneous surface. As they progress to become necrotic, ulcerations with thick indurated borders generally are seen. Although gummas usually respond dramatically to antibiotic therapy, those affecting the nasal septum or palate frequently result in a residual saddle-nose or cleft palate deformity.

Higouménakis' Sign. Unilateral thickening of the inner third or the clavicle is frequently described as a manifestation of late congenital syphilis. Since fracture of the middle third of the clavicle is the most common fracture occurring at birth, consequent healing and thickening of the involved bone often produces a clinical picture similar to that seen with Higouménakis' abnormality. This finding should therefore not be considered a reliable stigma of late congenital syphilis.

Syphilitic Arthritis. Arthritis may affect any of the larger joints (particularly the knees). Painless effusion into one or both knees may be known as *Clutton's joints*. Clutton's joints generally become apparent between 8 and 15 years of age, are not accompanied by fever, respond well to therapy or may involute spontaneously over several months or years, and leave no residual effects.

Paroxysmal Cold Hemoglobinuria. Characterized by shaking chills and voiding of dark urine within 8 hours following exposure to cold, paroxysmal cold hemoglobinuria may also occur as a manifestation of late congenital syphilis. This disorder is the result of autohemolysis following exposure to cold and generally is seen in patients with late congenital syphilis who did not receive treatment. Paroxysmal cold hemoglobinuria, in the absence of other definitive signs, although not pathognomonic, is highly suggestive of late congenital or untreated acquired syphilis.

Ocular Changes. Choroiditis, retinitis, and optic atrophy may also be seen as late manifestations of congenital syphilis. Optic atrophy, when present, is usually seen in conjunction with neurosyphilis.

Diagnosis. Early manifestations of congenital syphilis generally are so typical that the diagnosis of an infant with florid infection, once suspected, is usually not difficult. Unfortunately, the vast majority of infants frequently have minimal or no clinical evidence of infection. In such cases, early diagnosis often depends on the physician's index of suspicion and awareness of the possibility of the disorder.

Placental changes (consisting of focal villositis, endovascular and perivascular proliferation in villous vessels, and relative immaturity of villi) often assist in early diagnosis of congenital syphilis. Diagnosis may be confirmed by positive darkfield examination from the umbilical vein or from moist lesions of the skin or mucous membranes, by characteristic bone changes on radiographs, and by positive serologic tests for syphilis. Serologic tests, however, in the newborn must be interpreted with

caution since their results may be due to passive transfer of reaginic and IgG treponemal antibodies from the mother. The presence of these antibodies in the serum of the newborn merely indicates that the mother has or has had syphilis. A serologic titer in the newborn higher than that of the mother, however, is diagnostic. If no other indications of active infection are evident, with serologic titers equal to or lower than the maternal titer, infants should be followed closely (without treatment), with repeated titers taken at appropriate intervals. In cases of passive transfer of antibody, the neonatal titer should not exceed that of the mother and should revert to negative by the time the infant has reached 3 to 4 months of age.

Evaluation of infants suspected of having congenital syphilis should include a thorough examination for evidence of infection; darkfield microscopy or direct immunofluorescence on specimens from sites such as skin lesions, umbilicus, or placenta; nontreponemal reagin antibody (VDRL or rapid plasma reagin cord [RPR] test and automated reagin test [ART]); cerebrospinal fluid analysis for cells, protein, and VDRL; long-bone radiographs; other tests such as a chest radiograph as clinically indicated; and, if possible, a fluorescent treponemal antibody absorption (FTA-ABS) test. The nontreponemal antibody tests (VDRL, RPR, and ART) are useful for screening; the fluorescent treponemal antibody absorption test and microhemagglutination assay for antibodies to *T. pallidum* (MHA-TP) are used to substantiate the diagnosis; and quantitative nontreponemal antibody tests are used to assess the adequacy of therapy and to detect reinfection and relapse. Screening tests at delivery should be performed with maternal blood specimens, not cord blood. In cases in which the mother is infected late in pregnancy, both mother and child may be nonreactive at delivery. In such instances, clinical signs and rising titers during the ensuing weeks will confirm the diagnosis.

Treatment. Penicillin is the treatment of choice for all forms of congenital as well as acquired syphilis. Studies have demonstrated that 25 per cent of fetuses infected in utero die before birth and 30 per cent of infants with congenital syphilis, if not treated, will die shortly after delivery. Once there is evidence of disease, treatment should be instituted immediately. Although many treatment schedules differentiate between the treatment for infants with central nervous system involvement and those without, clinical experience shows that central nervous system involvement may be inapparent if the lumbar puncture is performed early. It is recommended, therefore, that infants with established or presumed diagnosis of congenital syphilis be treated by aqueous crystalline penicillin G in a dosage of 100,000 to 150,000 units/kg intramuscularly, or 50,000 units/kg administered intravenously every 8 to 12 hours, or procaine penicillin G in dosage of 50,000 units/kg administered intramuscularly once daily for 10 to 14 days. If daily injections cannot be administered, a single intramuscular injection of benzathine penicillin G (50,000 units/kg) may be satisfactory. Although failure of benzathine penicillin G in infants with early congenital syphilis without evidence of central nervous system involvement is rare,[96] infants so treated should have frequent follow-up evaluations and serologic nontreponemal tests 3, 6, and 12 months after the conclusion of treatment, or until they become unreactive. An asymptomatic newborn of a mother who received penicillin or one whose mother is adequately treated but remains seropositive need not be treated but should be clinically and serologically reevaluated at 1, 2, and 4 months.

Infants with evidence of central nervous system involvement should receive crystalline penicillin G daily (30,000 to 50,000 units/kg in two or three doses) or procaine penicillin G (50,000 units per kilogram in one daily dose) for a minimum of 2 weeks and preferably for a total of 3 weeks. Since studies with benzathine penicillin suggest inadequate penetration of the central nervous system of newborns when serum penicillin levels are low, the use of benzathine penicillin G for congenital syphilis with central nervous system involvement is probably inadequate and should not be recommended.

Cytomegalic Inclusion Disease

Cytomegalic inclusion disease in the newborn is a generalized infection caused by the cytomegalovirus (CMV), a DNA virus of the herpesvirus group. Endemic in nature, CMV may occur in 3.5 to 6.0 per cent of pregnant women in the United States. Of these, CMV excretion is found in only 0.5 to 2.0 per cent of newborns and only 1 in 3,000 develops the classic syndrome of cytomegalic inclusion disease.

Clinical Manifestations. Approximately 90 per cent of congenital CMV infections are asymptomatic. The remaining 10 per cent may have mild to severe, and occasionally fatal, cytomegalic inclusion disease. Although infection in infants is generally transmitted from a pregnant mother with inapparent infection across the placenta to the fetus late in gestation, it can also be transmitted by passage through an infected maternal genital tract at the time of delivery or by postnatal CMV-seropositive blood transfusion. Postnatal consumption of infected breast milk or colostrum can also transmit CMV, but presumably because of the presence of passively acquired antibody, most infants infected in this manner do not appear to be seriously ill. Most of the reported cases of congenital CMV infection are in premature infants or in those below average for their gestational age. Since most infections are asymptomatic, diagnosis is only made in the full-blown syndrome, one generally manifested by icterus, hepatosplenomegaly, and hemorrhagic diatheses.

Typical clinical findings include lethargy, the appearance of jaundice within the first 24 hours of life, hepatosplenomegaly, abdominal distention, anemia, thrombocytopenia, respiratory distress, protracted interstitial pneumonia, central nervous system depression, convulsions, and chorioretinitis. Cerebral calcifications (often paraventricular in location) may be noted on skull radiographs. Cutaneous manifestations include petechiae and purpura, a generalized maculopapular eruption, and, in some instances, a generalized papulonodular eruption with blueberry muffin lesions similar to those seen in infants with congenital rubella and neonatal toxoplasmosis. Although extremely rare, vesicular lesions have also been reported in infants with this disorder.[97]

Until recently, clinically apparent disease due to acquired rather than congenital CMV infection had not been recognized except in patients with primary or iatrogenic immune deficiency. It is now recognized, however, that in previously healthy older children and adults, CMV infection may result in a variety of abnormalities, including an infectious mononucleosis–like illness (CMV mononucleosis), infectious polyneuritis, hepatomegaly with abnormal liver function tests, and, particularly in those with a deficiency of cellular immunity, pneumonitis.

Most symptomatic cases of congenital cytomegalic inclusion disease are fatal within the first 2 months of life. Those who survive frequently manifest severe neurologic defects, namely microcephaly, mental retardation, deafness, spastic diplegia, convulsive disorders, chorioretinitis, optic atrophy, and blindness. Of the 90 per cent of CMV-infected infants who do not manifest clinical evidence of infection at birth, 5 to 15 per cent develop late-onset sequelae such as hearing loss, chorioretinitis, mental retardation, and neurologic defects.[98]

Diagnosis. Diagnosis of cytomegalic inclusion disease may be established by the finding of distinctive large cells containing intranuclear and cytoplasmic inclusions from the urine, liver biopsy specimens, gastric washings, or cerebrospinal fluid, or by direct isolation of the CMV from the pharynx, urine, or fibroblasts of cell cultures from affected infants. Since bacterial growth may interfere with viral cultures, efforts to prevent bacterial contamination must be made. Only urine specimens collected by a clean-catch technique or by aseptic suprapubic puncture should be used, and the specimens should be treated with antibiotics. Proof of congenital infection, however, depends on obtaining specimens within 3 weeks of birth. In that period viral recovery or a strongly positive test for serum IgM anti-CMV antibody is considered diagnostic. Later in infancy, differentiation between intrauterine and perinatal infection is difficult unless signs of intrauterine infection, such as chorioretinitis or ventriculitis, are present. When the diagnosis remains in doubt, persistent or rising complement-fixation titers may provide confirmatory evidence. Since IgM does not cross the placental barrier, specific fluorescence of CMV IgM antibody in the newborn is useful in the diagnosis of active congenital cytomegalic inclusion disease.

Management. There is no effective therapy for cytomegalic inclusion disease, and prognosis for the patient with severe involvement is poor. Although cytarabine and vidarabine have been used experimentally, there is no evidence that they have any lasting effect on the prognosis of this disorder. Ganciclovir (Cytovene), however, is beneficial in the treatment of retinitis and organ involvement of patients with acquired CMV infection and, although available studies are insufficient to establish safety in children, limited data suggest that efficacy is similar to that in adults.[99]

Congenital Epstein-Barr Virus Syndrome

Because the majority of young adults are Epstein-Barr virus seropositive, primary infection during pregnancy is uncommon. Although features of congenital Epstein-Barr virus infection such as micrognathia, cryptorchidism, cataracts, hypotonia, scaly erythematous rash, hepatosplenomegaly, transient lymphadenopathy, and persistent atypical lymphocytosis have been reported, the low frequency of Epstein-Barr virus infection in pregnancy makes it difficult to assess the full extent of this risk.[100]

Congenital Toxoplasmosis

Toxoplasmosis is a parasitic disorder that may affect infants and children as well as adults. Caused by *Toxoplasma gondii*, a tiny intracellular protozoan that may invade any tissue (with the exception of erythrocytes) of all mammals, many birds, and some reptiles, toxoplasmosis generally occurs as a clinically silent infection of the gravid woman. Estimated to affect 2 in 1,000 live births in the United States a year, toxoplasmosis is transmitted to the fetus by invasion of the bloodstream during a stage of maternal parasitemia and may result in a wide spectrum of clinical signs and symptoms. Acquired toxoplasmosis is a disorder of older children or adults accidentally infected either by ingestion of raw meat contaminated by *toxoplasma* cysts or by contact with soil containing resistant oocysts from the excreta of infected cats, dogs, or chickens.

Clinical Manifestations. In congenital toxoplasmosis the fetus may be stillborn, born prematurely, or born at full term. Illness apparent at birth or during the first few weeks of life may be characterized by malaise, vomiting, diarrhea, fever, a maculopapular rash, icterus, lymphadenopathy, hepatomegaly, splenomegaly, hydrocephaly, microcephaly, microphthalmos, cataracts, hypothermia, pneumonitis, abnormal bleeding or convulsions. Chorioretinitis in the region of the macula, seen in 80 to 90 per cent of infants with

congenital toxoplasmosis, is highly characteristic but not diagnostic of this disorder. Laboratory findings in patients with congenital toxoplasmosis reveal anemia, eosinophilia, thrombocytopenia, and, at times, severe leukopenia. The cerebrospinal fluid may be xanthochromic and may contain leukocytes, erythrocytes, and an elevated level of protein. Skull radiographs of affected infants frequently reveal diffuse punctate comma-shaped intracranial calcifications.

The cutaneous manifestations of congenital or acquired toxoplasmosis may consist of a generalized rubella-like maculopapular eruption that may be ecchymotic or purpuric and generally spares the face, palms, and soles. There may be a scarlatiniform eruption or subcutaneous nodules scattered over the trunk and extremities. Annular, urticarial pinkish papules or very rarely a vesicular rash or a micropapular typhus-like rash that spares the palms, soles, face, and scalp may also occur at times. In most severe cases, the rash develops during the first weeks of illness, perists for 1 to 6 days (rarely more than 1 or 2 weeks), and may be followed by desquamation or hyperpigmentation. In addition, congenital toxoplasmosis may be associated with dermal erythropoiesis, which presents clinically as localized or generalized bluish, hemorrhagic, infiltrated macules or as papular blueberry muffin lesions, similar to those seen in congenital rubella and cytomegalic inclusion disease.[101]

Diagnosis. The diagnosis of congenital toxoplasmosis is made on the basis of clinical evidence supported by demonstration of the organism in biopsy specimens of lymph node, liver, or spleen, or in Wright- or Giemsa-stained smears of centrifuged cerebrospinal or ventricular fluid. Isolation of the parasite in laboratory-reared animals (mice, hamsters, or rabbits proven free of *toxoplasma* prior to use) inoculated with blood, bone marrow, cerebrospinal fluid, saliva, or fresh suspensions of lymph node or other suspected tissue from biopsy or autopsy specimens is confirmatory. It should be noted, however, that although the Sabin-Feldman dye test is sensitive and specific, owing to technical difficulties this test has been abandoned in many countries. Since IgM does not cross the placental barrier, a more rapid and specific diagnosis can be established (as in cytomegalic inclusion disease) on a single infant serum sample by demonstration that the infant's antibodies are in the IgM fraction and, therefore, not of maternal origin. Here again a fluorescent antibody test for the detection of fetal IgM antibody to the *Toxoplasma* organism is valuable as a rapid confirmatory test. Other tests include a complement fixation test, indirect hemagglutination, latex agglutination, and enzyme-linked immunosorbent assay (ELISA) tests. Prenatal diagnosis is based on fetal blood sampling, amniocentesis, and ultrasound examination.

Management. Most cases of toxoplasmosis are subclinical or are associated with mild symptomatology. Although congenital infections may vary in their severity, chorioretinitis, residual brain damage, and fatalities are not uncommon. In the presence of an extremely high mortality rate in infants with fulminating infection, and because of the serious sequelae that may develop even in asymptomatic infants, once a diagnosis of congenital toxoplasmosis is established the patient should receive specific therapy whether or not the infection is clinically apparent or the patient is asymptomatic.

For severe congenital infection, sulfadiazine or trisulfapyrimidine, in combination with pyrimethamine (Daraprim), plus folinic acid appears to be effective. Treatment, however, must be individualized; and although optimal duration of treatment is not known, a minimum of 21 days is recommended and some authorities recommend that treatment be continued for 1 year.

The prognosis for infants with toxoplasmosis manifested at birth, particularly when it involves predominantly the liver and bone marrow, is poor. Although infants who become asymptomatic after a few weeks and who have predominantly central nervous system involvement often survive, their ultimate prognosis is poor. Many suffer from chorioretinitis and subsequent blindness and may become microcephalic or hydrocephalic and mentally defective. Infants with severe forms of congenital toxoplasmosis, accordingly, often require corticosteroids (prednisone in dosages of 1.5 mg/kg/day or its equivalent) until evidence of inflammatory processes, such as chorioretinitis and high cerebrospinal fluid protein levels, has subsided.[102]

DIAPER DERMATITIS

Diaper dermatitis (diaper rash) is perhaps the most common cutaneous disorder of infancy and early childhood. Seen most frequently in infants and children younger than 2 years of age, diaper dermatoses usually begin between the first and second months of life and, if not properly controlled, may recur at intervals until the child no longer wears diapers.

The term *diaper rash* is used all too frequently in a diagnostic sense, as though the diverse dermatoses that may affect the anogenital region of infants and young children constitute a single, specific clinical entity. In actuality, diaper dermatitis is not a specific diagnosis and is best viewed as a variable symptom-complex, a family of disorders initiated by a combination of factors, the most significant being prolonged contact with or irritation by urine and feces, maceration engendered by wet diapers and impervious diaper coverings, and, in a high percentage of cases, secondary infection with *Candida albicans*.[103]

Although frequently no more than a disagreeable nuisance, eruptions in this area may progress to secondary infection and ulceration, become complicated by other superimposed cutaneous disorders, or may be a source of confusion when a dermatologic disease of entirely different etiology arises in the anogenital region. The term *diaper dermatitis* reflects a variety of inflammatory disorders of the skin that occur on the lower aspect of the abdomen, genitalia, buttocks, and upper portions of the thighs in infants, young children, and incontinent or paralyzed individuals.

For years ammonia caused by bacterial breakdown of urea in the child's urine was believed to be a major factor in the etiology of diaper rash.[104] In 1921, when Cooke demonstrated that an aerobic gram-positive bacillus (*Bacillus ammoniagenes*) was capable of liberating ammonia from urea, this organism was seized on as the etiologic agent of most diaper dermatoses.[105] Recent studies, however, refute the role of urea-splitting bacteria in the etiology of this disorder and incriminate a combination of wetness, impervious diaper coverings, increase in pH as a result of liberation of urea by stool ureases, and *Candida albicans* as the primary factor in the initiation of most diaper eruptions in infants and small children. It is suggested that urinary wetness increases the permeability of the skin to irritants and the pH of the diaper environment, thus intensifying the activities of the fecal proteases and lipases, the major irritants responsible for this disorder.[106–108]

In some instances diaper dermatitis may be complicated by other superimposed conditions, and occasionally it may present as the first sign of a more severe or systemic disorder. In the absence of precise etiologic diagnosis, treatment based primarily on topographic distribution alone may fail to achieve satisfactory therapeutic results. All diaper eruptions, therefore, should be subjected to critical analysis prior to the initiation of definitive therapy.

Clinical Manifestations

Friction Dermatitis. The most prevalent form of diaper dermatitis is the chafing or friction dermatitis that affects most infants at some time. Generally present on areas where friction is the most pronounced (the inner surfaces of the thighs, the genitalia, buttocks, and the abdomen), the eruption tends to wax and wane quickly, is frequently aggravated by the use of harsh talcum preparations, consists of a mild erythema with a shiny glazed surface and occasional papules, and responds quickly to frequent diaper changes, avoidance of diapers whenever possible, and simple drying measures.

Irritant Dermatitis. Irritant or contact diaper dermatitis is usually confined to the convex surfaces of the buttocks, perineal area, lower abdomen, and proximal thighs, with sparing of the intertriginous creases (Fig. 2–27). The disorder may be attributable to contact with proteolytic enzymes and irritant chemicals, such as harsh soaps, detergents, and topical medications. Other significant factors appear to be excessive heat, moisture, and sweat retention associated with the warm subtropical environment produced by impervious diaper coverings.

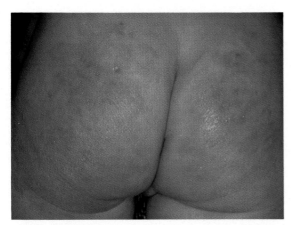

Figure 2–27. Irritant- or contact-type diaper dermatitis. The eruption is localized to convex surfaces with sparing of the intertriginous areas.

Allergic Dermatitis. Diaper dermatitis based on an allergic reaction, when present, may complicate an irritant diaper dermatitis or may arise de novo. It is frequently localized to the convex areas exposed to the contactants, with sparing of the intertriginous areas. True sensitization reactions, although relatively uncommon in infants, are generally attributable to detergent soap preparations, topical antibiotics, or topical medications aggravating a preexisting diaper dermatitis.

In mild diaper eruptions the skin may be diffusely reddened, with papules, vesicles, edema, and scaling of the involved areas. With beginning resolution a shiny, wrinkled parchment paper-like appearance may be noted. In more severe cases, papules, vesicles, psoriasiform lesions, annular plaques, secondary erosions, ulcerations, and infiltrated nodules may occur.

Jacquet's Dermatitis. The term *Jacquet's dermatitis* is often used to describe a severe papuloerosive eruption with umbilicated or crater-like appearance (Fig. 2–28). In male infants, ulceration

and crusting of the glans penis and urinary meatus may create difficulty or discomfort on micturition.

Intertrigo. Intertrigo is a common type of skin eruption in the diaper area, particularly in hot weather or when infants are overdressed. Usually well demarcated with maceration and oozing, intertrigo generally involves the inguinal region, the intergluteal area, and the fleshy folds of the thigh. Miliaria, caused by heat and sweat retention, is characteristic and often seen in association with intertrigo of the diaper area.

Seborrheic Dermatitis. Diagnosis of seborrheic dermatitis of the diaper area may be simplified by recognition of a characteristic salmon-colored greasy lesion with a yellowish scale and a predilection for intertriginous areas (Fig. 2–29). Coincident involvement of the scalp, face, neck, and postauricular and flexural areas helps establish the true nature of this eruption. Atopic dermatitis in the diaper area is not diagnostic in itself. When seen in association with typical lesions on the cheeks and antecubital or popliteal fossae and a family history of atopy, however, the correct diagnosis can generally be established.

Cutaneous Candidiasis. Candidal (monilial) diaper dermatitis is a commonly overlooked disorder and should be suspected whenever a diaper rash fails to respond to usual therapeutic measures. Cutaneous candidiasis is a common sequela to systemic antibiotic therapy and should be considered in any diaper dermatitis that develops during or shortly following antibiotic administration.

The typical candidal diaper rash presents as a more or less widespread erythema on the buttocks, lower abdomen, and inner aspects of the thighs. It has a vivid beefy red color, which develops as the result of specific irritant toxins elaborated by *Candida* organisms. The eruption is characterized by a raised edge, sharp marginization with white scales at the border of lesions, and pinpoint pustulo-

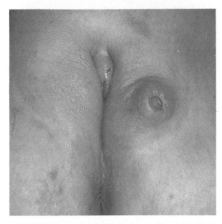

Figure 2–28. Papuloerosive eruption with crater-like appearance (Jacquet's dermatitis) on the labia majora.

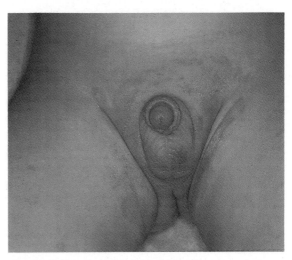

Figure 2–29. Seborrheic diaper dermatitis. Salmon-colored greasy lesions with a yellowish scale and predilection for intertriginous areas.

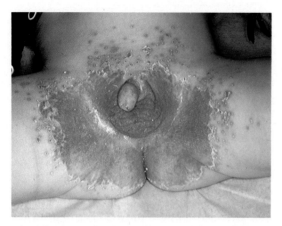

Figure 2–30. Candidal (monilial) diaper dermatitis with characteristic vivid red color, sharp margination, and pustulovesicular satellite lesions.

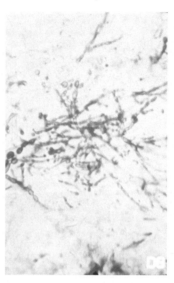

Figure 2–32. Budding yeasts with hyphae and pseudohyphae on microscopic examination of a cutaneous scraping. (Courtesy of Alfred Kopf, M.D.)

vesicular satellite lesions (the diagnostic markers of this disorder) (Fig. 2–30). Although cutaneous candidiasis frequently occurs in association with oral thrush (Fig. 2–31), commonly the mouth is bypassed and the infection is frequently confined exclusively to the diaper area. Infants harbor *Candida albicans* in the lower intestine, and it is from this focus that infected feces present the primary source for candidal diaper eruptions.

Occasionally the diagnosis of candidal diaper dermatitis may be verified by microscopic examination of skin scrapings with potassium hydroxide or by Gram stain or periodic acid–Schiff stain (Fig. 2–32). Although egg-shaped budding yeasts and hyphae or pseudohyphae may be identified by this relatively simple technique, a characteristic growth of white mucoid colonies of Sabouraud's or Nickerson's medium can confirm the diagnosis more consistently, usually within a mere 48- to 72-hour period (Fig. 2–33).

Dermatophyte Infection. Although *Candida albicans* is the fungus most commonly seen in the diaper area of infants and young children, dermatophyte infection is often overlooked as a possible cause of "diaper dermatitis" (Fig. 2–34). In such instances, a circinate annular configuration and scaly vesicular border is suggestive and microscopic examination of a potassium hydroxide preparation and fungal culture can confirm the diagnosis.[109]

Psoriasis. Psoriasis of the diaper area must also be considered in persistent diaper eruptions that fail to respond to otherwise seemingly adequate therapy (see Fig. 5–3). When this is the case, the presence of nail involvement and dark ruby-red

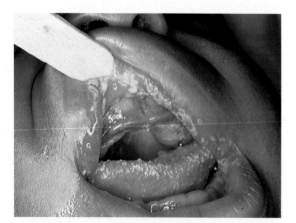

Figure 2–31. Oral candidiasis (thrush). Grayish white, often confluent, friable cheesy patches or plaques on the surface of the buccal mucosa, tongue, and gingiva.

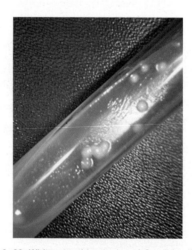

Figure 2–33. White mucoid colonies of *Candida albicans* on Sabouraud's medium.

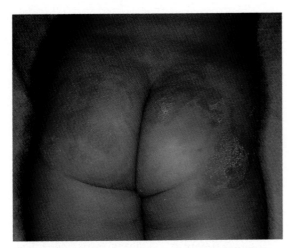

Figure 2–34. *Trichophyton rubrum* infection in the diaper area of a 15-month-old child.

well-marginated plaques with silvery mica-like scales on the trunk, face, or scalp, and a family history of psoriasis may help confirm this diagnosis.

Congenital Syphilis. Congenital syphilis usually begins between 2 and 6 weeks of age, with macules, papules, and bullous lesions of the anogenital region and an associated involvement of the palms and soles. Condylomata lata (large moist hypertrophic papules and flat nodules) may be seen about the anus, buttocks, other folds of the body, and angles of the mouth of infected infants. The color of the skin is often yellow or café au lait, hepatosplenomegaly is common, and there may be an associated anemia. The papular eruption in this disorder resembles that seen in acquired secondary syphilis, except that in the congenital disease lesions are usually larger, reddish brown, and more infiltrated.

Letterer-Siwe Disease. Letterer-Siwe disease (histiocytosis) may also have a characteristic predilection for the diaper area. The eruption (often seborrhea-like) is most frequently seen in the groin, axillae, and retroauricular areas. Characteristic lesions of this disorder consist of clusters of yellowish to reddish brown infiltrated papules, often with hemorrhagic or purpuric qualities. A hemorrhagic seborrhea-like eruption with chronic genitocrural ulceration should suggest the diagnosis of Letterer-Siwe disease (see Chapter 24, Figs. 24–3 and 24–4). Histiocytic infiltrate on cutaneous biopsy is diagnostic of this disorder.

Acrodermatitis Enteropathica. Acrodermatitis enteropathica in the diaper area often mimics candidal diaper dermatitis, with erythematous plaques suggesting severe candidiasis or psoriasis (see Chapter 22, Fig. 22–5). *Candida albicans* has been isolated from the skin and mucosal lesions in 20 per cent of cases; this association does not represent a primary etiologic factor but rather a sec-

ondary infection in these areas. Vesiculobullous eruptions of the periorificial areas, fingers, and toes; cachexia; alopecia; and diarrhea help differentiate this disorder.

Treatment. The management of diaper dermatitis is directed at keeping the area clean and dry and limiting irritation and maceration by avoidance of occlusive or impervious diaper coverings. Frequent diaper changes, especially at night, thorough cleansing with water or a mild soap, exposure to air whenever possible, and the judicious use of topical therapy may be sufficient to keep the infant free from this disorder. Dusting powders such as Caldesene (CIBA) or ZeaSorb (Stiefel), with appropriate precautions to avoid aspiration, can be used to reduce moisture and frictional injury to this area. Although for many years it was believed that corn starch could promote *Candida albicans* colonization, studies have shown that corn starch and talc powders help reduce moisture and frictional injury to this area and do not enhance the growth of yeast on human skin.[110] Although controversy still exists regarding the advantages and disadvantages of cloth and disposable diapers, recent studies appear to demonstrate a lower incidence of diaper dermatitis when cloth or disposable diapers containing absorbent gelling material are used.[111]

Severe secondarily infected dermatitis should be treated systematically with appropriate antibiotics. Candidal infection requires the topical application of an anticandidal agent (see Chapter 13), and severe cases often benefit from open, wet compresses of tap water or a 1:20 or 1:40 solution of aluminum acetate. This concentration can be prepared by the use of Domeboro packets or tablets (Miles); one packet or tablet in a pint of water will make a 1:40 solution of aluminum acetate. The proper method of using open wet dressings is described under the management of atopic dermatitis in Chapter 3. If *Candida* is resistant to topical therapy, or if there is evidence of *Candida* in the mouth as well as the perianal area, topical therapy may be supplemented by oral nystatin, available as Nilstat Oral Suspension (200,000 units four times a day) or Mycostatin Suspension (100,000 units four times a day) for 6 to 12 days. For recurrent diaper dermatitis, preparations such as 1-2-3 ointment (Rosen's ointment), made up of Burow's solution 10.0 cc, Aquaphor 20.0 g, and zinc oxide paste, plain, q.s. ad 60 g, are particularly useful.

Although topical corticosteroids such as hydrocortisone may be used for the inflammatory stage of the dermatitis, potent topical corticosteroids such as betamethasone dipropionate and clotrimazole (Lotrisone) and a combination of triamcinolone and nystatin (Mycolog) are not recommended because of the possibility of atrophy, telangiectasia, striae, or absorption (see Chapters 3, 13, and 25). In addition, although gentian violet has been used for decades for the treatment of oral candidiasis and candidal diaper dermatitis, reports of bacterial infection and hemorrhagic cystitis, in

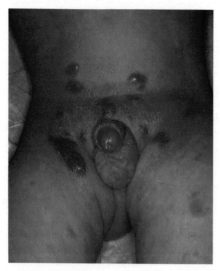

Figure 2–35. Granuloma gluteale infantum. Reddish purple granulomatous nodules in the diaper area.

addition to objectionable discoloration and staining associated with its use, suggest that gentian violet be avoided.[112, 113]

GRANULOMA GLUTEALE INFANTUM

Granuloma gluteale infantum is a benign disorder of infancy characterized by reddish purple granulomatous nodules that measure from 0.5 to 4.0 cm in diameter and occur in the groin and on the buttocks, lower aspect of the abdomen, penis, and at times the intertriginous areas of the axillae and neck (Fig. 2–35). Although the ominous appearance of these lesions may suggest a lymphomatous or sarcomatous process, the disorder appears to represent a unique cutaneous response to local inflammation, maceration, and secondary infection (usually *Candida albicans*).[114] Since lesions of granuloma gluteale infantum may resem-

ble early lesions of Kaposi's sarcoma and may involve areas other than those of the diaper region, other names suggested for this disorder include Kaposi's sarcoma-like granuloma and granuloma intertriginosum infantum.[115, 116]

Granulomas may arise in a variety of infections, such as tuberculosis, syphilis, and deep fungal infection; as allergic reactions to zirconium; in foreign body reactions; and in response to talcum or dusting powder, irritation, maceration, and infection in the intertriginous and diaper areas of infants, young children, and older or ill persons wearing diapers because of urinary or fecal incontinence.[117]

Although nodular lesions of granuloma gluteale infantum may at times suggest sarcomatous or lymphomatous processes or lesions of congenital fibromatosis (infantile myofibromatosis) (see Chapter 8, Fig. 8–44), they can be differentiated on the basis of clinical and histopathologic features. Light and electron microscopic examination of the nodular lesions of granuloma gluteale infantum reveal a hyperplastic epidermis with inflammatory cells (mainly neutrophils), a parakeratotic stratum corneum, and a dense inflammatory infiltrate throughout the depth of the cutis, with hemorrhage, neutrophils, lymphocytes, histiocytes, plasma cells, eosinophils, newly formed capillaries, and giant cells (Fig. 2–36).[118, 119]

Lymphomatous lesions of the skin reveal large masses of patchy accumulations of lymphoma cells or an inflammatory infiltrate mixed with lymphoma cells. Lesions of granuloma gluteale infantum lack the fibrous proliferative features, spindle cell formations, and mitoses that assist in the differentiation of this disorder from the more severe granulomatous processes.

Occasionally Kaposi's sarcoma may occur on various parts of the body of infants and children as well as adults or as a cutaneous marker of acquired immunodeficiency syndrome in adults (see Chapter 11). Classic (nonacquired immunodeficiency [AIDS]-related) Kaposi's sarcoma generally appears on the hands and feet of adults of central

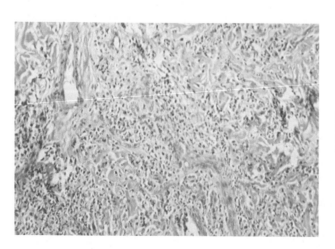

Figure 2–36. Dense inflammatory infiltrate of granuloma gluteale infantum (light micrograph). A lack of proliferative features, spindle cell formation, and mitoses assist in the differentiation of this disorder from sarcomatous and lymphomatous processes.

European or African origin. Rarely a disease of American or European children, Kaposi's sarcoma in African children infrequently affects the skin and usually occurs in the lymph nodes, salivary glands, and ocular glands. When seen in Bantu children of Africa, massive involvement of the lymph nodes (especially the cervical nodes), salivary glands, eyelids, and conjunctivae generally precedes the appearance of skin lesions.

Lesions of granuloma gluteale infantum resolve completely and spontaneously within a period of several months after treatment of the initiating inflammatory process with its associated maceration and secondary infection. Although the use of intralesional corticosteroid or impregnated flurandrenolide tape (Cordran tape [Dista]) may hasten resolution of lesions, such therapy is unnecessary and not recommended.[120]

References

1. Nachman RL, Esterly NB: Increased skin permeability in preterm infants. J. Pediatr. 79:628–632, 1971.

   Topical applications of 10 per cent Neo-Synephrine reveal rapid cutaneous blanching in premature infants of 28 to 34 weeks' gestation, a less dramatic response in infants 35 to 37 weeks', and generally no response to those of 38 to 42 weeks' gestation.

2. Barker N, Hadcraft J, Rutter N: Skin permeability in the newborn. J. Invest. Dermatol. 88:409–411, 1987.

   Studies of sodium salicylate transport across excised neonatal skin revealed absorption in preterm infants of 30 weeks' gestation or less to be 10^2 to 10^3 times greater than that of full-term infants.

3. Pearson HA, Cone TE Jr: Harlequin color change in young infants with tricuspid atresia. J. Pediatr. 50:609–612, 1957.

   Improvement of harlequin color change in a 3½-month-old infant with tricuspid atresia corrected by aorto-pulmonary artery anastomosis suggests unsaturation of arterial oxygen as a triggering mechanism for this phenomenon.

4. Onishi S, Itoh S, Isobe K, et al.: Mechanism of development of bronze baby syndrome in neonates treated with phototherapy. Pediatrics 69:273–276, 1982.

   A review of the bronze baby syndrome with studies of photobilirubin IXa and an unknown pigment produced during phototherapy of newborns with hyperbilirubinemia.

5. Ashley JR, Little CM, Burgdorf WHC, et al.: Bronze baby syndrome: Report of a case. J. Am. Acad. Dermatol. 12:325–328, 1985.

   A review of the bronze baby syndrome, its causes and differential diagnosis.

6. Purcell SM, Wians FH Jr, Ackerman NB Jr, et al.: Hyperbiliverdinemia in the bronze baby syndrome. J. Am. Acad. Dermatol. 16:172–177, 1987.

   A premature infant with hydrops fetalis treated by intrauterine transfusions developed biliverdinemia resulting in a bronze discoloration of the skin.

7. Ruiz-Maldonado R, Tamayo L, Fernández-Diez J: Universal acquired melanosis: The carbon baby. Arch. Dermatol. 114:775–778, 1978.

   A unique case of dark black pigmentation of undetermined origin that began on the face and limbs of a 15-day-old Mexican boy and gradually progressed to include his entire cutaneous surface and ocular and mucous membranes.

8. Craft AW, Brocklebank JT, Jackson RH: The "gray-toddler": Chloramphenicol toxicity. Arch. Dis. Child. 49:235–237, 1974.

   Report of three children with chloramphenicol toxicity (the "gray baby" syndrome).

9. Esterly NB, Elias S: Antenatal diagnosis of genodermatoses. J. Am. Acad. Dermatol. 8:655–662, 1983.

   Fetoscopy and fetal skin biopsy and their use in the antenatal diagnosis of hereditary cutaneous disorders.

10. Raimer SS, Raimer G: Needle puncture marks from midtrimester amniocentesis. Arch. Dermatol. 120:1360–1362, 1984.

    Report of an infant with two dimple-like scars on the back as a complication of mid-trimester amniocentesis.

11. Bruce S, Duffy JO, Wolf JE Jr: Skin dimpling associated with midtrimester amniocentesis. Pediatr. Dermatol. 2:140–142, 1984.

    Report of an 8-month-old infant with six dimple-like amniocentesis scars on the skin of the thigh, flank, and abdomen.

12. Plavidal FJ, Werch A: Fetal scalp abscess secondary to intrauterine monitoring. Am. J. Obstet. Gynecol. 125:65–70, 1976.

    Analysis of more than 7,000 infants revealed a 0.4 per cent incidence of scalp abscesses (1 in 230 intrauterine monitored infants).

13. Siddiqi SF, Taylor PM: Necrotizing fasciitis of the scalp: A complication of fetal monitoring. Am. J. Dis. Child. 136:226–228, 1982.

    Two infants with extensive necrosis following an anaerobic infection at the site of intrauterine scalp electrode placement.

14. Ashkenazi S, Metzker A, Merlob P, et al.: Scalp changes after fetal monitoring. Arch. Dis. Child. 60:227–269, 1985.

    In a review of scalp electrode fetal monitoring in which 41 per cent of 535 infants had scalp changes, most were superficial lacerations that resolved without complication.

15. Boyle RJ, Oh W: Erythema following transcutaneous PO_2 monitoring. Pediatrics 65:333–334, 1980.

    A review of complications of transcutaneous PO_2 monitoring.

16. Golden SM: Skin craters—a complication of transcutaneous oxygen monitoring. Pediatrics 67:514–516, 1981.

    Two premature infants developed persistent hyperpigmented cutaneous craters as a complication of transcutaneous oxygen monitoring.

17. Sell EJ, Hansen RC, Struck-Pierce S: Calcified nodules on the heel: A complication of neonatal intensive care. J. Pediatr. 96:473–475, 1980.

    A premature infant developed multiple calcified cutaneous nodules following diagnostic heel sticks.

18. Wiley HE III, Eagelstein WE: Calcinosis cutis in children following electroencephalography. JAMA 242:455–466, 1979.

    A report of seven children in whom calcinosis cutis developed at the sites of electroencephalogram electrode placement.

19. Kellum RE, Ray TL, Brown GR: Sclerema neonatorum: Report of case analysis of subcutaneous and epidermal-dermal lipids by chromatographic methods. Arch. Dermatol. 97:372–380, 1968.

    Increase in the saturated-unsaturated ratio of fatty acids in subcutaneous triglycerides of a patient with sclerema neonatorum suggests defective fatty acid mobilization as the cause of this disorder.

20. Horsefield GI, Yardley HJ: Sclerema neonatorum. J. Invest. Dermatol. 44:326–332, 1965.

Increased ratio of saturated to unsaturated fatty acids may be related to poorly developed enzyme systems in newborns with sclerema.

21. Kendall N, Ledis S: Sclerema neonatorum successfully treated with corticotropin (ACTH). Am. J. Dis. Child. 83:52–53, 1952.

Apparent successful treatment of sclerema suggests further trial of corticotropin for infants with this disorder.

22. Wickes IG: Sclerema neonatorum: Recovery with cortisone. Arch. Dis. Child. 31:419–421, 1956.

Apparent success of corticosteroid therapy in sclerema neonatorum appears to justify its use for infants with this potentially fatal disorder.

23. Blake HA, Goyette EM, Lytes CS, et al.: Subcutaneous fat necrosis complicating hypothermia. J. Pediatr. 46:78–80, 1965.

Subcutaneous fat necrosis follows the use of hypothermia in cardiac surgery.

24. Duhn R, Schoen EJ, Siu M: Subcutaneous fat necrosis with extensive calcification after hypothermia in two newborn infants. Pediatrics 41:661–664, 1968.

Hypothermia as therapy for neonatal asphyxia appeared to cause subcutaneous fat necrosis.

25. Thomsen RJ: Subcutaneous fat necrosis of the newborn and idiopathic hypercalcemia: Report of a case. Arch. Dermatol. 116:1155–1158, 1980.

A report of a newborn and a review of 14 other infants with anoxia, subcutaneous fat necrosis, and hypercalcemia.

26. Norwood-Galloway A, Lebwohl M, Phelps RG, et al.: Subcutaneous fat necrosis of the newborn with hypercalcemia. J. Am. Acad. Dermatol. 16:435–439, 1987.

A report of a newborn infant with subcutaneous fat necrosis and hypercalcemia with a review of the literature.

27. Silverman AK, Michels EH, Rasmussen JE: Subcutaneous fat necrosis in an infant occurring after hypothermic cardiac surgery: Case report and analysis of etiologic factors. J. Am. Acad. Dermatol. 15:331–336, 1986.

A report of an infant with extensive subcutaneous fat necrosis following induced hypothermia during cardiac surgery and a review of factors in neonatal skin and fat metabolism that may predispose infants to the development of this disorder.

28. Steiness I: Subcutaneous fat necrosis of the newborn and maternal diabetes mellitus (adiponecrosis subcutanea neonatorum). Acta Med. Scand. 170:411–416, 1961.

A report of two infants with subcutaneous fat necrosis in which one mother had diabetes mellitus and the other was believed to be prediabetic suggested that a metabolic disturbance or endocrine imbalance resulted in ischemia, tissue hypoxia, and the subsequent development of subcutaneous fat necrosis.

29. Levy HL, Cothran F: Erythema toxicum neonatorum present at birth. Am. J. Dis. Child. 103:617–619, 1962.

Erythema toxicum noted at the time of delivery.

30. Marino LJ: Toxic erythema present at birth. Arch. Dermatol. 92:402–403, 1965.

An additional report of erythema toxicum noted at birth supports the concept that this disorder may occur in utero.

31. Taylor WB, Bondurant CP: Erythema neonatorum allergicum: A study of the incidence in two hundred newborn infants and a review of the literature. Arch. Dermatol. 76:591–594, 1957.

The reported incidence of erythema toxicum varies because of the fleeting nature of this disorder and a disparity of clinical observations on the part of clinicians.

32. Carr JA, Hodgman JD, Freeman RI, et al.: Relationship between toxic erythema and infant maturity. Am. J. Dis. Child. 112:129–134, 1966.

The incidence of erythema toxicum appears to increase with gestational age.

33. Eitzman DV, Smith RT: The non-specific inflammatory cycle in the neonatal infant. Am. J. Dis. Child. 97:326–334, 1959.

Eosinophilia appears to be a normal newborn response to injury.

34. Keitel HG, Yadav V: Etiology of toxic erythema. Am. J. Dis. Child. 106:306–309, 1963.

Toxic erythema: a transient reaction of newborn skin to mechanical or thermal stimulation?

35. Ramamurthy RS, Riveri M, Esterly NB, et al.: Transient neonatal pustular melanosis. J. Pediatr. 88:831–835, 1976.

A previously undescribed skin eruption of newborns consisting of transient vesiculopustules and pigmented macules.

36. Barr RJ, Globerman LM, Werber FA: Transient neonatal pustular melanosis. Int. J. Dermatol. 18:636–639, 1979.

In a careful review of 602 infants only one child was found to have transient neonatal pustular melanosis.

37. Merlob P, Metzker A, Reisner SH: Transient neonatal pustular melanosis. Am. J. Dis. Child. 136:521–522, 1982.

Over a period of 17 months, transient neonatal pustular melanosis was diagnosed in 13 of 5,267 infants.

38. Cohen BA, Esterly NB, Nelson PF: Congenital erosive and vesicular dermatosis healing with reticulated supple scarring. Arch. Dermatol. 121:361–367, 1985.

A report of three children with an apparently newly described disorder characterized by an erosive dermatosis at birth that healed with reticulated scarring.

39. Gupta AK, Rasmussen JE, Headington JT: Extensive congenital erosions and vesicles healing with reticulate scarring. J. Am. Acad. Dermatol. 17:369–376, 1987.

A report of two children with severe neurologic abnormalities and congenital erosions and vesicles that healed with reticulate scarring.

40. Plantin P, Delaire P, Guillois B, et al.: Congenital erosive dermatosis with reticulated supple scarring: First neonatal report. Arch. Dermatol. 126:544–546, 1990.

A report of a newborn with a widespread erythematous dermatosis that resembled scalded skin and subsequently healed with erosive reticulated cutaneous scars.

41. Shuster S: The aetiology of dandruff and the mode of action of therapeutic agents. Br. J. Dermatol. 111:235–242, 1984.

Studies suggest that *Pityrosporon ovale* may play a role in the pathogenesis of seborrheic dermatitis.

42. Ford GP, Farr PM, Shuster S: Response of seborrheic dermatitis to ketoconazole. Br. J. Dermatol. 111:603–607, 1984.

A double-blind trial of ketoconazole in 19 patients with seborrheic dermatitis suggests that *Pityrosporon ovale* may be a secondary factor rather than a primary cause of this disorder.

43. Skinner RB, Noah PW, Taylor RM, et al.: Double-blind treatment of seborrheic dermatitis with 2% ketoconazole cream. J. Am. Acad. Dermatol. 12:852–856, 1985.

A report of a 75 to 95 per cent or better response to ketaconazole cream in 18 of 20 patients with seborrheic dermatitis.

44. Leyden JJ: The pathogenic role of microbes in seborrheic dermatitis. Arch. Dermatol. 122:16–17, 1986.

Studies suggest that *Pityrosporon* plays a secondary rather than primary role in the pathogenesis of seborrheic dermatitis.

45. Glover MT, Atherton DJ, Levinsky RJ: Syndrome of erythroderma, failure to thrive, and diarrhea in infancy: A manifestation of immunodeficiency. Pediatrics 81:66–72, 1988.

A review of five infants with erythroderma, diarrhea, and failure to thrive suggests that the disorder described in the past as Leiner's disease may represent a clinical manifestation of an underlying immunodeficiency disorder.

46. Jacobs JC, Miller ME: Fatal familial Leiner's disease: A deficiency of the opsonic activity of serum complement. Pediatrics 49:225–232, 1972.

Two patients with a deficiency of phagocytosis enhancement (opsonization) related to dysfunction of the fifth component of serum complement (C_5).

47. Miller ME, Koblenzer PJ: Leiner's disease and deficiency of C_5. J. Pediatr. 80:879–880, 1972.

Children with a deficiency of opsonic activity of the fifth component of serum complement (C_5) and a clinical course similar to that of Leiner's disease improved dramatically following infusion with fresh frozen plasma..

48. Amman AJ, Wara DW, Cowan MJ, et al.: The DiGeorge syndrome and the fetal alcohol syndrome. Am. J. Dis. Child. 136:906–908, 1982.

A review of four infants with a history of maternal alcoholism and clinical and laboratory features of the DiGeorge syndrome.

49. Crain LS, Fitzmaurice NE, Mondry C: Nail dysplasia and fetal alcohol syndrome: Case report of a heteropaternal sibship. Am. J. Dis. Child. 137:1069–1072, 1983.

A report of dysplasia of fingernails and toenails in four siblings with features of the fetal alcohol syndrome and a literature review in which nail dysplasia was found to be present in more than 20 per cent of individuals affected by this congenital disorder.

50. Hanson JW, Smith DW: The fetal hydantoin syndrome. J. Pediatr. 87:285–290, 1975.

Five children born to women on hydantoin anticonvulsants during pregnancy were found to have a syndrome characterized by craniofacial anomalies, nail and digital hypoplasia, prenatal-onset growth deficiency, and mental deficiency.

51. Verdeguer JM, Ramon D, Moragon M, et al.: Onychopathy in a patient with fetal hydantoin syndrome. Pediatr. Dermatol. 5:56–57, 1988.

A report of an infant with fetal hydantoin syndrome with ungual abnormalities (detachment of the nail plates, distal hyperpigmentation, and Beau's lines).

52. Zakai EH, Melman WT, Neiderer B: The fetal trimethadione syndrome. J. Pediatr. 87:280–284, 1975.

A report of three children with similar dysmorphic features, poor speech, and developmental retardation born to mothers who took trimethadione for the control of petit mal seizures during their pregnancies.

53. Hurwitz S, Klaus SN: Congenital hemihypertrophy with hypertrichosis. Arch. Dermatol. 103:98–100, 1971.

Since approximately 50 per cent of individuals with hemihypertrophy have associated anomalies, affected persons should be carefully evaluated for other congenital malformations and neoplasms of liver, adrenal cortex, and kidneys.

54. Peer LA, Duyn JV: Congenital defect of the scalp. Plast. Reconstr. Surg. 3:722–726, 1948.

An infant with aplasia cutis with a large scalp defect (2.5 × 6 × 10 cm) died at 12 weeks of age as a result of necrosis, inflammation, and ulceration of the involved area, with hemorrhage due to rupture of the sagittal sinus.

55. Resnick SS, Koblenzer PJ, Pitts FW: Congenital absence of the scalp with associated vascular anomaly. Clin. Pediatr. 4:322–324, 1965.

A 4-day-old newborn with aplasia cutis in association with an anomalous superficial scalp vein. Ligation of the vessel was performed to prevent hemorrhage and facilitate early closure of the defect.

56. Frieden IJ: Aplasia cutis congenita: A clinical review and proposal for classification. J. Am. Acad. Dermatol. 14:646–660, 1986.

A comprehensive review of aplasia cutis congenita and a classification based on clinical patterns, causes, associated anomalies, and modes of inheritance.

57. Levin DL, Nolan KS, Esterly NB: Congenital absence of the skin. J. Am. Acad. Dermatol. 2:203–206, 1980.

A report of a 5-day-old girl with infarction of the placenta and congenital absence of the skin suggests a degenerative rather than an aplastic or traumatic origin of congenital aplasia cutis.

58. Setleis H, Kramer B, Valcarel M, et al.: Congenital ectodermal dysplasia of the face. Pediatrics 32:540–548, 1963.

A review of five children of three families with clinical defects confined to the face, believed to be due to the multiple effects of a single gene.

59. Rudolph RI, Schwartz W, Leyden JJ: Amendation to "bitemporal aplasia cutis congenita." Arch. Dermatol. 110:636, 1974.

"Bitemporal aplasia cutis congenita" and "congenital ectodermal dysplasia of the face" appear to be the same disorder.

60. Marion RW, Chitagat D, Hutcheon G, et al.: Autosomal recessive inheritance in the Setleis bitemporal "forceps marks" syndrome. Am. J. Dis. Child. 141:895–897, 1987.

A report of two children with the Setleis syndrome suggests an autosomal recessive form of inheritance in individuals with this disorder.

61. Powell KR, Cherry JD, Hougen TJ, et al.: A prospective search for congenital dermal abnormalities of the craniospinal axis. J. Pediatr. 87:744–750, 1975.

A study of 1,997 consecutive term newborns revealed one or more abnormalities of the craniospinal axis in 3 per cent.

62. Pauli RM, Hall JG: Lip pits, cleft lip and/or palate, and congenital heart disease. Am. J. Dis. Child. 134:293–295, 1980.

Report of three infants with lip pits, cleft lip or cleft palate, and congenital heart disease.

63. Ray M, Hendrick SJ, Raimer SS, et al.: Amniotic band syndrome. Int. J. Dermatol. 27:312–314, 1988.

A patient with amniotic band syndrome and a review of the disorder and its associated abnormalities.

64. Christensen P, Barr RJ: Wattle: An unusual congenital anomaly. Arch. Dermatol. 121:22–23, 1985.

A report of a 12-year-old boy with an elongated skin-colored lesion on the anterior aspect of his neck.

65. Camisa C: Accessory breast on the posterior thigh of a man. J. Am. Acad. Dermatol. 4:367–369, 1981.

A 74-year-old man with a lesion on his posterior thigh that, although not substantiated by histopathology (the patient refused biopsy), resembled a female breast in every clinical respect.

66. Hersh JH, Bloom AS, Cromer AO, et al.: Does a supernumerary nipple/renal field defect exist? Am. J. Dis. Child. 141:989–991, 1987.

A review of 65 patients with supernumerary nipples concludes that this anomaly in an otherwise normal individual does not appear to be a marker of urinary tract malformation.

67. Cooper LZ, Green RH, Krugman S, et al.: Neonatal thrombocytopenic purpura and other manifestations of rubella contracted in utero. Am. J. Dis. Child. 110:416–427, 1965.

A study of 200 infants with congenital rubella syndrome reveals a broad spectrum of associated abnormalities.

68. Leads from the MMWR (Morbidity and Mortality Weekly Report): Increase in rubella and congenital rubella. J.A.M.A. 265:1076–1077, 1991.

A failure to vaccinate susceptible individuals appears to be a major cause of the dramatic increase in the incidence of rubella in 1990.

69. Schwartz JL, Maniscalco WM, Lane AT, et al.: Twin transfusion syndrome causing cutaneous erythropoiesis. Pediatrics 4:527–529, 1984.

A review of two cases of twin transfusion syndrome in which prolonged intrauterine anemia resulted in "blueberry muffin" lesions as a manifestation of dermal erythropoiesis.

70. Paryani SG, Arvin AM: Intrauterine infection with varicella-zoster virus after maternal varicella. N. Engl. J. Med. 314:1542–1546, 1986.

In a study of pregnancies complicated by varicella-zoster infection, 4.9 per cent of infants of mothers with intrauterine varicella infection in the first trimester were found to have abnormalities and none of 14 infants born to mothers with herpes zoster infection during gestation had evidence of morbidity or sequelae as a result of intrauterine infection.

71. Preblud SR, Cochi SL, Orenstein WA: Correspondence: Risk of abnormalities consistent with congenital varicella infection. N. Engl. J. Med. 315:1416–1417, 1986.

A review of four studies revealed that only 2.3 per cent (3 of 131 infants) of mothers infected with varicella during the first trimester of pregnancy had evidence of congenital varicella and 0.6 per cent of infants (3 of 461) born to mothers infected during the total period of gestation had evidence of this disorder.

72. Prober CG, Gershon AA, Grose C, et al.: Consensus: Varicella-zoster infections in pregnancy and the perinatal period. Pediatr. Infect. Dis. J. 9:865–869, 1990.

An authoritative review of the management of varicella and its complications during pregnancy and the perinatal period.

73. Frey HM, Bialkin G, Gershon AA: Congenital varicella: Case report of a serologically proved long-term survivor. Pediatrics 59:110–112, 1977.

Report of a female infant with chorioretinitis and cicatricial cutaneous scars attributed to varicella infection of the mother in the second trimester of pregnancy.

74. Asha Bai PV, John TJ: Congenital skin ulcers following varicella in late pregnancy. J. Pediatr. 94:65–67, 1979.

Skin ulcers in an infant born to a mother who had varicella in the third trimester of pregnancy suggest that the spectrum of disease in the affected fetus is related to the time that varicella was acquired in utero.

75. Strabstein JC, Morris N, Larke RPB, et al.: Is there a congenital varicella syndrome? J. Pediatr. 84:239–243, 1974.

A report of an infant with multiple congenital anomalies (microphthalmia, cataracts, chorioretinitis, micrognathia, encephalomyelitis, pneumonitis, hypotrophic leg with flexion contractures, and cutaneous scars) ascribed to maternal varicella infection early in pregnancy.

76. Overall JC Jr: Viral infections of the fetus and neonate. In Feigin RD, Cherry JD (Eds.): Textbook of Pediatric Infectious Diseases, 2nd ed. W. B. Saunders Co., Philadelphia, 1987, 966–1007.

Congenital viral infections of the newborn, their diagnosis and management.

77. Ogilvie MM, Stephen JRD, Larkin M: Letters to the editor: Chickenpox in pregnancy. Lancet 1:915–916, 1986.

Because of uncertainty regarding the most effective dose of ZIG required to protect infants born to mothers who have varicella within 4 days on either side of delivery, the authors recommend an increase in dosage from 125 to 250 mg.

78. Whitley R, Arvin A, Prober C, et al: Predictors of morbidity and mortality in neonates with herpes simplex virus infections. N. Engl. J. Med. 324:450–454, 1991.

A controlled study revealed no difference in outcome between vidarabine and acyclovir in the treatment of neonatal herpes simplex virus infection.

79. Komorous JM, Wheeler CE, Briggaman RA, et al.: Intrauterine herpes simplex infections. Arch. Dermatol. 113:918–922, 1977.

A report of two infants with documented herpes simplex infection in utero and associated congenital malformations.

80. Francis DP, Hermann KL, McMahon JR, et al.: Nosocomial and maternally acquired herpesvirus hominis infections. A report of four fatal cases in neonates. Am. J. Dis. Child. 129:889–893, 1975.

Of four fatal cases of infantile herpes simplex infection, three infants appeared to have been infected in utero or at delivery; the fourth infant did not develop signs of illness until age 6 weeks, suggesting possible infection by indirect contact with one of the other three infants.

81. Prober CG, Sullender WM, Yasukawa LL, et al.: Low risk of herpes simplex virus infections in neonates exposed to the virus at the time of vaginal delivery to mothers with recurrent genital herpes simplex virus infections. N. Engl. J. Med. 316:240–244, 1987.

Studies of 34 infants exposed to HSV type 2 concluded that the low incidence of herpes simplex infection in neonates born to mothers with recurrent genital herpes infections is probably related to the presence of neutralizing antibodies in the cord or newborn infant's blood during the first 2 weeks of life.

82. Arvin AM, Hensleigh PA, Prober CG, et al.: Failure of antepartum maternal cultures to predict the infant's risk of exposure to herpes simplex at delivery. N. Engl. J. Med. 315:796–800, 1986.

A study of 414 pregnant women with a history of recurrent genital herpes infection suggests that antepartum maternal vaginal cultures do not reflect the true risk of neonatal herpes simplex virus.

83. Montgomery JR, Flanders RW, Yow MD: Congenital anomalies and herpesvirus infection. Am. J. Dis. Child. 126:364–366, 1973.

Report of an infant with early intrauterine type 2 herpesvirus infection manifested by chorioretinopathy, psychomotor retardation, intrauterine growth retardation, cardiac abnormalities, short digits, and cutaneous findings.

84. Hutto C, Arvin A, Jacobs R, et al.: Intrauterine herpes simplex virus infections. J. Pediatr. 110:97–101, 1987.

A review of 13 infants with clinical manifestations of intrauterine HSV infection.

85. Jarratt M: Editorial: Herpes simplex infection. Arch. Dermatol. 119:99–103, 1983.

A review of genital herpes simplex virus infection with an emphasis on its epidemiologic characteristics, diagnosis, and therapy.

86. Honig PJ, Brown D: Congenital herpes simplex virus infection initially resembling epidermolysis bullosa. J. Pediatr. 101:958–960, 1982.

A report of an infant with congenital herpes simplex virus infection with multiple bullous and erosive lesions resembling those of epidermolysis bullosa.

87. Music SI, Fine EM, Yasushi T: Zoster-like disease in the newborn due to herpes-simplex virus. N. Engl. J. Med. 284:24–26, 1971.

On the basis of this report, viral cultures of lesions in the newborn must be obtained before any etiologic factor can be ascribed to a zoster-like distribution of vesicles in the neonate.

88. Binkin NJ, Koplan JP, Cates W Jr: Preventing neonatal herpes: The value of weekly viral cultures in pregnant women with recurrent genital herpes. J.A.M.A. 251:2816–2821, 1984.

A review of maternal genital tract viral cultures during the last 4 to 8 weeks of pregnancy suggests that cesarean section has limitations in the prevention of neonatal herpes.

89. Sullivan-Bolyai JZ, Fife KH, Jacobs RF, et al.: Experience and reason: Disseminated neonatal herpes simplex virus type I from a maternal breast lesion. Pediatrics 71:455–457, 1983.

An infant with disseminated herpes acquired from a maternal breast lesion emphasizes the importance of neonatal protection from open herpetic lesions.

90. Anand A, Gray ES, Brown T, et al.: Human parvovirus infection in pregnancy and hydrops fetalis. N. Engl. J. Med. 316:183–186, 1987.

In a review of an epidemic of human parvovirus infection, two of six women with serologic evidence of viral exposure had mid-trimester abortions in which both fetuses were grossly hydropic and profusely anemic.

91. Torök TJ: Human parvovirus B19 infection in pregnancy. Pediatr. Infect. Dis. J. 9:772–776, 1990.

A comprehensive review of fetal morbidity and mortality after maternal human parvovirus B19 infection.

92. Mascola L, Pelosi R, Blount JH, et al.: Congenital syphilis revisited. Am. J. Dis. Child. 139:575–580, 1985.

A review of 50 cases of early congenital syphilis in Texas.

93. Mascola L, Pelosi R, Blount JH, et al.: Congenital syphilis: Why is it still recurring? J.A.M.A. 252:1719–1722, 1984.

Minority groups and young and unmarried mothers who receive poor or no prenatal care appear to be major factors contributing to the resurgence of congenital syphilis.

94. Harter CA, Benirschke K: Fetal syphilis in the first trimester. Am. J. Obstet. Gynecol. 124:705–711, 1976.

Examinations of 9- and 10-week-old fetuses disprove the concept that T. pallidum does not cross the placenta before the fourth month of pregnancy.

95. Fojaco RM, Hensley JT, Moskowitz L: Congenital syphilis and necrotizing funisitis. J.A.M.A. 261:1788–1790, 1989.

A report of 16 infants with necrotizing funisitis, a frequently overlooked finding that the authors believe is virtually diagnostic of congenital syphilis.

96. Beck-Sague C, Alexander ER: Failure of benzathine penicillin G treatment in early congenital syphilis. Pediatr. Infect. Dis. J. 6:1061–1064, 1987.

A report of two infants with congenital syphilis without evidence of central nervous system infection who developed periostitis (one infant also developed asymptomatic neurosyphilis) despite apparently adequate benzathine penicillin G therapy.

97. Blatt J, Kastner O, Hodes, DS: Cutaneous vesicles in congenital cytomegalovirus infection. J. Pediatr. 92:509, 1978.

Although vesicles are unusual in congenital cytomegalovirus infection, the disorder must be considered in the differential diagnosis of cutaneous vesicular lesions in the neonate.

98. Stagno S, Whitley RJ: Current concepts: Herpesvirus infections of pregnancy: I. Cytomegalic and Epstein-Barr virus infections. N. Engl. J. Med. 313:1270–1274, 1985.

A comprehensive review of cytomegalovirus and Epstein-Barr virus infections and fetal problems that can arise as a result of maternal herpesvirus infection during pregnancy.

99. Hocker JR, Cook LN: Ganciclovir therapy for congenital cytomegalovirus pneumonia. Pediatr. Infect. Dis. J. 9:743–744, 1990.

A report of a premature infant with congenital cytomegalovirus pneumonia treated with ganciclovir, 5 mg/kg intramuscularly every 12 hours for 12 days, who, despite therapy, died at 3 months of age of respiratory failure (cultures of urine and respiratory tract secretions failed to yield cytomegalovirus once ganciclovir therapy was begun).

100. Goldberg GN, Fulginiti VA, Ray G, et al.: In utero Epstein-Barr virus (infectious mononucleosis) infection. J.A.M.A. 246:1579–1581, 1981.

Features of a congenital Epstein-Barr virus syndrome in an infant born to a mother who had infectious mononucleosis during the fifth to sixth weeks of gestation.

101. Sever JL, Ellenberg JH, Ley AC, et al.: Toxoplasmosis: Maternal and pediatric findings in 23,000 pregnancies. Pediatrics 82:181–192, 1988.

A comprehensive review of maternal and pediatric findings in patients with toxoplasmosis.

102. Wilson CR, Remington JS: Toxoplasmosis. In Feigen RD, Cherry JD (Eds.): Textbook of Pediatric Infectious Diseases, 2nd ed. W.B. Saunders Co., Philadelphia, 1987, 2067–2078.

An authoritative and comprehensive review of toxoplasmosis, its diagnosis and management in infancy and childhood.

103. Leyden JJ, Katz S, Stewart R, et al.: Urinary ammonia and ammonia-producing organisms in infants with and without diaper dermatitis. Arch. Dermatol. 113:1678–1680, 1977.

Microbiological and experimental studies reveal Candida albicans (not ammonia liberated by microorganisms) as a primary factor in the initiation of diaper dermatitis.

104. Zahorsky J: The ammoniacal diaper in infants and young children. Am. J. Dis. Child. 10:436–440, 1915.

In the early 1900s physicians came to view urinary ammonia as an important etiologic factor in diaper dermatitis.

105. Cooke JV: The etiology and treatment of ammonia dermatitis of the gluteal region of infants. Am. J. Dis. Child. 22:481–492, 1921.

Isolation of a gram-positive urea-splitting organism from stools of a number of infants led to the assumption that an etiologic relationship existed between this organism, the presence of ammonia in the diaper, and diaper dermatitis.

106. Leyden JJ, Kligman AM: The role of microorganisms in diaper dermatitis. Arch. Dermatol. 114:56–59, 1978.

Studies on forty infants with no history of diaper dermatitis and 100 infants with diaper rash refute the concept that microorganisms and ammonia play a central role in the pathogenesis of this disorder.

107. Zimmerer RE, Lawson KD, Calvert CJ: The effects of wearing diapers on skin. Pediatr. Dermatol. 3:95–101, 1986.

Studies show that skin wetness in diaper-covered infants increases coefficient of friction, cutaneous permeability, and susceptibility to abrasion damage and microbial growth.

108. Berg RW, Buckingham KW, Stewart RL: Etiologic features in diaper dermatitis: The role of urine. Pediatr. Dermatol. 3:102–106, 1986.

Studies in hairless mice suggest that urine increases the pH of the diaper environment (by breaking down urea in the presence of fecal urease), thus increasing the activity of fecal proteases and lipases that tend to damage the skin.

109. Jacobs AH, O'Connell BM: Tinea in tiny tots. Am. J. Dis. Child. 140:1034–1038, 1986.

This report of a variety of tinea infections in infants and young children serves as a reminder that dermatophyte infections should not be overlooked as a cause of cutaneous eruption in youngsters.

110. Leyden JJ: Corn starch, Candida albicans and diaper rash. Pediatr. Dermatol. 1:322–325, 1984.

Contrary to previous misconceptions, corn starch and talc powders on the skin of human volunteers provide protection against frictional injury and do not promote the growth of yeasts.

111. Lane AT, Rehder PA, Helm K: Evaluation of diapers containing absorbent gelling material with conventional disposable diapers in newborn infants. Am. J. Dis. Child. *144:*315–318, 1990.

An evaluation of 149 infants revealed a significantly lower incidence of diaper dermatitis in infants using diapers containing absorbent gelling material than those wearing conventional cellulose core disposable diapers.

112. Safranek TS, Jarvis WR, Carson LA: *Mycobacterium chelonae* after plastic surgery employing contaminated gentian violet skin marking. N. Engl. J. Med. *317:*197–201, 1987.

Severe skin and soft tissue *M. chelonae* infections developed in eight patients following plastic surgery in which contaminated gentian violet was used for preoperative skin-marking purposes.

113. Walsh C, Walsh A: Hemorrhagic cystitis due to gentian violet. Br. Med. J. *293:*732, 1986.

Although generally regarded as innocuous, gentian violet applied topically to the vaginal mucosa for the treatment of vaginal candidiasis resulted in hemorrhagic cystitis and extensive urinary bladder irritation.

114. Tappeiner J, Pfleger L: Granuloma gluteale infantum. Hautarzt *22:*383–388, 1971.

Report of a previously undescribed nodular eruption in six infants.

115. Uyeda K, Nakayasu K, Takaishi Y, et al.: Kaposi sarcoma-like granuloma on diaper dermatitis: A report of five cases. Arch. Dermatol. *107:*605–607, 1973.

Since lesions on five infants resembled early lesions of Kaposi sarcoma, "Kaposi sarcoma-like granuloma" is suggested as the name for this disorder.

116. Hamada T: Letters to the editor: Granuloma intertriginosum infantum (Granuloma gluteale infantum). Arch Dermatol. *111:*1072–1073, 1975.

Due to its association with irritation and candidal infection of the intertriginous regions of the neck and genitocrural region in a 3-month-old girl, granuloma intertriginosum infantum is suggested as the name for this eruption.

117. Maekawa Y, Sazaki Y, Hayashibara T: Diaper area granuloma of the aged. Arch. Dermatol. *114:*382–383, 1978.

A report of nine incontinent elderly women with diaper dermatitis and granuloma gluteale.

118. Uyeda K, Nakayasu K, Takaishi Y, et al.: Electron microscopic observations of the so-called granuloma gluteale infantum. J. Cutan. Pathol. *1:*26–32, 1974.

Electron microscopic examination of lesions revealed three types of giant cells: in the first type, the cells had widely enlarged endoplasmic reticulum, in the second they phagocytized erythrocytes, in the third they had vesicles and granules and were similar to histiocytes.

119. Bonifazi E, Garofalo L, Lospalluti M, et al.: Granuloma gluteale infantum with atrophic scars: Clinical and histologic observations in eleven cases. Clin. Exp. Dermatol. *6:*23–29, 1981.

A review of the clinical and histopathologic features of 11 patients with granuloma gluteale infantum.

120. Kikuchi I, Jono M: Letters to the editor: Flurandrenolide-impregnated tape for granuloma gluteale infantum. Arch. Dermatol. *112:*564, 1976.

Two cases of granuloma gluteale infantum showed early resolution of lesions following topical application of flurandrenolide-impregnated tape; one patient developed an associated steroid-induced atrophy.

3

ECZEMATOUS ERUPTIONS IN CHILDHOOD

Atopic dermatitis, one of the most common skin disorders seen in infants and children, is a source of frustration to parents and presents a challenge to immunologists, pediatricians, and dermatologists. Affecting 10 to 15 per cent of the childhood population, this disorder is confusing from several aspects. Confusion frequently exists because the terms *dermatitis* and *eczema* are often used synonymously and interchangeably. To the pediatrician the term *eczema* generally denotes a chronic fluctuating skin eruption occurring in atopic individuals. To the dermatologist *eczema* refers not to a disease but to a symptom-complex consisting of an acute form of inflammatory eruption characterized by itching, redness, papules, vesicles, edema, serous discharge, and crusts. In this context it fails to cover the chronic, thickened, leathery hyperpigmented forms. A modifying adjective is then added to the term *dermatitis* to specify the particular form of eruption under consideration, hence the terms *contact dermatitis, seborrheic dermatitis, nummular dermatitis,* and *atopic dermatitis.*

ATOPIC DERMATITIS

Atopic dermatitis is the most common cause of eczema in children. Any discussion of the etiology of this disorder presents obvious difficulties, stemming in part from the complexity of the disorder and our ignorance of many of the basic mechanisms of the disease.

The concept of "atopy" (the word is derived from the Greek *atopia,* meaning "different" or "out of place") was originated by Coca and Cooke in 1923.[1] They described it as a form of hypersensitivity based on a hereditary influence. Although they placed only asthma and hay fever in this category, they believed that eventually eczema, too, would be included. Shortly thereafter, in 1933, Wise and Sulzberger coined the term *atopic dermatitis* as it is used today.[2] This term is useful since it can be used to include the subacute and chronic, as well as the acute, forms of this disorder. By this designation a predisposition to asthma and hay fever is also implied, since 30 to 50 per cent of children with atopic dermatitis (infantile eczema) will go on to develop one of these forms of atopy. This is in contrast to the normal population in which the incidence of atopy is only 10 per cent of individuals. It must be remembered, however, that the term *atopic dermatitis* does not necessarily imply that the skin lesions of this disorder are caused by a union of antigen and antibody.

Stigmata Associated with Atopic Dermatitis. Although the cause of atopic dermatitis is not known, it has become evident that patients with this disorder have many systemic and cutaneous abnormalities besides their chronic pruritis and skin eruptions. Common associated findings include a tendency toward dry skin, a lower threshold to pruritic stimuli, keratosis pilaris, increased palmar markings, and atopic pleats.

Dryness and Itching. Atopic skin has an increased tendency to dryness and a peculiar itching response often referred to as a "spreading itch." Cutaneous dryness and itching are the outstanding symptoms of atopic dermatitis and appear to hold a key to the pathogenesis of this disorder. This tendency to dry skin is particularly noticeable on the extensor surfaces of the arms and legs; and in many patients, ichthyosis vulgaris is seen in association with this disorder (Fig. 3–1). Although more than 50 per cent of atopic patients have dry skin, the true frequency of ichthyosis is unknown because of the varied incidence with which the ichthyotic component has been diagnosed.

Characteristically the skin of patients with atopic dermatitis is worse during the winter months, owing to a low relative humidity aggravated by heating of the home and frequent bathing. The water-binding properties of stratum corneum appear to be due to hygroscopic water-soluble lipoprotein complexes. If these lipid materials are removed by solvents, the stratum corneum loses its capacity to act as a water barrier. Excessive bathing seems to remove lipoprotein complexes that hold water in the stratum corneum and seems to aggravate this loss of moisture. Transepidermal water loss has been demonstrated to be greater in patients with atopic dermatitis than in controls and might contribute to the inability of many individuals with atopic dermatitis to maintain soft and pliable skin and may explain the cutaneous dryness common to

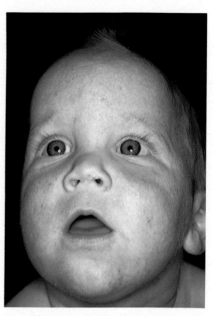

Figure 3–2. Atopic dermatitis on the face of a 6-month-old infant. Note the atopic pleats, the long luxuriant eyelashes, and the pallor of the paranasal and buccal areas.

many patients with atopic dermatitis. Such skin is easily chapped and split, particularly when the relative humidity of the atmosphere falls below 50 per cent.

Damage consequent to rubbing or scratching of this highly sensitive skin is particularly aggravating, triggers the pruritic cycle, and initiates rubbing and scratching, which results in the characteristic eczematoid reaction seen in patients with this disorder. This pruritis can be self-perpetuating by means of the "itch-scratch-itch" cycle (a phenomenon in which pruritus stimulates a bout of scratching) resulting in renewed irritation and further pruritus.[3] In susceptible persons a phenomenon of sweat retention also complicates the picture and may precipitate the itch-scratch-itch cycle.

Sites of Predilection. The sites of predilection are perhaps the best known peculiarity of the patient with atopic dermatitis. The face is favored in young infants (Fig. 3–2), extensor surfaces of the arms and legs in the crawling ages of 8 to 10 months, and the antecubital and popliteal fossae (Fig. 3–3), face, and neck in older children, adolescents, and adults (Fig. 3–4).

Keratosis Pilaris. Another associated finding is the follicular hyperkeratosis or chicken-skin appearance known as keratosis pilaris (Fig. 3–5). These lesions, most prominent on the trunk, buttocks, and outer aspects of the arms and legs, represent large cornified plugs in the upper part of the hair follicles. This cornification with a state of contraction of the erector pili muscles gives the skin a stippled appearance resembling gooseflesh or plucked chicken skin. Keratosis pilaris, a disorder

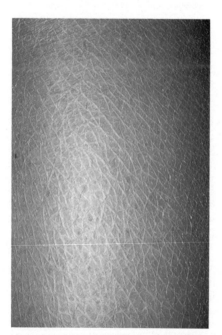

Figure 3–1. Ichthyosis vulgaris. Note large plate-like scales on the pretibial aspect of the lower leg. About 50 per cent of persons with autosomal dominant ichthyosis vulgaris show one or more atopic manifestations.

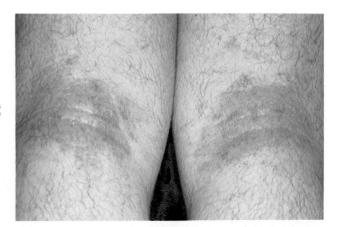

Figure 3–3. Atopic dermatitis. Oozing eczematous lesions in the popliteal fossae, a characteristic site of predilection.

whose treatment is discussed in Chapter 7, is not seen at birth, is very common from early childhood onward, and is an early and often persistent manifestation of ichthyosis vulgaris and atopic dermatitis.

Accentuated Palmar Creases. Many atopic patients exhibit an increased number of fine lines and accentuated markings of the palms (Fig. 3–6), which are usually present at birth and persist throughout life. Partially due to xerosis, they may result from thickening of the skin and may convey a poor prognosis as to the duration and severity of the disorder.

Lichenification. Also seen is the characteristic thickened, leathery, hyperpigmented lichenification, which is pathognomonic of chronic atopic dermatitis when it occurs on the wrists, ankles, and popliteal and antecubital fossae of atopic children and adolescents (Fig. 3–7).

Atopic Pleats. Atopic individuals also have a distinct tendency toward an extra line or groove of the lower eyelid, the so-called atopic pleat (Fig. 3–8).

The atopic pleat, seen just below the lower lid of both eyes, is present at birth, or shortly thereafter, and is retained throughout life. This groove (frequently referred to as Morgan's fold, Dennie's pleat, or a mongolian line), appears to be related to edema of the lower eyelids and represents a feature of the atopic diathesis rather than a pathognomonic marker of atopic dermatitis.[4]

Personality Disorders. Children with atopic dermatitis have been found to have characteristic personality traits. They are noted to be active, restless, irritable, and aggressive individuals, frequently precocious and bright, with a forceful, driving personality. If the dermatitis becomes worse and uncontrolled, the affected children often become

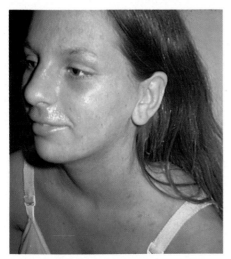

Figure 3–4. Excoriated infected atopic dermatitis on the face, neck, and chest, which are common areas of involvement in older children, adolescents, and adults.

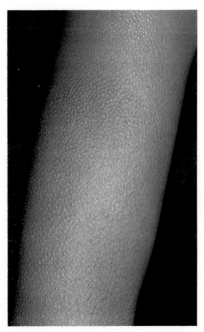

Figure 3–5. Keratosis pilaris. Fine keratotic papules most prominently seen on the trunk, buttocks, and lateral aspects of the upper arms and thighs. This is an early and often persistent manifestation of ichthyosis vulgaris and atopic dermatitis.

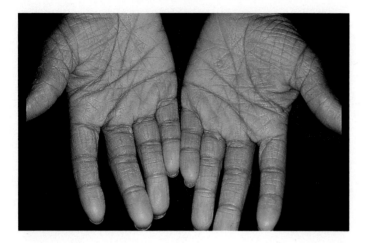

Figure 3–6. Accentuated palmar creases that are usually present at birth and persist throughout life are a common stigma of ichthyosis and atopic dermatitis.

selfish, dominating, and spoiled (Fig. 3–9). Such patients tend to lose their leadership qualities, often become frustrated or depressed, and occasionally go on to develop deep-rooted emotional disturbances. Today, with our better understanding of the nature of the disorder and more effective therapeutics, it is gratifying to see that this reaction is less common than it was in the past.

Pallor. Patients with atopic dermatitis also have various unexplained physiologic abnormalities and paradoxical responses to various stimuli. They are prone to cold hands and generalized pallor, particularly about the nose, mouth, and ears (Fig. 3–10). This phenomenon, formerly considered to be a manifestation of vasoconstriction, is now believed to be caused by capillary dilation and an increased vascular permeability, resulting in edema and blanching of the surrounding tissues.

White Dermographism. When the skin of most individuals without atopic dermatitis is stroked firmly with a pointed but not sharp instrument, the triple response of Lewis and Grant (sometimes called the triple response of Lewis) follows. *Dermographism*, a manifestation of the triple response

of Lewis said to occur in approximately 5 per cent of the normal population, is characterized by a red line, flare, and wheal reaction. A red line develops within 15 seconds at the exact site of stroking. This is followed, generally within 15 to 45 seconds, by an erythematous flare (due to an axon-reflex vasodilatation of arterioles). The response finally eventuates in a wheal (due to transudation of fluid from the injured capillaries in the original stoke line) 1 to 3 minutes later.

Individuals with atopic dermatitis demonstrate a paradoxical blanching of the skin termed *white dermographism*. The initial red line develops but is replaced, generally within a period of 10 seconds, by a white line without an associated wheal, hence the term *white dermographism*. This reaction also may occur in nonatopic individuals with allergic contact dermatitis. Although this phenomenon is not pathognomonic of either disorder, it is frequently helpful in the diagnosis of atopic dermatitis.

Delayed Blanching. Another unusual reaction frequently associated with atopic dermatitis is known as the delayed blanching phenomenon. In

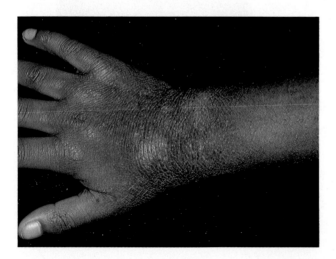

Figure 3–7. Lichenification. This hyperpigmented thickened leathery reaction to persistent rubbing and scratching characteristically occurs in patients with chronic atopic dermatitis.

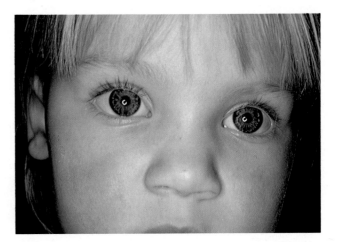

Figure 3–8. Atopic pleats (Morgan's folds, Dennie's lines). Accentuated lines or grooves are seen below the margin of the lower eyelids of both eyes.

this phenomenon the normal red flare occurs, only to be followed by an abnormal white blanching of the skin after acetylcholine injection. The delayed blanch phenomenon is seen in the skin of 70 per cent of patients with atopic dermatitis. Although uncommon in normal adults, this response occurs in newborns, patients with contact dermatitis, and young children who appear to be normal, but it, too, is nonspecific and therefore not diagnostic of atopic dermatitis.[5]

Cataracts and Keratoconus. A peculiar association of atopic dermatitis is the tendency toward early development of cataracts reportedly seen in 4 to 12 per cent of patients with this disorder. These cataracts appear at a much earlier period of life than senile cataracts. They mature rapidly; are usually bilateral, central, and shield shaped; and involve the posterior or the anterior superficial cortex, or both, rather than the peripheral and medullar areas as seen in persons with senile cataracts. Usually asymptomatic, they are generally seen only by slit lamp examination. Although the development of cataracts has been associated with long-term use of potent topical and systemic corticosteroids, atopic cataracts were described long before 1952 when compound F was released, and recent studies have shown that the long-term use of potent corticosteroids is not the cause of this phenomenon in patients with atopic dermatitis.[6, 7]

Keratoconus (elongation of the corneal surface),

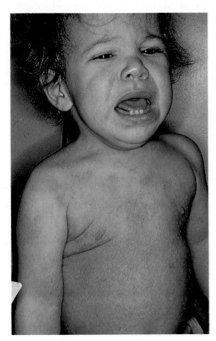

Figure 3–9. Characteristic facies of an infant with atopic dermatitis.

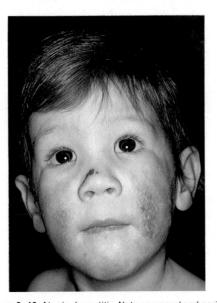

Figure 3–10. Atopic dermatitis. Note paranasal and periorbital pallor.

although uncommon, has been reported in about 1 per cent of patients with atopic dermatitis and seems to develop independently of cataracts. Keratoconus has been considered to be the result of continuous rubbing of the eyes or as a degenerative change in the cornea. Onset is in childhood. After a period of some years the disease is arrested, and contact lenses are frequently beneficial.

Altered Cell-Mediated Immunity. Patients with atopic dermatitis have evidence of altered cell-mediated immunity. Perhaps the most obvious result of this is the susceptibility to unusual cutaneous infections, especially viral, such as disseminated vaccinia (eczema vaccinatum) and herpes simplex (eczema herpeticum). Atopic individuals may also have an increased susceptibility to warts, molluscum contagiosum, and fungi (*Trichophyton rubrum*). Other studies have indicated a lowered incidence of allergic contact dermatitis in patients. Whereas *Rhus* (poison ivy) sensitivity is noted in 61 per cent of controls, studies reveal an incidence of sensitivity in only 15 per cent of individuals with atopic dermatitis.

Other Features. Other recognizable physiologic abnormalities seen in a high percentage of individuals with atopic dermatitis include a tendency toward abnormally flat glucose tolerance curves, an increased predisposition to hypotension, and a hyperactive cold pressor reaction. The latter phenomenon, an abnormal blood pressure elevation induced by immersion of a hand in ice water, is probably associated with vasoconstriction of the peripheral vascular system.

Slate-gray to violaceous infraorbital discoloration ("allergic shiners"), with or without swelling, is also seen in allergic patients and in patients with atopic dermatitis. Believed to be a manifestation of vascular stasis, induced by pressure on underlying venous plexuses by edema of the nasal and paranasal cavities, the swelling and discoloration become more prominent as a result of repeated rubbing of the eyes and melanocytic stimulation.

Another clinical feature, an exaggerated linear nasal crease caused by frequent rubbing of the nasal tip (the so-called nasal salute), although not a specific sign of atopic dermatitis, can also serve as a cutaneous clue to the possibility of an atopic diathesis and allergic rhinitis. Geographic tongue (benign migratory glossitis) is a disorder in which the dorsum of the tongue shows irregularly shaped red patches, loss of filiform papillae, and discrete brightly erythematous areas surrounded by elevated, grayish white exudative borders that change in configuration from day to day. Not necessarily a specific feature of atopic dermatitis, histologic changes of geographic tongue have also been described in patients with psoriasis.

Pathogenesis. Although the cause of atopic dermatitis remains unknown, evidence suggests that the underlying basis is a constitutional predisposition to develop pruritis. The itching leads to scratching, skin trauma, and chronic cutaneous changes characteristic of this disorder. The skin is more easily irritated than normal integument, and when pruritis occurs it initiates a "spreading" itch, thus producing more irritation, further pruritis, and the so-called itch-scratch-itch cycle. Although the pathogenesis remains unclear, the pruritus may be related to the inherent tendency toward dryness of the skin and various unexplained paradoxical physiologic responses to pharmacologic stimuli seen in individuals with this disorder.

The role of specific allergens in the pathogenesis of atopic dermatitis remains controversial. Although atopic eczema may indeed have an allergic component, particularly in infants, the antigen–antibody union is probably not directly responsible for the rash that develops in this condition.[9, 10] Allergic reactions may induce urticaria and itching, but the skin lesions themselves appear to develop in response to the rubbing and scratching induced by this reaction; and eosinophils, long overlooked in atopic dermatitis, also appear to have a role in the pathogenesis of this disorder.[11, 12]

As yet there is no satisfactory inclusive theory of atopy, one that could explain its peculiar immunologic features as well as the abnormal responses to pharmacologic agents. An interesting hypothesis is based on the β-adrenergic theory of atopy first suggested by Szentivanyi in 1968.[13] When applied to the skin, the theory of β-adrenergic blockade relates the peculiar irritability of the skin to an imbalance in the autonomic nervous system. It is postulated that in atopy there is reduced function of the β-adrenergic system. This autonomic imbalance induces a reduction in activity or blockade of the β-adrenergic receptor (adenyl cyclase), or perhaps an increase in activity of α-receptors, with a resultant dysfunction of cyclic adenosine monophosphate. As a result of this phenomenon there is an increased release of the pharmacologic mediators (histamine, bradykinin, and slow-reacting substance of anaphylaxis). These mediators produce vasodilatation, increased vascular permeability, edema, and urticaria, which in turn may be responsible for the pruritus and inflammatory cutaneous changes characteristic of atopic dermatitis. This theory may also explain the mechanism by which psychic stimuli, infection, mechanical injury, and immunologic reactions play a role in the exaggerated skin irritability of these individuals.

The role of hypersensitivity in atopic dermatitis remains controversial. Ishizaka's discovery of immunoglobulin E, the reaginic antibody, in 1966, however, adds credibility to Szentivanyi's theory.[14, 15] The union of antibody and antigen appears to precipitate mast cell release of pharmacologic mediators (histamine, bradykinin, and slow-reacting substance of anaphylaxis); this induces the itching, rubbing, and scratching that lead to the cutaneous lesions characteristic of this disorder. Juhlin and Johannsen have demonstrated elevated serum IgE levels in 82 per cent of patients with atopic dermatitis,[16] and Ogawa and others subsequently demonstrated a relationship between IgE levels and the severity of the dermatitis,[17] thus adding further credibility to this theory.

In addition, since the skin of patients with atopic dermatitis often contains high concentrations of *Staphylococcus aureus*, it has been shown that an immune reaction between bacteria on the skin and antibacterial IgE on dermal mast cells, and other abnormalities such as IgE overproduction, diminished cell-mediated immunity, and a T-cell defect of inadequate interferon-gamma production combined with excessive interleukin production may account for many of the immune and inflammatory defects associated with this disorder.[11, 18, 19]

For years pediatricians and dermatologists disagreed on the relationship between allergy to food protein and atopic dermatitis in children. Whereas dermatologists frequently minimized the role of diet in this disorder, pediatricians often suggested a close association between food ingestion (namely, egg white, wheat, milk, and citruses) and atopic dermatitis, particularly in children younger than 1 year of age. This controversy was probably related to the fact that most children seen by dermatologists were those who did not respond to hypoallergenic dietary regimens initiated by the pediatrician. Thus, it is now quite apparent that foods may at times act as allergens and that reactions to food in atopic dermatitis could be due to the release of physiologic mediators with resultant vasodilatation and possibly to effects on sweat secretion and, after puberty, on the pilosebaceous apparatus. Pruritis, therefore, may well be the primary connecting link between foods and the symptoms and cutaneous manifestations of atopic dermatitis.

Studies by Sampson and others have now clearly demonstrated that food sensitivity (particularly to milk, eggs, nuts, soy, wheat, and seafood) in some individuals may aggravate, precipitate, or perpetuate their dermatitis and that patients with severe unresponsive dermatitis deserve consideration of food as a possible cause or precipitating factor for their dermatosis.[20, 21] Recent developments in our understanding of late-phase allergic reactions may shed additional information on the role of foods in atopic dermatitis. Thus, although allergic reactions are frequently perceived as self-limiting, they may at times persist, even in the absence of reexposure to the allergen that precipitated the reaction.[22] It should be emphasized, however, that a high percentage of eczematous skin eruptions in infants and children are not caused by ingestants, nor are they cured by the removal of certain foods from the diet. It is probably just as much an error, therefore, to overlook the possible role of allergy in this age group as it is to attribute all manifestations of the disease to foods and ingested allergens.

Clinical Manifestations. Atopic dermatitis may be divided into three phases based on the age of the patient and the distribution of lesions. These arbitrary divisions may be referred to as the infantile, childhood, and adult forms of this disorder.

The infantile form of atopic dermatitis usually begins between the period of 2 and 6 months of age and, in 50 per cent of patients, clears by 2 to 3 years of age (see Figs 3–2, 3–9, and 3–10). It is characterized by intense itching, erythema, papules, vesicles, oozing, and crusting. In infants, it usually begins on the cheeks, forehead, or scalp and then extends to the trunk or extremities in scattered, often symmetrical, patches. Although infants with atopic dermatitis have a somewhat increased incidence of diaper dermatitis, lesions of atopic dermatitis generally spare the groin and diaper area during infancy. This may be due, at least in part, to protection by the diaper, but it is more likely related to increased hydration in these areas, keeping the stratum corneum barrier flexible and intact.[11] Although scaling and crusting of the scalp may suggest a diagnosis of seborrheic dermatitis, the severe itching, a personal or family history of atopy, and the character and distribution of lesions help differentiate the two disorders. In children 1 year of age or older, lesions often take on the appearance of nummular eczema, with sharply defined oval scaly eruptions on the face, trunk, and extremities.

The childhood phase of atopic dermatitis may follow the infantile stage without interruption and usually occurs during the period from 4 to 10 years of age. Affected persons in this age group are less likely to have exudative and crusted lesions and have a greater tendency toward chronicity and lichenification. Eruptions are characteristically more dry and papular and often occur as circumscribed scaly patches. The classic areas of involvement in this group are the wrists, ankles, and antecubital and popliteal regions (Fig. 3–11). Pruritus is frequently severe, and infection and irritation from scratching often modify the lesions. Again, remission may occur at any time before the prepubertal age, or the eruption may go on to merge into the succeeding adolescent and adult phase of this disorder.

The adolescent and adult stage of atopic der-

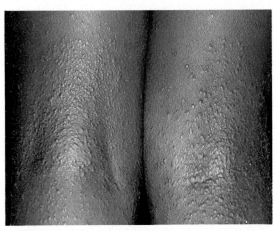

Figure 3–11. Papular atopic dermatitis, particularly common in the antecubital and popliteal areas of darkly pigmented individuals.

matitis begins at the age of 12 and frequently continues onward into the early 20s. Predominant areas of involvement include the flexor folds, the face and neck, the upper arms and back, and the dorsa of the hands, feet, fingers, and toes. The eruption is characterized by dry and thick lesions, confluent papules, and the formation of large lichenified plaques. Weeping, crusting, and exudation may occur, but they are usually the result of superimposed external irritation or infection.

Seventy-five per cent of individuals with atopic dermatitis improve by 10 to 14 years of age, and 25 per cent of patients continue to have difficulty during their adult life. Cases persisting or beginning after the middle 20s are the most difficult to manage and usually have little tendency to spontaneous cure. Fortunately, these are relatively rare.

Diagnosis. The diagnosis of atopic dermatitis is based on the evaluation of the aggregate of signs, symptoms, stigmata, course, and associated familial findings. Typical cases may be recognized easily. Atypical ones, however, may require long study and a careful differential diagnosis. Thus, the application of the diagnostic criteria summarized in Table 3–1 can be used to help distinguish atopic dermatitis from other eczematous disorders.

The disease is characterized by spasmodic itching and its consequences. Clinically, it is recognized as a pruritic, erythematous, papular, and vesicular eruption, with edema, serous discharge, and crusting. An important diagnostic feature is the fact that the borders of lesions of atopic dermatitis tend to gradually merge into the surrounding skin (Fig. 3–12) and, except in chronic cases of lichen simplex chronicus (neurodermatitis), are generally not well marginated.

Sites of predilection, a well-recognized peculiarity of the patient with atopic dermatitis, frequently are helpful and can aid in determining the true

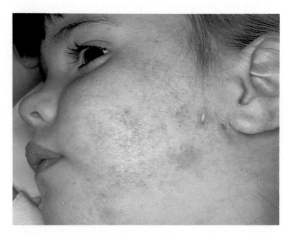

Figure 3–12. Atopic dermatitis. Eczematoid lesions merge into the surrounding skin.

nature of the eruption. In chronic forms of this disorder, scaling, lichenification, hyperpigmentation, thickening, and fissuring are characteristic and at times pathognomonic (see Fig. 3–7).

When the diagnosis remains in doubt, histopathologic examination of cutaneous lesions will at times help to ascertain the true nature of the eruption. Acute lesions of infantile atopic dermatitis reveal hyperkeratosis, parakeratosis, and hyperplasia of the epidermis, with an absence or diminution of the granular cell layer. Essential diagnostic features include increased intercellular and intracellular accumulation of fluid (spongiosis), with migration of leukocytes (exocytosis) through the epidermis.

Chronic lesions of atopic dermatitis are characterized by increased hyperkeratosis with areas of parakeratosis and papillomatosis (upward proliferation of dermal papillae). Although these chronic changes may at times resemble those of psoriasis, the fact that there is more edema and a lack of clubbing of the rete ridges in lesions of atopic dermatitis helps differentiate these two disorders.

Differential Diagnosis. Atopic dermatitis is a chronic fluctuating disease. The distribution and morphology of lesions vary with age, but itching remains as the cardinal symptom of this disorder. Although many skin conditions may occasionally resemble atopic dermatitis, certain characteristics assist in their differentiation.

Seborrheic dermatitis is characterized by a greasy yellow or salmon-colored scaly eruption that may involve the scalp, cheeks, trunk, extremities, and diaper area (see Chapter 2, Figs. 2–11 through 2–13). The major differentiating features include a tendency toward earlier onset, characteristic greasy yellowish or salmon-colored lesions with a predisposition for intertriginous areas (Figs. 3–13 and 3–14), a generally well-circumscribed eruption, and a relative absence of pruritus.

Contact dermatitis can be divided into irritant contact dermatitis and allergic contact dermatitis. *Primary irritant dermatitis* is frequently seen in

---

Table 3–1. CRITERIA FOR THE DIAGNOSIS OF ATOPIC DERMATITIS IN CHILDREN

A. Major Features (must have three)
  1. Pruritus
  2. Typical morphology and distribution
    a. Facial and extensor involvement during infancy and early childhood
    b. Flexural lichenification by adolescence
  3. Chronic or chronically relapsing dermatitis
  4. Personal or family history of atopy
B. Minor or Less Specific Features
  1. Xerosis
  2. Periauricular fissures
  3. Ichthyosis, hyperlinear palms or keratosis pilaris
  4. IgE reactivity (increased serum IgE, RAST, or prick test positivity)
  5. Hand or foot dermatitis
  6. Cheilitis
  7. Scalp dermatitis (cradle cap)
  8. Susceptibility to cutaneous infections (especially *Staphylococcus aureus* and herpes simplex)
  9. Perifollicular accentuation (especially in pigmented races)

Modified from Hanifin JM: Atopic dermatitis in infants and children. Pediatr. Clin. North Am. 38:763–789, 1991.

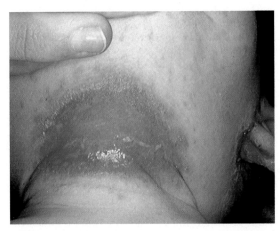

Figure 3–13. Intertrigo of the neck in an infant with seborrheic dermatitis.

infants and young children. In this disorder the site of eruption varies with the etiologic agent. It commonly is seen on the cheeks and the chin (owing to salivary secretion and associated rubbing of the involved areas), the extensor surfaces of the extremities (as a result of harsh soaps, detergents, or rough sheets), and the diaper area (from urine, feces, soaps, detergents, and the irritation associated with harsh talcum powder preparations). Primary irritant dermatitis is generally milder, less pruritic, and not as eczematoid as the eruptions seen in association with atopic dermatitis.

Allergic contact dermatitis, although relatively uncommon in the first few months of life, can mimic almost any type of eczematous eruption and is characterized by a well-circumscribed pruritic, erythematous, papular and vesicular eruption. Although such eruptions involute spontaneously on identification and removal of the cause, this disorder often requires a carefully detailed history and prolonged observation before the true causative agent is identified.

Nummular dermatitis (derived from the Latin, meaning "coin-like") is a distinctive disorder characterized by coin-shaped lesions. Measuring 1 cm or more in diameter, lesions of nummular dermatitis develop on dry skin (especially during winter months in heated homes with low humidity). The eruption begins with minute vesicles and papules that enlarge by confluence or peripheral extension, thus forming the discrete erythematous coin-like lesions studded with papules and vesicles characteristic of this disorder (Fig. 3–15). Although in the past nummular eczema has been believed by many to be a manifestation of atopic dermatitis, studies of IgE levels in patients with this disorder suggest nummular eczema to be a manifestation of dry skin (xerosis) and ichthyosis rather than a characteristic of atopy and atopic dermatitis.[23]

Psoriasis, another common skin disease of children as well as adults, must also be included in the differential diagnosis of infants and children with atopic dermatitis. The fully developed lesion of psoriasis has a full, rich, red hue and a loosely adherent silvery micaceous ("mica-like") scale. Psoriatic lesions are usually well defined, with a sharply delineated edge, and have a predilection for the extensor surfaces (particularly the elbows and knees), the scalp, and the genital regions.

A valuable clue in the diagnosis of psoriasis is the frequent presence of nail involvement. Seen in 25 to 50 per cent of patients, pitting or small punctate dimpling of the nail plate is the most common nail finding and results from an intermittent psoriatic defect in the matrix as the nail is formed. Although pitted nails may also be seen in atopic dermatitis and alopecia areata, the nail pits seen in atopic dermatitis (due to cutaneous eczematous changes in the areas of the nail matrix) are usually larger and more irregular. Nail pits seen in association with alopecia areata frequently are grid-like and less deep than those seen in patients with psoriasis.

Scabies in infants and children is commonly

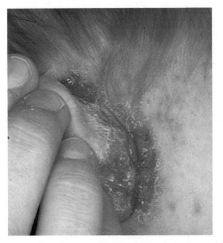

Figure 3–14. Infected postauricular seborrheic dermatitis.

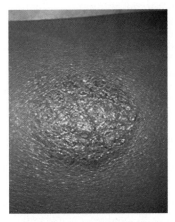

Figure 3–15. Nummular eczema. A well-circumscribed papulovesicular coin-shaped lesion on the pretibial area in a patient with ichthyosis vulgaris.

complicated by eczematous changes due to scratching and rubbing of involved areas or topical therapeutic agents. The diagnosis of scabies is best made by the history of itching, a characteristic distribution of lesions, the recognition of primary lesions (particularly the pathognomonic burrow when present), positive identification of the mite on microscopic examination of skin scrapings, and the presence of infestation among the patient's family or associates (see Chapter 14).

Letterer-Siwe disease, seen at the severe fulminating end of the histiocytosis spectrum, usually occurs during the first year of life and is almost exclusively limited to children up to 3 years of age (see Chapter 24). In this disorder the skin eruption generally begins with a scaly, erythematous seborrhea-like eruption on the scalp, behind the ears, and in the intertriginous regions. On close inspection the presence of reddish brown or purpuric papules or vesicular or crusted papules (in infants) is characteristic. When the diagnosis is indeterminate, cutaneous biopsy may confirm the true nature of the eruption.

Acrodermatitis enteropathica is a hereditary disorder characterized by vesiculobullous eczematoid lesions of the acral and periorificial areas, failure to thrive, diarrhea, alopecia, nail dystrophy, and frequent secondary bacterial or candidal infection. The characteristic distribution of lesions, accompanied by listlessness, diarrhea, failure to thrive, and low serum zinc levels, differentiate lesions of acrodermatitis enteropathica from those of atopic dermatitis.

Wiskott-Aldrich syndrome, an X-linked recessive disorder that occurs in male infants, is characterized by severe eczematous dermatitis, thrombocytopenic purpura, increased susceptibility to infection, bloody diarrhea, purpuric lesions, and defects in cellular and humoral immunity.

Phenylketonuria is a hereditary disorder characterized by mental retardation, seizures, diffuse hypopigmentation, blond hair, eczema, and photosensitivity. Caused by a defect in the enzyme phenylalanine hydroxylase, an elevated blood phenylalanine concentration of 15 mg/dl is usually accepted as presumptive evidence of this disorder (see Chapter 22).

Complications. *Secondary infection* is the most common complication seen in atopic dermatitis. Usually associated with group A β-hemolytic streptococci and, even more frequently, *Staphylococcus* organisms, studies suggest that the skin of patients with atopic dermatitis may be inherently favorable for *Staphylococcus aureus* colonization.[24] Whether this is related to chronic excoriation, depressed phagocytic function, or T-cell abnormality is as yet undetermined, but studies reveal a *Staphylococcus* carrier rate of 93 per cent in lesions of atopic dermatitis, 76 per cent in uninvolved (normal) skin, and 79 per cent from the anterior nares.[25] Pyoderma associated with atopic dermatitis is usually manifested by erythema with exudation and crusting, greasy moist scales, and small pustules in the advancing edge (Fig. 3–16). This complication must be considered whenever a flare of chronic atopic dermatitis develops or fails to respond to appropriate therapy.[26] In addition, osteomyelitis has also been described as a complication in children with infected atopic dermatitis.[27] In view of these factors, there is strong evidence endorsing the practice of adding an antibiotic, either topical if the dermatitis is localized, or systemic if the dermatitis is widespread or unresponsive to other conventional therapy. Penicillin G is generally the drug of choice in the treatment of known group A streptococcal skin infections. When the cause is not known immediately and when *S. aureus* is a distinct consideration, erythromycin or a semisynthetic penicillin, such as nafcillin, oxacillin, or dicloxacillin, should be used. If the secondary infection is due to group A β-hemolytic *Streptococcus*, treatment should be continued for at least 10 days, and for patients who demonstrate frequent or recurrent infection, I generally prefer a course of systemic antibiotics for a period of 3 weeks or more. Although systemic antibiotics may be valuable in the elimination of cutaneous streptococci, they do not appear to prevent glomerulonephritis due to streptococcal cutaneous infection. In areas in which nephritogenic M strains of streptococci are endemic, urinalysis should be performed and it has been recommended that patients be observed for signs of glomerulonephritis for at least 7 weeks after treatment.[28] When patients with asthma and infected atopic dermatitis are treated concomitantly, one must recognize the fact that erythromycin and ciprofloxacin (the latter is not recommended for children or pregnant women) can cause a reduction in theophylline clearance, thus causing elevated serum theophylline concentrations.[29] An analogous situation has also been reported in patients who take erythromycin concomitantly with carbamazepine (Tegretol), an anticonvulsant and analgesic used for the treatment of trigeminal neuralgia,[30] and patients taking the antihistamines terfenadine (Seldane) or astemizole (Hismanal).

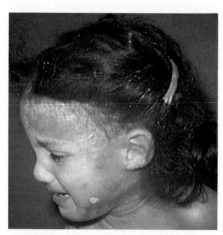

Figure 3–16. Infected atopic dermatitis.

Kaposi's varicelliform eruption is another, even more severe, complication of atopic dermatitis. It is caused by the virus of herpes simplex or vaccinia and may be referred to as eczema herpeticum or eczema vaccinatum. Heretofore eczema vaccinatum occasionally followed smallpox vaccination of an eczematoid child but was more frequently contracted by accidental contact with a recently vaccinated individual. Now that vaccination is no longer compulsory and the threat of smallpox appears to have been eliminated, eczema vaccinatum should not continue to be a problem for individuals with atopic dermatitis.

The explosive development of a vesicular eruption in an atopic individual should raise the possibility of Kaposi's varicelliform eruption. Umbilication of the vesicles is characteristic (Figs. 3–17 and 3–18), and the diagnosis can be verified by viral culture or the Tzanck test. In this test a cytologic examination is made of scraped vesicles with a search for multinuclear virus "giant cells," balloon cells, and, on rare occasion, intranuclear inclusions on a Giemsa-stained smear (see Chapter 2, Fig. 2–24).

The treatment of eczema herpeticum is symptomatic; requires maintenance of adequate hydration, control of fever, and prevention of secondary bacterial infection; and generally runs its course within 2 to 3 weeks. For severe cases, oral acyclovir (Zovirax, 25 to 30 mg/kg/day, up to 200 mg five times a day for older children and adults) or intravenous acyclovir (5 mg/kg every 8 hours or 1.5 g/m² per day) for a period of 5 to 10 days have been found to be effective.[31–34]

Management

Reduction of Dryness and Pruritis. The treatment of atopic dermatitis is dependent on the management of dry and itching skin. The problem is particularly troublesome in winter when it is aggravated by heat in the house and low humidity. Patients should be instructed to limit bathing and to use lubricants that help moisten and rehydrate the skin. This diminishes the tendency toward dryness and pruritus that seems to be critically involved in the pathogenesis of this condition. A mild soap (such as Dove or Neutrogena) may be used, and when lubricant is applied, it is best administered over slightly moistened skin. This seals in the moisture; rehydrates, lubricates, and moisturizes the skin; and thus diminishes the inherent dryness and itchiness that appear to trigger the eczematoid eruptions seen in patients with atopic dermatitis.

A hydrophilic lotion such as Cetaphil (Owen/Galderma) may be used as a cleansing and lubricating agent for individuals with dry skin. This may be applied liberally and rubbed gently over the skin (*without water*) until a light foaming occurs. Following removal by light wiping with a soft cotton cloth, diaper, or cleansing tissue, a protective film of stearyl alcohol and propylene glycol remains.

Bubble baths are contraindicated. When bathing is allowed, it is recommended that water be tepid or at room temperature (hot water stimulates vasodilatation and subsequent pruritus). Bath oils are only slightly beneficial and since they tend to make the tub slippery, should be used sparingly and cautiously, if at all, particularly with children.[11, 35]

The most important exacerbant to dryness is overbathing and inadequate hydration and emolliation.[35] Since excessive bathing will dry the skin unless an emollient is applied within 3 minutes of exiting the bath or shower, an effective alternative to the limited or no bathing Scholz-type regimen is a technique in which the patient can bathe frequently (every day, and in acute or severe circumstances, even two or three times a day). When this method is used, the patient can soak in a tepid or lukewarm bath for 20 minutes and apply an emollient, such as petrolatum (Vaseline) or Aquaphor (Beiersdorf), just before getting out of the bath (while still in the water) or immediately after getting out of the water, while the skin is still damp. I call these *Vaseline* or *Aquaphor* baths and find them to be extremely helpful for children who are older, have to be bathed more frequently, and can stay in a tub bath for the prescribed period. Furthermore, since topical corticosteroid penetration is 10-fold greater through hydrated skin, prompt application of corticosteroid after the bath can be extremely helpful. In addition, when repeated cutaneous infections present a problem, a household bleach (such as Clorox, 2 teaspoons per gallon of

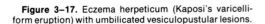

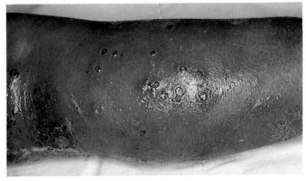

Figure 3–17. Eczema herpeticum (Kaposi's varicelliform eruption) with umbilicated vesiculopustular lesions.

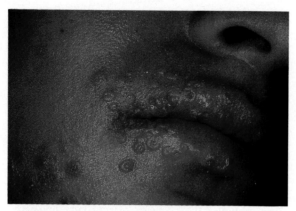

Figure 3–18. Umbilicated vesicular lesions of eczema herpeticum (Kaposi's varicelliform eruption) on the lips and chin of a young woman with atopic dermatitis.

water) can help reduce the incidence of recurrent cutaneous bacterial infection. Children may at times complain about sitting in a tub bath because of stinging, particularly during acute exacerbations. In such instances, the addition of 1 cup of table salt will help make the bath more tolerable.

Attention to clothing is also important. Soft cotton clothing is recommended over wool or other harsh materials, which tend to precipitate itching and scratching. The smoking of cigarettes in homes of children with atopic dermatitis, since it can lead to an increase in irritation and pruritus, and may also increase the tendency toward subsequent development of asthma, should also be avoided. Feather pillows, fuzzy toys, stuffed animals, and pets such as cats and dogs should also be avoided because of their potential allergenicity and the predisposition of patients with atopic dermatitis to develop respiratory allergies, particularly asthma. In households where pets cannot be eliminated, the pets should, if possible, be kept outside or restricted to areas of the house where the child will not be exposed to the animal, its dander, or saliva.

Reduction of perspiration is helpful since many patients have considerable difficulty adjusting to hot and humid weather owing to eccrine sweating and sweat retention. Air conditioning is sometimes helpful during the summer, and frequent airing of the bedroom and humidification helps to relieve the adverse effects of excessive skin dryness during the winter.

Wet Compresses. Topical treatment of the acute stage of atopic dermatitis is aided by open wet compresses. When properly applied, open wet compresses have a soothing, antipruritic, and cleansing action on acutely inflamed skin. They tend to dry weeping or oozing lesions, clean crusts, assist in the rehydration of dry skin, and, through evaporation of water, afford cooling to inflamed and irritated tissue. Aluminum acetate (as in Burow's solution, 1:20 or 1:40) is germicidal and, by precipitation of protein, suppresses the weeping and oozing of acutely inflamed lesions. Burow's solution, 1:40, is prepared by dissolving one

packet or effervescent tablet (Domeboro effervescent tablets or packets [Miles]) in a pint of cool or tepid tap water.

For the best results, wet dressings are applied during the acute stage of the disorder for a period of up to 5 days with a soft cloth such as a man's handkerchief, a thin diaper, or strips of bed sheeting. Gauze squares are contraindicated because of their tendency to adhere to skin and cause irritation. Washcloths and heavy toweling interfere with evaporation and therefore are not as effective for this purpose.

Solutions should be tepid, lukewarm, or at body temperature. If too hot, vasodilatation occurs with resulting weeping and pruritus; if too cold, vasoconstriction occurs. This may relieve warmth and pruritus temporarily, but secondary vasodilatation soon develops, thus reversing the process. Compresses should be moderately wet, not dripping, and should be remoistened at intervals. Following the compress, a topical corticosteroid may be applied and, in severe cases, the topical agent may be applied both before and after the compress. The hydration by the wet compress relieves the dryness of the skin, breaks the skin surface barrier, and facilitates the penetration and action of the applied corticosteroid preparation.

Dietary Restrictions. Although benefit from dietary restrictions may be interpreted with skepticism, many physicians advocate the elimination of specific foods in the management of atopic dermatitis during the first 1 or 2 years of life. It is important to realize that in some instances specific foods may indeed produce a visible or clinically imperceptible urticarial reaction, vasodilatation, and possible effects on sweat secretion that may initiate pruritus and an associated exacerbation of a preexisting dermatitis. For such infants, milk, eggs, tomatoes, citrus fruits, chocolate, wheat products, spiced foods, fish, and nuts or peanut butter may be eliminated, at least on a trial basis, until the disorder is controlled by frequent lubrication, topical corticosteroids, and appropriate antipruritic agents.

As the child grows older, food reactivity (said to occur in up to 10 to 15 per cent of children younger than age 5) frequently diminishes and the importance of inhalant allergens increases. In the older child, therefore, although food elimination is less often of value, a careful dietary history will occasionally reveal important information. Effective therapy requires a careful history, observation of ingestants that might trigger an exacerbation, particularly during the first 1 or 2 years of life, at least a temporary elimination of suspected food allergens, and, of primary consideration, judicious management of the dry and itching skin characteristic of this disorder.

Early exposure to cow's milk has been believed by many to be a major factor in the development of atopic disease in infancy. Therefore, most allergy prevention programs recommend the prophylactic elimination of cow's milk from infants predisposed to atopy and atopic dermatitis. Since the first suggestion that prolonged breast feeding might prevent atopic dermatitis, studies have produced conflicting results. Despite this controversy,[36-38] current studies suggest that it may be prudent to recommend the delay of potential allergenic foods such as cow's milk, eggs, fish, chocolate, nuts, and citrus fruits from infants' diets for 6 to 12 months.[39-42]

House Dust Mites and Atopy. Studies have also shown that exposure to house dust mites, particularly *Dermatophygoides farinae* in the United States and *D. pteronyssinus* in Europe, may also be responsible for exacerbations and chronicity of atopic dermatitis (Fig. 3–19).[43, 44] Although it is extremely difficult to eliminate house dust mites from the home environment, weekly washing of the bedding, regular vacuuming of carpets and curtains, and the use of plastic mattress and pillow covers will help reduce house dust mite population. When mite sensitivity is suspected, skin testing may provide a clue to this possibility and the presence of household mites may be assessed by microscopic identification of vacuumings of household dust. Although further studies are required to determine the value of house dust mite avoidance in patients with mite sensitivity and atopic dermatitis, natamycin (Tymosil), a fungicidal spray used in Europe to kill *Aspergillus penicillinoides* (the fungus that digests the lipids in the epidermal scales on which house dust mites feed), and benzyl benzoate (Acarosan), an acaricidal agent applied to carpets in bedrooms and other areas where children may have high contact with mites, may be helpful.[45]

Skin Tests and Hyposensitization. Although patients with atopic dermatitis often demonstrate reactions to a variety of allergens, hyposensitization does not appear to be of value in the treatment of this disorder. Skin tests are often unreliable and not recommended for the majority of infants and children with atopic dermatitis, but they may occasionally provide clues to the cause of persistent or recurrent eruptions not responsive to the usual rational therapy.

Standards for skin testing in young children are poor, irritant reactions are frequent, and in children younger than 8 years of age, false-negative and false-positive reactions are common. When hyposensitization for respiratory allergies is performed in a child with atopic dermatitis, care must be exercised to avoid flares of the dermatitis, which occasionally occur as the dose of extract is increased.

As an alternative to skin tests, an in vitro test, the radioallergosorbent test (RAST) for serum IgE specific antigen, is currently commercially available. RAST may be more sensitive than prick or scratch skin tests but is less sensitive than intradermal testing and is substantially more expensive. Another test, the radioimmunosorbent technique (RIST), has also become available. Although raised total IgE levels can be determined by the RIST and circulating reagins can be detected by the RAST, the value of these tests in the management of atopic dermatitis requires further investigation. Prick or scratch skin tests, therefore, are generally recommended when allergy testing is used in an attempt to identify possible offending allergens,[46] and RAST or RIST tests can be used for individuals with extensive dermatitis in whom skin testing is not feasible.

Topical Corticosteroids. Potent corticosteroid preparations are most effective in the treatment of atopic dermatitis. There is a science, however, to their use. It involves the selection of the correct strength corticosteroid in the proper formulation for the particular disease process and specific areas of involvement.

The potency of topical corticosteroids is related to their vehicle as well as to their chemical formulation. In general, gels penetrate more effectively, are somewhat more drying, are well accepted in hairy areas such as the scalp, and are particularly effective in the management of acute weeping or vesicular lesions. Corticosteroid ointments afford the advantage of occlusion, more effective penetration, and in general greater efficacy than equivalent cream or lotion formulations. They are particularly effective in the management of dry, lichenified, or plaque-like areas of dermatitis. Ointment formulations, however, tend to occlude eccrine pores, may induce sweat retention and pruritus, and accordingly are not as well tolerated during the summer months when heat, perspira-

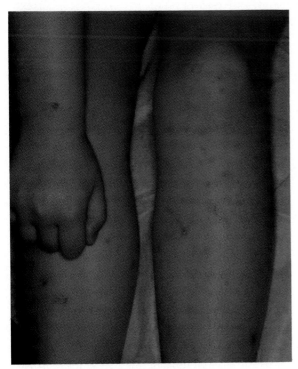

Figure 3–19. Excoriated atopic dermatitis on the legs of a young girl with house dust mite sensitivity.

tion, and high humidity are significant. Creams and lotions are generally less potent than gel and ointment formulations. They, however, afford the advantages of greater convenience and acceptability during hot weather and in intertriginous or hairy areas. It should be remembered that gels and lotions are drying and, except for wet or oozing lesions, are generally not indicated in the management of atopic dermatitis.

The use of corticosteroid-impregnated polyethylene film, available as Cordran tape (Dista), or the occlusion of treated areas with polyethylene film, such as Saran wrap, appears to enhance the penetration of corticosteroids up to 100-fold. This mode of therapy is particularly effective for short periods of time (8 to 12 hours a day on successive days) for patients with chronic lichenified or recalcitrant plaques of dermatitic skin. Occlusive techniques, however, are contraindicated for prolonged periods of time, are not recommended in acute infected or intertriginous areas, and occasionally may result in local infection, miliaria, folliculitis, and, with prolonged use, an increased incidence of atrophy and striae. Occlusive corticosteroid dressings, accordingly, should be used for relatively short periods of time, with appropriate admonition regarding overuse and potential adverse reactions.

Many practitioners erroneously associate fluorination of glucocorticosteroids with biologic potency and consider hydrocortisone formulations to be of low potency. However, hydrocortisone butyrate (Locoid) and a valerate derivative of hydrocortisone (Westcort) are effective mid-potency hydrocortisone preparations. Conversely, certain fluorinated agents, such as betamethasone alcohol, fluocinolone alcohol, and dexamethasone, are less effective than some of the more highly potent topical formulations. In Table 3–2 a summary of topical corticosteroid potency based on vasoconstrictor assays is presented.

In general, group I corticosteroids are not recommended for patients younger than the age of 12 years, should not be used in intertriginous areas or under occlusion, and require a rest period after 14 days of use. Although the package insert for diflorasone diacetate ointment (Psorcon) does not require this rest period, and does not specifically prohibit occlusion or use in patients younger than the age of 12 years, this agent should still be used with extreme caution. Furthermore, since vasoconstrictor assays reveal that generic formulations tend to vary in their clinical activity, and their vehicles may at times contain agents differing from those of brand name formulations, many authorities recommend that generic corticosteroid formulations be avoided until this situation has been rectified.[47]

Considering the wide use of topical corticosteroids, there have been relatively few reports of adverse reaction due to their absorption. When applied over large areas of dermatitic skin, or when used under occlusion, the possibility of systemic

Table 3–2. ORDER OF POTENCY OF TOPICAL CORTICOSTEROIDS (FROM MOST TO LEAST POTENT)

I. Diprolene Gel or Ointment	0.05%
Psorcon Ointment	0.05%
Temovate Cream or Ointment	0.05%
Ultravate Cream or Ointment	0.05%
II. Cyclocort Ointment	0.1%
Diprolene AF Cream	0.05%
Diprosone Ointment	0.05%
Elocon Ointment	0.1%
Florone Ointment	0.05%
Halog Cream	0.1%
Lidex Cream, Gel, and Ointment	0.05%
Maxiflor Ointment	0.05%
Maxivate Ointment	0.05%
Topicort Cream and Ointment	0.25%
Topicort Gel	0.05%
III. Aristocort Ointment	0.1%
Cutivate Ointment	0.05%
Diprolene Cream or Lotion	0.05%
Diprosone Cream	0.05%
Florone Cream	0.05%
Halog Ointment	0.1%
Lidex E Cream	0.05%
Maxiflor Cream	0.05%
Maxivate Cream and Lotion	0.05%
Valisone Ointment	0.1%
IV. Cordran Ointment	0.05%
Cutivate Cream	0.05%
Cyclocort Cream	0.05%
Elocon Cream and Lotion	0.1%
Kenalog Cream	0.1%
Synalar Ointment	0.025%
Topicort LP Emollient Cream	0.05%
Westcort Ointment	0.2%
V. Aristocort Cream	0.1%
Cloderm Cream	0.1%
Cordran Cream	0.05%
Diprosone Lotion	0.05%
Kenalog Lotion	0.1%
Locoid Cream	0.1%
Synalar Cream	0.025%
Valisone Cream	0.1%
Westcort Cream	0.2%
VI. Aclovate Cream and Ointment	0.05%
DesOwen Cream	0.05%
Locorten Cream	0.03%
Synalar Cream and Solution	0.01%
Tridesilon Cream	0.05%
Valisone Lotion	0.05%
VII. Topicals with hydrocortisone, dexamethasone, flumethalone, prednisolone, and methylprednisolone	

Group I is the super-potent category; groups II and III are high-potency, groups IV and V are mid-potency, and groups VI and VII are low-potency corticosteroids.

Modified from Stoughton RB, Cornell RC: Review of super-potent steroids. Semin. Dermatol. 6:72–76, 1987.

absorption, however, must be considered, particularly in infants and small children, and suppression of the pituitary-adrenal axis, although relatively uncommon, has been documented.[48–51]

Other potential side effects of potent topical corticosteroids, particularly when used under occlusion or for long periods of time, include cutaneous atrophy, steroid rosacea, striae (Fig. 3–20), and telangiectasia. Potent topical corticosteroids, however, may be used in small areas for short periods of time with little risk of absorption. Once the disorder is under control, it is advisable to taper the

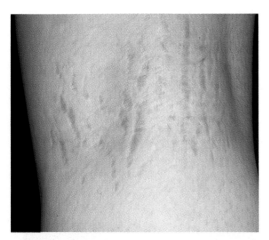

Figure 3–20. Atrophic striae. Shallow linear depressed lesions in the popliteal fossae from prolonged use of potent topical corticosteroids.

therapy to a moderately potent topical corticosteroid and, as the disorder continues to improve, to one of the milder potency hydrocortisone formulations. This gradual reduction of topical corticosteroid potency over a period of weeks is advisable in an effort to avoid a rebound phenomenon that tends to occur with too rapid discontinuation of topical corticosteroids. Following this gradual reduction of topical corticosteroids, the dermatitis can frequently be relatively well maintained by a regimen of limited or vaseline baths, frequent lubrication, and antipruritics (as needed) in an effort to minimize the dryness and itchiness inherent in this disorder.

Tar Preparations. Although tar preparations have been replaced to a certain degree by topical corticosteroids, they are still effective in the management of subacute, chronic, and lichenified forms of dermatitis. The mechanism by which tar formulations act on abnormal skin is not known, but they appear to have vasoconstrictive, astringent, disinfectant, and antipruritic properties and help correct abnormal keratinization by a decrease in epidermal proliferation and dermal infiltration. Heretofore, many patients found tar formulations to be cosmetically objectionable. Cosmetically acceptable preparations such as AquaTar (Herbert), Estar (Westwood-Squibb), Fototar (Elder), Psorigel (Owen), and T/Derm Tar Emollient (Neutrogena), and an extract of coal tar (liquor carbonis detergents, 2 to 5 per cent in a vanishing cream base or zinc oxide ointment) appear to be well tolerated and are useful as adjunctive therapy in patients with chronic dermatitis. Prolonged use of tar preparations, however, may be associated with the production of folliculitis; and since tars tend to promote photosensitivity, they should be used with some degree of caution in sun-exposed areas. The incidence of this reaction, however, has probably been overstated and is extremely uncommon.

Urea and α-Hydroxy Acids. Urea-containing preparations have a softening and moisturizing effect on the stratum corneum and thus provide a therapeutic effect on dry skin, atopic dermatitis, and the pruritus associated with these disorders. Because of an occasional tendency toward stinging, 10 per cent rather than 20 or 25 per cent urea concentrations are frequently advisable in young children, particularly in those with acute or fissured dermatoses.

Urea may be formulated with topical corticosteroids or with emollient creams or lotions. Some of the presently available urea preparations include Aqua Care cream or lotion (Menley and James) and Ureacin Creme (Pedinol). α-Hydroxy lactic-acid containing preparations such as Aqua Lacten Lotion (Herald), Lacticare or Lacticare-HC Lotion (Stiefel), Lac-Hydrin Lotion (Westwood-Squibb), and Nutraderm 30 (Owen) can also be used in the treatment of dry skin, ichthyosiform dermatoses, and atopic dermatitis. Since they, too, may tend to cause stinging, care should be exercised when they are used in the treatment of young children and patients with atopic dermatitis, particularly those with acute, abraded, or fissured dermatoses.

Antipruritic Agents. For proper management of the eczematous eruptions in atopic dermatitis, it is imperative that pruritus be controlled. Although various antihistamines have been used, their mode of action appears to be related to their sedative action as well as to their antihistaminic qualities. Hydroxyzine (Atarax or Vistaril) has excellent antihistaminic and antipruritic qualities, with less of a tendency to sedation. Benadryl and Phenergan are valuable when sedation is desirable. In addition, topical formulations containing pramoxine (such as Prax or Pramosone [Ferndale] or PrameGel [GenDerm]), or Sarna Foam or Lotion (Stiefel), which contains camphor and menthol, offer an effective topical approach to the management of pruritus. Again it should be noted that in dermatitic or irritated skin, formulations containing camphor, menthol, and/or phenol may cause a temporary stinging sensation.

A variety of other pharmacologic agents have also been suggested in an attempt to control the pruritus and manifestations of atopic dermatitis. These include caffeine, a phosphodiesterase inhibitor used topically in 30 per cent concentrations, oral primrose oil, papaverine hydrochloride, and topical and oral cromoglycate. Although initial studies suggested some degree of success, subsequent trials offer contradictory results.[52–59]

Thymic hormones such as thymopoietin pentapeptide (TP-5, 50 mg subcutaneously three times a week) and thymostimulin (TP-1) that induce maturation of thymocytes and influence T-cell and B-cell differentiation, azathioprine, cyclophosphamide, recombinant interferon gamma-1b (50 μg/m^2, 2 to 3 million units/day), thalidomide, and cyclosporine (4 to 5 mg/kg/day) have also been used for the treatment of individuals with severe recalcitrant forms of atopic dermatitis. Although further clinical trials and evaluation are required, their efficacy, at least in some patients, supports the hypothesis that T-helper cell function plays an important role in the pathogenesis of atopic dermatitis, and short-term use may at times be beneficial in the treatment of resistant forms of atopic dermatitis.[60–62] In addition, ultraviolet radiation (ultraviolet B, a combination of ultraviolet A and ultraviolet B, and PUVA therapy) have been beneficial for patients with long-term recalcitrant forms of the disorder.[63, 64]

Sedatives. For patients unable to sleep despite appropriate topical and antipruritic therapy, chloral hydrate is a valuable sedative and soporific. For children and infants it is available as a syrup that contains 500 mg per teaspoonful. The sedative dose of chloral hydrate for children is 10 to 20 mg/kg/dose, repeated, if necessary, at intervals of 6 to 8 hours.

Systemic Corticosteroids. Appropriate antibiotics are important in the treatment of secondary infection. Systemic corticosteroids, however, should be reserved for only those few extremely severe cases that cannot be controlled by other means. Long-term corticosteroid administration is seldom justified and frequently results in severe side effects. An added problem following the use of systemic corticosteroids is the difficulty in weaning patients from this form of therapy without severe and recurrent exacerbations. Therapy with lubrication, effective antipruritics, and potent topical corticosteroids seldom makes this form of therapy necessary. Proper management, therefore, can usually control atopic dermatitis, even in the most severe cases, without necessitating the use of systemic corticosteroids with their serious side effects, associated difficulties, and complications.

PITYRIASIS ALBA

Pityriasis alba is a common cutaneous disorder characterized by discrete asymptomatic hypopigmented patches on the face, neck, upper trunk, and proximal extremities of children and young adults. Individual lesions vary from 1 cm or more in diameter and have sharply delineated margins and a fine branny scale (Fig. 3–21).

The cause is unknown, but this disorder appears to represent a nonspecific dermatitis (possibly a mild form of atopic dermatitis). Most cases appear following sun exposure and result from a disturbance in pigmentation of the affected areas. This lack of pigment, formerly attributed to a screening effect by the thickened stratum corneum, appears to be related to interference in melanization of the epidermal cells.

Differential diagnosis includes tinea corporis, tinea versicolor, vitiligo, the white macules seen in association with tuberous sclerosis, and postinflammatory hypopigmentation secondary to atopic

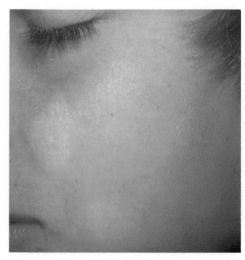

Figure 3–21. Pityriasis alba. Circumscribed scaly hypopigmented lesions are seen on the cheek.

dermatitis, psoriasis, or pityriasis rosea. Topical corticosteroids and lubrication followed by sun exposure appear to diminish the dry skin and fine scaling, allowing repigmentation of involved areas, generally within several weeks.

HYPERIMMUNOGLOBULIN E (HYPER-IgE) AND THE JOB SYNDROME

The hyperimmunoglobulin E syndrome (hyper-IgE syndrome) is a rare primary immunodeficiency disorder characterized by recurrent cutaneous and systemic (often sinopulmonary) infections, chronic dermatitis, and markedly elevated serum IgE levels. Symptoms begin in the first 3 months of life with recurrent infections, an eczematous dermatitis (particularly involving the face and extensor surfaces), or both. With advancing age, patients develop coarse facial features with an irregularly proportioned jaw and cheeks, a broad nasal bridge, and prominent nose (a result of recurrent facial abscesses). They have a lifelong history of severe recurrent streptococcal or staphylococcal infections involving the skin, lungs, joints, and other sites; exceptionally high serum IgE concentrations (usually 10 times, often 100 times, that of normal levels); eosinophilia of the blood and sputum; an intermittent chemotactic defect in circulating neutrophils; and a personal or family history of atopy (often with a pruritic eczematoid dermatitis mimicking but not typical of that seen in patients with atopic dermatitis).[65, 66] Serum levels of IgE greater than 2,000 IU/ml are common but not pathognomonic.

Although the pathogenesis of this disorder remains speculative, reports of familial cases suggest that it occurs in a sporadic manner or as an autosomal dominant disorder with incomplete penetration. IgE antibodies to *Staphylococcus aureus* suggest an impaired regulation of humoral function, and a diminished neutrophil chemotaxis may explain the recurrent bacterial infections seen in individuals with this disorder.

The *Job syndrome* is a term that refers to a subgroup of patients, usually women of Italian descent, who, in addition to displaying the major features of the hyper IgE syndrome, have red hair, fair skin, hyperextensible joints, blue eyes, freckles, atrophic or dystrophic nails, and a tendency to develop huge chronic and recurrent staphylococcal abscesses (cold abscesses) that deform and distort the body contour. The term *Job syndrome* is taken from the biblical story of Job, who is said to have been "smitten with boils from head to toe" and is believed to have suffered from chronic furunculosis. A defective erythema response may explain the lack of redness, heat, or pain ordinarily associated with abscesses (hence the term *cold*) in such patients.

Symptoms of this disorder generally begin in the first year of life with a persistent seborrheic eruption of the scalp, ears, periorbital areas, and inguinal regions. Scalp folliculitis, vesicular eruptions clinically indistinguishable from herpetic lesions, recurrent respiratory tract infections, otitis media, pneumonia, and abscesses of the lung and liver are commonly seen in this disorder. Although the Job syndrome was originally believed to be an autosomal recessive form of chronic granulomatous disease, it currently is believed to be a variant of the hyper-IgE syndrome.[66, 67]

WISKOTT-ALDRICH SYNDROME

The Wiskott-Aldrich syndrome is a rare X-linked recessive disorder seen almost exclusively in young boys, characterized by a recalcitrant eczematous dermatitis, platelet dysfunction, thrombocytopenia, recurrent pyogenic infections, and suppurative otitis media.[68] Affected infants have a deficiency of a glycoprotein (sialophorin) on the surface of lymphocytes and platelets, defects in cell-mediated and humoral immunity, low or absent antibodies to blood group antigens A and B (isohemagglutinins), deficient IgM levels (with compensatory increases in levels IgA and IgE), impaired delayed hypersensitivity, and impaired or absent antibody response to virus infections and bacterial antigens.

The syndrome has its onset from the time of birth to 4 months of age, and its first clinical features usually include petechiae, a purpuric dermatitis or a bleeding episode (usually in the first 6 to 12 months of life), and an eczematoid eruption that resembles atopic dermatitis usually beginning on the scalp, face, buttocks, and antecubital and popliteal fossae. Splenomegaly, hepatomegaly, and cervical adenopathy are present, and affected infants are susceptible to a variety of bacterial, fun-

gal, and virus infections, of which otitis media is the most prominent.

Until recently, death usually occurred early in life, and almost always before the age of 5 to 7 years, from overwhelming infection, hemorrhage, or both. As in other immunoglobulin deficiency states there is a high incidence of lymphoreticular malignancy in children who survive early childhood.

Treatment of the Wiskott-Aldrich syndrome consists of genetic counseling, appropriate topical therapy for the eczematoid eruption, antibiotics, periodic plasma transfusions, or bone marrow transplantation following ablation of the patient's marrow with chemotherapeutic agents to supplement the child's immunologic system. Vigorous antibiotic therapy, plasma and fresh platelet transfusions, and the recent introduction of transfer factor also appear to offer a more optimistic outlook for this severe and previously unresponsive disorder.

LICHEN SIMPLEX CHRONICUS

Lichen simplex chronicus (circumscribed neurodermatitis) is a localized, chronic pruritic disorder characterized by patches of dermatitis that result from repeated itching, scratching, and rubbing of the involved area. Although the etiology of this disorder is unknown, lesions are produced and perpetuated by rubbing and scratching. The pruritus may begin in an area of normal-appearing skin or may be initiated in a preexisting lesion of atopic, seborrheic, or contact dermatitis, lichen planus, or psoriasis.

Lesions of lichen simplex chronicus, rarely seen in young children, generally occur in adolescents or adults (particularly women), with a peak incidence in adults between 30 and 50 years of age. The disorder may develop at any location on the body, but the most common areas of involvement are those that are easily reached and may be scratched unobtrusively (particularly during periods of tension and concentration). These include the nape or sides of the neck, wrists, ankles, and pretibial areas (Fig. 3–22). Other common sites of involvement include the inner aspects of the thighs, vulva, scrotum, and perianal areas.

The clinical features of lichen simplex chronicus include single or multiple oval plaques with a long axis measuring anywhere from 5 to 15 cm in diameter. During the early stages the skin is reddened and slightly edematous and normal markings are somewhat exaggerated. Older lesions are characterized by well-circumscribed patches of dry, thickened, scaly, pruritic hyperpigmented or hypopigmented plaques. At times flat-topped confluent excoriated papules may be seen in the center of lesions.

The diagnosis of lichen simplex chronicus is dependent on the presence of pruritic lichenified plaques in the characteristic sites of predilection. Lesions of tinea corporis may be differentiated by a

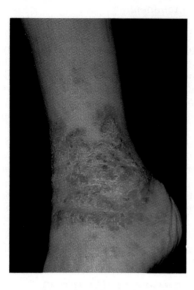

Figure 3–22. Infected lichen simplex chronicus (neurodermatitis).

lack of lichenification, by the presence of a vesicular or scaly border (often with clearing in the center), by demonstration of hyphae on microscopic examination of skin scrapings, and by fungal culture. Psoriatic plaques generally may be differentiated by a characteristic thick, adherent white or silvery scale, their underlying deep red hue, and characteristic areas of involvement. Lesions of atopic dermatitis may be differentiated by history, the presence of atopic stigmata, and a tendency toward involvement in antecubital and popliteal areas.

The histopathologic appearance of lesions of lichen simplex chronicus is that of a chronic dermatitis. It is characterized by hyperkeratosis, areas of parakeratosis, acanthosis, and elongation of the rete ridges. Spongiosis may be present, but vesiculation does not occur. Dermal papillae are broad and elongated, and there is a chronic perivascular inflammatory infiltrate accompanied by fibroblasts and fibrosis in the dermis.

The successful management of lichen simplex chronicus depends on an appreciation of the itch-scratch-itch cycle and the associated scratching and rubbing that accompany and perpetuate this disorder. Topical application of potent corticosteroids, under occlusion if necessary, and the administration of systemic antipruritics (antihistamine or hydroxyzine) will usually induce remission of the pruritus and the eruption within a period of several weeks. Open wet compresses with tepid tap water or Burow's solution will hasten resolution of chronic as well as acutely inflamed lesions. In par-

ticularly stubborn lesions, occlusive dressings and the use of an intralesional corticosteroid (triamcinolone acetonide diluted with isotonic saline or lidocaine to a concentration of 5 mg/ml) may be necessary.

SEBORRHEIC DERMATITIS

Seborrheic dermatitis is a term used to refer to an erythematous, scaly, or crusting eruption that occurs primarily in the so-called seborrheic areas (those with the highest concentration of sebaceous glands), namely the scalp, face, and postauricular, presternal, and intertriginous areas. Although the specific etiology of seborrheic dermatitis remains unknown, it appears to be related to an inflammatory reaction of the skin in constitutionally predisposed individuals. Many attempts have been made to relate infection with *Pityrosporum ovale* (*Malassezia furfur, Malassezia ovalis*) to the etiology of this disorder, and the observation that some cases improve with topical or systemic ketoconazole (Nizoral) suggests that this yeast infection may, at least in some instances, play a primary or secondary role in the pathogenesis of this disorder.[69, 70]

Seborrheic dermatitis is most commonly seen in infants and adolescents. It appears in infancy between the second and tenth weeks of life (usually the third or fourth) and, although it may continue throughout life, it usually clears spontaneously by 8 to 12 months and generally does not recur until the onset of puberty. Infantile seborrheic dermatitis often begins with a noneczematous erythematous scaly dermatitis of the scalp (termed *cradle cap*) or the diaper area and is manifested by thin dry scales or sharply defined round or oval patches covered by thick, yellowish brown greasy crusts (see Figs. 2–11 through 2–13). Although infantile seborrheic dermatitis has many features in common with seborrheic dermatitis of adolescence and adult life, it lacks the presence of follicular lesions and clinically evident seborrhea normally seen in association with seborrheic dermatitis as occurs in older individuals.

Diagnosis. The disorder commonly begins and may be confined to the scalp in infants but may progress and spread downward over the forehead, ears, eyebrows, nose, and back of the head. Erythematous greasy salmon-colored scaly lesions may involve other parts of the body, particularly the intertriginous and flexural areas of the body (see Fig. 3–13), the postauricular areas (see Fig. 3–14), the trunk, umbilicus, anogenital areas, and groin (see Fig. 2–13). Pruritus is slight or absent, and the disorder usually lacks the stigmata generally associated with atopic dermatitis. The prognosis of seborrheic dermatitis, even without treatment, is usually good, and most cases clear spontaneously, usually within several weeks or months. Although infantile seborrheic dermatitis may at times be succeeded by atopic dermatitis such cases may result from a chance occurrence.

To date there is no evidence that these two disorders are constitutionally or genetically related.

The diagnostic features of infantile seborrheic dermatitis are its early onset, lack of pruritus and stigmata of atopy, a greasy yellowish or salmon-colored scale, the generally well-circumscribed nature of the lesions, and its predisposition for the scalp and intertriginous regions. Differentiation of this disorder from Letterer-Siwe disease is predicated on the lack of purpura, hepatosplenomegaly, lymphadenopathy, anemia, thrombocytopenia, and osseous lesions, and, if the diagnosis remains in doubt, histopathologic examination of cutaneous lesions.

The histopathologic picture of seborrheic dermatitis is not diagnostic. The pathologic findings are those of a low-grade inflammatory process, with parakeratosis, moderate acanthosis, some elongation of the rete ridges, and slight intracellular edema and spongiosis. Although the histologic picture has features of both psoriasis and chronic dermatitis, the presence of spongiosis generally is lacking in lesions of psoriasis, thus helping in the histopathologic differentiation of these two disorders.

In infants, when the erythema and scaling of seborrheic dermatitis becomes severe, generalized, and exfoliative, the diagnosis of *Leiner's disease* must be considered. Infantile seborrheic dermatitis may be differentiated from Leiner's disease by a lack of constitutional findings (diarrhea, fever, inanition), alopecia, a lack of associated infections, and the relatively benign nature of seborrheic dermatitis (see Leiner's Disease in Chapter 2 and Fig. 2–14).

Between puberty and middle age, seborrheic dermatitis may appear on the scalp as a dry fine flaky desquamation commonly known as pityriasis sicca or dandruff. This disorder is an extreme form of normal desquamation in which scales of the scalp become abundant and visible. Erythema and scaling of various degrees may also involve the supraorbital areas between the eyebrows and above the bridge of the nose, nasolabial crease, lips, pinna, retroauricular areas, and aural canal.

Occasionally a patient may have an eruption that has clinical features of both seborrheic dermatitis and psoriasis. Such eruptions may be termed *seborrhiasis* or *sebopsoriasis*. Lesions of seborrheic dermatitis can be differentiated from those of psoriasis by a lack of the characteristic vivid red hue, micaceous scale, a predisposition toward flexural rather than extensor aspects of the extremities, and the fact that lesions of seborrhea generally tend to remain within the confines of the hairline. Lesions of psoriasis (or seborrhiasis) frequently extend beyond the hairline and, in general, are more resistant to standard antiseborrheic therapy.

Blepharitis is a form of seborrheic dermatitis in which the eyelid margins are red and covered with small white scales. Seborrheic dermatitis may also involve the sideburns, beard, and mustache areas, with diffuse redness, greasy scaling, and pustulation. The severity and course of seborrheic eruptions of the eyelids and bearded areas are variable and have a tendency to chronicity and recurrence.

Treatment. The therapy for seborrheic dermatitis depends on the nature, severity, and location of the disorder. If one concentrates on clearing the scalp lesions in infantile seborrheic dermatitis, the remainder of the eruption usually responds rapidly to medium- to low-potency topical corticosteroid preparations. The scalp should be treated with an antiseborrheic shampoo. Those containing sulfur or salicylic acid, or both, are generally satisfactory. If the scale is extremely thick and adherent, it can be loosened by warmed mineral oil massaged into the scalp or by the use of P and S Liquid (Baker/Cummins). When used, P and S Liquid should be allowed to remain on the scalp for 8 to 12 hours, followed by scrubbing with the fingers or a soft brush in an effort to loosen the scales prior to an appropriate shampoo. In stubborn cases, a topical corticosteroid lotion, with or without 3 to 5 per cent sulfur precipitate or salicyclic acid, or both, may be used on the scalp one or three times daily.

Adolescents with seborrhea of the scalp may use similar antiseborrheic shampoos. Those with more stubborn involvement may use shampoos containing zinc pyrithione such as Head and Shoulders, DHS Zinc, Zincon, or X Seb Shampoo; selenium sulfide (Exsel or Selsun); corticosteroids (FS Shampoo); tar shampoos; or, if believed to be associated or related to infection with *Pityrosporum ovale*, ketoconazole (Nizoral 2 per cent Shampoo). For patients with associated erythema or pruritus, topical corticosteroid lotions or sprays may be used; and for individuals with associated pruritus, a topical lotion combining fluocinolone and pramoxine (Derma-Smoothe/FS) can be beneficial.

Blepharitis may be managed by warm water compresses, gentle cleansing with a dilute solution of a nonirritating or baby shampoo, mechanical removal of scales when necessary, and topical sulfacetamide ointment (Sulamyd) or sulfacetamide with 0.5 per cent prednisolone (Metimyd). Corticosteroids on the eyelids, or eyelid margins, however, should be used with caution.

Complications. Seborrheic dermatitis of the intertriginous or diaper areas occasionally may be complicated by secondary candidal or bacterial infection. In such instances, preparations containing anticandidal or antibacterial agents, or both, are generally helpful. For patients refractory to topical treatment or for those with extensive secondary bacterial infection (*infectious eczematoid dermatitis*, Fig. 3–23), bacterial cultures and appropriate systemic antibiotics are frequently necessary.

INTERTRIGO

Intertrigo is a superficial inflammatory dermatitis that occurs in areas where the skin is in apposition (see Fig. 3–13). As a result of friction, heat,

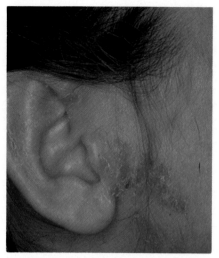

Figure 3–23. Infectious eczematoid dermatitis of the preauricular area. The clinical picture is that of impetigo associated with and spreading beyond the preceding eczematous or seborrheic lesions.

and moisture, the affected areas become erythematous, macerated, and secondarily infected by bacteria or fungi.

Treatment is directed toward elimination of the macerated skin. Open wet compresses, dusting powders (ZeaSorb [Stiefel]), topical corticosteroid lotions, and, when indicated, appropriate antibiotics or fungicidal agents may be used.

POMPHOLYX

Pompholyx (dyshidrotic eczema) is a term used to describe a nonspecific acute recurrent or chronic eczematous eruption of the palms, soles, and lateral aspects of the fingers. Of unknown etiology, it is characterized by deep-seated vesicles in various inflammatory stages, hyperhidrosis, and, at times, an associated burning or itching. The distribution of lesions generally is bilateral and somewhat symmetrical. Attacks usually last a few weeks but, because of frequent relapses, may persist for longer periods of time.

Although the cause of dyshidrotic eczema is unknown, it occurs chiefly in nervous individuals and, in many instances, emotional stress appears to be a provocative factor. Attacks of pompholyx are characterized by the sudden appearance of crops of clear "sago-grain"–like vesicles. The contents are commonly clear or colorless; occasionally they may become straw colored or purulent. Vesicles rapidly become confluent and, at times, may present as large bullae.

When unilateral or only affecting one area of the hands, pompholyx may be confused with contact dermatitis. "Id" reactions, pustular psoriasis, and primary fungal infections must be considered in the differential diagnosis of this disorder. The true diagnosis can be differentiated, however, on the basis of fungal culture and histopathologic examination of lesions. Histologic examination of biopsied lesions reveals intraepidermal vesicles with balloon cells, usually little or no inflammatory changes, and varying degrees of spongiosis.

The natural course of pompholyx is one of frequent recurrence (often several times a year). Although not a disorder of eccrine glands, per se, the use of 20 per cent topical aluminum chloride, available as Drysol (Persōn and Covey) is at times helpful in the control of this disorder. Open wet compresses tend to macerate and open the vesicles, and applications of topical corticosteroid creams, although not curative, help to relieve the manifestations of this disorder. When stress or nervousness appears to be a factor, sedative or mild tranquilizing agents may be helpful and, when infection is present, antibiotics may be administered topically or systemically.

LICHEN STRIATUS

Lichen striatus is a self-limiting, usually unilateral, linear dermatitis of unknown origin that usually occurs in children. It consists of discrete and confluent, minute, slightly raised lichenoid papules that evolve suddenly, usually on an extremity, but occasionally may involve the face, neck, trunk, or buttocks. It may occur early in infancy, generally affects children between the ages of 5 and 10 years, and, on occasion, has been reported in older individuals.

Girls appear to be affected two to three times as frequently as boys. The eruption is asymptomatic, reaches its maximum extent within several days to a few weeks, and generally regresses spontaneously within 3 months to 1 year, and occasionally longer. Seen primarily along Blaschko's lines, the involved area varies from several millimeters to 1 or 2 cm in width and is characterized by a linear band of small flat-topped pink or flesh-colored papules, occasionally surmounted by a fine silvery scale (Fig. 3–24). In dark-skinned or tanned individuals the eruption may appear as a scaly or papular band-like area of hypopigmentation (Fig. 3–25). Although the band is usually continuous, it may occasionally be interrupted by or interspersed with coalescent plaques several centimeters in diameter along the area of linear configuration.

The differential diagnosis of lichen striatus is not difficult if the disorder is kept in mind. It may be recognized by its highly characteristic linear appearance. The differential diagnosis includes nevus unius lateris, linear lichen planus, psoriasis, tinea corporis, and verruca plana. When the diagnosis remains in doubt, histopathologic examination of a cutaneous biopsy specimen will help exclude other possible linear eruptions.

The histologic changes of lichen striatus are sim-

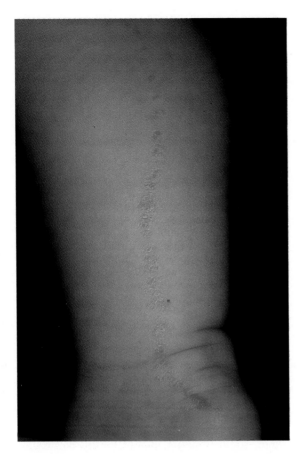

Figure 3–24. Lichen striatus. A self-limiting, usually unilateral linear dermatitis generally seen on the extremities of children.

ilar to those of a chronic dermatitis. The primary feature of this disorder is a dense, usually perivascular, but occasionally band-like, lymphohistocytic infiltrate of the dermis. The epidermis may show slight invasion by lymphocytes, with focal areas of acanthosis, parakeratosis, and spongiosis, and occasionally dyskeratotic cells resembling the grains and corps ronds of Darier's disease may be seen in the granular layer.

Lichen striatus usually resolves spontaneously within 3 to 12 months, but occasionally lasts longer (sometimes 1 or 2 years), and often leaves an area of hypopigmentation that also disappears. Although therapy is not necessary, for those who for cosmetic reasons or otherwise prefer treatment, corticosteroids applied topically, alone or under occlusion, or injected intralesionally may hasten resolution.

FRICTIONAL LICHENOID DERMATITIS

Frictional lichenoid dermatitis (frictional lichenoid eruption, juvenile papular dermatitis, re-

current summertime pityriasis of the elbows and knees) is a recurring cutaneous disorder affecting children, especially boys, between 4 and 12 years of age. Most cases are seen in the spring and summer when outdoor activities are common, and many cases have been associated with playing in sandboxes (sandbox dermatitis). The eruption is characterized by aggregates of discrete lichenoid papules, 1 or 2 mm in diameter, which occur primarily on the elbows, knees, and backs of the hands of children in whom such areas are subject to minor frictional trauma without protection of clothing (Fig. 3–26). Lesions may be hypopigmented, and pruritus is occasionally but not necessarily present. Although its etiology is unknown, it is believed to be related to frictional trauma and occurs in children with a predisposition to atopy.[71-73]

Histopathologic changes are nonspecific and include hyperkeratosis, a moderate degree of acanthosis, and areas of lymphocytic infiltration in the upper dermis. The differential diagnosis of this disorder includes psoriasis and the Gianotti-Crosti syndrome (a disorder of young children characterized by clustered flesh-colored lichenoid papules, 1 to 5 mm in diameter, on the legs, thighs, buttocks, extensor aspects of the arms and, finally, the face, which appears to represent a host response to a variety of infectious agents, and generally resolves spontaneously within 6 weeks) (Fig. 3–27).

The management of frictional lichenoid dermatitis includes avoidance of frictional trauma to the

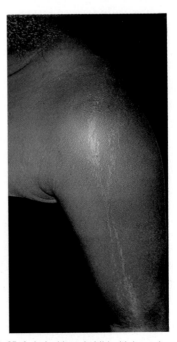

Figure 3–25. A dark-skinned child with hypopigmented linear papular lesions of lichen striatus.

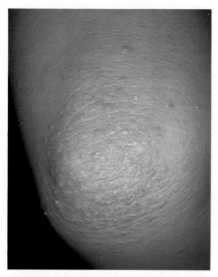

Figure 3–26. Frictional lichenoid dermatitis. Aggregates of lichenoid papules occur primarily on the elbows, knees, knuckles, and backs of the hands of children.

involved areas (as might occur with leaning on elbows and knees) and the use of topical corticosteroids and lubricating creams, with or without the addition of 10 to 20 per cent urea.

NUMMULAR ECZEMA

Nummular eczema is a cutaneous eruption characterized by discoid or coin-shaped plaques of eczema. The name is derived from the Latin word *nummulus*, which refers to its coin-like size and configuration.

Lesions of nummular eczema are composed of minute papules and vesicles, which enlarge by peripheral extension to form discrete, round or oval, erythematous, often lichenified and hyperpigmented plaques varying from 1 cm or more in diameter (see Fig. 3–15). They usually occur on the extensor surfaces of the hands, arms, and legs as single or multiple lesions on dry or asteatotic skin. Pruritus is variable. Occasionally the face and trunk may be involved.

The specific etiology of this disorder is unknown; however, it seems to appear in a cold or dry environment and is aggravated by excessive bathing and local irritants such as wool or harsh or drying soaps. There have been conflicting reports in the literature regarding the association of nummular eczema with atopic dermatitis. This relationship has been refuted by a lack of increase in the incidence of atopy and relatively normal IgE levels in patients with this eruption. Nummular eczema is a scaly dermatosis that appears related to dry skin rather than to atopy. Since pathogenic staphylococci have been cultured from lesions of nummular eczema and since, at times, the disease appears to improve with antibiotic administration, it has been suggested that microorganisms may contribute to the pathogenesis and persistence of this disorder.

Nummular eczema must be differentiated from allergic contact dermatitis, atopic dermatitis, psoriasis, and superficial dermatophyte infections of the skin. This disorder is characterized by pinpoint vesicles and generally shows the histologic picture of a subacute dermatitis with acanthosis and scattered intradermal vesicles at various levels of the epidermis surrounded by spongiosis.

Effective therapy depends on limited baths, frequent lubrication, and potent topical corticosteroids, preferably in an ointment base or under occlusion (assuming, of course, that associated secondary infection is controlled).

WINTER ECZEMA

Winter eczema (eczema hiemalis), also known as asteatotic eczema, eczema craquelée, or xerotic eczema, is a subacute eczematous dermatitis charac-

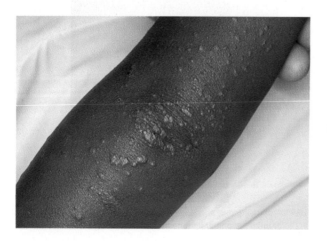

Figure 3–27. Gianotti-Crosti disease. Papular acrodermatitis of childhood.

terized by pruritic scaly erythematous patches, usually associated with dryness and dehydration (asteatosis) of the epidermis. Generally seen on the extremities and occasionally on the trunk, these changes are most frequent during winter when the humidity is low, particularly in older individuals and adolescents who bathe or shower frequently with harsh or drying soaps. Frequent bathing with incomplete drying and resultant evaporation of moisture causes dehydration of the epidermis, with redness, scaling, and fine cracking that may resemble cracked porcelain (hence the term *eczema craquelée*).

The diagnosis of winter eczema is established by the characteristic eczematous, occasionally fissured, patches of dermatitis overlying dry (xerotic) skin in individuals with a history of frequent bathing or showering and exposure to low temperatures and low humidity.

The treatment of winter eczema is centered around the maintenance of proper hydration of the stratum corneum and is dependent on the routine use of emollients or lubricating creams or lotions, limitation of bathing (with mild soaps such as Dove or Neutrogena), the use of humidifiers when feasible, and topical therapy with corticosteroids (preferably those in an ointment base) for individual lesions.

INFECTIOUS ECZEMATOID DERMATITIS

Infectious eczematoid dermatitis is a term used to describe a distinct clinical form of dermatitis in which secondary bacterial infection is superimposed on lesions of atopic, nummular, or seborrheic dermatitis (see Fig. 3–23). In this disorder the dermatitis extends from preceding lesions and is characterized by circumscribed eczematous plaques, with vesicles, pustules, exudation, and/or crusting on an erythematous base. Coagulase-positive *Staphylococcus aureus* is the organism most frequently associated with this disorder.

Infectious eczematoid dermatitis is best managed by appropriate systemic antibiotics based on bacterial culture and sensitivities, open wet dressings, and topical application of corticosteroids. In cases that are not severe, topical antibiotics and topical corticosteroids without systemic antibiotics may be adequate. When systemic antibiotics are used, the concomitant use of topical antibiotics is generally not necessary.

FIXED DRUG ERUPTION

Fixed drug eruption is a term used to describe a sharply localized, circumscribed round or oval dermatitis that characteristically recurs in the same site or sites each time the offending drug is administered. Lesions are solitary at first, but with repeated attacks new lesions usually appear and ex-

isting lesions may tend to increase in size. The lesions tend to be erythematous and dusky at their onset with well-defined borders. At times they may become bullous, with subsequent desquamation or crusting and a residual hyperpigmentation that may persist for months (Fig. 3–28).

The mechanism of the production of fixed drug eruptions remains unknown. Phenolphthalein is the most common of the long list of drugs capable of causing this disorder. Other causative preparations include barbiturates, penicillin, tetracycline, erythromycin, trimethoprim, streptomycin, sulfonamides, antipyrine, quinine and its derivatives, salicylates, potassium iodide, metronidazole (Flagyl), pseudoephedrine hydrochloride (an agent widely used in cold remedies and nasal decongestants), tetrahydrozoline (an imidazole derivative used in eyedrops for the vasoconstriction of conjunctival vessels), quinacrine (Atabrine), emetine (Ipecac), gold salts, phenylbutazone, acetaminophen, chlordiazepoxide (Librium), phenytoin (Dilantin), and various food substitutes and flavorings.[74, 75]

In the early stages of fixed drug eruption, histopathologic examination of lesions may reveal subepidermal bullae with degeneration of the detached portion of the epidermis (not unlike the picture seen in erythema multiforme). In the late stages, melanin may be seen within macrophages in the upper dermis, and there is an increase in the

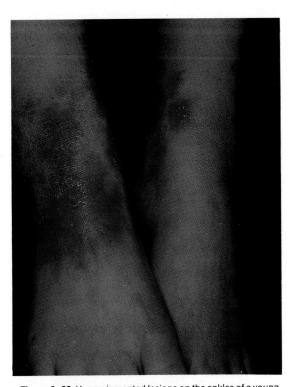

Figure 3–28. Hyperpigmented lesions on the ankles of a young woman with a fixed drug eruption.

amount of melanin in the basal layers of the epidermis.

CONTACT DERMATITIS

Contact dermatitis may be defined as an eczematous eruption produced either by local exposure to a primary irritating substance or by an acquired allergic response to a sensitizing substance (Fig. 3–29). When the dermatitis is due to a nonallergic reaction of the skin, it is termed an *irritant contact dermatitis;* when a manifestation of delayed hypersensitivity to a contact allergen, it is termed *allergic contact dermatitis.* An eczematous allergen is defined as a substance that is not primarily irritating on a first exposure, but with repeated exposure causes an allergic sensitization of the delayed type. A primary eczematous irritant, on the other hand, may be defined as a substance that produces an eczematous response on the basis of irritation rather than by immunologic means.

Primary Irritant Dermatitis

The skin in infancy is thin and highly vascularized, reddens quickly when irritated, and appears to be more resistant to contact sensitization than that of older children and adults. Common substances that produce primary irritant dermatitis include harsh soaps, bleaches, detergents, solvents, acids (Fig. 3–30), alkalis, fiberglass particles, baby oils containing antiseptics such as oxy-

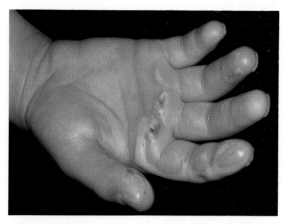

Figure 3–30. Primary irritant dermatitis due to hydrochloric acid with blistering.

quinoline sulfate, bubble baths, certain foods, saliva, talcum particles, urine, feces, and intestinal secretions. The only variation in the severity of the dermatitis from person to person, or from time to time in the same person, is a result of the condition of the skin at the time of exposure, the strength of the irritant, the location of the eruption, the cumulative effect of repeated exposures to the irritating substance, and local factors such as perspiration, maceration, and occlusion.[76]

In children, the lips and adjacent skin frequently become dry and, as a result of a licking habit, inflamed and irritated (lip-licker's dermatitis) (Fig. 3–31). In addition, saliva frequently becomes trapped between the thumb and mouth of thumb-suckers, and a similar reaction is commonly seen in toddlers who continue to use pacifiers for long periods of time. Occlusive pastes such as zinc oxide ointment or 1–2–3 paste (see Chapter 2, Diaper Dermatitis), moisturizing creams, and low- to medium-potency topical corticosteroid creams or ointments are helpful in the management of this disorder.

Allergic Contact Dermatitis

The incidence of allergic contact dermatitis in children is less (approximately one eighth) than that seen in adults, with figures of 1.5 per cent in the former as compared with 13 per cent in older age groups. The process responsible for contact sensitization appears to be deficient at birth and matures more slowly than other processes of resistance and immunity such as phagocytosis and circulating antibody formation.

Although infants younger than the age of 1 year have a depressed ability to react to allergens, newborns and infants have demonstrated allergic contact dermatitis from vinyl identification bands, nickel in earrings and umbilical cord clips, neomycin, ethylenediamine, thimerosal (Merthiolate), merbromin (Mercurochrome), balsam of Peru (a

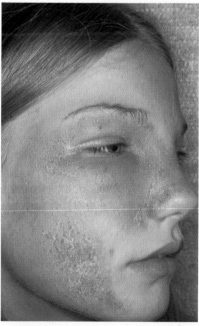

Figure 3–29. Contact dermatitis caused by exposure to poison ivy (*Rhus* dermatitis).

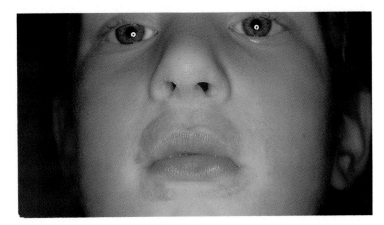

Figure 3–31. Lip-licker's dermatitis.

product in diaper preparations such as Balmex [Macsil]), antioxidants such as mercaptobenzothiazole and tetramethylthiuram (Fig. 3–32), plasticizers or softeners in rubber products, and poison ivy. The decreased reactivity of infant skin to potential allergens, although not completely understood, appears to be related to the decreased exposure of infants and young children to potential sensitizing allergens, a decreased function of cell-mediated immune mechanisms in this age group, and the fact that the process responsible for contact sensitization matures more slowly than other mechanisms of resistance and immunity. Although

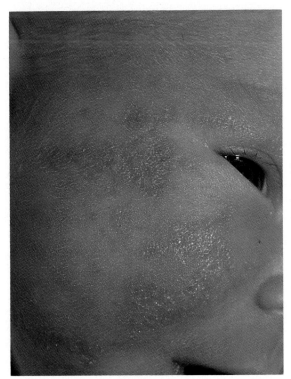

Figure 3–32. Contact dermatitis from an oxygen face mask in a newborn. (Courtesy of William Weston, M.D.)

sensitivity to allergic contact allergens is less common in childhood, it still manages to account for up to 20 per cent of all dermatitis in childhood.[76–78]

The mechanism of sensitization, although not well understood, is probably under genetic control and represents a type IV immunologic (delayed hypersensitivity or cell-mediated) reaction in which sensitized tissue, lymphocytes, and Langerhans cells act as mediators.[79]

Allergic contact dermatitis may develop within 7 to 10 days following initial exposure to a sensitizing substance, or exposure may continue for months or even years before manifestations of allergy develop. Once the area has become sensitized, however, reexposure to the offending allergen may result in an acute dermatitis within a relatively brief period (generally 8 to 12 hours following exposure to the sensitizing allergen).

The diagnosis of allergic contact dermatitis is made on the appearance and distribution of skin lesions, aided, when possible, by a history of contact with an appropriate allergen. Acute eczematous lesions are characterized by an intense erythema accompanied by edema, papules, vesiculation (sometimes bullae), oozing, and a sharp line of demarcation between the involved and normal skin (Figs. 3–33 through 3–35). In the subacute phase, vesiculation is less pronounced and is mixed with crusting, scaling, and thickening of the skin. Chronic lesions, conversely, are characterized by lichenification, fissuring, scaling, and little or no vesiculation.

Clinically, the distribution of lesions is characterized by the mode of sensitization. In the infant and young child, circumoral dermatitis may appear as a response to a primary irritant, or as an allergic contact dermatitis from foods such as tomatoes, oranges, carrots, shrimp, other seafoods, or spinach. Here the dermatitis is caused by direct contact with the skin, not from ingestion of the offending food substances. This may be aggravated by regurgitation of food particles, dribbling of saliva, and rubbing of the involved areas.

The histopathologic picture of eczematous allergic contact dermatitis is generally not pathogno-

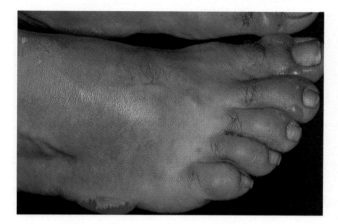

Figure 3–33. Contact dermatitis due to the dye in a sandal made of the hide of the water buffalo (water buffalo sandal dermatitis).

monic of this condition and seldom permits differentiation from primary irritant dermatitis or other forms of eczema. The histologic description for acute, subacute, and chronic dermatitis, therefore, applies in general to both forms of contact dermatitis.

PATCH TESTING

The patch test, a valuable aid in the diagnosis of contact skin sensitivity in older children and adults, is frequently unreliable in children younger than the age of 1 year and (as a consequence of the fact that normal adult reactivity is not reached until 7 to 8 years of age) often difficult to interpret in children younger than the age of 8 years. Although it has been suggested that except for nickel, formaldehyde, and dichromate children can generally be tested with concentrations similar to those used in adults, Fisher recommends that one half of the concentration be used in the patch testing of children younger than 5 years of age.[76, 80]

When patch testing is performed, patches should be placed on grossly normal, nonhairy skin. Patch testing should be deferred in the presence of extensive active dermatitis, at which time the entire skin may be irritated, false-positive reactions may be obtained, and a strongly positive patch-test reaction may cause acute exacerbation of the dermatitis. The systemic administration of cortico-

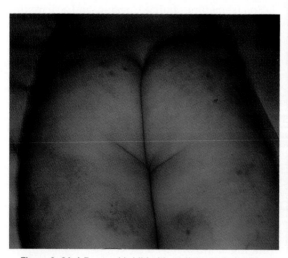

Figure 3–34. A 7-year-old child with a toilet seat–induced contact dermatitis.

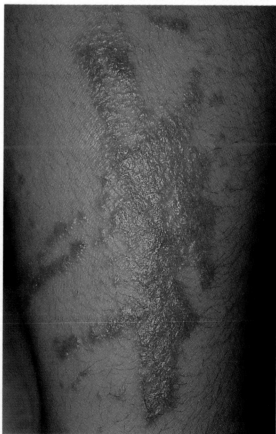

Figure 3–35. A characteristic linear vesicular eruption on the forearm of a young man with poison ivy (*Rhus*) dermatitis.

steroids (in contrast to antihistamines) is not a contraindication to patch testing and, although patch testing of patients while they are on corticosteroid therapy might tend to mask weak patch test responses (which are of little clinical significance), it generally will not mask or alter significant reactions to allergens applied in standard concentrations.

Patch tests generally should be kept in place for 48 hours, and a reading can be made after an interval of 20 to 60 minutes following removal of the patch. This brief time interval is required to allow the skin to recover from the effects of pressure, which may produce mild transient erythema or a temporary blanching effect, resulting in false reactions. Doubtful reactions should be read again after a period of 24 hours. Unless testing for weak sensitizers (such as fabrics or cosmetics), a doubtful reaction (faint macular erythema only) is usually of no significance. A 1 plus (1+) reaction is characterized by erythema, infiltration, and possibly papules. The addition of vesicles to this response indicates a 2 plus (2+) reaction, and a bullous reaction is read as 3 plus (3+).

Occasionally, positive reactions may have no clinical significance. Similarly, the offending material may not give rise to a positive reaction at the site of the test but may show a positive test if carried out on an area of skin closer to the point of the previously existing dermatitis. The value of patch tests is corroborative and should be used only as a guide in an attempt to confirm a suspected allergen. Furthermore, scratch and intracutaneous tests are not indicated in contact dermatitis, since this condition is neither mediated by nor associated with skin-sensitizing antibodies.

POISON IVY (RHUS DERMATITIS)

The major sources of contact allergy in children are metals, shoes, preservatives or fragrances used in cosmetics and topical medications, and plants. In the United States, poison ivy, poison oak, and poison sumac produce more cases of allergic contact dermatitis than all other contactants combined. The plants causing poison ivy dermatitis are included under the botanical term *Rhus*. Poison ivy and poison oak are the principal causes of *Rhus* dermatitis in the United States.

The poison ivy plant, with its characteristic three leaflets more or less notched at the edge, grows luxuriantly as a tall shrub or woody rope-like vine in vacant lots, among grasses, and on trees or fences throughout all sections of the United States except the extreme southwest. Poison sumac grows as a shrub or tree, never as a vine. It has 7 to 13 leaflets (arranged in pairs along a central stem) with a single leaflet at the end, is relatively uncommon, grows less abundantly, and is found only in woody or swampy areas primarily east of the Mississippi River. Poison oak, conversely, grows as an upright shrub, is most prominent on the west coast,

and is not a problem in the eastern United States. Although *Rhus* dermatitis is more common in the summer, the eruption may occur at any time of year by direct contact with the sensitizing allergen from the leaves, roots, or twigs of plants.

No matter which of the *Rhus* plants produces the eruption there is no difference in the antigen or clinical appearance of the dermatitis. Furthermore, since the *Rhus* group belongs to the family of plants known as Anacardiaceae, cross-reactions may occur with chemicals and nuts from related plants, namely furniture lacquer derived from the Japanese lacquer tree, oil from the shell of the cashew or Brazil nut, the fruit pulp of the gingko tree (a large ornamental tree of China and Japan), the rind of the mango, and the marking nut tree of India, from which a black "ink" used to mark wearing apparel is produced. The allergic contact dermatitis to this ink is termed *dhobi itch*.

Pathogenesis. The eruption produced by poison ivy and related plants is a delayed contact hypersensitivity reaction to an oleoresin (urushiol) of which the active sensitizing ingredient is pentadecylcatechol. It is characterized by itching, redness, papules, vesicles, and bullae (see Fig. 3–29). A linear distribution, the Koebner reaction, with an irregular spotty distribution is highly characteristic of the eruption (see Fig. 3–35). When contact is indirect, such as from a pet that has the oleoresin on its fur, the dermatitis is often diffuse, thus making the diagnosis more difficult unless the true nature of exposure is suspected. In the fall, when brush and leaves are burned, it must be remembered that the sensitizing oil may be vaporized and transmitted by smoke to exposed cutaneous surfaces.

Rhus dermatitis usually appears, in susceptible individuals, within 1 to 3 days after contact with the sensitizing oleoresin; in highly sensitive individuals it may occur within 8 hours of exposure. Such temporal differences are probably due to the degree of exposure, individual susceptibility, and regional variation in cutaneous reactivity.

About 70 per cent of the population of the United States would acquire *Rhus* dermatitis if exposed to the plants or the sensitizing oleoresin contained in its leaves, stems, and roots. The result is an acute eczematous eruption, which, barring complications or reexposure to the offending allergen, persists for a variable period of 1 to 3 weeks. In addition, since the sap from plants of the *Toxicodedron* species turns black when exposed to dry surfaces and skin, it is not unusual to see dramatic black lacquer- or enamel-like deposits on the skin of individuals exposed to poison ivy or other urushiol-containing plants.[81]

Management. The best prophylaxis, as with any type of allergic contact dermatitis, is complete avoidance of the offending allergen. Patients should be instructed in how to recognize and avoid members of the poison *Rhus* group. Unfortunately, no topical measure is totally effective in the prevention of poison ivy dermatitis. When poison ivy is present in the garden or children's play areas, chemical destruction or physical removal is indicated.

In an effort to minimize the degree of dermatitis, individuals with known exposure should wash thoroughly as rapidly as possible so that removal of the oil is accomplished, preferably within 5 to 10 minutes of exposure. If the oleoresin is not carefully removed shortly after exposure, the allergen may be transmitted by the fingers to other parts of the body (particularly the face, forearms, or male genitalia). Contrary to popular belief, however, the fluid content of vesicles and bullae is not contagious and does not produce new lesions. Thus, unless the sensitizing antigen is still on the skin, the disorder is neither autoinoculable nor contagious from one person to another.

Complete change of clothing is advisable, and, whenever possible, contaminated shoes and clothing should be washed with soap and water or cold water mixed with alcohol. This helps remove the urushiol, which dries and remains antigenic indefinitely unless washed off within a few minutes after exposure.[76] Harsh soaps and vigorous scrubbing offer no advantage over simple soaking and cool water. Thorough washing may not prevent a severe dermatitis in highly sensitive persons. It may, however, reduce the reaction and prevent spread of the oleoresin. When early washing is not feasible, it is worthwhile to wash at the first opportunity in an effort to remove any oleoresin remaining on the skin or clothing and thus prevent its transfer to other parts of the body.

In the management of mild *Rhus* dermatitis, treatment with an antipruritic "shake" lotion such as calamine lotion is helpful. Topical preparations containing potential sensitizers such as antihistamines[82] or benzocaine and zirconium, however, should be avoided. As in other acute eczematous eruptions, cool compresses with plain tap water or Burow's solution are soothing, help remove crusts, and relieve pruritus. Administration of potent topical corticosteroids and systemic use of antihistamines and antipruritic agents are helpful. Antihistamines, however, are used primarily for their antipruritic rather than antihistaminic effect, and topical corticosteroids are only partially effective in the acute stages of *Rhus* dermatitis. Thus, they help suppress the pruritic manifestations and give temporary relief but do little to hasten involution of individual lesions. Aerosol-type sprays, gels, or lotions are often helpful. Because they cover the acutely involved areas more easily and have a drying tendency, they appear to be beneficial in the management of acute weeping and bullous lesions. Aseptic aspiration of large vesicles or bullae is frequently helpful and assists in the relief of discomforting symptoms associated with such lesions.

In severe and incapacitating cases of *Rhus* dermatitis, short-term systemic corticosteroid treatment may be indicated. Systemic corticosteroid therapy may be initiated with dosages in the range of 20 to 30 mg of prednisone or its equivalent with gradually tapering dosages over a period of 2 to 3 weeks. Premature termination of systemic corticosteroids may result in a rapid rebound, with return of the dermatitis to its original intensity. The use of systemic corticosteroids in injectable form should be discouraged, however, since temporary atrophy may occur and the dosage can be neither modified nor terminated in the event of adverse reaction or need for change in therapy (Fig. 3–36).

Desensitization to the oleoresin of poison ivy by systemic administration of *Rhus* antigen is unreliable, is frequently disappointing, and should be reserved only for extremely sensitive individuals who cannot avoid repeated exposure to the antigen. Standardization of material is difficult, and systemic reactions are not uncommon with the use of hyposensitization procedures. For those cases in which hyposensitization is deemed advisable, a reliable active oleoresin is supplied by Hollister-Stier Laboratories. Although heretofore a satisfactory barrier cream has not been available to prevent *Rhus* dermatitis, Ivy Shield (Interpro), Hollister Moisture Barrier, Hydropil, and a polyamine salt of a linoleic acid dimer (Stoko-Gard Outdoor Cream; available from Stockhausen, Inc., Greensboro, NC) offer some degree of protection.[83, 84]

HOUSE PLANT AND FLOWER DERMATITIS

Common flowers and house and garden plants present a common source for contact dermatitis in adults as well as children. Of the many plants and flowers capable of causing dermatitis, chrysanthemums, orchids, tulips, tulip bulbs, alstroemeria (Peruvian lilies), asters, various types of daisies, a variety of primrose (*Primula obconica*), and *Euphorbia myrsinites* (a garden plant referred to as creeping spurge or donkey tail) appear to be among the most frequent offenders.[85–87] Prolonged and repeated contact, however, is necessary, and florists, horticulturists, and gardeners rather than

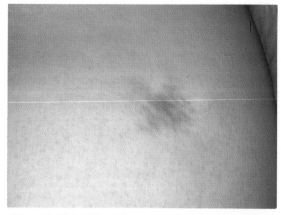

Figure 3–36. Local atrophy of buttock due to intramuscular corticosteroid injection (most cases fortunately resolved spontaneously, generally within a period of 6 to 14 months).

children appear to be the most frequently affected by this form of sensitization.

Among the common house plants, philodendrons, geraniums, poinsettias, and diffenbachia are frequent causes of contact dermatitis. In this form of contact dermatitis the hands and arms are involved (since exposure to the plant generally takes place when the patient washes, oils, or plucks the leaves).

Contact dermatitis may also be caused by handling other plants and flowers, namely the buttercup, foxglove, lilac, lady slipper, magnolia, daffodil, and narcissus. In addition, capsicum, a common condiment used as a component of tear gas, in antimugger aerosol sprays, on nipples of women desiring to terminate nursing, on nails of individuals to discourage nail biting, in cases of child abuse, and as a cause of "Hunan hand syndrome" (a dermatitis predominantly seen in individuals who process chili peppers and persons living along the Mexican border of the United States) may also cause dermatitis. Treatment of the contact dermatitis to plants and flowers is similar to that outlined for *Rhus* dermatitis.

POLLEN DERMATITIS

Dermatitis caused by plant pollens, particularly ragweed, is a fairly common cause of contact dermatitis in children as well as adults. The ragweed pollens contain two antigens: (1) an aqueous protein fraction that may produce asthma, hay fever, and occasionally an atopic-type dermatitis and (2) an oleoresin capable of producing sensitization and eczematous contact dermatitis.

Air-borne pollen dermatitis generally involves the exposed surfaces of the face, neck, arms, legs, and "V" area of the chest. Although pollen dermatitis may at times resemble a photosensitivity dermatitis due to plants, drugs, or topical preparations, the lines of demarcation produced by pollen contact dermatitis are not as sharp as those seen in eruptions due to photosensitivity. This lack of sharp delineation in pollen dermatitis is due to the fact that pollen grains often get inside the clothing, thus extending the area of dermatitis to include the upper chest, shoulders, and upper back.

CLOTHING DERMATITIS

Although nonspecific irritation from fabrics, rubber, dyes, and cleaning solutions is not uncommon, eczematoid contact dermatitis due to true sensitization to fabrics is rarely seen in childhood. Dermatitis from cotton is virtually nonexistent (except for the fact that the sizing used in cotton to stiffen or glaze the material occasionally may sensitize the skin and produce a dermatitis). Silk is an occasional sensitizer, and wool is usually a primary irritant rather than a true contact sensitizer. In recent years, primarily as a result of formaldehyde or formaldehyde resins used in their manufacture, "drip-dry" and crease-resistant fabrics have been responsible for many cases of contact dermatitis. This type of dermatitis is more likely to occur in individuals whose clothes are tight-fitting and close to the skin. The inner thighs and popliteal fossae are particularly susceptible to formaldehyde contact sensitivity.

Instances of irritation or dermatitis attributable to dyes in wearing apparel are remarkably few. The incidence of dermatitis from a dye is generally increased, however, if the dye "bleeds" readily from the fabric. Certain individuals tolerate light colors in clothing but may, on occasion, acquire a dermatitis from dark clothing, particularly that dyed black or dark blue (since the concentration of dyes in dark clothing is much higher than that of dyes in light-colored clothing, and dark colors tend to "bleed" more readily than dyes of lighter hue). Whenever washable garments are suspected of causing dermatitis, such clothes should be washed before they are worn again. This frequently will result in removal of irritants and sensitizers, thus occasionally allowing them to be worn without further difficulty.

Spandex is a nonrubber stretchable polyurethane fiber used in girdles, brassieres, and support hose. Although not a problem in spandex manufactured in the United States, allergic contact dermatitis has been reported in foreign-made spandex girdles and brassieres (owing to the presence of the potent sensitizer mercaptobenzothiazole).

Other causes of clothing dermatitis include contact dermatitis to epoxy resin in a knee-patch adhesive,[88] elastic or rubber waist bands on underclothing, purpuric pressure-induced dermatitis ("pants-pressure purpura," a disorder that occurs in individuals who wear rubber or elasticized underwear or tight-fitting slacks, jeans, or dungarees),[89] and clothing washed with fiberglass-contaminated materials (fiberglass dermatitis). Washing new underclothing with a mild soap will frequently help control dermatitis from elasticized or rubber waistbands of underclothing.

SHOE DERMATITIS

Shoe dermatitis is an extremely common form of contact dermatitis in childhood. This dermatosis, frequently misdiagnosed as tinea pedis (a disorder that, although it may occur, is much less common in children prior to puberty), usually begins over the dorsal surface of the base of the great toe, may remain localized to that area indefinitely, and spreads by extension to the dorsal surfaces of the feet and other toes (Fig. 3–37). There is erythema, lichenification, and in severe cases, weeping and crusting. A valuable diagnostic feature of shoe dermatitis is the fact that the interdigital spaces, except in severe cases, remain relatively normal in appearance. This is in contrast to the maceration, scaling, and occasional vesiculation of the interdigital webs, particularly those between the fourth and fifth and, at times, the third and fourth toes of either or both feet, usually associated with tinea

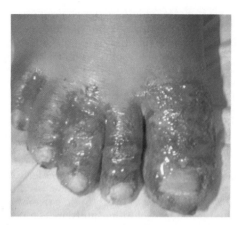

Figure 3–37. Infected foot eczema. This common dermatosis should not be confused with tinea pedis, a disorder that is relatively uncommon in prepubertal children.

pedis. The thick skin of the plantar surfaces is generally more resistant but may at times demonstrate a keratotic dermatitis over the distal areas, the instep, or at times the entire plantar surface.

Pathogenesis. A variety of factors play a role in the pathogenesis of shoe dermatitis. The occlusive effect of hosiery and shoes inhibits the evaporation of moisture, which tends to "leach" out the chemicals in shoes and increase the percutaneous penetration of potentially irritating and sensitizing agents contained therein. Particularly in children, the dermatitis may become sharply localized to the dorsal aspect of the toes as a result of friction and irritation from ill-fitting shoes rather than from allergic sensitization to agents contained in shoes or sneakers.

The most common causes of shoe dermatitis are rubber, adhesives and cements, tanning agents, and dyes. Seventy-five per cent of cases of shoe dermatitis are due to rubber that contains accelerators (mercaptobenzothiazole and tetramethylthiuram monosulfide) or rubber antioxidants (monobenzyl ether of hydroquinone). Adhesive agents are also common sources for sensitization. Here, rubber, ether, plasticizers, esters that improve the plasticity of rubber, and phenolic resins may be implicated. Tanning agents toughen collagen in leather and allow it to resist wear, water, putrefaction, and changes due to heat.

Of the various agents used in the manufacture of shoes, the dichromates appear to be the most frequently implicated as sources of shoe dermatitis. Leather dyeing is usually done with azoaniline dyes. These dyes are well "fixed" to the leather, rarely leach out, and accordingly are relatively uncommon causative factors in the pathogenesis of shoe dermatitis.

Management. Patients with shoe sensitivity should avoid shoes whenever possible, and the control of hyperhidrosis of the feet will frequently aid in the management of individuals with this disorder. Open sandals should be worn, if tolerated, and children should be encouraged to change their socks frequently and remove their shoes whenever possible. Practical shoe substitutes include canvas-topped tennis sneakers, unlined sewn leather moccasins, wooden clogs, or plastic jellies (Happy Feet). In addition, polyvinyl shoes, although they increase the tendency to perspiration, frequently lack many of the potential sensitizers seen in regular shoes; Bass Weejuns loafers and vinyl tennis shoes are frequently acceptable substitutes. Since the inner sole is a frequent source of contact sensitization, removal and replacement with cork insoles, Dr. Scholl's Air Foam Pads, or Johnson's Odor-Eaters, held in place with a nonrubber adhesive such as Elmer's glue, are frequently helpful.

The management of active shoe dermatitis, as in other eczematous disorders, is aided by the use of open wet compresses, topical corticosteroids, and antipruritic agents. Since hyperhidrosis is usually responsible for the "leaching" out of potential sensitizing agents, utilization of measures that minimize excessive perspiration of the feet is advisable. The topical use of aluminum chloride, available as Drysol (Persōn and Covey) or tannic acid soaks (2 tea bags in 1 quart of water), once or twice weekly will frequently assist in the control of hyperhidrosis, and noncaking agents such as Zea-Sorb powder (Stiefel) dusted freely into shoes and hosiery not only tend to lessen perspiration but may also act as a mechanical barrier, thus limiting contact with potential allergens and irritants. When painful fissures are present, soaking the foot in water for 20 minutes at bedtime followed by the application of 30 per cent tincture of benzoin in zinc oxide ointment into the fissured areas and the use of topical corticosteroids and emollient creams, frequently with occlusion at night by Saran Wrap or "baggies," will hasten resolution and lessen discomfort.

JUVENILE PLANTAR DERMATOSIS

Juvenile plantar dermatosis (dermatitis plantaris sicca, "sweaty sock dermatitis") is a common dermatosis of infancy and childhood localized to the distal aspect of the soles and toes, particularly the great toes, but sparing the interdigital spaces. Associated with hyperhidrosis and believed to represent a frictional contact dermatitis in children who have a tendency to atopic dermatitis, the disorder is manifested by a symmetrical, smooth, red, glazed appearance with fissuring, loss of epidermal patterns, and fine scaling (Fig. 3–38). Similar changes have also been reported on the fingertips in up to 5 per cent of patients with excessive perspiration. Untreated juvenile plantar dermatosis generally tends to persist for several years and, although there is no seasonal pattern, some patients report slight worsening of the condition during the summer and in cold weather.

Histopathologic features consist of a psoria-

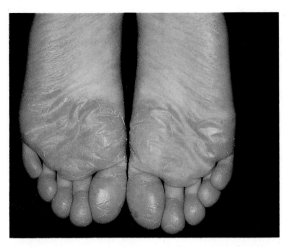

Figure 3–38. A characteristic smooth, glazed dermatosis on the skin of the toes and distal plantar surfaces of the feet of a child with juvenile plantar dermatosis ("sweaty sock dermatitis").

siform acanthosis, focal loss of the granular layer, uniform parakeratosis, inflammatory changes within the epidermis (mainly around sweat ducts), paranuclear vacuolization of epidermal keratinocytes, intracellular edema of the malpighian layer, and spongiotic vesiculation similar to that seen in other eczematous disorders.[90,91] Although treatment is not always completely successful, children with hyperhidrosis of the feet should wear all-cotton socks and avoid occlusive footwear whenever possible, remove their shoes when indoors, change their socks whenever they are damp, dust an absorbent powder such as ZeaSorb (Stiefel) into shoes and hosiery (to help lessen perspiration), and use an emollient cream as soon as the shoes and socks are removed.

METAL AND METAL SALT DERMATITIS

The most common forms of contact dermatitis to metals are those caused by sensitivity to nickel, chromates, and mercury. Most objects containing metal or metal salts are combinations of several metals, some of which may have been used to plate the surface, thus enhancing its attractiveness, tensile strength, or durability.

Since we all are constantly exposed to nickel, nickel dermatitis is one of the most common causes of metal contact sensitivity (Fig. 3–39). In teenage girls and women wearing earrings, ear lobe dermatitis is a cardinal sign of nickel dermatitis; other causes include metal snaps and nickel-containing buttons on blue jeans, zippers, belt buckles, clothing hooks, and fasteners. Many consumers and even jewelers do not realize that most metal alloys, including those of gold and silver, contain nickel.

Patch testing for nickel sensitivity can be per-

formed with a five-cent coin, provided that World War II nickels made up of silver, copper, and manganese are not used and that nonspecific pressure effects are not confused with true allergic eczematous eruptions. If a substance is suspected of containing free nickel, application of a test solution of dimethylglyoxime in a 10 per cent aqueous solution of ammonia to the suspected item will cause the suspected metal to turn pink. The dimethylglyoxime spot test may be obtained from Allerderm Laboratories, P.O. Box 931, Mill Valley, CA 94941. It should be recognized, however, that this test is not sensitive enough to detect all nickel-containing metals and that although nickel levels as low as 0.05 μg have at times been shown to elicit dermatitis in highly sensitive individuals, nickel-containing alloys in general only test positive when 10 μg or more is released.[92]

Nickel sensitivity occurs eight to ten times more frequently in women than men, and individuals who have pierced ears have a nickel sensitivity as high as 15 per cent (this is in contrast to the 2 per cent sensitivity seen in those without pierced ears). Since piercing of ears is responsible for an increased tendency to sensitization to nickel and nickel products, ear piercing should be done with a stainless steel needle, and persons undergoing this procedure should be advised to wear only stainless steel earrings until the earlobes are completely healed. Although stainless steel may contain sensitizing metals, such as chromium, nickel, and occasionally cobalt, the nickel is firmly bound and since it does not leach out with ordinary contact generally does not prove to be a problem.

Once the presence of hypersensitivity to nickel has been established, the hypersensitivity usually lasts for years. Patients, therefore, must be taught how to avoid contact with nickel objects through the use of proper substitutes. Periodic coating of the offending metal with clear nail polish, application of an adhesive moleskin on the back of a watch, or the use of topical aerosol dexamethasone (Decaspray) on both the skin of the individual and

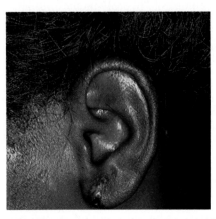

Figure 3–39. Earlobe dermatitis—a cardinal sign of nickel dermatitis.

that portion of the nickel-plated object that comes into contact with the skin, may be helpful for those who prefer to continue to wear potentially allergenic jewelry. The combination of dexamethasone and the film formed by the isopropyl myristate is necessary for successful prophylaxis, since corticosteroid alone or isopropyl myristate alone does not protect nickel-sensitive patients. Both the skin and the nickel-plated object should be sprayed twice at 5-minute intervals, and in warm weather and for patients who perspire profusely (since perspiration tends to release the bound nickel), dexamethasone spray may have to be repeated after a period of 6 hours.[93]

COSMETIC DERMATITIS

The most common cosmetic agents causing allergic contact dermatitis are hair dyes, lipsticks, antiperspirants, paraphenylenediamine (a popular oxidation-type hair dye), substances in commercial and home permanent wave formulations, lanolins, acrylics, nail lacquers, thimerosal (Merthiolate) or benzalkonium and ascorbic acid in contact lens solutions, fragrances (perfumes), sunscreening agents, and a number of preservatives (parabens, quaternium-15, diazolidinyl or imidazolidinyl urea, bronopol, and formaldehyde) used in cosmetics. Since early use of cosmetics adds to this problem, it is recommended that cosmetics be avoided in young children.

In many instances, the eyelids are affected not only by cosmetics applied to the lids and lashes but also by preparations applied to the scalp, face, and nails. Generally, cutaneous allergic reactions take on the form of an eczematous dermatitis. However, antiperspirants and poison ivy preparations containing zirconium may produce allergic granulomatous reactions. Although the incidence of lanolin (wool wax, wool grease, and wool fat) sensitivity obtained from the fleece of sheep is very low, lanolin and its derivatives may be present under many different names and guises. Should patients be found to have allergic sensitivity to lanolin, the manufacturers of "hypoallergenic" cosmetics can furnish lanolin-free products.

In the United States, parabens (compounds containing p-hydroxybenzoic acid) are frequently added in low concentrations to creams, lotions, and cosmetics in an attempt to retard microbial growth. Since the concentration of paraben in topical preparations is too low (below 0.5 per cent) to produce a positive patch test to the medications, patch tests for paraben sensitivity should be performed with a 5 per cent concentration of paraben in petrolatum.

REACTIONS TO TOPICAL MEDICATIONS AND PREPARATIONS

A variety of topical prescription and over-the-counter formulations are capable of producing con-

tact and, at times, systemic contact reactions. Of these, ethylenediamine, benzocaine and its derivatives, tars, parabens, balsam of Peru, and perfumes (including those in a variety of baby care products) are the most common.[78] Although the incidence of cutaneous reactions to topically applied antihistamines is difficult to assess,[82] 12 of 117 cases of dermatitis medicamentosa seen in England in 1 year were due to a formulation containing calamine and diphenhydramine.[76]

Neomycin, a tropical antibiotic incorporated into many topical preparations, is reported to have a high incidence of allergenicity. The majority of contact allergies to this agent, however, are seen in older individuals, particularly those with chronically inflamed skin. In view of the frequent topical use of neomycin in children (without evidence of sensitization), when adults and individuals with chronic dermatoses are excluded the incidence of neomycin sensitivity appears to be appreciably lower, approximately 1 in 100,000 uses rather than the frequently cited 3.0 to 6.0 per cent.[94] When neomycin sensitivity is considered, patch testing requires the use of appropriate material (20 per cent concentrations in aqueous solution or petrolatum, rather than the lower levels seen in most proprietary formulations). Although neomycin and bacitracin are not chemically related, they frequently co-react; and it is not unusual for patients to become sensitized to both antibiotics. Polysporin ointment, although free of neomycin, contains bacitracin and thus may not always be a safe alternative for neomycin-sensitive individuals. Safe substitutes in such instances include Garamycin, which at times can also become sensitizing, erythromycin (Ilotycin) ointment, and mupirocin (Bactroban).

Ethylenediamine, a compound stabilizer seen in various topical preparations, cross-reacts with antihistamines and aminophylline and is a potent sensitizer capable of producing an eczematous contact-type dermatitis. Adequate patch testing requires a 1 per cent concentration, approximately five times that found in commercial products. This sensitizer joins neomycin and the parabens as an agent that may cause dermatitis but yet may produce a negative patch-test response when the commercially available topical preparation is used in patch testing. Antihistamines that are ethylenediamine derivatives are particularly active topical sensitizers and may produce systemic eczematous contact dermatitis when administered to individuals previously sensitized by topical application of ethylenediamine.

Aminophylline, frequently used in the treatment of asthma, contains theophylline and ethylenediamine (the ethylenediamine renders the theophylline soluble so that it can be injected). Although a number of theophylline preparations without ethylenediamine can be given orally to ethylenediamine-sensitive individuals, in an emergency situation where intravenous or intramuscular theophylline is required, an ethylenediamine-free intravenous theophylline preparation (available from Travenol Labs, Inc., Deerfield, IL 60015) or an ethylenediamine-free intramuscular formulation (dyphylline [Lufyllin; Wallace Laboratories, Cranbury, NJ 08512]) may be used.[76]

ADHESIVE TAPE DERMATITIS

Although most cutaneous reactions related to the wearing of adhesive tape are of a mechanical rather than contact sensitivity type, allergic reactions may be due to the rubber compounds (rubber accelerators or antioxidants) that have been incorporated into the adhesive or the vinyl backing of the adhesive. Dermicel (Johnson and Johnson), Steristrips or Microspore surgical tape (3 M Company), and nonrubber "acrylate" are helpful for those individuals allergic to or irritated by ordinary adhesive tapes.

VIDEO DISPLAY TERMINAL DERMATITIS

With our ever-increasing technology a facial eruption (termed *video display dermatitis*) has been reported following exposure to computer video display units. Described as a rosacea-like or seborrheic dermatitis predominantly seen over the zygomatic and upper buccal regions of the face, and occasionally the dorsal aspect of the hands and distal aspects of the forearms, it develops within 2 hours and up to 2 or 3 days following exposure to video display units.

Whether or not this cutaneous eruption is a true entity is controversial. If it truly exists, it is believed to be related to an electrostatic field between the operator and the video display terminal screen in a room with low humidity causing suspended particles in the air to be deposited on the operator's skin. Adjusting the humidity in the workspace of computer operators may help eliminate the problem.[95]

FIBERGLASS DERMATITIS

Fiberglass particles frequently cause intense pruritus because the fine glass fiber particles from fiberglass insulation panels or drapes can penetrate the skin and cause an eruption consisting of small erythematous follicular papules. At times clothes washed in a washing machine in which fiberglass materials have been washed are also capable of inducing this cutaneous reaction (Fig. 3–40).

Fiberglass dermatitis clinically appears to represent a patchy folliculitis or subacute dermatitis. Microscopic examination of skin scrapings of involved areas or suspected articles of clothing may reveal pale, greenish, granular rod-like fibers one to two times the width of a hair.

Patients with fiberglass dermatitis respond to removal of exposure to the offending agents, topical corticosteroids, systemic antipruritics, and, when necessary, epidermal stripping to facilitate removal of embedded particles.[96]

AUTOSENSITIZATION DERMATITIS

Autosensitization is a term used to describe a clinical disorder created by sensitization of the body by circulating antibody or by specifically activated lymphocytes (delayed hypersensitivity) to constituents of its own tissues. Frequently referred to as an "id" reaction, the disorder is characterized by an acute papulovesicular eruption that appears on the forearms, flexor aspects of the upper arms, the extensor aspects of the upper arms and thighs, and, less commonly, the face and trunk (Fig. 3–41). The disorder usually appears acutely over a few days and nearly always is preceded by an exacerbation of the preexisting dermatitis by infection, rubbing, or inappropriate therapy. The eruption is nearly always symmetrical but may demonstrate an isomorphic response (the Koebner phenomenon)

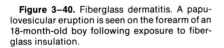
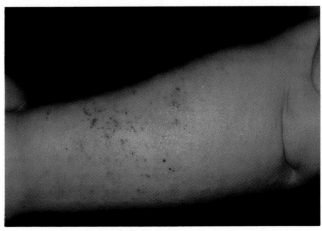

Figure 3–40. Fiberglass dermatitis. A papulovesicular eruption is seen on the forearm of an 18-month-old boy following exposure to fiberglass insulation.

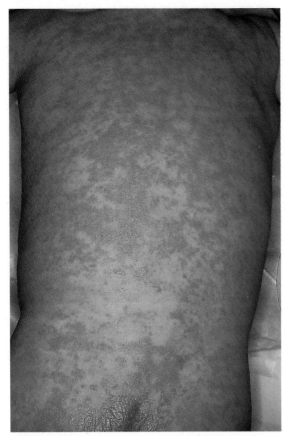

Figure 3–41. Autosensitization dermatitis ("id" reaction) on the back of a young boy.

or light sensitivity. Lesions begin as discrete edematous papules or papulovesicles and are generally associated with a moderate to severe degree of pruritus.

The acute eruption may subside spontaneously in a few weeks if the primary dermatitis is controlled. Relapses, however, are common, particularly when the initial local lesion flares and is followed by a further disseminated eruption.

The diagnosis of autosensitization dermatitis (autoeczematization) is made clinically on the basis of a generalized papulovesicular eruption that develops in the wake of a preexisting eczematoid dermatitis. Treatment depends on open wet compresses, antihistamines, and the use of topical corticosteroid preparations. Control of the primary lesion is important to prevent further or recurrent antigenic stimulation. Although seldom indicated, a 2- to 3-week course of systemic corticosteroids may at times be necessary in cases that are unresponsive to more conservative therapy.

References

1. Coca AF, Cooke RA: On the classification of the phenomenon of hypersensitiveness. J. Immunol. 8:163–182, 1923.

A discussion of hypersensitivity and its classification into normal and abnormal groups.

2. Wise F, Sulzberger MB: Year Book of Dermatology and Syphilology. Year Book Medical Publishers, Inc., Chicago, 1933, 59.

The term *atopic dermatitis* permits inclusion of the eruption from its acute eczematous form to the chronic lichenified lesions that technically fail to merit the term *eczema*.

3. Cormia FE: The basis of itching (discussion). J. Pediatr. 66:207–209, 1965.

Itching is a modified form of pain carried on slow afferent fibers, the intensity varying with the number of free nerve endings in the affected area.

4. Morgan DB: A suggestive sign of allergy. Arch. Dermatol. Syph. 57:1050, 1948.

The terms *Morgan's fold* and *Dennie's pleat* are used to describe a definite wrinkle that appears just beneath the margin of the lower eyelids (originally described by Dr. Charles C. Dennie, who first called the attention of students to the sign, which he believed rather pathognomonic for patients with allergy).

5. Uehara M, Ofugi S: Abnormal vascular reactions to atopic dermatitis. Arch. Dermatol. 113:627–629, 1977.

White dermographism, nicotinic acid blanching, and delayed blanching with metacholine occur in atopic dermatitis and in nonatopic patients with allergic contact dermatitis.

6. Dunand P, Chai H, Weltman D, et al.: Posterior polar cataracts and steroid therapy in children. J. Allergy Clin. Immunol. 55:123, 1975.

Slit-lamp studies of 92 children on long-term corticosteroid therapy revealed 10 children (10.8 per cent) with evidence of cataracts.

7. Sevel D, Weinberg MB, Van Niekirk CH: Lenticular complications of long-term steroid therapy in children with asthma and eczema. J. Allergy Clin. Immunol. 60:215–217, 1977.

Of 42 children with chronic asthma (including 10 with associated eczema) on long-term oral corticosteroids, only 1 was found to have cataracts commensurate with corticosteroid therapy, but the authors emphasize that children on long-term corticosteroid therapy be examined for possible posterior capsular cataracts..

8. Jones HE, Lewis CW, McMarlin SL: Allergic contact sensitivity in atopic dermatitis. Arch. Dermatol. 107:217–222, 1973.

Comparison studies of poison ivy sensitivity revealed an incidence of 15 per cent reactivity in patients with atopic dermatitis as compared with 61 per cent in the control group.

9. Strauss JS: Atopic allergy and atopic dermatitis—a discussion of their relationship. NY State J. Med. 59:53–58, 1959.

Specific protein antigens may cause exacerbations of atopic dermatitis.

10. Strauss JS, Kligman AM: The relationship of atopic allergy and dermatitis. Arch. Dermatol. 75:806–811, 1957.

Inhalant and ingested allergens probably are secondary rather than primary factors in the causation of dermatitic flares.

11. Hanifin JM: Atopic dermatitis in infants and children. Pediatr. Clin. North Am. 38:763–789, 1991.

An authoritative review of atopic dermatitis, its pathogenesis, clinical features, and management.

12. Kapp A, Czech W, Krutman J, et al.: Eosinophilic cationic protein in sera of patients with atopic dermatitis. J. Am. Acad. Dermatol. 24:555–558, 1991.

Studies suggest that eosinophils and their secretory products may contribute to the immunologic alterations and pathogenesis of atopic dermatitis.

13. Szentivanyi A: The beta-adrenergic theory of the atopic abnormality in bronchial asthma. J. Allergy 42:203–232, 1968.

A theory of atopy based on a cellular control system mediated through adenyl cyclase and cyclic adenosine monophosphate.

14. Ishizaka K, Ishizaka T: Physicochemical properties of reaginic antibody: I. Association of reaginic activity with an immunoglobulin other than gamma A or gamma C-globulin. J. Allergy 37:169–185, 1966.

Sera from atopic patients fractionated by chromatography reveal a unique immunoglobulin (IgE) capable of passive sensitization of normal skin.

15. Ishizaka K, Ishizaka T: Identification of gamma E-antibodies as a carrier of reaginic activity. J. Immunol. 99:1187–1198, 1967.

Evidence supports the concept that IgE is the reaginic antibody against antigen E.

16. Juhlin C, Johannssen SGO: Immunoglobulin E. Arch. Dermatol. 100:12–16, 1969.

Elevated serum levels of IgE detected in 82 per cent of patients with atopic dermatitis.

17. Ogawa M, Berger PA, McIntyre OR, et al.: IgE in atopic dermatitis. Arch. Dermatol. 103:575–580, 1971.

The mean serum IgE levels in atopic dermatitis are higher than those of control groups; a strong correlation exists between this level and the severity of dermatitis.

18. Dahl MV: Staphylococcus aureus and atopic dermatitis. Arch. Dermatol. 119:840–846, 1983.

A review of Staphylococcus aureus colonization and its possible role in the pathogenesis of atopic dermatitis.

19. Hanifin JM: Atopic dermatitis. J. Am. Acad. Dermatol. 6:1–13, 1982.

A comprehensive review of the clinical and epidemiologic aspects of atopic dermatitis.

20. Sampson HA, Jolie PL: Increased plasma histamine concentration after food challenges in children with atopic dermatitis. N. Engl. J. Med. 311:372–376, 1984.

In a study of 33 patients with severe atopic dermatitis, positive responses to skin-prick tests and increased histamine concentrations following food challenges add credence to the hypothesis that food allergies may at times have a positive role in the pathogenesis of atopic dermatitis.

21. Sampson HA, McCaskill CC: Food hypersensitivity in atopic dermatitis: Evaluation of 113 patients. J. Pediatr. 107:669–675, 1985.

In a study in which 56 per cent of 113 selected patients with severe atopic dermatitis experienced positive responses to food challenges, egg, peanut, and milk accounted for 72 per cent of the hypersensitivity reactions.

22. Berman BA, Kniker WT, Cohen GA: An allergist's view of atopic dermatitis. Dermatol. Clin. 4:55–66, 1986.

An overview of the pathophysiology, clinical aspects, and management of atopic dermatitis.

23. Kreuger GG, Kahn G, Weston WL, et al.: IgE levels in nummular eczema and ichthyosis. Arch. Dermatol. 107:56–58, 1973.

Significantly lower IgE levels in 26 patients with nummular eczema suggest that nummular eczema is not a manifestation of atopic dermatitis.

24. Leyden JJ, Marples RR, Kligman AM: Staphylococcus aureus in the lesions of atopic dermatitis. Br. J. Dermatol. 90:525–530, 1974.

Staphylococcus aureus was isolated from 90 per cent of 50 patients with chronic atopic dermatitis.

25. Aly R, Maibach HI, Shinefield HR: Microbial flora of atopic dermatitis. Arch. Dermatol. 113:780–782, 1977.

Studies of the skin and anterior nares of 39 patients with atopic dermatitis reveal a 93 per cent incidence of Staphylococcus aureus carriage in cutaneous lesions, a 76 per cent incidence in noninvolved skin, and a 79 per cent carriage rate in the anterior nares.

26. David TG, Cambridge GC: Bacterial infection and atopic dermatitis. Arch. Dis. Child. 61:20–23, 1986.

In a 2½-year study of 190 children with atopic dermatitis, 76 (40 per cent) had exacerbations attributed to bacterial infection and 32 per cent of these developed a repeat infection within 3 months.

27. Boiko S, Kaufman RA, Lucky AW: Osteomyelitis of the distal phalanges in three children with severe atopic dermatitis. Arch. Dermatol. 124:418–423, 1988.

A report of three children with severely infected atopic dermatitis and osteomyelitis of the distal phalanges.

28. Lasch EE, Frankel V, Pardy PA, et al.: Epidemic glomerulonephritis in Israel. J. Infect. Dis. 124:141–147, 1971.

Early treatment of streptococcal infection does not appear to prevent the development of acute nephritis.

29. LaForce CF, Miller MF, Chai H: Effect of erythromycin in theophylline clearance in asthmatic children. J. Pediatr. 99:153–156, 1981.

Since erythromycin interferes with the metabolic breakdown of theophylline, increased theophylline levels may at times prove to be a problem for asthmatic children who receive erythromycin for the treatment of infected atopic dermatitis.

30. Wrobleski BA, Singer MD, Whyte J: Carbamazepine–erythromycin interaction. J.A.M.A. 255:1165–1167, 1986.

Four patients taking carbamazepine concomitantly with erythromycin developed significantly elevated serum carbamazepine levels.

31. Woolfson H: Oral acyclovir in eczema herpeticum. Br. Med. J. 288:531–532, 1984.

A report of two children with eczema herpeticum successfully treated with oral acyclovir.

32. Jawitz JC, Hines HC, Moshell AN: Treatment of eczema herpeticum with systemic acyclovir. Arch. Dermatol. 121:274–275, 1985.

Intravenous acyclovir was well tolerated and effective in the treatment of eczema herpeticum in a 9-month-old infant.

33. David TJ, Longson M: Herpes simplex infections in atopic eczema. Arch. Dis. Child. 60:338–343, 1985.

Four severely ill children with eczema herpeticum showed a rapid response to intravenous acyclovir.

34. Atherton DJ, Harper JI: Management of eczema herpeticum. J. Am. Acad. Dermatol. 18:757–758, 1988.

High-dose intravenous acyclovir therapy (1.5 g/m²/day) is suggested as an appropriate form of therapy for children with severe eczema herpeticum.

35. Hanifin JM: Atopic dermatitis. In Greer KE (Ed.): Common Problems in Dermatology. Year Book Medical Publishers, Inc., Chicago, 1988, 42–49.

Helpful hints for the management of patients with atopic dermatitis.

36. Grulee CG, Sanford HN: The influence of breast and artificial feeding on infantile eczema. J. Pediatr. 9:223–225, 1936.

An authoritative study of breast feeding and cow's milk avoidance and their role in minimizing the risk of atopic dermatitis for infants at high risk.

37. Karmer MS, Moroz B: Do breast-feeding and delayed introduction of solid foods protect against subsequent atopic dermatitis? J. Pediatr. 98:546–550, 1981.

A study of 636 infants, in which 36 per cent of breast-fed and 26 per cent of non-breast-fed infants developed atopic dermatitis, questions the value of breast-feeding and delayed introduction of solid foods as prophylaxis against atopic dermatitis.

38. Gruskay FL: Comparison of breast, cow, and soy feedings in

the prevention of onset of allergic disease: A 15-year prospective study. Clin. Pediatr. 21:486–491, 1982.

A 15-year study of 328 children comparing breast-fed, cow's milk–fed, and soy formula–fed children revealed little difference in the various feeding regimens and the subsequent risk of atopic dermatitis.

39. Moore W, Midwinter R, Morris A, et al.: Infant feeding and subsequent risk of atopic eczema. Arch. Dis. Child. 80:722–726, 1985.

A review of infants genetically predisposed to atopic dermatitis suggests that exclusive breast feeding can indeed help reduce the risk of severe atopic dermatitis.

40. Kajosaari M, Saarinen UM: Prophylaxis of atopic disease by 6 months total solid elimination: Evaluation of 135 exclusively breast-fed infants of atopic families. Acta Pediatr. Scand. 72:411–418, 1983.

A study of 135 exclusively breast-fed infants with atopic backgrounds showed that although 35 per cent of those who received early solid foods developed atopic dermatitis, only 10 per cent of those fed exclusively on breast milk went on to develop this disorder.

41. Fergusson DM, Horwood J, Shannon FT: Early solid feeding and recurrent childhood eczema: A 10-year longitudinal study. Pediatrics 86:541–546, 1990.

A 10-year study revealed that children exposed to four or more different types of solid food before the age of 4 months had a 2.9 times greater risk of recurrent or chronic eczema than infants not exposed to early solid feeding.

42. Cavagni G, Paganelli G, Caffarelli C, et al.: Passage of food antigens into circulation of breast-fed infants with atopic dermatitis. Ann. Allergy 621:361–365, 1989.

Studies of IgE levels for cow's milk and egg antigens in 13 exclusively breast-fed infants with atopic dermatitis provide firm evidence of maternal milk food antigen transfer to the infant's circulation.

43. Carswell F, Thompson S: House dust mites and atopy. Does natural sensitization in eczema occur through the skin? Lancet 2:13–15, 1986.

Studies appear to confirm the hypothesis that eczema can at times be aggravated by house dust mite exposure.

44. Coloff MJ, Lever RS, McSharry C: A controlled trial of house dust mite eradication using natamycin in homes of patients with atopic dermatitis. Br. J. Dermatol. 121:199–208, 1989.

A study on natamycin, an antifungal agent that works as an acaricide by killing house dust fungi (which digest lipids on human skin scales, the food of the house dust mite), failed to demonstrate the value of this agent, vacuuming, or both, in the management of patients with atopic dermatitis.

45. Van Bronswijk JEMH, Schober G, Kniest FM: The management of house dust mite allergies. Clin. Ther. 12:221–226, 1990.

Although further studies are required to determine the value of house dust mite avoidance in patients with suspected mite-induced atopic dermatitis, studies suggest that miticidal agents help sensitive individuals control the concentration of mite allergens in their environment.

46. Burks AW, Mallory SB, Williams LW, et al.: Atopic dermatitis: Clinical relevance of food hypersensitivity reactions. J. Pediatr. 113:447–451, 1988.

Of 46 patients with mild to severe atopic dermatitis, 61 per cent demonstrated positive skin-prick reactions confirming that although food hypersensitivity is not the only cause of atopic dermatitis, it can, at least in selected cases, be a major contributing factor.

47. Stoughton RB: Are generic formulations equivalent to trade name topical glucocorticosteroids? Arch. Dermatol. 123:1312–1314, 1987.

Studies comparing generic and brand name topical corticosteroids reveal that generic preparations often contain agents differing from those of trade name formulations and frequently vary in their clinical efficacy.

48. Weston WL, Sams WM Jr, Morris HG, et al.: Morning plasma cortisol level in infants treated with topical fluorinated glucocorticoids. Pediatrics 65:103–106, 1980.

A report of temporary suppression of morning plasma cortisol levels in 17 infants treated with topical corticosteroids.

49. Stoppolino G, Prisco F, Santinelli R, et al.: Potential hazards of topical steroid therapy. Am. J. Dis. Child. 137:1130–1131, 1983.

A report of a 4½-month-old infant who developed Cushing's syndrome following 3 months of topical clobetasole proprionate usage.

50. Bode HH: Dwarfism following long-term topical corticosteroid therapy. J.A.M.A. 244:813–814, 1980.

A report of a 13-year-old boy in whom short stature began at the age of 18 months (when betamethasone ointment 2 per cent, 45 g a week, was initiated for his atopic dermatitis).

51. Bartorelli A, Rimondini A: Severe hypertension in childhood due to prolonged topical application of corticosteroid ointment. Hypertension 6:586–588, 1984.

A report of a 9-year-old boy with atopic dermatitis who developed severe hypertension (230/160 mm Hg) while on treatment with fluroprednisolone ointment (100 mg/day).

52. Kaplan RJ, Daman L, Rosenberg EW, et al.: Topical use of caffeine with hydrocortisone in the treatment of atopic dermatitis. Arch. Dermatol. 114:60–62, 1978.

In a study of 83 patients, a combination of 30 per cent caffeine and 0.5 per cent hydrocortisone appeared to help relieve the pruritus associated with atopic dermatitis.

53. Haider SA: Treatment of atopic eczema in children: Clinical trial of 10 per cent cromolyn ointment. Br. Med. J. 1:1570–1572, 1977.

In a double-blind randomized study, 16 of 21 children with atopic dermatitis treated with 10 per cent sodium cromoglycate in a white soft paraffin appeared to benefit from the therapy.

54. Molkhou P, Waguet J-C: Food allergy and atopic dermatitis in children: Treatment with oral sodium cromoglycate. Ann. Allergy 47:173–175, 1981.

Oral sodium cromoglycate (100 to 600 mg/day) appeared to help 23 children with atopic dermatitis.

55. Atherton DJ, Soothill JF, Elvidge J: Controlled trial of oral sodium cromoglycate in atopic eczema. Br. J. Dermatol. 106:681–685, 1982.

A double-blind study of 29 children with atopic dermatitis treated with 100 mg of oral disodium cromoglycate four times a day failed to demonstrate any significant effect on itching, sleep disturbance, corticosteroid applications, or antihistamine use.

56. Wright S, Burton JL: Oral evening primrose oil improves atopic dermatitis. Lancet 2:1120–1122, 1982.

Administration of evening primrose oil showed a 30 per cent improvement in overall severity in 43 per cent of 99 patients (60 adults and 39 children) with atopic dermatitis.

57. Bamford JT, Gibson RW, Renier CM: Atopic dermatitis unresponsive to evening primrose oil (linoleic and gamma-linoleic acids). J. Am. Acad. Dermatol. 13:959–965, 1985.

A double-blind placebo-controlled crossover study of 123 patients with atopic dermatitis failed to demonstrate any significant effect on erythema, scale, excoriation, lichenification or overall severity of the dermatitis.

58. Skogh M: Atopic eczema unresponsive to evening primrose oil (linoleic and gamma-linoleic acids). J. Am. Acad. Dermatol. 15:114–115, 1986.

In a study of eight patients with a long history of severe atopic dermatitis, evening primrose oil (identical to that used in the

1982 report) showed no convincing effect on the course of the dermatitis.

59. Baer RL: Papaverine therapy in atopic dermatitis. J. Am. Acad. Dermatol. 13:806–808, 1985.

Papaverine hydrochloride, in a dosage of 100 mg four to six times a day (or 150-mg time-release capsules two or three times a day), appeared to relieve itching in patients with atopic dermatitis.

60. Kang K, Cooper KD, Hanifin JM: Thymopoietin pentapeptide (TP-5) improves clinical parameters and lymphocyte populations in atopic dermatitis. J. Am. Acad. Dermatol. 8:372–377, 1982.

Preliminary evidence suggests a beneficial effect of thymic hormone thymopoietin pentapeptide (TP-5) in patients with atopic dermatitis.

61. Harper JI, White IR, Staughton RCD, et al.: Thymostimulin (TP-1) therapy for atopic eczema. Br. J. Dermatol. 119:14, 1988.

A double-blind controlled study of twice-weekly injections of TP-1 in 29 patients with atopic dermatitis showed a 20 per cent reduction in the clinical severity of the disorder.

62. Van Joost T, Stolz E, Huele F: Efficacy of low dose cyclosporine in severe atopic dermatitis. Arch. Dermatol. 123:166–167, 1987.

Near-complete remission of two patients with severe atopic dermatitis treated with cyclosporine supports the hypothesis that not only does T-helper cell function play an important role in the pathogenesis of this disorder but also that short-term use may prove to be beneficial in the treatment of resistant forms of atopic dermatitis.

63. Jekler J, Larkö O: Combined UVA-UVB versus UVB phototherapy for atopic dermatitis: A paired-comparison study. J. Am. Acad. Dermatol. 22:49–53, 1990.

In a paired comparison study of 30 patients with atopic dermatitis, the combination of UVA and UVB appeared to be significantly more effective than UVB alone in the treatment of patients with this disorder.

64. Atherton DJ, Carabolt F, Glover MT, et al.: The role of psoralen photochemotherapy (PUVA) in the treatment of severe atopic dermatitis in adolescents. Br. J. Dermatol. 118:791–795, 1988.

Ten to 25 weeks of PUVA (oral psoralen photochemotherapy) achieved nearly complete clearance of the cutaneous lesions in 14 of 15 patients with severe persistent atopic dermatitis.

65. Buckley RH, Wray BB, Belnaker EZ: Extreme hyperimmunoglobulinemia E and undue susceptibility to infection. Pediatrics 49:59–70, 1972.

Clinical and immunologic features of two adolescent boys with recurrent pyogenic infections are judged to constitute a new syndrome characterized by recurrent bacterial and fungal infections, impaired cell-mediated immunity, and exceptionally high serum IgE concentrations.

66. Stiehm ER: Immunological Disorders of Infants and Children, 3rd ed. W.B. Saunders Co., Philadelphia, 1989.

A comprehensive review of immunologic disorders in infancy and childhood.

67. Kamei R, Honig PJ: Neonatal Job's syndrome featuring a vesicular eruption. Pediatr. Dermatol. 5:75–82, 1988.

A report of a newborn with a vesicular eruption who eventually developed classic features of Job's syndrome.

68. Aldrich RA, Steinberg AG, Campbell DD: Pedigree demonstrating a sex-linked recessive condition characterized by draining ears, eczematoid dermatitis and bloody diarrhea. Pediatrics 13:133–139, 1954.

A severe recalcitrant dermatitis, thrombocytopenia, and sex-linked recessivity are seen as part of a disorder initially described by Wiskott in 1937.

69. Ruiz-Maldonado R, López-Martinez R, Pérez Chavarria EL, et al.: Pityrosporum ovale in infantile seborrheic dermatitis. Pediatr. Dermatol. 6:16–20, 1989.

A study of four groups of infants (aged 1–24 months) revealed that the presence of P. ovale was significantly more frequent in infants with seborrheic dermatitis than healthy infants or those with other dermatoses, and the effectiveness of topical ketoconazole therapy suggested that this organism may play a pathogenic role in some infants with seborrheic dermatitis.

70. Hickman JG: Nizoral (ketoconazole) shampoo therapy in seborrheic dermatitis. J. Int. Postgrad. Med. 2:14–17, 1990.

A study comparing selenium sulfide 2.5 per cent shampoo and ketoconazole 2 per cent shampoo showed both to be equally effective in the treatment of patients with moderate to severe seborrheic dermatitis of the scalp.

71. Waisman M, Sutton RL: Frictional lichenoid eruption in children: Recurrent pityriasis of the elbows and knees. Arch. Dermatol. 94:592–593, 1966.

A distinctive scaly lichenoid eruption of the extremities, particularly the elbows and knees, in children 4 to 12 years of age.

72. Goldman L, Kitzmiller KW, Richfield DF: Summer lichenoid dermatitis of the elbows in children. Cutis 13:836–838, 1974.

In seven children a pruritic eruption of the elbows and knees during the summertime seemed to clear with the advent of cool weather.

73. Patrizi A, di Lernia V, Ricci V, et al.: Atopic background of a recurrent papular eruption of childhood (frictional lichenoid eruption). Pediatr. Dermatol. 7:111–115, 1990.

A high proportion of atopy (atopic dermatitis, allergic rhinitis, and/or asthma) in 45.7 per cent of 35 children with frictional lichenoid dermatitis appears to confirm the hypothesis that an underlying atopy may predispose to the development of this disorder.

74. Seghal VN, Gangwani OP: Fixed drug eruptions: Current concepts. Int. J. Dermatol. 26:67–74, 1987.

A comprehensive review of fixed drug eruptions, their pathophysiology and clinical features.

75. Shelley WB, Shelley ED: Nonpigmenting fixed drug eruption as a distinctive reaction pattern: Examples caused by sensitity to pseudoephedrine hydrochloride and tetrahydrozoline. J. Am. Acad. Dermatol. 17:403–407, 1987.

A report of three patients with fixed drug eruptions caused by a nighttime cold remedy, a children's cough syrup, and vasoconstricting eyedrops.

76. Fisher AA: Contact Dermatitis, 3rd ed. Lea & Febiger, Philadelphia, 1986.

A classic review by a leading authority in contact dermatitis.

77. Weston WL, Weston JA: Allergic contact dermatitis in children. Am. J. Dis. Child. 138:932–936, 1984.

An overview of allergic contact dermatitis as manifested in childhood.

78. Fisher AA: Allergic contact dermatitis in early infancy. Cutis 35:315–316, 1985.

A review of contact dermatitis in newborns and infants.

79. Bergstresser PR: Contact allergic dermatitis: Old problems and new techniques. Arch. Dermatol. 125:276–279, 1989.

A comprehensive review of our current knowledge of allergic contact dermatitis and the role of Langerhans cells and T-lymphocyte subsets.

80. Pevny I, Brennenstuhl M, Rzinskas G: Patch testing in children: I. Collective test results: Skin testability in children. Contact Dermatitis 11:201–206, 1984.

Ten years of patch testing in children between the ages of 3 and 16 years revealed that positive patch tests are relatively infrequent in children and that, except for nickel, formaldehyde, and dichromate, children generally can be tested with the same patch test concentrations as those used for adults.

81. Mallory SB, Miller OF III, Tyler WB: *Toxicodendron radicans* dermatitis with black lacquer deposit on the skin. J. Am. Acad. Dermatol. 6:363–368, 1982.

A report of four patients who developed black lacquer-like deposits at the sites of *Rhus* oleoresin deposition.

82. Patranella P: Diphenhydramine toxicity due to topical application of Caladryl. Clin. Pediatr. 25:163, 1986.

A 4-year-old boy developed hyperactivity, irregular eye movements, hallucinations, disorientation, ataxia, tongue rolling, and combative behavior following the topical application of diphenhydramine hydrochloride in calamine lotion (Caladryl).

83. Orchard S, Fellman JH, Storrs FJ: Poison ivy/oak dermatitis: Use of polyamine salts of a linoleic acid dimer for topical prophylaxis. Arch. Dermatol. 122:783–789, 1986.

Polyamine salts of a linoleic acid dimer were found to be effective in the prevention of *Rhus* dermatitis in individuals at risk for this dermatosis.

84. Grevelink SA, Murrell DF, Olsen EA: Effectiveness of various barrier preparations in preventing and/or ameliorating experimentally produced *Toxicodendron* dermatitis. J. Am. Acad. Dermatol. 27:182–188, 1992.

In a study of seven barrier preparations for the prevention or amelioration of experimentally induced *Rhus* dermatitis, Stokogard, Hollister Moisture Barrier, and Hydropil were 59%, 53%, and 48% effective, respectively. The remaining four barrier preparations (Ivy Shield, Shield Skin, Dermofilm, and Uniderm) were not as effective (their percentage reductions in dermatitis severity were read as 22%, 13%, 3%, and −9%, respectively).

85. Thiboutot DM, Hamory BH, Marks JG Jr: Dermatoses among floral shop workers. J. Am. Acad. Dermatol. 22:54–58, 1990.

Alstroemeria, a common flower containing tuliposide A recently popularized in the United States, along with chrysanthemums, currently appears to be a leading cause of hand dermatitis of workers in the floral industry.

86. Gette MT, Marks JE Jr: Tulip fingers. Arch. Dermatol. 126:203–205, 1990.

Allergic contact dermatitis of the fingers in five workers who packaged and sorted tulip bulbs.

87. Spoerke DG, Temple AR: Dermatitis after exposure to a common garden plant (*Euphorbia myrsinites*). Am. J. Dis. Child. 133:28–29, 1979.

A report of six children with erythematous papulovesicular eruptions following exposure to *Euphorbia myrsinites*.

88. Taylor JS, Bergfeld WF, Guin JD: Contact dermatitis to a knee patch adhesive in boys' jeans: A nonoccupational cause of epoxy resin sensitivity. Cleve. Clin. Q. 50:123–127, 1983.

A report of three boys who developed eczematous dermatitis of the knees from an epoxy resin contained in a knee patch adhesive.

89. Fisher AA: Purpuric contact dermatitis. Cutis 33:346, 351, 359, 1984.

A review of petechial and purpuric eruptions from contact with wool, formaldehyde resin, fiberglass, optical whitener, tight-fitting pants, rubber and rubber-antioxidants, and cobalt.

90. Weston JA, Hawkins K, Weston WL: Foot dermatitis in children. Pediatrics 72:824–827, 1983.

A review of 34 children with foot dermatitis and a discussion of dermatoses of the dorsal and plantar aspects of the foot in childhood.

91. Carrefero G, Sanchez J, Fernandez E, et al.: Juvenile plantar dermatosis: A histopathologic study. Actas Dermo-Sif. 78:85–90, 1987.

Histopathologic features of eight patients with juvenile plantar dermatosis.

92. Fischer T, Fregert S, Gruvberger B, et al.: Nickel release from earpiercing kits and earrings. Contact Dermatitis 10:39–41, 1984.

Although the amount of nickel released to the skin necessary to sensitize individuals has not been clearly established, levels as low as 0.05 μg have been shown to elicit dermatitis.

93. Fisher AA: Steroid aerosol spray in contact dermatitis: Prophylactic use with particular reference to nickel hypersensitivity. Arch. Dermatol. 89:841–843, 1967.

A combination of dexamethasone and a film formed by isopropyl myristate in Decadron spray affords protection to patients with nickel sensitivity.

94. Leyden JJ, Kligman AM: The case for topical antibiotics. Prog. Dermatol. 7:11–14, 1973.

Neomycin appears to be far less a sensitizer than most studies seem to indicate.

95. Berg M, Lidén S: Skin problems in video display terminal users. J. Am. Acad. Dermatol. 17:682–683, 1987.

A review of the controversy regarding computer video display terminals and facial dermatitis.

96. Parlette HL: Fiberglass dermatitis. Bull. Assoc. Milit. Dermatol. 22:53–55, 1974.

A patchy pruritic dermatitis of the wrists, forearms, and shins of a young man working with fiberglass insulation panels.

PHOTOSENSITIVITY AND PHOTOREACTIONS

Reactions to the sun's rays have become increasingly common in recent years, owing not only to the ever-expanding number of photosensitizers in the environment but also to much of the public's obsession with sunbathing. Sunlight emits a wide spectrum of radiation energy, extending from radio waves through infrared, visible, and ultraviolet (UV) light to x-rays. The unit used to specify the wavelength of light is the nanometer (1 nanometer [nm] is equal to 10 Ångstroms). Visible light is in the range of 400 to 800 nm and is relatively harmless. From 800 to 1,800 nm is the infrared range. It is the UV wavelengths (290 to 400 nm) that cause most cutaneous reactions. Since wavelengths less than 220 nm are absorbed by atmospheric gases, including oxygen and nitrogen, and those less than 290 nm are absorbed by the atmospheric ozone layer, it is the middle ultraviolet (UVB) wavelengths of 290 to 320 nm that primarily produce sunburn, suntan, and skin cancer. Long-wave ultraviolet light (UVA, 320 to 400 nm) may augment these cutaneous reactions. It is in this range that most drug-induced or chemical-induced photosensitivity reactions occur.

An important factor in sun exposure is the fact that UV light also reaches the skin through reflection from snow (80 to 85 per cent), sand (17 to 25 per cent), water (5 per cent, but up to 100 per cent when the sun is directly overhead), sidewalks, and turf, and that UV exposure increases 4 per cent for every 1,000 feet elevation above sea level. It must be remembered that on a bright cloudy day with thin cloud cover it is possible to receive 60 to 85 per cent of the amount of UV radiation that is present on a bright clear day, that hats and umbrellas provide only a moderate degree of protection, and that surfaces with reflectivity greatly increase sunlight exposure.

TANNING AND SUNBURN REACTIONS

A deepening pigmentation due to increased melanization of the skin (referred to as a tan) occurs following UV exposure. Sunburn is caused by UV light with wavelengths between 290 and 320 nm. Wavelengths from 290 to 400 nm are mainly responsible for tanning. Immediate pigmentary darkening occurs within minutes of sun exposure and fades within 6 to 8 hours, and the major pigmentary change occurs within 48 to 72 hours, reaching its maximum intensity in 2 to 3 weeks.

Sunburn may be defined as a cutaneous erythema caused by sun exposure at wavelengths between 290 and 320 nm of sufficient degree to cause discomfort. Reactivity may range in severity from a mild asymptomatic erythema to a more intense reaction, with redness accompanied by tenderness, pain, edema, and, at times, vesiculation and bulla formation. Sunburn-induced erythema and edema appear to be mediated by prostaglandin D, histamine, and arachidonic acid. Systemic reactions (chills and fever) appear to be induced by an increase in keratinocyte-released serum interleukin-1 activity.[1, 2]

Clinical Manifestations. Mild reactions from sunlight begin 6 to 12 hours after the onset of exposure, reach a peak intensity within about 24 hours, begin to decline gradually over 3 to 5 days, and usually result in a tan that reaches its maximum 2 to 3 weeks after exposure. Intense reactions begin in a similar manner. Signs and symptoms, however, are more intense and continue to progress, generally reaching their peak on the second day, at which time large blisters may form in the most severely affected areas. After several days the erythema and edema subside and are soon followed by a degree of desquamation relative to the intensity of the clinical reaction. If the sunburned area is extensive, constitutional symptoms may include nausea, malaise, headache, fever, chills, delirium, and, in some cases, even prostration.

Histopathologic features of sunburn damage include damaged keratinocytes, resembling dyskeratotic cells seen in other conditions, epidermal cells with homogeneous eosinophilic cytoplasm and pyknotic nuclei ("sunburn cells"), vacuolization of melanocytes and Langerhans cells, and a reduction in number of Langerhans cells. Dermal changes include vascular dilatation, perivenular edema, the presence of perivascular mononuclear and polymorphonuclear cells, and endothelial swelling (leading to partial occlusion of superficial blood vessels).

Management. Treatment for sunburn depends primarily on the utilization of measures that reduce exposure to strong sunlight. This is especially important for fair-skinned individuals, particularly blue-eyed persons, redheads, blonds, and those with freckles who withstand actinic exposure poorly, burn easily, and, over the years, tend to suffer chronic effects of light exposure. Prophylactic measures include timing of outdoor activities to avoid peak UV light exposure between 10 AM and 3 PM in the warm seasons of the year. Broad-rimmed hats and long-sleeved clothing help reduce the impact of harmful UV rays. However, the possibility of reflection must be considered, and it should be recognized that light-textured materials such as T-shirts (especially when wet) give only partial protection.

Sunscreens occupy an important position in the management of UV light exposure. The most common misconception (particularly among teenagers) is the belief that certain preparations can induce or promote a suntan. Sunscreens are topical preparations designed to protect the skin from the effects of UV light. They act as "screens" that absorb the light at particular wavelengths or as opaque "sun-blocking" agents that act as "barriers" and impede the passage of UV light. Since tanning and sunburn both result from the same UV waveband, it is difficult to promote one without promoting the other.

It should be noted that many commercially available preparations that claim to promote tanning afford little or no UV protection. The most effective and widely used sunscreens contain *p*-aminobenzoic acid (PABA) and its esters, benzophenones, anthranilates, and cinnamates in suitable vehicles that provide penetration of and adherence to the cutaneous surface. Ideally, sunscreens should be applied at least 30 minutes before the onset of sun exposure and reapplied after swimming, periods of excessive perspiration, frequent washing, or showering.

Sunscreens may be divided into three types depending on the wavelengths of sunlight they block. *Short UV sunscreens* screen the sunburn spectrum (290–320 nm). The most effective agents in this group are the formulations of PABA and its esters. One disadvantage of the PABA sunscreens is the fact that they may result in contact or photocontact dermatitis. It should be noted, however, that this can also be true of cinnamates, benzophenones, and other sunscreen ingredients.[3] PABA-free formulations are available for individuals who are sensitive to PABA or its ingredients. An open patch test on an area such as the patient's volar wrist prior to the use of any sunscreen is a reasonable precautionary measure.

Full-spectrum UV sunscreens screen a wider spectrum that includes both UVB (290–320 nm) and UVA (320–400 nm) wavelengths. In addition to their photoprotection against UVB sunburn, sun damage, and photocarcinogenesis, their advantage is the added protection from photosensitivity reactions and sun damage induced by UVA wavelengths.[4, 5]

Full-spectrum UV and *visible light sunscreens* are opaque formulations that block out all wavelengths between 290 and 700 nm. These include zinc oxide ointment, titanium oxide formulations, and red petroleum formulations (RVP, RVPaque, and RV Plus).

The use of sunscreens has been simplified by a classification based on sun protective factor (SPF) ratings. The SPF rating can be determined by dividing the least amount of time it takes to produce erythema on sunscreen-protected skin by the time it takes to produce the same erythema without sunscreen protection. Thus, individuals using a sunscreen with an SPF of 15 who normally burn following unprotected sun exposure can theoretically stay out 15 times longer before getting the same degree of erythema.

The degree to which a person sunburns or tans depends on genetic factors and the natural protection of the skin. Skin types, accordingly, are ranked from skin type I, the most sensitive, to skin type VI, the least sensitive to sun damage (Table 4–1). Since sun damage begins in children and sun damage is cumulative, it is strongly recommended that everyone adopt a program of sun protection and daily sunscreen use, preferably with an SPF of 15 or greater from early childhood on.[6, 7] Individuals with extreme photosensitivity should use sunscreens with levels higher than SPF 15. For blacks, who already have protective mela-

Table 4–1. SKIN TYPES AND PHOTOSENSITIVITY

Skin Type	Reactivity to Sun	Examples
I	Very sensitive: always burn easily and severely, tan little or not at all	Individuals with fair skin; blond hair, blue or brown eyes, and freckles
II	Very sensitive: usually burn easily, tan minimally or lightly	Individuals with fair skin; red, blond, or brown hair; and blue, hazel, or brown eyes
III	Moderately sensitive: burn moderately, tan gradually and uniformly	Average white individuals
IV	Moderately sensitive: burn minimally, tan easily	Individuals with dark brown hair, dark eyes, and white or light brown skin
V	Minimally sensitive: rarely burn, tan well and easily	Brown-skinned (middle Eastern and Hispanic) individuals
VI	Deeply pigmented: almost never burn, tan profusely	Blacks and others with heavy pigmentation

nin levels, sunscreens with an SPF of 6 or 8 may be adequate.

Treatment of sunburn consists of cool compresses or cool tub baths in colloidal oatmeal Aveeno [Rydell], baking soda, or cornstarch; topical formulations such as Prax or Pramosone (Ferndale), PrameGel (GenDerm), or Sarna foam or lotion (Stiefel); topical corticosteroid formulations; an emollient cream; and systemic preparations with analgesic and anti-inflammatory properties such as aspirin that diminish the untoward effects of prostaglandin. When symptoms are severe, a short course of systemic corticosteroids (oral prednisone, or its equivalent, in dosages of 20 to 60 mg, with tapering after a period of 4 to 8 days) will abort severe reactions and afford added relief. It should be noted that treatment of sunburn is not listed among the manufacturer's indications for the use of indomethacin, that conditions for its use in childhood have not been established, and that this preparation should not be prescribed for pregnant women, nursing mothers, or children younger than 14 years of age.

PHOTOSENSITIVITY REACTIONS

Photosensitivity is a broad term used to describe abnormal or adverse reactions to sunlight energy in the skin. Photosensitivity reactions may be phototoxic or photoallergic and endogenous or exogenous. Phototoxic reactions are common and can be likened to a primary irritant reaction. Photoallergy is relatively uncommon and presumably is dependent on antigen–antibody or cell-mediated hypersensitivity.

Phototoxic reactions refer to a nonimmunologic exaggerated sunburn or sunburn-like reaction characterized by erythema (and, at times, edema), occurring within a few minutes to several hours (usually within a period of 2 to 6 hours) after exposure to sunlight and followed by hyperpigmentation and desquamation confined to the exposed areas. This type of sensitivity usually occurs with the first exposure to the photosensitizing substance, when the systemic or percutaneous absorption of the sensitizing substances is in high enough

concentration to result in a photo-induced cutaneous reaction.

Histopathologic examination of phototoxic reactions reveals epidermal necrosis, epidermal cell degeneration, and dermal edema, with a mild to moderate infiltrate consisting mostly of polymorphonuclear leukocytes.

Photoallergic reactions are defined as an acquired delayed hypersensitivity dermatitis caused by light energy alone or by the presence of a photosensitizing substance plus sunlight. Photoallergic reactions are relatively uncommon and develop on initial occurrence after an incubation or refractory period of about 9 days. Instead of sunburn-type reactions, photoallergic responses are generally characterized by immediate urticarial or delayed papular or eczematoid lesions that are not followed by hyperpigmentation. After the first sensitization, subsequent photoallergic reactions generally appear within 24 hours after even very brief periods of exposure.

Histopathologic features of photoallergic reactions include spongiosis, intraepidermal vesiculation, infiltration of the epidermis by lymphocytes, and a characteristic, but not necessarily diagnostic, dense perivascular round cell infiltrate.

Immediate Photoallergic Responses (Solar Urticaria)

Solar urticaria is a relatively uncommon type I IgE-mediated type of sensitivity characterized by pruritus and erythema. It appears either during or within a few minutes of sunlight exposure and is followed almost immediately by a localized urticarial reaction (without pseudopods) confined to the exposed areas and an irregular flare reaction that extends onto unexposed skin (Fig. 4–1). After several hours the involved skin returns to its normal appearance and new lesions will not develop for 12 to 24 hours, even if subsequent exposure to sunlight occurs. Although the reaction is generally transient and usually fades within 15 or 30 minutes to 1 or 2 hours, scratching and rubbing may lead to secondary eczematization with persistent cutaneous changes.

Figure 4–1. Solar urticaria. A localized urticarial reaction occurred on the back of a 25-year-old woman within a few minutes following a 20-minute exposure to sun.

The disorder usually does not manifest until the third or fourth decade of life, and females are affected three times more often than males. It has been reported, however, as early as 3 years of age and, at times, may occur during later childhood or adolescence.

Solar urticaria represents a characteristic clinical phenomenon apparently due to or dependent on a variety of mechanisms.[8] An inborn error of protoporphyrin metabolism (erythropoietic protoporphyria), however, is responsible for some cases, and several categories of reactivity can be differentiated, namely, those sensitive to wavelengths in the UVB (290–320 nm), UVA (320–400 nm), and visible light (400–700 nm) ranges; the majority of patients react within the range of 290 to 480 nm. Passive transfer and reverse passive transfer tests have been positive in most case studies in the UV range shorter than 370 nm, thus supporting a proposed allergic nature of the process in this group. The mechanism of response in the other groups, however, remains uncertain.

The diagnosis of solar urticaria is based on the clinical picture and induction of lesions by natural or artificial light under controlled conditions. The differential diagnosis includes all agents capable of causing urticaria. The relationship to light, and the fact that lesions are confined solely to light-exposed areas, however, are helpful in establishing the true nature of this disorder.

In patients with mild forms of solar urticaria (those in whom the threshold is high) the disorder may be controlled simply by appropriate sunscreens and avoidance of prolonged unprotected sun exposure. Those individuals highly sensitive to sunlight, however, must completely avoid daytime exposure. Antihistamines, antimalarials, adrenocorticosteroids, and plasmapheresis have been beneficial in some patients; and in some individuals it is possible to build up sun tolerance slowly by carefully metered exposures to natural or artificial light or the oral administration of a psoralen followed by UVA (PUVA) radiation.[9–13] This procedure stimulates pigmentation and possibly depletes the UV-induced mediators of urticaria responsible for the clinical features seen in this disorder. In most patients treated in this manner tolerance can be maintained for 24 to 48 hours by brief, once or twice a week, 10- to 20-minute exposures administered alone or in combination with oral terfenadine (Seldane).

Delayed Photoallergic Reactions (Polymorphous Light Eruption)

Polymorphous light eruption is a term that was introduced in 1929 to describe a group of inflammatory disorders characterized by a delayed response to light (Fig. 4–2). Although its etiology remains unknown, it appears to be associated with a phototoxic reaction to UV rays in the 290- to 480-nm range, with the predominant activity (85 per cent of cases) in the sunburn range (290–320 nm).[14] Although the mechanism or mechanisms of the process have not been established, the clinical patterns, reaction time, histology, and flares of previously involved areas following exposure at distant sites suggest a delayed hypersensitivity response. The fact that this disorder is extremely common in Native Americans also suggests a possible genetic factor in some individuals.[15] Hereditary polymorphic light eruption occurs in Native Americans of both North and South America. Onset is in childhood, and female patients outnumber male patients 2:1. There is a positive family history in 75 per cent of cases, and an autosomal dominant mode of transmission is proposed. The eruption appears in spring, subsides in winter, and involves only exposed areas of the skin (Figs. 4–3 and 4–4).

Diagnosis. Despite conflicting results in individual studies, there appears to be no sex predisposition in this disease. Seen in children as well as adults, the disorder usually begins in young and middle-adult life, but it may occur at any age and appears to be the most common childhood-onset photodermatosis.[16, 17] Often referred to as "sun al-

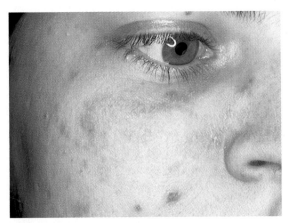

Figure 4–2. Polymorphous light eruption. Erythematous papulovesicular and plaque-like lesions with a characteristic distribution on the sun-exposed area of the cheek.

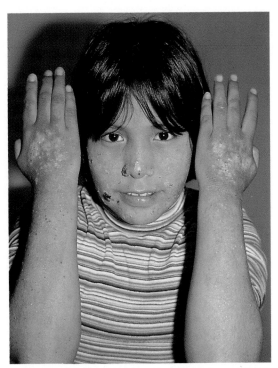

Figure 4–4. Papulovesicular and urticarial lesions on the face and sun-exposed areas of the arms and hands of a young girl with polymorphous light eruption. (Courtesy of Lincoln Krochmal, M.D.)

lergy," "sun poisoning," or actinic prurigo, the clinical eruption consists of a group of pleomorphic or polymorphic lesions that occur 1 to 2 days after sunlight exposure on exposed cutaneous areas. The lesions may range from small papular, urticarial, vesicular, or eczematous reactions to large papules, plaques, or patterns resembling erythema multiforme. The areas of the body most commonly involved include the face, the sides of the neck, and the arms, hands, legs, and feet. In children it most commonly begins on the face as an acute, erythematous, eczematous eruption with small papules (see Fig. 4–2). Pruritus, although relatively rare, may be severe. Lesions usually in-

volute spontaneously in 1 to 2 weeks, provided no additional exposure to sunlight occurs.

The diagnosis of polymorphous light eruption is suggested by the character of the lesions, their distribution, and their relationship to sun exposure. When the diagnosis remains in doubt, phototesting assists confirmation of the diagnosis and helps differentiate polymorphous light eruption from photocontact reactions and erythropoietic porphyria. This technque consists of exposing uninvolved skin of the forearm to three to five minimal erythema doses of UVB (rays shorter than 320 nm) every 24 to 72 hours for up to five exposures (this repeated exposure phototest is positive in 70 to 80 per cent of patients with polymorphous light eruption). Some patients with lupus erythematosus (LE), particularly those with systemic LE, acquire sun-induced lesions indistinguishable from those of polymorphous light eruption. Examination for evidence of systemic LE and fluorescent microscopic studies for basement membrane immunofluorescence and antinuclear antibodies, however, serve to differentiate these two disorders.[14]

Microscopic findings in all forms of polymorphous light eruption feature dense perivascular accumulations of round cells in the upper dermis and mid-dermis, with epidermal edema, spongiosis, and vesicle formation in urticarial, eczematous, and papular forms of this disorder. In the vesicular form, subepidermal blisters are present; in the

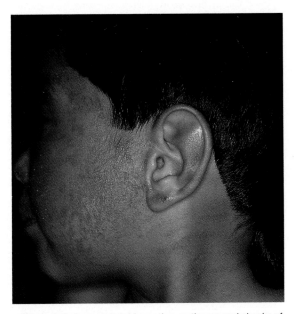

Figure 4–3. An eczematoid eruption on the ear and cheeks of an 8-year-old child from Colombia (polymorphous light eruption of the American Indian).

plaque type, histologic lesions are indistinguishable from early lesions of chronic discord LE.

Management. The treatment of polymorphous light eruption consists of sunscreens, appropriate clothing, and the avoidance of midday sun exposure. If patients severely affected by this disorder anticipate intense or prolonged sun exposure, synthetic antimalarials such as chloroquine, hydroxychloroquine (Plaquenil), and quinacrine (Atabrine) are extremely effective. Because of ocular complications associated with these preparations, however, their use should be reserved for severe cases involving short courses of therapy.

Beta-carotene, a carotenoid pigment that appears naturally in green and yellow vegetables, is available as Solatene (Roche). This preparation absorbs the visible spectrum of light (in the 360- to 600-nm range), with maximum absorption at 450 to 475 nm, and it has been found to be beneficial for patients with this disorder.[18] The usual dose for children younger than 14 years of age is 30 to 150 mg (1 to 5 capsules) per day, taken with meals; for adults it is 30 to 300 mg (1 to 10 capsules a day). The therapeutic dosage is adjusted to achieve serum beta-carotene levels of 600 to 800 μg/dl. The only side effects appear to be a slightly yellowish discoloration of the skin, first seen as yellowness of the palms and soles, orange-colored stools, and occasional gastrointestinal upset. Other forms of therapy include topical and systemic corticosteroids for acute exacerbations, oral nicotinamide, topical indomethacin, thalidomide, and the oral ingestion of a psoralen followed by UVA light exposure (PUVA therapy). Possible long-term effects of thalidomide (not available in the United States) and PUVA, however, suggest caution in their use for the treatment of this disorder in children.[19–22]

Photosensitivity Induced by Exogenous Sources

Exogenous photosensitizers may reach the skin by topical or systemic routes, and the reactions induced by them may be phototoxic or photoallergic.

Topical photosensitizers include furocoumarin-containing cosmetic preparations (e.g., Shalimar perfume); fluorescein derivatives, as in indelible lipsticks; and blankophores (optical brighteners) added to detergents.

Coal-tar preparations are time-honored topical therapies for childhood dermatoses. Although these preparations carry a warning regarding possible photosensitivity, documentation of childhood photosensitization from such products is uncommon, and most reports of photosensitivity involve adults contacting coal-tar preparations in industrial settings.

Clinical Manifestations

Salicylanilide Reactions. Since 1960, halogenated salicylanilides and related antibacterial and antifungal compounds were the most important

contact allergenic, photosensitizing agents. They were responsible for the vast majority of reactions reported in that decade, with an estimated 10,000 cases presumably caused by tetrachlorosalicylanilides in England between 1960 and 1962. Although tetrachlorosalicylanilides have been removed from general use, a number of related photosensitizers have been incorporated into soaps and other vehicles to combat infection, reduce body odor, and destroy fungi. These include hexachlorophene, dichlorophene, certain carbanilides, and antifungal agents chemically related to bithionol and tribromosalicylanilide (Figs. 4–5 and 4–6). Photosensitivity to salicylanilides probably represents a true delayed hypersensitivity phenomenon, appearing predominantly in 40- to 60-year-old men, and is relatively uncommon in childhood.[23, 24]

Sunscreens also, at times, may induce photoallergic-type reactions. One of these, padimate A, is capable of provoking phototoxic reactions.[25] Photoallergic reactions to blankophores (optical brighteners added to certain detergents) have also been reported by European observers but, fortunately, their use has been largely discontinued in the United States.

The hallmark of sunlight-induced photoreaction, whether toxic or allergic, is its characteristic distribution. The exposed areas of the face, neck, upper extremities, and, in women, the anterior aspects of the legs and proximal dorsal areas of the feet are most prominently affected.

Lesions are similar to an exaggerated sunburn reaction. Edema and vesiculation are prominent, and other cutaneous lesions include eczematous, morbilliform, papulovesicular, urticarial, and lichen planus–like reactions. The clinical course is brief, and elimination of the offending drug or sunlight exposure usually results in improvement. In

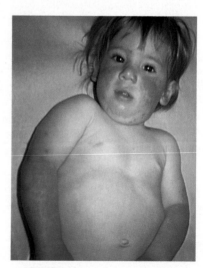

Figure 4–5. Drug-induced photosensitivity. Photoallergic dermatitis is seen on sun-exposed areas of an infant following topical use of hexachlorophene.

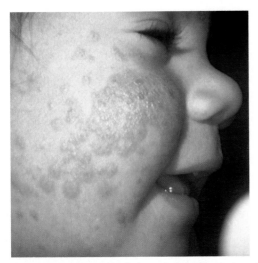

Figure 4–6. Papulovesicular lesions of photoallergic dermatitis due to hexachlorophene.

unusual cases, however, the photosensitivity may persist for months after the last known exposure to the offending chemical. Such individuals are known as *persistent light reactors.* Generally seen in middle-aged or older persons (usually men older than age 40), the eruption (more aptly termed *chronic actinic dermatitis*) ranges from a chronic dermatitis initially restricted to sun-exposed surfaces to thickened hyperpigmented plaques. Hypotheses presented to account for this condition include the possibilities that affected individuals continue to react because the photoallergen or a cross-reacting substance remains in the patient's environment, that the chemical may persist in the skin long after the original contact, and that a constituent of the skin has become altered and capable of eliciting the reaction.[26]

The action spectrum of topical and systemic photosensitizers is usually in the UVA range (320 to 400 nm). The upper eyelids, subnasal and submental areas, flexures of the wrist, and antecubital fossae (areas generally not as well exposed to sunlight) tend to be spared. Since UVA light passes through plate glass, the eruption may be accentuated on the left side of the face and left arm of drivers who drive automobiles from the left front seat position. Although clothing generally provides protection, reactions can also be produced by penetration of rays through light fabrics worn in summer.

Plant-Induced Photosensitivity (Phytophotodermatitis). Plant-induced photosensitivity (phytophotodermatitis) may at times be responsible for a number of dermatologic reactions. The large majority are phototoxic reactions due to the presence of furocoumarin compounds (psoralens) used in the treatment of psoriasis and vitiligo and found widely in such plants as parsnips, carrots, dill, parsley, figs, meadowgrass, giant hogweed, lemons, limes, mangos, wheat, clover, cocklebur, but-

tercups, Shepherd's purse, pigweed, and celery (particularly but not necessarily celery infected with a fungus that causes pink rot disease).[27, 28] Psoralens can also reach the skin following ingestion, such as noted in a report of grocery workers who developed phototoxic reactions following the ingestion of celery and subsequent outdoor and tanning salon UV light exposure.[28]

The light-induced eruption usually begins the day after exposure to the furocoumarin and sunlight, ranges in severity from mild erythema to severe blistering, and eventuates in a characteristic dense inflammatory hyperpigmentation (Figs. 4–7 through 4–9). A bizarre linear streaking configuration of the dermatitis, with subsequent hyperpigmentation, especially on the face, chest, hands, and lower legs of children, is characteristic and highly diagnostic of this disorder and, if unrecognized, may at times lead to a misdiagnosis of child abuse.[29]

Berloque (Berlock) Dermatitis. Several perfumes and colognes contain oil of bergamot, which is extracted from the peel of small oranges that grow in southern France and southern Italy. Oil of bergamot contains a furocoumarin (5-methylpsoralen), a potent photosensitizer; Shalimar perfume, containing 5- and 8-methoxypsoralen, is a common cause of berloque dermatitis.

Hyperpigmentation occurs in bizarre configurations according to areas of application, hence the drop-like or pendant-like configuration and the name *berloque* (misspelled from the French word *breloque*) or *Berlock* (German), meaning trinket or pendant. This dermatitis is seen most frequently

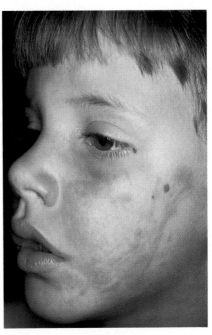

Figure 4–7. Plant-induced photosensitivity (phytophotosensitivity). Linear hyperpigmentation on the face of a child following exposure to limes and sunlight.

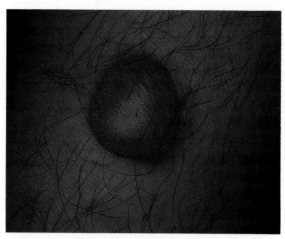

Figure 4–8. Photocontact dermatitis. A bullous lesion appeared on the forearm of a 15-year-old following exposure to sun and chemicals used while grooming a horse.

logic and histologic means. Photoallergic testing, however, is particularly valuable in the diagnosis of photoallergic contact dermatitis. By this method duplicate patch tests using suspected photoallergens are applied. One set is uncovered and irradiated with a window glass–filtered UV light source (one emitting only long-wave UV light rays) 24 hours after application. The following day a comparison is made of the covered and irradiated sites. A positive test reproduces the clinical eczematous lesion at the phototest site.

Management. The management of acute photosensitivity reactions consists of removal (whenever possible) of the offending agent. Protective clothing and full-spectrum sunscreens afford the greatest degree of protection against exposure. In addition, patients should minimize their exposure to natural sunlight, use broad-spectrum sunscreens that provide total (UVA as well as UVB) protection, and avoid unnecessary exposure to lamp sources with irradiance in the UV or visible light spectrum. These include fluorescent bulbs as well as UV sun lamps.

on the sides of the neck and in the retroauricular areas, shoulders, breasts, hands, and face of women. When seen in men, the disorder usually occurs on the bearded area and is related to oil of bergamot or related substances present in aftershave lotions.

Systemic Sources of Photosensitization. Systemic photosensitizers include systemic antibacterial agents (namely, demethylchlortetracycline and doxycycline and only rarely tetracycline, sulfonamides, or nalidixic acid); antifungal preparations (griseofulvin); phenothiazine derivatives, particularly chlorpromazine (Thorazine); sulfo-nylurea hypoglycemic agents; anovulatory drugs; antihistamines (particularly the phenothiazine congeners); furosemide; nonsteroidal antiinflammatory preparations such as naproxen (Naprosyn)[30]; the antiarrhythmic drug amiodarone (Cordarone)[31]; quinine; isoniazid; thiazide diuretics; and certain dyes (acridine, methylviolet, and eosin).

Diagnosis. Generally the diagnosis of photoallergic sensitization reactions depends on morpho-

Juvenile Spring Eruption

Juvenile spring eruption is a term used to describe a disorder of unknown etiology. Perhaps a sunburn reaction of children with light complexions, a mild photosensitivity or polymorphous light reaction, or possibly a form of erythema multiforme, the disorder has been described in England, particularly in boys (sometimes girls) aged 5 to 12 in the early spring on unprotected areas following exposure to sunlight. Most commonly affecting the helix of the ears (Fig. 4–10) and occasionally the dorsa of the hands and the trunk, the disorder is characterized by dull-red edematous papules, many of which become vesicular and crusted. The lesions heal within a week, without scarring, unless secondary infection develops. Topical corticosteroids may relieve itching, but sunscreens do not appear to prevent recurrences of this disorder.

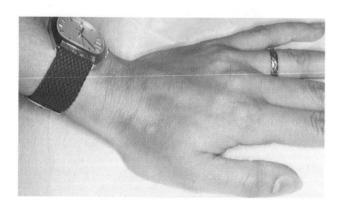

Figure 4–9. Hyperpigmentation on the dorsal aspect of the hands following the use of limes and sunlight exposure.

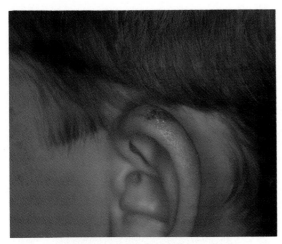

Figure 4–10. Juvenile spring eruption. A vesicular eruption on the superior aspect of the pinna of the ear of a fair-complected child occurred following sun exposure in the early spring.

Hydroa Aestivale and Hydroa Vacciniforme

Hydroa aestivale (summer prurigo of Hutchinson) and hydroa vacciniforme are rare, possibly related disorders that tend to appear each summer in children on uncovered parts of the body following exposure to sunlight. Boys are more often affected than girls in a ratio of 2 : 1. Although the role of heredity has not been clarified, these disorders appear to be transmitted as genetic recessive traits and are believed by some authorities to represent variants of polymorphous light eruption. Whereas some researchers believe hydroa vacciniforme to be a more severe form of hydroa aestivale, others use both terms interchangeably and consider distinctions between these disorders to be ambiguous and unnecessary.[32–34]

The mechanism of this disorder has not been clarified. Most current studies suggest a delayed erythema-type reaction to a UV action spectrum in the UVB (290–320 nm), UVC (254 nm), and, at times, UVA (320–400 nm) spectra (Fig. 4–11). The primary lesion is a pruritic edematous papule, vesicle, or bulla that occurs within hours or days on uncovered surfaces exposed to sunlight. Lesions tend to appear on the face, the sides of the neck, and extensor surfaces of the extremities and are arranged symmetrically over the nose, cheeks, ears, and dorsal surfaces of the hands. The vesicles or bullae usually develop on an erythematous base and initially are rather tense. These are followed by progressive necrosis that leads to healing with a varioliform scar. Although vesicular forms of polymorphous light eruption are rare, it should be noted that their clinical presentation may at times mimic hydroa aestivale and hydroa vacciniforme. Itching and burning as well as mild constitutional symptoms may precede the outbreak of the cutaneous lesions. The vesicles and bullae generally dry up after 3 to 4 days with the resultant formation of adherent brown crusts. The course of the disease is usually characterized by recurrent flares after sun exposure, and, in most instances, the disorder involutes spontaneously by the late teenage years.

Histopathologic examination of lesions reveals epidermal vesicles, areas of hyperkeratosis with acanthosis, and a perivascular, predominantly lymphocytic and polymorphonuclear infiltrate in the dermis.

Treatment of hydroa aestivale and hydroa vacciniforme consists of preventive measures such as appropriate sunscreens, proper clothing, and avoidance of midday sun exposure. Although antimalarial drugs and p-aminobenzoic acids have been used with some therapeutic success, because of potential ophthalmic complications antimalarial agents must be used with extreme caution, particularly in children.[33] Although not fully studied in children, beta-carotene (Solatene) appears to offer relief for individuals with this disorder.[34]

GENETIC DISORDERS ASSOCIATED WITH PHOTOSENSITIVITY

Xeroderma Pigmentosum

Xeroderma pigmentosum is a severe, rare autosomal recessive disease characterized by cutaneous photosensitivity, a decreased ability to repair DNA damaged by UV radiation, and a tendency to early development of cutaneous malignancies.

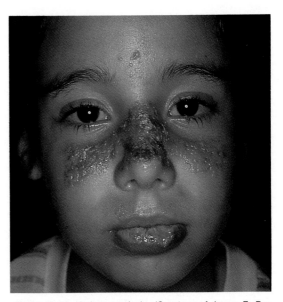

Figure 4–11. Hydroa aestivale. (Courtesy of James E. Rasmussen, M.D.)

The cardinal features of this disorder include sensitivity to light at wavelengths in the UVB spectrum, primarily 290 to 320 nm; premature aging of the skin accompanied by dystrophy, pigmentary changes, and the development of epithelial neoplasms; severe eye involvement; progressive neurologic degeneration in some patients; and malignancy.

Estimated to occur in a frequency of 1 in 250,000 individuals in the United States and Europe, and with a higher 1 in 40,000 incidence in Japan, the basic abnormality is attributed to a defect in endonuclease, an enzyme that recognizes UV light–damaged regions of DNA and excises damaged thymine dimers so that other enzymes (DNA polymerase and polynucleotide ligase) may initiate DNA repair. Recent techniques have led to the identification of at least eight different forms of DNA repair defects (complementation groups A through G, plus a "variant" form).[35, 36]

Clinical Manifestations. Children with xeroderma pigmentosum develop erythema, freckling, and increased pigmentation after exposure to sunlight. Most cases begin in early childhood. In 75 per cent of cases the first symptoms appear between 6 months and 3 years of age and reach the tumor stage (basal cell carcinoma, angiosarcoma, fibrosarcoma, keratoacanthoma, and malignant melanoma) before age 20.

In the acute form the first manifestations appear very early, sometimes shortly after birth or during the first weeks of life, after the first exposure to sun. Initial clinical findings include photophobia, erythema (which sometimes progresses to vesiculation and bulla formation), freckled hyperpigmentation of exposed parts, and subsequent papillomatous or verrucous lesions followed by degenerative and eventual malignant changes (Fig. 4–12).

Many authors have reported the presence of neurologic complications in patients with this disorder. In addition to their cutaneous manifestations, those with the most severe form of xeroderma pigmentosum (termed the *DeSanctis-Cacchione* syndrome) have microcephaly with mental deficiency, premature closure of the sutures, retarded growth and sexual development, choreoathetosis, cerebellar ataxia, shortening of the Achilles tendons, and, at times, sensorineural deafness.[37]

Once the possibility of xeroderma pigmentosum is suspected, the clinical features are so distinctive that diagnosis is usually obvious. The characteristic clinical features include erythema, freckling, both hyperpigmentation and depigmentation, an appearance of premature aging, telangiectasias, hyperkeratoses, ulcerations, keratoacanthomas, and, after a relatively short period of time, skin cancers. Areas of skin ordinarily protected by clothing remain relatively normal or may eventually show similar features, but to a lesser degree. Conjunctivitis, keratitis, corneal opacities and ulcerations, photophobia, blepharitis, crust-

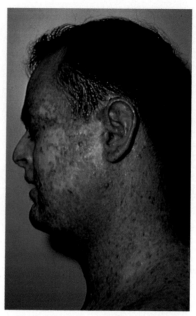

Figure 4–12. Xeroderma pigmentosum. Freckled hyperpigmentation and papillomatous and verrucous lesions on the face and neck. (Courtesy of Department of Dermatology. Yale University School of Medicine.)

ing of the eyelids, symblepharon, and ectropion are highly characteristic and are said to occur in 60 to 90 per cent of individuals with this disorder.

Management. When present at an early age, xeroderma pigmentosum usually presents a relentless course with irreversible skin damage. Although the severity of the disease varies, those individuals with severe forms frequently die before they reach the age of 10 years, and two thirds of affected children die before the age of 20. Treatment consists of genetic counseling; vigorous avoidance of UV light exposure; methylcellulose eye drops to keep the corneas moist and soft contact lenses to protect against mechanical trauma in individuals whose eyelids are severely deformed; corneal transplantation for patients with severe keratitis and corneal opacity; destruction of individual premalignant and malignant tumors by topical antimetabolite agents such as 5-fluorouracil; removal of malignant lesions; and dermabrasion of actinically damaged skin, or resurfacing of severely damaged skin, by dermatome shaving with homografts from less severely involved cutaneous surfaces.[38] Although the use of high-dose oral isotretinoin has been successful in the prevention of new skin cancers, withdrawal of therapy results in reversal of its chemoprophylactic effect.[39] Treatment of this defect is not yet available, but prenatal diagnosis can be reassuring if the fetus is free of chromosomal aberrations, or it can afford an opportunity to elect termination of pregnancy if abnormalities are present.[40]

Hartnup Disease

Hartnup disease (named after the family in whom the disorder was first reported) is a rare autosomal recessive light-sensitive disorder characterized by a pellagra-like cutaneous eruption, neurologic abnormalities, and a specific aminoaciduria (due to a defect in the cellular transport of a group of monoamino-monocarboxylic acids). The basic defects appear to be a failure in the absorption of tryptophan from the gastrointestinal tract and a renal tubular defect causing inadequate reabsorption of amino acids, including tryptophan. These result in reduced levels of available tryptophan and, accordingly, nicotinic acid, which in turn may be responsible for the pellagra-like photosensitivity.

The biochemical defect (aminoaciduria) is a constant feature of Hartnup disease. Clinical manifestations, however, are intermittent, recurrent, and quite variable. The cutaneous eruption usually appears in the spring and summer. It may be present in early childhood, occasionally during early infancy, and, when present, is usually seen in children between 3 and 9 years of age, with symptoms generally becoming milder with increasing age. The cutaneous manifestations consist of a symmetrical distribution of inflammatory macules that tend to coalesce and eventuate in well-marginated red scaly lesions over light-exposed parts of the face, neck, uncovered areas of the arms, inframammary and perineal folds, elbows, knees, dorsal aspects of the hands, wrists, and lower legs; once they appear, they usually persist for weeks or months.

Acute dermatitis and blistering with secondary crusting and scarring frequently occur following sun exposure. These changes, together with marked hyperpigmentation, are similar to the findings seen in pellagra. Malnutrition and intercurrent infections frequently aggravate the dermatitis, and glossitis, angular stomatitis, vulvovaginitis, diffuse hair loss and fragility, and nail abnormalities (longitudinal streaking) may also be seen. In many patients, the cutaneous manifestations become milder with subsequent sun exposure, and some individuals may occasionally tolerate the sun without any difficulty. The reason for this inconsistency is not known.

Cerebellar ataxia is the predominant neurologic feature of Hartnup disease. Seen in over two thirds of those afflicted with this disorder, it seems to occur during periods when the rash is most prominent or following acute episodes of febrile illness. The gait is broad-based and unsteady, and patients have both nystagmus and an intention tremor. Ocular abnormalities include diplopia and ptosis, and some patients have mental retardation, emotional lability, or frank psychosis.

The diagnosis of Hartnup disease is based on the clinical picture and demonstration of specific amino acid and indole excretion patterns (not the total amino acid excretion). Treatment consists of avoidance of sunlight exposure and prolonged oral administration of high doses (40 to 200 mg) of nicotinic acid or nicotinamide. Since nicotinamide does not cause the flushing generally associated with administration of nicotinic acid, the former is generally the drug of choice. Although the eruption and ataxia seem to improve when patients are on this regimen, assessment of therapy is difficult since the natural history of the disorder is one of spontaneous remission and exacerbation.

Pellagra

Pellagra is a systemic disturbance caused by a cellular deficiency of niacin due to inadequate dietary intake of nicotinic acid or its precursor (tryptophan) or the ingestion of certain antinicotinic substances, such as hydantoin derivatives used in the therapy for epilepsy or the antituberculosis drug isoniazid. This nicotinamide deficiency state may be seen in all ages, but as a result of current nutritional standards and vitamin supplementation, it is relatively rare in infancy and in children in most parts of the world. It still occurs, however, as a result of dietary insufficiency in children as well as adults, in chronic alcoholics, in malnourished homeless persons, in adolescents with anorexia nervosa, in patients with malabsorption syndromes, and in individuals maintained on diets high in corn.[41, 42]

Characterized by seasonal recurrences and a classic triad of dermatitis, diarrhea, and dementia, at the onset of the disorder there is weakness, loss of appetite, abdominal pain, mental depression, and photosensitivity. In later stages, nervous symptoms may predominate to such a degree that the cutaneous lesions may be overlooked. The most prominent cutaneous lesions of pellagra are precipitated by the sun and, although not always present, begin as asymptomatic or pruritic symmetrical erythematous eruptions on areas exposed to sunlight, heat, friction, or pressure. The usual sites of involvement include the face, neck, dorsal surface of the hands, arms, feet, inguinal region, and, particularly in infants and small children, the diaper area. The eruptions begin as well-marginated erythema and superficial scaling on sun-exposed areas resembling sunburn (with or without vesiculation or blister formation) that gradually subside leaving a dusky brown-red discoloration (Fig. 4–13). In acute cases the lesions may progress to vesiculation, ulceration, exudation, cracking, and, at times, secondary infection. With chronicity, lesions become more livid, thickened, scaly, and ultimately fissured, atrophic, and deeply pigmented (Fig. 4–14). About the lower neck the eruption may appear as a broad collarette of dermatitis known as *Casal's necklace*. In cases in which the "necklace" is incomplete, the lesions maintain their symmetrical and otherwise characteristic appearance.

The nose has a fairly distinctive appearance with a dull erythema of the nasal bridge, slight scaling,

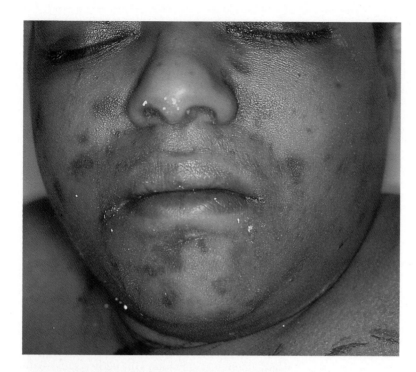

Figure 4–13. Pellagra. Symmetrical erythematous eruption on the face was precipitated by sun exposure. (Hurwitz S: The Skin and Systemic Disease in Children. Year Book Medical Publishers, Inc., Chicago, 1985.)

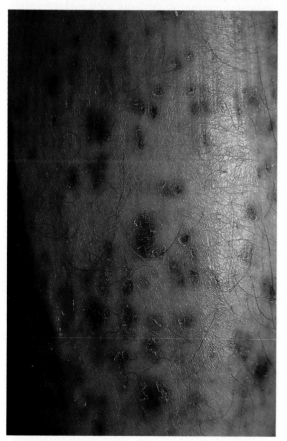

Figure 4–14. Pellagra. Well-marginated eruptions are seen on the sun-exposed aspect of the leg. (Courtesy of Charles Samuel Fulk, M.D.)

and a powdery appearance. Mucous membrane involvement, when present, consists of painful fissures and ulceration. The lips and cheeks are thin and pale, the mouth is dry, and the tongue is red, swollen, and, at times, darkened (the so-called black tongue). Aphthous ulcers, fissuring, and angular cheilitis are also common.

Neurologic manifestations may appear with or without involvement of the skin and digestive tract. In mild cases they consist of weakness, anorexia, and depression. In more severe cases, delirium, amentia, posterolateral spinal cord degeneration, and pyramidal and peripheral nerve involvement may be noted. The disease tends to be progressive and, if untreated, may eventuate in death within a period of several years.

Diagnosis. The characteristic skin lesions, with or without gastrointestinal and neurologic manifestations, should suggest the diagnosis. This can be aided by an abnormal dietary history or a history of therapy with antinicotinic substances such as hydantoin or isoniazid. When the diagnosis is suspected, measurement of the urinary excretion of N_1-methylnicotinamide and/or pyridone (metabolites of niacin) is helpful. Histopathologic examination of cutaneous lesions of pellagra is nonspecific. Early lesions present as a chronic inflammatory infiltrate in the upper dermis and, at times, as subepidermal or intraepidermal vesicles or bullae. Older lesions are characterized by hyperkeratosis, parakeratosis, and a moderate degree of acanthosis. Melanin is increased in the basal layer of the epidermis, and the dermis may show fibrosis in addition to the chronic inflammatory infiltrate. Although the histologic picture of pellagra is frequently not diagnostic and may merely present as a chronic dermatitis, in the end-stages of the disorder, atrophy of the stratum malpighii and hyperkeratosis with areas of parakeratosis, increased melanin in the basal layer of the epidermis, dermal fibrosis, and chronic inflammation may help differentiate this disorder from other forms of chronic dermatitis.

Treatment. Treatment of pellagra consists of a high-protein diet and nicotinic acid or nicotinamide in dosages of 100 to 400 mg/day supplemented by vitamin B complex. If a good diet can be maintained, complete recovery is the rule.

Rothmund-Thomson Syndrome (Poikiloderma Congenitale)

Poikiloderma congenitale (Rothmund-Thomson syndrome) is a rare autosomal recessive disorder, with only 121 cases reported in the English literature, characterized by atrophy, pigmentation, and telangiectasia of the skin in association with juvenile cataracts, shortness of stature, partial or total alopecia, defects of the nails and teeth, and hypogonadism.[43–45]

Although the skin may be involved at birth, cutaneous changes generally make their appearance between the third and sixth months of life. Cutaneous features include diffuse erythema and, at times, edema and vesiculation of the cheeks, forehead, chin, ears, buttocks, and extensor surfaces of the arms and legs. As the erythema resolves, the skin begins to show a reticulated pattern of telangiectasia and alterations in pigmentation (both hypopigmentation and hyperpigmentation) with areas of atrophy. Children may at times develop bullae after sun exposure (this tendency appears to subside as patients grow older); a small percentage of patients develop verrucous hyperkeratoses on the hands, feet, knees, and elbows at puberty or during adolescence. Although photosensitivity is a feature of many cases and exposure to sunlight may extend the distribution of the eruption, they probably are not responsible for the poikilodermatous appearance that develops on unexposed as well as light-exposed areas.

Patients are frequently short, and some have a characteristic facies with saddle nose, frontal bossing, wide forehead, and narrow chin, giving a triangular configuration to the face. Hypotrichosis with sparse or absent eyebrows or eyelashes (and sometimes involvement of the scalp, face, and body) occurs in 50 per cent of patients. Hypogonadism occurs in one fourth of patients (female patients may be amenorrheic; male patients may have undescended testes), and affected individuals may exhibit premature graying and loss of hair.

Cataracts occur in about 40 per cent of reported cases, and defective bone development, which predominantly involves the long bones, occurs in about two thirds of affected individuals (absence,

hypoplasia, or other dysplasias of bones are most common at the distal portions of the limbs). Other deformities include absence or shortening of digits, cleft hand or foot, an asymmetry in length of limbs, and cystic lesions, osteoporosis, and sclerotic areas on radiographic examination of the long bones and pelvic areas. Nail changes (rough, ridged, heaped-up, small, or atrophic nails) and dental abnormalities (microdontia, malformation, and failure of teeth to erupt) may be seen, and, as in patients with radiodermatitis, carcinomatous changes may develop in some adults with this disorder.

The disorder has been seen at times with features of epidermolysis bullosa (this is known as the Kindler or Weary-Kindler syndrome), and some authorities separate the Rothmund-Thomson syndrome into two variants. In the *Rothmund* variant consanguinity of parents is frequent, juvenile cataracts are generally present, cutaneous lesions appear to be more degenerative and atrophic, depressed striae and marked diminution of eyebrows and eyelashes may be present, and patients frequently have a saddle nose and frontal bossing. In the *Thomson* variant consanguinity of parents is infrequent, cataracts are absent, cutaneous changes are characterized by fine punctate pitting, hypotrichosis of the eyebrows and eyelashes is less apparent, a triangular facies with a wide disproportionate forehead and narrow chin is present, and congenital anomalies such as dystrophy or absence of distal portions of the limbs may be noted.

Individuals with the Rothmund-Thomson syndrome have a normal life span, and there is no effective treatment except for the use of sunscreens, prophylactic avoidance of sunlight, and surgical attention to keratoses and carcinomas of the skin.

Bloom's Syndrome

Bloom's syndrome (congenital telangiectatic erythema) is a rare autosomal recessive disorder characterized by a triad of telangiectatic erythema, photosensitivity, and severe intrauterine and postnatal growth retardation.[46] In this disorder, erythema of the cheeks, often resembling lesions of lupus erythematosus, appears, between the second and third week of life, and typically spreads with exposure to sunlight to involve the nose, eyelids, forehead, ears, and lips. Eighty per cent of affected children are male, and 50 per cent are of Ashkenazic Jewish ancestry.[47]

Affected patients are born at term with reduced body weight and size. They have small narrow faces with prominent features and, although physical growth is stunted, intellectual and sexual development is normal. The cutaneous changes include facial erythema in a butterfly distribution that develops after exposure to sunlight. Although this light sensitivity eventually disappears, erythema, telangiectasia, mottled pigmentation, scarring, and atrophy of these sites remain as prominent features. Other findings may include café au lait spots, defective dentition, prominent ears, dolichocephaly, polydactyly, clinodactyly, syndactyly, cryptorchidism, shortened lower extremities, clubbed feet, reduced levels of immunoglobulins (especially of IgA and IgM), a high incidence of nonspecific chromosomal breakage, and increased predisposition to neoplastic disease, particularly Wilms' tumor and leukemia, lymphosarcoma, and carcinomas of the alimentary tract (the mouth and esophagus) during the second and third decades of life.[48, 49] Patients also develop serious and sometimes fatal gastrointestinal and respiratory tract bacterial infections early in life as a result of defects of both humoral and cellular immune function. With increasing age, however, resistance to infection tends to become more normal.

The diagnosis of Bloom's syndrome may be suggested by a history of low birth weight and the presence of facial telangiectasia and photosensitivity in a child of small stature of Ashkenazic Jewish heritage, and can be confirmed by chromosomal abnormalities (an increased rate of chromosomal breakage and sister chromatid exchange in cultured leukocytes and fibroblasts).

Although there is no specific treatment, avoidance of sun exposure and protection by sunscreens can help prevent some of the cutaneous eruptions associated with photosensitivity. Appropriate antibiotics for gastrointestinal and respiratory tract bacterial infections are frequently helpful in the management of patients with this disorder, and, since life expectancy may be shortened by malignancy, periodic evaluation for possible neoplastic disease is advisable.

Cockayne's Syndrome

Cockayne's syndrome (trisomy 10) is a rare, recessively inherited disorder, generally seen in persons of English lineage, characterized by dwarfism, bird-like facies, sunken eyes, large eyes and nose, disproportionately large extremities, a "senile" appearance in childhood due to diffuse loss of subcutaneous fat, telangiectasia, photosensitivity, quick bird-like movements, and a 4 : 1 male preponderance.[50]

Children with Cockayne's syndrome appear to be normal during infancy and develop signs of the disorder during the second year of life. The cutaneous changes include facial erythema in a butterfly distribution that develops after exposure to sunlight. Although this light sensitivity eventually disappears, erythema with telangiectasias characteristic of photosensitivity, mottled pigmentation, scarring, and atrophy of these sites remain as prominent features. Loss of subcutaneous fat produces a "bird-like" facies; a tendency toward progressive ataxia, long limbs (the upper extremities are long in proportion to body length), quick bird-like movements, disproportionately large hands and feet, progressive contractures of the joints, and large protruding ears suggest a "Mickey Mouse"–like appearance.

Affected individuals are generally below the tenth percentile for height, and other abnormalities include thickened skull bones, sunken eyes, intracranial calcification, hypertension and renal disease in some individuals, retinal pigmentation, optic atrophy, cataracts, deafness, and mental retardation. The skin becomes atrophic and develops striae, and scalp and body hair are sparse. There is no effective treatment for patients with this disorder, and most patients die in the second or third decade of life as a result of arteriosclerotic vascular disease, profound neurologic deterioration, or both.

KWASHIORKOR

Kwashiorkor, a clinical syndrome that results from a severe deficiency of protein (and less than adequate caloric intake), is the most serious and prevalent form of malnutrition in the world today. Seen primarily in industrially underdeveloped countries, the inadequate protein intake results in amino acid (phenylalanine and tyrosine) deficiency, pellagrous cutaneous changes, hair abnormalities, impaired growth, mental and gastrointestinal features, and, in the absence of proper dietary treatment, a high mortality rate.

The clinical picture generally occurs in children between 6 months and 5 years of age and consists of a conspicuous dermatosis that begins as an erythema that blanches on pressure, rapidly followed by small dusky purple patches that do not blanch. The eruption has a sharply marginated edge raised above the surrounding skin, much as enamel paint that is lifting up and about to peel off. In contrast to lesions of pellagra, the dermatosis seldom appears on areas exposed to sunlight and tends to spare the feet and dorsal areas of the hands. Photosensitivity, purpura, and excessive bruisability may also be present. Other associated features include changes in mental behavior, anorexia, apathy, irritability, growth retardation, fatty infiltration of the liver with hypoproteinemia, and, as a result, edema of the face, feet, and abdomen with a characteristic potbelly appearance.

In mild cases the cutaneous eruption is associated with a superficial desquamation; in severe cases there are large areas of erosion. As the disease progresses, the entire cutaneous surface develops a reddish or coffee-colored hue, hence the term *red children*. Other associated features include circumoral pallor, loss of pigmentation (especially after minor trauma), and depigmentation of the hair from its normal black color in African children to a reddish yellow, gray, or straw color. Edema, xerosis, fine branny desquamation, dyschromia with hypopigmentation (perhaps due to phenylalanine deficiency), and cracking along Langer's lines that produces a "mosaic" or "cracked" appearance of the skin complete the cutaneous picture. When periods of malnutrition alternate with intervals of adequate dietary intake, alternating bands of light and dark color (the flag sign) are produced in the hair.[51]

Children afflicted with kwashiorkor are extremely ill, and if they are not treated the mortality rate can be 30 per cent or more. In areas where the disorder is common, since even small amounts of milk provide many of the necessary nutriments lacking in the local diet, breast feeding should be encouraged and continued for longer periods of time than is customary. Treatment of affected individuals consists of administration of a high-protein diet, vitamin supplementation, and correction of dehydration and electrolyte imbalance.

THE PORPHYRIAS

The porphyrias comprise a group of genetically determined or acquired disorders of porphyrin, the chemical precursor for hemoglobin synthesis. Porphyrins, the only well-established photosensitizers made by the human body, are substances that produce photodynamic types of phototoxic reactions with a primary action spectrum in the 400-nm range. There are two main categories of porphyric disease in humans. Based on the tissue in which the biochemical abnormality is experienced, they are classified into erythropoietic or hepatic forms. The erythropoietic porphyrias are divided into erythropoietic porphyria and erythropoietic protoporphyria; the hepatic porphyrias include acute intermittent porphyria, porphyria cutanea tarda, hepatoerythropoietic porphyria, hereditary coproporphyria, and a combination of acute intermittent porphyria and porphyria cutanea tarda (porphyria variegata).[52]

Erythropoietic Porphyrias

CONGENITAL ERYTHROPOIETIC PORPHYRIA

Erythropoietic porphyria (congenital erythropoietic porphyria, EP, Günther's disease) is an extremely rare porphyric disorder. The only porphyria inherited in an autosomal recessive manner and with fewer than 200 cases reported in the world literature, it is characterized by the appearance of red urine during infancy, severe photosensitivity that occurs in the first 2 or 3 years of life, splenomegaly, and hemolytic anemia.

Photosensitivity is frequently absent in the neonatal period but generally becomes apparent during the first years of life as exposure to the sun increases. Recurrent vesicobullous eruptions on sun-exposed areas of the skin eventually result in mutilating ulceration, scarring, and loss of acral tissues, such as the ears, tip of the nose, distal phalanges, and nails. Other common clinical features include hypertrichosis manifested as fine

blond lanugo hair over the face and extremities, conjunctivitis, keratitis, brown-stained teeth that fluoresce under exposure to Wood's light, hyperpigmentation, hemolytic anemia, growth retardation, and bone fragility due to encroachment of the hyperplastic marrow on the cortex. The legendary werewolves of the middle ages, with fluorescent teeth and nails, mutilated and deformed ears, nose, and eyelids, and nocturnal habits due to their sensitivity to light, may have been persons afflicted with congenital erythropoietic porphyria.

The biochemical disturbance in this disorder appears to be a deficiency of the enzyme uroporphyrinogen cosynthetase III (urocosyn III), resulting in marked overproduction of uroporphyrin I and coproporphyrin I in circulating erythrocytes and bone marrow cells.

The diagnosis of erythropoietic porphyria can be made by the clinical features that appear early (usually in the first few months of life): vesicular or bullous photosensitivity, pinkish red urine, fluorescence of the teeth and nails under black light examination, and sharply elevated levels of uroporphyrin I (20 to 50 times greater than normal) in erythrocytes, plasma, urine, and feces. When the diagnosis is suspected, screening tests with the aid of a Wood's light may reveal reddish orange porphyrin fluorescence in urine or aqueous suspensions of feces and red fluorescence in thin smears of peripheral erythrocytes examined under a fluorescent microscope. Prenatal diagnosis is possible by means of analysis of amniotic fluid and cells. Splenomegaly, an almost constant feature of this disorder, may remain undetected during the neonatal period only to appear as the child grows older. In the majority of reported cases hemolytic activity is indicated by normochromic anemia, elevated reticulocyte levels, circulating normoblasts, normoblastic hyperplasia of the bone marrow, and increased excretion of fecal urobilinogen. The anemia is believed to be due to hemolysis secondary to an intracorpuscular defect and ineffective erythropoiesis. The color of the urine of patients may vary from faint pink to burgundy or port-wine, depending on the concentration of uroporphyrin derived from the oxidation of uroporphyrinogen.

Since the skin lesions are the same in all types of porphyria with cutaneous lesions, and differences are based on the severity rather than the type of porphyria, skin biopsies are helpful but cannot be relied on for a definitive diagnosis. Histopathologic examination may reveal subepidermal bullae and an atrophic epidermis with destruction of adnexal glands and fibrosis in patients with advanced disease. Other features include varying degrees of inflammatory change and periodic acid–Schiff-positive staining hyaline material around small vessels in the papillary dermis.

The prognosis of erythropoietic porphyria is poor, with few patients surviving into the fourth or fifth decade. Death, when it occurs, is frequently associated with hemolytic anemia. Treatment includes avoidance of sun exposure and trauma, with resolution of cutaneous manifestations, anemia, and splenomegaly often occurring with protection from light at wavelengths below 510 nm. Splenectomy, although frequently recommended, and chronic transfusion regimens, in an effort to suppress the endogenous bone marrow activity, have had variable success.[52, 53] Window glass and ordinary sunscreen preparations do not protect against light waves absorbed by porphyrins. Therefore, appropriate clothing and wide-spectrum sun protectants should be used (indoors as well as outdoors) for appropriate topical protection. Oral beta-carotene (Solatene), in doses of 30 to 150 mg/day, also appears to be an effective photoprotective agent.[54]

ERYTHROPOIETIC PROTOPORPHYRIA

Erythropoietic protoporphyria (EPP), the most common form of porphyria, is an autosomal dominant disorder with variable expressivity characterized by photosensitivity, eczematization and inflammation of exposed skin, and high concentrations of protoporphyrin in erythrocytes, plasma, and feces. The primary biochemical defect appears to be related to a deficiency of ferrochelatase, the enzyme that accelerates the incorporation of iron into protoporphyrin. Approximately 300 cases have been reported, but frequent subtlety of clinical signs and symptoms and the absence of increased levels of protoporphyrin in urine (due to the relative insolubility of this porphyrin in water) predispose toward frequent failure of recognition.[52]

Erythropoietic protoporphyria usually becomes symptomatic between the ages of 2 and 5 years. It may present clinically as burning, tingling, or itching of the exposed skin (often manifested by the child's crying when placed in sunshine) following short periods of sunlight exposure. This burning sensation may be followed by pruritic reddened edematous plaques that return to normal within 24 hours, occasionally papulovesicular and petechial eruptions that may persist for longer periods, and chronic changes such as hypopigmentation, hyperpigmentation, and a papular thickening that gives a cobblestone appearance to the skin. Despite the severely painful acute symptoms, chronic skin manifestations tend to be mild, ranging from grossly undetectable lesions to shallow linear or elliptical pits on the face, linear furrows around the lips, thickened hyperkeratotic skin, and a weatherbeaten, leathery, or pebbly appearance, particularly over the knuckles (Figs. 4-15 through 4-17). In a few patients, hypersplenism with associated anemia (which responds favorably to splenectomy) has been reported. Liver biopsy specimens from patients with erythropoietic protoporphyria reveal portal and periportal fibrosis and deposition of pigment in bile canaliculi and bile ducts with terminal hepatic failure (in a small number of patients). Cholecystitis and cholelithiasis have also been reported (in up to 12 per cent of

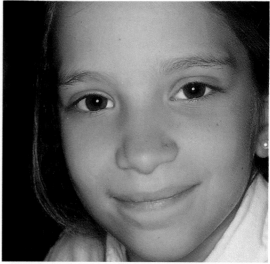

Figure 4–15. Erythematous pruritic lesions on the nasal area of a 6-year-old girl with erythropoietic protoporphyria.

patients), with gallstones consisting of almost pure protoporphyrin IX. It now appears that this disease is much more common than previously suspected and may account for many undiagnosed light-sensitive reactions. Laboratory findings include abnormally high protoporphyrin levels in circulating erythrocytes, bone marrow cells, and plasma. Fluorescence of the erythrocytes can be demonstrated by Wood's light or fluorescence microscopy.[55] In contrast to erythropoietic porphyria, fluorescence of teeth and nails is not present and there is no increase in fecal or urinary levels of uroporphyrins.

As in congenital erythropoietic porphyria, window glass does not protect patients with this disor-

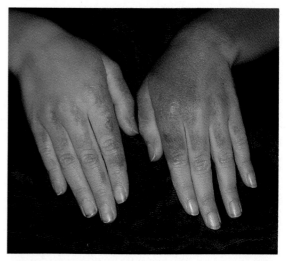

Figure 4–16. Painful purpuric edematous plaques following sun exposure on the dorsal aspect of the hands of a 6-year-old girl with erythropoietic protoporphyria.

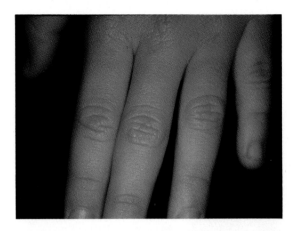

Figure 4–17. Thickened hyperkeratotic skin with a pebbly texture over the knuckles is a subtle, frequently overlooked clinical clue to the diagnosis of erythropoietic protoporphyria in an 8-year-old girl with this disorder.

der. The management of erythropoietic protoporphyria, accordingly, is dependent on limited exposure to sunlight, use of opaque sunscreens, administration of beta-carotene (Solatene), and hypertransfusion and exchange transfusion techniques.[52, 56] Other therapeutic approaches include the oral administration of cholestyramine, which helps prevent reabsorption of protoporphyrin excreted into the intestinal lumen,[57] or pyridoxine[58]; and, for patients with progressively deteriorating liver function, liver transplantation can be used as an option of last resort.[52]

Hepatic Porphyrias

ACUTE INTERMITTENT PORPHYRIA

Acute intermittent porphyria (AIP) is a rare autosomal dominant disorder characterized by overproduction of porphyrin precursors (aminolevulinic acid and porphobilinogen); episodes of abdominal pain associated with vomiting; constipation; peripheral paresis or paralysis; and psychological manifestations or psychoneuroses provoked by barbiturates, sulfonamides, dapsone, griseofulvin, anticonvulsive agents, sulfonylurea compounds, and estrogens. Although the disease never manifests before puberty, the disorder is included here as a matter of completeness. Women seem to have a greater predisposition than men to develop this disorder, and photosensitivity is not reported. Freshly voided urine may be colorless and only darkens on standing; and, except for possible laparotomy scars from previous abdominal surgery, cutaneous lesions are absent.

The fundamental problem of diagnosis is the differentiation of acute intermittent porphyria from medical or surgical cases of an acute abdomen and from other organic, psychiatric, or neurologic disease. The classic triad of abdominal pain, urine that darkens on standing, and neuropsychiatric symptoms, particularly when associated with multiple laparotomy scars from previous surgery, should raise suspicion of this disorder. Diagnosis can be made by the demonstration of elevated aminolevulinic acid and porphobilinogen levels during attacks and by the demonstration of porphobilinogen in the urine by the Watson-Schwartz test.

There is no effective treatment for acute intermittent porphyria. Drugs that are known to precipitate attacks of porphyria should be avoided. Bromides have been used with success, propoxyphene (Darvon) is tolerated well, chlorpromazine (Thorazine) is useful for the treatment of acute abdominal pain, and meperidine (Demerol) is effective for severe pain.

PORPHYRIA CUTANEA TARDA

Porphyria cutanea tarda (PCT), the most common form of porphyria, appears to be an inborn error of metabolism characterized by the excretion of excessive uroporphyrin and coproporphyrin in both urine and feces. Estimated to have an incidence of 1 in 25,000, it is most common in adults during the third and fourth decades of life. This disorder has also been seen in children (three cases have been reported in children younger than 15 years of age, with one as young as 2 years of age) and has a high incidence among the Bantus in Africa, where home-brewed alcohol or beer with high iron content is ingested.[59]

Basically a disease of the liver, porphyria cutanea tarda has been shown to be associated with a deficiency in the activity of uroporphyrinogen decarboxylase and, as a result, excessive production and accumulation of 8-carboxy porphyrins. The primary cutaneous lesion of porphyria cutanea tarda is a photosensitivity to the uroporphyrin deposited in the skin. Light in the 400-nm range is necessary for production of cutaneous lesions. Skin lesions in this disease consist of vesicles or blisters on light-exposed cutaneous surfaces, especially the dorsal aspect of the hands (Fig. 4–18). The blisters vary markedly from 1 mm to 2 to 3 cm across, with small blisters often being overlooked. They are most commonly filled by clear or slightly turbid liquid, soon rupture, turn into erosions, and frequently become infected. On healing, the blister sites may scar or evolve into milia (rounded, yellowish or pale-colored intraepidermal inclusions 1 to 2 mm or more in diameter). Other features include increased fragility of the skin, with erosions and ulcerations as the result of relatively minor trauma, and hypertrichosis and melanosis of the face that appear to be related to sun exposure.

Porphyria cutanea tarda can be precipitated by estrogen therapy, alcoholic cirrhosis, and accidental ingestion of the fungicide hexachlorobenzene (this is not to be confused with the insecticide gamma benzene hexachloride used for the treatment of scabies and pediculosis) responsible for an

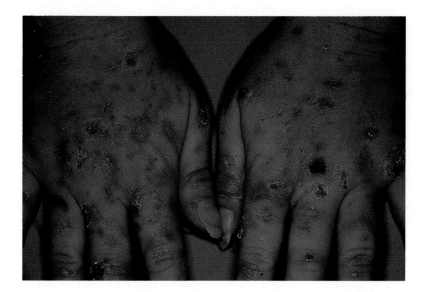

Figure 4–18. Vesicles, erosions, and ulcerations on the dorsal aspect of the hands of a patient with porphyria cutanea tarda. (Courtesy of the Department of Dermatology, Yale University School of Medicine.)

epidemic of porphyria cutanea tarda in Turkey.[60] Although diabetes mellitus is present in 25 to 50 per cent of patients with porphyria cutanea tarda, the reason for this high association is unknown.

Confirmation of the clinical diagnosis of porphyria cutanea tarda can be made by increased levels of uroporphyrin, slightly elevated fecal coproporphyrin and protoporphyrin levels, and positive fluorescence of the patient's urine with a Wood's light. Skin biopsy specimens of vesicular lesions show subepidermal bullae with dermal papillae arising irregularly from the floor of the bulla into its cavity. Immunofluorescent studies show deposition of IgG and, less commonly, IgM or complement at the dermal-epidermal junction and around the upper dermal vessels. Electron microscopic examination reveals reduplication of the basal lamina of the upper dermal vessels and dermal-epidermal junction, suggesting repeated injury to the endothelial and basal cells. Since similar observations can be made in other forms of porphyria, none of the above findings is pathognomonic.

Treatment is dependent on the elimination of alcohol, estrogen, or iron ingestion and on phlebotomy, with the number and frequency of phlebotomies dependent on clinical response, hemoglobin levels, and urinary porphyrin levels. Low-dose chloroquine therapy, alone or in combination with phlebotomy, has also been recommended as an effective form of therapy. The therapeutic effect proposed for chloroquine in this disorder appears to be related to chloroquine destruction of hepatocyte mitochondria and the formation of a water-soluble complex with porphyrin that can be excreted by the kidneys.

HEPATOERYTHROPOIETIC PORPHYRIA

In hepatoerythropoietic porphyria, an extremely rare disorder considered to be equivalent to a homozygous and more severe form of porphyria cutanea tarda, the disease is usually manifest before 2 years of age with dark urine being the most frequently observed sign. Skin lesions appear in childhood, and the activity of uroporphyrinogen decarboxylase in all organs is usually decreased to less than 10 per cent of normal. The disorder is characterized by excessive porphyrin production in the liver and bone marrow, increased erythrocyte prophyrin levels, severe photosensitivity, vesicles, bullae, crusts and erosions, skin fragility, hypertrichosis that begins in infancy and early childhood, mutilating scarring deformities similar to those of congenital erythropoietic porphyria, and scleroderma-like changes in skin that is exposed to the sun. The face and dorsal aspect of the hands are the most severely affected areas of involvement, malar hypertrichosis may be striking, and patients present with erythrodontia (reddish brown teeth) that fluoresce when exposed to a Wood's lamp. In addition to clinical features similar to those of erythropoietic porphyria, hepatoerythropoietic porphyria has biochemical abnormalities suggestive of porphyria cutanea tarda and erythropoietic protoporphyria. Cutaneous photosensitivity of a bullous, erosive, or mutilating type that begins at an early age suggests the disorder, and diagnosis is confirmed by findings of increased levels of erythrocyte protoporphyrin, urinary uroporphyrin, and fecal coproporphyrin. Although porphyria cutanea tarda and hepatoerythropoietic porphyria may both present in the first few years of life, the photosensitivity seems to diminish with age and is followed by hypertrichosis, hyperpigmentation, and scleroderma-like scarring.[61, 62]

HEREDITARY COPROPORPHYRIA

Hereditary coproporphyria is an exceedingly rare form of hepatic porphyria with a female predominance seen in adults and characterized by acute attacks of abdominal pain identical to those of acute intermittent porphyria and porphyria variegata. Approximately 30 per cent of patients also have photocutaneous sensitivity, and when skin lesions are present they resemble those of porphyria cutanea tarda. This disease, inherited as an autosomal dominant trait, is associated with a defect of coproporphyrinogen oxidase, resulting in accumulation of coproporphyrinogen III and its oxidized form coproporphyrin III. Cutaneous eruptions occur concurrently with attacks of abdominal pain and psychiatric symptoms and are precipitated by barbiturates, glipizide (Glucotrol, an oral blood glucose–lowering drug of the sulfonylurea class), and agents similar to those that induce acute intermittent porphyria and porphyria variegata.[63] The diagnosis is made by demonstration of elevated levels of coproporphyrin III in both urine and feces, and treatment is similar to that of patients with acute intermittent porphyria and porphyria variegata (variegate porphyria).

PORPHYRIA VARIEGATA

Porphyria variegata (variegate porphyria, congenital cutaneous hepatic porphyria) is an autosomal dominant disorder that represents a combination of acute intermittent porphyria and porphyria cutanea tarda. This disease, not seen in young children, has its onset after puberty and generally appears in the fourth to fifth decades of life.

Clinical features include sun sensitivity in adult life, with vesicles or blisters on light-exposed surfaces, hyperpigmentation, a weather-beaten or waxy complexion with excessive furrowing of the forehead, cutis rhomboidalis frontalis, scars on the back of the neck and frontal hair margin, milia, and scleroderma-like plaques (Fig. 4–19). The urinary findings overlap those of both acute intermittent porphyria and porphyria cutanea tarda. Treatment consists of avoidance of hepatotoxic agents and sun exposure, repeated phlebotomies, low-dose chloroquine therapy, and, in some patients, the administration of beta-carotene.[64]

PSEUDOPORPHYRIA

Pseudoporphyria is a term used to describe a syndrome in which increased cutaneous fragility and vesiculobullous eruptions similar to those of porphyria cutanea tarda occur despite normal lev-

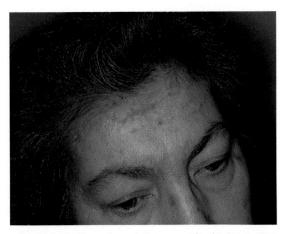

Figure 4–19. Hyperpigmentation, a weather-beaten appearance, and excessive furrowing of the forehead in porphyria variegata.

els of porphyrin in individuals receiving dapsone, furosemide, nalidixic acid, naproxen (Naprosyn), sulfonamides, or tetracyclines. A similar if not identical disorder has also been described in patients receiving long-term UVA radiation and hemodialysis. A nonimmunologically mediated phototoxicity reaction with histopathologic features similar to those of patients with porphyria, a careful history, and the presence of normal porphyrin levels in serum, erythrocytes, urine, and feces will generally establish the true nature of this disorder.[65, 66]

References

1. Gilchrest BA, Soter NA, Stoff JC, et al.: The human sunburn reaction: Histologic and biochemical studies. J. Am. Acad. Dermatol. 5:411–422, 1981.

   Studies of ultraviolet-induced erythema provide the first data that histamine may mediate the early phase of human sunburn reaction.

2. Ansel J, Luger T, Green I: Fever and increased serum IL-1 activity, a systemic manifestation of acute phototoxicity in New Zealand white rabbits. J. Int. Dermatol. 89:32–36, 1987.

   Studies in New Zealand white rabbits demonstrate a 5- to 10-fold increase in serum interleukin-1 activity following ultraviolet light exposure.

3. Knobler E, Almeida L, Ruzkowski AM, et al.: Photoallergy to benzophenone. Arch. Dermatol. 125:801–804, 1989.

   A report of photoallergy to oxybenzone in four individuals serves as a reminder that benzophenones as well as PABA and its esters must be considered as possible sources of allergic sunscreen reactions.

4. Pathak MA: Sunscreens and their use in the preventive treatment of sunlight-induced skin damage. J. Dermatol. Surg. Oncol. 13:739–350, 1987.

   A discussion of the nature of solar radiation and guidelines for the prevention of sunburn, cutaneous photoaging and skin cancer.

5. Gange RW, Soparker A, Matzinger E, et al.: Efficacy of a sunscreen containing butyl methoxydibenzoylmethane against ultraviolet A radiation in photosensitized subjects. J. Am. Acad. Dermatol. 15:494–499, 1986.

Topical formulations containing Parsol 1789 offer broad-spectrum sunscreen for the protection from UVA as well as UVB radiation.

6. Hurwitz S: The sun and sunscreen protection: Recommendations for children. J. Dermatol. Surg. Oncol. 14:657–660, 1988.

A review of ultraviolet radiation, its effect on the skin, and recommendations for the protection of children as well as adults.

7. Council on Scientific Affairs: Harmful effects of ultraviolet radiation. J.A.M.A. 262:380–384, 1989.

A comprehensive report of the harmful effects of cosmetic tanning and ultraviolet radiation photodamage (photoaging, photocarcinogensis, phototoxicity, and photoallergy).

8. Sams WM Jr, Epstein JH, Winkelmann RK: Solar urticaria: Investigation of pathogenetic mechanisms. Arch. Dermatol. 99:390–397, 1969.

A 29-year-old man with solar urticaria with an action spectrum between 250 and 330 nm.

9. Duschet P, Leyen P, Schwarz T, et al.: Solar urticaria: Effective treatment by plasmapheresis. Clin. Exp. Dermatol. 12:185–188, 1987.

Successful plasmapheresis of a patient with solar urticaria suggests that elimination of a circulating serum factor apparently essential to the pathogenesis of solar urticaria may provide a long-lasting form of therapy for this disorder.

10. Ramsay SA: Solar urticaria treatment by inducing tolerance to artificial radiation and natural light. Arch. Dermatol. 113:1222–1225, 1977.

Repeated exposures to small doses of artificial and natural light, presumably by depletion of mast cell mediators, can induce tolerance to sunlight exposure in individuals with solar urticaria.

11. Bernhard JD, Jaenicke K, Momtaz T-K, et al.: Ultraviolet A phototherapy in the prophylaxis of solar urticaria. J. Am. Acad. Dermatol. 10:29–33, 1984.

Ultraviolet A phototherapy helped three of five patients with solar urticaria increase their tolerance to sunlight.

12. Ragatanavin N, Bernhard JD: Solar urticaria: Treatment with terfenadine. J. Am. Acad. Dermatol. 18:574, 1988.

A patient with treatment-resistant solar urticaria obtained marked improvement by the use of up to 180 mg of terfenadine 30 minutes prior to going outdoors.

13. Parrish JA, Jaenicke KF, Morison, WL, et al.: Solar urticaria: Treatment with PUVA and mediator inhibitors. Br. J. Dermatol. 106:575–580, 1982.

Incremental suburticarial UVA exposure 2 hours after oral methoxsalen (three times a week for 4 to 8 weeks) was able to induce a tolerance to solar urticaria in six patients with this disorder.

14. Fisher DA, Epstein JH, Kay D, et al.: Polymorphous light eruption and lupus erythematosus: Differential diagnosis by fluorescent fluoroscopy. Arch. Dermatol. 101:458–461, 1970.

Polymorphous light eruptions confirmed by phototest techniques.

15. Birt AR, Davis RA: Hereditary polymorphic light eruption of American Indians. Int. J. Dermatol. 14:105, 1975.

An autosomal dominant form of polymorphous light eruption in Native Americans (from mid-Canada to South America).

16. Jansén CT: Photosensitivity in childhood. Acta Derm. Venereol. Suppl. 95:54–57, 1981.

In a study of 95 childhood-onset photodermatoses 78 (82 per cent) were found to be related to polymorphous light eruptions.

17. Draelos ZK, Hansen RC: Polymorphic light eruption in pediatric patients with Native American ancestry. Pediatr. Dermatol. 3:384–389, 1986.

A review of polymorphous light eruption in 11 pediatric patients of Native American ancestry.

18. Nordlund JJ, Klaus SN, Mathews-Roth MM, et al.: New therapy for polymorphous light eruptions. Arch. Dermatol. 108:710–712, 1973.

Carotenes offer protection for patients with light sensitivity in the 360- to 600-nm range.

19. Neumann R, Rappold E, Pohl-Markl H: Treatment of polymorphous light eruption with nicotinamide: A pilot study. Br. J. Dermatol. 115:77–80, 1986.

Ingestion of nicotinamide (3 g/day for 2 weeks) allowed 25 of 42 patients with polymorphous light eruption to remain clear of their disorder despite extensive sun exposure.

20. Farr PM, Diffey BL: Effect of indomethacin on UVB- and UVA-induced erythema in polymorphic light eruption. J. Am. Acad. Dermatol. 21:230–236, 1989.

Although 13 patients showed a beneficial response to topical indomethacin, ten patients developed an abnormal augmentation of UVB- and UVA-induced erythema, suggesting that polymorphous light eruption may embrace at least two disease states with different mechanisms of photosensitivity.

21. Saul A, Flores O, Navales J: Polymorphous light eruption: Treatment with thalidomide. Aust. J. Dermatol. 17:17–21, 1976.

Although not available in the United States, thalidomide was successfully used for the treatment of some patients with polymorphous light eruption.

22. Ortel B, Tanew A, Wolff K, et al.: Polymorphous light eruption: Action spectrum and photoprotection. J. Am. Acad. Dermatol. 14:748–753, 1986.

Sixty-four per cent of 51 patients receiving PUVA treatment for polymorphous light eruption reported total protection, 26 per cent reported partial protection, and 10 per cent were not protected from photoreaction following periods of summer outdoor activity.

23. Freeman RG, Knox JM: The action spectrum of photocontact dermatitis caused by halogenated salicylanilides and related compounds. Arch. Dermatol. 97:130–136, 1968.

Nineteen patients with photocontact dermatitis due to tetrachlorosalicylanilide and related compounds.

24. Epstein JH, Wuepper KD, Maibach HI: Photocontact dermatitis to halogenated salicylanilides and related compounds. Arch. Dermatol. 97:236–244, 1968.

Twenty-six patients with photocontact dermatitis associated with halogenated salicylanilides and related compounds.

25. Kaidbey KH, Kligman AM: Phototoxicity to a sunscreen ingredient: Padimate A. Arch. Dermatol. 114:547–549, 1978.

Amyl paradimethylaminobenzoic acid (padimate), an ester of para-aminobenzoic acid (PABA) found in popular proprietary sunscreens, was found to produce phototoxicity.

26. Kaidbey KH, Messenger JL: The clinical spectrum of the persistent light reactor. Arch. Dermatol. 120:1441–1448, 1984.

An analysis of eight men who had chronic recurrent photodermatitis for periods of 5 to 19 years despite apparent lack of re-exposure to photosensitizing agents.

27. Knudsen EA: Seasonal variations in the content of phototoxic compounds in giant hogweed. Contact Dermatitis 9:281–284, 1984.

Studies of phytophotocontact dermatitis to hogweed suggest that the pathogenesis of photocontact dermatitis requires a certain amount of the phototoxic substance in the plant and a sufficient degree of skin contact as well as exposure to ultraviolet A.

28. Seligman PJ, Mathias CGT, O'Malley MA, et al.: Phytophotodermatitis from celery among grocery store workers. Arch. Dermatol. *123*:1478–1482, 1987.

Outdoor sunlight exposure during working hours and tanning salon use during nonworking hours resulted in phytophotodermatitis in 19 grocery store workers; the celery incriminated in this study was not infected with the pink rot fungus.

29. Coffman K, Boyce WT, Hansen RC: Phytophotodermatitis simulating child abuse. Am. J. Dis. Child. *139*:239–240, 1985.

Two children with bizarre hyperpigmented skin lesions initially attributed to child abuse actually had a phytophotodermatitis following sun exposure and direct or indirect contact with limes used in the preparation of mixed drinks.

30. Kaidbey KH, Mitchell FN: Photosensitizing potential of certain nonsteroidal anti-inflammatory agents. Arch. Dermatol. *125*:783–786, 1989.

A review of the photosensitizing potentials of a variety of nonsteroidal anti-inflammatory agents.

31. Alinovi A, Riverberi C, Melissari M, et al.: Cutaneous hyperpigmentation induced by amiodarone hydrochloride. J. Am. Acad. Dermatol. *12*:563–566, 1985.

Amiodarone-induced slate-gray hyperpigmentation in light-exposed areas was believed to be the result of phototoxic-induced lysosomal damage.

32. Eramo LR, Garden JM, Esterly NB: Hydroa vacciniforme: Diagnosis by repetitive ultraviolet-A phototesting. Arch. Dermatol. *122*:1310–1313, 1986.

Lesions of hydroa vacciniforme were reproduced in an 8-year-old boy by repetitive phototesting with UVA.

33. Goldgeier MH, Nordlund JJ, Lucky AW, et al.: Hydroa vacciniforme: Diagnosis and therapy. Arch. Dermatol. *118*:588–591, 1982.

A 15-year-old boy with hydroa vacciniforme, when treated with hydroxychloroquine sulfate, was able to tolerate summer sun exposure for the first time in 8 years.

34. Bickers DR, Demar LK, DeLeo V, et al.: Hydroa vacciniforme. Arch. Dermatol. *114*:1193–1196, 1978.

Two children with hydroa vacciniforme effectively treated with beta-carotene (Solatene).

35. Cleaver JE: DNA damage and repair in light-sensitive human skin disease. J. Invest. Dermatol. *54*:181–195, 1970.

Studies demonstrate the defect in xeroderma pigmentosum to be that of endonuclease, an enzyme that recognizes and initiates repair of an ultraviolet-light–damaged region of DNA.

36. Kraemer KH, Lee MM, Scotto J: Xeroderma pigmentosum: Cutaneous, ocular, and neurologic abnormalities in 830 published cases. Arch. Dermatol. *123*:241–250, 1987.

In a review of 830 patients with xeroderma pigmentosum, basal cell or squamous cell carcinomas were found in 45 per cent, melanomas were seen in 5 per cent, ocular abnormalities developed in 40 per cent, and neurologic abnormalities were present in 18 per cent of patients afflicted with this disorder.

37. Reed WB, Sugarman GI, Mathis RA: DeSanctis-Cacchione syndrome: A case report with autopsy findings. Arch. Dermatol. *113*:1561–1563, 1977.

The DeSanctis-Cacchione syndrome, a form of xeroderma pigmentosum with neurologic complications.

38. Epstein EH Jr, Burk P, Cohen IK, et al.: Dermatome shaving in the treatment of xeroderma pigmentosum. Arch. Dermatol. *105*:589–590, 1972.

Dermabrasion of severely sun-damaged skin in a patient with xeroderma pigmentosum retarded the development of malignant tumors.

39. Kraemer KH, DiGiovanna JJ, Moshell AN, et al.: Prevention of skin cancer in xeroderma pigmentosum with the use of oral isotretinoin N. Engl. J. Med. *318*:1633–1637, 1988.

Although studies showed that high doses of oral isotretinoin (2 mg/kg/day for 2 years) could help prevent new skin cancers in patients with xeroderma pigmentosum, in three of five patients withdrawal of therapy resulted in rapid reversal of isotretinoin's chemoprophylactic effect.

40. Ramsay CA, Coltart TM, Blunt C, et al.: Prenatal diagnosis of xeroderma pigmentosum: Report of first successful case. J. Invest. Dermatol. *63*:392–396, 1974.

Amniotic fluid studies at 16 weeks' gestation in a mother with a previous child afflicted with xeroderma pigmentosum revealed a 78 per cent reduction in DNA repair synthesis, thus allowing termination of the pregnancy by prostaglandin and oxytocin infusion.

41. Rappaport MJ: Pellagra in a patient with anorexia nervosa. Arch. Dermatol. *121*:255–257, 1985.

A report of a 20-year-old woman with anorexia nervosa who developed pellagra as a result of her dietary idiosyncrasy.

42. Stratogos JD, Katsambasa A: Pellagra: A still existing disease. Br. J. Dermatol. *96*:99–106, 1977.

Malabsorption syndromes, chronic alcoholism, diets high in corn, and a variety of chemotherapeutic agents are incriminated as causes of pellagra.

43. Silver HK: Rothmund-Thomson syndrome: An oculocutaneous disorder. Am. J. Dis. Child. *111*:182–190, 1966.

A review of Rothmund-Thomson syndrome in two brothers.

44. Berg E, Chuang T-Y, Cripps D: Rothmund-Thomson syndrome: A case report, phototesting and literature review. J. Am. Acad. Dermatol. *17*:332–338, 1987.

A report of a 25-year-old woman with Rothmund-Thomson syndrome who developed a basal cell epithelioma and a review of the literature.

45. Collins P, Barns L, McCabe M: Poikiloderma congenitale: Case report and review of the literature. Pediatr. Dermatol. *8*:58–60, 1991.

A report of an 8-year-old girl with poikiloderma congenitale (Rothmund-Thomson syndrome) and a review of the literature.

46. Bloom D: Congenital telangiectatic erythema resembling lupus erythematosus in dwarfs. Am. J. Dis. Child. *88*:754–758, 1954.

Three children with facial telangiectatic erythema, photosensitivity, and dwarfism (Bloom's syndrome).

47. Gretzula JC, Hevia O, Weber PJ: Bloom's syndrome. J. Am. Acad. Dermatol. *17*:479–488, 1987.

A review of four patients with Bloom's syndrome and studies indicating a specific defect in immunoglobulin production in patients with this disorder.

48. Van Kerkhove CW, Cueppens JL, Vanderschuren-Lodeweyckx M, et al.: Bloom's syndrome: Clinical features and immunologic abnormalities in four patients. Am. J. Dis. Child. *142*:1089–1093, 1988.

Studies in four patients with Bloom's syndrome indicate that patients with this disorder have a specific defect in immunoglobulin production.

49. Cairney AEL, Greenberg M, Smith D, et al.: Wilms' tumor in three patients with Bloom syndrome. J. Pediatr. *111*:414–416, 1987.

A review of Wilms' tumor in three patients suggests that this neoplasm should be added to the list of neoproliferative disorders manifested in individuals with Bloom's syndrome.

50. Andrews AD, Barrett SF, Yoder FW, et al.: Cockayne's syndrome fibroblasts have increased sensitivity to ultraviolet light but normal rates of unscheduled DNA synthesis. J. Invest. Dermatol. 70:237–239, 1978.

Studies of fibroblasts from nine patients with Cockayne's syndrome reveal markedly decreased post–ultraviolet light fibroblast colony formation.

51. McLaren DS: Skin in protein energy malnutrition. Arch. Dermatol. 123:1674–1676a, 1984.

A comprehensive review of protein malnutrition and its relationship to marasmus and kwashiorkor.

52. Poh-Fitzpatrick MB: Porphyria. In Greer KE (Ed.): Common Problems in Dermatology. Year Book Medical Publishers, Inc., Chicago, 1988, 309–317.

An authoritative review of the porphyrias, their clinical manifestations and management.

53. Bechtel MA, Bertolone SJ, Hodge SJ: Transfusion therapy in a patient with erythropoietic porphyria. Arch. Dermatol. 117:99–101, 1981.

Washed, packed red blood cell transfusions in an 8-year-old boy with erythropoietic porphyria produced a decline in free erythrocyte protoporphyrin levels and a notable increase in sunlight tolerance.

54. Moshell AN, Bjornson L: Photoprotection in erythropoietic porphyria: Mechanism of photoprotection by beta carotene. J. Invest. Dermatol. 68:157–160, 1977.

Although protection from light in the 400-nm range may be the mechanism by which beta-carotene helps patients with erythropoietic porphyria, it is suggested that free radical trapping and singlet oxygen quenching may be the primary mechanism of its photoprotection in patients with this disorder.

55. Poh-Fitzpatrick MB, Piomelli S, Young P, et al.: Rapid quantitative assay for erythrocyte porphyrins: Rapid quantitative microfluorometric assay applicable to diagnosis of erythropoietic protoporphyria. Arch. Dermatol. 110:225–230, 1974.

A quantitative assay for free erythrocyte porphyrins allows a rapid diagnosis of erythropoietic protoporphyria (EPP).

56. DeLeo VA, Poh-Fitzpatrick M, Mathews-Roth M, et al.: Erythropoietic protoporphyria: Ten years' experience. Am. J. Med. 60:8–22, 1976.

In a review of clinical and laboratory findings in 32 patients with erythropoietic protoporphyria, 19 of 23 patients showed a significant response to beta-carotene treatment.

57. Bloomer JR: Pathogenesis and therapy of liver disease in protoporphyria. Yale J. Biol. Med. 52:39–48, 1979.

Cholestyramine resin (Questran) and vitamin E for 11 months dramatically reduced a lifelong problem of photosensitivity in a 26-year-old woman with protoporphyria.

58. Ross JB, Moss MA: Relief of photosensitivity of erythropoietic protoporphyria by pyridoxine. J. Am. Acad. Dermatol. 22:340–342, 1990.

Two children (4 and 7 years of age) with erythropoietic protoporphyria only moderately responsive to beta-carotene and sunscreen use had a successful therapeutic response following the administration of pyridoxine in dosages of 150 to 1,000 mg/day.

59. Kasky A: Porphyria cutanea tarda in a two-year-old girl. Br. J. Dermatol. 90:213–216, 1974.

A 2-year-old girl with small vesicles, crusts, and scars on the face with biochemical findings compatible with a diagnosis of porphyria cutanea tarda.

60. Cam C, Nigogosyan G: Acquired toxic porphyria cutanea tarda due to hexachlorobenzene. J.A.M.A. 183:89–91, 1963.

A report of 348 of an estimated 5,000 cases of porphyria cutanea tarda due to accidental consumption of wheat treated with the fungicide hexachlorobenzene (C_6Cl_6).

61. Czarnecki DB: Hepatoerythropoietic porphyria. Arch. Dermatol. 116:307–311, 1980.

A patient with hepatoerythropoietic porphyria with onset in infancy had spontaneous resolution of the photosensitivity by the age of 7 years.

62. Lim HW, Poh-Fitzpatrick MB: Hepatoerythropoietic porphyria: A variant of childhood-onset porphyria cutanea tarda. J. Am. Acad. Dermatol. 11:1103–1111, 1984.

A report of hepatoerythropoietic porphyria in two children and a comprehensive review of the disorder.

63. Moder KG, Schwenk NM: A coproporphyria-like syndrome induced by glipizide. Mayo Clin. Proc. 66:312–316, 1991.

A report of a patient with a 1-month history of severe episodic abdominal pain associated with glipizide, an oral hypoglycemic agent of the sulfonylurea class.

64. Muhlbauer JE, Pathak MA, Tishler PV, et al.: Variegate porphyria in New England. J.A.M.A. 247:3095–3102, 1982.

A review of five families with variegate porphyria.

65. Murphy GM, Wright J, Nicholls DSH, et al.: Sunbed-induced porphyria. Br. J. Dermatol. 120:555–562, 1989.

A report of four patients with porphyria-like tissue damage after exposure to UVA sunbed tanning over a long period of time.

66. Levy ML, Barron KS, Eichenfield A, et al.: Naproxen-induced pseudoporphyria: A distinctive photodermatitis. J. Pediatr. 117:660–664, 1990.

A porphyria-like dermatosis in 22 children (21 with juvenile rheumatoid arthritis and one with systemic lupus erythematosus) who presented with erythema, vesiculation, and skin fragility after sun exposure while being treated with naproxen.

PAPULOSQUAMOUS AND RELATED DISORDERS

CHILDHOOD PSORIASIS

Psoriasis is a common inherited disorder characterized by erythematous scaly papules or plaques with a predisposition for the scalp, elbows, knees, extensor surfaces of the limbs, genitalia, and lumbosacral area. Affecting 1 to 3 per cent of the population, it is uncommon in Japanese, Native Americans, and blacks, particularly those of African origin who comprise the bulk of the American black population. It usually follows an irregularly chronic course marked by remissions and exacerbations of unpredictable onset and duration.

Despite continuing research and investigation, the etiology of psoriasis remains unknown. Although early studies suggested autosomal dominant transmission with incomplete penetrance, it is apparent that genetic transmission of the psoriatic tendency is more complicated than previously suspected and probably reflects the presence of subpopulations involving different genetic loci. Of interest in this regard are studies linking HLA-B13, HLA-B17, HLA-Bw16, HLA-B37, and HLA-Cw6 with psoriasis and the fact that approximately one third of patients have a family member with the disease (the risk of a child developing psoriasis is stated to be 17 per cent if one sibling has the disorder, 25 per cent if one parent has psoriasis, 31 per cent if one parent and one sibling have the condition, and 60 to 75 per cent if both parents have psoriasis). In addition, it is recognized that patients with HLA-B17 develop psoriasis at an earlier age than those with HLA-Bw16; individuals with HLA-Bw17 appear to have a higher familial incidence and more extensive skin involvement; those with HLA-Bw13 seem to have a milder more reversible disease and are more likely to give a history of antecedent streptococcal infection; and patients with HLA-B27, HLA-B38, HLA-A26, HLA-Cw6, and HLA-DRw7 appear to be more likely candidates for the development of psoriatic arthritis.[1, 2]

For years it has been stated that psoriasis is uncommon in childhood and rare in children younger than 3 years of age. Statistical studies, however, reveal that 37 per cent of patients first develop the disease before the age of 20. Twenty-seven per cent of affected individuals develop the disorder before age 15; 10 per cent have the onset of lesions before age 10; 6.5 per cent develop lesions before age 5; 2 per cent have lesions before age 2; and patients with active lesions present at birth (congenital psoriasis) have been documented (Figs. 5–1 through 5–3).[3–5] In adults the disorder occurs with equal frequency in both sexes. In childhood forms, however, the ratio of females to males is 2 : 1.[3, 4] Of these, one third have at least one relative with the disorder. Although studies of twins may be open to criticism on the basis of selective reporting, up to 72 per cent of identical twins appear to be concordant for this disorder.[6]

The basic cause of psoriasis appears to be related to defective inhibitors of epidermal proliferation with shortening of the epidermal cell cycle, excessive cell proliferation, and a marked increase in epidermal cell turnover. Although the

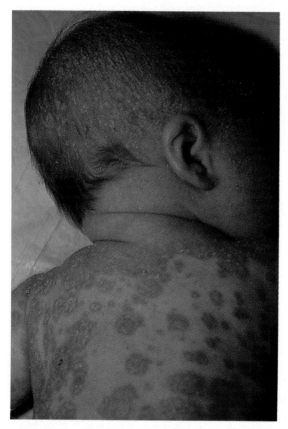

Figure 5–1. Congenital psoriasis in a newborn. (Courtesy of Dr. Jonathan A. Schneider.)

factors that initiate this process remain unknown, this increased production and proliferation of psoriatic epidermis appears to be responsible for the scaling and thickening characteristic of psoriatic lesions.

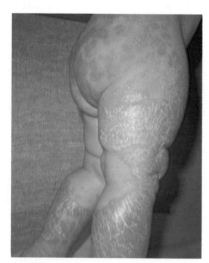

Figure 5–2. Childhood psoriasis in a 10-month-old infant (this patient had the onset of her disorder at 3½ months of age).

Despite the fact that the majority of patients with psoriasis give no history of a precipitating or provocative influence, stress, trauma, infection (particularly streptococcal disease in children), endocrine factors, climate, and a variety of medications such as lithium, β-adrenergic blocking agents (e.g., propranolol), antimalarials, phenylbutazone derivatives, nonsteroidal anti-inflammatory agents, and tetracycline have been incriminated at one time or another in this regard. The precise mechanism by which they exert this response, however, requires further study and clarification.[7–11]

Clinical Manifestations. Classic lesions of psoriasis consist of round, erythematous, well-marginated patches with a full, rich, red hue covered by a characteristic grayish or silvery-white scale. Lesions almost invariably begin as small, reddish, pinpoint to pinhead-sized papules surmounted by fine scales. These papules coalesce and form patches or plaques that measure 1 cm or more in diameter (Fig. 5–4).

The disorder may present as solitary lesions or countless patches of plaques distributed over wide areas of the body. Although exceptions occur, lesions generally are seen in a bilaterally symmetrical pattern with a distinct predilection for the scalp, elbows, knees, and lumbosacral and anogenital regions. Central portions of the patches may heal and involute so that nummular, annular, gyrate, arcuate, or circinate figures may be produced. Although the classic distribution of psoriasis characteristically occurs on the extensor surfaces (the elbows, knees, and lumbosacral regions), lesions may also be found in a flexural distribution with involvement of the axillae, groin, perineum, central chest, and umbilical region. This variant, termed *psoriasis inversus,* may be seen alone, without involvement of extensor surfaces, in 2.8 to 6.0 per cent of patients, or in association with other regional involvement (in 30 per cent of patients).

The hallmark of psoriasis is the silvery micaceous (mica-like) scale that is generally attached at the center rather than the periphery of lesions. Removal of this scale results in fine punctate bleeding points. This phenomenon (termed *Auspitz's sign*) is highly characteristic but not exclusively diagnostic of this disorder and is related to rupture of capillaries high in the papillary dermis of lesions (Fig. 5–5). Although generally attributed to be and believed by some researchers to be pathognomonic, this clinical feature can also be seen in Darier's disease, actinic keratosis, clear cell acanthoma, acrokeratosis neoplastica of Basex (an uncommon disorder seen primarily in middle-aged adult males characterized by psoriasiform lesions on the helices of the ears, nasal bridge, cheeks, hands, feet, knees, and, at times, the scalp, neck, elbows, and lower legs; palmoplantar keratosis; atrophoderma and malignant neoplasms of the pulmonary and upper gastrointestinal tracts; and metastatic cervical adenopathy), and

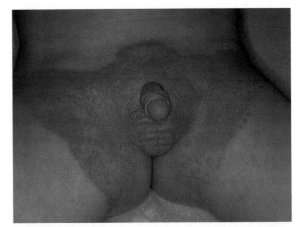

Figure 5–3. Psoriasis in the diaper area of a 3-month-old infant.

Flegel's disease (hyperkeratosis lenticularis perstans), an autosomal dominant psoriasiform dermatosis seen primarily on the arms and feet of men in their 30s or 40s.[12]

The Koebner phenomenon, a special feature seen in psoriasis as well as in certain other skin disorders (verrucae, *Rhus* dermatitis, lichen planus, lichen nitidus, Darier's disease, and pityriasis rubra pilaris), is seen as skin lesions that occur at sites of local injury. While the precise mechanism of the Koebner phenomenon is unknown, it appears to represent a reaction to trauma (an isomorphic response) that follows simple irritation such as a scratch or sunburn, a surgical scar, or a preexisting disease such as seborrheic or atopic dermatitis. In addition to its clinical value as a diagnostic sign, this phenomenon is frequently seen as a precipitating cause of psoriasis and should be emphasized to all patients afflicted with this disorder.

Guttate Psoriasis. The Koebner phenomenon is particularly significant in childhood psoriasis when drop-like (guttate) lesions appear suddenly over a large part of the body surface (Fig. 5–6). This variant, termed *guttate psoriasis*, may be the first manifestation of the disorder, which is generally, but not necessarily, streptococcal in origin. Two thirds of patients with guttate psoriasis give a history of an upper respiratory tract infection 1 to 3 weeks before the onset of an acute flare of the disorder. Seen in 14 to 17 per cent of the population, guttate forms of psoriasis generally occur in children and young adults. Lesions are round or oval, measure from 2 to 3 mm to 1 cm in diameter, and generally occur in a symmetrical distribution over the trunk and proximal aspects of the extremities (occasionally the face, scalp, ears, and distal aspects of the extremities). Although the precise relationship of streptococcal infection and acute

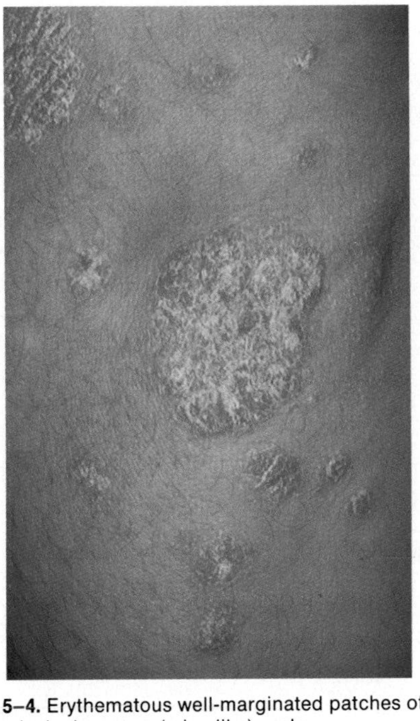

Figure 5–4. Erythematous well-marginated patches of psoriasis with typical micaceous (mica-like) scale.

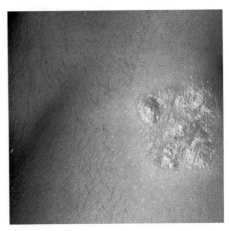

Figure 5–5. Psoriasis inversus in popiteal fossa. Note mica-like scale and fine punctate bleeding points (Auspitz's sign).

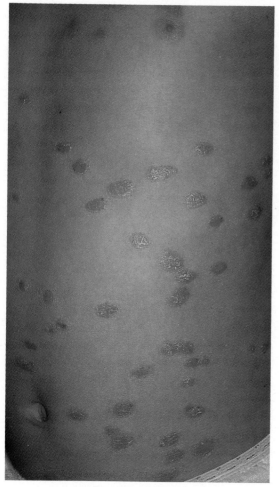

Figure 5–6. Guttate (drop-like) psoriasis.

Whereas lesions of seborrhea generally remain within the hairline, lesions of psoriasis frequently extend beyond the confines of the hairline onto the forehead, preauricular, postauricular, and nuchal regions (Fig. 5–7). When the true nature of the disorder remains in doubt, appropriate diagnosis may be aided by the fact that lesions particularly resistant to appropriate treatment for seborrhea are more likely to prove to be psoriatic rather than seborrheic.

Pityriasis Amiantacea (Tinea Amiantacea). Another variant of psoriasis of the scalp is known as *pityriasis* or *tinea amiantacea* (asbestos-like). This disorder is unrelated to fungus infection of the scalp and refers to forms of seborrhea or psoriasis of the scalp generally seen in children or adolescents in which crusts are firmly adherent and asbestos-like (Fig. 5–8). When seen as a manifestation of psoriasis, tinea amiantacea frequently is persistent and somewhat resistant to therapy.

Nail Involvement. Although statistics vary, the nails appear to be affected in 25 to 50 per cent of patients with psoriasis. Pitting is probably the best known and most characteristic nail change in psoriasis. Generally seen as small, irregularly spaced depressions measuring less than 1 mm in diameter, larger depressions or punched-out areas of the nail plate may also be noted. These pits, formed during the process of keratinization of the nail, probably represent small intermittent lesions in the part of the matrix that forms the superficial layers of the nail plate.

Although psoriatic pitting, when present, is highly characteristic, it must be differentiated from nail pitting seen in alopecia areata and atopic dermatitis. That of atopic dermatitis has a

guttate psoriasis is not completely understood, it has been hypothesized that a specific streptococcal proliferative factor, with an effect on epidermal keratinocytes and circulating T cells, produces a Koebner phenomenon and may be responsible for subsequent flares of the disorder.[13] To further substantiate this role, some patients with refractory psoriasis have been shown to improve following tonsillectomy for the treatment of chronic and recurring streptococcal infection.[14]

Seborrhiasis. The scalp is frequently seen as the initial site of psoriatic involvement. Although psoriatic lesions of the scalp, eyebrows, and ears (the superior and postauricular folds and external auditory meatus) may present as well-demarcated erythematous plaques with thick adherent silvery scales similar in appearance to those on other parts of the body, lesions often tend to be greasy, soft, and salmon colored, suggesting a diagnosis of seborrhea. In this variant, often termed *seborrhiasis* (*sebopsoriasis*), lesions may present with features of both seborrhea and psoriasis.

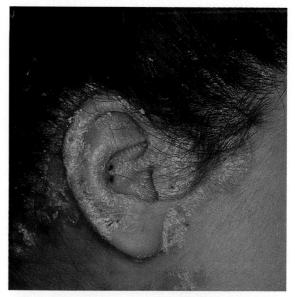

Figure 5–7. Seborrheic psoriasis (seborrhiasis). Lesions of seborrhea generally remain within the hairline; lesions of psoriasis frequently extend beyond the confines of the hairline.

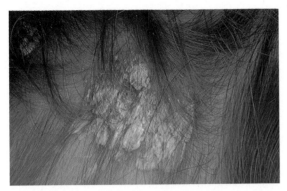

Figure 5–8. Tinea (pityriasis) amiantacea. In this severe form of psoriasis of the scalp the scales are strongly adherent (asbestos-like).

coarse irregular appearance and frequently is associated with nail dystrophy, roughening and discoloration of the nail surface, and a history of recent paronychia or dermatitis of the fingers. Although pitting is said to be an infrequent manifestation of childhood psoriasis, in actuality it is far more common than is realized. This impression is substantiated by a study of 14 infants and small children with psoriasis younger than age 2 in which 79 per cent (11 children) manifested psoriatic pitting of the nails. Of these, one actually displayed pitting of the nails at the time of birth.[15]

Other psoriatic nail changes include discoloration, subungual hyperkeratosis, crumbling and grooving of the nail plate, and onycholysis (separation of the nail plate from the nail bed) (Figs. 5–9A and 5–9B). Onycholysis, also seen in other diseases (onychomycosis, congenital ectodermal defects, hypothyroidism, photo-onycholysis due to tetracycline), may be differen-

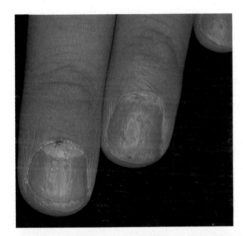

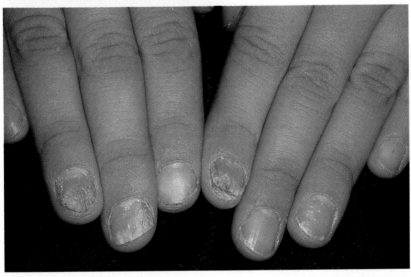

Figure 5–9. A. Nail psoriasis with pitting, discoloration, subungual keratin, and onycholysis. B. Psoriasis of the nail with dystrophy, discoloration, and crumbling of the nail plate.

tiated by a yellow or brown band that separates the white free edge from the normal pink color of the attached portion of the nail. This yellow band, when present, is a particularly valuable clinical feature in the differentiation of psoriasis from onychomycosis (tinea involvement of the nail) and appears to be related to accumulation of large amounts of glycoprotein associated with psoriatic involvement of the hyponychium and nail bed. Subungual keratosis is a common source of secondary bacterial and fungal infection. Bacterial or candidal infections, therefore, are frequently seen in association with psoriasis of the nails (see Fig. 5–10).

Diagnosis. The diagnosis of psoriasis can be made on the basis of clinical findings alone or in combination with histologic findings. The histopathologic features of psoriasis include epidermal thickening (acanthosis with elongation of the rete ridges); elongation and edema of the dermal papillae, with thinning of the suprapapillary portions of the epidermis; increased mitoses in the basal layer and lower malpighian layers of the epidermis (in contrast to the presence of mitoses only in a single basal cell layer of normal skin); the presence of immature nucleated cells (parakeratosis) in the stratum corneum, with a diminished or absent stratum granulosum; inflammatory infiltrate (usually lymphocytic or monocytic) in the superficial corium; and focal collection of neutrophils in the stratum corneum or subcorneal layer (Munro's microabscesses) (Fig. 5–11).

Course. The course of psoriasis in general is prolonged, chronic, and unpredictable. In most patients the disease is not severe and remains confined to localized cutaneous regions. Remissions and exacerbations are the rule in most patients, with a marked tendency to improvement in summer, particularly during long periods of sun exposure. In some patients the disease may undergo spontaneous improvement; in others exacerbations may occur without apparent cause. Although sunlight generally is beneficial, an occasional patient may be photosensitive with resultant exacerbation of lesions in areas exposed to the sun. At times the disorder may remain relatively unchanged for years, but with appropriate therapy satisfactory control of the disease is possible in a majority of patients.

Topical Therapy. Although studies suggest that childhood psoriasis usually portends a more severe course in adult life,[3] spontaneous remissions lasting for variable time periods occur in 38 per cent of patients and most patients generally respond well to presently available therapeutic measures.[4, 16] Whatever therapeutic approach is chosen, patients and their families should receive some degree of instruction as to the pathophysiology and natural course of the disease, with reassurance that most patients, with a little bit of effort, can do much to control the cutaneous aspects of their disorder.

Since psoriasis is a chronic dermatosis characterized by periods of exacerbation, and individual response to therapy frequently varies, it is wise to have a variety of therapeutic modalities available. The nature of the disorder and the lack of a specific cure can be discouraging to the patient, the patient's family, and the physician. It is imperative, therefore, that the patient and family of the patient understand the treatment and the rationale for its use. The approach to medication should be made as simple as possible, since therapy is time consuming, burdensome, and easily rejected. It is important to let the patient learn day-to-day care and, whenever possible, to carry out the routine as independently as possible.

Corticosteroids. Frequently producing dramatic resolution of lesions, corticosteroids are often the mainstay of topical therapy. Although high-potency topical corticosteroids are invaluable in short-term management of severe recalcitrant lesions, many patients with psoriasis respond quite well to moderate or low-potency corticosteroid formulations. Since there is a science to the use of topical corticosteroids, which involves selection of the correct-strength corticosteroid in the proper formulation for particular disease processes and specific areas of involvement, an appreciation of the approximate ranking of the potency of these compounds and a review of the pharmacology of these agents are invaluable (see Chapter 3, Table 3–2).

Formulations of topical corticosteroids are available as creams, ointments, gels, lotions, and sprays. Gel formulations are generally more effective than ointments; corticosteroids in ointment base have greater biologic activity than those incorporated into creams or lotions; creams generally are more effective than lotions. On the scalp, clear solutions (gels, lotions, or sprays) are preferable to ointments and creams; creams or lotions are preferred in the intertriginous areas; creams or ointments are more convenient and ef-

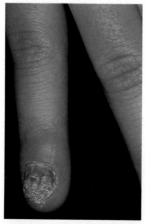

Figure 5–10. Psoriasis of the nail with dystrophy, discoloration, crumbling of the nail plate, and associated secondary candidal infection.

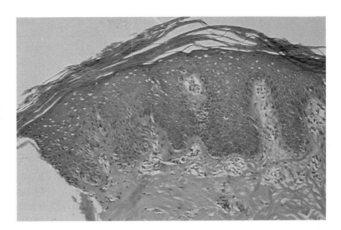

Figure 5-11. Psoriasis. Histologic features include hyperkeratosis, parakerotosis, diminished granular layer, acanthosis, elongation of rete ridges, vascular dilatation, and inflammatory round cell infiltrate.

fective on exposed areas. In recent years occlusive dressings using corticosteroid creams under polyethylene film (Saran Wrap) or as flurandrenolide tape (Cordran Tape [Dista]) have been used to augment the effectiveness of topical therapy. By means of these occlusive dressings the scales soften and the medication can penetrate 10 to 100 times more readily into the skin. Such occlusive dressings are usually used only during sleeping hours (for periods of 6 to 12 hours). Since folliculitis, telangiectases, and atrophic striae may result from prolonged use of corticosteroids under occlusion, care and appropriate precautions should be advised when this form of therapy is recommended.

Prompt resolution of small persistent psoriatic plaques can also be accomplished by intralesional injection of corticosteroid suspension (through a small 30-gauge needle or by dermojet). The corticosteroid most commonly used for intralesional therapy is triamcinolone acetonide (Kenalog) diluted with sterile saline or a local anesthetic (to minimize the pain of injection) to concentrations of 2.5 to 5.0 mg/ml. Frequently, only one or two injections may produce satisfactory clearing at the sites of injection. Limitation, however, must be placed on size and number of injections because of associated discomfort and the possibility of corticosteroid atrophy, telangiectasia, or systemic absorption (fortunately, atrophy due to intralesional corticosteroids usually disappears spontaneously, frequently within a period of 6 to 9 months).

Psoriatic nails are extremely distressing to the patient, respond slowly to therapy, and are frequently difficult to treat. This disorder can be treated with triamcinolone acetonide suspension (10 mg/ml) injected into the nail fold just proximal to the diseased matrix by a 30-gauge needle or dermojet (two or three times) at intervals of 2 to 6 weeks. Although uncomfortable to a certain degree, this regimen is beneficial at times and can produce some cosmetic improvement. One per cent 5-fluorouracil in propylene glycol or a combination of benzoyl peroxide gel and a potent topical corticosteroid applied twice daily into the cuticle of chronically involved nails for periods of 4 to 6 months is also reported to be somewhat beneficial. Patients with severe arthropathy or active psoriasis of the nail fold are less likely to respond to 5-fluorouracil therapy, and individuals with onycholysis should not be treated with this modality (since an increased tendency to onycholysis occurs in individuals on this form of therapy).

Tar Preparations. Although topical corticosteroids to a great extent have replaced tar in the treatment of many forms of dermatitis, tars still remain a highly effective therapeutic modality, particularly in the management of psoriasis and other chronic dermatoses. The exact mechanism by which tar exerts its therapeutic effect remains unclear, but it appears to be related to its anti-inflammatory effect and its ability to decrease epidermal proliferation. Cosmetically acceptable tar preparations are now available for baths (Balnetar [Westwood-Squibb], Polytar Bath [Stiefel], Zetar Emulsion [Dermik]) and as creams, gels, oils, or lotions (Estar Gel [Westwood-Squibb], Fototar [Elder], Neutrogena T/Derm Oil, and P & S Plus [Baker/Cummins]).

Removal of Scalp Lesions. The scalp frequently presents mechanical difficulties to patients with thick encrustations and scaling. Removal of scales can be facilitated by the use of P and S Liquid (Baker/Cummins), a mixture of phenol and sodium chloride in a mineral oil, glycerin, and water formulation. This preparation is highly effective when applied to scalp lesions with a cotton pledget once or twice a day followed 6 to 8 hours later by an appropriate antiseborrheic tar or corticosteroid shampoo (FS Shampoo [Hill Dermaceuticals]). In stubborn or persistent cases, the use of a corticosteroid lotion once or twice a day in conjunction with the above regimen is also beneficial. When scaling and crusting are particularly thick and resistant to therapy, the use of a plastic shower cap over the corticosteroid lotion for several hours or overnight and the incorporation of 3 to 5 per cent salicylic acid into the corticosteroid lotion are helpful.

Sunlight. Most psoriatic patients are benefited by exposure to sunlight and accordingly are frequently better during the summer months. Advantage should be taken of this in planning the summer activities of the psoriatic child. Appropriate sunburn precautions, however, must be used since sudden overexposure may result in sufficient epidermal injury to cause exacerbation of the disorder. For those who can arrange exposure to sunlight on a regular basis, this can be an important aspect of therapy, alone or in combination with crude coal tar preparations or their derivatives. Again caution is recommended in an effort to reduce sunburn and photosensitization. Although natural sunlight is easier and less aggressive than artificial ultraviolet therapy, ultraviolet treatment, under proper precautions, may be used as an adjunct to therapy. Care must be exercised, however, to protect the eyes and to avoid overexposure resulting in sunburn or exacerbation of the disorder. When natural sunlight is used, a sunscreen with a sun protective factor (SPF) of 15 or more on uninvolved areas and one with an SPF of 6 or 8 on affected areas are beneficial in blocking out ultraviolet light in the UVB (sunburn) range while still allowing exposure to the UVA tanning rays. Application of an emollient cream, mineral oil, or petrolatum to the affected areas during periods of sun exposure helps maximize the UVA effect.

The Goeckerman Regimen. Since first introduced over 60 years ago, the Goeckerman regimen has been a highly effective treatment for severe recalcitrant forms of psoriasis.[17] The Goeckerman procedure consists of crude coal tar (Zetar emulsion) or one of its derivatives (Estar gel, T/Derm Tar Emollient) applied to the entire body at bedtime. In the morning the excess tar is removed with mineral oil and the patient receives ultraviolet light therapy to the entire body (after first testing the patient for the minimal erythema dose to minimize the tendency for sunburn or exacerbation in light-sensitive persons). The amount of ultraviolet light exposure is increased gradually (generally by 1 minute a day) to an erythema or suberythema dose. When properly used, the Goeckerman regimen is safe, is highly effective, and within 2 or 3 weeks results in clinical remissions for most patients for periods lasting 6 to 8 months. Variations and modifications of this technique include a double Goeckerman regimen (in which therapy is performed on a twice-a-day treatment schedule), office or home Goeckerman routines, and modifications of the regimen by use of anthralin instead of tar (as in the Ingram technique). Complications of the Goeckerman regimen include folliculitis, sunburn, and occasional aggravation of the disease (if the patient is sensitive to tar or if therapy is too aggressive).

Anthralin and the Ingram Technique. The Ingram method, a therapeutic regimen popularized in Great Britain, includes a daily tar bath followed by exposure to a suberythema dose of ultraviolet light and subsequent application of a zinc paste containing anthralin (dioxyanthranol). In a modification of this regimen, 0.2 per cent anthralin can be incorporated into Lassar's paste with 0.4 per cent salicylic acid (anthralin is unstable in the absence of salicylic acid). Yellowish brown to brownish purple staining of the skin, a side effect of anthralin, generally disappears within a week following discontinuation of this modality or, if desired, may be removed by the use of a salicylic acid ointment.[18] Although economical and highly effective, it is often difficult to get the patient to use this regimen on a routine outpatient basis.

As an alternative, commercially available forms of anthralin (Anthra-Derm Ointment or Drithocreme [Dermik]) can be applied for shorter periods of time, starting with the lowest concentration and gradually increasing the concentration (depending on the patient's tolerance), and removed after 10 to 30 minutes by washing or showering. By using this short-contact technique, alone or in combination with ultraviolet light therapy, there is less likelihood of staining. Patients and their family, however, should be cautioned to use rubber or latex gloves when applying anthralin formulations, and contact with the eyes should be avoided.[19, 20]

Systemic Therapy. Most drugs given internally for psoriasis have potentially harmful side effects and should not, in general, be given to children with this disorder. Systemic corticosteroids should not be used in the routine care of psoriasis. They have a role in the management of persistent, otherwise uncontrollable erythroderma but generally are contraindicated in the treatment of children. Methotrexate, a folic acid antagonist, although highly effective in the management of severe recalcitrant psoriasis, has serious side effects (ulceration of the mucous membranes of the mouth and throat, gastrointestinal disturbances, lowering of leukocyte and platelet counts, and fibrosis and fatty changes in the liver). Because of its associated side effects, methotrexate, except in special circumstances, should not be used in children.

Photochemotherapy (PUVA) is a form of systemic therapy that combines the use of 8-methoxypsoralen and high-intensity long-wave ultraviolet light in the 320- to 400-nm spectrum (UVA). In this outpatient form of therapy, the interaction of a drug (8-methoxypsoralen) and UVA light produces biologic changes of the skin, including the conjugation of psoralen with DNA and the inhibition of DNA synthesis.[21] Methoxsalen, at a dosage of approximately 0.6 mg/kg, is given orally 2 hours before a measured exposure to long-wave ultraviolet light. After the psoriasis has cleared, maintenance therapy is required to prevent recurrence. Although the effectiveness and acceptance of this form of therapy are now well established, this regimen is generally not recommended for children and long-term follow-up is necessary because of possible long-term effects such as cataracts, premature actinic damage, or skin cancer. In addition, UVA-blocking wrap-around eyeglasses should be worn while patients are outdoors for a 24-hour period after ingesting the psoralen in an effort to eliminate the risk of possible eye damage or cataract formation. When indoors and under bright fluorescent lights, the same type of protective eyewear is recommended.

Oral retinoids (isotretinoin and etretinate) have also been used for the treatment of recalcitrant psoriasis. Particularly helpful in treating severe pustular, erythrodermic, and plaque types of psoriasis, oral retinoids should be avoided, in adults as well as children, when the disease can be controlled by less toxic modalities. When oral retinoids are deemed necessary, they are particularly effective in combination with topical corticosteroids, anthralin, methotrexate, and ultraviolet or PUVA therapy.[22–24] In addition, acitretin (a carboxylic acid metabolite of etretinate),[25] immunosuppressive agents such as cyclosporine[26] and sulfasalazine (Azulfidine),[27] and Tacrolimus (FK506), a new immunosuppressive investigational therapeutic agent, have also been found to be effective. Since etretinate is excreted extremely slowly and has a long half-life (120 days), and serum concentrations have been detected 2 and 3 years after its discontinuation, discretion should be used whenever its use is considered for women with future or present child-bearing potential.[28]

The National Psoriasis Foundation, 6443 S.W. Beaverton Highway, Suite 210, P.O. Box 9009, Portland, Oregon 97221 (1-800-562-0606) is available as a support group for patients and families of patients with psoriasis.

PSORIATIC ARTHRITIS

Arthritis occurs in 5 to 7 per cent of patients with psoriasis. It has its peak incidence in individuals between 30 and 50 years of age; the peak onset in children occurs between 9 and 12 years of age.[2, 29] Although it is often stated that psoriatic arthritis affects women more frequently than men, this apparent preponderance may be attributed to a female predilection for a pattern of rheumatoid arthritis frequently indistinguishable from psoriatic arthritis. The course and pathogenesis of psoriatic arthritis are unknown, but hereditary factors, abnormalities in cell-mediated immunity, immunologic reactions to streptococcal or staphylococcal antigens, and vascular and mechanical factors have been suggested.[2, 30]

In the majority of patients the onset of psoriasis precedes the onset of arthritis by 2 or more years. Although severe cases may be rapidly progressive and incapacitating, the course of psoriatic arthritis in most patients is mild and intermittent, and its long-term prognosis is usually good.[29] Although the classic pattern of psoriatic arthritis is said to involve the distal interphalangeal joints of the hands and feet (Fig. 5–12), this pattern occurs in less than 5 per cent of patients, and approximately 70 per cent of patients have asymmetric oligoarticular arthritis involving two or three joints at a time. In the acute stage of distal interphalangeal psoriatic arthritis the involved joint is red, tender, and swollen. The swelling often includes the juxta-articular tissue, resulting in a blunt "sausage-shaped" appearance of the involved fingers or toes. With long-standing disease, flexure deformities and severe bone destruction may occur with osteoporosis and shortening of the involved distal phalanx. As the lesions progress there is a "whittling" away and tapering of the bones. On radiologic examination this resembles a sharpened pencil (the so-called pencil-in-cup or pencil-and-goblet deformity) at the metatarsophalangeal and metacarpophalangeal joints. Sacroiliitis and ankylosing spondylitis may also be seen as minor manifestations of psoriatic arthritis.

The psoriatic skin lesions in patients who develop arthritis are identical to those seen in patients who do not manifest joint disease, and there is no relationship between the severity of the cutaneous disease and the development of joint disease.

Clinicians generally have little difficulty in the diagnosis of typical cases of psoriatic arthritis. In less typical cases, however, the disorder must be differentiated from rheumatoid arthritis or systemic lupus erythematosus. Compared with rheumatoid arthritis the onset is generally, but not invariably, monoarticular and subacute. It tends to

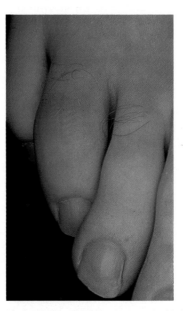

Figure 5–12. Psoriatic arthritis in a teenager with inflammatory involvement of the interphalangeal joint.

be less painful, and flexural deformity (rather than ulnar deviation) is characteristic of this disease. Psoriatic arthritis is frequently associated with nail changes and severe psoriasis or psoriatic erythroderma. The erythrocyte sedimentation rate is usually elevated but not specific for psoriatic arthritis. There are no subcutaneous nodules, and latex fixation, bentonite flocculation, and sheep cell agglutinations are negative.

Therapy for psoriatic arthritis, similar to that for rheumatoid arthritis, consists primarily of heat, physical therapy, and aspirin or other nonsteroidal anti-inflammatory agents. Although etretinate and folic acid antagonists, particularly methotrexate, have been used with great success in the treatment of severe juvenile and adult forms of psoriasis and psoriatic arthritis, these preparations are generally not recommended in children.

PUSTULAR PSORIASIS

There are two conditions to which the term *pustular psoriasis* is generally applied. These include localized pustular psoriasis of the palms and soles (pustulosis palmaris et plantaris), a bilaterally symmetric, chronic pustular eruption that occurs on the palms and soles but is not necessarily associated with evidence of psoriasis on others parts of the body, and generalized pustular psoriasis, a severe explosive disorder associated with high fever, severe toxicity, poor prognosis, and frequent relapses. In addition, a rare variant, annular pustular psoriasis, characterized by annular or circinate lesions and pustular eruptions on a ring-like erythema sometimes resembling erythema annulare centrifugum may occur. This disorder runs a cyclical recurrent course that may at times span decades. Although reputedly rare in childhood, there are many case reports of pustular psoriasis in infants and children (of these, 27 per cent occurred during the first year of life and the majority were of the generalized von Zumbusch type).[31-33]

Localized Pustular Psoriasis

Also termed *pustulosis of the palms and soles* (pustulosis palmaris et plantaris), localized pustular psoriasis is a chronic disorder characterized by deep-seated 2- to 4-mm sterile pustules that develop within areas of erythema and scaling on the palms, soles, or both. Often referred to as *pustular bacterid of Andrews* or *pustular psoriasis of the palms and soles of Barber,* these two terms probably imply clinical variants of the same cutaneous process rather than separate clinical entities. The primary lesion is a subcorneal or intraepidermal pustule or a vesicle that becomes pustular within a few hours. Within several days the pustules resolve and leave a dark yellow or

brown scale that is shed, generally within 1½ to 2 weeks. Stages of quiescence and exacerbation are characteristic. Before the brown crusts of preceding lesions exfoliate, crops of fresh pustules often appear and recurring crops of pustules frequently occur. Accordingly, exfoliating crusted lesions and newly developing pustules may be seen at the same time in the same patient (Figs. 5–13 and 5–14). Although the etiology of pustulosis of the palms and soles remains unknown, the presence of psoriatic nail changes and lesions in other areas of some affected individuals suggests that this disorder may represent a clinical variant or predisposition to psoriasis vulgaris.

The histologic picture of pustulosis palmaris et plantaris does not resemble that of psoriasis. The chief histologic feature is that of large intraepidermal unilocular pustules containing polymorphonuclear leukocytes (the spongiform pustules of Kogoj) with little if any surrounding spongiosis or inflammation. Although staphylococcal infection may at times occur as a secondary complication, bacterial cultures of these abscesses usually remain sterile throughout the course of the disorder.

Pustulosis of the palms and soles tends to pursue a chronic course characterized by periods of quiescence and exacerbation. Local applications of wet dressings with Burow's solution 1:40 or potassium permanganate 1:5,000 (one crushed 65-mg tablet to 250 ml of water) frequently help relieve acute flares of the pustular aspect of this disorder. Topical or intralesional corticosteroids often produce temporary subsidence of lesions. Topical tar and anthralin preparations, although at times helpful in chronic forms of this disorder, are

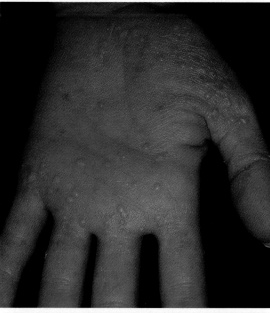

Figure 5–13. Localized pustular psoriasis of the palms.

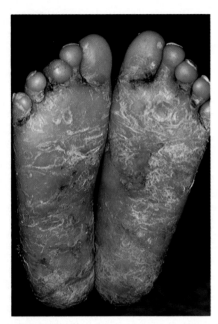

Figure 5–14. Pustular psoriasis of the soles. These lesions generally are raised, horny, quite hard, and covered by a white or grayish white scale.

plaques suddenly develop erythematous halos that soon become studded with superficial pinpoint to 2- to 3-mm pustules (Fig. 5–15). Sheets of erythema and pustulation spread to involve unaffected skin, with a particular predisposition to the flexures, genital regions, webs of the fingers, and regions about the fingernails. The nails often become thickened or separated by subungual lakes of pus. Mucous membrane lesions in the mouth and tongue are common (Fig. 5–16). The dermatitis progresses from discrete sterile pustules to shallow subcorneal layers of pus, to dry brownish crusts, and finally to a generalized exfoliative dermatitis. The disease is cyclic and associated with complete clearance of the pustular phase and unexplained exacerbations. Relapses are common and become progressively more severe, often with poor prognosis.

The histologic picture of generalized pustular psoriasis, as in pustulosis palmaris et plantaris, shows a characteristic spongiform pustule in the upper epidermis (the spongiform pustule of Kogoj). Aside from the presence of spongiform pustules the epidermal changes are very much like those of psoriasis, with parakeratosis and elonga-

generally not as effective as topical corticosteroids. Methotrexate, etretinate, acitretin, and cyclosporine have also met with encouraging results. Their benefit, particularly in childhood forms of the disorder, however, must be carefully weighed against the risk of side effects.

Generalized Pustular Psoriasis

Often termed the *von Zumbusch variety, acrodermatitis continua of Hallopeau,* or *impetigo herpetiformis,* generalized pustular psoriasis is a relatively rare, sometimes fatal, severe form of psoriasis characterized by an explosive generalized eruption associated with high fever, leukocytosis, and toxicity. Although the cause is unknown, precipitating agents such as hydroxychloroquine, lithium, sulfonamides, sulfapyridine, propranolol, phenylbutazone, procaine, morphine, iodides, salicylates, progesterone, or penicillin; hypocalcemia; discontinuation of systemic corticosteroids; acute infection; pregnancy; and emotional upset may be related to the transformation of ordinary psoriasis to the generalized pustular form of this disorder.[33–38] Generalized pustular psoriasis can occur in infants and children, and a frequent history of antecedent seborrheic dermatitis suggests possible linkage between seborrheic dermatitis and generalized pustular psoriasis in this age group.[31]

Attacks of generalized pustular psoriasis are often preceded by a sensation of burning associated with high fever, leukocytosis, chills, malaise, and polyarthralgia. Previously quiescent psoriatic

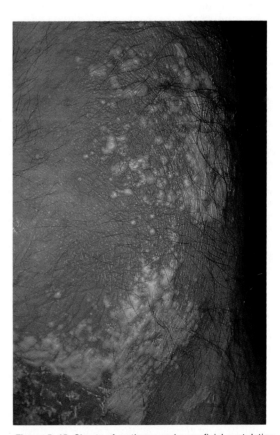

Figure 5–15. Sheets of erythema and superficial pustulation on the leg of a patient with generalized pustular psoriasis of von Zumbusch. (Courtesy of Department of Dermatology, Yale University School of Medicine.)

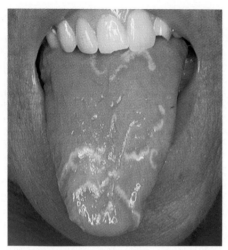

Figure 5–16. Annulus migrans. Psoriasis of the mucous membranes of the tongue in a patient with generalized pustular psoriasis (Zumbusch variety).

tion of rete ridges, an infiltrate of lymphocytes and neutrophils in the upper dermis, and neutrophils migrating from the dermis into the epidermis.

Therapy for the acute phase of generalized pustular psoriasis is best managed with soothing, moist compresses and general supportive measures. Although true infection is uncommon, death secondary to overwhelming sepsis, fluid loss, electrolyte imbalance, and general debility can occur. Periodic cultures of the skin, blood, and urine, therefore, should be performed. Occlusive ointments and dressings are contraindicated. Childhood forms of generalized pustular psoriasis appear to carry a better prognosis than adult forms of this disorder and are more likely to resolve spontaneously within a few weeks following bland topical therapy and good general nursing and medical care.[31] As acute stages of this disorder subside, the Goeckerman regimen, PUVA therapy, or topical corticosteroids often hasten the involution of stubborn pustules. Systemic corticosteroids are generally ineffectual and may predispose to severe complications, particularly infection; methotrexate and etretinate should be reserved for children with extreme, debilitating, or life-threatening disease.

ERYTHRODERMIC (EXFOLIATIVE) PSORIASIS

Erythrodermic or exfoliative psoriasis is a severe generalized disorder that occurs in a small percentage of adults and, on rare occasions, children with psoriasis. Although it may occur spontaneously as an initial manifestation of the disease, it generally occurs in chronic forms of psoriasis following sunburn, phototherapy complications or excessive ultraviolet exposure, or as a compli-

cation of excessive topical therapy, severe emotional stress, excessive alcohol consumption, or systemic viral or bacterial disease.[39]

The skin is almost totally involved with deep erythema, massive exfoliation, and associated abnormalities of temperature and cardiovascular regulation. Erythrodermic psoriasis, therefore, is a serious complication that necessitates hospitalization and skilled management. Although methotrexate and systemic retinoids have been recommended for adult forms of this disorder, the hazards inherent in the use of folic acid antagonists in childhood suggest these agents be employed only in cases where less hazardous measures are ineffective.[40]

ACROPUSTULOSIS OF INFANCY

Acropustulosis of infancy (infantile acropustulosis) is a disease of infancy and childhood that generally appears in black infants with an onset between birth and 2 years of age; it persists, with periods of remission and exacerbation, for about 2 years (Fig. 5–17).[41, 42] This disorder, seen in infants without family histories of atopy or psoriasis, is characterized by crops of intensely pruritic papulopustular or vesiculopustular lesions that appear for 7 to 10 days, after which time the eruption generally remits for 2 or 3 weeks prior to recurrences. The condition is about four times as common in males and in blacks than winter. The lesions begin as pinpoint erythematous papules and enlarge into well-circumscribed discrete pustules within 24 hours. They are concentrated on the palms and soles and appear in lesser numbers on the dorsal aspect of the hands, feet, wrists, and ankles, and less often on the face and scalp. New lesions are accompanied by intense pruritus, restlessness, and fretfulness. The eruption is unresponsive to potent topical corticosteroids, the pruritus is re-

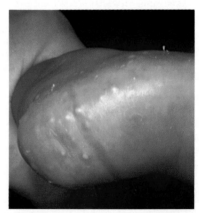

Figure 5–17. Acropustulosis of infancy (infantile acropustulosis). Recurrent pruritic papulopustular lesions occurred on the feet of a 9-month-old black girl.

lieved only by soporific doses of antihistamine, and the disease resolves spontaneously by the time the patient is 2 to 3 years of age.[42]

The differential diagnosis of this disorder includes dyshidrotic eczema, pustular psoriasis, toxic erythema of the newborn, transient neonatal pustular melanosis, scabies, impetigo, and subcorneal pustular dermatosis. The histopathologic features of infantile acropustulosis include large, well-circumscribed subcorneal or intraepidermal pustules filled with polymorphonuclear leukocytes. The initial histopathologic event in patients with this disorder appears to be related to necrolysis of keratinocytes followed by intraepidermal vesiculation and invasion by neutrophils, eosinophils, or both.[43–46]

Suggested treatment for infantile acropustulosis includes systemic antibiotics such as erythromycin or sulfones. Although this disorder requires further study, some believe that dapsone in a dosage of 2 mg/kg/day may be more effective than erythromycin in the management of infantile acropustulosis.[41]

REITER'S DISEASE

Reiter's disease is a disorder of unknown etiology characterized by a triad of urethritis, arthritis, and nonbacterial conjunctivitis. The classic triad, however, is seen in only one third of patients, and the presence of seronegative, oligoarticular, asymmetric arthritis with urethritis or cervicitis has been proposed as sufficient to establish the diagnosis. In 50 to 80 per cent of patients cutaneous lesions that mimic or closely resemble psoriasis may be seen. Generally recognized as a disorder that primarily affects young men, particularly those between 20 and 40 years of age, it also can affect young children, the youngest reported case being that of a 9-month-old infant. In children the disorder seems to be less severe but otherwise similar to that in adults and, although there are relatively few reports of the disease in this age group, a total of 39 childhood cases have been reported.[47–51]

Isolated cases can occur in females, but more than 90 per cent of reported cases have been in males. The syndrome has been associated with an antecedent, apparently infectious dysenteric or urethritic episode, possibly due to *Shigella flexneri*, *Salmonella typhimurium*, *Yersinia*, *Chlamydia*, or *Mycoplasma* organisms that enter the body through inflamed membranes (either intestinal or urethral). The disorder has also been seen in patients with the acquired immunodeficiency syndrome. Diarrhea is initially present in 90 per cent of children but in only one third of adults with this disorder. HLA typings suggest that heredity plays a significant role in the predisposition of affected individuals to the development of this disorder.[52, 53]

The cutaneous manifestations of Reiter's disease may develop in association with, or independently of, the other features of the disorder. The most characteristic lesions are those that appear over the glans penis, palms, soles, and toes. Discrete lesions may also be found on the limbs, scrotum, trunk, and scalp. They begin as pinpoint vesicular or macular lesions that become purulent and eventuate in red scaly psoriasiform lesions (Fig. 5–18). The term *keratoderma blennorrhagicum* refers to the thickened hyperkeratotic, often psoriasiform, yellowish scaly lesions on an erythematous base that have a predilection for the palms, soles, and toes (Fig. 5–19).

Oral lesions consist of painless erythema, shallow erosions, and small pustules that may occur on the buccal mucosa, gums, lips, palate, and tongue and generally resolve spontaneously after a period of several days. Lesions on the tongue, particularly when thickly coated, may simulate a geographic tongue.

The ocular lesions of Reiter's disease are seen in at least 50 per cent of patients. They consist of conjunctivitis, iritis, and, at times, keratitis. Arthritis, the predominant feature of this syndrome, resembles rheumatoid arthritis. It is usually polyarticular and generally involves the sacroiliac joints, knees, ankles, and, less frequently, joints of the upper extremities.

Diagnosis of this disorder is aided by the presence of the classic triad, with or without the presence of cutaneous or mucosal lesions. The clinical and histopathologic appearance of cutaneous lesions of Reiter's disease may be identical to or similar to those of psoriasis but may be differentiated by the presence of ocular, arthritic, and urethral lesions, by HLA testing, and by a lack of family history of psoriasis.

Treatment consists primarily of bed rest and salicylates for the arthritis; topical corticosteroids for cutaneous lesions; broad-spectrum antibiotics, particularly tetracycline, for the associated urethritis; and, for patients with severe unresponsive

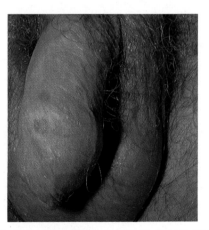

Figure 5–18. Psoriasiform lesions of Reiter's syndrome. When several penile lesions coalesce into a circinate form, it is termed *balanitis circinata*.

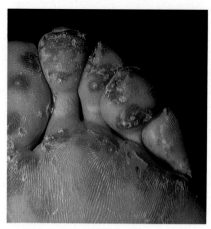

Figure 5–19. Keratoderma blennorrhagicum. Thickened hyperkeratotic psoriasiform lesions occur on the foot of a patient with Reiter's disease.

disease, immunosuppressive agents (6-mercaptopurine or methotrexate). Although deaths have been reported in children as well as adults with Reiter's syndrome, the prognosis is generally better in childhood.[50, 51] Systemic or intra-articular corticosteroids may be used if symptoms are severe, but, since they may aggravate the cutaneous manifestations, they should generally be avoided. In view of the usual excellent prognosis in children, treatment in this age group is symptomatic and consists primarily of bed rest and analgesics.

PITYRIASIS RUBRA PILARIS

Pityriasis rubra pilaris is a chronic skin disorder characterized by small follicular papules, disseminated yellowish pink scaly plaques surrounding islands of normal skin, and hyperkeratosis of the palms and soles. The papules are an important diagnostic feature of this disorder. They are fine, firm, and conical and topped by a central keratotic plug. They are pinpoint sized, arise at the mouth of hair follicles, may or may not be pierced by a central hair, and vary from normal skin color to a yellowish pink or red.

Available evidence suggests two distinct variants of this disorder: a familial type and an acquired variety. The familial form is inherited as an autosomal disorder that may present at birth or have its onset during infancy or childhood. The acquired type may appear at any age and is generally seen in individuals older than 15 years of age. Although the acquired form has no known genetic tendency, many authorities believe that this variant may show mild, easily overlooked features at an early stage and accordingly may merely represent a delayed expression of the inherited form of this disorder. Based on clinical characteristics, age at onset, and prognosis, five types of pityriasis rubra pilaris have been recognized (Table 5–1).[54, 55]

The cause of pityriasis rubra pilaris is unknown. It appears to represent a disturbance in keratinization in which the precise defect is as yet undetermined. Skin lesions, both clinically and histologically, are suggestive of those seen in phrynoderma (vitamin A deficiency). Vitamin A levels, however, are variable, and the role of vitamin A, if any, remains obscure.

Although little is known about the pathophysiology of this disease, it has been speculated that the involved areas reflect an underlying abnormality in epidermal cell kinetics (decreased transit time and accelerated epidermal proliferation) as a significant pathogenetic factor.[56] Some patients have also been reported to have low serum levels of retinol-binding protein. Further studies, however, are required to substantiate this finding and its significance.

Clinical Manifestations. Pityriasis rubra pilaris, particularly in children, frequently starts gradually with a generalized scaling of the scalp and forehead and a diffuse erythema of the face and ears. In adults the onset is often more acute, and a generalized erythroderma may develop over the course of a few days. The characteristic fine eruption usually appears first on the hands and feet, particularly over the dorsal aspects of the first and second phalanges, wrists, knees, elbows, sides of the neck, and trunk. On the dorsal aspect of the fingers the papules remain distinctly follicular and pathognomonic. In other areas, as new le-

Table 5–1. CLASSIFICATION OF PITYRIASIS RUBRA PILARIS

Types	Clinical Features	Approximate Frequency
I Classic adult	Majority of cases; generally clears in 3 years; entire cutaneous surface may become erythrodermic	50% to 55%
II Atypical adult	Rare; of long duration (lesions gradually develop over a decade or more); involvement of the legs is more ichthyosiform, other areas are more eczematous	5%
III Classic juvenile	Early onset (generally in first 2 years of life), slow clearing, clinically similar to classic adult type I	10%
IV Circumscribed juvenile	Prepubertal children; often persists into adult life; affects elbows, knees, and other bony prominences; less than 50% clear spontaneously	25% (approximately 60% of childhood cases)
V Atypical juvenile	Rare, with largely familial onset; begins in first few years of life and tends to run a lifelong course	5%

sions occur, they tend to coalesce and form sharply marginated patches (much like plucked chicken skin) and thickened psoriasiform plaques with a coarse texture similar to the surface of a nutmeg grater. The plaques are generally symmetrical and diffuse and contrast sharply to islands of normal skin that occur within the affected areas (Fig. 5–20).

In adults, at times the eruption can progress to an exfoliative dermatitis with associated systemic symptoms of malaise, chills, fever, and diarrhea. Facial involvement may be seen as a heavy waxy scaling and an associated ectropion of the eyelids. Painful fissures can occur in involved areas of the skin, but pruritus is usually not a prominent feature.

Thickened hyperkeratotic skin frequently develops on the palms and soles. When seen on the soles, this has been referred to as a "keratodermic sandal." The nails are often thickened and opaque, with transverse striations and subungual debris. The characteristic pitting of nails seen in psoriasis, however, is not a feature of this disorder.

The diagnosis of pityriasis rubra pilaris is based primarily on the acuminate follicular papules with keratotic plugs that appear on the backs of fingers, sides of the neck, and extensor surfaces of the limbs. Salmon-colored scaling plaques, islands of normal skin in the midst of the eruption, and hyperkeratosis of the palms and soles help confirm the clinical impression.

The histologic picture is similar to that of vitamin A deficiency and keratosis pilaris. Although not pathognomonic, it is fairly characteristic and consists of follicular keratosis, diffuse hyperkeratosis, irregular mild acanthosis, and inconstant patchy parakeratosis (particularly near the hair follicles). Liquefactive degeneration of the basal layers of the epidermis with extension along the hair follicles is often present. A mild chronic inflammatory infiltrate in the upper dermis, particularly around hair follicles and superficial vessels, helps complete the histopathologic picture.

The clinical course of pityriasis rubra pilaris is variable. In most cases a protracted clinical course may be anticipated. In 25 to 50 per cent of cases spontaneous clearing may develop after a period of time varying from several months to years. In childhood forms, however, the disorder frequently tends to be persistent and may be characterized by spontaneous remissions and exacerbations.

Treatment. Treatment of pityriasis rubra pilaris depends on suppression of hyperkeratinization; mild forms may require only emollients, topical corticosteroids, and keratolytic agents (formulatons containing urea, salicylic acids, α-hydroxy acid and topical retinoic acid). In adults, success has been achieved with large doses of oral vitamin A, varying from 150,000 to 600,000 units/day. In children a lower dose (50,000 units twice a day and dosages up to 150,000 to 300,000 units/day) has been used with complete remission after 6½ weeks of therapy.[57] Adequate therapeutic trial requires treatment for a period of at least 3 to 6 weeks. If effective, it can be continued for months before signs of hypervitaminosis A (anorexia, pruritus, dry skin, hair loss, subcutaneous swellings, painful hyperostoses, liver toxicity, hypertriglyceridemia, neurologic abnormalities, prolonged clotting time, reduced prothrombin time, abdominal pain, dizziness, visual disturbances, sluggishness, irritability, sleepiness, and polyarthralgia) occur. After several months of continuous therapy, in an effort to avoid signs of toxicity, oral vitamin A may be discontinued for periods of 2 to 3 months or more. Although oral vitamin A therapy is frequently supplanted by the use of systemic retinoids, complications associated with the prolonged administration of aromatic retinoids frequently preclude their use in children. Oral retinoids, if used, should be carefully monitored and reserved for only those patients with chronic, resistant, or severely disabling forms of the disorder.[58]

Because of their ability to inhibit DNA synthesis and cell division, folic acid antagonists

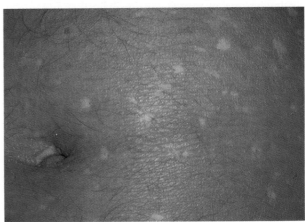

Figure 5–20. Pityriasis rubra pilaris. Islands of normal skin are surrounded by areas of erythema.

(aminopterin and methotrexate) have also been suggested in the therapy for this disorder. Because of potential toxicity associated with these agents, adequate precautions should be taken and folic acid antagonists should be avoided or given with great caution to children, women during the child-bearing period, and patients with renal or hepatic disease.

PITYRIASIS LICHENOIDES

Pityriasis lichenoides is a distinctive cutaneous eruption of children and young adults characterized by crops of macules, papules, or papulovesicles that tend to develop central necrosis and crusts soon after they arise. Originally described by Mucha of Vienna in 1916, and later by Habermann in Germany in 1921, the disorder appears in two forms and may be seen at any age: (1) an acute form (acute guttate parapsoriasis, parapsoriasis varioliformis, pityriasis lichenoides et varioliformis acuta, Mucha-Habermann disease) seen mainly in children and young adults and (2) a chronic form (pityriasis lichenoides chronica, guttate parapsoriasis of Juliusberg) more commonly noted in adolescents and young adults.

Acute pityriasis lichenoides (pityriasis lichenoides acuta et varioliformis, PLEVA) is a polymorphous eruption that usually begins as symmetrical 2- to 3-mm, oval or round, reddish brown macules and papules. The papules occur in successive crops and rapidly evolve into vesicular, necrotic, and sometimes purpuric lesions (Figs. 5–21 and 5–22). These develop a fine crust and gradually resolve, with or without a varioliform scar. Occasionally temporary hypopigmentation or hyperpigmentation may result. Although the eruption is usually the first manifestation of the disease, occasionally fever and constitutional symptoms may precede or accompany the cutaneous eruption. Lesions may involve the entire body but are most pronounced on the trunk, thighs, and upper arms, especially the flexor surfaces. The face, scalp, mucous membranes, palms, and soles are frequently spared or may be involved to a lesser degree.[59, 60] The course usually lasts for periods of a few weeks to several months; and although recurrences may continue for periods of 2 or 3 years, despite an occasional prolonged and stormy course, except for a report of two children in which the disorder apparently evolved into cutaneous T-cell lymphoma, the prognosis is generally good.[61]

Chronic pityriasis lichenoides (pityriasis lichenoides chronica) may begin de novo or may evolve from pityriasis lichenoides acuta. The course of chronic pityriasis lichenoides is variable and may last for periods of 6 months to several years. It begins with smooth or slightly firm, reddish brown papules that measure several millimeters to a centimeter in diameter. Scales, when present, are adherent, are slightly thicker in the

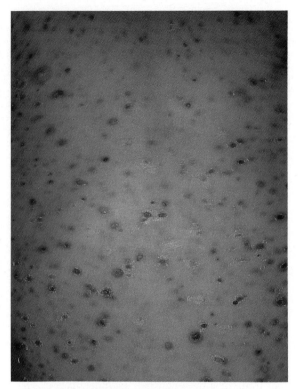

Figure 5–21. Pityriasis lichenoides et varioliformis acuta (PLEVA). Symmetrical oval and round reddish brown macular, papular, necrotic, and crusted lesions on the chest and abdomen of an 8-year-old child.

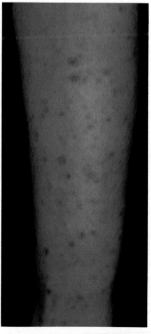

Figure 5–22. Mucha-Habermann disease. Acute pityriasis lichenoides (pityriasis lichenoides et varioliformis acuta, PLEVA).

center, and can be detached by gentle scraping to reveal a shiny brown surface (a diagnostic feature of this disorder). Over a period of several weeks the individual papules recede, the scale separates spontaneously, and a hyperpigmented or hypopigmented macule results and eventually fades (usually without residual scar). Although sequelae are uncommon, in occasional cases the lesions may progress to form nodules with highly atypical cells, which on histopathologic examination suggest a malignant cutaneous lymphoma. The subsequent clinical course, evolution, and morphology of lesions confirm the benign character of the disorder. Cases that histologically mimic lymphoma have been classified by some authorities as a separate disorder termed *lymphomatoid papulosis* (Fig. 5–23).[62]

In the early stages pityriasis lichenoides may be mistaken for chickenpox, arthropod bites, impetigo, pityriasis rosea, allergic vasculitis, or scabies; chronic forms may be confused with psoriasis, lichen planus, and secondary syphilis. The duration of the eruption (often in crops), the presence of macules and papules interspersed with vesicular, crusted, or hemorrhagic lesions with or without varioliform scarring, and subsequent hypopigmentation or hyperpigmentation help differentiate pityriasis lichenoides from other conditions. When the diagnosis remains in doubt, histopathologic examination of a skin biopsy specimen will often substantiate the proper diagnosis.

The histology of pityriasis lichenoides varies with the stage, intensity, and extent of the reaction. The prominent feature is a heavy, primarily lymphocytic and histiocytic perivascular infiltrate. Diapedesis of erythrocytes occurs in the dermis, and severe intercellular and intracellular edema in the epidermis lead to intraepidermal vesicle formation, necrosis of the epidermis, and finally erosions and eventual crusting.

A number of theories have been proposed concerning the etiology of pityriasis lichenoides, but all are unsubstantiated. The clinical and histologic features suggest a vasculitis. Some authors suggest an autoimmune process, a hypersensitivity reaction triggered by various etiologic factors, or an exanthem of viral or rickettsial etiology.[63]

Owing to the undetermined etiology and variable nature of this disease, there is no well-established form of therapy. Antipruritics, nonsteroidal anti-inflammatory agents, and lubricants may be helpful in ameliorating the symptoms, and topical corticosteroids, tar preparations, sun exposure, ultraviolet light, and PUVA phototherapy have been effective for the treatment of persistent or chronic forms of the disorder.[64–67] Tetracycline in high doses (2 g/day for older children and adults) and erythromycin (30 to 50 mg/kg/day, with a maximum of 1 or 2 g/day for older children and adults) for several weeks to 2 months are frequently helpful, particularly in the acute forms of the disorder; however, results are variable, and tetracycline should not be administered to children younger than 8 years of age or to pregnant women.[68, 69] Methotrexate, in dosages of 7.5 to 20 mg weekly by mouth, has resulted in improvement in persistent cases.[70] Relapse, however, usually follows discontinuance of treatment and, again, this form of therapy is not generally recommended, particularly in children or pregnant women.

LYMPHOMATOID PAPULOSIS

Lymphomatoid papulosis is a recurrent self-healing papulonecrotic, nodular, and occasionally plaque-like dermatosis with histologic features suggesting malignant lymphoma.[62] Although its nosologic status remains unclear, the disorder has been considered to be a variant of pityriasis lichenoides, a pseudolymphoma, or a cutaneous T-cell lymphoma of low-grade malignancy.

The disorder is manifested by numerous reddish brown papules and by vesiculopustules that may have a smooth surface, scales, crusts, ulcers, small scars, and hyperpigmentation over the trunk and proximal portions of the extremities and occasionally the hands and feet, scalp, and genitalia. Lesions characteristically develop hemorrhagic necrotic centers and crusting, which gradually involute with residual hyperpigmentation or hypopigmentation. Occasionally varioliform scars or large ulcerating nodules, plaques, or papules occur that do not ulcerate. Although individual lesions evolve over a period of several weeks to 1 month or more, tend to appear in crops, and sometimes disappear spontaneously within 3 to 6 weeks, the entire course of the disorder may be prolonged and last for years. Except perhaps for mild pruritus, the disorder is generally asymptomatic. Of particular significance is the fact that in 10 to 20 per cent of patients, usually adults, a malignant lymphoma such as cutaneous T-cell lymphoma, Hodgkin's disease, or non-Hodgkin's

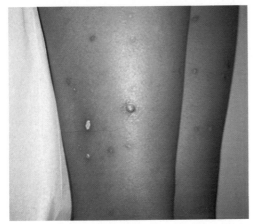

Figure 5–23. Crusted and necrotic varioliform lesions of parapsoriasis lichenoides chronica.

lymphoma may develop.[71–73] Lymphomatoid papulosis, however, is relatively rare in children and usually does not occur in association with malignant disease.

The histopathologic picture of lymphomatoid papulosis is characterized by moderately dense, mixed cell infiltrates that, although usually wedge-shaped, are band-like in the upper part of an edematous dermis. The infiltrate consists of lymphocytes, histiocytes, plasma cells, eosinophils, neutrophils, and strikingly atypical lymphocytes with convoluted nuclei similar to and at times indistinguishable from those of cutaneous T-cell lymphoma (mycosis fungoides).

Despite the fact that recurrences may persist for many years, 80 to 90 per cent of patients have a benign clinical course. Because of the risk of malignancy, particularly in adults, patients, especially those with large, destructive, or atypical lesions, require careful long-term follow-up examinations.[74] Individual patients have responded to systemic corticosteroids, antibiotics (erythromycin or tetracycline), sulfones, electron beam therapy, PUVA therapy, and chemotherapeutic agents such as methotrexate (5 to 25 mg once a week), but the response to treatment is inconsistent and frequently unsatisfactory.[75, 76]

PITYRIASIS ROSEA

Pityriasis rosea is an acute benign self-limiting disorder that affects males and females equally, with a peak incidence in adolescents and young adults. Although uncommon in children younger than 5 years of age, I have seen it in an 8-month-old infant and it has been reported in an infant as young as 3 months of age.[77] The disorder appears to be more common during the fall, winter, and spring and is believed to have a slight female preponderance. Except for a prodrome that may at times consist of headache, malaise, pharyngitis, and lymphadenitis, and occasional reports of mild constitutional symptoms, there is no evidence of systemic involvement, complications, or sequelae. Although the etiology of pityriasis rosea remains unknown, a viral disorder is suggested by the occasional presence of prodromal symptoms, the course of the disease, epidemics with seasonal cluster, reports of simultaneous occurrence in closely associated individuals, and a tendency to life-long immunity in 98 per cent of cases.[78, 79]

The eruption follows a distinctive pattern, and 70 to 80 per cent of cases start with a single isolated lesion, the so-called herald patch (Fig. 5–24). It may occur anywhere on the body, most commonly on the trunk, upper arms, neck, and thighs. This characteristic initial lesion is seen as a sharply defined oval area of scaly dermatitis (2 to 5 cm in diameter) with a flat, pink or brown center and a red, finely scaled, and slightly elevated border. After an interval of 5 to 10 days a secondary generalized eruption appears in crops, character-

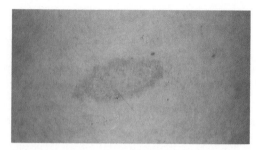

Figure 5–24. Herald patch (pityriasis rosea). Oval lesion with finely scaled elevated border, occasionally misdiagnosed as tinea corporis.

istically sparing the face (in 85 per cent of individuals), scalp, and distal extremities. These clinically distinctive lesions resemble the herald patch in morphology but are smaller and generally more ovoid. They may appear as small, pink, finely scaled macules that measure 2 to 10 mm in diameter or as slightly larger, dull pink, round or oval patches that measure 0.5 to 3.0 cm in diameter. On the thorax the long axis of individual lesions runs parallel to the lines of skin cleavage in what has been described as a "Christmas-tree" pattern (Fig. 5–25). Typical of these secondary lesions is a fine scaly edge with a characteristic cigarette paper–like "collarette" scale (Fig. 5–26).

Occasionally, particularly in young children, lesions may be predominantly papular, vesicular, pustular, urticarial, or even purpuric, particularly during the early stages of the eruption (see Fig. 5–25); and in some instances bullous or lichenoid lesions have been noted. The papular variety is more common in young children, blacks, and pregnant women. Less commonly, some patients, particularly children, may show an inverse distribution of lesions on the face, wrists, and extremities, which may or may not spread centrally to include the trunk. This atypical form of pityriasis rosea may be particularly difficult to diagnose if there is no history of a herald patch and if the characteristic morphology of lesions goes unrecognized.

The head and face are frequently affected in children, and the face and neck are occasionally involved in blacks. Involvement of the oral mucous membranes, often overlooked, is unusual but may be seen as red patches that, at times, may appear to be erosive, hemorrhagic, or bullous. Other reported oral manifestations include large erythematous plaques covering the entire palate, multiple hemorrhagic puncta scattered over the buccal and palatal mucosae, confluent white erosions on the buccal mucosa, annular lesions with clear centers and raised borders, and mild desquamation. In about 25 per cent of cases a moderate itching, particularly in secondary lesions, may be noted. Malaise, headache, adenopathy, low fever, and joint pains have been reported but appear to be rare. Once the secondary cutaneous eruption begins to appear it usually reaches its

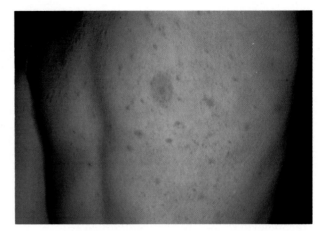

Figure 5–25. Pityriasis rosea. Christmas-tree pattern in lines of cleavage. Note papulovesicular lesions occasionally seen in childhood forms of this disorder.

height within a few days to a week. Healing generally begins after 2 to 4 weeks, first in lesions that appeared earliest, and is usually complete by 6 to 14 weeks. Postinflammatory hypopigmentation (Fig. 5–27) or hyperpigmentation may frequently be noted, particularly in dark-skinned individuals, and may persist for weeks to months after healing is complete.

Diagnosis of pityriasis rosea depends on recognition of the characteristic appearance and distribution of the oval lesions with their fine peripheral or "collarette" scales. The herald patch may be mistaken for tinea corporis, and the full-blown eruption must be differentiated from lesions of secondary syphilis (a frequent misdiagnosis), drug eruption, Mucha-Habermann disease, seborrheic dermatitis, nummular eczema, and psoriasis (particularly the guttate variety).

The histologic features of pityriasis rosea are not diagnostic and resemble those of a subacute or chronic dermatitis with vascular dilatation, edema, a superficial lymphohistiocytic dermal infiltrate, acanthosis, epidermal spongiosis, mild exocytosis, and, at times, patchy parakeratosis.

Most patients require no treatment beyond re-

assurance as to the nature and prognosis of the disorder. Pruritus, if present, usually responds to topical antipruritics (calamine lotion, with 0.5 to 1 per cent phenol if desired, Sarna lotion [Stiefel], and Pramoxine-containing formulations such as Prax [Ferndale], PrameGel [GenDerm], or Pramosone [Ferndale]), oral antihistamines, colloidal starch or oatmeal baths, and mild topical corticosteroid formulations. Exposure to ultraviolet light or sunshine generally tends to hasten resolution of lesions, and in the summertime it is not uncommon to see patients with pityriasis rosea under covered areas with little to no evidence of the eruption on sun-exposed regions.[80]

LICHEN PLANUS

Lichen planus is a relatively common subacute or chronic dermatosis of unknown etiology that occurs in persons of all ages. Although 66 to 85 per cent of cases occur in adults between 30 and 70 years of age, the disorder has also been recorded in an infant 3 weeks of age and 2 to 3 per cent of the reported cases occur in children

Figure 5–26. Pityriasis rosea. Note fine peripheral "collarette" scale.

Figure 5–27. Postinflammatory hypopigmentation following resolution of pityriasis rosea.

younger than age 20.[81, 82] The etiology of lichen planus is unknown, but current evidence suggests a cell-mediated immune response and perhaps, in some patients at least, a genetic predisposition. In familial cases the disorder appears to have an earlier age at onset, increased severity, a greater likelihood of chronicity, and an increased incidence of erosive, linear, ulcerative, and hypertrophic forms.[83–86]

The primary lesion is a small shiny flat-topped polygonal reddish or violaceous papule (Fig. 5–28). Individual papules vary from 2 mm to 1 cm or more, may be closely aggregated or widely dispersed, and are generally intensely pruritic. The disorder is usually limited to a few areas, with the flexural surfaces of the wrists, legs, genitalia, and mucous membranes as the sites of predilection. In chronic forms, the sites of predilection are the flexor surfaces of the wrists, the forearms, and the inner aspects of the knees and thighs.

At times one may detect small grayish puncta or streaks that form a network over the surface of papules. These delicate white lines, termed *Wickham's striae*, become more visible under magnification with a hand lens or by application of a drop of oil, which renders the horny layers of lesions more transparent. Occasionally, lesions may coalesce to form plaques or a linear configuration (the Koebner phenomenon) over sites of minor trauma such as scratch marks (Fig. 5–29).

Mucous membrane involvement is seen in 50 to 70 per cent of patients. When present, lesions are usually seen as pinhead-sized white papules forming annular or linear lace-like patterns on the inner aspects of the cheeks (Fig. 5–30). Lesions on the palate, lips, and tongue are less characteristic and, except for their reticulated appearance, may easily be mistaken for areas of leukoplakia. On the lips the papules are more often annular, there is adherent scaling similar to that seen in lupus erythematosus (Fig. 5–31), and, in some in-

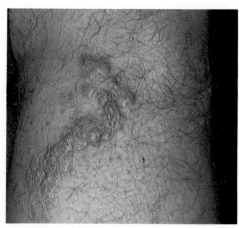

Figure 5–29. Thickened papular lesions of hypertrophic lichen planus with a Koebner phenomenon.

stances, painful ulcerative lesions have been found on the tongue (Fig. 5–32), oral mucous membranes, and mucosal surfaces of the pharynx, esophagus, gastrointestinal tract, vulva, and vagina.[87, 88]

Up to 10 per cent of patients with lichen planus demonstrate nail involvement, but lichen planus of the nail without skin lesions is rare. Apparently associated with inflammation of the nail matrix and nail fold, such lesions may involve one, several, or all nails. Occasionally violaceous lines or papules in the nail bed may be seen through the nail plate. Although not pathognomonic of the disorder, nail dystrophy is highly characteristic. It consists of loss of luster, thinning of the nail plate, longitudinal ridging or striation, splitting or nicking of the nail margin, atrophy, overlapping skin folds (pterygia), marked subungual hyperkeratosis, lifting of the distal nail plate, red or brown discoloration, and, at times, complete and permanent loss of the nail. Reviews suggest that twenty-nail dystrophy may, in some cases at least, represent a variant of lichen planus.

Variants. Although lichen planus is considered to be papulosquamous, many variations in morphology and configuration may be noted. These

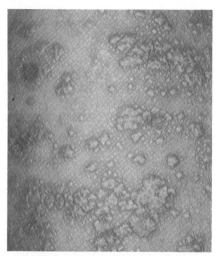

Figure 5–28. Lichen planus. Papules are shiny, flat-topped, violaceous, and polygonal.

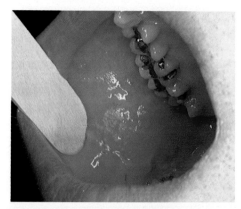

Figure 5–30. White papules of lichen planus in a linear lace-like reticulated pattern on the buccal mucosa.

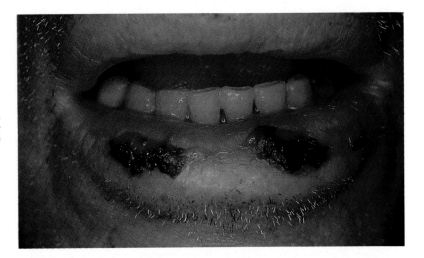

Figure 5–31. Crusted lesions of lichen planus on the lips. (Courtesy of Department of Dermatology, Yale University School of Medicine.)

variations include vesicular, bullous, actinic, annular, hypertrophic, atrophic, linear, erythematous, and follicular forms.

Vesicular and Bullous Forms. Lesions may appear in part as vesicles or bullae located on top of pre-existing papules (bullous lichen planus). Occasionally bullous lesions may also appear on otherwise normal skin (lichen planus pemphigoid). When other characteristic lesions are not apparent, this variant may be confused with other bullous disorders such as pemphigus vulgaris or dermatitis herpetiformis.

Actinic Lichen Planus. This variant is generally seen in children and young adults of Asian heritage. Often confined to individuals in tropical and subtropical regions, sun-exposed areas are principally involved and pruritus may be mild or absent. Lesions may be pigmented, dyschromic, or

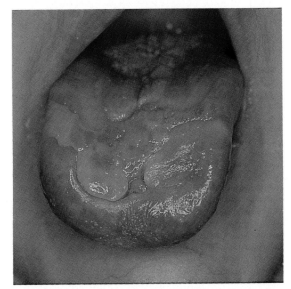

Figure 5–32. Lichen planus. Oral lesions on the tongue. (Courtesy of Department of Dermatology, Yale University School of Medicine.)

resemble granuloma annulare and may be confused with lupus erythematosus. In such cases, individual lesions, course, and histologic features are similar to those of true lichen planus. Whether these lesions truly represent lichen planus has not been determined.

Annular Lichen Planus. Annular lichen planus, seen in 10 per cent of affected individuals, is a variant that evolves from chronic forms of the disorder and results in a ring-like grouping of lesions. It commonly occurs on the penis and lower trunk but may occur anywhere. Lesions of granuloma annulare may at times resemble this variant, but few other conditions simulate this disorder.

Hypertrophic (Verrucous) Lichen Planus. Hypertrophic lichen planus is characterized by verrucous plaques covered with fine adherent scales. This variant may involve any region of the body but most commonly appears on the pretibial areas of the legs and ankles. Lesions may appear as isolated or multiple plaques, or they may be confluent and cover the entire anterior tibial area. Although superficial inspection may suggest a diagnosis of psoriasis, careful examination may reveal small flat-topped polygonal papules that reveal the true nature of the disorder.

Lichen Planus Atrophicus. In this variant, lesions tend to be few and atrophy may be the result of resolved annular or hypertrophic lesions.

Linear Lichen Planus. Linear or zosteriform lesions are occasionally seen as an uncommon variant of lichen planus.[89] In this extremely pruritic variant, lesions extend along an extremity or on the trunk, often overlying thrombosed veins and along the course of nerves. Although no explanation for this variant has been satisfactory, it is thought that this form of the disorder may be the result of trauma or that it may follow dermatomal segments of the skin or distribution of peripheral nerves.

Erosive and Ulcerative Lichen Planus. Bullous, erosive, and ulcerative lesions of lichen planus may at times be seen on the mucous membranes, palms, and soles. When present on the plantar surfaces, lesions can be extremely painful and at times disabling. Although malignant transformation of oral lichen planus has been reported, leading some to suggest that oral lichen planus is premalignant, case reports fail to substantiate claims that oral lesions, except perhaps atrophic lesions associated with chronic irritation, local trauma, or carcinogens such as tobacco, arsenic, or radiation, present malignant potential.[90, 91]

Lichen Planus Erythematosus. Discrete vivid red, soft, nonpruritic lesions of lichen planus that measure 5 to 10 mm in diameter and blanch on pressure may arise on the trunk of affected individuals. Although this variant may at times be associated with mucosal or nail changes and shows typical histologic features of this disorder, the question of whether this is a true form of lichen planus is uncertain.

Lichen Planopilaris (Follicular Lichen Planus). This follicular type of lichen planus, also termed *folliculitis decalvans of Graham Little*, is seen more frequently in women and generally consists of spinous or acuminate (conical) follicular lesions with typical cutaneous and mucosal lichen planus, follicular lesions and alopecia of the scalp (with or without atrophy), an increased incidence of nail involvement, and erosion of mucous membrane lesions. The end stage of this disorder may be indistinguishable from pseudopelade (a cicatricial form of alopecia of unknown origin) (see Chapter 17).

Lichenoid Drug Eruptions. Many drugs produce an eruption very similar or identical to lichen planus, and it is highly probable, at least in some cases, that drugs may precipitate attacks of lichen planus. For years it had been realized that certain drugs (gold and arsenicals) could produce lichenoid eruptions. Not until World War II when large numbers of troops taking quinacrine (Atrabrine) developed drug eruptions was it recognized how closely these disorders resembled typical lichen planus. Subsequent studies revealed that soldiers who developed such lichenoid drug eruptions were those with a deficiency of glucose-6-phosphate dehydrogenase.[92] Other drugs known to cause lichenoid eruptions include antituberculous preparations (*p*-aminosalicylic acid and isoniazid), streptomycin, quinidine, chlorpropamide (Diabinese), tetracycline, the phenothiazines, benzodiazepines such as chlordiazepoxide (Librium), carbamazepine (Tegretol), β-blocking agents (propranolol), furosemide (Lasix), gold salts, naproxen (Naprosyn), D-penicillamine, dapsone, and paraphenylenediamine salts in color film developers.[93]

When lesions of lichenoid drug eruption closely resemble those of lichen planus, the histologic picture generally also resembles that of lichen planus. Parakeratosis in the stratum corneum and eosinophils in the cellular infiltrate, neither of which is seen in lesions of lichen planus, help differentiate the two disorders.

Diagnosis. Diagnosis of lichen planus depends on the recognition of typical papules of this disorder or one of its variants in location, clinical pattern, or morphology. When the diagnosis is in doubt, histopathologic examination of a cutaneous lesion will generally help to establish the proper diagnosis. The histopathologic picture of lichen planus is that of hyperkeratosis, a thickened granular layer without parakeratosis, destruction of the basal cell layer (liquefactive degeneration), saw-toothing of the rete pegs, and a band-like lymphocytic infiltrate that hugs and invades the lower epidermis.

Although cases of lichen planus occasionally clear in a few weeks, two thirds of affected individuals with acute forms display spontaneous resolution within 8 to 15 months. In most patients the lesions tend to flatten but are often replaced by an area of pigmentation that may persist for months or years. Occasionally the disorder may persist for years, and 10 to 20 per cent of patients suffer one or more recurrences of their disorder.

Treatment. There is no specific treatment for lichen planus. Symptomatic relief, however, may be obtained by systemic antihistamines, ataractics such as hydroxyzine (Atarax or Vistaril) in dosages of 10 to 25 mg or more three or four times a day, or sedatives (particularly in individuals in whom stress may be a precipitating factor). Symptomatic relief may also be obtained by colloidal oatmeal or corn starch baths. Since drug-induced lichen planus may at times present a problem, medications should be discontinued or substituted whenever possible. Local symptomatic treatment with topical corticosteroid preparations is helpful; in lesions that are recalcitrant or hypertrophic, occlusive dressings over topical corticosteroids, Cordran Tape (Dista) or intralesional corticosteroids may be beneficial; on rare occasions (perhaps in 1 of 20 patients) a brief 2- to 6-week course of systemic corticosteroids may be necessary. When traditional forms of therapy fail, systemic antibiotics, griseofulvin, PUVA therapy, oral retinoids, and cyclosporine have been shown to be effective in selected cases.[94–97]

Mucous membrane lesions usually require no therapy. When they are symptomatic, eroded, or ulcerated, however, topical anesthetics such as diphenhydramine (Benadryl) elixir, lidocaine (Xylocaine) viscous, topical corticosteroids (Kenalog in Orabase), or intralesional corticosteroids may be beneficial. Since erosive forms of oral lichen planus may have an increased risk of malignant transformation, patients with oral lesions should avoid carcinogenic factors (such as tobacco) and receive periodic follow-up examinations and biopsy of suspicious lesions.[90, 91]

LICHEN NITIDUS

Lichen nitidus is a relatively uncommon benign dermatosis that affects individuals of all ages and is most commonly seen in children of preschool and school age. Although the etiology remains unknown, association with lichen planus has been reported and many authorities consider lichen nitidus to be a variant of this disorder.[98]

Individual papules of lichen nitidus are sharply demarcated, pinpoint to pinhead sized, round or polygonal, and usually flesh colored (Fig. 5–33). Surfaces of individual lesions are flat, shiny, and slightly elevated, often with a central depression. The eruption is arranged in groups primarily located on the trunk, genitalia, abdomen, and forearms of affected individuals. Linear lesions (Koebner reaction) in lines of trauma are common, and minute grayish flat papules on the buccal mucous membrane have been described. The course is variable. It occasionally clears spontaneously after a period of several weeks to months (usually 1 year or less) but frequently lasts much longer (occasionally years) with little or no response to treatment.[99]

The histologic features of lichen nitidus are pathogonomonic and consist of circumscribed nests of lymphocytes and histiocytes, and occasionally epithelioid and Langhans giant cells in the uppermost dermis. The overlying epidermis is compressed, occasionally with an area of detachment from the dermis above the center of the lesion, with a characteristic claw-like projection of the rete ridges as though in an attempt to encircle the infiltrate in the manner of a hand clutching a ball.

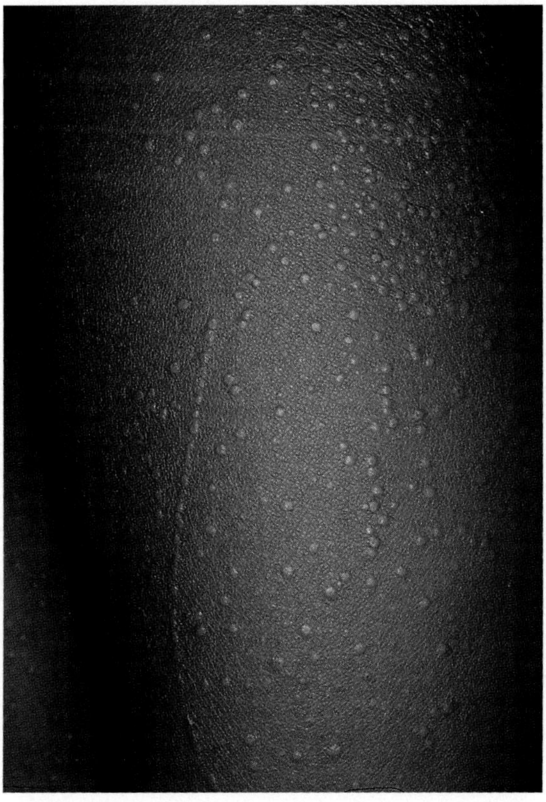

Although the lack of symptoms in lichen nitidus and the tendency for spontaneous healing have made evaluation of therapy difficult, in selected cases oral antihistamines, topical antipruritics, and topical corticosteroids may be helpful.[100]

KERATOSIS LICHENOIDES CHRONICA

Keratosis lichenoides chronica is a rare, chronic, asymptomatic dermatosis characterized by reticulated erythema; scaling and telangiectasia of the face; keratotic purplish papules, nodules, and plaques distributed in linear patterns on the trunk and extremities (Figs. 5–34 and 5–35); and at times infiltration of the epiglottis resulting in hoarseness.[101–103] Nail changes include yellowish brown discoloration, thickening of the nail plate, longitudinal ridging, onycholysis, fragmentation of the free margin, splinter hemorrhages, and hyperkeratosis of the nail bed and periungual areas.[104] Although the histologic picture may resemble that of lichen planus, its clinical features and the presence of parakeratosis, alternating areas of atrophy and acanthosis, and a heavier infiltrate than that usually seen in lichen planus may help differentiate the two disorders.

Keratosis lichenoides chronica may persist for many years and is unresponsive to corticosteroid therapy. Ultraviolet light exposure, PUVA therapy, and retinoids such as etretinate, however, alone or in combination, may at times be beneficial.[104]

Figure 5–33. Pinhead-sized flesh-colored shiny elevated papules of lichen nitidus. Note the linear Koebner reaction over a site of trauma.

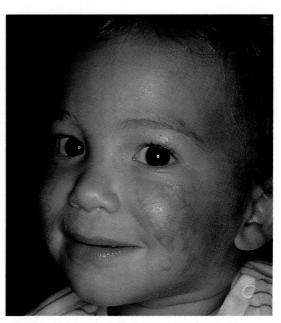

Figure 5–34. Reticulated erythema, scaling, and telangiectasia on the cheeks of a 1½-year-old boy with keratosis lichenoides chronica.

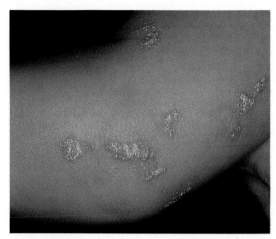

Figure 5–35. Keratosis lichenoides chronica. Red to violaceous hyperkeratotic lesions are seen in a linear configuration on the arm.

PAPULAR ACRODERMATITIS OF CHILDHOOD

Papular acrodermatitis of childhood (Gianotti-Crosti syndrome) is a distinctive, self-limiting dermatosis of childhood characterized by the abrupt onset of nonpruritic lichenoid papules on the face, buttocks, and extremities, generally lasting about 20 days (occasionally longer), with at times mild constitutional symptoms and acute, usually anicteric, hepatitis. First recognized in Milan in 1953 and described by Gianotti in 1955 and later by Crosti and Gianotti in 1956, the term *infantile papular acrodermatitis* was coined in 1957.[105, 106]

Since its original description it now appears that this frequently unrecognized disorder is worldwide in distribution. The disease begins abruptly, and the eruption is often preceded by an upper respiratory tract infection, generalized lymphadenopathy, hepatomegaly and occasionally splenomegaly, and mild constitutional symptoms. Although adults have also been afflicted by this disorder, children between 3 months and 15 years of age are usually affected, with a peak incidence between the years of age 1 and 6.

The clinical features of papular acrodermatitis of childhood are quite distinctive. The eruption consists of monomorphous, nonpruritic, generally but not necessarily symmetrical, flat-topped 1- to 10-mm, flesh-colored, pale pink, or coppery red papules that appear in crops and involve the face, buttocks, extremities, palms, soles, and occasionally the upper aspect of the back (Figs. 5–36 through 5–38 and, in Chapter 3, Fig. 3–27). Although the trunk is generally spared, a transient eruption may be seen in this region during the initial early phase of the disorder. The rash develops in a few days and lasts for 15 to 20 days or more (occasionally up to 8 weeks or more). In infancy the lesions are generally large (5 to 10 mm

in diameter); in older children the eruption is often micropapular (1 to 2 mm in diameter). At times the lesions may have a purpuric appearance and, on occasion, a coarse infiltrated tumor-like appearance has been noted. As the rash progresses, lesions frequently tend to become confluent and, particularly on areas subject to trauma, may merge to form plaques of flat-topped lichenoid papules.

Constitutional symptoms and systemic manifestations include malaise, low-grade fever, mild generalized lymphadenopathy, hepatomegaly, splenomegaly, and, at times, diarrhea. Hepatitis, when present, begins at the same time or 1 or 2 weeks after the onset of the cutaneous eruption, tends to last for approximately 2 months, and only rarely progresses to chronic liver disease. The rash resolves spontaneously after a variable period of 2 to 8 weeks (usually 15 to 20 days). The lymphadenitis, which is mainly inguinal and axillary, generally lasts 2 to 3 months; and hepatomegaly, when present, generally persists for 3 months.

Although leukopenia with a relative increase in monocytes (up to 20 per cent) and a mild hypochromic anemia have been reported, laboratory findings generally consist of a normal leukocyte count and normal erythrocyte sedimentation rate. Abnormal liver function studies with elevation of aspartate aminotransferase, alanine aminotransferase, lactate dehydrogenase, alkaline phosphatase, and Bromsulphalein retention without abnormal bilirubin levels have been noted; and liver biopsies done during the dermatitis phase of

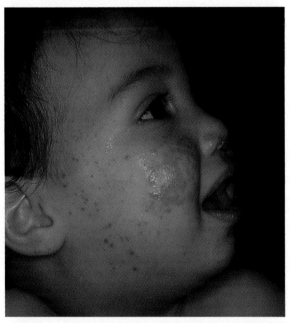

Figure 5–36. Flat-topped symmetrical lichenoid papules on the face of a child with papular acrodermatitis of childhood (Gianotti-Crosti syndrome).

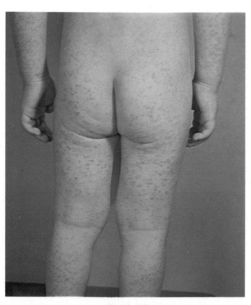

Fig. 5–37

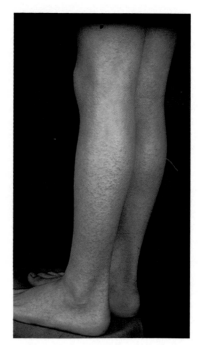

Fig. 5–38

Figures 5–37 and 5–38. Flat-topped symmetrical lichenoid papules of papular acrodermatitis of childhood (Gianotti-Crosti syndrome). (Courtesy of Professor Ferdinando Gianotti.)

the disorder, at least in patients with associated hepatitis, reveal a histologic picture indistinguishable from that of acute viral hepatitis.[105]

In 1973 the association with Australian antigen was reported,[105] and in 1976 in Japan an epidemic of the syndrome associated with a very high incidence of hepatitis B surface antigen (subtype ayw, an uncommon subtype in Japan) was reported.[107] Australian antigen, when present, is generally detectable 10 days or more after the onset of the skin eruption and persists for 2 months to several years. Evidence of hepatitis manifested by hepatomegaly, elevated serum enzyme levels, virus-like particles in liver and lymph node specimens, and detection of elevated

serum levels of hepatitis B surface antigen in some patients suggested a viral etiology. Since the disorder subsequently has also been associated with infection with Epstein-Barr virus, parainfluenzavirus, coxsackievirus A16 respiratory syncytial virus, poliovirus vaccine, other enteroviruses, cytomegalovirus, and group A β-hemolytic streptococci, papular acrodermatitis of childhood may actually represent a host response to a variety of infectious agents.[108–114]

Gianotti has also described a similar disorder that generally affects children of a more limited age group (2 to 6 years) not associated with hepatomegaly or hepatitis virus B surface antigenemia.[115, 116] This disorder, termed *papulove-*

Figure 5–39. Microscopic features of Gianotti-Crosti disease. Hyperkeratosis, acanthosis, focal spongiosis, exocytosis, liquefaction and degeneration of basal layer, and lymphomonocytic and histiocytic dermal infiltrate. (Courtesy of Professor Ferdinando Gianotti.)

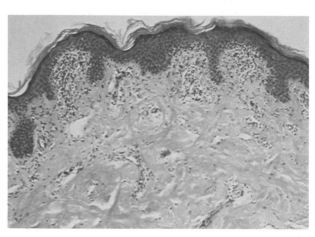

sicular acrolocalized syndrome (papulovesicular acrolocated syndrome), is characterized by small, 1- to 5-mm, alabaster to rose-pink or purple, spherical or hemispherical, vesicular papules that are often covered with a hemorrhagic crust. The eruption is symmetrically located on the cheeks, ears, buttocks, and extremities. Pruritus is common, splenomegaly is absent, results of liver function studies are normal, and hepatitis virus B surface antigenemia is absent. Whether this disorder warrants separate classification remains uncertain.

The diagnosis of papular acrodermatitis of childhood is dependent on the characteristic clinical findings and histopathologic examination of cutaneous lesions. Microscopic features of the cutaneous eruption include mild acanthosis, hyperkeratosis, focal spongiosis with extensive exocytosis of mononuclear cells, liquefactive degeneration of the basal layer, a dense perivascular lymphomonocytic and histiocytic dermal infiltrate, swelling of the vascular endothelium, and dilatation of dermal capillaries (Fig. 5–39).

Since this syndrome is benign and self-limiting (with a low incidence of familial involvement), treatment with other than symptomatic measures is unnecessary. It should be noted, however, that corticosteroid creams may have an adverse effect on the cutaneous eruption.[117]

References

1. Krulig L, Farber EM, Grumet FC, et al.: Histocompatibility (HL-A) antigens in psoriasis. Arch. Dermatol. *111*:857–860, 1975.

    Studies of 101 psoriatic patients suggest that the HLA locus (w17 and w16) may be a marker for hereditary factors affecting susceptibility to psoriasis.

2. Perlman SG: Psoriatic arthritis in children. Pediatr. Dermatol. *1*:283–287, 1984.

    A review of the clinical features of psoriatic arthritis in childhood with emphasis on genetics, pathophysiologic mechanisms, clinical manifestations, and treatment.

3. Farber EM, Carlsen RA: Psoriasis in childhood. Calif. Med. *105*:415–420, 1966.

    Of 1,000 patients with psoriasis 27 per cent developed the disorder at or before age 15. Females were affected in a 2 : 1 ratio over males in childhood, and patients seemed to be more severely involved in adult life if the disorder had its onset during childhood.

4. Farber EM, Bright RD, Nall ML: Psoriasis. A questionnaire survey of 2144 patients. Arch. Dermatol. *98*:248–259, 1968.

    A computerized analysis of 2,144 individuals with psoriasis.

5. Lerner MR, Lerner AB: Congenital psoriasis. Arch. Dermatol. *105*:598–601, 1972.

    Case histories of three patients with congenital psoriasis, one of whom developed severe crippling psoriatic arthritis before age 13.

6. Farber EM, Nall MA: Genetics of psoriasis. Twin study. In Farber EM, Cox AJ (Eds.): Psoriasis, Proceedings of the International Symposium. Stanford University Press, Stanford, CA, 1971, 7–14.

    A review of the status of genetic knowledge about psoriasis.

7. Hutton KP, Oranberg EK, Jacobs AH: Childhood psoriasis. Cutis *39*:26–27, 1987.

    A comprehensive review of psoriasis as manifested in the childhood age group.

8. Kavli G, Forde OH, Arneson E, et al.: Psoriasis: Familial predisposition and environmental factors. Br. Med. J. *291*:999–1000, 1985.

    A questionnaire study of almost 15,000 Norwegians confirms a family predisposition but is unable to verify an environmental influence in the pathogenesis of psoriasis.

9. Kreuger GC, Eyre RW: Trigger factors in psoriasis. Dermatol. Clin. *2*:373–381, 1984.

    Stress and local trauma are implicated as common precipitants to exacerbations of psoriasis.

10. Rasmussen JE: Psoriasis in children. Dermatol. Clin. *4*:99–106, 1986.

    A review of the incidence, genetics, inciting factors, and clinical features of psoriasis in over 200 children.

11. Tzankov N, Botev-Zlatkov N, Lazarova AZ, et al.: Psoriasis and drugs: Influence of tetracycline in the course of psoriasis. J. Am. Acad. Dermatol. *19*:629–632, 1988.

    Tetracycline appeared to represent a precipitating or aggravating factor in 76 (16 per cent) of 462 patients with psoriasis.

12. Bernhard JD: Auspitz sign is not sensitive or specific for psoriasis. J. Am. Acad. Dermatol. *22*:1079–1081, 1990.

    A study in which the Auspitz sign was present in only 41 of 234 patients suggests that this clinical phenomenon lacks sensitivity as a diagnostic sign of psoriasis.

13. Rasmussen EO, Wuepper KD: Purification and characterization of streptococcal proliferative factor. J. Invest. Dermatol. *77*:246–269, 1981.

    In vivo studies suggest a streptococcal proliferative factor as the cause of guttate flares of psoriasis.

14. Nyfors A, Rasmussen PA, Lemholt K, et al.: Improvement of refractory psoriasis vulgaris after tonsillectomy. Dermatologica *151*:216–222, 1975.

    Improvement in the course of psoriasis in 71 of 74 patients after tonsillectomy confirms the etiologic role of streptococcal infection in the persistence and exacerbation of lesions in individuals with this disorder.

15. Farber EM, Jacobs AH: Infantile psoriasis. Am. J. Dis. Child. *131*:1266–1269, 1977.

    A report of 14 children younger than 2 years of age with psoriasis vulgaris.

16. Farber EM, Mullen RH, Jacobs AH, et al.: Infantile psoriasis: A follow-up study. Pediatr. Dermatol. *3*:237–243, 1986.

    Examination of nine children with infantile psoriasis 6 to 13 years after their initial presentation revealed that the majority of these children had relatively mild courses of their disorder and that two patients remained completely clear of disease after the initial resolution of their dermatosis.

17. Perry HO, Soderstrom CW, Schulze RW: The Goeckerman treatment of psoriasis. Arch. Dermatol. *98*:178–182, 1968.

    Excellent results with Goeckerman regimen, with remissions varying from 6 to 18 months.

18. Comaish S: Ingram method of treating psoriasis. Arch. Dermatol. *92*:56–58, 1965.

    An attempt to introduce this effective therapeutic regimen to American dermatologists.

19. Lowe NJ, Ashton RE, Koudsi H, et al.: Anthralin for psoriasis: Short-contact anthralin therapy compared with

topical steroid and conventional anthralin. J. Am. Acad. Dermatol. *10*:69–72, 1984.

Short-contact anthralin therapy was shown to be just as effective as long-term (8-hour) topical anthralin or 0.05 per cent diflorasone diacetate ointment in the treatment of patients with psoriasis.

20. Swinehart JM, Lowe NJ: UVABA therapy for psoriasis: Efficacy with shortened treatment times with the combined use of coal tar, anthralin, and metal halide ultraviolet machines. J. Am. Acad. Dermatol. *24*:594–597, 1991.

Rapid clearing of psoriasis in a psoriasis treatment center was obtained with a combination of short-contact coal tar phototherapy consisting of UVA and UVB, and short-contact high-potency anthralin therapy (UVABA).

21. Parrish JA, Fitzpatrick TB, Tannenbaum L, et al.: Photochemistry of psoriasis with methoxsalen and long-wave ultraviolet light. N. Engl. J. Med. *291*:1207–1211, 1974.

An experimental approach (8-methoxypsoralen and high-energy long-wave UVA light) is extremely effective in clearing severe and extensive psoriasis.

22. Ellis CN, Voorhees JJ: Etretinate therapy. J. Am. Acad. Dermatol. *16*:267–291, 1987.

An overview of etretinate and its use (alone or in combination with other modalities) for psoriasis and other disorders of keratinization.

23. Shelnitz LS, Esterly NB, Honig PJ: Etretinate therapy for generalized pustular psoriasis in children. Arch. Dermatol. *123*:230–233, 1987.

Two 19-month-old children with recalcitrant debilitating pustular psoriasis were shown to have a good clinical response to etretinate.

24. Lowe NJ, Roenigk H, Voorhees JJ: Etretinate: Appropriate use in severe psoriasis. Arch. Dermatol. *124*:527–528, 1988.

An overview of etretinate with guidelines for its use in patients with severe psoriasis.

25. Lowe NJ, Prystkowsky JH, Bourget T, et al.: Acitretin plus UVB therapy for psoriasis. J. Am. Acad. Dermatol. *24*:591–594, 1991.

Combined acitretin and UVB therapy was shown to be of value in the treatment of patients with recalcitrant, extensive, or hyperkeratotic forms of psoriasis. Unlike etretinate, however, acitretin is cleared from the body within 48 hours after it is discontinued.

26. Gupta AK, Ellis CN, Nickoloff BJ, et al.: Oral cyclosporine in the treatment of inflammatory and noninflammatory dermatoses. Arch. Dermatol. *126*:339–350, 1990.

A report of 24 patients successfully treated with short-term cyclosporine (6 mg/kg/day) for periods of 5 to 30 weeks for a variety of dermatoses including psoriasis.

27. Gupta AK, Ellis CN, Siegel MT, et al.: Sulfasalazine improves psoriasis: A double-blind analysis. Arch. Dermatol. *126*:487–493, 1990.

An 8-week double-blind study showed sulfasalazine (Azulfidine) to be effective for patients with moderate to severe psoriasis whose disease severity did not justify the risks associated with more potentially toxic forms of therapy.

28. DiGiovanna JJ, Zech LA, Ruddel ME, et al.: Etretinate: Persistent serum levels after long-term therapy. Arch. Dermatol. *125*:246–251, 1989.

In a study of 47 patients who received long-term etretinate therapy, serum concentrations were detected for periods of up to 244 weeks after the discontinuation of therapy.

29. Shore A, Ansell BM: Juvenile psoriatic arthritis: An analysis of 60 cases. J. Pediatr. *100*:529–535, 1982.

In a review of 60 patients with juvenile psoriatic arthritis, 15 per cent had the onset of their cutaneous and joint involvement at about the same time, 43 per cent developed arthritis prior to the onset of their cutaneous features, and in 42 per cent of the patients the arthritis was preceded by the cutaneous eruption.

30. Finzi AF, Gibelli E: Psoriatic arthritis. Int. J. Dermatol. *30*:1–7, 1991.

A comprehensive review of psoriatic arthritis, theories of pathogenesis, clinical manifestations, and management.

31. Beylot C, Bioulac P, Grupper C, et al.: Generalized pustular psoriasis in infants and children: Report of 27 cases. In Farber EM, Cox AJ (Eds.): Psoriasis, Proceedings of the Second International Symposium. Yorke Medical Books, New York, 1976, 171–179.

A description of 27 cases of generalized pustular psoriasis in children with emphasis on clinical aspects and therapy.

32. Rosen RM: Annular pustular psoriasis induced by UV radiation from tanning salon use. J. Am. Acad. Dermatol. *25*:336–337, 1991.

A report of a patient with chronic stationary plaque psoriasis who developed annular pustular psoriasis following an ultraviolet burn received in a tanning salon.

33. Zelicksen BD, Muller SA: Generalized pustular psoriasis in childhood. J. Am. Acad. Dermatol. *24*:186–194, 1991.

In a report of 13 children with generalized pustular psoriasis, most patients were controlled with topical therapy alone.

34. Baker H, Ryan TJ: Generalized pustular psoriasis: A clinical and epidemiologic study of 104 cases. Br. J. Dermatol. *80*:771–793, 1984.

A study of 104 patients with generalized pustular psoriasis suggested that in at least half of the patients the disorder was precipitated by a withdrawal of systemic corticosteroids.

35. Lowe NJ, Ridgway HB: Generalized pustular psoriasis precipitated by lithium carbonate. Arch. Dermatol. *114*:1788–1789, 1978.

A woman with a 22-year history of psoriasis developed a generalized pustular form of the disorder when started on lithium for a manic-depressive psychosis.

36. Friedman SJ: Pustular psoriasis associated with hydroxychloroquine. J. Am. Acad. Dermatol. *16*:1256–1257, 1987.

A 60-year-old man developed pustular psoriasis 3 weeks after starting hydroxychloroquine for the treatment of his rheumatoid arthritis.

37. Stewart AF, Battaglini-Sabetta J, Milstone L: Hypocalcemia-induced pustular psoriasis of von Zumbusch. Ann. Intern. Med. *100*:677–680, 1984.

In a report of a patient with generalized pustular psoriasis, apparently precipitated by hypocalcemia following surgical hypoparathyroidism, the disorder cleared rapidly following the initiation of oral calcium with vitamin D supplementation.

38. Katz M, Seidenbaum M, Weinrauch L: Penicillin-induced generalized pustular psoriasis. J. Am. Acad. Dermatol. *17*:918–920, 1987.

Severe generalized pustular psoriasis was induced by penicillin on at least four separate occasions in a 26-year-old woman with recalcitrant psoriasis.

39. Boyd AS, Menter A: Erythrodermic psoriasis: Precipitating factors, course, and prognosis in 50 patients. J. Am. Acad. Dermatol. *21*:985–991, 1989.

A review of 50 patients with psoriatic erythroderma seen in a psoriasis day-care center over a period of 9½ years.

40. Scott RB, Surana R: Erythrodermic psoriasis in childhood. Am. J. Dis. Child. *116*:218–221, 1968.

Psoriatic erythroderma in a child whose disease began at about 18 months of age and terminated fatally following chickenpox complicated by staphylococcal pyoderma and sepsis while on methotrexate therapy.

41. Kahn G, Rywlin AM: Acropustulosis of infancy. Arch. Dermatol. *115*:831–833, 1979.

   Two infants with acropustulosis of infancy, a disorder believed to be distinct from all other disorders of infancy, with pruritic lesions on hands, feet, and face.

42. Jarrat M, Ramsdell W: Infantile acropustulosis. Arch. Dermatol. *115*:834–836, 1979.

   Clinical and histologic features in 10 children with infantile acropustulosis.

43. Jennings JL, Burrows WM: Infantile acropustulosis. J. Am. Acad. Dermatol. *9*:733–738, 1983.

   A review of clinical and histopathologic features in four infants with infantile acropustulosis.

44. Vignon Pennamen M-D, Wallach D: Infantile acropustulosis. Arch. Dermatol. *122*:1155–1160, 1986.

   In a review of the clinical and histopathologic features of infantile acropustulosis in six infants and children, the authors auggest that necrolysis of the keratinocytes is the initial microscopic feature of this disorder.

45. Findlay RJ, Odom RB: Infantile acropustulosis. Am. J. Dis. Child. *137*:455–457, 1983.

   A report of a 22-month-old black infant with infantile acropustulosis who manifested sporadic recurrences at 2- to 4-week intervals over a period of 10 months.

46. Lucky A, McGuire JS: Infantile acropustulosis with eosinophilic pustules. J. Pediatr. *100*:428–429, 1982.

   In a report of a 5½-month-old white infant with acropustulosis in whom the disorder was characterized by an eosinophilic vesicular eruption, the authors suggest that an initial eosinophilic response of infancy eventually changes to one that is neutrophilic.

47. Jacobs A: A case of Reiter's syndrome in childhood. Br. Med. J. *2*:155, 1961.

   A 9-year-old boy with Reiter's disease manifested by urethritis, conjunctivitis, and arthritis (without cutaneous findings) following a bout of dysentery.

48. Margileth AM: Reiter's syndrome in children: Case report and review of the literature. Clin. Pediatr. *1*:148–151, 1962.

   A 6-year-old boy with conjunctivitis, urethritis, and arthritis.

49. Moss JS: Reiter's disease in childhood. Br. J. Venereol. Dis. *40*:166–169, 1964.

   Review of 27 cases of Reiter's disease in children, the youngest child being 1 year and 9 months of age.

50. Sehgal VN, Koranne RV, Prasad ALS: Unusual manifestations of Reiter's disease in a child. Dermatologica *170*:77–79, 1985.

   A 9-year-old boy with Reiter's disease, who initially improved on a regimen of prednisolone, erythromycin, and gentamicin, eventually died of septicemia and cardiac failure.

51. Rosenberg AM, Petty R: Reiter's disease in children. Am. J. Dis. Child. *133*:394–398, 1979.

   A report of three boys (2 to 15 years of age) with Reiter's disease and a review of previous reports of this disorder in children.

52. Brewerton DA, Caffrey M, Nicholls A, et al.: Reiter's disease. Lancet *2*:996–998, 1973.

   HLA antigen found in 25 (76 per cent) of 33 patients with Reiter's disease.

53. Morris R, Metzger AL, Bluestone R, et al.: HL-A: Clue to diagnosis and pathogenesis of Reiter's syndrome. N. Engl. J. Med. *290*:554–556, 1974.

Ninety-six per cent of patients with Reiter's syndrome were HLA-w27–positive.

54. Griffiths A: Pityriasis rubra pilaris: Etiologic considerations. J. Am. Acad. Dermatol. *10*:1086–1088, 1984.

   A review of 93 patients with pityriasis rubra pilaris and a classification of the disorder into five subgroups.

55. Gelmetti C, Schiuma AA, Cerri D, et al.: Pityriasis rubra pilaris in childhood: A long-term study of 29 cases. Pediatr. Dermatol. *3*:446–451, 1986.

   A review of pityriasis rubra pilaris in 29 children.

56. Porter D, Shuster S: Epidermal renewal and amino acids in psoriasis and pityriasis rubra pilaris. Arch. Dermatol. *98*:339–343, 1968.

   Increased transit times and rapid epidermal turnover in lesions of psoriasis and pityriasis rubra pilaris.

57. Huntley CC: Pityriasis rubra pilaris. Am. J. Dis. Child. *122*:22–23, 1971.

   Complete remission in a 16-month-old child with pityriasis rubra pilaris after 50,000 units of oral vitamin A twice a day for 6½ weeks.

58. Goldsmith LA, Weinrich AE, Shupack J: Pityriasis rubra pilaris response to 13-*cis*-retinoic acid (isotretinoin). J. Am. Acad. Dermatol. *6*:710–715, 1982.

   Forty-five patients with pityriasis rubra pilaris treated with isotretinoin manifested marked improvement in the degree of erythema, induration, and scaling within a period of 4 weeks.

59. Longley J, Demar L, Feinstein RP, et al.: Clinical and histologic features of pityriasis lichenoides in children. Arch. Dermatol. *123*:1335–1339, 1987.

   Clinical and histopathologic features of acute pityriasis lichenoides in five children.

60. Luberti AA, Rabinowitz LG, Ververeli KO: Severe febrile Mucha-Habermann's disease in children: Case report and review of the literature. Pediatr. Dermatol. *8*:51–57, 1991.

   A report of a 12-year-old boy with the febrile ulceronecrotic form of Mucha-Habermann disease.

61. Fortson JS, Schroeter AL, Esterly NB: Cutaneous T-cell lymphoma (parapsoriasis en plaque): An association with pityriasis lichenoides et varioliformis acuta in young children. Arch. Dermatol. *126*:1449–1453, 1990.

   A report of two children with pityriasis lichenoides that eventually evolved over a period of several years into cutaneous T-cell lymphoma.

62. Macaulay WL: Lymphomatoid papulosis: A continuing self-healing eruption, clinically benign, histologically malignant. Arch. Dermatol. *97*:23–30, 1968.

   "Lymphomatoid papulosis." Is this a distinct disorder or merely a manifestation of Mucha-Habermann disease?

63. Muhlbauer JE, Bhan AK, Harrist TJ, et al.: Immunopathology of pityriasis lichenoides acuta. J. Am. Acad. Dermatol. *10*:783–795, 1984.

   Direct immunofluorescence and immunoperoxidase studies of 11 biopsy specimens from four patients with pityriasis lichenoides acuta suggest that cell-mediated immunity plays a role in the pathogenesis of this disorder.

64. Levine ML: Phototherapy of pityriasis lichenoides. Arch. Dermatol. *119*:378–380, 1983.

   Minimally erythemogenic doses of ultraviolet B radiation administered three to five times a week, with an average of 29 treatments, gave complete clearing of all exposed lesions in 11 patients with pityriasis lichenoides et varioliformis acuta.

65. Tham SN: UV-B phototherapy for pityriasis lichenoides. Aust. J. Dermatol. *26*:9–13, 1985.

   Fourteen (82 per cent) of 18 patients (17 with chronic pityriasis lichenoides and one with the acute form of the disorder) were shown to have a good to excellent response to UVB phototherapy.

66. Takado Y, Irasawa K, Kawada A: Heliotherapy of pityriasis lichenoides chronica. Jpn. J. Dermatol. 4:91–97, 1977.

In 87 per cent of 15 patients with chronic pityriasis lichenoides, sunbathing was shown to be extremely beneficial and hastened resolution of the cutaneous disorder.

67. Powell FC, Muller SA: Psoralens and ultraviolet A therapy of pityriasis lichenoides. J. Am. Acad. Dermatol. 10:59–64, 1984.

Three men with pityriasis lichenoides resistant to other therapeutic modalities showed good clinical responses to PUVA therapy.

68. Shelley WB, Griffith RF: Pityriasis lichenoides et varioliformis acuta: A reported case controlled by high dosage of tetracycline. Arch. Dermatol. 100:596–597, 1969.

Two grams of tetracycline a day appeared to have a suppressive effect on the course of pityriasis lichenoides.

69. Truhan AP, Hebert AA, Esterly NB: Pityriasis lichenoides in children: Therapeutic response to erythromycin. J. Am. Acad. Dermatol. 15:66–70, 1986.

Although it often took as long as 2 months before significant therapeutic results were noted, 13 (87 per cent) of 15 children had remission or partial improvement of pityriasis lichenoides with oral erythromycin therapy.

70. Cornelison RL Jr, Knox JM, Everett MA: Methotrexate for treatment of Mucha-Habermann disease. Arch. Dermatol. 106:507–514, 1972.

Improvement of six patients with Mucha-Habermann disease with low dosages of oral methotrexate.

71. Rogers M, DeLauney J, Kemp A, et al.: Lymphomatoid papulosis in an 11-month-old infant. Pediatr. Dermatol. 2:124–130, 1984.

An 11-month-old boy with a 5-week history of multiple skin lesions on the trunk is believed to be the youngest patient with lymphomatoid papulosis reported to date.

72. Ashworth J, Paterson WD, Mackie RM: Lymphomatoid papulosis/pityriasis lichenoides in two children. Pediatr. Dermatol. 4:238–241, 1987.

A report of two children, ages 3 and 6 years, with lymphomatoid papulosis who, until the correct diagnosis was established, were thought to have aggressive lymphomas.

73. Hellman J, Phelps RG, Baral J, et al.: Lymphomatoid papulosis with antigen deletion and clonal arrangement in a 4-year-old boy. Pediatr. Dermatol. 7:42–47, 1990.

A report of a young child with lymphomatoid papulosis in whom antigen deletion and clonal rearrangement indicated an immunoproliferative disease suggests that childhood forms of lymphomatoid papulosis require the same careful follow-up evaluations as adult forms of this disorder.

74. Sánchez NP, Pittelkow MR, Muller SA, et al.: The clinicopathologic spectrum of lymphomatoid papulosis: Study of 31 cases. J. Am. Acad. Dermatol. 8:81–94, 1983.

Six patients with clinical features of Mucha-Habermann disease who had infiltrates composed primarily of atypical lymphoid cells and subsequently went on to develop malignant lymphomas.

75. Lange Wantzin G, Thomen K: PUVA treatment in lymphomatoid papulosis. Br. J. Dermatol. 107:687–690, 1982.

A report of five patients with lymphomatoid papulosis who responded to PUVA therapy.

76. Everett MA: Treatment of lymphomatoid papulosis with methotrexate. Br. J. Dermatol. 111:631, 1984.

Low-dose oral methotrexate cleared the lesions of lymphomatoid papulosis in four of eight patients in 6 to 12 months.

In the other four patients, intermittent methotrexate therapy was required for a longer period of time.

77. Hyatt HW SR: Pityriasis rosea in a 3-month-old infant. Arch. Pediatr. 77:364–368, 1960.

A 3-month-old infant with pityriasis rosea is believed to represent the youngest patient reported to date with this disorder.

78. Marschall J: Pityriasis rosea. A review of its clinical aspects and a discussion of its relationship to pityriasis lichenoides et varioliformis acuta and parapsoriasis guttata. S. Afr. Med. J. 30:210–217, 1956.

A review of pityriasis rosea, its epidemiology, clinical appearance, and histopathologic features.

79. Parsons JM: Pityriasis rosea update: 1986. J. Am. Acad. Dermatol. 15:159–167, 1986.

An extensive review suggests that pityriasis rosea may represent a nonspecific, possibly cell-mediated, immunologic cutaneous reaction precipitated by a number of causes.

80. Arndt KA, Paul BS, Stern RS, et al.: Treatment of pityriasis rosea with UV radiation. Arch. Dermatol. 119:381–382, 1983.

A comparison study of 20 patients with extensive symptomatic pityriasis rosea treated with unilateral UVB phototherapy showed a substantial decrease in pruritus and extent of disease on the treated side. The response was particularly pronounced in those who initiated their treatment early (during the first week of the disorder).

81. Pusey W: Lichen planus in an infant less than six months old. Arch. Dermatol. 19:671–672, 1929.

A report of a 9-month-old girl with lichen planus in whom lesions of this disorder were first noted when she was 3 weeks of age.

82. Kanwar AJ, Kaur S, Rajagopalan M, et al.: Lichen planus in an 8-month-old. Pediatr. Dermatol. 6:358–359, 1989.

A report of lichen planus in an 8-month-old infant in whom lesions apparently began when she was approximately 5 months of age.

83. Kofoed ML, Wantzin GL: Familial lichen planus: More frequent than previously suggested? J. Am. Acad. Dermatol. 13:50–54, 1985.

A study in which 15 of 140 patients with lichen planus had familial forms of their disorder suggests, at least in some patients, the probability that a genetic form of this disorder exists.

84. Mahood JM: Familial lichen planus: A review of nine cases from four families with a review of the literature. Arch. Dermatol. 119:292–294, 1983.

Studies suggest that familial forms of lichen planus have an earlier onset, a greater tendency to chronicity, increased severity, and a more frequent predisposition to hypertrophic, erosive, linear, and ulcerative forms of the disorder.

85. Lowe NJ, Cudworth AG, Woodrow JC: HL-A antigens in lichen planus. Br. J. Dermatol. 95:169–171, 1976.

In a study of 57 patients with lichen planus, 54 per cent (as compared to 29.7 per cent of the control population) were found to have HLA_3 chromosomal linkage.

86. Gibstine CF, Esterly NB: Lichen planus in monozygotic twins. Arch. Dermatol. 120:580, 1984.

A report of 11-year-old monozygotic twin sisters who concurrently developed lichen planus.

87. Sheehan-Dare RA, Coterill JA, Simmons AV: Esophageal lichen planus. Br. J. Dermatol. 115:729–730, 1986.

A woman with severe oral lichen planus and dysphagia was subsequently found to have erosive esophageal lesions.

88. Pelisse M: The vulvo-vaginal-gingival syndrome: A new

form of erosive lichen planus. Int. J. Dermatol. 28:381–384, 1989.

A report of 19 patients with erosive or desquamative lesions of lichen planus on the gingiva and mucosal surfaces of the vulva and/or vagina.

89. Gupta AK, Gorsulowsky DC: Unilateral lichen planus: An unusual presentation. Arch. Dermatol. 123:295–296, 1987.

A report of a patient with lichen planus in whom the disorder began at the site of nitroglycerin patches on the arm and gradually spread in a unilateral distribution to the upper and lower extremities and trunk.

90. Silverman S Jr, Gorsky M, Lozada-Nur F: A prospective follow-up of 570 patients with oral lichen planus: Persistence, remission, and malignant association. Oral Surg. 60:30–34, 1985.

In a review of 570 patients with oral lichen planus, 1.2 per cent were found to develop malignant transformation of the lesions (this complication usually occurred in those with erosive forms of the disease).

91. Massa MC, Greaney V, Kron T, et al.: Malignant transformation of oral lichen planus: Case report and review of the literature. Cutis 45:45–47, 1990.

In a report of a patient with oral lichen planus and squamous cell carcinoma of the oral cavity, the authors suggest that exposure to tobacco carcinogens accounts for malignant transformation in patients with erosive oral forms of this disorder.

92. Cotton DWK, Van den Hurk JJMA, Van der Staak WBJM: Lichen planus, an inborn error of metabolism. Br. J. Dermatol. 87:341–346, 1972.

A group of patients with congenital deficiency of glucose-6-phosphate dehydrogenase with drug-induced attacks of lichen planus.

93. Boyd AS, Neldner KH: Lichen planus. J. Am. Acad. Dermatol. 25:593–619, 1991.

A comprehensive overview of lichen planus and miscellaneous lichenoid dermatoses.

94. Brice SL, Barr RJ, Rattet JP: Childhood lichen planus: A question of therapy. J. Am. Acad. Dermatol. 3:370–376, 1980.

A report of an 8-year-old boy with lichen planus and a review of therapeutic options with emphasis on the efficacy and risk factors in childhood forms of this disorder.

95. Gonzalez E, Momtaz TK, Freedman S: Bilateral comparison of generalized lichen planus treated with psoralens and ultraviolet light. J. Am. Acad. Dermatol. 10:958–961, 1984.

Five of 10 patients with generalized lichen planus treated by PUVA cleared completely; 3 of the remaining 5 patients improved at least 50 per cent and 2 patients developed exacerbations of their disorder while receiving treatment.

96. Staus ME, Bergfeld WF: Treatment of oral lichen planus with low-dose isotretinoin. J. Am. Acad. Dermatol. 11:527–528, 1984.

A patient with a 14-year history of unremitting erosive painful oral lichen planus was successfully treated with isotretinoin.

97. Ho VC, Gupta AK, Ellis CN, et al.: Treatment of lichen planus with cyclosporine. J. Am. Acad. Dermatol. 22:64–68, 1990.

Two patients with severe chronic lichen planus treated with oral cyclosporine (6 mg/kg/day) had complete clearing of the disorder after 8 weeks of treatment.

98. Aram H: Association of lichen planus and lichen nitidus. treatment with etretinate. Int. J. Dermatol. 27:117, 1988.

Coexistence of lichen planus and lichen nitidus in a 35-year-old woman.

99. Lapins NA, Willoughby C, Helwig EB: Lichen nitidus: A study of forty-three cases. Cutis 2:634–637, 1978.

Although 43 patients with lichen nitidus improved spontaneously, usually within 1 year, in one patient the disorder persisted for 8 years.

100. Wright S: Successful treatment of lichen nitidus. Arch. Dermatol. 120:155–156, 1984.

Fluocinonide 0.05 per cent cream applied topically twice a day for 1 month completely cleared lichen nitidus lesions that had been present for 12 years in a 24-year-old woman.

101. Margolis MH, Cooper GA, Johnson SAM: Keratosis lichenoides chronica. Arch. Dermatol. 105:739–743, 1972.

A 36-year-old patient with a 15-year history of keratosis lichenoides chronica had persistent hoarseness as a manifestation of the disorder.

102. Petrozzi JW: Keratosis lichenoides chronica: Possible variant of lichen planus. Arch. Dermatol. 112:709–711, 1976.

Clinical and histologic features suggest that keratosis lichenoides chronica may represent a variant of lichen planus.

103. Nabai H, Mehregan AH: Keratosis lichenoides chronica: Report of a case. J. Am. Acad. Dermatol. 2:217–220, 1980.

Clinical and histopathologic features of a 37-year-old woman suggest that keratosis lichenoides chronica may represent a clinical variant of lichen planus.

104. Baran R, Panizzon R, Goldberg L: The nails in keratosis lichenoides chronica: Characteristics and response to treatment. Arch. Dermatol. 120:1471–1474, 1984.

A report of nail changes seen in three patients with keratosis lichenoides chronica.

105. Gianotti F: Papular acrodermatitis of childhood: An Australian antigen disease. Arch. Dis. Child. 48:794–799, 1973.

A report of 39 children with papular acrodermatitis of childhood, all of whom demonstrated the presence of Australian hepatitis antigen.

106. Gianotti F: Papular acrodermatitis of childhood: An Australian antigen disease. Mod. Probl. Paediatr. 17:180–189, 1975.

A review of papular acrodermatitis of childhood presented at the 1st International Symposium on Pediatric Dermatology (Mexico City, 1973).

107. Ishimaru Y, Ishimaru H, Toda G, et al.: An epidemic of infantile papular acrodermatitis (Gianotti's disease) in Japan associated with hepatitis-B surface antigen subtype ayw. Lancet 1:707–709, 1976.

Ninety-three per cent of patients with infantile papular acrodermatitis of childhood with hepatitis B surface antigen subtype ayw suggested this disorder to be a manifestation of hepatitis B virus infection in children younger than age 3.

108. Schneider JA, Poley JR, Millunchik EW, et al.: Papular acrodermatitis (Gianotti-Crosti syndrome) in a child with anicteric hepatitis B, virus subtype adw. J. Pediatr. 101:219–222, 1982.

An 18-month-old boy with Gianotti-Crosti syndrome demonstrates a variability in the viral antigens responsible for this disorder.

109. James WD, Odom RB, Hatch MH: Gianotti-Crosti–like eruption associated with coxsackievirus A-16 infection. J. Am. Acad. Dermatol. 6:862–866, 1982.

Culture and serum confirmation of coxsackievirus A16 associated with Gianotti-Crosti syndrome in a 2-year-old boy.

110. Berant M, Naveh Y, Weissman I: Papular acrodermatitis with cytomegalovirus hepatitis. Arch. Dis. Child. 58:1024–1025, 1983.

Cytomegalovirus is incriminated as a potential precipitating factor of Gianotti-Crosti syndrome in a 1-year-old boy in Israel.

111. Spear KL, Winkelmann RK: Gianotti-Crosti syndrome: A review of ten cases not associated with hepatitis B. Arch. Dermatol. *120:*891–896, 1984.

A report of 10 patients with papular acrodermatitis of childhood suggests that this disorder can represent a self-limiting cutaneous response to a number of infections, including hepatitis B, Epstein-Barr, coxsackievirus, and parainfluenza virus infections.

112. Iosub S, Santos C, Gromisch DS: Papular acrodermatitis with Epstein-Barr virus infection. Clin. Pediatr. *23:*33–34, 1984.

A report of a 9-month-old infant with Gianotti-Crosti syndrome in whom Epstein-Barr virus titers rose from 0 to 160 over a period of 3 weeks.

113. Draelos ZK, Hansen RC, James WD: Gianotti-Crosti syndrome associated with infections other than hepatitis B. J.A.M.A. *256:*2386–2388, 1986.

In a report of nine children with Gianotti-Crosti syndrome, all were negative for hepatitis B surface antigen, two had viral culture or serologic evidence of respiratory syncytial virus infection, one revealed a poliovaccine-induced enterovirus, and two had evidence of group A β-hemolytic streptococcal infection.

114. Tieb A, Plantin P, DuPasquier P, et al.: Gianotti-Crosti syndrome: a study of 26 cases. Br. J. Dermatol. *115:*49–59, 1986.

A review of 26 patients with Gianotti-Crosti syndrome in which one patient's dermatosis was associated with hepatitis B, two patients had recently been immunized, Epstein-Barr virus was found in seven, coxsackievirus B was found in three, and cytomegalovirus B was found in three patients appears to support the hypothesis that non-HBS virus may be more common than HBS virus in patients with this disorder.

115. Gianotti F: Infantile papular acrodermatitis: Acrodermatitis papulosa and infantile papulovesicular acrolocalized syndrome. Hautarzt *27:*467–472, 1976.

A review of infantile papular acrodermatitis and "acrolocalized infantile papulovesicular syndrome."

116. Gianotti F: Papular acrodermatitis of childhood and other papulovesicular acro-located syndromes. Br. J. Dermatol. *100:*49–59, 1979.

A review of papular acrodermatitis (Gianotti-Crosti syndrome) suggests that the term *papulovesicular acrolocalized syndrome* should be reserved for cases in which there is no known etiologic agent.

117. Hjorth N, Kopp H, Osmundsen PE: Gianotti-Crosti syndrome: Papular eruption of infancy. Trans. St. John's Hosp. Derm. Soc. *53:*46–56, 1967.

A review of 117 patients with Gianotti-Crosti syndrome.

6

DISORDERS OF THE SEBACEOUS AND SWEAT GLANDS

DISORDERS OF THE SEBACEOUS GLANDS
Acne Vulgaris

Although the basic cause of acne vulgaris remains unknown, considerable data concerning its pathogenesis accumulated in recent years allow a rational and therapeutically successful approach to the management of this disorder. Acne therefore should never be dismissed as being of no consequence, with mere reassurance that the patient will outgrow it, because the psychological scars and trauma are often deeper and more disastrous than the blemishes displayed on the cutaneous surface. There is no single treatment for acne. The choice of therapy must be individualized for each patient, with appropriate modifications as the activity of the disease fluctuates. The success of therapy depends on the cooperation of the patient and the interest, enthusiasm, and careful selection of medications on the part of the physician (Fig. 6–1).

Acne vulgaris, a disorder of the pilosebaceous apparatus, is the most common skin disorder of the second and third decades of life and for years has been a perplexing enigma to patients and physicians. Recent scientific advances have finally dispelled much of its mystique and mythology, allowing a rational and highly successful approach to the therapy for this disorder. Its name is attributed to the Greek and Latin words *akmē* and *acme*, respectively, no doubt owing to the fact that this condition is most prominent during adolescence, the so-called peak of life. The word *vulgaris* is derived from the Latin adjective meaning "ordinary or common" and denotes an average form of acne rather than a disorder with a coarse or derogatory connotation.

Incidence. The tendency to develop acne is often familial and is thought to be inherited as an autosomal dominant trait. However, because of the high prevalence of this disorder, its exact genetic pattern remains undetermined. Actually we know very little about the genetics and epidemiology of acne. Hereditary influences can easily be appreciated by taking histories and looking for scars among first-order relatives; yet, except for Nierman's study showing 98 per cent concordance for the presence of acne in identical twins, controlled data are lacking.[1] Acne therefore probably represents a polygenic disorder in which the clinical

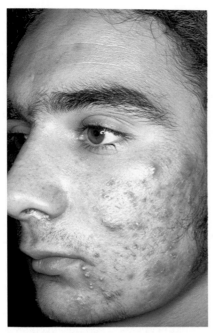

Figure 6–1. Comedones, papules, pustules, cysts, and nodules on the face of a 20-year-old man with acne vulgaris.

expression represents the sum of the action of many genes.[2]

Adolescence is the period of life between childhood and adulthood. It begins with puberty, which may appear at any time between 9 and 17 years of age. The physiologic mechanism that triggers the changes associated with the onset of puberty is unknown, but it appears to involve the release of gonadotropic hormone from the anterior pituitary, which in turn stimulates ovarian secretion of estrogen and the production of androgen by the testes, ovaries, and adrenal cortex. These steroid hormones are responsible for the production of the secondary sex characteristics as well as the cutaneous disorders associated with adolescence.

Although acne may be present at birth, as the result of hormonal stimulation of sebaceous glands that have not yet involuted to their childhood state of immaturity (neonatal acne), it is frequently not until puberty that acne becomes a common problem. It may develop as early as the fifth to the eighth year of life, and in girls may precede menarche by more than a year. In girls its peak is reached between the ages of 14 and 17; in boys the greatest severity is noted between 16 and 19 years of age. It is seen slightly more often in boys than in girls, the disparity between the sexes becoming more apparent as the severity of the disorder increases. Depending on one's definition of acne, approximately 85 per cent of high school students between 15 and 18 years of age have some degree of this disorder,[3] Mild forms, however, appear to be so prevalent that if one considers an occasional comedo and papule as acne, the disorder might be regarded as a physiologic phenomenon with estimates of its presence reaching almost 100 per cent of individuals.[4] In 80 per cent of patients, the incidence and severity of acne appear to decline at about 22 to 23 years of age; in 10 per cent of patients active lesions may occur even into the 30s or 40s, and by the age of 50 to 59 years, 6 per cent of the men and 8 per cent of women may still demonstrate varying degrees of the disorder.[5]

Etiology. An understanding of the physiologic basis of acne can simplify one's therapeutic approach and can produce results far better than heretofore have been attainable. Acne usually begins 1 or 2 years prior to the onset of puberty as a result of androgenic stimulation of the sebaceous glands and is attributable to an abnormal keratinization process that results in obstruction of the pilosebaceous unit. Sebaceous glands are present in all human skin except the palms, soles, dorsa of the feet, and perhaps the lower lip. The highest concentrations are noted on the face, chest, and back, with a total of 15,000 to 20,000 glands on the face alone. Each gland is composed of several lobules that lead into a common excretory duct. These holocrine glands are devoid of motor innervation and depend solely on androgenic stimulation.

Studies have demonstrated that the increasing flux of circulating testosterone is taken up by the sebaceous gland and converted to dihydrotestosterone by the enzyme 5α-reductase. Current research suggests that dihydrotestosterone is the tissue androgen that causes hypertrophy of the sebaceous gland and an increased production of sebum associated with this disorder. Acne patients appear to convert testosterone to dihydrotestosterone more readily than unaffected individuals. In boys the testes are the major source of androgen for sebaceous gland development. In girls, androgens, in normal amounts, are derived from the ovary and adrenal gland. The androgenic stimulation of sebaceous glands does not imply a hormonal imbalance, merely a normal physiologic phenomenon that sets the stage for the subsequent changes seen in acne. In girls the endogenous androgen secretion is approximately two thirds that of boys, with acne accordingly less common and less severe in girls than it is in boys.[6]

In addition to excessive sebum production, patients with acne have one other major abnormality of the sebaceous follicle, namely, a change in the process of keratinization. Acne thus develops in the sebaceous follicles and is initiated by an altered keratinization process of the follicular canal that results in obstruction of the pilosebaceous unit. The cause of this abnormality of keratinization is unknown, although patients with a predisposition to acne appear to have a tendency for irritation of the follicular wall by free fatty acids.[7] When the normal flow of sebum onto the skin surface is obstructed by this follicular hyperkeratosis, microcomedones are formed, thus initiating the process of acne (Fig. 6–2).

In terms of pathogenesis, two types of comedones are formed: open comedones (black-

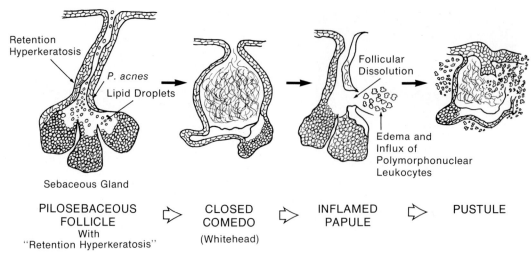

Retention
Hyperkeratosis

P. acnes

Lipid Droplets

Sebaceous Gland

Follicular
Dissolution

Edema and
Influx of
Polymorphonuclear
Leukocytes

PILOSEBACEOUS   CLOSED   INFLAMED   PUSTULE
FOLLICLE   COMEDO   PAPULE
With   (Whitehead)
"Retention Hyperkeratosis"

Figure 6–2. The pathogenesis of acne. (Adapted from Hurwitz S: Acne vulgaris. Current concepts of pathogenesis and treatment. Am. J. Dis. Child. *133*:536–544, 1979.)

heads) and closed comedones (whiteheads) (Figs. 6–3 and 6–4).[8] The open comedo is composed of an epithelium-lined sac filled with keratin and lipid, with a widely dilated orifice. For years there has been much speculation regarding the genesis of the blackened tip of the open comedo. Contrary to popular misconception, the color is not caused by exogenous dirt or lack of hygiene. Although various theories suggest compaction and oxidation of the keratinous material at the follicular orifice as the cause of the brown to black discoloration, histochemical and histologic studies suggest that melanin also plays a role in the etiology of open comedones.[9, 10] Blackheads, although unsightly, are easily managed and rarely create problems in acne. The contents of the open comedones easily escape to the skin surface; follicular disruption and inflammation, therefore, rarely occur, except when the comedones are traumatized by the patient.

Conversely, it is the whitehead, or closed comedo, that is responsible for the problems seen in acne. These lesions are seen as small, skin-colored, slightly elevated papules just beneath the skin surface (their visualization may be enhanced by a slight stretching of the overlying skin) (see Fig. 6–3). The closed comedo has a microscopic opening that keeps its contents from escaping. It continues to form keratin and some sebum; and when the follicular wall ruptures, it acts as a veritable time bomb and expels sebum into the surrounding dermis, thus initiating the inflammatory process.[8] The clinical appearance of the resulting inflammatory lesion is dependent not only on the size of the comedo in which the rupture occurs but also on the location of the inflammatory reaction in the dermis. Thus, if the inflammatory nidus is close to the surface, the lesion will usually be a pustule; deeper inflammation results in a larger papule or nodule.

Some authors believe that stressful events such as emotional tension, lack of sleep, and menses in the female patient result in increased sebum for-

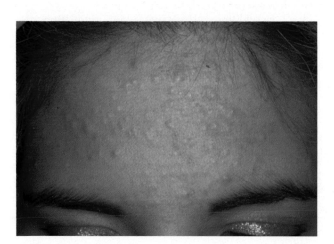

Figure 6–3. Closed comedones (whiteheads) and papules on the forehead of a patient with acne vulgaris.

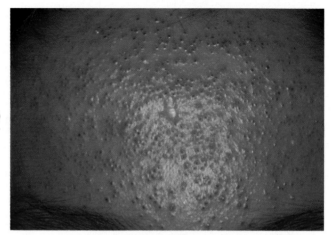

Figure 6–4. Multiple open comedones (blackheads) on the forehead of a 14-year-old boy with acne vulgaris.

mation that tips the balance and creates a breach in the follicular epithelium. This break permits leakage of the irritating follicular contents, thus initiating the inflammatory reaction within the dermis. The explanation for the worsening of acne vulgaris after stressful situations is unclear, but it appears to be related to an increased adrenocortical response by way of the pituitary-adrenal pathway.

Sebum is made up of a mixture of triglycerides, wax esters, squalene, and sterol esters. Currently, free fatty acids, particularly those with short chains (C_8 to C_{14}), are believed to play an important role in comedogenesis and the formation of inflammatory lesions.[11] Free fatty acids, however, are not found in the lipids normally present within the sebaceous canal. Their release appears to be the result of hydrolysis of triglycerides within the pilosebaceous follicles (to diglycerides, monoglycerides, and finally glycerol) by lipases, with release of physiologically active molecules of free fatty acids at each step of the process. An ordinarily harmless bacterium, the anaerobic *Propionibacterium acnes* (formerly termed *Corynebacterium acnes*), appears to be the major source of lipolytic enzymes within the pilosebaceous follicle. These organisms produce phosphatases, hyaluronidase, proteases, and neuraminidase, which may increase the permeability of the follicular epithelium. *P. acnes* also produces a low-molecular-weight chemotactic factor that recruits polymorphonuclear leukocytes and in the process of phagocytizing bacteria releases hydrolases that further disrupt the integrity of the follicular wall, thus intensifying the inflammatory reaction characteristically seen in individuals with this disorder.[12, 13]

Clinical Manifestations. Acne usually presents as a variety of lesions in which the comedo is pathognomonic. In its mildest form it is limited to open comedones (blackheads) and closed comedones (whiteheads) (see Figs. 6–3 and 6–4). As the disorder increases in severity, patients may develop papules, pustules, nodules, or cysts (Figs. 6–1, 6–5, and 6–6). The term *cyst* is actually a

misnomer; in this case it denotes a large nodular lesion that has undergone suppuration, thus resembling an inflamed cyst.

The primary sites of acne are the face, chest, back, and shoulders. There is often a seasonal variation, with acne being least active in summer and most severe in winter. As acne lesions resolve they are frequently followed by temporary postinflammatory redness and hyperpigmentation. Although patients commonly regard these as active lesions and potential scars, this discoloration gradually subsides once the condition is controlled. In the more severe pustular and cystic forms of acne,

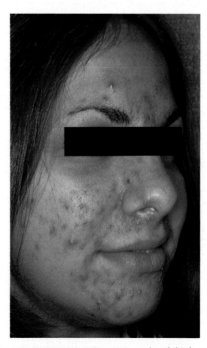

Figure 6–5. Papules, pustules, cysts, and nodules in a 16-year-old girl with acne vulgaris.

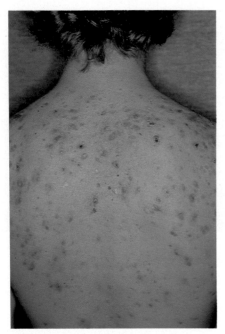

Figure 6–6. Severe acne vulgaris with scarring on the back.

sheaths of epithelium from remaining follicular walls tend to encapsulate the inflammatory areas with subsequent fibrous contraction and eventual cicatricial formation. The scars usually present as sharply punched-out pits or as hypertrophic and keloid scars (Figs. 6–7 and 6–8). The severity of the scarring depends on the depth and intensity of the inflammation and on the patient's susceptibility to cicatrization.

Treatment. For years the treatment of acne was hindered by mythical concepts of etiology, a lack of concern for the physical and psychological trauma of those affected with severe forms of this disorder, and the perpetuation of ineffective therapeutic regimens based on misconception and misinformation. No concerned physician should fail to recognize the deep emotional trauma suffered by patients with acne, nor should he or she ignore the tremendous benefits, both physical and emotional, that today's effective therapeutics can evoke. It is indeed a grievous injustice for either parent or physician to regard acne as evanescent or untreatable, because the psychological scars that accompany this disorder can frequently be far more devastating and destructive than the visible cutaneous aberrations caused by the disease itself.[14, 15]

As yet there is no single treatment for acne vulgaris. Therapy must be individualized with appropriate variations and modifications as the degree or severity of the disorder fluctuates. Success of acne therapy depends on (1) prevention of follicular hyperkeratosis, (2) reduction of *P. acnes* and free fatty acids, and (3) elimination of comedones and the papules, pustules, cysts, and nodules that result from them. Today this goal can be achieved by proper selection of available medications, coupled with the cooperation of the patient, and the knowledge, continued interest, and enthusiasm of the physician, usually within 6 to 12 weeks of treatment. Once this has been accomplished, therapy must be continued faithfully for as long as the tendency toward acne persists. Unfortunately, as with so many long-term programs, patients occasionally develop a false sense of security and tend to modify their therapy, often with regrettable effects. To achieve the best long-term results, patients should be forewarned of this possibility and encouraged to continue treatment as long as their tendency to develop acne persists.

Diet. Controlled studies refute the value of dietary restrictions imposed on acne patients. For years the elimination of various foods such as chocolate and cola drinks, sweets, milk, ice cream, fatty foods, shellfish, and iodides dominated many of the futile approaches to acne control. The misconception that iodine is injurious to patients with acne originated with the concept that iodides administered orally as medication occasionally initiate a papulopustular acneiform eruption (iodism). A large-scale epidemiologic investigation of over 1,000 North Carolina high school students revealed that dietary iodine exerts no influence on either the prevalence or the severity of acne.[16] The concept that chocolate exerts an adverse effect on acne has also been challenged. In a carefully controlled double-blind study, it was found that this too failed to affect either the course of acne vulgaris or the composition of sebum.[17] For those patients who attest to flares following certain foods, it is

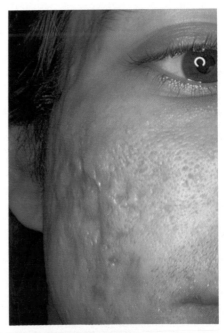

Figure 6–7. Keloidal and atrophic "ice-pick" scars on the cheek of a boy with acne vulgaris.

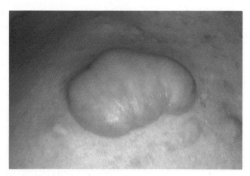

Figure 6–8. Keloidal acne scarring on the shoulder of a 16-year-old boy with acne vulgaris.

judicious to eliminate the suspicious agents until their true influence can be appropriately and individually assessed.

Topical Therapy. Appropriate topical therapy is essential to the successful management of acne. With presently available pharmacologic agents, frequently topical drugs are the only modalities necessary for therapy of even some of the most severe forms of acne vulgaris. For years various drying and exfoliating agents (abrasive soaps, astringents, ultraviolet light, sulfur, resorcinol, and salicylic acid), alone or in various combinations, were the focus of acne therapy. Whereas such preparations may indeed cause drying and peeling, remove oils from the surface of the skin, and suppress individual lesions to a limited degree, they fail in the effective prevention of new lesions and actually impede the proper utilization of the effective topical agents currently available for the treatment of acne vulgaris.

P. acnes organisms are the source of lipases responsible for the breakdown of sebum into irritating free fatty acids. These anaerobic diphtheroids live beneath the skin surface, within the pilosebaceous follicle, where they are inaccessible to most previously available topical antibacterial agents. Therefore, soaps containing hexachlorophene and other antibacterial agents are also probably ineffective in the therapy of acne vulgaris.

Of the available topical agents, those that have had the greatest popularity include sulfur, resorcinol, salicylic acid, benzoyl peroxide, topical antibiotics, and vitamin A acid (tretinoin). Sulfur and resorcinol have been used in varying concentrations of from 1 to 5 per cent and 1 to 10 per cent, respectively. Their efficacy is limited and seems to be related to their capacity to produce erythema and desquamation. They tend to help dry and peel existing comedones, papules, and pustules but fail in attempts to limit the formation of closed comedones (whiteheads) and the lesions that result from them.

Benzoyl peroxide and vitamin A acid, although potential irritants, appear to be the most effective topical agents. Based on our current understanding of the pathogenesis of acne, these two agents offer a highly effective therapeutic approach that can be

tailored to each patient. Although success in the management of acne vulgaris can be achieved by the use of topical vitamin A acid or benzoyl peroxide alone, under proper management the therapeutic effect can be increased substantially by the use of the two agents in combination.[18, 19]

Salicylic Acid. Salicylic acid is categorized as a "keratolytic" agent and has been used in a wide variety of cutaneous disorders. The concentration of salicylic acid in most proprietary acne preparations, however, is often too low, or it is formulated with other agents that may handicap its activity. When used in the treatment of acne, it may be used in concentrations of 5 to 10 per cent salicylic acid in equal parts of 85 per cent ethanol and propylene glycol, as 5 per cent salicylic acid in a hydroalcoholic gel (Saligel [Stiefel]), or as SalAc Acne Medication Cleanser (GenDerm). Although somewhat less effective than tretinoin or benzoyl peroxide, salicylic acid formulations may be used for patients with mild comedonal acne and individuals who have difficulty with or prefer not to use tretinoin.

Benzoyl Peroxide. In 1934, topical benzoyl peroxide was first introduced in the therapy for acne vulgaris. Unfortunately, a lack of appreciation of the role of the vehicle in delivery of medication to the skin prevented consistently effective results and more widespread use of this modality. During the 1960s this chemotherapeutic agent was introduced, initially in lotion form, and then in a series of more potent gel formulations. With these newer vehicles, the benzoyl peroxide appears to penetrate the pilosebaceous follicle more effectively. Benzoyl peroxide is currently available in lotions, creams, or gels ranging in concentrations from 2.5 to 10 per cent. The gels are generally considered more active, and water-based gels are less irritating than alcohol- or acetone-based formulations. Although the precise mechanism of action of benzoyl peroxide is not fully understood, these preparations offer more than a form of epidermal irritation. They produce a mild degree of comedolytic activity, are bactericidal for *P. acnes*, inhibit triglyceride hydrolysis, and decrease inflammation of acne lesions (Table 6–1).

Benzoyl peroxide is potentially irritating and drying, particularly when used excessively or in association with abrasive soaps or astringents or both. Therapy must be individualized and initiated gradually, particularly in fair-skinned or atopic individuals. A relatively low incidence of irritant or allergic contact dermatitis (probably less than 1 per cent) suggests a certain degree of caution in its use in the treatment of acne (Fig. 6–9).[19, 20] A test for possible allergic contact der-

Table 6–1. ACTION OF BENZOYL PEROXIDE

1. Irritant and keratolytic
2. Suppresses *Propionibacterium acnes*
   a. Inhibits triglyceride hydrolysis
   b. Lowers free fatty acids
   c. Decreases inflammation in acne lesions

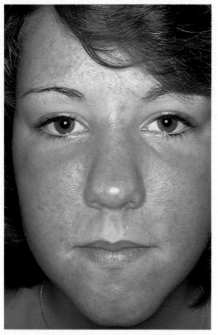

Figure 6–9. Allergic contact dermatitis due to the use of benzoyl peroxide in the treatment of acne vulgaris.

matitis, perhaps by an open patch test on the volar aspect of the patient's wrist, prior to the initiation of therapy, therefore, appears to be a sensible precautionary measure.

Following an initial test application, benzoyl peroxide should be applied as a thin film, initially every day or every other day, and rubbed in gently, gradually increasing the frequency and strength of the preparations as tolerance is developed (generally within a period of 2 or 3 weeks). To best achieve this, a small pea-sized dot should be divided into three dots and then gently rubbed into each affected area (the cheek, forehead, and chin and, if needed, chest or back) (Figs. 6–10 and 6–11). If irritation or excessive dryness develops, the preparation may be discontinued for several days. Lubricants may then be used for 1 to several days until the irritation resolves. Once the irritation or dryness disappears, therapy can be resumed gently and cautiously as tolerance is established. Although clinical dryness and exfoliation were thought to be helpful and resulted in a more effective therapeutic response, when benzoyl peroxide is applied properly in a thin film (with a certain degree of care and caution) most patients will achieve success without the unpleasant side effects of dryness, redness, or irritation. Most problems with benzoyl peroxide, accordingly, appear to be related to overzealous or improper application of the prescribed formulations.

Vitamin A Acid (Retinoic Acid, Tretinoin). For years, vitamin A has been administered orally to patients with acne vulgaris in the hope of reducing hyperkeratosis of the sebaceous follicle. Unfor-

tunately, therapeutic effect requires dosage in the toxic range of 400,000 to 700,000 units/day.[21] In an effort to find a way of delivering a substantial dose of this drug to the target area without exacting the penalty of systemic toxicity, the use of topical vitamin A acid in the therapy for acne vulgaris was proposed in 1969.[22]

Available as Retin-A, in liquid (0.05 per cent), cream (0.025, 0.05, and 0.1 per cent), and gel (0.01 or 0.025 per cent) formulations, topical vitamin A acid seems to have several beneficial effects on the skin of patients with acne vulgaris. Included among these benefits are an increased cell turnover within the pilosebaceous ducts and a decreased cohesiveness of epidermal cells. This stimulates dehiscence of horny cells, which results in a thinning of the horny layer, an increased cell turnover, a decreased comedo formation, a sloughing and expulsion of existent comedones from their sebaceous follicles, a reduction of inflammatory lesions arising from comedones, and enhanced transepidermal penetration of benzoyl peroxide and topical antibiotics (Table 6–2).[19, 22]

It is unfortunate that vitamin A acid, perhaps the single most effective topical remedy for acne, is potentially irritating and improperly used by many patients. Because of its known capacity to cause severe irritation and peeling, topical vitamin A acid therapy should be initiated conservatively on an alternate-day or occasionally on an every-third-day regimen, again using the three-dot method (see Figs. 6–10 and 6–11), preferably with the less irritating gel or cream formulation. If tolerated, the patient may then gradually use the more potent cream, gel, or liquid preparations. Patients should be instructed to wash with a mild soap, no more than two or three times a day, and to wait at least 30

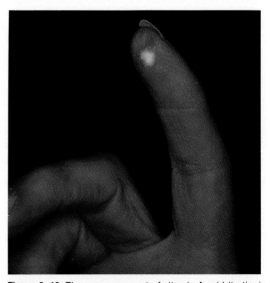

Figure 6–10. The proper amount of vitamin A acid (tretinoin, Retin-A) or benzoyl peroxide is a small pea-sized dot. This, divided into three smaller dots, can then be used to cover one treatment area such as the cheek.

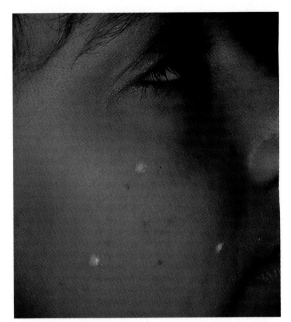

Figure 6–11. Application of vitamin A acid (tretinoin, Retin-A) or benzoyl peroxide by dividing a small pea-sized dot into three smaller dots and then gently rubbing the preparation into the skin to cover an area such as the cheek.

minutes after washing (to ensure that the skin is completely dry) before applying the vitamin A acid.[23] A problem frequently cited in the literature is heightened susceptibility to sunburn and sun damage in patients using topical vitamin A acid. Patients should therefore be cautioned about excessive sun exposure and advised to use a noncomedogenic sunscreen with a sun protective factor (SPF) of 15 or greater.[24, 25]

Vitamin A Acid and Benzoyl Peroxide. The art of medicine is predicated on the physician's ability to balance side effects against the potential benefits of various pharmacologic agents. Although success in the management of acne vulgaris can be achieved by the use of vitamin A acid or benzoyl peroxide alone, the therapeutic effect is substantially increased by the use of the two agents in combination. When the two agents are used in combination (one in the morning and one at night), there appears to be less irritation than when vitamin A acid is used alone, the use of systemic antibiotics can be decreased and often eliminated, and dramatic therapeutic success can be achieved in a relatively short period of time in a high percentage

of patients, even those with severe pustulocystic forms of this disorder.[18, 19]

In 1972 the combination of vitamin A (tretinoin) acid and benzoyl peroxide was suggested for the topical therapy of acne vulgaris.[18] In addition to its keratolytic effect, it was proposed that benzoyl peroxide could suppress *P. acnes*, inhibit triglyceride hydrolysis, and lower free fatty acid levels in sebum; vitamin A acid would simultaneously thin the epidermis, lessen follicular hyperkeratosis, and enhance penetration of benzoyl peroxide. It was theorized that this combination of two potent topical medications could produce an additive, possibly synergistic, effect and could result in a more effective therapeutic approach to the management of acne vulgaris. In an attempt to test this hypothesis, I treated 1,207 patients having varying degrees of acne vulgaris with topical vitamin A acid in combination with benzoyl peroxide.[19] Of these patients, 847 (70.2 per cent) had moderate to severe cases of acne vulgaris, many of them unresponsive to previous conventional therapeutic regimens (Table 6–3); 512 (42.4 per cent) were treated simultaneously with antibiotics; and 695 (57.6 per cent) received no antibiotics. Having stood the test of time, this approach is recommended as a treatment of choice for topical acne therapy.[12] The steps taken in the regimen I use are as follow:

Step 1. Most patients are initially seen at 6- to 7-week intervals and then less frequently as their acne responds to therapy. Education of the patient prior to the initiation of treatment is essential. A careful history, therefore, should be taken, the nature of the disease explained, potential pitfalls discussed, and the treatment outlined in detail.

Step 2. Vitamin A acid (tretinoin, retinoic acid) can be used in the form of Retin-A cream (0.025, 0.05, or 0.1 per cent), Retin-A gel (0.01 or 0.025 per cent), or Retin-A swabs (0.05 per cent), depending on the complexion of the patient, his or her tolerance to the medication, and the degree of acne. For persons with potentially irritable skin (particularly light-complected girls and women with blond or red hair), Retin-A cream is initiated on an alternate-day or occasionally on an every-third-day regimen. For those with a more ruddy complexion, Retin-A gel in a 0.1 per cent concentration is employed. As tolerance develops the frequency of administration can be increased to daily application with gradual introduction to the higher concentration cream, gel, or liquid formulations as deemed necessary.

Table 6–2. ACTION OF VITAMIN A ACID (TRETINOIN)

1. Thins epidermis
   a. Increased cell turnover
   b. Decreased cohesiveness of epidermal cells
2. Reverses comedo formation
   a. Increased cell turnover in pilosebaceous ducts
   b. Sloughing and expulsion of existing comedones
3. Increases transepidermal penetration

Table 6–3. SEVERITY OF ACNE ACCORDING TO SEX IN A 5-YEAR STUDY OF COMBINATION THERAPY

	Mild	Moderate	Severe	Total
Males	105	336	86	527 (43.7%)
Females	255	367	58	680 (56.3%)
	360	703	144	1207

Hurwitz S: The combined effect of vitamin A acid and benzoyl peroxide in the treatment of acne. Cutis *17*:585–590, 1976.

To minimize possible adverse cutaneous reactions, all recommended precautions for vitamin A acid are carefully emphasized and strictly implemented. Patients are instructed to wash gently with a mild soap (such as Dove, Neutrogena, or Purpose)[26] no more than two or three times a day and to wait at least 30 minutes after washing (to ensure that the skin is completely dry) before the application of the Retin-A. Only noncomedogenic cosmetics are allowed, and excessive sun exposure is limited. If sun exposure is anticipated, patients are cautioned to use an appropriate noncomedogenic sun-protective preparation.

Step 3. Benzoyl peroxide is used as benzoyl peroxide gel, in a 2.5 to 10 per cent or 20 per cent concentration (the latter is available as Syoxin Gel [Syosset]), but not before testing for possible allergy by an open or closed patch test on the volar aspect of the wrist. Since it has been suggested that benzoyl peroxide might oxidize vitamin A acid if the two preparations are applied simultaneously, patients are instructed to apply the two medications separately (one in the morning and the other at night).

Step 4. Topical or oral antibiotics may be prescribed in combination with the above regimen for patients with severe pustular or cystic forms of acne vulgaris. Once the inflammatory aspect improves, the oral antibiotic dose is reduced and, if possible, discontinued.

Step 5. To ensure a minimum of complications, patients are instructed to maintain close telephone communications, particularly during the first weeks of treatment. At each office visit therapy is reviewed, comedones are extracted, liquid nitrogen is gently applied to individual lesions, and pustulocystic lesions are treated by intralesional corticosteroid injection. If irritation occurs, patients are instructed to discontinue treatment for a few days, use a noncomedogenic moisturizer for 1 or 2 days, and then reinstitute treatment, slowly and cautiously as tolerated. Careful re-evaluation at each visit reveals that most side effects, when present, are associated with excessive or inappropriate application of the medication, or medications, or failure to follow the precautions outlined at the onset of therapy.

Although success in the management of acne vulgaris can often be achieved by the use of topical vitamin A acid or benzoyl peroxide alone, the therapeutic effect can be substantially increased by the use of the two agents in combination (Figs. 6–12 through 6–15 and Tables 6–3 and 6–4), frequently without the need for systemic antibiotics.

Antibiotics

Systemic Antibiotics. Systemic antibiotic therapy suppresses *P. acnes* and inhibits bacterial lipases, causing a reduction in the concentration of free fatty acids (the primary irritant of sebum). For years, broad-spectrum antibiotics have been invaluable in the treatment of inflammatory pustules, nodules, and cystic lesions. Today, however, the

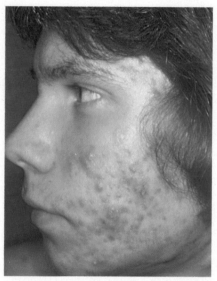

Figure 6–12. Sixteen-year-old boy with grade III–IV acne (large papules, pustules, and cystic lesions) before treatment with vitamin A acid and benzoyl peroxide.

use of systemic antibiotics can be decreased and often eliminated as experience and sophistication in the use of effective topical agents are developed.[19] Since little or no improvement can be expected with noninflammatory lesions, antibiotics are unnecessary in patients in whom these lesions appear as the sole manifestation of their acne problem.

When antibiotics are considered necessary, tetracycline, the antibiotic most frequently pre-

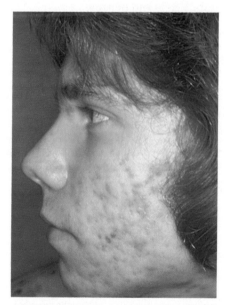

Figure 6–13. Same patient as in Figure 6–12 after 6 weeks of treatment with vitamin A acid gel (0.025%) in the morning and benzoyl peroxide gel (10%) in the evening.

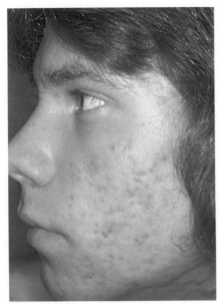

Figure 6–14. Appearance of same patient as in Figures 6–12 and 6–13 after 9 weeks of treatment.

scribed, is effective, inexpensive, and relatively free of side effects. Erythromycin, clindamycin, doxycycline, minocycline, dapsone, and sulfamethoxazole-trimethoprim (Bactrim, Septra) are also beneficial when inflammatory and pustular lesions fail to respond to oral tetracycline. Of these alternative agents, erythromycin is the least expensive and has the fewest complications.

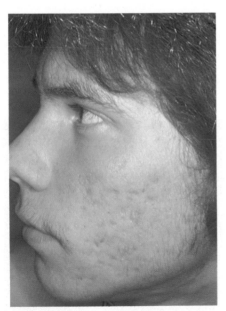

Figure 6–15. Appearance of same patient as in Figures 6–12 through 6–14 after 14 weeks of treatment. Patient received systemic tetracycline (500 mg two times a day initially, with gradual reduction and eventual discontinuation).

Table 6–4. RESULTS OF 5-YEAR STUDY OF COMBINED TRETINOIN AND BENZOYL PEROXIDE THERAPY

Extent of Clearing	Number	Per Cent
Excellent (90–98%)	737	61.1
Good (80–90%)	338	28.0
Fair (60–80%)	80	6.6
Poor (less than 60%)	5	0.4
Lost to follow-up	47	3.9
Total	1207	100.0

Long-term systemic use of clindamycin is not recommended owing to the possibility of induced pseudomembranous ulcerative colitis. This complication of clindamycin appears to be due to a toxin that is liberated by *Clostridium difficile*, which is able to grow in large numbers in the intestinal tract of some patients who receive clindamycin or other antibiotics. In such individuals it has been found that the problem responds rapidly to the administration of vancomycin or metronidazole.

Minocycline, a second-generation tetracycline derivative, achieves a very high intrafollicular concentration and produces a more prolonged effect than tetracycline. It has an added advantage in that it can be administered with food, including milk, but not ferrous sulfate, and it has a much lower risk of onycholysis and photosensitivity.[27, 28] Its disadvantages are its expense and its affinity for the central nervous system, with a resulting high incidence of headache and dizziness. This problem can frequently be eliminated by administration of minocycline in small dosages at mealtime. Other adverse reactions include ototoxicity, bluish gray hyperpigmentation in sites of previous inflammation such as acne lesions and acne scars (Fig. 6–16), occasional staining of the teeth or gums, fixed drug eruptions, erythema nodosum, erythema multiforme, and Stevens-Johnson syndrome. The mucosal and cutaneous pigmentary changes fortunately tend to resolve within a period of several months to a year after discontinuation of therapy. Of additional clinical significance is the fact that, although tetracycline staining of the teeth occurs when it is administered to children younger than the age of 8 years, minocycline-induced dental discoloration may on rare occasions occur when it is administered during adolescence and adulthood.[29–35]

Sulfones (diaminodiphenylsulfone) and sulfamethoxazole-trimethoprim (Bactrim, Septra) may be used for the management of severe, resistant nodulocystic and conglobate acne. Sulfones, however, should be used with extreme caution, with full awareness of the risk of hemolytic anemia, leucopenia, peripheral neuropathy cyanosis, and methemoglobinemia, and sulfamethoxazole-trimethoprim may result in erythema multiforme, Stevens-Johnson syndrome, toxic epidermal necrolysis, hepatic necrosis, agranulocyto-

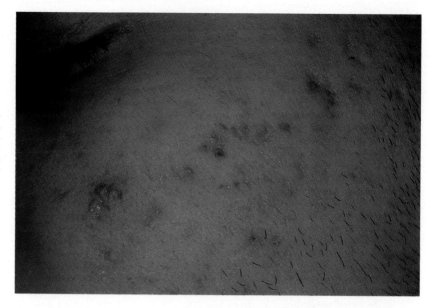

Figure 6–16. Minocycline pigmentation. Blue-gray areas of pigmentation at sites of previous inflammation appear on the cheek of a patient who had been receiving oral minocycline for the treatment of acne vulgaris.

sis, aplastic anemia, and other blood dyscrasias. I therefore generally try to avoid the use of these agents, whenever possible, and, when I do use them I advise careful monitoring for possible side effects. Penicillin and its derivatives appear to be ineffective in the treatment of acne. Sulfa drugs have been used, but their clinical results are not as favorable as those of the broad-spectrum antibiotics.

Tetracycline therapy generally begins with a dosage of 500 to 1,000 mg/day. This is gradually decreased to the lowest optimal level, usually to a dosage of 250 mg/day or every other day, until clinical improvement allows its discontinuation. The capacity for tetracycline to bind to certain types of cells and to intracellular organelles is well documented; however, it takes several weeks to develop an effective level of tetracycline in the skin. Antibiotic treatment, therefore, should be used for a minimum of 3 to 4 weeks before results are appreciable. Tetracyclines are incompletely absorbed from the gastrointestinal tract and may be impaired by food, iron supplements, milk, aluminum hydroxide gel, and calcium-magesium salts. To ensure optimal absorption, patients should be instructed to take this medication on an empty stomach, preferably 1 hour before or 2 hours after mealtime.

Low-dosage tetracycline therapy may be continued for many months with relatively few side effects. The most frequent complication of antibiotic therapy in female patients is vaginal candidiasis. This complication, less frequently seen in young adolescents, is proportionally more common in women who take oral contraceptives concomitantly with their systemic antibiotics. Patients taking tetracycline occasionally manifest gastrointestinal irritation (epigastric distress, anorexia, nausea, or vomiting) after ingestion of tetracycline or its derivatives (this may often be obviated by

the substitution of tetracycline tablets rather than capsules), and on occasion esophageal ulcerations have been associated with its use.[37] Enteric symptoms (cramps and diarrhea) are believed to result from alteration of normal intestinal flora, with overgrowth of yeasts and resistant bacteria. Complications based on antigen–antibody mechanisms (urticaria, angioneurotic edema, erythema multiforme, and fixed eruptions), although reported, are relatively rare.

The incidence of photoreactivity to oral tetracycline is unknown but appears to be extremely low, except for doxycycline and demethylchlorotetracycline (Declomycin, in which photosensitivity appears to develop in about 20 per cent of cases). Reports also describe brown discoloration and onycholysis as well as an unusual porphyria-like photosensitivity with bullae on the hands of patients on tetracycline or doxycycline therapy (Fig. 6–17).[38–41]

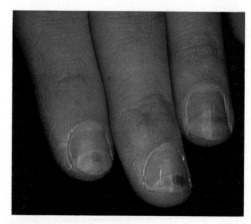

Figure 6–17. Photo-onycholysis as a complication of oral tetracycline hydrochloride therapy for acne vulgaris.

Patients on long-term antibiotic therapy may at times develop a gram-negative folliculitis due to *Escherichia coli, Klebsiella,* and at times *Pseudomonas, Enterobacter,* or *Proteus* overgrowth.[42, 43] This complication, manifested by a pustular folliculitis along the ala nasi or deep nodulocystic lesions of the face (Fig. 6–18), can be treated by discontinuation of the antibiotics that altered the patient's gram-positive flora, by topical compresses with a 1 per cent acetic acid solution (which can be approximated by the addition of 4 or 5 teaspoons of white vinegar to a pint of water), or by povidone-iodine (Betadine) compresses, 0.1 per cent aqueous gentamicin compresses,[44] topical antibiotics such as polymyxin B–bacitracin (Polysporin), gramicidin, or mupirocin (Bactroban), and oral antibiotics such as ampicillin, amoxicillin, trimethoprim-sulfamethoxazole, or carbenicillin (the choice of antibiotic should be governed by the results of bacterial culture sensitivity studies). For patients with gram-negative folliculitis unresponsive to the above regimen, a 4- to 5-month course of isotretinoin (Accutane) will generally result in rapid, complete, and prolonged remissions.[45]

The possibility that tetracycline will stain the teeth precludes its use for children younger than 8 years of age and tetracycline and its derivatives should not be used in pregnant women. The deposition of the drug in the teeth is thought to be the result of its chelating properties, with the formation of a tetracycline-calcium orthophosphate complex. In time, exposure to light results in slow oxidation with a change in color of affected teeth from yellow to a cosmetically objectionable grayish brown or gray (Fig. 6–19). The ingestion of outdated tetracycline may cause severe toxicity. It is particularly dangerous in patients who use "leftover" medication and who start and stop therapy on their own without proper medical guidance. Other reported complications of tetracycline therapy include drug eruptions, hyperpigmentation,

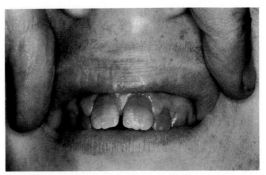

Figure 6–19. Staining of teeth due to the oral administration of tetracycline hydrochloride during early childhood.

hemolytic anemia,[46] erythema multiforme, intracranial hypertension (pseudotumor cerebri),[47, 48] and the possibility that broad-spectrum antibiotics may interefere with oral contraceptive efficacy. Evidence supporting this interaction, however, is primarily anecdotal and its incidence (if it does exist) is probably extremely low. Nevertheless, physicians should be aware of this possibility, and when oral antibiotics are prescribed for women who may be taking oral contraceptives, discussion of this theoretical possibility and consultation with a gynecologist prior to the initiation of concurrent antibiotic and oral contraceptive therapy are advisable.[49]

Although many questions have been raised concerning the safety of long-term use of tetracycline or erythromycin in acne, in general these drugs appear to be relatively safe, with no evidence of significant deleterious effect. Nevertheless, complete blood cell counts and screening studies for hepatic and renal function every 6 to 12 months appear to be good precautionary measures when long-term use is contemplated.

Topical Antibiotics. Despite their relative safety, it is desirable to avoid oral or systemic therapy in the treatment of acne if an equally potent topical agent can be used. Thus, topical antibiotics such as clindamycin, erythromycin, or meclocycline sulfosalicylate, although not as effective as benzoyl peroxide gel formulations, can be used for those who are allergic or sensitive to benzoyl peroxide, alone, or in combination with vitamin A acid, benzoyl peroxide, or both.[50, 51] When clindamycin was introduced for the topical treatment of acne vulgaris, the question was raised as to whether pseudomembranous colitis might occur in individuals who were treated with the drug. Although this complication is indeed quite rare, patients should be made aware of this possibility.[52–55]

Oral Retinoids. Isotretinoin (13-*cis*-retinoic acid), released in the United States in September 1982 as Accutane, is currently the most effective drug for the treatment of severe, recalcitrant nodulocystic acne unresponsive to effective conventional therapy. Although the precise mechanism of action is unknown, its beneficial effects appear to

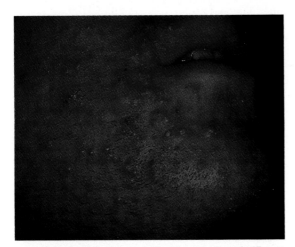

Figure 6–18. Gram-negative folliculitis on the face of a 17-year-old young man with acne.

be related to marked inhibition of sebum synthesis, lowering of *P. acnes* concentration, inhibition of neutrophil chemotaxis, and its comedolytic and anti-inflammatory effects. Most patients treated with isotretinoin achieve excellent results with a dosage of 1 mg/kg/day for 12 to 20 weeks. For those with severe or persistent side effects, however, the dosage may be reduced to 0.5 mg/kg/day; and for those with severe involvement of the trunk (particularly the back), 2 mg/kg/day may be required.[56–58] Since its initial release, the use of isotretinoin has been expanded to include patients with acne conglobata (a severe rapidly spreading disease that is likely to result in significant scarring), severe forms of rosacea, and gram-negative folliculitis. Since isotretinoin is teratogenic, however, it must not be administered to women who are pregnant or are likely to become pregnant while taking it or within 1 month after its use has been discontinued.[59]

Other side effects of oral isotretinoin include cheilitis, conjunctivitis, and xerosis; dry eyes, chapped lips, epistaxis, dermatitis, pruritus, fragility and easy bruisability of the skin; palmoplantar desquamation; muscular stiffness and muscular aches and pains; headaches; corneal opacities, myopia, and difficulties with dark adaptation and night vision acuity; paronychias and pyoderma; appetite changes; hair changes or increased shedding of the scalp hair; increased susceptibility to sunburn; leukopenia; neutropenia; hypertriglyceridemia; increase in erythrocyte sedimentation rate and cholesterol, alanine aminotransferase, aspartate aminotransferase, and alkaline phosphatase levels; exuberant granuloma-like granulation tissue; depression; urticaria, vasculitis, and erythema nodosum; acne flare in the early weeks of treatment; hyperostoses and bone-growth arrest and premature epiphyseal closure (in children receiving high dosages over a prolonged period of time); and gastrointestinal intolerance to the medication, and perhaps regional ileitis, peptic ulceration, or ulcerative colitis. Since pseudotumor cerebri has been reported, particularly in patients concomitantly receiving tetracycline or minocycline, patients with headache, nausea, vomiting, or visual disturbances should be evaluated for possible papilledema.[59–67]

Since teratogenic effects are seen in approximately 25 per cent of women exposed to the drug during pregnancy,[68–71] use of oral isotretinoin should be restricted to only those patients who meet the criteria for its use who are not pregnant or likely to become pregnant while taking it (or within 1 month after its use). It also should not be given to women who are breast feeding and it should not be administered by physicians who are not well versed in the pharmacokinetics of this agent. Since the half-lives of isotretinoin and its metabolite oxotretinoin are 10 to 20 hours and 20 to 29 hours, respectively, there is no demonstrable risk of embryopathy 1 month after the drug has been discontinued.[72]

Topical Acne Therapy and Pregnancy. Physicians are frequently consulted regarding the safety of acne treatment in women who are pregnant, may become pregnant, or are breast feeding an infant. Although there are no long-term studies on the use of topical antibiotics during pregnancy, erythromycin, which is the drug of choice for systemic treatment in pregnant patients who are allergic to penicillin, is safe for topical use during pregnancy. Since it is estimated that approximately 5 per cent of topically applied clindamycin can be absorbed, this drug is probably best avoided for women who are breast feeding, are pregnant, or are contemplating becoming pregnant. Although approximately 5 per cent of topically applied benzoyl peroxide is absorbed through the skin, since it is rapidly metabolized to benzoic acid within the skin, enters the dermal blood vessels as benzoate, and is then transported to the kidneys and excreted in the urine, this agent also appears to be safe during pregnancy. Despite the fact that topical vitamin A acid also appears to be safe, and there are no reports of fetal malformation or measurable plasma concentrations associated with its use, the ultimate decision as to whether to use topical vitamin A acid during pregnancy should probably be left to the discretion of the patient and her obstetrician.[73, 74]

Estrogens. Although acne is not listed among the manufacturers' indications for use of anovulatory drugs, these preparations have been useful in the treatment of women older than 16 years of age with severe, recalcitrant, pustulocystic acne. These agents produce good results, but not without a certain element of potential risk. Anovulatory drugs suppress the androgenic stimulation of sebum production, and when adequate amounts of estrogen are used they are beneficial in 50 to 70 per cent of patients.

It is important to weigh the risks and benefits when the use of estrogens is contemplated in the treatment of acne. Side effects to be considered include nausea, weight gain, candidal vaginitis, chloasma, hypertension, and thromboembolic phenomena. I prefer to restrict the use of estrogens to those few female patients, older than 16 years of age, with severe recalcitrant pustulocystic acne, or to those who elect a course of anovulatory drugs for reasons other than their acne. Estrogens should never be prescribed for male patients, since the dose required for sebum suppression will produce feminizing side effects, nor should they be administered to patients younger than the age of 16 when possible bone growth inhibition is a consideration.

Although some patients will respond to lower dosages of estrogen (50 μg of ethinyl estradiol or its 3-methyl ether derivative, mestranol), a more consistent response follows the use of higher daily dosages, 80 to 100 μg (i.e., 0.1 mg of ethinyl estradiol or mestranol). Because of the potential androgenicity of norethindrone and norgestrel, however, oral contraceptives containing these progestational agents are best avoided. Although sebum production occasionally decreases during the first or second cycle of drug administration, it usually takes three or four cycles (12 to 16 weeks) for a maximum effect to be achieved. In two thirds of patients a temporary acne flare may occur during the first two cycles of therapy. Patients should be forewarned of this possibility and reassured that this effect is only temporary.[75]

Other Agents. Azaleic acid, a topical dicarboxylic acid formulation with antibacterial activity against *P. acnes*, and cyproterone acetate, an oral antiandrogen that when given in combination with estrogen can reduce sebaceous gland secretion in women, are still being evaluated and are currently unavailable in the United States.

Zinc Therapy. In 1977 it was suggested that oral zinc in a dosage of 0.2 g (200 mg) daily might be effective for the treatment of patients with moderate to severe forms of acne vulgaris. In a double-blind study of 64 patients a substantial reduction of papules, pustules, and infiltrates was noted by the end of 4 weeks of therapy.[76] Another study suggests that zinc may have a beneficial effect on pustules, but not on comedones, papules, infiltrates, or cysts. However, the effect of placebo in acne varies between 19 and 56 per cent improvement according to the literature, so the 37 per cent improvement in pustules attributed to zinc in this study may prove to be a placebo effect.[77]

A subsequent double-blind study of 22 patients with acne who received 411 mg of zinc sulfate monohydrate or a lactose placebo daily showed no statistical difference in lesion counts (papules, pustules, open comedones, and closed comedones) between the 12 zinc-treated and the 10 lactose placebo–treated patients despite evidence of zinc absorption in serum and urine samples of the treated patients.[78] Furthermore, it should be noted that as little as one 220-mg capsule of zinc sulfate a day has caused high plasma zinc levels with nausea and vomiting and that anemia secondary to a bleeding gastric erosion has been reported in a 15-year-old girl following the use of 220 mg of oral zinc sulfate twice a day for 1 week for the treatment of acne vulgaris.[79, 80] The divergence of results among various clinical studies may reflect the difficulties inherent in the characteristics of patient populations or differences in design study, or perhaps the form of zinc sulfate may be significant. In addition, since studies support the use of a topical formulation of zinc and erythromycin,[81] further evaluation should determine what role if any zinc has in the pathogenesis or management of this disorder.

Acne Surgery. Acne surgery, the mechanical removal of comedones, pustules, and cysts, although time consuming, is extremely important for the rapid involution of individual acne lesions. This procedure is helpful only when properly done. The removal of open comedones does not materially influence the course of acne. However, it is desirable that they be removed for cosmetic purposes. Closed comedones should be removed to prevent rupture and spilling of their inflammatory contents into the surrounding dermis. For stubborn lesions, the procedure may be assisted by nicking the surface of the lesion with a sharp needle and expressing the contents with a comedo extractor. When improperly performed, inaccurate placement of the comedo extractor or overzealous manipulation may cause damage and irritation to the overlying skin, or rupture of the comedo wall with escape of sebum and further formation of inflammatory lesions.

Intralesional Acne Therapy. When cystic lesions are drained, a slightly larger incision is occasionally necessary. Whenever possible a small-gauge sterile needle is preferred over a scalpel blade in an effort to minimize potential scarring. Intralesional corticosteroid injection usually results in rapid involution of nodular and cystic lesions. The injection of 0.1 to 0.3 ml of triamcinolone acetonide (in a concentration of 0.625 to 10.0 mg/ml) or betamethasone sodium phosphate (Celestone Soluspan suspension, [Schering]), diluted to a concentration of 1 to 2 mg/ml, is recommended. With proper use of intralesional corticosteroid injection, incision and drainage of lesions is rarely required, and scars can frequently be avoided. Extreme caution should be exercised, since atrophy of the skin may occur when the injection is high in the dermis, particularly when the amount or concentration of triamcinolone acetonide is excessive (Fig. 6–20). This atrophy fortunately generally disappears spontaneously within 6 months to 1 year. When intralesional corticosteroid formulations are mixed, those diluted with sterile saline or lidocaine are less painful when injected intradermally than those diluted in distilled water.[82]

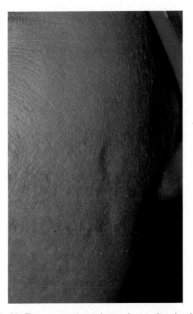

Figure 6–20. Temporary dermal atrophy on the cheek following intralesional corticosteroid injection in the treatment of pustulocystic acne vulgaris.

Phototherapy. The value of ultraviolet light is debatable. Its major effect is to give the patient a feeling of well-being, mild erythema, desquamation, and a resultant tan, which helps to conceal acne lesions. The risk of overexposure and conjunctival inflammation from failure to shield the eyes suggests caution and a limitation on the use of ultraviolet light as a method of home therapy. Of particular note are studies suggesting that long-term ultraviolet light may result in increased sebum production and acceleration of follicular hyperkeratosis, thus leading to comedo formation.[83] It appears, therefore, that the adverse effects of ultraviolet light may outweigh its benefit as a possible adjunct to acne therapy.

Radiation Therapy. Once widely employed in the treatment of acne, the use of x-ray has been abandoned as more effective forms of therapy have developed. Superficial irradiation has been shown to reduce the size of sebaceous glands; however, acne often recurs when the glands regenerate after 3 to 4 months.

Cryotherapy. Cryotherapy appears to be helpful in the hands of some dermatologists. Erythema and desquamation may be produced by a carbon dioxide "slush," made of powdered dry ice and acetone. A piece of gauze held in a clamp is used to apply the slush by lightly brushing the skin. Involution of isolated persistent acne lesions may also be accelerated by local application of solid carbon dioxide dipped in acetone or by liquid nitrogen on a simple cotton-tipped applicator applied carefully to individual lesions. This technique effectively hastens involution of small pustular lesions; more vigorous liquid nitrogen application (10 to 30 seconds or more), particularly when used in combination with intralesional triamcinolone acetonide injection, appears to help resolution of cystic lesions and keloidal scars, particularly those measuring 1.0 to 1.5 cm in diameter or less.

Scar Removal. Acne scars may improve spontaneously to a surprising degree over a period of 2 to 3 years, but often the patient's final appearance is less than desirable. Topical chemotherapy with 20 to 30 per cent trichloroacetic acid appears to help some patients with persistent pitting.

Dermabrasion offers hope for improvement for those with residual scarring and persistent nodular lesions. It is important, however, to note that following dermabrasion a small percentage of individuals who pigment easily occasionally develop hyperpigmentation, which may be more unattractive than the original scars. Other possible complications of dermabrasion include infection, further scarring, occasional hypopigmentation, or an inability to tan properly over treated areas.

Medical-grade liquid silicone (dimethyl polysiloxane) has been found to be of value in the reconstruction of deep pits and atrophic scars, but its use is no longer authorized in the United States. Other useful techniques include implants of injectable bovine collagen (Zyderm or Zyplast [Collagen Corp.]) or Fibrel gelatin (a derivative of fibrin foam), cutaneous punch-graft excision with full-thickness graft replacement, and surgical excision and plastic revision of epithelialized sinus tracts.[84, 85]

Neonatal and Infantile Acne

Occasionally infants develop an eruption that resembles acne vulgaris as seen in adolescents. Although the etiology of neonatal and infantile acne is not clearly defined, they appear to develop as a result of hormonal stimulation of sebaceous glands that have not yet involuted to their childhood state of immaturity. Although testosterone synthesis occurs in the fetal testis and adrenal gland between the 9th and 15th weeks of intrauterine life, steroid synthesis in the fetal ovary is relatively limited. This disparity may explain the apparent higher incidence of acne neonatorum (neonatal acne) and infantile acne in male infants.[86, 87]

Lesions of acne neonatorum may be present at birth or may appear in early infancy. Lesions characteristically present as erythematous papules or pustules, and rarely as comedones, usually confined to the cheeks and occasionally affecting the chin and forehead. In contrast to adolescent acne, the chest and back are not affected.

The term *infantile acne* has also been applied to a more serious type of acne that generally does not make its appearance until the infant is 3 or 4 months of age, or sometimes older (Fig. 6–21). This disorder deserves a separate designation. Lesions may be fairly numerous, and comedones (mainly on the cheeks) often predominate. Indi-

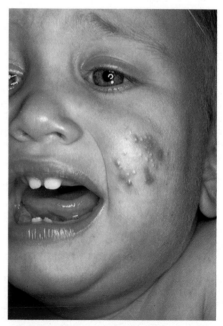

Figure 6–21. An infant with comedonal and papular acne on the cheek (infantile acne).

vidual lesions may be quite inflammatory, papules and pustules are common, and, at times, nodules (occasionally healing with scar formation) may be apparent.[4]

The course of infantile acne varies considerably. The lesions may be limited to a few comedones that clear after a few weeks. Most cases disappear within the first 2 or 3 years of life; others reportedly have persisted for up to 11 years. Cases with early onset and strong family history are generally the most persistent and are subject to severe resurgence at puberty. Infants with acne neonatorum or infantile acne generally have no evidence of sexual precocity; those with persistent involvement, however, should be investigated for evidence of precocity or abnormal virilization. If endocrine abnormality is suspected, 17-ketosteroid excretion should be evaluated. During the first few weeks of life excretion of 17-ketosteroids may normally be elevated. A level of 0.5 mg in a 24-hour urine sample after 2 weeks of age, however, should be considered excessive, suggesting further investigation for gonadal or adrenal cortex hyperfunction.

Acne neonatorum must be differentiated from milia of the newborn, which is a disorder manifested by multiple, 1- to 2-mm white or yellowish white follicular papules (Fig. 6–22). Milia of the newborn usually occurs on the face, particularly the nose, cheeks, chin, and forehead, as a normal phenomenon in up to 40 per cent of full-term infants and children during the first years of life.

In mild cases of acne neonatorum and infantile acne, therapy is generally unnecessary; daily cleansing with soap and water may be all that is required. Exogenous oil such as baby oils and lotions may aggravate this disorder and should be avoided. Occasionally mild keratolytic agents containing 3 to 5 per cent sulfur, salicylic acid, or resorcinol may be helpful. In the more severe cases of infantile acne, benzoyl peroxide gels or lotions may be used. Although topical vitamin A acid can be used for severe cases of neonatal acne, this preparation is potentially irritating, and most parents of children with this disorder prefer to use milder therapeutic agents. Management, therefore, should be determined by the degree of peeling or irritation and individual tolerance to available preparations.

Drug Acne

Corticosteroid acne, although not commonly seen in small children, occasionally occurs in older children and adults following the administration of adrenocorticotropic hormone (ACTH) and corticosteroids. Identical lesions can also be produced by application of potent topical corticosteroid formulations.[88] The lesions represent a folliculitis rather than a stimulation of the sebaceous glands. Lesions consist of dull red, smooth, dome-shaped papules or small pustules and are seen primarily on the upper trunk, arms, and neck. The face may be involved, but to a lesser degree (Fig. 6–23).

Iodides and bromides, particularly after long periods of administration, may induce an inflammatory acneiform eruption composed chiefly of follicular pustules in the typical acne areas (face and upper trunk), as well as elsewhere. Usually this eruption is caused by the iodine content of therapeutic agents rather than the use of iodized salt. Antituberculous drugs such as isoniazid may also cause an acneiform eruption, starting with the face and spreading to the trunk and even beyond, without pustule or comedo formation. It consists primarily of reddish brown papules somewhat resembling those of corticosteroid acne. Anticonvulsive drugs (phenytoin and trimethadione) and antidepressants (lithium-containing compounds) after a month or so of therapy are also known to exacerbate acne in susceptible persons (Fig. 6–24).

Androgen Excess and Acne

It is well recognized that androgens may precipitate or aggravate acne in both men and women. Thus, acne may be produced or aggravated by increased adrenal gland production in response to stress, adrenal tumors, ACTH, and ovarian androgen excess such as that which occurs in patients with polycystic ovarian disease or the Stein-Leventhal syndrome. Women with severe, persistent, or recalcitrant forms of acne, and women who have the onset or recurrence of acne during the third decade of life or later, therefore, even if they do not manifest other signs of androgen excess, should be screened for this possibility by the measurement of free testosterone and dehydroepiandrosterone sulfate. Additional evaluation may include measurement of 17-hydroxyprogesterone,

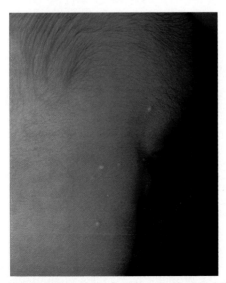

Figure 6–22. Milia neonatorum. One- to 2-mm white follicular papules over the cheeks and forehead (a common phenomenon seen in up to 40 per cent of full-term infants).

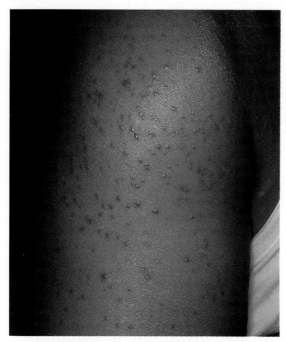

Figure 6–23. Steroid acne (steroid folliculitis). Smooth dome-shaped papules on the arm of a patient who had been receiving systemic corticosteroids.

follicle-stimulating hormone, luteinizing hormone, and prolactin levels. When abnormalities are detected, patients should have a complete endocrinologic evaluation and their acne can be treated by oral estrogens (generally in the form of an oral contraceptive containing 0.05 mg or more of estrogen), low-dose glucocorticosteroids (2.5 to

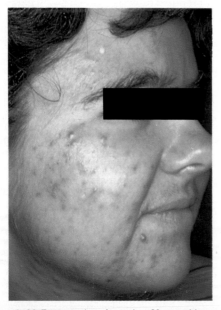

Figure 6–24. Exaggeration of acne in a 20-year-old woman on anticonvulsant drug therapy.

7.5 mg of prednisone or 0.25 to 0.5 mg of dexamethasone), or cyproterone acetate (not available in the United States except as Cyproteron, an orphan drug [Berlex Laboratories, Wayne, NJ 07470]) alone or in combination with estrogen, or a mineralocorticoid androgen antagonist such as spironolactone (Aldactone) in a dosage of 50 to 200 mg/day, preferably by an endocrinologist, gynecologist, or physician experienced in hormonal abnormalities and their regulation.[89-92]

Rosacea

Acne rosacea is a chronic vascular inflammatory disorder usually limited to the face that is characterized by erythema, telangiectasia, papules and pustules, and, at times, hyperplasia of the sebaceous glands and the soft tissues of the nose (rhinophyma). Primarily a disease of adults between the ages of 30 and 50, it may also appear as early as the second decade of life, at times coexisting with acne vulgaris (Fig. 6–25); a variety of ocular lesions may also be seen as a complication in 5 per cent of patients.[93] The latter complication, termed *ocular rosacea*, is characterized by blepharitis, conjunctivitis, episcleritis, iritis, keratitis, and, at times, corneal ulceration and subsequent opacity.

Although the etiologies of rosacea and ocular rosacea are not well understood, affected individuals should avoid factors that may provoke facial vasodilatation, namely, exposure to extremes of heat and cold and excessive sunlight and the ingestion of hot liquids, alcohol, highly seasoned foods, and spices. Complete clearing is rarely achieved, but reasonably satisfactory control can usually be accomplished by the use of systemic tetracycline or metronidazole (Flagyl) and topical formulations containing benzoyl peroxide, sulfur, topical antibiotics, and metronidazole cream (MetroGel [Curatek]). Oral isotretinoin has been effective in patients with severe rosacea, predominantly of the granulomatous type. The telangiectasia may be treated by electrodesiccation or tunable dye laser therapy, and rhinophyma can be treated by shaving the excess tissue with a scalpel blade, dermabrasion, electrocautery with bipolar cutting current, carbon dioxide or argon laser surgery, or surgical excision and skin grafting.

Lupus Miliaris Disseminatus Faciei

Lupus miliaris disseminatus faciei is a self-limiting papular eruption of unknown etiology characterized by asymptomatic papular or papulopustular lesions symmetrically distributed in the central portion of the face. Believed by some to represent a variant of "lupoid" rosacea or a tuberculid dermatitis of unknown cause, the disorder appears to be associated with a granulomatous reaction to breakdown products of pilosebaceous units occurring primarily in adolescents and young

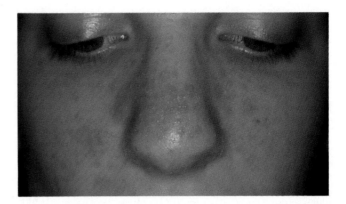

Figure 6–25. Acne rosacea on the nose and cheeks of a 17-year-old girl.

adults characterized by bright red, soft papules that later turn brown with gentle pressure with a glass slide (diascopy).

Histopathologic examination of lesions reveals well-defined tubercle-like structures composed of epithelioid cells and some giant cells, usually showing in their center a large area of caseation necrosis. Although tetracycline and dapsone therapy may at times be beneficial and response to oral isotretinoin (Accutane) has been reported,[94] the disorder may leave small pitted scars and usually resolves spontaneously after several months to a few years.

Pomade Acne

A variety of external agents can induce acne-like eruptions on repeated exposure to the skin of susceptible persons. These include greasy or oily suntan preparations, heavy makeup bases, and grooming agents. An acneiform eruption induced by various grooming substances used on the scalp has been termed *pomade acne*.[95] This disorder, seen chiefly on the forehead and temples in blacks, consists of closely set, rather uniform, closed comedones. The cheek and chin may also be involved if the pomade is rubbed over the entire face. In more advanced cases, papular or papulopustular lesions may be noted (Fig. 6–26). They improve with discontinuation of the offending comedogenic preparation and the use of appropriate topical keratolytic agents. Currently available pomades and oils with reduced comedogenicity for patients with black skin include Jojoba Hair Oil, Posner-Lite Touch, TCB Hair Oil, Finisheen, and Vitapoint.

Occupational Acne

Acnegenic agents such as relatively unrefined oils, greases, and waxes derived from petroleum (such as insoluble cutting oils and chlorinated hydrocarbons), coal tar derivatives, and animal and vegetable oils produce eruptions in workers in gas stations, garages, and restaurants, particularly those specializing in hamburgers and french fries. The eruption appears at the sites of contact, particularly the face, back, upper extremities, and neck.

Acne Cosmetica

Acne cosmetica is a variant of acne described in women, usually older than 20, as a result of the frequent or heavy use of cosmetics,[96] particularly those containing lanolin, petrolatum, certain vegetable oils, butyl stearate, isopropyl myristate, sodium lauryl sulfate, lauryl alcohol, and oleic acid. Lesions are predominantly small, scattered, closed comedones on the face and should be differentiated from acne vulgaris that may persist into adult life. Although common in women who never had acne vulgaris, women with a history of adolescent acne seem to be the most susceptible. A prominent feature is a coarse facial appearance associated with dark prominent follicles that is often more distressing to the patient than the actual acne-like lesions seen in this disorder. The most extensive eruptions are seen in women who attempt to mask the lesions under a heavy coating of cosmetics.

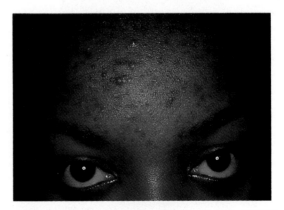

Figure 6–26. An 18-year-old black girl with multiple comedones, papules, and hyperpigmented postinflammatory lesions on the forehead caused by the use of a grooming substance on the hair and scalp ("pomade acne").

Fortunately, most cosmetic companies today are aware of the problem of comedogenicity and many cosmetics are currently marketed as non-comedogenic or nonacnegenic.

Acne Excoriee des Jeunes Filles

Acne excoriee des jeunes filles is a form of acne most frequently seen in adolescent girls. Often associated with various degrees of emotional stress, acne excoriee occasionally may be seen in boys, but to a lesser degree. Excoriating or squeezing of acne lesions may vary from mild irritation to severe scarring and occasional gross mutilation (Fig. 6–27). In the mild forms a simple explanation and local therapy may be all that is required to control the situation. In severe forms intensive psychiatric therapy may be required to control the underlying psychiatric basis of this disorder.

Pyoderma Faciale

Pyoderma faciale is a relatively uncommon form of acne usually seen in women in their early 20s. It is characterized by a sudden fulminating onset of pyoderma localized to the face with superficial or deep abscesses intercommunicating with one another through channels or sinus tracts. The condition is marked by a reddish cyanotic color of the involved areas with sharply demarcated borders, an absence of comedones, and strict localization to the face. Keloidal scars are often seen as a prominent feature of this disorder.

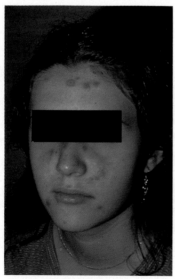

Figure 6–27. A 16-year-old girl with excoriated acne vulgaris (acne excoriee des jeunes filles).

Acne Conglobata

Acne conglobata is another suppurative form of acne vulgaris that is usually chronic and seen in men from 18 to 30 years of age. It is characterized by cysts, abscesses, and burrowing sinus tracts. Healing often results in cosmetically disfiguring keloidal scars.

Acne With Facial Edema

Acne may at times be associated with an inflammatory edema of the middle third of the face (cheeks, forehead, periorbital areas, base of the nose, and glabella). Although its pathogenesis is unknown, the disorder is believed to be a manifestation of chronic cutaneous inflammation and edema, analogous to that of the legs in patients with recurrent cellulitis and venous insufficiency. The disorder, which is unresponsive to high-dose oral antibiotics or topical therapy, responds to oral corticosteroids and isotretinoin.[97]

Perioral Dermatitis

A relatively common distinctive skin eruption resembling acne occurs primarily in young women. It was originally described by Frumess and Lewis in 1957 under the title of "light-sensitive seborrheid."[98]

The eruption consists of discrete, 1- to 3-mm erythematous papules, papulovesicles, and papulopustules. The eruption is symmetrical and affects the chin and nasolabial folds, sparing a clear zone around the vermilion border (Fig. 6–28). As the papules resolve they are often replaced by a diffuse redness or erythematous scale; itching is rare and never severe, but a sensation of burning is frequently noted. Histologic features include nonspecific inflammation and parakeratotic scaling around the follicular opening.

The etiology of this disorder is uncertain, but the eruption is distinctive owing to its peculiar localization and sex and age distribution. Marks and Black suggest an external irritant, possibly cosmetics or topical corticosteroids, as provoking or perpetuating stimuli of this disorder.[99] Its clinical resemblance to acne, the fact that potent topical corticosteroids can induce or aggravate the disorder, and its response to tetracycline therapy and mild topical keratolytic agents suggest that it is a distinctive acne variant.

Granulomatous perioral dermatitis is a term used to describe a self-limiting granulomatous perioral, perinasal, and periorbital dermatitis, seen primarily in children and young adults, that is believed by some researchers to represent a variant of perioral dermatitis in which focal disruption of the follicular walls of the sebaceous glands incites a granulomatous response (Fig. 6–29). Although therapy is not invariably successful, oral erythro-

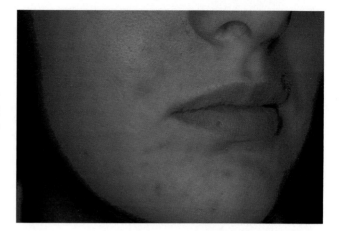

Figure 6–28. A 17-year-old girl with perioral dermatitis-discrete erythematous papules, papulovesicles, and pustules on the chin, upper lip, and the lower aspect of the cheeks, with sparing of the vermilion border of the lips.

mycin and topical application of 2 per cent sulfur in hydrocortisone cream can be beneficial, and patients and parents can generally be reassured by the fact that the disorder frequently undergoes spontaneous resolution within a period of several months to a year.[100]

Fordyce's Spots

Fordyce's spots (Fordyce's condition, Fordyce's disease) is a commonly observed benign condition characterized by minute yellowish macules and globoid papules that may form large plaques. Frequently symmetrical and generally found on the vermilion border of the lips and oral mucosa and, at times, the glans penis or labia minora, the disorder, a manifestation of aberrant or ectopic sebaceous glands, is uncommon in young children, becomes more apparent during adolescence, and increases to an incidence of 70 to 80 per cent in older adults. The disorder is asymptomatic, and treatment, which is generally unsuccessful, is unnecessary.

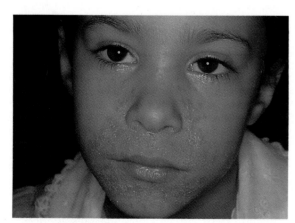

Figure 6–29. Granulomatous perioral dermatitis on the face of a 6½-year-old girl. The disorder developed several days after the use of Halloween makeup.

DISORDERS OF THE APOCRINE GLANDS

Fox-Fordyce Disease

Fox-Fordyce disease (apocrine miliaria) is a chronic itching papular eruption of apocrine gland–bearing areas, principally the axillae, the mammary areolae, and the pubic and perineal regions. Seen primarily in young women, this disorder is of unknown etiology but appears to be a form of apocrine sweat retention associated with obstruction and rupture of the intraepidermal portions of the affected apocrine glands. The disease is more common in women, with an estimated female-to-male ratio of 9 or 10:1. It has its onset between 13 and 35 years of age and is not seen before puberty owing to prepubertal quiescence of the apocrine glands.

Lesions of Fox-Fordyce disease are small, usually smooth and rounded papules that are principally follicular (Fig. 6–30). Itching, often paroxysmal and aggravated by emotional stress, is a prominent symptom of this disorder. The histologic picture is characterized by obstruction of the apocrine duct at its entrance into the follicular wall and an inflammatory infiltrate that surrounds the upper third of the hair follicles in involved areas.

The management of this disorder is less than satisfactory. Topical corticosteroids have limited value. Intralesional corticosteroids are helpful and can produce a temporary remission for periods of 6 to 8 months. Surgical excision of the affected areas with plastic repair, although effective, is rarely justified. Estrogen therapy (Premarin in a 1.25-mg dose daily), although not universally successful, appears to be beneficial in some women with this disorder.

Hidradenitis Suppurativa

Hidradenitis suppurativa is a chronic suppurative and cicatricial disease of the apocrine sweat glands in the axillary, inguinal, and anogenital re-

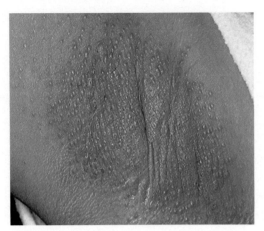

Figure 6–30. Fox-Fordyce disease (apocrine miliaria). Small round follicular papules are seen in the axilla of an adolescent girl.

gions. The disease affects blacks and females more often than whites or males, usually develops after puberty, and appears to be related to keratinous plugging of the apocrine duct, associated bacterial infection, and rupture of the involved area with extension of the infection to adjacent areas.

The earliest clinical sign of hidradenitis suppurativa is a painful, inflammatory abscess-like swelling, usually 0.5 to 1.5 cm in diameter, in the affected apocrine areas. Within a period of hours to days the abscess frequently enlarges and, if untreated, will often perforate the overlying skin. There is then a seropurulent drainage. The abscess heals by deep fibrosis, resulting in intercommunicating sinus tracts and band-like or bridge-like hypertrophic scars (Fig. 6–31).

Bacteriologic study of early lesions usually reveals coagulase-positive staphylococci or streptococci, probably representing secondary infection and not the cause of hidradenitis. Occasionally

Escherichia coli, Bacillus proteus, or *Pseudomonas aeruginosa* contaminates the flora.

In the early stages of hidradenitis suppurativa, sections of the skin show keratinous obstruction of the apocrine duct and often of the associated hair follicle orifice, ductal and tubal dilation, and associated inflammatory changes. As the process becomes more chronic there is fibrosis and scarring, with destruction of the apocrine gland, eccrine gland, and pilosebaceous apparatus. In the healing stage, one sees deep tortuous invaginations of the epidermis filled with keratin and representing the sinus tracts.

Optimal therapy for hidradenitis suppurativa depends on early and accurate diagnosis, prolonged antibacterial therapy, intralesional corticosteroids, incision and drainage of abscesses, and, in recalcitrant cases, total excision of the affected region. Early in the disease, broad-spectrum antibiotics and elimination of the local factors might reverse the process, but in the chronic phase surgery remains the only curative mode of therapy. Repeated incision and drainage of abscesses and incomplete excision of infected tracts, however, are often harmful since they permit extension of the infection and an increase in fibrosis and tract formation. Advanced cases, therefore, have a more pessimistic outlook. In such cases both recurrence and complication rates are lowest after total excision of the hair-bearing area, followed by coverage with a split-thickness skin graft.

DISORDERS OF THE ECCRINE GLANDS

The eccrine sweat glands are distributed over the entire skin surface and are found in greatest abundance on the palms and soles and in the axillae. They represent the principal means of maintaining homeostatic balance by evaporation of water. Their secretion depends on their sympathetic nerve supply, which is controlled by stimuli of three types: thermal, mental, and gustatory. By these mechanisms the quantity and quality of sweat may be varied.

Hyperhidrosis

Hyperhidrosis is a disorder characterized by an excessive production of perspiration in response to heat or emotional stimuli. Topical and systemic therapy can be temporarily suppressive but are basically unsatisfactory. Treatment with systemic anticholinergic agents (atropine, 0.01 mg/kg every 4 to 6 hours, or Pro-Banthine, 1.5 mg/kg/24 hr), effective to variable degrees, is limited by side effects such as mucous membrane dryness, blurred vision, and mydriasis. Sedative or tranquilizing drugs appear to be beneficial for axillary or palmar hyperhidrosis, as are aluminum salts applied locally (10 to 25 per cent aluminum chloride in distilled water). Drysol (Persōn and Covey), a solu-

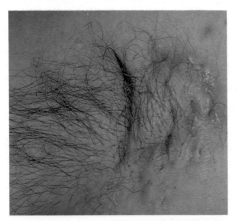

Figure 6–31. Hidradenitis suppurativa. Painful inflammatory abscess-like swellings with deep fibrosis, intercommunicating sinus tracts, and hypertrophic scars are evident in the axilla.

tion of 20 per cent aluminum chloride in alcohol, is cosmetically acceptable and beneficial for most patients with this disorder.

In palmar hyperhidrosis, local astringents of value are those that inhibit the production of perspiration (Burow's soaks 1:40 or potassium permanganate 1:4,000). Dusting powders, such as Zeasorb (Stiefel), may be helpful. Plantar hyperhidrosis may be suppressed with a solution of 10 per cent glutaraldehyde buffered with sodium bicarbonate to a pH of 7.5 (1.65 g of NaHCO$_3$ per milliliter) applied topically daily or every other day. This solution causes staining and therefore is not a useful modality for treatment of the palms.

For individuals unresponsive to other forms of therapy, a portable iontophoretic device (the Drionic unit [General Medical Company, Los Angeles, CA]) has been suggested as a less aggressive approach to therapy.[101, 102] Although surgical techniques such as selective removal of overactive axillary eccrine glands and cervicothoracic sympathectomy have been suggested for patients with intractable or disabling hyperhidrosis of the palms, soles, or axillae, the disorder can generally be controlled reasonably well without resorting to surgery.

Dyshidrosis

Dyshidrosis (pompholyx) is a term applied to a condition of recurring vesiculation of the palms and soles in which hyperhidrosis and retention of sweat precede the eruption. Although this condition may not be a disorder of the sweat glands per se, hyperhidrosis is an important accessory factor; treatment directed toward the hyperhidrosis may prove beneficial. Topical corticosteroid formulations and efforts to minimize excessive perspiration are helpful in controlling this disorder.

Anhidrosis

Anhidrosis is an abnormal absence of perspiration from the surface of the skin in the presence of appropriate stimuli, often resulting in hyperthermia. This condition may be caused by a deficiency or abnormality of the sweat glands (as in hypohidrotic ectodermal dysplasia) or of the nervous pathways from the peripheral or central nervous system leading to the sweat glands (as in syringomyelia, leprosy, anticholinergic drug therapy, or sympathectomy). Cool baths, air conditioning, light clothing, and reduction of the causes of normal perspiration help to relieve symptoms.

Bromhidrosis

Bromhidrosis is an embarrassing malodorous condition in which an excessive, usually offensive, odor emanates from the skin. It may be of two types: (1) apocrine, resulting from bacterial degradation of apocrine sweat, and (2) eccrine, from the microbiologic degradation of stratum corneum softened by excessive eccrine sweat.

The human skin is populated with two distinct types of sweat glands: the eccrine and apocrine glands. Apocrine glands are found in only a few areas: in the axillae, the perianal region, and the areolae of the breasts. They are poorly developed in childhood but, triggered by androgen production, begin to enlarge with the approach of puberty. Apocrine secretion is sterile and odorless when it initially appears on the cutaneous surface.[103] The term *apocrine bromhidrosis* refers to an exaggeration of the axillary odor normally noted by all postpubertal individuals. Short-chain fatty acids, products of bacterial degradation of this secretion by gram-positive organisms (coagulase-negative staphylococci and diptheroids), are responsible for the odor associated with this disorder.[103, 104] *Eccrine bromhidrosis* refers to the excessive odor produced by bacterial action on the stratum corneum when it becomes macerated by eccrine sweat. This disorder occurs on the plantar surfaces of the feet and intertriginous areas, particular the inguinal region.

Bromhidrosis is best managed by regular thorough cleansing, preferably with an antibacterial soap; the use of commercial deodorants; the application of topical antibiotics and dusting powder to the affected areas; and frequent changes of clothing. Topical application of aluminum salts (10 to 25 per cent aluminum chloride in alcohol or distilled water) may help relieve the hyperhidrosis often associated with this disorder. Oral anticholinergic drugs (Pro-Banthine, 1.5 mg/kg/day) may help axillary eccrine hyperhidrosis, but there is little evidence of their effect on apocrine gland secretion.

Plantar bromhidrosis is managed by careful and scrupulous hygiene, preferably with germicidal soaps, the use of dusting powders (Zeasorb [Stiefel]) to absorb excessive perspiration, topical aluminum chloride preparations (Drysol [Persōn and Covey]) to limit hyperhidrosis, and the avoidance of shoes and sneakers whenever possible. Disagreeable odors may be reduced by soaks with Burow's solution (1:40) or potassium permanganate (1:4000).

Miliaria

Miliaria, a common dermatosis caused by sweat retention, is characterized by a vesicular eruption secondary to prolonged exposure to perspiration, with subsequent maceration and obstruction of the eccrine ducts. The pathophysiologic events that lead to this disorder are keratinous plugging of eccrine ducts followed by disruption of the duct and escape of the eccrine sweat into the skin below the level of obstruction. Studies suggest that increased perspiration causes hydration of the horny layer with an increase in the aerobic bacterial flora.[105] Subsequent release of a "toxin" secreted by these aerobic cocci injures luminal cells and precipitates a cast within the lumen. Cell membranes subsequently become more permeable and allow extravasation of sweat through the damaged sweat ducts, resulting in the clinical picture of miliaria rubra. Thereafter, as reparative processes come into play, the occluding mass moves upward, finally occupying the coils of ducts within the horny layer. These observations explain the sequence of miliaria crystallina, rubra, and profunda.

Thus we see three forms of this disorder: miliaria crystallina (sudamina), miliaria rubra (prickly heat), and miliaria profunda (a more severe form of miliaria rubra commonly seen in the tropics). Although frequently seen in children, adolescents, and adults, the incidence of miliaria is greatest in the first few weeks of life, owing to a relative immaturity of the eccrine ducts that favors poral closure and sweat retention.

In infants miliaria is seen as crops of crystal-clear, pinpoint superficial vesicles without an inflammatory areola as miliaria crystallina (sudamina) or as miliaria rubra ("prickly heat"), which is characterized by small discrete erythematous, often pruritic papules, vesicles, or papulovesicles (see Chapter 2, Fig. 2–5).

MILIARIA CRYSTALLINA

Characterized by clear, thin-walled vesicles, 1 to 2 mm in diameter, miliaria crystallina develops in crops on otherwise normal-appearing skin. The vesicles are asymptomatic and occur most frequently in intertriginous areas, particularly on the neck and axillae, or on parts of the trunk covered by clothing.

Lesions of miliaria crystallina are highly characteristic and easily differentiated from other vesicular diseases. When the diagnosis is in doubt, rupture of vesicles with a fine needle results in release of the clear, entrapped sweat. In miliaria crystallina the obstruction is quite superficial; histopathologic examination of lesions reveals vesicles either within or directly beneath the stratum corneum. On serial sectioning the vesicles can be seen to be in direct communication with ruptured sweat ducts.

MILIARIA RUBRA

"Prickly heat" is the most frequently seen and most important clinical form of miliaria (see Chapter 2, Fig. 2–5). Lesions have a predilection for the covered parts of the skin, especially where there is friction from clothing, particularly the forehead, upper trunk, volar aspects of the arms, and body folds. They are characterized by pruritic, discrete, but closely aggregated, small papules, vesicles, or papulovesicles surrounded by erythema. The fact that lesions of miliaria rubra are always extrafollicular helps in the differentiation of this disorder

from the papules or pustules of folliculitis. Miliaria rubra, therefore, can be differentiated by close inspection, expecially under slight magnification with a hand lens, by typical papules or vesicles surrounded by an erythematous areola, without penetrating hairs, which characterize the eruption seen in lesions of folliculitis. Histologic examination of lesions of miliaria rubra reveals varying degrees of spongiosis and vesicle formation within the epidermal sweat duct and adjacent epidermis, with or without a hyperkeratotic or parakeratotic plug above the area of spongiosis.

Miliaria pustulosa is a variant of miliaria rubra consisting of distinct superficial pustules not associated with hair follicles. Lesions tend to occur in areas of skin that have had previous inflammation and frequently appear coexistent with lesions of miliaria rubra.

MILIARIA PROFUNDA

A more pronounced form of miliaria, miliaria profunda is uncommon except in the tropics. This disorder nearly always follows repeated attacks of miliaria rubra and is characterized by firm, whitish, 1- to 3-mm papules. Lesions are most prominent on the trunk, but they may also be seen on the extremities. The deep location of the sweat retention in miliaria profunda results in papular rather than vesicular lesions. Erythema and pruritus are not seen in association with this disorder. Although miliaria profunda may at times resemble cutis anserina ("goose flesh"), the nonfollicular location of lesions of miliaria profunda helps in the differentiation of these two disorders. Histologic examination of lesions of miliaria profunda demonstrates rupture of the sweat duct in the upper dermis, with or without surrounding edema and inflammatory infiltrate.

The key to the management of miliaria is avoidance of excessive heat and humidity. In infants, generally all that is required is reassurance and advice on proper clothing and temperature regulation. Cool baths, light clothing, and air conditioning are invaluable. Calamine lotion, with or without 0.25 per cent menthol and 0.5 per cent phenol, is effective but has a tendency to cause excessive dryness; when this occurs, emollient creams or lotions may be helpful. Resorcinol, 3 per cent in alcohol, or Cetaphil lotion is therapeutically beneficial in this disorder.

Granulosis Rubra Nasi

Granulosis rubra nasi is a rare chronic disease that occurs on the nose (occasionally the cheeks and chin) of prepubertal children, with the highest reported incidence between the ages of 7 and 15 years. It is characterized by diffuse redness, persistent hyperhidrosis, and discrete pinpoint to pinhead-sized red or brownish red macules and soft papules on an erythematous base. Vesicles and small cystic lesions have also been seen in some patients with this disorder.[106]

The etiology of granulosis rubra nasi is unknown, but it appears to represent an inherited disorder. The role of the sweat glands and cutaneous vasculature is obscure, although occasionally this disease is associated with hyperhidrosis of the palms and soles.

Histologic examination of a cutaneous biopsy specimen is characterized by dilatation of the dermal blood vessels and lymphatic channels with an inflammatory infiltrate about the sweat ducts, sometimes associated with occlusion and dilatation and cyst formation.

No effective local or systemic therapy is available for this disorder, although simple drying lotions, tinted to help obscure the erythema, may provide symptomatic and cosmetic relief. Although granulosis rubra nasi may sometimes persist into later years, reassurance that the disorder usually disappears at puberty is helpful.

References

1. Nierman H: Bericht über 230 Zwillinge mit Hautkrankheiten. Z. Menschl. Vererb. Knostitutional. *34*:483–487, 1958.

   A study of 230 twins reveals 98 per cent concordance of acne in identical twins.

2. Kligman AM: An overview of acne. J. Invest. Dermatol. *62*:268–287, 1979.

   A critical appraisal of acne vulgaris with emphasis on its anatomy and pathophysiology.

3. Emerson GW, Strauss JS: Acne and acne care: A trend survey. Arch. Dermatol. *105*:407–411, 1972.

   A statisitcal survey and analysis of acne, its incidence, and severity in 1,023 high school students.

4. Plewig G, Kligman AM: Acne: Morphogenesis and Treatment. Springer-Verlag, New York, 1975.

   A richly illustrated treatise on acne depicting gross and microscopic features and therapeutic strategies to aid in the management of this disorder.

5. Cunliffe WJ, Gould DJ: Prevalence of facial acne in late adolescence and in adults. Br. Med. J. *1*:1109–1110, 1979.

   A survey of 1,066 healthy women and 1,089 healthy men between 17 and 70 years of age showed that clinical acne can at times persist until late adulthood.

6. Strauss JS, Kligman AM, Pochi P: The effect of androgens and estrogens on human sebaceous glands. J. Invest. Dermatol. *39*:139–155, 1962.

   Studies on the effect of estrogens and androgens on human sebaceous glands.

7. Van Scott EJ, McCardle RC: Keratinization of the duct of the sebaceous gland and growth cycle of the hair follicle in the histogenesis of acne in the human skin. J. Invest. Dermatol. *27*:405–429, 1956.

   Hyperkeratinization of the excretory duct of the sebaceous gland is shown to be the earliest histologic change in acne.

8. Strauss JS, Kligman AM: The pathologic dynamics of acne vulgaris. Arch. Dermatol. *82*:729–790, 1960.

   A classic study in the pathogenesis of acne vulgaris.

9. Blair C, Lewis CA: The pigment of comedones. Br. J. Dermatol. *82*:572–583, 1970.

   Histochemical techniques confirm the presence of melanin granules within the horny compacted cells of the tips of blackheads.

10. Kaidbey KH, Kligman AM: Pigmentation in comedones. Arch. Dermatol. *109*:60–62, 1974.

    Melanocytes as the source of color in blackheads (open comedones).

11. Kellum RE: Acne vulgaris: Studies in pathogenesis: Relative irritancy of free fatty acids from C_2 to C_{16}. Arch. Dermatol. *97*:722–726, 1968.

    Repeated applications of free fatty acids to human skin under occlusive patch tests revealed a greater irritancy and penetration by the C_8 to C_{14} range of fatty acids.

12. Shalita AR, Leyden JE Jr, Pochi PE, et al.: Periodic synopsis: Acne vulgaris. J. Am. Acad. Dermatol. *16*:410–412, 1987.

    A comprehensive overview of recent advances and concepts of pathogenesis and management of acne.

13. Winston MH, Shalita AR: Acne vulgaris, pathogenesis and management. Pediatr. Clin. North Am. *38*:889–903, 1991.

    An authoritative update on acne vulgaris, its pathogenesis and management.

14. Schachter RJ, Pantel E: Acne vulgaris and psychological impact on high school students. N.Y. State J. Med. *71*:2886–2890, 1971.

    A study of 1,254 high school students with acne and an analysis of the emotional and psychological handicaps of individuals afflicted by this disorder.

15. Van der Meeren HLM, van de Schaar WW, van den Hurk LMAM: The psychological impact of severe acne. Cutis *36*:84–86, 1985.

    An analysis of anxieties, depression, and neuroses seen in individuals with severe forms of acne.

16. Hitch JM, Greenburg BG: Adolescent acne and dietary iodine. Arch. Dermatol. *89*:898–911. 1961.

    Although iodine in medications can cause an acneiform eruption, dietary iodine appears to have little effect on the prevalence or severity of acne.

17. Fulton JE, Plewig G, Kligman AM: The effect of chocolate on acne vulgaris. J.A.M.A. *210*:2071–2074, 1969.

    Ingestion of large amounts of chocolate influences neither the production nor composition of sebum, nor does it affect the course of acne vulgaris.

18. Fulton JE Jr, Farzad-Bakeshandeh A, Bradley S: Studies on the mechanism of action of topical benzoyl peroxide and vitamin A acid in acne vulgaris. J. Cutan. Pathol. *1*:191–200, 1974.

    Although systemic tetracycline remains the most frequent treatment for acne vulgaris, this report indicates that topical therapy can clear the majority of cases within the initial 3 months of therapy.

19. Hurwitz S: The combined effect of vitamin A acid and benzoyl peroxide in the treatment of acne. Cutis *17*:585–590, 1976.

    The combination of vitamin A acid and benzoyl peroxide, when used properly, offers a well-tolerated, extremely effective therapeutic approach to the topical management of acne vulgaris.

20. Cunliffe WJ, Burke B: Benzoyl peroxide: Lack of sensitization. Acta Derm. Vernereol. *62*:458–459, 1982.

    A long-term prospective study of 445 patients in which only one instance of true contact dermatitis to benzoyl peroxide was found confirms the hypothesis that the vast majority of problems associated with benzoyl peroxide are related to improper application rather than true contact dermatitis.

21. Lynch FW, Cook, CD: Acne vulgaris treated with vitamin A. Arch. Dermatol. *55*:355–357, 1947.

Oral vitamin A, even when given in dosages of 100,000 units/day, was not effective in the treatment of a group of university students with acne.

22. Kligman AM, Fulton JE Jr, Plewig G: Topical vitamin A acid in acne vulgaris. Arch. Dermatol. *99:*469–476, 1969.

    Topical vitamin A acid, when used properly, can be most beneficial for the treatment of patients with extensive comedopapular acne.

23. Kligman AM, Mills OH Jr, Leyden JJ, et al.: Letters to the Editor: Postscript to vitamin A acid therapy for acne vulgaris. Arch. Dermatol. *107:*296, 1973.

    Appropriate precautionary instructions to patients can relieve the irritation formerly associated with vitamin A acid therapy.

24. Kligman LH, Akin FJ, Kligman AM: Sunscreens prevent ultraviolet photocarcinogenesis. J. Am. Acad. Dermatol. *3:*30–35, 1980.

    Sunscreens tested on hairless albino mice appear to prevent tumor formation over a 30-week period.

25. Epstein JH, Grekin DA: Inhibition of ultraviolet-induced carcinogenesis by all-*trans*-retinoic acid. J. Invest. Dermatol. *76:*178–180, 1981.

    Studies suggest that topical retinoic acid, when used with appropriate sun protection, is not only safe but may indeed be helpful in the prevention of cutaneous tumor formation.

26. Frosch PJ, Kligman AM: The soap chamber test: A new method for assessing the irritancy of soaps. J. Am. Acad. Dermatol. *1:*35–41, 1979.

    Studies of irritancy (scaling, redness, and fissuring) of 18 well-known toilet soaps contrast to a number of previous studies that failed to show differences among soaps or concluded that soaps are innocuous.

27. Hubbell CG, Hobbs ER, Rist T, et al.: Efficacy of minocycline compared with tetracycline in the treatment of acne vulgaris. Arch. Dermatol. *118:*989–992, 1982.

    In a double-blind evaluation of 49 patients, those treated with minocycline achieved and maintained improvement of their acne status in less time than those treated with tetracycline.

28. Leyden JJ: Absorption of minocycline hydrochloride and tetracycline hydrochloride: Effect of food, milk and iron. J. Am. Acad. Dermatol. *12:*308–312, 1985.

    Studies demonstrate that minocycline absorption, when given with milk or food, was considerably better than that of tetracycline. The absorption of both antibiotics, however, when taken with ferrous sulfate, was significantly reduced.

29. Simons JJ, Morales A: Minocycline and generalized cutaneous pigmentation. J. Am. Acad. Dermatol. *3:*244–247, 1980.

    A report of a patient who developed a generalized dark blue-gray cutaneous pigmentation while taking oral minocycline.

30. Fenske NA, Millns LJ: Cutaneous pigmentation due to minocycline hydrochloride. J. Am Acad. Dermatol. *3:*308–310, 1980.

    A report of discoloration of the gums, teeth, fingernails, and lower legs that occurred in a 42-year-old woman who had been taking oral minocycline.

31. Poliak SC, DiGiovanna JJ, Gross EG, et al.: Minocycline-associated tooth discoloration in young adults. J.A.M.A. *25:*2930–2932, 1985.

    A report of four patients who developed discoloration of the teeth following treatment with minocycline during or after adolescence.

32. Berger RS, Mandel EB, Hayes TJ, et al.: Minocycline staining of the oral cavity. J. Am. Acad. Dermatol. *21:*1300–1301, 1989.

    In a report of patients with bluish gray minocycline-induced staining of the teeth, pigmentary changes of the skin, gingi-

val hyperpigmentation, and staining of the alveolar bones, the authors hypothesize that dental staining may be related to oxidation of minocycline excreted in gingival fluid.

33. LePaw MI: Fixed drug eruption due to minocycline: Report of one case. J. Am. Acad. Dermatol. *8:*263–264, 1983.

    A report of a male in whom a fixed drug eruption of the scrotum and glans penis occurred on three separate occasions after taking minocycline.

34. Shogi A, Sumeda Y, Hamada T: Stevens-Johnson syndrome due to minocycline therapy. Arch. Dermatol. *123:*18–20, 1987.

    A report of a patient who developed Stevens-Johnson syndrome 4 days after the initiation of minocycline hydrochloride for an influenza-like illness.

35. Bridges AJ, Graziano FM, Calhoun W, et al.: Hyperpigmentation, neutrophilic alveolitis, and erythema nodosum resulting from minocycline. J. Am. Acad. Dermatol. *22:*959–962, 1990.

    A report of hyperpigmentation of the trunk, arms, and legs, erythema nodosum, and pulmonary infiltration with eosinophilia associated with minocycline ingestion.

36. Sato S, Murphy GF, Bernhard JD, et al.: Ultrastructural and x-ray microanalytic observations of minocycline-related hyperpigmentation of skin. J. Invest. Dermatol. *77:*264–271, 1981.

    Studies confirm that dermal iron deposition and dermal and perivascular minocycline–hemosiderin complexes are responsible for the cutaneous hyperpigmentation associated with minocycline administration.

37. Crowson TD, Head LH, Ferrante WA: Esophageal ulcers associated with tetracycline therapy. J.A.M.A. *235:*2747–2748, 1976.

    Three patients with esophageal ulceration presumably associated with the ingestion of tetracycline or its derivative doxycycline (Vibramycin).

38. Frank SB, Cohen HJ, Minkin W: Photo-onycholysis due to tetracycline hydrochloride and doxycycline. Arch. Dermatol. *103:*520–521, 1971

    Three patients on tetracycline and doxycycline developed photosensitivity and onycholysis.

39. Kestel JL Jr: Tetracycline-induced onycholysis unassociated with photosensitivity. Arch. Dermatol. *106:*766, 1972.

    Two patients while on tetracycline developed discoloration and separation of the nails without sun exposure.

40. Epstein JH, Tuffanelli DL, Seibert JS, et al.: Porphyria-like cutaneous changes induced by tetracycline. Arch. Dermatol. *112:*661–666, 1976.

    Blisters similar to those seen in porphyria can develop as a complication of tetracycline therapy.

41. Cravens TR: Onycholysis of the thumbs probably due to a phototoxic reaction from doxycyline. Cutis *27:*53–54, 1981.

    Three members of a party climbing Mt. Kilimanjaro developed photo-onycholysis from grasping of their hiking sticks and prolonged exposures of their thumbs to sunlight while taking doxycyline prophylactically during their climb.

42. Fulton JE Jr, McGinley K, Leyden J, et al.: Gram-negative folliculitis in acne vulgaris. Arch. Dermatol. *98:*349–353, 1968.

    A previously unrecognized complication of tetracycline therapy in acne.

43. Leyden J, Marples RR, Mills OH, et al.: Gram-negative folliculitis: A complication of antibiotic therapy in acne vulgaris. Br. J. Dermatol. *88:*533–538, 1973.

    Fifty cases of gram-negative folliculitis in a series of 1200 patients with acne vulgaris.

44. Kinney JP, Frank RR: Topical treatment of gram-negative bacterial superinfection in acne. Arch. Dermatol. *116:*597, 1980.

Gram-negative folliculitis due to *Staphylococcus epidermidis* and *Pseudomonas aeruginosa* responded to 0.1 per cent aqueous gentamicin compresses and topical benzoyl peroxide gel in a 10 per cent formulation within a period of 6 weeks.

45. James WD, Leyden JJ: Treatment of gram-negative folliculitis with isotretinoin: Positive clinical and microbiological response. J. Am. Acad. Dermatol. *12*:319–324, 1985.

    Serial microbiologic evaluations of 32 patients with gram-negative folliculitis revealed rapid, complete, and prolonged remissions following 5 months of isotretinoin therapy.

46. Mazza JJ, Kryda MD: Tetracycline-induced hemolytic anemia. J. Am. Acad. Dermatol. *2*:506–508, 1980.

    A 28-year-old man developed hemolytic anemia on two occasions following ingestion of oral tetracycline.

47. Stuart BH, Litt IF: Tetracycline-associated intracranial hypertension in an adolescent: A complication of systemic acne therapy. J. Pediatr. *92*:679–680, 1978.

    In a report of a 14-year-old girl who developed pseudotumor cerebri while receiving 1 g of tetracycline daily for the treatment of her acne, all signs and symptoms resolved within 2 weeks after discontinuation of therapy.

48. Walter BNJ, Gubbary SS: Tetracycline and benign intracranial hypertension: Report of five cases. Br. Med. J. *282*:19–20, 1981.

    A report of five patients who developed benign intracranial hypertension while receiving oral tetracycline or minocycline; two patients were also taking vitamin supplements containing vitamin A.

49. Fleischer AB Jr, Resnick SD: The effect of antibiotics on the efficacy of oral contraceptives: A controversy revisited. Arch. Dermatol. *125*:1562–1564, 1989.

    A review of the controversy regarding the possible interaction of antibiotics and oral contraceptives.

50. Fulton JE Jr, Pablo G: Topical antibacterial therapy for acne. Arch. Dermatol. *110*:83–86, 1974.

    Two per cent erythromycin base applied three or four times daily in 10 patients produced a decrease in papules and pustules in 2 weeks and a reduction of comedones after 2 months.

51. Fulton JE Jr, Bradley S: The choice of vitamin A acid, erythromycin, or benzoyl peroxide for the topical treatment of acne. Cutis *17*:560–564, 1976.

    Retinoic acid, benzoyl peroxide, and topical erythromycin (their advantages and disadvantages) in the treatment of acne.

52. Milstone EB, McDonald AJ, Scholhamer CF Jr: Pseudomembranous colitis after topical application of clindamycin. Arch. Dermatol. *117*:154–155, 1981.

    A report of a patient with a facial port-wine stain who developed pseudomembranous colitis 5 days after starting topical 1 per cent clindamycin hydrochloride for the treatment of acne.

53. Barza M, Goldstein JA, Kane A, et al.: Systemic absorption of clindamycin hydrochloride after topical application. J. Am. Acad. Dermatol. *7*:208–214, 1982.

    A study of serum levels and urinary excretion of clindamycin suggests that an average of 4 to 5 per cent of topically applied clindamycin hydrochloride enters the circulation.

54. Siegle RJ, Fekety R, Sarbone PD, et al.: Effects of topical clindamycin on intestinal microflora in patients with acne. J. Am. Acad. Dermatol. *15*:180–185, 1986.

    A study of 32 patients suggested that the commercially available clindamycin phosphate formulations are safer and less likely to be absorbed systemically than extemporaneously prepared formulations containing the hydrochloride form of topical clindamycin.

55. Parry MF, Rha CK: Pseudomembranous colitis caused by topical clindamycin phosphate. Arch. Dermatol. *122*:583–584, 1986.

    The first proven case of pseudomembranous colitis associated with the topical administration of clindamycin phosphate.

56. Peck GL, Olsen TG, Yoder FW, et al.: Prolonged remissions of cystic and conglobate acne with 13-*cis*-retinoic acid. N. Engl. J. Med. *300*:329–333, 1979.

    Complete resolution of severe, chronic, treatment-resistant cystic and conglobate acne in 13 of 14 patients treated with oral 13-*cis*-retinoic acid and the apparent persistence of this beneficial effect for periods lasting for as long as 20 months after discontinuation of therapy.

57. Shalita AR, Cunningham WJ, Pochi PE, et al.: Isotretinoin treatment for acne and related disorders: An update. J. Am. Acad. Dermatol. *9*:629–638, 1983.

    A comprehensive review of isotretinoin, its use, efficacy, and complications.

58. Strauss JS, Rapini RP, Shalita AR, et al.: Isotretinoin therapy for acne: Results of a multicenter dose-response study. J. Am. Acad. Dermatol. *10*:490–496, 1984.

    A comparison study of three dosage schedules of isotretinoin and their efficacy in the management of patients with severe recalcitrant forms of pustulocystic acne.

59. Bigby M, Stern RS: Adverse reactions to isotretinoin: A report from the adverse drug reporting system. J. Am. Acad. Dermatol. *18*:543–552, 1988.

    A comprehensive review of adverse reactions reported in 93 patients who received Accutane.

60. Milstone LM, McGuire J, Ablow RC: Premature epiphyseal closure in a child receiving oral 13-*cis*-retinoic acid. J. Am. Acad. Dermatol. *7*:663–666, 1982.

    A report of a 4½-year-old patient who developed radiographic evidence of partial closure of the proximal epiphysis of the tibia following 6-month periods of isotretinoin therapy with an average dosage of 3.5 mg/kg/day over a period of 2½ years.

61. Marini JC, Hill S, Zasloff MA: Dense metaphyseal bands and growth arrest assoicated with isotretinoin therapy. Am. J. Dis. Child. *142*:316–318, 1988.

    A report of dense metaphyseal bands and arrest of bone growth in a 9-year-old boy treated with high-dose isotretinoin (5 mg/kg/day) for fibrodysplasia ossificans progressiva.

62. Pittsley RA, Yoder FW: Retinoid hyperostosis: Skeletal toxicity associated with long-term administration of 13-*cis*-retinoic acid for refractory ichthyosis. N. Engl. J. Med. *308*:1012–1014, 1983.

    Four of nine patients receiving long-term isotretinoin for ichthyosis developed an ossification disorder resembling diffuse idiopathic skeletal hyperostosis (the DISH syndrome).

63. Ellis CN, Madison KC, Pennes DR, et al.: Isotretinoin therapy is associated with early skeletal radiographic changes. J. Am. Acad. Dermatol. *10*:1024–1029, 1984.

    Six of eight patients treated with isotretinoin with an average dosage of 2 mg/kg/day for 9 months showed small but unequivocal radiographic evidence of skeletal hyperostoses.

64. Kilcoyne RF, Cope R, Cunningham W, et al.: Minimal spinal hyperostosis with low-dose isotretinoin therapy. Invest. Radiol. *21*:41–44, 1986.

    Radiographic studies reveal small asymptomatic spurs on the anterior margins of the cervical, thoracic, or lumbar vertebral bodies in 10 of 96 patients treated for acne vulgaris with isotretinoin in a dosage range of 1.0 to 2.0 mg/day.

65. DiGiovanna JJ, Helfgott R, Gerber LH, et al.: Extraspinal

tendon and ligament calcification after long-term isotretinoin therapy. J. Invest. Dermatol. 88:485, 1987.

In a study of 12 patients treated with isotretinoin over an 8-year period, 11 developed extraspinal tendon calcifications in the pelvis, knee, or shoulder; 10 had spurring of the spine; and 5 had bridging of two or more vertebral bodies.

66. Elpern DJ: Atypical pyoderma as a side effect of isotretinoin. J. Am. Acad. Dermatol. 13:1045–1046, 1985.

A report of a 16-year-old boy who developed a mixed infection of group A β-hemolytic streptococcal and coagulase-positive staphylococcal infection of the nose while on isotretinoin therapy for acne vulgaris.

67. Leyden JJ, James WD: *Staphylococcus aureus* infection as a complication of isotretinoin therapy. Arch. Dermatol. 123:606–608, 1987.

In a study of 18 patients who developed S. *aureus* infection during or shortly after therapy with isotretinoin, twice-daily application of a topical antibiotic to the anterior nares significantly reduced S. *aureus* colonization and the risk of cutaneous infection.

68. Benke JP: The isotretinoin teratogen syndrome. J.A.M.A. 251:3267–3269, 1984.

A report of two infants with prominent frontal bossing, hydrocephalus, microphthalmia, and small malformed low-set ears born to women who took isotretinoin during the first trimester of their pregnancies.

69. De La Cruz E, Sun S, Vangvanichyakorn K, et al.: Multiple congenital malformations associated with maternal isotretinoin therapy. Pediatrics 74:428–430, 1984.

Microcephaly, rudimentary pinnae, hydrocephalus, and major heart defects in an infant born to a mother who took isotretinoin for 8 days between the fourth and sixth weeks of gestation.

70. Lammer EJ, Chen DT, Hoar RM, et al.: Retinoic acid embryopathy. N. Engl. J. Med. 313:837–841, 1985.

In a review of 154 pregnancies with fetal exposure to isotretinoin, 21 mothers were delivered of malformed infants, 95 women had elective abortions, and in a subset of 154 pregnancies observed prospectively, there were 23 normal infants, 5 malformed infants, and 8 spontaneous abortions.

71. Vorhees CV: Retinoic acid embryopathy. N. Engl. J. Med. 315:262–263, 1986.

Oral retinoids can act as central nervous system teratogens, thus resulting in mental deficiency, hearing disability, and behavioral dysfunction in offspring of mothers who are on oral retinoids during pregnancy.

72. Dai WS, Hsu M-A, Itri LM: Safety of pregnancy after discontinuation of isotretinoin. Arch. Dermatol. 125:362–365, 1989.

A review of 88 pregnancies revealed no evidence of statistically significant risk of congenital malformation in women who had completed or discontinued isotretinoin 1 month or more prior to conception.

73. Rothman KF, Pochi PE: The use of oral and topical agents for acne in pregnancy. J. Am. Acad. Dermatol. 19:431–442, 1988.

An authoritative discussion of topical and oral agents and their use for the treatment of acne vulgaris in pregnant women.

74. Kligman AM: Retin-A teratogenicity. J.A.M.A. 259:2916, 1988.

Since topically applied tretinoin is rapidly metabolized from the skin and there are no reports of fetal abnormality after nearly 20 years of use by millions of patients, it is concluded that topical application of this agent probably does not present a risk of fetal teratogenicity.

75. Strauss JS, Pochi PE: Effect of cyclic progestin-estrogen therapy on sebum and acne in women. J.A.M.A. 190:815–819, 1964.

Drugs containing estrogen in the management of recalcitrant pustulocystic acne in women.

76. Michaelsson G, Juhlin L, Vahlquist A: Effect of oral zinc and vitamin A in acne. Arch. Dermatol. 113:31–36, 1977.

In a study of 64 patients with acne, the number of acne lesions was significantly decreased in the zinc-treated group. Although data appear to support the efficacy of zinc therapy in acne, further double-blind studies are required to substantiate this finding.

77. Weimar VM, Puhl SC, Smith WH, et al.: Zinc sulfate in acne vulgaris. Arch. Dermatol. 114:1776–1778, 1978

In a study of 40 patients, oral zinc appeared to have a somewhat beneficial effect on pustules but not on comedones, papules, infiltrates, or cysts.

78. Orris L, Shalita AR, Sibulkin D, et al.: Oral zinc therapy of acne. Arch. Dermatol. 114:1018–1020, 1978.

In a double-blind controlled study of 22 male subjects that lasted 8 weeks there was no statistically significant difference in lesion counts in the zinc-treated and lactose placebo–treated patients.

79. Glover SC, White MI: Zinc again. Br. Med. J. 2:640–641, 1977.

A warning of potential side effects due to oral zinc sulfate and nonphysiologic zinc level concentrations in human plasma.

80. Moore R: Bleeding gastric erosion after oral zinc sulphate. Br. Med. J. 1:754, 1978.

Epigastric discomfort and gastrointestinal bleeding in a 15-year-old English girl developed within 1 week after the initiation of 220 mg of oral zinc sulfate twice a day for the treatment of acne.

81. Schachner L, Eaglstein W, Kittles C, et al.: Topical erythromycin and zinc therapy for acne. J. Am. Acad. Dermatol. 22:253–260, 1990.

A double-blind study of a topical formulation containing 1.2 per cent zinc acetate and 4 per cent erythromycin documents the safety and efficacy of this combination in the management of patients with acne vulgaris.

82. Sperling LC, Weber CB, Rodman OG: Toward less painful anesthesia: Water, saline, lidocaine. J. Dermatol. Surg. Oncol. 7:730–731, 1981.

Physiologic saline and lidocaine are less painful than distilled water when injected intradermally.

83. Mills OH, Porte M, Kligman AM: Enhancement of comedogenic substances by ultraviolet radiation. Br. J. Dermatol. 98:145–150, 1978.

Solar-simulating irradiation enhancement of the degree of follicular hyperkeratosis suggests that the adverse effects of sunbathing and ultraviolet light outweigh their benefit in the treatment of acne.

84. Klein AW: Implantation techniques for injectable collagen: Two and one-half years of personal clinical experience. J. Am. Acad. Dermatol. 9:224–228, 1983.

The art of injectable collagen implantation.

85. Cohen IS: Fibrel. Semin. Dermatol. 6:228–237, 1987.

When compared with collagen implantation, although Fibrel has the advantage of a lower incidence of adverse reaction, its long preparation time and need for venipuncture in preparation for its utilization offer significant disadvantages to its use in the treatment of facial scarring.

86. Giknis FL, Hall WK, Tolman MM: Acne neonatorum. Arch. Dermatol. 66:717–721, 1952.

A case of acne neonatorum with onset at 7 weeks, with a review of 17 patients with this disorder.

87. Pochi PE, Strauss JS: Endocrinologic control of the development and activity of the human sebaceous gland. J. Invest. Dermatol. *62*:191–201, 1974.

The fetal endocrine system and sebaceous gland development in acne neonatorum.

88. Plewig G, Kligman AM: Induction of acne by topical steroids. Arch. Dermatol. Forsch. *247*:29–52, 1973.

Potent topical corticosteroids can produce "steroid acne."

89. Lucky AW, McGuire J, Rosenfield RL, et al.: Plasma androgens in women with acne vulgaris. J. Invest. Dermatol. *81*:70–74, 1983.

A study of 46 young adult women with acne revealed that many women with acne, hirsutism, or both may have hyperandrogenism and yet not necessarily have abnormal menses associated with their endocrine abnormality.

90. Reingold SB, Rosenfield RL: The relationship of mild hirsutism or acne in women to androgens. Arch. Dermatol. *123*:209–212, 1987.

A study of 62 women comparing their clinical features with their plasma-free testosterone levels suggests that hyperandrogenemia may be found in about 50 per cent of women with mild hirsutism and one third of those with mild acne.

91. Hammerstein J, Moltz L, Schwartz U: Antiandrogens in the treatment of acne and hirsutism. J. Steroid Biochem. *19*:591–597, 1983.

A review of spironolactone and cyproterone acetate, antiandrogens that inhibit androgen production and receptor site binding, in the treatment of 71 patients with acne.

92. Muhlemann MF, Carter GD, Cream JJ, et al.: Oral spironolactone: An effective treatment for acne vulgaris in women. Br. J. Dermatol. *115*:227–232, 1986.

Spironolactone in a dosage of 200 mg/day over a 3-month period significantly improved acne vulgaris in 21 women.

93. Drolet B, Paller AS: Childhood rosacea. Pediatr. Dermatol. *9*:22–26, 1992.

A report of three children with rosacea who responded dramatically to systemic and topical antibiotics.

94. Berbis P, Privat Y: Lupus miliaris disseminatus faciei: Efficacy of isotretinoin. J. Am. Acad. Dermatol *16*:1271–1272, 1987.

A report of a 27-year-old man with lupus miliaris disseminatus faciei successfully treated with isotretinoin.

95. Plewig G, Fulton JE, Kligman AM: Pomade acne. Arch. Dermatol. *101*:580–584, 1970.

The physician should be alert to this disorder, which is seen particularly on the forehead in blacks using greasy hair grooming formulations.

96. Kligman AM, Mills OH: "Acne cosmetica." Arch. Dermatol. *106*:843–850, 1972.

Low-grade acneiform eruptions can be attributed to cosmetics.

97. Friedman SJ, Fox BJ, Albert HL: Solid facial edema as a complication of acne vulgaris: Treatment with isotretinoin. J. Am. Acad. Dermatol. *15*:286–289, 1986.

A 20-week course of isotretinoin was found to be beneficial in the treatment of a patient with solid facial edema and severe pustulocystic acne vulgaris.

98. Frumess GM, Lewis HM: Light-sensitive seborrheid. Arch. Dermatol. *75*:245–248, 1957.

This unique perioral eruption was initially believed to be a light-sensitive disorder.

99. Marks R, Black MM: Perioral dermatitis: A histologic study of 26 cases. Br. J. Dermatol. *84*:242–247, 1971.

Histologic findings suggest external irritants as provocative or perpetuating stimuli to perioral dermatitis.

100. Frieden IJ, Prose NS, Fletcher V, et al.: Granulomatous perioral dermatitis in children. Arch. Dermatol. *125*:369–373, 1989.

A report of five children with a distinctive perioral, perinasal, and periorbital rash with granulomatous features suggests that granulomatous perioral dermatitis may represent a variant of perioral dermatitis in children.

101. Stolman LP: The treatment of excess sweating of the palms by iontophoresis. Arch. Dermatol. *123*:893–896, 1987.

A report of 18 patients with palmar hyperhidrosis treated successfully by tap water iontophoresis.

102. Akins DL, Meisenheimer JL, Dobson RL: Efficacy of the Drionic unit in the treatment of hyperhidrosis. J. Am. Acad. Dermatol. *16*:828–832, 1987.

Twenty-two patients treated with a portable iontophoretic device for persistent axillary palmar and/or plantar hyperhidrosis.

103. Shelley WB, Hurley HJ, Nichols AC: Axillary odor: Role of bacteria, apocrine sweat, and deodorants. Arch. Derm. Syph. *68*:430–446, 1953.

Axillary microorganisms are responsible for axillary odor.

104. Shehadeh NH, Kligman AM: Bacteria responsible for axillary odor. J. Invest. Dermatol. *41*:3, 1963.

Gram-positive organisms, coagulase-negative staphylococci, and diphtheroids generate axillary odor.

105. Hölzle E, Kligman AM: The pathogenesis of miliaria rubra: Role of the resident microflora. Br. J. Dermatol. *117*:99–137, 1978.

Studies demonstrate that the degree of sweat suppression and miliaria after a thermal stimulus was directly proportionate to the increase in density of resident aerobic bacteria, notably cocci.

106. Aram H, Mohagheghi AP: Granulosis rubra nasi. Cutis *10*:463–464, 1972.

A case of granulosis rubra nasi of 4 years' duration in a 12-year-old girl.

7

HEREDITARY SKIN DISORDERS: THE GENODERMATOSES

The genodermatoses represent a group of cutaneous disorders dependent on genetic as opposed to environmental causes. In this chapter, the significant hereditary dermatoses including ichthyoses, ectodermal dysplasias, and disorders of collagen and elastic tissue are discussed, with emphasis on aids to clinical recognition, recent concepts of pathophysiology, and advances in therapeutics.

ICHTHYOSIS

Ichthyosis refers to hereditary cutaneous conditions characterized by dryness and scaling. Initially, the classification of the ichthyoses relied on primarily descriptive and confusing clinical and histologic criteria, which offered little understanding of etiology or pathogenesis. The introduction of reliable measurements of cellular kinetics, a better understanding of abnormalities of lipid metabolism, and clinical, histologic, and genetic criteria currently allow these disorders to be divided into four major classes[1]:

1. Ichthyosis vulgaris, the most common variant, transmitted as an autosomal dominant trait
2. Sex-linked ichthyosis (recessive X-linked ichthyosis), expressed only in males and transmitted as an X-linked recessive trait
3. Epidermolytic hyperkeratosis (bullous con-

genital ichthyosiform erythroderma), inherited as an autosomal dominant disorder

4. Lamellar ichthyosis, inherited as an autosomal recessive trait, with two variants (classic lamellar ichthyosis and nonbullous congenital ichthyosiform erythroderma)

In the past, lamellar ichthyosis and epidermolytic hyperkeratosis have been designated as the nonbullous and bullous congenital ichthyosiform erythrodermas, respectively. Williams and Elias, however, have subdivided lamellar ichthyosis into two entities: classic lamellar ichthyosis and the milder erythrodermic form of nonbullous congenital ichthyosiform erythroderma.[2, 3] These designations have found wide acceptability and are used in this discussion.

Pathogenesis of the ichthyoses appears to involve (1) an increased rate of arrival of cells at the skin surface (this has been determined by epidermal mitotic activity and cellular transit time); (2) a decrease in the rate of cell removal (increased adhesiveness of the stratum corneum); (3) an abnormal transepidermal water loss[4]; and (4) abnormalities of protein and lipid composition and metabolism affecting the corneocytes and intercellular matrix.[2, 3]

Appropriate studies, however, have not been performed for many of the ichthyoses. It is therefore not possible to classify all ichthyoses in this manner. Division of the stratum corneum into a two-compartment system analogous to a brick wall in which the corneocytes (or "bricks") are surrounded by a matrix (the "mortar") can help one visualize the mechanisms of normal and abnormal desquamation. In this context, the keratin-filled corneocytes are responsible for the resilience and water-holding capacity of the skin and the lipid-enriched intercellular matrix is responsible for the relative impermeability to water.[5]

All four major types of ichthyosis demonstrate abnormalities of the third mechanism—an increased transepidermal water loss with resultant loss of suppleness and moisture content of the integument. Excessive scaling seen in ichthyosis vulgaris and X-linked ichthyosis is probably related to the second mechanism (increased adhesiveness of the cells of the stratum corneum with normal cellular transit rates). The cause of the retention hyperkeratosis in X-linked ichthyosis is associated with a deficiency or an absence of steroid sulfatase activity. In lamellar ichthyosis and epidermolytic hyperkeratosis the thickening of the stratum corneum appears to be related to cellular kinetics (a decreased transit time of the epidermal cells from the basal layer to the stratum corneum); in the nonbullous congenital ichthyosiform erythrodermic form of lamellar ichthyosis it has been suggested that an inborn error of lipid metabolism in the epidermis may account for the increased rate of epidermal turnover.[2, 3]

Ichthyosis Vulgaris

Ichthyosis vulgaris, transmitted as an autosomal dominant trait, is the mildest, most common form of ichthyosis (Table 7–1). Often overlooked and undiagnosed, it is estimated to occur in approximately 1 in 300 persons.

This disorder, which is not present at birth, is first noted in childhood, usually after the first 3 months of life. It is often milder and more localized than other types of ichthyosis. Scales are most prominent on the extensor surfaces of the extremities particularly in cold and dry weather (Figs. 7–1 through 7–3). Scales on the pretibial and lateral aspects of the lower leg are large and plate-like, resembling fish scales; the flexural areas are characteristically spared. In other areas small, white, bran-like scales may be seen. Scaling of the forehead and cheeks, common during childhood, generally diminishes and clears with age.

Keratosis pilaris, which is frequently associated with ichthyosis vulgaris and atopy (see Chapter 3, Fig. 3–5), is most predominant over the upper arms, buttocks, and thighs. The palms and soles may show a moderate degree of chapping with accentuation of palmar markings (see Fig. 3–6), and a discrete hyperkeratosis may occur on the elbows, knees, and ankles. Patients with ichthyosis often reveal an atopic background with a tendency toward eczema, asthma, or hay fever.

Skin biopsy is helpful for differentiating this disorder from other forms of ichthyosis. A moderate thickening of the stratum corneum is characteristically present; the granular layer is usually reduced or absent in contrast to the normal stratum granulosum of other ichthyoses.

Ichthyosis vulgaris generally improves with age, in summer, and in warm moist environments and can usually be managed with frequent application of emollients and appropriate topical keratolytic agents.

Sex-linked Ichthyosis (Recessive X-linked Ichthyosis)

Sex-linked ichthyosis, transmitted as an X-linked recessive trait, is seen primarily in males. Although an affected homozygous female has been described, female carriers generally do not develop the full clinical picture but may manifest partial abnormalities. This phenomenon appears

---

Table 7–1. ICHTHYOSIS VULGARIS

1. Incidence approximately 1 : 300 (250–1,000)
2. Develops after 3 months
3. Large lamellar scales
   a. Face, back, extensors
   b. Spares flexures
4. Favorable course (improves with age)
5. *Histopathology:* Hyperkeratosis of stratum corneum with decrease in granular layer

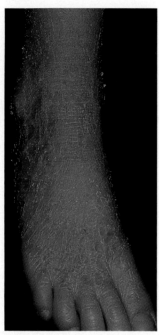

Figure 7–1. Large plate-like scales on the ankle and dorsal aspect of a foot in a patient with ichthyosis vulgaris.

to be explained by the Lyon principle (formerly the Lyon hypothesis). In this hypothesis one X chromosome in each cell of a normal XX female carrier of an X-linked recessive trait shows a reduced level of the gene product, which is not fully expressed. Accordingly the phenotypes of such heterozygous females may present only mild manifestations of the X-linked disorder.

The prevalence of this dermatosis is unknown; Wells and Kerr's study in England, however, esti-

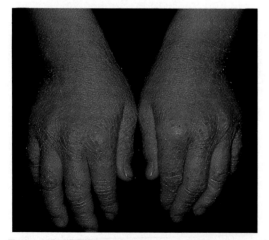

Figure 7–2. Ichthyosis vulgaris on the extensor aspect of hands and fingers.

mated the incidence at approximately 1 in 6,000 males.[6] Although the exact biochemical basis of recessive X-linked ichthyosis is not fully understood, it has been shown that affected individuals have a deficiency of arylsulfatase C and steroid sulfatase.[7] Unlike lamellar ichthyosis and epidermolytic hyperkeratosis, epidermal cell kinetics in X-linked ichthyosis are normal. It has been postulated that cholesterol sulfate, which is located in the intercellular membrane region, plays a role in stratum corneum adhesion.

Recessive X-linked ichthyosis begins early in infancy, usually within the first 3 months of life and occasionally as late as 1 year. Some infants have a collodion-like membrane at birth (Fig. 7–4). This form of ichthyosis generally involves the entire body with accentuation on the posterior neck, abdomen, back, front of the legs, and feet, with sparing of the palms and soles, central face, and flexural areas.

Scales are small to large and light or yellowish brown (Fig. 7–5) to black, with invariable involvement of the sides of the neck giving the patient an unwashed appearance (this gave rise to the name ichthyosis nigricans). Patients may shed or molt their scales episodically, particularly in the spring and fall (Table 7–2). Individuals with X-linked ichthyosis also appear to have an increased predisposition to hypogenitalism and cryptorchidism and, independent of the latter, an increased risk for testicular cancer.[8]

Since placental sulfatase syndrome and recessive X-linked ichthyosis represent prenatal and postnatal consequences of a deficiency of the same enzyme (steroid sulfatase), women with the gene for X-linked ichthyosis have a deficiency of placental steroid sulfatase (this is reflected by low maternal urinary estriol and elevated sulfated steroid levels) and tend to have a difficult or prolonged labor, often requiring intervention by cesarean section.

Deep corneal opacities may be found in almost all affected males and, with less consistency, in female carriers of this disorder. The opacities are discrete and diffusely located near Descemet's membrane or deep in the corneal stroma. On slit lamp examination the opacities appear as gray-white filaments, commas, dots, or coronas in the deep stroma and do not affect vision. Slit lamp examination of the eyes, therefore, is useful for identification of individuals with this dermatosis.

Skin biopsy is of value for differentiation of sex-linked ichthyosis from the dominant form of ichthyosis vulgaris. In the sex-linked disorder, there is a moderately increased stratum corneum, granular layer, and stratum malpighium. In the autosomal dominant form the granular layer is reduced or absent. X-linked ichthyosis can also be diagnosed by measuring the mobility of β-lipoproteins, which is increased owing to the high amounts of cholesterol sulfate, and by the finding of increased amounts of cholesterol sulfate in the serum, stratum corneum, or nails.[9–11]

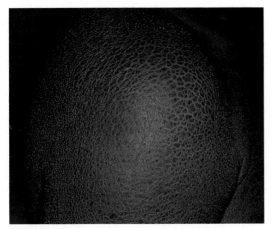

Figure 7–3. Ichthyosis vulgaris. Typical large adherent scales on the shoulder.

Lamellar Ichthyosis

Lamellar ichthyosis is a severe autosomal recessive form of ichthyosis characterized by congenital onset. Infants are frequently born with a parchment-like collodion membrane that desquamates over the next 10 to 14 days (hence the term *collodion baby* (see Fig. 7–4). Although most authorities previously grouped patients with lamellar ichthyosis under a single designation, the disorder has recently been divided into two recessive disorders: a more severe form of the disease (classic lamellar ichthyosis) and a milder erythrodermic variant (congenital or nonbullous congenital ichthyosiform erythroderma) (Table 7–3).[2, 12] In ad-

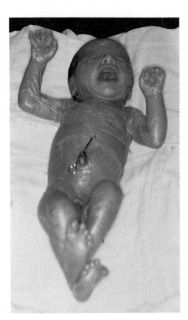

Figure 7–4. "Collodion baby." Note parchment-like membrane with beginning cracking and desquamation. (Courtesy of Department of Dermatology, Yale University School of Medicine.)

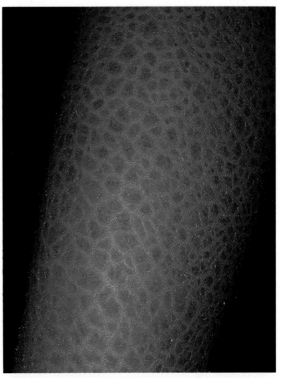

Figure 7–5. Sex-linked (recessive X-linked) ichthyosis. Small to large, firmly adherent, light brown scales are separated by narrow zones of apparently normal skin, with truncal involvement and, to some degree, relative sparing of the antecubital flexures (probably as a result of friction or increased hydration in these areas).

dition, reports of vertical transmission through three generations suggest the possibility of an additional autosomal dominant variant.[13]

CLASSIC LAMELLAR ICHTHYOSIS

Classic lamellar ichthyosis, which is estimated to occur in 1 in 200,000 individuals, is a severe skin disorder characterized by large lamellar plate-like scales, ectropion (eversion of an edge or margin of the eyelid resulting in exposure of the palpebral conjunctiva), eclabium (eversion of the lips), a relatively mild, barely perceptible erythroderma beneath the large scales, and hyperkeratosis of the palms and soles (Table 7–4). In this disorder a

Table 7–2. X-LINKED ICHTHYOSIS

1. Affects males
2. First 3 months (collodion membrane)
3. Ichthyosis nigricans
   a. Large yellow to black scales
   b. All body surfaces (except palms and soles)
   c. Central face, neck, and flexures
4. Corneal opacities (males, and female carriers)
5. Same or worse with age
6. *Histopathology:* hyperkeratosis with increased granular layer

Table 7–3. COMPARISON OF TYPES OF LAMELLAR ICHTHYOSIS

	Classic Lamellar Ichthyosis	Nonbullous Congenital Ichthyosiform Erythroderma
Scales	Thick, plate-like	Fine, white, smaller
Erythroderma	Mild	Prominent
Ectropion	Severe	Mild (variable)
Alopecia	Not a prominent feature	Occasionally
Course	Progressive	Variable
Histology	Thicker stratum corneum	More acanthosis, parakeratosis, hypergranulosis; less prominent capillaries
n-Alkanes	5%	25%

Adapted from Williams ML, Elias PM: Heterogeneity in autosomal recessive ichthyosis: Clinical and biochemical differentiation of lamellar ichthyosis and nonbullous congenital ichthyosiform erythroderma. Arch. Dermatol. *121*:477–488, 1985. Copyright © 1985, American Medical Association.

collodion or parchment-like membrane is usually present at birth; on occasion, however, skin findings are not evident until approximately 3 months of age. The cutaneous covering dries out and is gradually shed in large sheet-like layers, leaving a residual redness and hyperkeratosis. Collodion babies, although frequently associated with lamellar ichthyosis, are not specific for this disorder. They are discussed in greater detail later in this chapter.

Lamellar scales are large, quadrangular, yellow to brown-black, often thick, and centrally adherent with raised edges resembling armor plates (hence the term *lamellar ichthyosis*) (Fig. 7–6). Scales are most prominent over the face, trunk, and extremities, with a predilection for the flexor areas. Cheeks are often red, taut, and shiny; more scales appear on the forehead than on the lower portion of the face. The scalp is often scaly with partial hair loss. Ectropion is common, but the eye itself remains unaffected (Fig. 7–7).[14]

The palms and soles are almost always affected in lamellar ichthyosis; severity varies from increased palmar markings to a thick keratoderma with fissuring. Involvement of the nails is variable. They may be stippled, pitted, ridged, or thickened, often with a collection of subungual keratin.

Classic lamellar ichthyosis is a severe unremitting disorder that persists throughout the affected individual's lifetime. Although a partial remission may occur during the summer, because of obstruction of eccrine glands by the overlying hy-

perkeratosis, severely affected patients tend to experience hyperpyrexia, heat intolerance, difficulty with perspiration, and heat exhaustion during periods of warm or hot humid weather and vigorous physical exercise.

Histology of lamellar ichthyosis is similar to that of the sex-linked form of ichthyosis. The epidermis shows marked hyperkeratosis with occasional patchy parakeratosis, increased thickness of the granular layer, acanthosis, and variable papillomatosis. Studies of epidermal kinetics suggest that an increased mitotic activity and an associated rapid epidermal transit time are responsible for the skin changes seen in this disorder.

Table 7–4. CLASSIC LAMELLAR ICHTHYOSIS

1. Rare (1 : 200,000)
2. At birth or soon after (collodion baby, ectropion in one third)
3. Large lamellar scales
   a. Grayish brown
   b. Adherent in center
   c. Face, trunk, flexures, palms, and soles
4. Hair normal, but scalp infection may lead to alopecia; nails may be dystrophic
5. Decreased sweating (hyperpyrexia and heat exhaustion common with exertion)
6. Same or worse with age
7. *Histopathology:* Marked hyperkeratosis, prominent granular cell layer

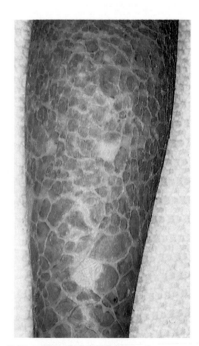

Figure 7–6. Large, thick, centrally adherent quadrangular scales with raised edges (resembling armor plates) on the leg of a patient with lamellar ichthyosis.

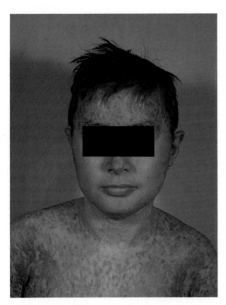

Figure 7–7. Lamellar ichthyosis. Prominent quadrangular scales are evident on the forehead and chest. Note contrasting shiny cheeks. (Courtesy of Sidney Hurwitz.)

NONBULLOUS CONGENITAL ICHTHYOSIFORM ERYTHRODERMA

Nonbullous congenital ichthyosiform erythroderma, estimated to occur in 1 in 100,000 individuals, is milder and more variable with respect to severity than classic lamellar ichthyosis. Patients have a much more prominent erythrodermic component; platelike scales on the extensor surfaces of the legs and fine white scales on the face, scalp, and trunk; mild or variable ectropion; and a milder degree of palmoplantar keratoderma. Cicatricial alopecia and thickening and ridging of the nails are common; although mild growth retardation may occur in severely erythrodermic patients, most patients exhibit normal growth and developmental patterns (Figs. 7–8 and 7–9).

The histology of both forms of lamellar ichthyosis is characterized by parakeratosis, increased thickness of the granular layer, and variable papillomatosis. Patients with classic lamellar ichthyosis display a thicker stratum corneum and less acanthosis than seen in patients with nonbullous congenital ichthyosiform erythroderma. Although research shows increased alkanes in the skin of patients with nonbullous congenital ichthyosiform erythroderma (suggesting the possibility of an inborn error in lipid metabolism), because long-chain alkanes are ubiquitous in our environment further studies are required to ascertain if these findings are endogenous or exogenous and what role they play in barrier function and intercellular cohesion.[3]

Epidermolytic Hyperkeratosis

Epidermolytic hyperkeratosis (bullous congenital ichthyosiform erythroderma) is a distinctive, dominantly inherited form of ichthyosis characterized by verruciform scales particularly prominent in the flexural area. Affecting approximately 1 in 300,000 individuals, cases in 50 per cent of patients appear to represent new mutations. The skin is red, moist, and tender at birth, and bullae generally appear within the first week of life (often within a few hours after delivery) (Fig. 7–10); hyperkeratosis often appears from the third month on (Fig. 7–11). The presence of bullae is highly characteristic of this disorder. The blisters occur in crops and vary from 0.5 cm to several centimeters in diameter. They are superficial, tender, and frequently painful, and when ruptured, they discharge clear fluid and leave raw denuded areas. Secondary infection with β-hemolytic Streptococci or *Staphylococcus aureus* is commonly associated with this disorder (Table 7–5).

Thick grayish brown scales cover most of the skin surface; the flexural creases and intertriginous areas show marked involvement, often with furrowed hyperkeratosis (Fig. 7–12). Palms and soles are frequently affected and may show varying degrees of hyperkeratosis and scaling (Fig. 7–13).[14] This hyperkeratosis is often generalized, with a thick covering of prominent verruciform scales over the flexural areas, hands, feet, wrists, and ankles (Figs. 7–14 and 7–15). Facial involvement may occur, but ectropion does not; although scalp involvement may result in nit-like encasement of

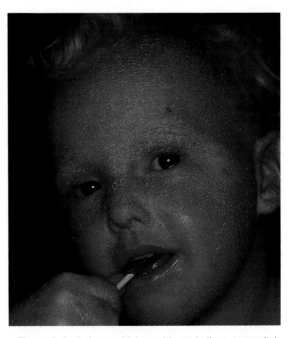

Figure 7–8. A 2-year-old boy with nonbullous congenital ichthyosiform erythroderma (NBCIE) manifesting as scaling of the scalp and fine white scales and erythema of the face.

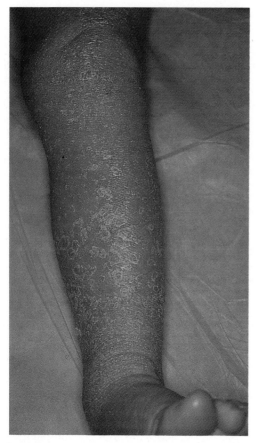

Figure 7–9. Nonbullous congenital ichthyosiform erythroderma. Note plate-like scales on the legs and an underlying erythroderma.

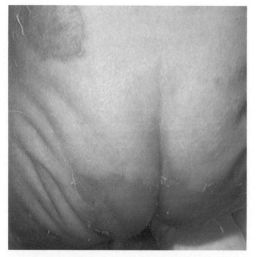

Figure 7–10. Epidermolytic hyperkeratosis (bullous congenital ichthyosiform erythroderma). The presence of bullae (present here in a 2-day-old infant) helps differentiate this disorder from other types of ichthyosis.

hair shafts, the hair, eyes, teeth, and nails are normal. A disagreeable body odor is frequently associated with severe forms of this disorder. Histologically, linear epidermal nevi and their systematized variant, nevus unius lateris, appear to be closely related to localized variants of this disorder. When this involvement is extensive or bilateral, it is frequently termed *ichthyosis hystrix* (Fig. 7–16).

As in lamellar ichthyosis, the epidermal turnover has been described as six times that of normal epidermal tissue.[1] Skin biopsy specimens show distinctive histologic changes. An extreme degree of hyperkeratosis is associated with vacuolization (due to intracellular edema) of epidermal cells in the upper and midportions of the stratum malpighium.[15] Vacuolization or ballooning of the squamous cells is responsible for their dehiscence, which often results in formation of microvesicles and bullae.

Collodion Baby

The *collodion baby* is a descriptive term used to describe infants who are born with a membrane-like covering resembling collodion or oiled parchment (see Fig. 7–4). The collodion baby is not a disease entity but is a phenotype common to several disorders. Most collodion babies (i.e., two thirds or more) are infants with congenital ichthyosiform erythroderma. Less often, in affected infants the disorder may evolve into lamellar ichthyosis, Netherton's syndrome, Conradi's disease, and, at times, trichothiodystrophy, Sjögren-Larsson syndrome, recessive X-linked ichthyosis, and ichthyosis vulgaris; some infants (5 to 6 per cent) with otherwise apparently normal skin may also present in this manner.[16] Although the pathogenesis of the collodion membrane is unknown, the disorder appears to represent a physiologic variant caused by increased cohesiveness of corneal cells normally shed in utero and during the first days of life.

At birth collodion babies are completely covered by a cellophane or oiled parchment-like membrane that, by its tautness, may distort the facial features and extremities. Thus, peripheral edema, flattened ears, and bilateral eversion of the eyelids, lips, and at times the vulva frequently cause affected infants to resemble one another during the first few days of life. The major problems facing these infants are an inability to suck properly, respiratory difficulty due to restriction of chest expansion by the thick membrane, cutaneous and systemic infection, temperature instability, pneumonia, and, since the thickened stratum corneum does not function well as a permeability barrier, increased water loss leading to hypernatremic dehydration.[17]

Supportive care is of primary importance in the management of collodion babies. They are best managed in a humidified incubator, with special attention given to the prevention of temperature instability, sepsis, and fluid and electrolyte imbal-

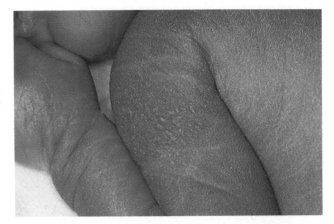

Figure 7–11. Epidermolytic hyperkeratosis. Thick verruciform scales in the patient in Figure 7–10 at 6 months of age.

ance. Cultures should be obtained from fissured areas and appropriate antibiotic therapy initiated if infection is detected. Manual debridement, however, should be avoided (gradual sloughing of the membrane is recommended); also, since greasy emollient creams may contribute to the risk of cutaneous or systemic infection, topical therapy should be restricted to the use of light emollient preparations. Keratolytic agents, however, should be avoided since cutaneous permeability may be increased and, if these agents are absorbed, systemic toxicity may result.[18]

Harlequin Fetus

The term *harlequin fetus* refers to a severe and dramatic form of congenital ichthyosis. Whereas mild and moderately severe forms of ichthyosis are relatively common disorders, this represents a rare condition with less than 100 cases described in the world's literature. Because of the rarity of this condition and the short life span of most affected infants (6 weeks or less), the place of this disorder in the spectrum of icthyoses remains controversial. The presence of familial cases and consanguinity among the parents of some of the patients suggest that the disorder is inherited as an autosomal recessive trait. Although the nature of the abnormality is not clear, x-ray diffraction analysis of the stratum corneum in one case revealed the presence of an unusual fibrous protein, suggesting a defect in epidermal keratin. On the basis of x-ray diffraction

studies, keratins have been found to exist in two forms, α and β. In this disorder cross–β-fibrous protein (rather than the usual α-fibrous protein of normal keratin) appears as a major component of the stratum corneum,[19] and a defect in epidermal lipid metabolism has been postulated as the biochemical abnormality in the skin.[20]

The disorder is manifested by a gross appearance and severe hyperkeratosis characterized by deep reddish brown or purple fissures that divide the thickened gray- or yellow-colored skin into polygonal, triangular, or diamond-shaped plaques that simulate the traditional costume of a harlequin. The skin is dry and hard and has been likened to that of a baked apple, the bark of a tree, morocco leather, and tortoise, elephant, and crocodile skin. Rigidity of the skin about the eyes results in marked ectropion, everted O-shaped lips with a gaping fishmouth deformity, and a distorted, flat-

Table 7–5. EPIDERMOLYTIC HYPERKERATOSIS

1. Generally at birth, with bullae in first week
2. Secondary infection common
3. Hyperkeratosis after third month
   a. Flexures (furrowed hyperkeratosis)
   b. Elbows, knees, wrists, ankles
   c. Palms and soles
4. Same or worse with age
5. *Histopathology:* Marked hyperkeratosis, thickened granular layer, vacuolization of epidermal cells

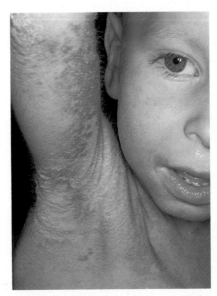

Figure 7–12. Epidermolytic hyperkeratosis. Thick grayish brown scales in flexural creases.

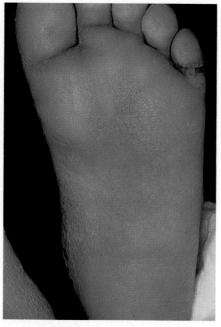

Figure 7–13. Plantar hyperkeratosis in a patient with epidermolytic hyperkeratosis.

Therapy for this most severe form of ichthyosis is generally ineffective, and most infants are stillborn or die during the neonatal period (usually during the first few hours or days of life) of prematurity, pulmonary infection (associated with hypoventilation due to thoracic rigidity), poor feeding, excessive fluid loss, poor temperature regulation, or sepsis as a result of cutaneous infection. Prenatal diagnosis by fetoscopic biopsy is possible,[21] and prolonged survival has been achieved in a few cases by intensive supportive measures, emollients, and oral administration of etretinate.[22–24] Although etretinate and intensive cutaneous care can at times allow survival, the quality of life of affected survivors often tends to suffer because of a lack of effective control of the severe life-long ichthyosis.

Erythrokeratodermia Variabilis

Erythrokeratodermia variabilis is an uncommon, dominantly inherited ichthyosis characterized by two distinct types of lesions: (1) symmetrically distributed, sharply marginated areas of erythema that undergo changes in size, shape, and distribution during a period of days and (2) plaques with thick, yellow-brown scales that occur in most of the erythematous areas. Lesions may be found on the face, trunk, or extremities and have a chronic course with variable remissions and exacerbations. Although lesions are usually noted at birth or shortly thereafter during the first year of life, in a few individuals the onset has been noted during late childhood or early adulthood.[25] In rare cases, in a disorder (possibly a variant of erythrokeratodermia variabilis) termed *progressive symmetrical erythrokeratodermia*, only persistent erythematous hyperkeratotic plaques are noted. Not present at birth, this disorder is limited to the extremities, buttocks, and face; begins in infancy; tends to stabilize after 1 or 2 years; and may partially regress at puberty.[26] Although autosomal dominant transmission has been documented in most patients with erythrokeratodermia variabilis, sporadic cases as-

tened, and undeveloped appearance to the nose and ears, all of which add to the grotesque clown-like appearance of the infant.

The nails of the harlequin fetus may be hypoplastic or absent. Rigidity of the skin restricts respiratory movements, sucking, and swallowing. Extreme inelasticity of the skin is associated with flexion deformity of all joints of the limbs. The hands and feet are ischemic, hard, and waxy, often with poorly developed digits and an associated rigid and claw-like appearance.

Histopathologic examination of the skin of affected infants is characterized by perforation of the epidermis by distorted and fragmented hair shafts, extreme hyperkeratosis, a grossly deficient or absent granular layer, and plugging of eccrine sweat ducts and sebaceous follicles by hyperkeratotic debris.

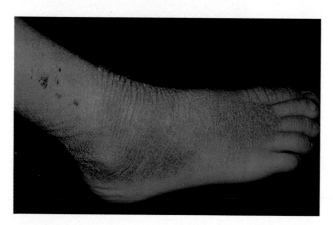

Figure 7–14. Epidermolytic hyperkeratosis. Verruciform scales are seen on the dorsal aspect of the foot.

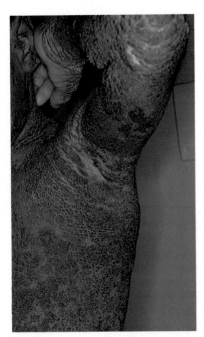

Figure 7–15. Thick grayish brown verruciform scales (epidermolytic hyperkeratosis).

Netherton's Syndrome

Netherton's syndrome is a rare condition described as a combination of ichthyosis, atopy, and hair shaft deformities (usually trichorrhexis invaginata, occasionally trichorrhexis nodosa or pili torti). Although the number of reported cases is too small for a thorough genetic analysis, the syndrome is thought to be determined by an autosomal recessive gene of variable expressivity. The ichthyotic changes have usually been described as ichthyosis linearis circumflexa; however, it has been noted that individuals may also manifest lamellar ichthyosis or ichthyosis vulgaris in combination with their hair shaft abnormality.[30]

Refsum's Disease

Refsum's disease is a rare autosomal recessive disorder with ichthyosis, retinitis pigmentosa, and chronic polyneuritis with deafness, progressive flaccid paralysis, and ataxia. Other ocular findings include night blindness, concentric constriction of

sociated with consanguinity also suggest a recessive form of this disorder.

The histopathologic features of erythrokeratodermia variabilis are not specific. In the hyperkeratotic plaques they consist of acanthosis, hyperkeratosis, focal parakeratosis, a normal or prominent granular layer, and papillomatosis with suprapapillary thinning.[27] The disorder may partially regress at puberty and tends to improve in summer with exacerbations from exposure to heat, cold, and wind, from emotional factors, and during high estrogen states (such as pregnancy or the taking of oral contraceptives) in women.[28] Aromatic retinoids have been shown to be beneficial in some patients but, since relapses occur when treatment is discontinued, are generally not recommended.[29]

Ichthyosis Linearis Circumflexa

Ichthyosis linearis circumflexa is an autosomal recessive disorder characterized by migratory, polycyclic scaly lesions with a peripheral double-edged scale (Fig. 7–17). Partial remissions have been noted, but there is little tendency to spontaneous resolution. In a survey of 15 patients with ichthyosis and structural defects of the hair shaft it appears that ichthyosis linearis circumflexa is frequently seen in association with Netherton's syndrome, but all patients with ichthyosis linearis circumflexa do not have hair shaft abnormalities.[30]

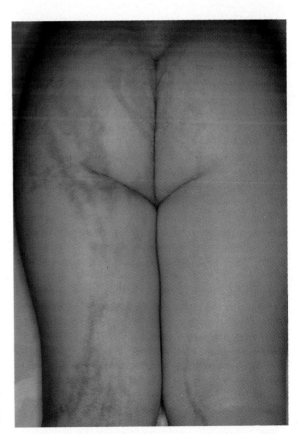

Figure 7–16. Linear epidermal lesions in a segmental pattern (ichthyosis hystrix) in a 3-year-old boy. Histopathologic features of this disorder are similar to those of patients with epidermolytic hyperkeratosis.

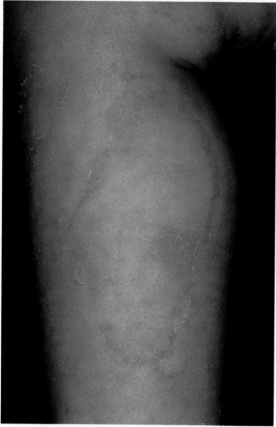

Figure 7–17. Peripheral double-edged polycyclic scaly eruption of ichthyosis linearis circumflexa on the leg of a 17-month-old boy.

the visual fields, nystagmus, cataracts, and, rarely, photophobia. Mild scaling of the skin is variable, and a generalized branny desquamation of dirty-brown scale appears to be the most characteristic cutaneous change in individuals with this disorder.

A block in the degradation pathway of phytanic acid appears to be the significant metabolic defect.[31] The diagnosis is based on the demonstration of increased levels of phytanic acid in the patient's serum, tissue, or urine. Therapy consists of a chlorophyll-free diet and avoidance of phytanic acid–containing foods.

Rud's Syndrome

Rud's syndrome is a rare recessive disorder characterized by ichthyosis, mental deficiency, epilepsy, dwarfism, and sexual infantilism. The cutaneous findings vary from a mild, generalized, branny desquamation to a severe ichthyosis resembling "snakeskin" with predilection for the extensor surfaces of the extremities.

Frequent and recurring seizures prove to be a difficult management problem, and patients usu-

ally require institutional care because of severe mental retardation. Other associated anomalies include arachnodactyly, structural defects of the hands and feet, hypoplastic or absent teeth, alopecia, nerve defects, and various ophthalmologic defects (strabismus, retinitis pigmentosa, cataracts, ptosis, blepharospasm, and nystagmus).

Sjögren-Larsson Syndrome

Sjögren-Larsson syndrome is a rare autosomal recessive disorder that combines generalized ichthyosis, spastic paralysis, mental retardation, and, at times, retinitis pigmentosa and epilepsy. Ichthyosis is present at birth and is characterized by a generalized fine scaling with accentuation in the flexures, a varying degree of erythroderma, and hyperkeratosis of the palms and soles.[32, 33] Other prominent features include dysarthria, enamel hypoplasia, skeletal anomalies, and retinopathy (glistening dots on the macula). As in Rud's syndrome, the cutaneous findings are relatively insignificant in comparison to the neurologic defects. The histologic features are consistent with those observed in patients with lamellar ichthyosis (hyperkeratosis, acanthosis, and papillomatosis of the epidermis, and a normal to slightly increased granular layer).

Although the pathogenesis of this disorder is unknown, defective metabolism of long-chain fatty acids has been suggested. Prenatal diagnosis has been made by fetoscopic biopsy[34]; detection of fatty alcohol (hexanol) dehydrogenase in keratinocytes, cultured fibroblasts, leukocytes, and jejunal mucosa may be used as a marker in prenatal and postnatal diagnosis and in identification of carriers.[35, 36]

Conradi's Disease

Conradi's disease is a rare congenital disorder of variable expression also termed *chondrodysplasia punctata* and *chondrodysplasia congenita punctata*. Estimated to occur in 1 in 500,000 new births, about one fourth of affected persons with this multisystemic disorder are characterized by ichthyosis of the skin similar to that of the collodion baby at birth, followed by hyperkeratotic yellow-white adherent scales arranged in whorl and swirl patterns on the trunk and limbs, rough and erythematous intervening skin, and hyperkeratosis of the palms and soles. The erythema and ichthyosiform dermatosis generally disappear by 3 to 6 months of age only to be followed, in some cases, by blotchy pigmentation in the pattern of incontinentia pigmenti, follicular atrophoderma, and patchy cicatricial alopecia. Follicular atrophoderma is a late manifestation and seems to occur at sites previously affected with hyperkeratosis, and the hyperpigmented changes seen in some patients may represent postinflammatory changes rather than true incontinentia pigmenti.[37, 38]

Associated skeletal changes include shortening of the femur and humerus, dwarfism, and flexion contraction of large joints, due not only to shortening of the bone but also to replacement of muscle by fibrous tissue. Bilateral cataracts with or without optic atrophy, microphthalmia, microcornea, glaucoma, dislocated lenses, rubeosis iridis (new formation of vessels and connective tissue on the surface of the iris), synechiae of the iris to the cornea or lens, partly normal and partly coarse lusterless hair, nasal bone dysplasia with saddle-nose deformity, and high-arched palate constitute other features of this disorder.

Three major types of chondrodysplasia punctata (stippling of the epiphyses detectable on radiologic examination) with different prognoses, radiologic changes, and modes of inheritance have been distinguished. These have been described as type 1, the Conradi-Hünermann syndrome; type 2, the X-linked dominant type (Happle); and type 3, rhizomelic dwarfism. Type 1 has been associated with advanced paternal age and appears to follow an autosomal dominant inheritance. Type 2, inherited in an X-linked dominant fashion, is lethal in males and seen only in females (most patients with chondrodysplasia punctata and skin lesions will be in this group). Type 3, the rhizomelic form, is associated with psychomotor retardation and spasticity; although approximately 25 per cent of patients with type 3 are believed to have skin changes, these are not well defined and may not be characteristic.[39]

Treatment of Ichthyosis

The management of all types of dry skin consists of retardation of water loss, rehydration and softening of the stratum corneum, and alleviation of scaliness and associated pruritus. Ichthyosis vulgaris and recessive X-linked ichthyosis can be managed quite well by topical application of emollients and the use of keratolytic agents to facilitate removal of scales from the skin surface. Limited baths with a mild soap and hydration of dry skin by frequent use of lubricating creams or lotions over moisture are helpful. Urea, in concentrations of 10 to 20 per cent (in a cream, lotion, or ointment base), has a softening and moisturizing effect on the stratum corneum and is helpful in the control of dry skin and pruritus. Propylene glycol (40 to 60 per cent in water), applied overnight under plastic occlusion, hydrates the skin and causes desquamation of scales.

Salicylic acid is an effective keratolytic agent and at concentrations between 3 and 6 per cent promotes shedding of scales and softening of the stratum corneum. When it is used to cover large surface areas for prolonged periods, however, care should be taken to ensure that salicylate toxicity does not occur. A keratolytic gel containing salicylic acid and proplyene glycol, available as Keralyt gel (Westwood-Squibb), a proprietary preparation containing 6 per cent salicylic acid in propylene glycol, is frequently helpful following hydration of the involved area. This preparation, when used either alone or under occlusive polyethylene wrapping, has been most successful in patients with ichthyosis vulgaris and X-linked ichthyosis. α-Hydroxy acid preparations such as lactic, glycolic, and pyruvic acids appear to be particularly helpful in the treatment of patients with ichthyosis and dry skin.[40] Lactic acid is available in Epilyt, Lacticare, or Lacticare-HC lotion (Stiefel) and Lac-Hydrin lotion (Westwood-Squibb), and glycolic acid is available as Aqua-Glycolic lotion and Aqua-Glycolic shampoo (Herald).

The treatment of lamellar ichthyosis by frequent lubrication or the addition of urea, salicylic acid, or lactic acid to lubricating creams or lotions, although encouraging, is not as effective as in the treatment of ichthyosis vulgaris and X-linked ichthyosis. The treatment of epidermolytic hyperkeratosis is similar to that of lamellar ichthyosis, with the exception that topical or systemic antibiotics are frequently required to control secondary infection, particularly in young individuals. Oral vitamin A has been used in the treatment of lamellar ichthyosis but appears to be ineffective except in large doses. The hazards of toxicity, therefore, preclude its use in infants and small children with this disorder. Topical vitamin A acid (Retin-A), althouth potentially irritating, is beneficial in the treatment of lamellar ichthyosis (Fig. 7–18).[14]

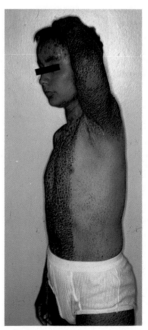

Figure 7–18. Lamellar ichthyosis. The patient's left side was treated with topical tretinoin (vitamin A acid). (Courtesy of Sidney Hurwitz.)

Oral retinoids such as isotretinoin (Accutane) and etretinate (Tegison) have been beneficial for patients with lamellar ichthyosis, X-linked ichthyosis, epidermolytic hyperkeratosis, erythrokeratodermia variabilis, and for the harlequin fetus. Since long-term management, however, is necessary, complications generally preclude their routine use for patients with ichthyosis.

Other Ichthyotic Disorders and Syndromes

In addition to inherited or congenital forms of ichthyosis, there are a number of clinical disorders and syndromes that include ichthyosis as a constant or variable feature and acquired forms of ichthyosis may at times be seen as clinical markers of other underlying disorders. These include pityriasis rotunda, the CHILD and KID syndromes, neutral lipid storage disease (the Dorfman-Chanarin syndrome), peeling skin syndrome, nutritional disorders such as hypovitaminosis or hypervitaminosis A, hypothyroidism, dermatomyositis, chronic debilitating disorders, leprosy, neoplastic disorders such as Hodgkin's disease, non-Hodgkin's lymphoma, cutaneous T-cell lymphoma (mycosis fungoides), multiple myeloma and carcinomatosis, and acquired immunodeficiency syndrome (AIDS).

PITYRIASIS ROTUNDA

A rare variant of acquired ichthyosis, pityriasis rotunda is characterized by asymptomatic, circular or oval, brown scaly patches on the trunk or extremities. Seen primarily in Japanese and in African and West Indian blacks, and at times in Egyptians and Koreans, its occurrence in whites is extremely rare. The disorder may at times signify an internal malignancy (e.g., cancer, leukemia, lymphoma, and myeloma), a chronic illness (e.g., dysentery, tuberculosis, leprosy, sarcoidosis), a nutritional deficiency, diabetes with ketoacidosis, of gynecologic disease or may follow pregnancy. Reports of familial forms of this disorder suggest a genetic predisposition in some affected patients. [41-44] The condition is resistant to treatment and, although partial remissions have occasionally been noted, its course is chronic and it tends to improve only when the underlying disorder is treated.

CHILD SYNDROME

The CHILD syndrome is a congenital disorder characterized by *c*ongenital *h*emidysplasia, *i*chthyosiform erythrodema, and *l*imb *d*efects. Also known as unilateral congenital ichthyosiform erythroderma, the hallmark of the disorder, which encompasses abnormalities of several organ systems (viz., the skin, musculoskeletal system, viscera, and occasionally the central nervous system), is the sharp midline demarcation and its unilateral cutaneous features.[45, 46] Although incomplete penetrance may account for skipped generations reported in the literature, the pattern is consistent with that of an X-linked dominant disorder lethal to males. Unilateral alopecia and severe nail dystrophy with claw-like nails are reported; the face is spared; and limb defects, ranging in severity from hypoplasia of the fingers to complete agenesis of an extremity, are ipsilateral to the ichthyosis. Although some degree of improvement of the cutaneous features with aromatic retinoids such as etretinate has been reported, treatment is generally unsatisfactory.[45, 46]

KID SYNDROME

The KID syndrome (previously known as Senter's syndrome) is a rare autosomal recessive disorder characterized by *k*eratitis, congenital *i*chthyosis, and neurosensory *d*eafness. Patients can generally be identified by their similar peculiar facial appearance, ichthyosis with a predilection for the formation of plaques on the extensor surfaces characterized by diffusely hyperkeratotic skin with fine spiny papules, vascularizing keratitis (although not always present) leading to visual impairment or blindness, acral keratoderma, sensorineural deafness, immunologic disorders, and an increased incidence of cutaneous infections and neoplasms.[48-50]

NEUTRAL LIPID STORAGE DISEASE WITH ICHTHYOSIS

Neutral lipid storage disease with ichthyosis, the Dorfman-Chanarin (or Chanarin-Dorfman) syndrome, is a rare autosomal recessive disorder seen primarily in individuals of Middle Eastern or Mediterranean descent. The disorder is characterized by a nonbullous congenital ichthyosiform erythroderma, vacuolated leukocytes, myopathy, and other systemic involvement such as fatty liver, central nervous system disorders, deafness, ocular abnormalities, a malabsorption syndrome with villous atrophy, and neural tumors of the posterior mediastinum. Believed to be related to a defect in intracellular triglyceride metabolism with deposition of neutral lipids in multiple organs, the diagnosis can be established by the demonstration of cytoplasmic lipid vacuoles within most granulocytes and monocytes by direct examination of a peripheral blood smear and by demonstration of cytoplasmic lipid vacuoles in the basal and granular cell layers of the epidermis, eccrine ducts, pilosebaceous epithelium, macrophages, fibroblasts, and mast cells.[51-53]

PEELING SKIN SYNDROME

The peeling skin syndrome is an unusual congenital ichthyosis probably inherited as an autosomal recessive disease characterized by life-long peeling of the epidermis, easy mechanical separation of the stratum corneum, pruritus, short stature, and easily removable anagen hairs. Histopathologic features include a psoriasiform dermatitis with hyperkeratosis, parakeratosis, intraepidermal separation between the stratum corneum and the stratum granulosum, acanthosis with elongation of rete ridges, and a chronic perivascular infiltrate in the dermis. Patients with this disorder often demonstrate a moderate generalized aminoaciduria and low tryptophan levels, which may be biochemical markers.[54]

OTHER HYPERKERATOTIC DISORDERS

Keratosis Pilaris

Keratosis pilaris is an autosomal dominant disorder common among persons with dry skin. Starting in early childhood, between the ages of 2 and 3, continuing through adolescence, and then subsiding in adulthood, keratosis pilaris is characterized by minute keratotic follicular papules over the lateral aspects of the upper arms (see Fig. 3–5), the fronts and sides of the thighs, and, at times, the cheeks and buttocks. Characterized by cornified plugs in the upper part of the hair follicles, which gives the skin a stippled appearance resembling gooseflesh or plucked chicken skin, the disorder is often seen in individuals with atopy and dry skin as a manifestation of ichthyosis vulgaris or erythrokeratodermia variabilis and in individuals with a deficiency of vitamin A (hypovitaminosis A, phrynoderma). Because lesions are associated with and accentuated by dry skin, they generally are more prominent during the winter and tend to improve during the summer.

Treatment, although not completely satisfactory, consists of frequent use of emollients (particularly those containing urea or lactic or glycolic acid), increasing the humidity in the sleeping quarters, application of 5 to 10 per cent salicylic acid in a moisturizing cream such as Aquaphor or a 20 per cent formulation of urea available as Ureacin Creme (Pedinol Pharmacal) intermittent application of Keralyt Gel (under occlusion, if tolerated), and gentle exfoliation by a pumice stone, washcloth, loofah sponge, or Buf-Puf (a polyester sponge available from Home Products Division of 3M).

Lichen Spinulosis

Lichen spinulosis is a disorder characterized by hyperkeratotic spiny follicular papules grouped into 2- to 5-cm, skin-colored plaques or patches, seen primarily in children, especially blacks and more frequently boys, during the second decade of life. Lesions tend to occur in crops and are minute, closely set, follicular papules grouped into large patches with round or polycyclic contour, often appearing in a symmetrical distribution on the nuchal area, back, abdomen, buttocks, and extensor surfaces of the extremities. Histopathologic changes are similar to those of keratosis pilaris; and, although pruritus may be seen as a feature of this disorder, lesions are generally asymptomatic, come and go spontaneously, and usually tend to involute over a period of time. Treatment is similar to that for keratosis pilaris.

Palmar and Plantar Hyperkeratosis

Palmar and plantar hyperkeratosis (palmoplantar keratoderma, keratoderma of the palms and soles) describes a diffuse or localized thickening of the stratum corneum of the palms and soles that may appear alone or as part of a more generalized disorder such as congenital ichthyosiform erythroderma, epidermolytic hyperkeratosis, Sjögren-Larsson syndrome, Conradi's syndrome, pityriasis rubra pilaris, psoriasis, Reiter's syndrome, hypohidrotic ectodermal dysplasia, or tyrosinemia II.

Keratosis palmaris et plantaris (palmoplantar keratoderma of Unna-Thost), first described by Thost in 1880 and further delineated by Unna in 1883, is an autosomal dominant generally bilateral disorder with variable expressivity characterized by sharply circumscribed congenital thickening of the palms and soles. The palms may have a smooth, waxy appearance or a dry surface with fissures, and most patients have hyperhidrosis, which may lead to maceration and fissuring and an increased incidence of dermatophytosis.[55] Other variants of palmoplantar keratoderma include the Vörner type, a clinically indistinguishable disorder characterized by vacuolization of the epidermal cells similar to that seen in patients with epidermolytic hyperkeratosis, and a familial disorder characterized by palmoplantar keratoderma, diffuse scleroatrophy and sclerodactyly, and, at times, nail changes and squamous cell carcinomas in the atrophic skin (Huriez's syndrome). *Vohwinkel's syndrome* (mutilating palmoplantar keratoderma) is an uncommon autosomal dominant mutilating form of palmoplantar hyperkeratosis characterized by polygonal starfish-shaped hyperkeratoses on the dorsal aspects of the hands and feet and irregular linear hyperkeratoses on the elbows and knees; occasionally these patients may have scarring alopecia, high-frequency hearing loss, or autoamputation of fingers or toes.[56]

Mal de Meleda (keratosis palmoplantaris transgrediens) is an extremely rare autosomal recessive disorder described in individuals living on the Adriatic island of Meleda characterized by hyperkeratosis of the palms and soles with spillover at times, hence the term *transgrediens*, to the dorsal aspects of the hands and feet.

The *Papillon-Lefèvre syndrome* is an autosomal recessive disorder that, starting in the first 6 months of life, is manifested by redness and diffuse sometimes localized hyperkeratosis of the palms and soles, which usually extends to the dorsal aspects of the hands and feet. Psoriasiform lesions occur on the knees and elbows. Gingivitis and periosteal changes of the alveolar bone (juvenile periodontitis) result in loss of both deciduous and permanent teeth. At times, the patient may have intracranial calcification of the falx cerebri and choroid plexus, arachnodactyly, mental retardation, and increased susceptibility to infection.[57]

The *Olmstead syndrome* is a rare disorder characterized by progressive, diffuse, symmetrical, sharply marginated, mutilating palmoplantar keratoderma with spread onto the dorsal surfaces of the hands and feet, linear or star-shaped keratoses similar to those seen in patients with Vohwinkel's syndrome, and constriction of the digits. There may also be linear keratotic streaks on the flexural aspects of the wrists, onychodystrophy, and periorificial keratoderma.[58]

Keratosis punctata palmaris et plantaris, a rare autosomal dominant disorder seen almost exclusively in young black adults, is characterized by discrete keratoses of the palms and soles. Confined to the palmoplantar creases and volar aspects of the fingers (Fig. 7–19), the central keratinous plug may be lost or can be picked out, leaving a shallow depressed pit with a keratotic base. Lesions can be particularly painful when walking or from pressure on the hands in persons who perform manual labor. The presence of gastrointestinal carcinomas in three members of a family with this disorder suggests a possible association between the two conditions.[59, 60]

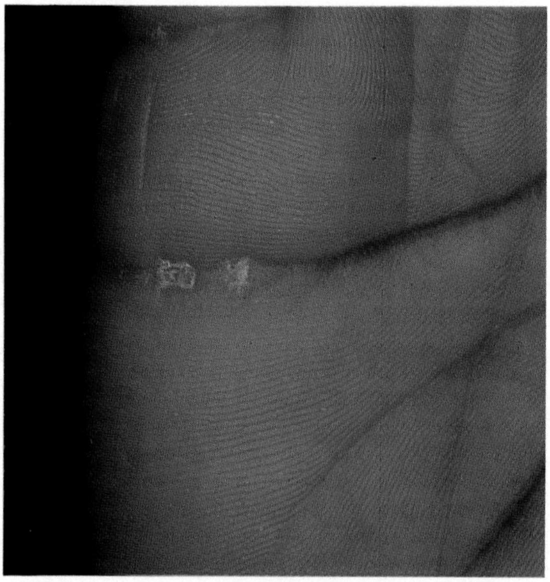

The *Howel-Evans syndrome* is a rare, dominantly inherited, diffuse form of keratoderma of the palms and soles that appears between the ages of 5 and 15 years. Carcinoma of the esophagus may occur in patients with this disorder in later life.

The treatment of all forms of hyperkeratosis of the palms and soles is generally palliative and consists of application of keratolytic formulations such as 10 to 20 per cent salicylic acid in an emollient cream such as Ureacin Creme (under occlusion at night if tolerated), intermittent use of Keralyt Gel or 40 per cent salicylic acid (Mediplast) plasters, periodic soaking of the affected area in water, and gentle removal of excessive keratinous material by a pumice stone, scalpel, or single-edged razor blade. Painful fissures can be treated by a formulation of 30 per cent tincture of benzoin in zinc oxide, or cryoglycate (Krazy Glue), followed by the application of a keratolytic formulation such as 10 to 20 per cent salicylic acid in Aquaphor, the wearing of comfortable shoes, and avoidance of pressure or friction to affected areas. Although oral retinoids are helpful, they are recommended only for short-term use for the temporary relief of individuals with significant disability (Fig. 7–20).

CONGENITAL ECTODERMAL DEFECTS

Ectodermal dysplasia is a descriptive term for an inherited group of defects involving the skin and its appendageal structures. These defects include hidrotic ectodermal dysplasia, hypohidrotic ectodermal dysplasia, and congenital aplasia cutis. Although these defects share involvement of similar structures (the integument and its appendages), they are distinct nosologic entities, with individual histologic and clinical manifestations. Genetically they are not related to one another.

Hidrotic Ectodermal Dysplasia

The hidrotic type of ectodermal dysplasia is an autosomal dominant disorder of keratinization characterized by dystrophy of the nails, hyperkeratosis of the palms and soles, and defects of the hair. Most cases have been reported in French-Canadian families. Unlike anhidrotic (hypohidrotic) ectodermal dysplasia, which is an X-linked recessive disorder and more common in males, hidrotic ectodermal dysplasia is of equal sex incidence, shows no abnormality of sweating, and although dental caries may be present, includes normal teeth and facies.

There is some evidence that hidrotic ectodermal dysplasia is caused by a defect in keratinization due to a molecular abnormality of keratin. In 30 per cent of individuals with this disorder, however, there may be no obvious defect other than dystrophy of the nails. Although nail dystrophy is the

Figure 7–19. Keratosis punctata palmaris in a 12-year-old black girl.

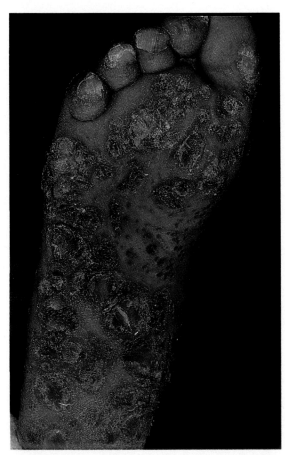

Figure 7–20. Severe painful hyperkeratotic lesions in patient with keratoderma plantaris.

which more than 90 per cent of affected patients have been male. Clinical features include absent or reduced sweating, hypotrichosis, and defective dentition. Abnormal absence of perspiration from the surface of the skin in the presence of an appropriate stimulus often results in hyperthermia. Patients may appear normal at birth but soon develop intermittent fevers during hot weather or following exercise or meals.

Affected persons often appear more like each other than like their own siblings; classic features may be present by the age of 1 year. Most have a distinctive pathognomonic facies—a square forehead with frontal bossing, saddle nose, large conspicuous nostrils, wide cheekbones with depressed cheeks, thick everted lips, and prominent chin. Ears may be small, satyr-like (pointed), low-lying, and anteriorly placed.

Skin is soft, thin, white, and shiny, often feminine-like in quality, with easily seen cutaneous vasculature. Alopecia is often the first feature to attract attention but is seldom complete. Nails are defective in 50 per cent of cases and may be thin, brittle, or ridged. Gross deformities are uncommon.

Dentition is generally delayed, and dental anomalies varying from complete to partial absence of teeth may be noted. Incisors and canines are often discolored, peg-shaped or conical, and pointed with inward curving. Occlusion is poor, and caries are common. General physical development is often stunted. Mental development is retarded in 30 to 50 per cent of cases, and life expectancy is normal or slightly reduced.[61]

Early diagnosis is helpful since even one episode of severe or prolonged hyperthermia can affect mental development.[62] Diagnosis can be assisted by direct visualization of fingertip skin for a decrease in the number of sweat pores, evaluation of sweat gland activity by skin imprint techniques using bromphenol blue, the starch/iodine test, or cutaneous biopsy demonstration of absence or hypoplasia of sweat glands. The starch/iodine test is done by drying the skin, painting it with 2 per cent iodine, allowing it to dry, and taping good quality paper to the skin overnight. By this technique, the starch in the paper reacts with iodine and sweat droplets can be seen as minute dark spots.[63–65]

Therapy is difficult and should be directed toward temperature regulation, restriction of excessive physical exertion, choice of suitable occupation, and avoidance of warm climates. Cool baths, air conditioning, light clothing, and the reduction of the causes of normal perspiration are beneficial. Regular dental supervision may help preserve teeth and reduce cosmetic disfigurement.

Other hypohidrotic ectodermal dysplasia syndromes include the following:

Rapp-Hodgkin syndrome, an autosomal dominant disorder characterized by variable clefts of the lip, palate, and uvula; small narrow dysplastic nails; hypodontia with small conical teeth; high

primary feature of this syndrome, various nail changes may occur, none of which is characteristic. Nails grow slowly and may appear thickened or thinned, striated, discolored, brittle, or hypoplastic. Paronychial infections are common and may result in partial to complete destruction of the nail matrix.

Body hair may be sparse; eyebrows and eyelashes may be thinned or absent, and the skin has a smooth texture. Scalp hair, generally normal during infancy and childhood, may become thin, fragile, or sparse to absent following puberty. Keratoderma (hyperkeratosis) of the palms and soles is common and occasionally extends to involve the sides and dorsa of affected hands and feet. Extreme hyperkeratosis of the palms and soles may be controlled to a degree by topical keratolytic agents (3 to 10 per cent salicylic acid or 10 to 20 per cent urea) in an emollient cream.

Hypohidrotic Ectodermal Dysplasia

Hypohidrotic ectodermal dysplasia (formerly termed *anhidrotic ectodermal dysplasia*) is believed to be a sex-linked recessive disorder in forehead; low nasal bridge; narrow nose; maxillary hypoplasia; and hypohydrosis

Ankyloblepharon–ectodermal dysplasia–clefting (AEC) syndrome, an autosomal dominant disorder characterized by ankyloblepharon (congenital fusion of the eyelids), hypotrichosis (sparse, predominantly blond wiry hair and sparse eyebrows and eyelashes), midfacial hypoplasia (small lips, nose, and ears), palmar and plantar keratoderma, hyperpigmentation, and partial hypohidrosis

Basan's syndrome, characterized by ectodermal dysplasia with hypohidrosis, hypotrichosis, defective teeth, and unusual dermatoglyphics

Friere-Mara syndrome, characterized by hypohidrosis, partial alopecia, follicular hyperkeratosis of the scalp, onychogryphosis, frontal bossing, saddle nose, oligophrenia, cataracts, and hyperchromic macules on the face

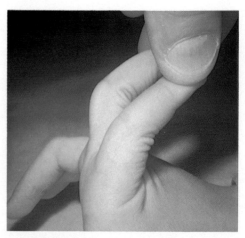

Figure 7–22. Hyperextensibility of the fingers in Ehlers-Danlos syndrome.

CONGENITAL DERMAL DEFECTS

Hereditary disorders of the dermal tissue generally involve one element of the connective tissue. Three types of fiber form the connective tissue of the dermis—collagen, reticulum, and elastin. The mucopolysaccharides are a major component of the ground substance between these fibers. Discussion in this section will include a disorder of collagen, the largest constituent of the connective tissue (Ehlers-Danlos syndrome), and some disorders of elastin (cutis laxa and pseudoxanthoma elasticum). The mucopolysaccharidoses are reviewed in Chapter 22.

Ehlers-Danlos Syndrome

Ehlers-Danlos syndrome consists of a group of inherited disorders of collagen characterized by increased cutaneous elasticity (Fig. 7–21), hyperextensibility of the joints (Fig. 7–22), and fragility

of the skin, with formation of pseudotumors and large gaping scars (Fig. 7–23). The collagenous defect appears to be the manner in which collagen bundles are joined to one another (a defective wickerwork arrangement), which results in increased mobility and rubber-like stretchability of the skin and joints. To date, although at least 11 varieties of Ehlers-Danlos syndrome have been recognized (Table 7–6), approximately 50 per cent of patients do not fit into one of the described subtypes (they are currently designated as type unspecified).[66–70]

In general, infants with Ehlers-Danlos syndrome are prone to premature birth because of early rupture of membranes (the placenta is determined entirely by the fetal genotype and therefore its membranes have the same fragility as other structures in this disorder). The skin of affected individuals is velvety and soft and on palpation has

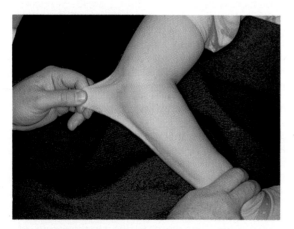

Figure 7–21. Hyperelasticity of skin overlying the elbow (Ehlers-Danlos syndrome). (Braverman IM: Skin Signs of Systemic Disease. W. B. Saunders Co., Philadelphia, 1970).

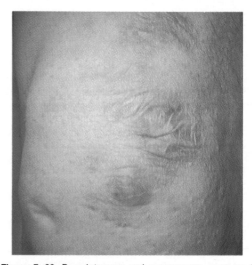

Figure 7–23. Pseudotumors and papyraceous scars on the knee in Ehlers-Danlos syndrome.

Table 7–6. EHLERS-DANLOS SYNDROMES

Type	Name	Inheritance	Clinical Features	Pathology and Tissue Defect
I	Gravis	Autosomal dominant	Prematurity associated with premature rupture of fetal membranes, soft velvety fragile hyperextensible skin, marked bruising, cigarette paper and fishmouth scars, marked hypermobility of joints	Large irregular collagen fibrils, biochemical defect unknown
II	Mitis	Autosomal dominant	Less severe, prematurity uncommon, moderately hypermobile joints, moderately hyperextensible skin, varicosities, hernias	Large irregular collagen fibrils, biochemical defect unknown
III	Benign hypermobile	Autosomal dominant	Minimal cutaneous manifestations, soft skin, marked joint hypermobility; floppy mitral valve may occur	Large irregular collagen fibrils, tissue defect unknown
IV	Ecchymotic, arterial, or Sack type	Autosomal dominant and recessive forms	Marked bruising, thin skin; arterial, gastrointestinal, and uterine rupture; elastosis perforans serpiginosa	Small collagen fibers, variable-sized fibrils, thin dermis, decreased type III collagen
V	X-linked	X-linked recessive	Similar to type II, skin highly extensible; floppy mitral valve may occur	Lysyl oxidase deficiency
VI	Ocular	Autosomal recessive	Intraocular bleeding; soft velvety skin; cigarette paper scars; severe scoliosis; markedly hyperextensible skin and joints	Small collagen bundles, fibrils similar to type I, lysyl hydroxylase deficiency
VII	Arthroclasis multiplex congenita	Autosomal recessive and autosomal dominant	Markedly lax joints with mobility and multiple dislocations; microcornea; moderate skin fragility	Aminoterminal procollagen peptidase deficiency with structural mutation of type I collagen
VIII	Periodontal	Autosomal dominant	Severe early periodontitis; aesthenic habitus; marked skin fragility, with pigmented scars, pretibial scarring; minimal joint hypermobility	Varied fibril diameter, biochemical disorder unknown
IX	Occipital horn syndrome (previously called X-linked recessive cutis laxa)	X-linked recessive	Hyperextensible skin; bony occipital horns; broad clavicles; hernias; bladder diverticula and rupture	Varied fibril diameter, lysyl oxidase deficiency, abnormal copper metabolism
X	Fibronectin deficient	Autosomal recessive	Striae; moderate extensibility of skin; hypermobility of joints; platelet dysfunction and easy bruisability	Variable fiber diameter, dysfunction of plasma fibronectin
XI	Familial joint laxity	Autosomal dominant	Normal skin; marked joint laxity and dislocation	Tissue defect unknown

a peculiar, doughy consistency. It is hyperelastic, yet not lax except in late stages. After being stretched it returns to its normal position as soon as released (see Fig. 7–21) and, in contrast to 10 per cent of apparently normal individuals, approximately 50 per cent of patients with Ehlers-Danlos can touch the tip of their nose with their tongue (Gorlin's sign). In addition, the skin of the hands, feet, and, at times, the elbows also tends to be lax and redundant, thus resulting in a loose-fitting glove- or moccasin-like appearance. A number of patients also have a tendency toward pressure induced herniation of subcutaneous fat on the medial or lateral aspect of the heels, evident when the patient is standing (piezogenic pedal papules) (Fig. 7–24), or wrists, a disorder at times seen in otherwise apparently normal individuals.

In addition to abnormal elasticity, the skin of patients with Ehlers-Danlos syndrome is ex-

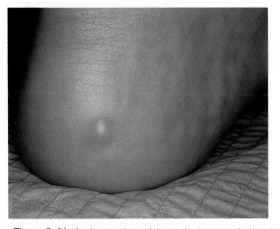

Figure 7–24. A piezogenic pedal papule (pressure-induced herniation of subcutaneous fat) on the heel of an otherwise normal person. The disorder becomes apparent when the patient is standing.

tremely fragile, and minor trauma may produce gaping "fishmouth" wounds. It has poor tensile strength and cannot hold sutures properly. This leads to frequent dehiscence, poor healing, and the formation of wide, papyraceous, wrinkled hernia-like scars, particularly over areas of trauma (such as the forehead, elbows, and knees). Blood vessels are fragile, resulting in hematomas. The resolution of hematomas is accompanied by fibrosis, which produces soft subcutaneous pseudotumors (see Fig. 7–23). Except for areas of skin that have been altered by trauma, histopathologic examination of the skin of persons with Ehlers-Danlos disease reveals no obvious alteration in either elastic or collagen fiber.

Hyperextensible joints may result in "double-jointed" fingers or frequent subluxation of larger joints (see Fig. 7–22). This may occur spontaneously or follow slight trauma. Muscle tone is often poor, and inguinal and diaphragmatic hernias are common. Anomalies of the heart and dissecting aortic aneurysms have been described, and although life expectancy is generally normal, premature deaths have occurred from gastrointestinal bleeding, rare bowel perforation, and rupture of cardiovascular defects.

The diagnosis of Ehlers-Danlos syndrome is made on the characteristic clinical, genetic, and biologic features of the disorder and its various subgroups. Except for areas of skin that have been altered by trauma, histopathologic examination generally reveals no obvious abnormalities either in thickness of the skin or in the appearance of collagen or elastic fibers. Some patients, however, may demonstrate thin collagen fibers that are not united to collagen bundles. In such cases, the skin may be reduced in thickness and a relative increase in elastic fibers may be noted.

Management is mainly supportive and should include genetic counseling. The cardiovascular status should be evaluated in all patients, particularly those suspected of having Ehlers-Danlos syndrome type IV, and patients with easy bruisability should be evaluated for specific bleeding disorders. The possibility of premature birth should be discussed, and cutaneous, skeletal, and ocular difficulties (possible retinal detachment and abnormalities of the lens) should be emphasized. Surgical procedures present problems because tissues are friable and difficult to suture. Edges of gaping wounds, therefore, should be kept approximated with appropriate sutures and adhesive closure to facilitate healing. Precautions must be taken to minimize trauma to the skin and joints. Pressure bandages over hematomas may help prevent pseudotumor formation.

Ascorbic acid stimulates collagen synthesis in tissues by serving as a cofactor for prolylhydroxylase and lysylhydroxylase, enzymes that catalyze the formation of hydroxyproline and hydroxylysine. Large doses of ascorbic acid, 2 to 4 g/day, therefore, have been used in some patients with type VI Ehlers-Danlos syndrome with apparent clinical response. Since one of the metabolites of ascorbic acid is oxalic acid, caution must be exercised when this modality is used in patients prone to kidney stone formation.[71]

Cutis Laxa

Cutis laxa (generalized elastolysis) is an extremely rare disorder of the elastic tissue characterized by inelastic, loose, and pendulous skin, which results in an aged, bloodhound-like appearance (Fig. 7–25). Although its pathogenesis is not well understood, current studies suggest a fragmentation and decrease in elastic tissue in the skin and rest of the body, increased collagenase expression of fibroblasts, and reduced messenger RNA levels, resulting in deficient collagen production in patients with this disorder.[72, 73] Cutis laxa can be acquired or congenital, with the genetic forms inherited as autosomal dominant, autosomal recessive, and X-linked recessive disorders (the latter has been reclassified as type IX Ehlers-Danlos syndrome; Table 7–7). Acquired forms of cutis laxa have been associated with other generalized disorders and may follow a febrile illness, an allergic reaction, urticaria, drug eruption, or erythema multiforme. They have also been described in a patient with multiple myeloma and may occur as a manifestation of an autosomal recessive form of pseudoxanthoma elasticum or an autosomal dominant form of amyloidosis.[74–77]

Patients with cutis laxa present a striking picture of loose inelastic redundant skin that sags and hangs in pendulous folds as if it were too large for the body. The drooping and ectropion of the eyelids, together with the sagging facial skin and ac-

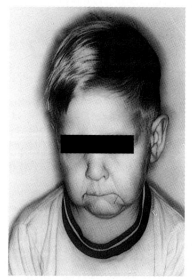

Figure 7–25. Sagging cheeks and bloodhound-like facies of a child with cutis laxa. (Courtesy of Sidney Klaus, M.D., *In* Braverman IM: Skin Signs of Systemic Disease. W. B. Saunders Co., Philadelphia, 1970.)

Table 7–7. CUTIS LAXA

Type	Defect	Clinical Features
Autosomal recessive	Abnormal collagen linkage with defect in lysyl oxidase	Relatively rare (more common in females); severe skin changes; progressive; vascular and pulmonary abnormalities and early death
Autosomal dominant	Unknown	May appear at any age; loose sagging skin with few systemic abnormalities, normal growth and life expectancy
X-linked recessive	Low lysyl oxidase activity and reduced levels of copper and ceruloplasmin	Relatively normal facies, mild cutaneous laxity, moderate hypermobility of joints, association with Ehlers-Danlos syndrome type IX
Acquired	Unknown	Cutaneous changes mild to moderate; occasional systemic involvement

centuation of the nasal, labial, and other facial folds, help produce the "bloodhound" or aged appearance (see Fig. 7–25). Although the skin is frequently prominent and, at times, almost grotesque, as children grow older they often grow into the skin abnormality and are not as severely affected in later life.

Systemic manifestations caused by weakened supportive tissue include aortic dilatation, pulmonary artery stenosis, pulmonary emphysema, diverticula of the gastrointestinal tract or urinary bladder, uterine or rectal prolapse, and ventral, hiatal, or inguinal hernias. In patients with the severe autosomal recessively inherited disease, the disorder is gradually progressive and death from pulmonary complications related to emphysema may occur early in infancy or, in many instances, in the second to fourth decades of life. The autosomal dominant form may appear at any age and presents as a cosmetic problem with few systemic changes. The acquired type has no genetic background, internal organs are frequently involved, and in about half the patients the symptoms are preceded or accompanied by a cutaneous eruption (urticaria, erythematous plaques, or a vesicular eruption).[78]

The skin in cutis laxa is extensible but, in contrast to that of Ehlers-Danlos syndrome, does not spring back to place on release of tension. In Ehlers-Danlos syndrome the hyperextensibility of the joints and pseudotumors of the skin with large atrophic scars are diagnostic. In pseudoxanthoma elasticum the lax skin is covered with characteristic soft yellowish papules and plaques. In neurofibromatosis (von Recklinghausen's disease), café au lait spots, Lisch nodules, and/or fibrous tumors indicate the true nature of the disorder.

Cutis laxa affects the elastic fibers of the skin as well as those throughout the entire body. Although no histologic abnormality is demonstrable with hematoxylin and eosin stain, elastic tissue stains reveal a decreased number of elastic fibers throughout the entire dermis and electron microscopy reveals a granular degeneration of elastic fibers. In cases in which an inflammatory infiltrate

is present, it may consist of a nonspecific chronic inflammatory infiltrate of lymphocytes and histiocytes and, at times, neutrophils. If vesicles are present, they are subepidermal and may show papillary microabscesses composed of neutrophils and eosinophils suggestive of dermatitis herpetiformis.[78]

Therapy for cutis laxa is limited, and prognosis in general is poor. Family members should be examined for the presence of cutis laxa or other heritable connective tissue disorders, and the determination of inheritance patterns, when possible, can guide genetic counseling. Surgery can correct diverticula, rectal prolapse, or hernias; pulmonary function studies may aid in the early detection of emphysema; and plastic surgery can make a dramatic improvement in patients, inevitably with important psychological benefit.

Pseudoxanthoma Elasticum

Pseudoxanthoma elasticum is a genetic disorder of the elastic tissue that involves the skin, eyes, and cardiovascular system. It is characterized by soft yellowish papules and polygonal plaques on the neck, below the clavicles, in the axillae, antecubital fossae, and periumbilical areas, and on the perineum and thighs (Fig. 7–26). There are two recessive and two dominant forms of this disorder. Most cases are autosomal recessive (Table 7–8). Pathogenesis is controversial and appears to be related to an abnormal proliferation of elastic fibers that prematurely calcify and fragment.

Skin lesions are a hallmark of this disorder. They are yellowish and xanthoma-like (hence the name pseudoxanthoma). They vary from several papules to linear plaques resembling plucked chicken skin, morocco leather, or orange skin (peau d'orange). Although lesions are seen in childhood, they may be overlooked because of their small size and the lack of symptomatology. As a result, the diagnosis frequently does not become apparent until the patient reaches the second or third decade of life.

Eye changes associated with this disorder are

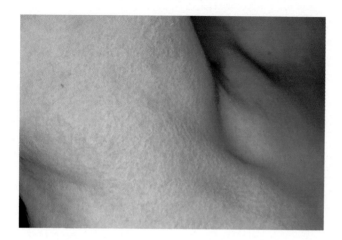

Figure 7–26. Soft yellowish papules and polygonal plaques in the axilla of a patient with pseudoxanthoma elasticum.

characteristic; they are slate gray to reddish brown linear bands (angioid streaks), caused by tears in Bruch's membrane and subsequent fibrosis, and are seen in 50 to 70 per cent of patients. Angioid streaks, however, are uncommon in young children and usually do not appear until the second or third decade of life. The association of skin lesions with angioid streaks is known as the Grönblad-Strandberg syndrome. Loss of central vision is the most frequent disability and may develop in more than 70 per cent of cases with this complication. These retinal changes are not pathognomonic, since they may also be found in patients with sickle cell anemia, Paget's disease of the bone, idiopathic thrombocytopenic purpura, acromegaly, Ehlers-Danlos syndrome, and lead poisoning.

Significant cardiovascular changes include peripheral artery disease with easy fatigability, intermittent claudication, hypertension, mitral valve prolapse, coronary artery involvement, and cerebral, gastrointestinal, or uterine hemorrhage.[79]

The diagnosis of pseudoxanthoma elasticum is based on the clinical findings and on histopathologic evidence of calcification in elastic tissue and basophilic degeneration of the elastic tissue in the middle and deeper zones of the dermis. Elastic tissue degeneration also affects connective tissue elements of the aorta and medium-sized muscular arteries in the heart, kidneys, gastrointestinal tract, and other organs.

There is no specific therapy for this disorder. Genetic counseling should be provided, and patients should be advised to avoid contact sports and heavy straining such as that which occurs with weight lifting. Since the disabling aspects of this disorder are slow but progressive, regular vascular survey (including careful auscultation and echocardiographic evaluation in an effort to rule out mitral valve prolapse) and ophthalmologic examinations are important.

Progeria

Progeria (Hutchinson-Gilford syndrome) is a rare disease characterized by a combination of dwarfism, generalized atrophy of the subcutaneous tissue and muscle, a high incidence of generalized atherosclerosis, and early onset of progressive senile degenerative changes. Although its presence in siblings and examples of parental consanguinity have been reported, suggesting an autosomal recessive basis for this disorder, affected individuals do not reproduce and there are far too few familial cases to draw definitive conclusions as to the heritability of this disorder.[80–83] There is no sex pre-

Table 7–8. PSEUDOXANTHOMA ELASTICUM

Type	Description
Dominant type 1	Classic peau d'orange (plucked chicken) skin; severe and early retinopathy with visual loss frequently leading to blindness; severe vascular disease with angina, claudication, hypertension; uterine and gastrointestinal bleeding common
Dominant type 2	Clinical features less severe than dominant type 1; a high incidence of blue sclerae with myopia and mild retinopathy; vascular changes minimal; arched palate, loose-jointedness, extensible skin, and marfanoid appearance common
Recessive type 1	Classic flexural lesions; hematemesis may occur but vascular and ocular changes only of mild to moderate severity
Recessive type 2	Extremely rare; universal cutaneous involvement with lax loose-fitting appearance; no systemic involvement

dilection, and rarely is more than one family member affected.

Affected children tend to have a reduced size and birth weight, and except for evidence of scleroderma-like cutaneous changes on the trunk, dusky mid-facial skin tone, and a small indentation on the tip of the nose, otherwise appear to be relatively normal during the first 6 to 12 months of life. The classic clinical picture consists of dwarfism; alopecia of the scalp, eyebrows, and lashes; prominent scalp veins; and generalized atrophy of muscle and subcutaneous tissue. Frequently there is nasolabial and circumoral cyanosis. The face is small, the chin is recessed, and the nose is thin and beaked, giving the face a bird-like appearance (Fig. 7–27). Although the head is usually 2 to 4 cm smaller in circumference than average, severe growth retardation and alteration of the facial structures resulting in a disproportionately small face with frontal and parietal bossing give the head a hydrocephalic appearance.

The skin generally becomes thin (except for areas with sclerodermatous plaques), dry, and wrinkled, with mottled brownish orange pigmentation. The underlying subcutaneous veins, especially those on the scalp and thighs, become plainly visible and more prominent. The nails become yellowish, thin, atrophic, and brittle, and resorption of bone leads to osteoporosis with a tendency to frequent fractures. The teeth become crowded, irregular in form, or deficient in number, and deciduous dentition is often retained. Speech becomes high pitched and squeaky, and intelligence is generally normal. The chest becomes narrow and the abdomen protuberant, and, owing to a mild flexion of the knees, a "horse-riding" stance becomes apparent.

Progeria should be distinguished from scleroderma, from Werner's, Hallermann-Streiff, Cockayne's, Bloom's, and Rothmund-Thomson syndromes, and from hypohidrotic ectodermal dysplasia. Atherosclerosis is early and severe. Cardiac murmurs frequently occur after the age of 5 years and are soon followed by hypertension, cardiomegaly, angina, myocardial infarction, and congestive heart failure. Death usually occurs during the second decade of life.

Werner's Syndrome

Werner's syndrome (progeria of the adult) is a rare autosomal recessive disorder characterized by premature graying of hair at the temples (which may develop as early as 8 years of age but generally occurs between the ages of 14 and 18), progressive alopecia, shortness of stature due to arrest of growth at puberty, bird-like facies, cataracts, and an apparent aged appearance. Cutaneous features include sclerodermoid changes of the skin of the extremities and, to a lesser degree, the face and neck; telangiectasias; mottled or diffuse pigmentation; keratoses; and indolent ulcers over pressure points, particularly on the soles and ankles.

Patients with adult progeria develop severe, often generalized vascular disease; diabetes mellitus (in 30 to 45 per cent of affected individuals); hypogonadism; loss of subcutaneous tissue; severe muscle wasting in the legs, arms, feet, and hands with large abdominal fat deposits (leading to a body habitus of a stocky trunk with spindly extremities); senile cataracts developing in the late 20s and 30s; diffuse bronze pigmentation of the skin; premature balding and graying of the hair; dystrophic fingernails; irregular tooth development; osteoporosis of the extremities and spine; soft tissue calcification; a high-pitched voice or hoarseness; and a predisposition to neoplastic disease (hepatoma, thyroid adenocarcinoma, ovarian carcinoma, fibrosarcoma, osteogenic sarcoma, and carcinoma of the breast).

Winchester's Syndrome

A rare autosomal recessive connective tissue disorder described only in the offspring of consanguineous parents, Winchester's syndrome is characterized by dwarfism, small joint destruction, corneal opacities, thickened leathery and hypertrichotic skin, gargoyle-like features, hypertrophic lips and gingivae, and severe osteoporosis. Although its pathogenesis is not clear, an abnormal function of fibroblasts is believed to be responsible for the cutaneous manifestations.

Dyskeratosis Congenita

Dyskeratosis congenita is a rare genetic disorder characterized by atrophy, telangiectasia, and reticular hyperpigmentation of the skin, by nail dystro-

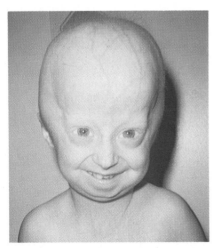

Figure 7–27. Progeria. Alopecia, subcutaneous atrophy, prominent scalp veins, and bird-like appearance. (Fleischmajer R, Nedwich A: Progeria [Hutchinson-Gilford]. Arch. Dermatol. 107:253, 1973. Copyright © 1973, American Medical Association.)

phy, and by leukokeratosis of the oral and, at times, anal mucosa. Almost all reported cases have been in males, and available pedigrees suggest it to be an autosomal recessive or X-linked disorder (Table 7–9).

Nail changes are usually the first to make their appearance (Fig. 7–28). Between the ages of 5 and 13 the nails become thin and dystrophic. In mild cases they develop ridging and longitudinal grooving; in severe forms they are shortened and, at times, almost nonexistent. Cutaneous changes may develop simultaneously or in a few years following the onset of nail changes and reach their full development within a subsequent period of 3 to 5 years. A fine reticulated grayish brown hyperpigmentation (surrounding hypopigmented and atrophic patches of uninvolved skin) on the face, neck, shoulders, upper back, and thighs is characteristic of this disorder (Fig. 7–29). Other cutaneous changes may include telangiectasia of the trunk; redness and atrophy of the face with irregular macular hyperpigmentation; acrocyanosis; palmoplantar hyperkeratosis; hyperhidrosis and bullae of the palms and soles; wrinkled atrophic skin over the elbows, knees, and penis; and a diffuse atrophic, transparent, and shiny appearance on the dorsal aspects of the hands and feet. The hair of the scalp, eyebrows, and eyelashes is often sparse and lusterless, and patients with this disorder frequently have atrophic changes of the mucles and bones of the feet and hands, giving a "cupped" appearance to the palms.

Mucous membrane changes consist of small blisters, erosions, and subsequent leukoplakia of the oral (Fig. 7–30) and anal mucosa, esophagus, and urethra. Similar changes of the tarsal conjunctiva may result in atresia of the lacrimal ducts, excessive lacrimation, chronic blepharitis, conjunctivitis, and ectropion. The teeth tend to be defective and subject to early decay. Periodontitis may develop, and affected persons have an increased incidence of cutaneous malignancy (predominantly epidermoid carcinoma) and a high incidence of carcinoma in the areas of leukoplakia.[84]

In some patients a severe hematologic disease resembling Fanconi's anemia has been reported. In these patients there is severe anemia with leukopenia (especially neutropenia), splenomegaly, and hypoplastic bone marrow; hemorrhagic diatheses are prominent. Other features include prenatal and postnatal growth retardation, mental retardation, elevated immunoglobulin levels, gastrointestinal hemorrhage, mucosal ulceration, intracranial calcification, cirrhotic changes of the liver, premature baldness, a hyposthenic build, joint deformities, incomplete closure of the vertebral arches, osteoporosis, bone fragility, radiolucent areas of the shafts of the long bones, coarse trabeculation in the metaphyses, aseptic necrosis of the hips, and clinical features of graft-versus-host disease.[85] Opportunistic infection, sepsis, leukemia, gastrointestinal bleeding, and generalized debilitation are common; and patients seldom survive beyond 50 years of age, with death generally being attributed to cancer, leukemia, hemorrhage, or sepsis.

The diagnosis is dependent on the clinical history and characteristic features, with nearly all patients eventually manifesting the diagnostic triad of cutaneous pigmentation, nail dystrophy, and leukoplakia. Management of patients consists of bougienage for esophageal stenosis; fulguration, curettage, and surgical excision of leukokeratosis of the buccal and anal mucosae; and regular supervision for early detection of mucosal or cutaneous carcinomas.

Focal Dermal Hypoplasia

Focal dermal hypoplasia (Goltz's syndrome) is characterized by linear areas of dermal hypoplasia with herniation of underlying tissue, telangiectasia, linear or reticular areas of hyperpigmentation or hypopigmentation, localized superficial fatty deposits in the skin, red papillomas of mucous membranes or periorificial skin, and anomalies of the extremities, including syndactyly, adactyly, and oligodactyly. This is primarily a disorder of females (90 per cent); available family histories suggest that this condition is caused by an X-linked dominant trait lethal to homozygous males.[86] When the disorder occurs in males, it probably represents a new mutation.

The cutaneous manifestations of focal dermal hypoplasia include widely distributed linear areas of hypoplasia of the skin; soft, yellowish, reddish yellow, or yellowish brown nodular outpouchings, often in a linear distribution (caused by herniation of the subcutaneous fat through the thinned dermis); and large cutaneous ulcers (due to congenital absence of skin) that gradually heal with atrophy. Additional abnormalities include lack of a digit, which may be associated with syndactyly and "lobster claw" deformities; colobomas of the eyes; hypoplasia of hair, nails, or teeth; streaky pigmentation, atrophy, and telangiectasia, usually present at birth over the trunk and extremities; red papillomatosis of the skin or mucosae of the oral, anal, or genital region; hypohidrosis; paper-thin nails; sparseness of the hair; lichenoid and follicular hyperkeratotic papules; keratotic lesions on the palms and soles; focal alopecia in areas of severe aplasia or atrophy; polydactyly; clinodactyly; ver-

---

Table 7–9. DYSKERATOSIS CONGENITA

1. A rare X-linked disorder (mostly males)
2. A triad of poikilodermatous lesions (atrophy, hyperpigmentation, and telangiectasia), nail dystrophy, and leukoplakia
3. Cutaneous malignancy (predominantly epidermoid carcinoma) and carcinoma in areas of leukoplakia (usually between third and fifth decades)
4. Atrophic changes of muscles and bones of the hands and feet

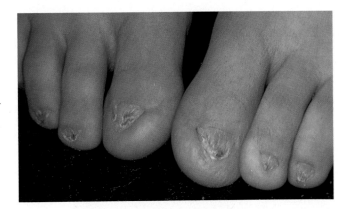

Figure 7–28. Dyskeratosis congenita. Thin dystrophic nails with longitudinal grooving.

tebral anomalies; scoliosis; spina bifida; and aplasia or hypoplasia of the "right" clavicle. Other associated abnormalities include umbilical or inguinal hernia, strabismus, colobomas, microphthalmia, hypodontia and hypoplasia of the dental enamel, cleft lip and/or cleft palate, and, in some affected individuals, microcephaly and mental retardation (Table 7–10).

Disorders included in the differential diagnosis of this condition include congenital ectodermal dysplasia, congenital poikiloderma (Rothmund-Thomson syndrome), incontinentia pigmenti, linear scleroderma, and nevus lipomatosus cutaneous superficialis of Hoffmann and Zurhelle (an extremely rare cutaneous nevus of localized groups of soft papules or nodules manifested in the newborn).

Virtually all cases of focal dermal hypoplasia reveal fine parallel linear striations in the metaphyses of long bones at or near epiphyseal junctions on radiographs. Although striations can be seen with other bony abnormalities, this linear change in the metaphyseal regions of the long bones (termed *osteopathia striata*) is a very useful index for the diagnosis of this disorder. When there is doubt, the diagnosis can be verified by biopsy of an affected area of the skin. Histopathologic features consist of absence or hypoplasia of dermal connective tissue with upward extension of the subcutaneous fat tissue almost to the normal epidermis.

Except for surgery for developmental defects such as syndactyly or polydactyly and removal of papillomas of the skin or mucous membranes, very little can be done for patients with this disorder.

Elastosis Perforans Serpiginosa

Elastosis perforans serpiginosa (perforating elastoma) is a disorder of elastic tissue characterized by an annular, arciform, or linear arrangement of keratotic papules with a predilection for the posterolateral aspects of the neck and occasionally the chin, cheeks, mandibular areas of the face, antecubital fossae, elbows, and knees. Affecting predominantly males, it appears to be a genetically determined disorder of transepidermal elimination and may act as a cutaneous marker for systemic disease. Up to 44 per cent of the reported cases have been seen in association with Down's syndrome, osteogenesis imperfecta, Ehlers-Danlos syndrome type IV, pseudoxanthoma elasticum, cutis laxa, Rothmund-Thomson

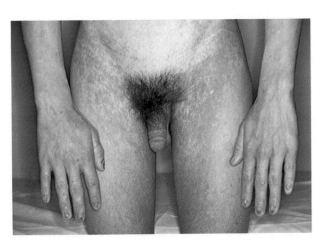

Figure 7–29. Dyskeratosis congenita. Fine, reticulated grayish brown hyperpigmentation of the thighs. (Courtesy of Department of Dermatology, Yale University School of Medicine.)

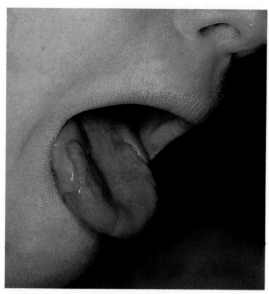

Figure 7–30. Leukoplakia on the tongue of a patient with dyskeratosis congenita.

syndrome, congenital berry aneurysm of the circle of Willis, renal disease, acrogeria, morphea, Marfan's syndrome, and, at times, as a complication of penicillamine therapy.[87, 88]

This cutaneous disorder primarily affects young persons, especially those in the second decade of life, and generally disappears spontaneously within 5 to 10 years. Characteristic features consist of deep red conical papules, 2 to 4 mm in diameter, arranged in a linear, circinate, horseshoe, or serpiginous fashion, varying from 1.0 to 2.5 cm to as much as 15 to 20 cm in overall length. The papules are generally capped by a distinctive keratotic plug, which when forcibly dislodged reveals a bleeding crateriform lesion. (Fig. 7–31).

Diagnosis depends on recognition of the characteristic keratotic plug-topped conicle papules in an annular, arciform, or linear arrangement and can be confirmed by the identification of hyphae-like fibers on microscopic examination of scraped hyperkeratotic lesions treated with 10 per cent potassium hydroxide followed by the use of Sedi-Stain, which can permit rapid diagnosis of this disorder often without the need for cutaneous biopsy.[89] The distinctive histopathologic features

---

Table 7–10. FOCAL DERMAL HYPOPLASIA (GOLTZ'S SYNDROME)

1. X-linked dominant, lethal to homozygous males
2. Linear hypoplasia of skin; soft reddish yellow fatty outpouchings of the skin in a linear distribution; large ulcers; syndactyly, "lobster-claw" deformities; colobomas of eyes; and hypoplasia of hair, nails, or teeth
3. Diagnosis:
   a. Hypoplasia or absence of dermal tissue with upward extension of subcutaneous fat
   b. Osteopathic striata (striations in metaphyses of long bones or near epiphyseal junctions)

---

consist of elongated tortuous channels within the epidermis, perforated by abnormal and degenerated elastic tissue that is extruded from the dermis.

The important feature of this disorder is recognition of the high incidence of associated systemic diseases. Although treatment, in most instances, is generally unsatisfactory and recurrences are common, stripping of the surface keratinous material by repeated application of Scotch tape has resulted in improvement of some lesions, and cryosurgical techniques may produce a satisfactory cosmetic result. Because of a high incidence of residual scar and keloid formation, removal by electrodesiccation and curettage or by surgical excision is not recommended.[87]

Keratosis Follicularis (Darier's Disease)

Keratosis follicularis (Darier's disease, Darier-White disease) is an autosomal dominant defect characterized by greasy crusted papules on the scalp, face, neck, seborrheic areas of the trunk, and flexures of the extremities (Fig. 7–32) and at times by guttate, perifollicular hypopigmentation. It typically has its onset between 8 and 15 years of age, and rarely before the age of 5 years, but the age at onset may vary from early childhood through adulthood. Although there does not appear to be any specific predilection for a particular race or sex, many authorities suggest that it occurs more frequently in males.

Lesions generally begin as pinhead- to pea-sized flesh-colored papules. Most papules are perifollicular, and as the disorder progresses, coalesce to form plaques covered with flesh-colored to yellowish brown greasy crusts that frequently tend to become purulent and malodorous. The sites of predilection are the seborrheic areas of the trunk, flanks, scalp, sides of the neck, and face (particularly the temples, forehead, ears, and nasolabial furrows). In 10 per cent of cases the lesions may occur in a zosteriform linear distribution confined to one side of the body.[90] Exacerbations during summer months and following ultraviolet exposure suggest photosensitivity as a precipitating factor in the etiology of this disorder.

Nail involvement, usually beginning as a red streak with subungual hyperkeratosis, accompanied by adjacent white steaks in the nail plate, is often the first sign of the disorder and may be the only manifestation in early childhood. Fragility, splintering, and fissuring of the nail and subungual splinter hemorrhages complete the nail changes of affected individuals. Lesions of the mucous membranes consist of small white papules or pebbly areas with verrucous white plaques simulating leukoplakia in up to 50 per cent of patients (particularly those whith a familial history of the disorder). As with nail abnormalities, lesions of the oral mucosa may be the only manifestation seen in childhood. A generalized thickening of the palms

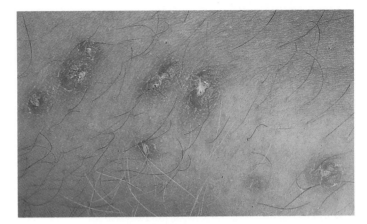

Figure 7–31. Elastosis perforans serpiginosa. Deep red conical papules appear in a linear configuration. When forcibly dislodged the distinctive keratotic plugs on individual papules reveal characteristic bleeding crateriform lesions. (Hurwitz S: The Skin and Systemic Disease in Children. Year Book Medical Publishers, Chicago, 1985.)

and soles (palmoplantar hyperkeratosis) is present in about 10 per cent of affected individuals, and punctate keratoses or minute pits may be seen on the palms and soles.

Indolent papules resembling flat warts on the dorsal aspect of the hands and feet, with lesser involvement of the volar surfaces, wrists, and ankles (a disorder termed *acrokeratosis verruciformis of Hopf*), have been described in association with Darier's disease. Although initially viewed as distinct entities, these disorders have been linked together by a growing number of observers. In its mildest form acrokeratosis verruciformis may be manifested by white nails with subungual hyperkeratosis or by punctate keratoses of the palms or soles. In its more intense form it is expressed as the more widespread changes characteristic of Darier's disease.[91]

Significant complications, including bacterial and viral infections (Kaposi's varicelliform eruption due to *Herpesvirus hominis* and coxsackievirus type A16), suggest local factors or a basic immunologic abnormality of T-cell function as the genesis of increased susceptibility to infection seen in individuals with this disorder.[92]

Warty *dyskeratomas* are benign keratotic lesions that occur as solitary verrucous nodules on the face, neck, scalp, mouth, or neck or in the axillae. Seen primarily in adults, the lesions appear as brownish red nodules that have a soft yellowish keratotic central plug. Although warty dyskeratomas are histologically indistinguishable from lesions of Darier's disease, warty dyskeratoma represents a distinct entity and there is no clinical resemblance between these two conditions.

The diagnosis of keratosis follicularis depends on recognition of the characteristic appearance and distribution of the eruption and can be confirmed by histopathologic examination of affected areas. The histopathologic changes of Darier's disease (and warty dyskeratoma) consist of intraepidermal suprabasal clefts or lacunae, a peculiar form of dyskeratosis that results in the formation of corps ronds and grains, and irregular upward proliferation of villi (papillae lined with a single layer of basal cells) into the lacunae. "Corps ronds" are cells with a basophilic nucleus surrounded by a clear halo, and "grains" are small dark cells with a pyknotic nucleus, generally seen in the stratum corneum of the skin of affected individuals.

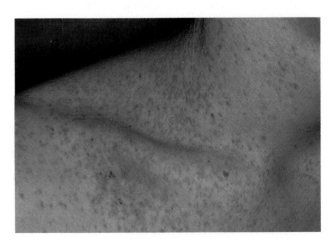

Figure 7–32. Keratosis follicularis (Darier's disease). Greasy crusted papules occur on the neck and supraclavicular areas.

At present there is no satisfactory specific therapy for Darier's disease. Patients should be instructed to avoid excessive sun exposure, heat, and humidity, since this disorder is characteristically more severe during summer and is aggravated by sunlight or ultraviolet exposure, perspiration, heat, and humidity. Large doses of oral vitamin A (200,000 to 300,000 units/day for a period of months) have been used with variable results. Because of possible toxicity with such dosages, this is generally not recommended for children. Topical vitamin A acid, although potentially irritating, has been helpful (the irritation can be minimized by use of adequate yet threshold concentrations or by the conjoint use of topical corticosteroids). Although isotretinoin and etretinate can produce dramatic and remarkable improvement for most patients, prolonged remissions are not seen and the potential toxicity of these agents limits their use in the treatment of this disorder.[93, 94]

Lipoid Proteinosis

Lipoid proteinosis (hyalinosis cutis et mucosae) is a rare chronic inherited disorder of lipid metabolism characterized by hoarseness and yellowish nodular infiltrates in the skin and mucous membranes. The exact cause of this disorder is unknown. It is an autosomal recessive trait and appears to be related to an abnormal deposition of hyaline material (believed to be a glycoprotein elaborated by fibrocytes) in the skin, mucous membranes, upper respiratory and gastrointestinal tracts, and other visceral organs, perhaps associated with an enzyme deficit of fibrocytes.[95–97]

Hoarseness secondary to vocal cord involvement is a clinical feature in virtually every case, and persons with this disorder can be recognized instantly because of their husky voice and thickened eyelids. The voice may be hoarse from birth or within the first few years of life and becomes progressively worse during early childhood. Further examination of such individuals commonly reveals hyperkeratotic plaques on elbows and knees, morphea-like plaques on the trunk, and papular infiltrates on the skin and mucous membranes.[97]

In a typical case the skin is yellow-white, resembling old ivory. Individual lesions, consisting of discrete or confluent 2- to 3-mm yellowish white to yellowish brown papules, are found most frequently on the face, eyelids, neck, and hands. In about 50 per cent of individuals a string of bead-like papules, often followed by a loss of cilia, appears on the free eyelid margins. Also characteristic are eversion of the lips (with their surfaces studded with tiny yellow nodules), hypertrophic or vegetative lesions at the corners of the mouth, and round papules just below the lip on the midline of the chin. Skin lesions, particularly in children, may also occur as vesicles, pustules, or bullae. Ulcerations; atrophic or varioliform scars; plaques simulating localized scleroderma; radiating fissures at the corners of the mouth; alopecia of the scalp, eyebrows, eyelashes, or bearded area; hypohidrosis; hypertrichosis; hypoplasia or aplasia of permanent teeth; a yellow waxy appearance with diffuse thickening of the skin (particularly in the flexures); parotid pain and recurrent parotid swelling as a result of obstruction of Stensen's duct; impaired nail growth; and multiple confluent papules seen as verrucous plaques on the elbows, knees, hands, and feet help complete the picture.

Because of hyaline deposition the tongue becomes thick, firm, and woody, is bound to the floor of the mouth, and is difficult to extrude; the soft palate, tonsils, uvula, and undersurface of the tongue show extensive irregular yellow-white infiltrations. Dysphagia caused by pharyngeal infiltration and respiratory obstruction as a result of severe laryngeal involvement can complicate the disorder. The abnormal glycoprotein has also been found in the stomach, intestine, trachea, lung, eye, pancreas, bladder, kidney, vagina, testis, lymph nodes, and striated muscle. A diabetic tendency has been stated to be part of the syndrome in 20 per cent of family members and affected individuals. This finding, however, requires further investigation and documentation. Central nervous system involvement has been associated with attacks of rage and psychomotor or grand mal epilepsy. Usually, however, the central nervous system involvement is restricted to asymptomatic calcification (seen in 70 per cent of patients older than 10 years of age), which can be seen on radiographic examination as bilateral bean-shaped opacities above the sella turcica.

Diagnosis is aided by a history of hoarseness from early childhood; thickening, stiffening, and difficulty in extrusion of the tongue; an impaired ability to swallow; characteristic involvement of the skin and mucous membranes; and histopathologic examination of involved tissue. Histologic features consist of thick homogeneous bands of eosinophilic, periodic acid–Schiff-positive, hyaline-like amorphous material in the upper dermis, with an associated patchy distribution surrounding blood vessels, sweat glands, and arrector pili muscles.

Lipoid proteinosis has a chronic but relatively benign course. Treatment is chiefly symptomatic and consists of surgical removal of laryngeal nodules or tracheostomy for laryngeal obstruction, and cosmetic measures such as dermabrasion or electrodesiccation and curettage for unappealing cutaneous lesions on the face or other exposed surfaces.

Marfan's Syndrome

Marfan's syndrome is a heritable disorder of connective tissue characterized by excessive length of long bones, ocular defects (particularly ectopia lentis), and cardiovascular defects. Inherited as an autosomal dominant trait with a high degree of penetrance and variable expressivity, it occurs in 1 in 15,000 to 20,000 persons, and up to 30 per cent of cases may represent new mutations. Skipped generations due to variable expressivity are common; and although the nature of the basic defect is unknown, the gene defect has been localized to the fibrillin gene on the long arm of chromosome 15. Studies of collagen metabolism suggest abnormalities of collagen function and cross-link formation in type I collagen, alterations in the synthesis of hyaluronic acid, and defects in the structural glycoprotein or glycoproteins of microfibrils as factors in the etiology of this complex clinical syndrome.[98, 99] Although most cases of Marfan's syndrome are diagnosed in adolescence or adulthood, a severe form of this disorder, with, at times, early fatality has also been recognized in infants during the first few months of life.[100, 101]

The chief manifestations of Marfan's syndrome are skeletal, ocular, and cardiovascular. Patients are often tall, with long extremities. The arm span characteristically is greater than the height, and after puberty the lower segment (pubis to sole) measurement is greater than that of the upper segment (vertex to pubis). Arachnodactyly, hyperextensible joints, kyphoscoliosis, pectus excavatum, and flat feet are commonly seen in patients with this disorder (Fig. 7–33). At times the great toes are elongated out of proportion to the others; the skull and face are elongated; and dolichocephaly, frontal bossing, high-arched palate, and large deformed ears are frequently seen.

Ocular abnormalities consist of ectopia lentis (the hallmark of ocular involvement, seen in 50 to 70 per cent of patients), myopia, heterochromia iridis, and retinal detachment. Cardiovascular defects, due to a defect in the media of the great vessels, consist of aneurysmal dilatation of the ascending aorta, dilatation of the aortic rings with aortic insufficiency, and dilatation of the mitral rings with mitral regurgitation. Contrary to previous emphasis, mental retardation is not a component of this syndrome. Studies suggest that Abraham Lincoln had Marfan's syndrome, and studies of some of his relatives show evidence of this disease or a forme fruste of it.[102] Cutaneous changes include a pronounced sparsity of sub-

cutaneous fat, striae (particularly over the pectoral and deltoid regions, the thighs, and abdomen), and elastosis perforans serpiginosa.

The prognosis depends on the extent and severity of cardiovascular defects. Dissection of the aorta, a frequent cause of death in children as well as adults, is common during the first decade of life and is most commonly seen during the 30s. Survival beyond the fifth decade is unusual. Although there is no specific treatment, propranolol (Inderal) has been shown to decrease myocardial contractility and to reduce the abruptness of ventricular ejection, thus limiting the progression of aortic dilatation. Surgical replacement of the aortic or mitral valve and excision of aortic aneurysms have been successful in some patients. Orthopedic surgery with casts and fusion have been beneficial for patients with kyphoscoliosis, and aspiration techniques appear to give improved results when lens extraction is necessary because of glaucoma or serious visual impairment.

Osteogenesis Imperfecta

The term *osteogenesis imperfecta* refers to a group of inherited connective tissue disorders characterized by osseous fragility, skeletal deformity, blue sclerae, impaired hearing, cutaneous fragility, hypermobility of the joints, and imperfect dentition. With an incidence of 1 in 25,000 to 30,000 births, osteogenesis imperfecta, a heterogeneous disorder in which four clinical groups have been described, along with Marfan's syndrome, ranks among the most common inherited disorders of connective tissue (Table 7–11). Abnormalities in the bone and other connective tissues of patients with the various forms of osteogenesis imperfecta suggest an abnormality of type I collagen synthesis and maturation, with secondary effects combining to produce the defects seen in patients with the various forms of this disorder.

In patients with the congenital form of osteogenesis imperfecta, multiple fractures may occur in utero or during delivery. These patients are usually stillborn or die early. Generally of low birth

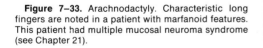
Figure 7–33. Arachnodactyly. Characteristic long fingers are noted in a patient with marfanoid features. This patient had multiple mucosal neuroma syndrome (see Chapter 21).

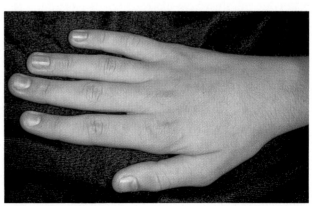

Table 7–11. OSTEOGENESIS IMPERFECTA

Group	Inheritance	Clinical Features
I Congenital (severe)	Autosomal recessive	Mild bony fragility; low birth weight; blue sclerae; deafness seldom present until adult life; severe micromelia; bowing of limbs; poorly mineralized bones with multiple fractures; dentogenesis imperfecta in some patients. Patients rarely survive infancy (beyond infancy the outlook for survival is good)
II Tarda (severe)	Heterogeneous, sporadic; some may be autosomal recessive, but new mutations may be involved	Normal birth weight; progressive deformities; prenatal short-limbed growth failure; poorly mineralized bones with recurrent fractures; blue or normal sclerae; dentogenesis imperfecta usually present; deafness uncommon; frequent neonatal deaths
III Tarda (mild)	Autosomal dominant	Fracture tendency mild (congenital fractures rare); blue sclerae; shortness, bowing and angulation of the limbs; dentogenesis imperfecta usually absent; deafness and family history of deafness common
IV Dentinogenesis imperfecta	Autosomal dominant	Patients are mildly affected; occasional fractures; normal sclerae; dentinogenesis imperfecta (cardinal feature); amber yellowish brown or a translucent bluish gray color to the teeth because of improper deposition of dentine; deafness not reported

weight, they have severe micromelia (abnormally small limbs) with bowing. Patients with the tarda variety often do not sustain fractures until later in life, generally when they are 1 or 2 years of age or older. Repeated fractures produce grotesque deformities (especially of the limbs and, in many patients, shortened stature) and affected individuals have bluish (China blue) (Fig. 7–34) to normal-colored sclerae. Patients with the dentinogenesis imperfecta form have normal sclerae, mild to moderate osteoporosis, and, occasionally, fractures.

The skin may be thin, atrophic, and somewhat translucent. Although wound healing may be normal, scars frequently are atrophic or hypertrophic. Wide fishmouth scars such as those seen in patients with Ehlers-Danlos syndrome have been described. The teeth are susceptible to caries, break easily, and have an abnormal color ranging from amber yellow to bluish gray. China-blue sclerae, when present, are a particularly distinctive feature of the disease and are seen in about 90 per cent of patients. Caused by the choroid pigment showing through the thin sclera, several hues of blue have been described. Blue sclerae, however, since they also may be seen in patients with Marfan's and Ehlers-Danlos syndromes, and at times in individuals with iron deficiency anemia, are not pathognomonic. Other features include otosclerosis with hearing loss, which may begin during the second or third decade of life, and cardiovascular lesions, including mitral and aortic valve dilatation with regurgitation, floppy mitral valve syndrome, and cystic medionecrosis of the aorta.

Diagnosis depends on the clinical manifestations and sometimes on the family history. Af-

fected bones show thinning of the cortex and trabeculae spongiosa, disorganization of collagen matrix, and poor organic bone matrix. Histopathologic examination of the skin shows a reduction in normal adult collagen fibers and an increase in argyrophilic fibers.

The treatment of osteogenesis imperfecta is difficult and frequently requires psychological as well as medical and surgical support. Since pregnancy presents a danger to an affected mother or infant, cesarean section is recommended in an effort to prevent fractures. Pinning and plating of fractures have been helpful, but immobilization

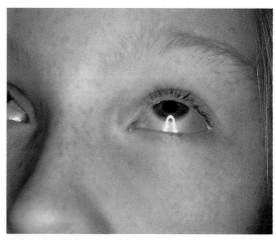

Figure 7–34. China-blue sclerae in a 12-year-old girl with osteogenesis imperfecta.

should be avoided since it results in further decrease in bone matrix. Promising results have been achieved in some cases with synthetic salmon calcitonin (Calcimar), a compound that directly inhibits bone absorption and enhances bone formation. The efficacy of this form of therapy, however, requires further confirmation.[103]

References

1. Frost P, Van Scott EJ: Ichthyosiform dermatoses. Arch. Dermatol. *94*:113–126, 1966.

   Separation of the ichthyoses on the basis of clinical and histologic features and observations of cellular kinetics.

2. Williams ML, Elias PM: Heterogeneity in autosomal recessive ichthyosis: Clinical and biochemical differentiation of lamellar ichthyosis and nonbullous congenital ichthyosiform erythroderma. Arch. Dermatol. *121*:477–488, 1985.

   Clinical, histologic, and biochemical findings allow differentiation of lamellar ichthyosis into a more severe form, classic lamellar ichthyosis, and a milder erythrodermic form, nonbullous congenital ichthyosiform erythroderma.

3. Williams ML: The ichthyoses—pathogenesis and prenatal diagnosis: A review of recent advances. Pediatr. Dermatol. *1*:1–24, 1983.

   An outstanding review of the ichthyoses and of disturbances in protein and lipid metabolism and their role in the pathogenesis of ichthyosis.

4. Frost P, Weinstein GD, Bothwell JW, et al.: Ichthyosiform dermatoses: III. Studies of epidermal water loss. Arch. Dermatol. *98*:230–233, 1968.

   Increased transepidermal water loss due to inefficient barrier function of the stratum corneum.

5. Williams ML: A new look at the ichthyoses: Disorders of lipid metabolism. Pediatr. Dermatol. *3*:476–486, 1986.

   Evidence linking aberrant lipid metabolism to the pathogenesis of ichthyosis.

6. Wells RS, Kerr CB: Clinical features of autosomal dominant and sex-linked ichthyosis in an English population. Br. Med. J. *1*:947–950, 1966.

   Separation of sex-linked ichthyosis from the autosomal dominant form of ichthyosis vulgaris.

7. Shapiro LJ, Weiss R, Webster D, et al.: X-linked ichthyosis due to steroid sulphatase deficiency. Lancet *1*:70–74, 1978.

   An assay of cultured fibroblasts identified several individuals with 3β-hydroxysteroid-sulfatase deficiency. All patients with this inborn error of metabolism had clinically apparent ichthyosis and a family history of this skin disorder compatible with an X-linked inheritance.

8. Lykkesfeldt G, Hoyer H, Lykkesfeldt AE, et al.: Steroid sulfatase deficiency associated with testicular cancer. Lancet *2*:1456, 1983.

   A report of two patients with recessive X-linked ichthyosis, steroid sulfatase deficiency, normally descended testes, and testicular cancer suggests that steroid sulfatase insufficiency may perhaps predispose patients with this disorder to testicular cancer.

9. Williams ML, Epstein EH Jr: Diagnostic tests for recessive X-linked ichthyosis. Pediatr. Dermatol. *5*:211, 1988; Hebert AA, Hood OJ: Diagnosis of X-linked ichthyosis. Pediatr. Dermatol. *5*:211–212, 1988.

   Letters to the editor review currently available diagnostic tests for recessive X-linked ichthyosis.

10. Marinkovic-Ilsen A, Wolthers BC, Jansen G, et al.: Early diagnosis of recessive X-linked ichthyosis: Elevation of cholesterol sulfate levels in placental sulfatase deficiency before the onset of skin symptoms. Pediatr. Dermatol. *3*:59–64, 1985.

    Studies of cholesterol sulfate levels in maternal blood, amniotic fluid, cord blood of infants born to women with placental sulfatae deficiency, and the cutaneous scales of patients with recessive X-linked ichthyosis.

11. Matsumoto T, Sakura N, Ueda K: Steroid sulfatase activity in nails: Screening for X-linked ichthyosis. Pediatr. Dermatol. *7*:266–269, 1990.

    A method of assaying steroid sulfatase activity in nails.

12. Hazell M, Marks R: Clinical, histologic and cell kinetic discriminants between lamellar ichthyosis and nonbullous congenital ichthyosiform erythroderma. Arch. Dermatol. *121*:489–493, 1985.

    A review of nine patients offers data to support the hypothesis that classic lamellar ichthyosis and nonbullous congenital ichthyosiform erythroderma are separate disorders.

13. Traupe H, Kolde G, Happle R: Autosomal dominant lamellar ichthyosis: A new skin disorder. Clin. Genet. *25*:42–51, 1984.

    A report of vertical transmission of lamellar-like ichthyosis in three generations suggests an autosomal dominant form of this disorder.

14. Mirrer E, McGuire JS: Lamellar ichthyosis—response to retinoic acid (tretinoin): A case report. Arch. Dermatol. *102*:548–551, 1972.

    Dramatic response of lamellar ichthyosis to tretinoin (vitamin A acid).

15. Klaus S, Weinstein GD, Frost P: Localized epidermolytic hyperkeratosis: A form of keratoderma of the palms and soles. Arch. Dermatol. *101*:272–275, 1970.

    A histopathologic relationship between epidermolytic hyperkeratosis and some forms of keratoderma.

16. Frenk E, de Techermann F: Self-healing collodion baby: Evidence for autosomal recessive inheritance. Pediatr. Dermatol. *9*:95–97, 1992.

    A report of five spontaneously healing collodion babies without other associated disease.

17. Garty BB, Metzker A, Nitzan M: Hypernatremia in congenital lamellar ichthyosis. J. Pediatr. *95*:814, 1979.

    A report of hypernatremic dehydration, which probably occurred as a result of water loss higher than expected, in two infants with lamellar ichthyosis.

18. Beverly DW, Wheeler D: High plasma urea concentrations in collodion babies. Arch. Dis. Child. *61*:696–698, 1986.

    Although urea is not a particularly toxic substance, this report describes two collodion babies with toxicity from topical formulations containing 10 per cent urea and 5 per cent lactic acid.

19. Craig JM, Goldsmith LA, Baden H: An abnormality of keratin in the harlequin fetus. Pediatrics *46*:437–440, 1970.

    X-ray diffraction analysis of the stratum corneum of a harlequin fetus revealed the presence of an unusual fibrous protein (cross-beta fibrous protein).

20. Buxbaum MM, Goodkin PE, Fahrenbach WH, et al.: Harlequin ichthyosis with epidermal lipid abnormality. Arch. Dermatol. *115*:189–193, 1979.

    Histochemical, biochemical, and electron microscopic changes in the epidermis of a child with harlequin ichthyosis who survived for 9 months suggest a defect in epidermal lipid metabolism as the biochemical abnormality in the skin of patients with harlequin ichthyosis.

21. Elias S, Mazur M, Sabbagha R, et al.: Prenatal diagnosis of harlequin ichthyosis. Clin. Genet. *17*:275–280, 1980.

    Intrauterine studies of an infant with harlequin ichthyosis.

22. Lawlor F: Progress of a harlequin fetus to nonbullous ichthyosiform erythroderma. Pediatrics *82*:870–873, 1988.

A report of two harlequin fetuses treated with retinoids who survived to 2½ years and 6 months of age, respectively.

23. Rogers M, Scarf C: Harlequin baby treated with etretinate. Pediatr. Dermatol. 6:216–221, 1989.

A report of a child 2 years of age who, born with the harlequin syndrome, showed a surprising degree of spontaneous improvement in the first 6 weeks of life and derived considerable improvement from etretinate treatment.

24. Roberts LJ: Long-term survival of a harlequin fetus. J. Am. Acad. Dermatol. 21:335–339, 1989.

A 9-year-old girl who, born as a harlequin fetus, survived and displayed clinical and histologic features similar to those of patients with nonbullous congenital ichthyosiform erythroderma.

25. Gewirtzman GB, Winkler NW, Dobson RL: Erythrokeratodermia variabilis: A family study. Arch. Dermatol. 114:259–261, 1978.

Studies of erythrokeratodermia variabilis in a family with 12 involved members in five generations.

26. Ruiz-Maldonado R, Tamayo L, DelCastillo V, et al.: Erythrokeratodermia progressive symmetrica. Dermatologica 164:133–141, 1982.

A report of 10 patients with symmetric progressive erythrokeratodermia.

27. Nazzaro V, Blanchet-Bardon C: Progressive symmetric erythrokeratodermia: Histological and ultrastructural study of a patient before and after treatment with etretinate. Arch. Dermatol. 122:434–440, 1986.

Report of a case of progressive symmetric erthrokeratodermia with clinical, histologic, and ultrastructural findings before and after treatment with etretinate.

28. Rand RE, Baden HP: The ichthyoses: A review. J. Am. Acad. Dermatol. 8:285–305, 1983.

A review of the ichthyoses with emphasis on their differentiation and management.

29. Rappaport IP, Goldes JA, Goltz RW: Erythrokeratodermia variabilis treated with isotretinoin: A clinical, histologic and ultrastructural study. Arch. Dermatol. 122:441–445. 1986.

A woman with erythrokeratodermia variabilis was successfully treated with isotretinoin but, as in other chronic disorders of keratinization, relapse ensued when treatment was discontinued.

30. Hurwitz S, Kirsch N, McGuire J: Re-evaluation of ichthyosis and hair shaft abnormalities. Arch. Dermatol. 103:266–271, 1971.

A patient with ichthyosis linearis circumflexa and a reappraisal of Netherton's syndrome, ichthyosis, and hair shaft abnormalities.

31. Herndon JH Jr, Steinberg D, Uhlendorf BS, et al.: Refsum's disease: Characterization of the enzyme defect in cell culture. J. Clin. Invest. 48:1017–1032, 1969.

Patients with Refsum's disease appear to be deficient in α-decarboxylase and therefore accumulate phytanic acid in their serum and tissues.

32. Sjögren T, Larsson T: A clinical and genetic study: Oligophrenia in combination with congenital ichthyosis and spastic disorders. Acta Psychiatr. Neurol. Scand. 32(suppl. 113):9–112, 1957.

All cases of this disorder appear to be explained by mutation of a recessive gene that occurred in a heterozygote in Northern Sweden in the 14th century.

33. Jagell S, Lidén S: Ichthyosis in Sjögren-Larsson syndrome. Clin. Genet. 21:243–252, 1982.

A description of Sjögren-Larsson ichthyosis based on a review of 36 patients.

34. Kousseff BG, Matsuoka LY, Stenn KS, et al.: Prenatal diagnosis of Sjögren-Larsson syndrome. J. Pediatr. 101:998–1001, 1982.

Studies demonstrate the value of fetoscopic biopsy for the prenatal diagnosis of Sjögren-Larsson syndrome.

35. Rizzo WB, Dammann AL, Craft DL, et al.: Sjögren-Larsson syndrome: Inherited defect in fatty alcohol cycle. J. Pediatr. 115:228–234, 1989.

Studies suggest that excess fatty alcohol or its metabolic products may be responsible for the pathologic changes in patients with the Sjögren-Larsson syndrome.

36. Judge MR, Lake BD, Smith VV, et al.: Depletion of alcohol (hexanol) dehydrogenase activity in the epidermis and jejunal mucosa in Sjögren-Larsson syndrome. J. Invest. Dermatol. 95:632–634, 1990.

A histochemical technique appears to offer a reliable test for the screening of patients with ichthyosis as well as, perhaps, carriers of the Sjögren-Larsson syndrome.

37. Bodian EL: Skin manifestations of Conradi's disease: Chondrodystrophia congenita punctata. Arch. Dermatol. 94:743–748, 1966.

A review of Conradi's disease and report of a newborn with classic features of this disorder.

38. Spranger JW, Opitz JM, Bidder U: Heterogeneity of chondrodysplasia punctata. Humangenetik. 11:190–212, 1971.

A review of reported cases of chondrodysplasia punctata and categorization of the disorder into two major forms with different modes of inheritance, radiologic changes, and prognosis.

39. Happle R: Cataracts as a marker of genetic heterogeneity in chondrodysplasia punctata. Clin. Genet. 19:64–66, 1981.

A review of type 2 (the X-linked dominant form of) chondrodysplasia punctata in which cataracts are often seen as markers.

40. Van Scott J, Yu RJ: Control of keratinization with alphahydroxy acids and related compounds: I. Topical treatment of ichthyotic disorders. Arch. Dermatol. 110:586–590, 1974.

Topical preparations containing α-hydroxy acids and closely related compounds in the management of ichthyosiform dermatoses.

41. Leibowitz MR, Weiss R, Smith EH: Pityriasis rotunda: A cutaneous sign of malignancy in two patients. Arch. Dermatol. 119:607–609, 1983.

A report of two South African blacks with pityriasis rotunda and malignant disease in whom the cutaneous lesions cleared when the malignancies were treated.

42. Rubin MG, Mathes B: Pityriasis rotunda: Two cases in black Americans. J. Am. Acad. Dermatol. 14:74–78, 1986.

A report of two patients with pityriasis rotunda (one had a metastatic adenocarcinoma; the other had diabetes mellitus with ketoacidosis).

43. Kahana M, Levy A, Ronnen M, et al.: Pityriasis rotunda in a white patient. J. Am. Acad. Dermatol. 15:362–365, 1986.

A report of a 19-year-old white woman with pityriasis rotunda.

44. Lodi A, Betti R, Chiarelli G, et al.: Familial pityriasis rotunda. Int. J. Dermatol. 29:483–485, 1990.

In a report of three patients with pityriasis rotunda in a Sardinian family, the authors suggest that this disorder be considered a minor form of acquired ichthyosis initiated by a debilitating illness in a genetically predisposed individual.

45. Happle R, Koch R, Renz W: The CHILD syndrome: Congenital hemidysplasia and ichthyosiform erythroderma and limb defects. Eur. J. Pediatr. 134:27–33, 1980.

A report of two patients and a review of 18 previously recorded individuals with the CHILD syndrome.

46. Christianson JV, Peterson HO, Sogaard H: Congenital hemidysplasia with ichthyosiform erythroderma and limb defects: A case report. Acta Derm. Venereol. 64:165–168, 1984.

A 3-year-old girl with the CHILD syndrome who, having a negative family history, was believed to represent a spontaneous mutation of the disorder.

47. Skinner BA, Greist MC, Norins AL: The keratitis, ichthyosis and deafness (KID) syndrome. Arch. Dermatol. 117:285–289, 1981.

A report of a patient with the KID syndrome and a review of 17 similar patients described under a variety of descriptive labels.

48. Harms M, Gilardi S, Levy PM, et al.: KID syndrome (keratitis, ichthyosis, and deafness) and chronic mucocutaneous candidiasis: Case report and review of the literature. Pediatr. Dermatol. 2:1–7, 1984.

A report of a girl with the KID syndrome and chronic mucocutaneous candidiasis.

49. Grob JJ, Breton A, Bonafe JL, et al.: Keratitis, ichthyosis and deafness (KID) syndrome: Vertical transmission and death from multiple squamous cell carcinomas. Arch. Dermatol. 123:777–782, 1987.

A report of a father and daughter with KID syndrome, the first report of vertical transmission of this disorder, demonstrates the hereditary nature and emphasizes its seriousness—in the case of the father, it was complicated by fatal cutaneous carcinomas.

50. Jurecka W, Aberer E, Mainitz M, et al.: Keratitis, ichthyosis and deafness with glycogen storage. Arch. Dermatol. 121:799–801, 1985.

A 7-year-old girl with the KID syndrome and glycogen storage disease.

51. Elias PM, Williams ML: Neutral lipid storage disease with ichthyosis: Defective lamellar body contents and intracellular dispersion. Arch. Dermatol. 121:1000–1008, 1985.

Studies of skin biopsy material from three family members of a kindred with the Chanarin-Dorfman syndrome provide strong support that lamellar body–derived lipids influence stratum corneum desquamation and that abnormalities of neutral lipid–alkane metabolism provoke the hyperplasia of the epidermis in patients with this disorder.

52. Srebrnik A, Tur E, Perluk C, et al.: Dorfman-Chanarin syndrome: A case report and a review. J. Am. Acad. Dermatol. 17:801–808, 1987.

A report of two sisters of Jewish-Iraqi origin with the Dorfman-Chanarin syndrome and a review of previously reported cases of patients with this disorder.

53. Venencie PY, Armengaude D, Foldés C, et al.: Ichthyosis and neutral lipid storage disease (Dorfman-Chanarin syndrome). Pediatr. Dermatol. 5:173–177, 1988.

A report of a family of a boy with the Dorfman-Chanarin syndrome suggests an autosomal recessive mode of inheritance.

54. Levy SB, Goldsmith LA: The peeling skin syndrome. J. Am. Acad. Dermatol. 7:606–613, 1982.

A report of two patients with the peeling skin syndrome.

55. Neilson PG: Hereditary palmoplantar keratoderma and dermatophytosis. Int. J. Dermatol. 27:223–231, 1988.

An increased incidence of dermatophytosis suggests a predisposition to dermatophyte infection in individuals with hereditary palmoplantar keratoderma.

56. Goldfarb MT, Woo TY, Rasmussen JE: Keratoderma hereditaria mutilans (Vohwinkel's syndrome): A trial of isotretinoin. Pediatr. Dermatol. 3:216–218, 1985.

Although an 8-year-old girl with Vohwinkel's syndrome achieved a modest degree of improvement following a 12-week course of isotretinoin, treatment was discontinued because of concern of risk of long-term therapy associated with the use of this modality.

57. Nguyen TQ, Greer KE, Fisher GB Jr, et al.: Papillon-Lefèvre syndrome: Report of two patients successfully treated with isotretinoin. J. Am. Acad. Dermatol. 15:46–49, 1986.

Keratoderma in two women with the Papillon-Lefèvre syndrome was greatly improved within 2 weeks after the initiation of isotretinoin therapy.

58. Poulin Y, Perry HO, Muller SA: Olmstead syndrome: Congenital palmoplantar and periorificial keratoderma. J. Am. Acad. Dermatol. 10:600–610, 1984.

A report of a patient with the Olmstead syndrome who initially presented with clinical features suggesting a diagnosis of acrodermatitis enteropathica.

59. Dilaimy MS, Owen WB, Sina B: Keratosis punctata of the palmar creases. Cutis 33:394–396, 1984.

A review of 19 patients with punctate keratoses of the palmar creases.

60. Bennion SD, Patterson JW: Keratosis punctata et plantaris and adenocarcinoma of the colon. J. Am. Acad. Dermatol. 10:587–591, 1984.

A review of three of eight family members with punctate keratoderma who developed gastrointestinal carcinomas suggests a possible association between the two disorders.

61. Sybert VP: Hypohidrotic ectodermal dysplasia: Argument against an autosomal recessive form clinically indistinguishable from X-linked hypohidrotic ectodermal dysplasia (Christ-Siemens-Touraine syndrome). Pediatr. Dermatol. 6:76–81, 1989.

A critical review of previously reported cases of presumed autosomal recessive hypohidrotic ectodermal dysplasia (HED) suggests that all sporadic instances of females with classic HED should be considered to be X-linked recessive.

62. Wassertail V, Bruce S: Fever and hypotrichosis in a newborn. Arch. Dermatol. 122:1325–1330, 1985.

A report of an infant with hypohidrotic ectodermal dysplasia and a review of the clinical features and management of this disorder.

63. Happle R, Frosch PJ: Manifestation of the lines of Blaschko in women heterozygous for X-linked hypohidrotic ectoderma dysplasia. Clin. Genet. 27:468–471, 1985.

The authors conclude that the results of sweat tests in the lines of Blaschko on the back may be a more reliable method of carrier detection than the search for a mosaic pattern of lyonization on the fingertips and the palms.

64. Kleinbrecht J, Degenhart K-H, Grubisic A, et al.: Sweat pore counts in ectodermal dysplasias. Hum. Genet. 57:437–439, 1981.

Sweat pore counts were found to be helpful in the diagnosis and genetic counseling of individuals with hypohidrotic ectodermal dysplasia.

65. Lambert WC, Bilinski DL: Diagnostic pitfalls in anhidrotic ectodermal dysplasia: Indications for palmar skin biopsy. Cutis 31:182–187, 1983.

Palmar skin biopsy is suggested as an aid to the diagnosis of hypohidrotic ectodermal dysplasia.

66. Cupo LN, Pyeritz RE, Olson JL, et al.: Ehlers-Danlos syndrome with abnormal collagen fibrils, sinus of Valsalva aneurysms, myocardial infarction, panacinar emphysema and cerebral heterotopias. Am. J. Med. 71:1051–1058, 1981.

A report of a woman with Ehlers-Danlos syndrome who failed to fit into any of the 10 previously described subtypes of this disorder.

67. Pinnell SR: Molecular defects in the Ehlers-Danlos syndrome. J. Invest. Dermatol. 79:90s–92s, 1982.

A review of the biochemical defects in Ehlers-Danlos syndrome types IV, V, VI, and VII.

68. Nelson DL, King RA: Ehlers-Danlos syndrome type VIII. J. Am. Acad. Dermatol. 5:297–303, 1981.

Three members of a family with features of Ehlers-Danlos syndrome type VIII.

69. Arneson MA, Hammerschmidt DE, Furcht LT, et al.: A new form of Ehlers-Danlos syndrome: I. Fibronectin corrects defective platelet function. J.A.M.A. *244*:144–147, 1980.

Fibronectin, platelet malfunction, and joint hypermobility are described as clinical features of patients with Ehlers-Danlos syndrome type IX.

70. Hammerschmidt DE, Arneson MA, Larson SL, et al.: Maternal Ehlers-Danlos syndrome type X: Successful management of pregnancy and parturition. J.A.M.A. *248*:2487–2488, 1982.

A report of a woman with fibronectin-deficient Ehlers-Danlos syndrome who gave birth to a normal infant demonstrates that normal pregnancies and childbirth are possible in individuals with Ehlers-Danlos syndrome type X.

71. Elsas LJ, Miller RL, Pinnell SR: Inherited human collagen lysyl hydroxylase deficiency: Ascorbic acid response. J. Pediatr. *92*:378–384, 1978.

Ascorbic acid appears to help reduce bruising of the skin in patients with type XI Ehlers-Danlos syndrome.

72. Goltz RW, Hult AM, Goldfarb M, et al.: Cutis laxa: Manifestations of generalized elastolysis. Arch. Dermatol. *92*:373–387, 1965.

A decrease in serum elastase inhibitor appears to cause increased fragmentation of elastic fibers in patients with cutis laxa.

73. Hatamochi A, Wada T, Takeda K, et al.: Collagen metabolism in cutis laxa fibroblasts: Increased collagenase gene expression associated with unaltered expression of type I and type III collagen. J. Invest. Dermatol. *97*:483–487, 1991.

Data suggest that increased collagenase expression of fibroblasts is related to the structural abnormality of dermal connective tissue in cutis laxa.

74. Sakati NO, Nyhan WL: Congenital cutis laxa and osteoporosis. Am. J. Dis. Child. *137*:452–454, 1983.

A report of a 16-month-old infant with cutis laxa who was incapacitated by osteoporosis.

75. Fisher BK, Page E, Hanna W: Acral localized acquired cutis laxa. J. Am. Acad. Dermatol. *21*:33–40, 1989.

A patient who developed an acral localized form of acquired cutis laxa at the age of 13 years.

76. Koch SE, Williams ML: Acquired cutis laxa: Case report and review of disorders of elastolysis. Pediatr. Dermatol. *4*:282–288, 1985.

A case report of a 10-year-old boy who developed cutis laxa while receiving isoniazid and a review of disorders of elastolysis.

77. Lewis PG, Hood AF, Burnett NK, et al.: Postinflammatory elastolysis and cutis laxa. J. Am. Acad. Dermatol. *22*:40–48, 1990.

The first report of postinflammatory elastolysis and cutis laxa, a disorder previously reported only in African and South American children, in a white child from North America.

78. Lever WR, Schaumburg-Lever G: Histopathology of the Skin, 7th ed. JB Lippincott Co., Philadelphia, 1990.

An authoritative review of dermatopathology.

79. Lebwohl MG, Distefano D, Prioleau PG, et al.: Pseudoxanthoma elasticum and mitral valve prolapse. N. Engl. J. Med. *307*:228–231, 1982.

In a review of 14 patients with pseudoxanthoma elasticum, 10 patients (71 per cent) had evidence of mitral valve prolapse.

80. Fleischmajer R, Nedwich A: Progeria (Hutchinson-Gilford). Arch. Dermatol. *107*:253–258, 1973.

A nine-year-old child with sclerodermatous lesions and typical features of progeria.

81. DeBusk FL: The Hutchinson-Gilford progeria syndrome. J. Pediatr. *80*:697–724, 1972.

A report of four patients with progeria and a comprehensive review of 60 patients with this disorder.

82. Badame AJ: Progeria. Arch. Dermatol. *125*:540–544, 1989.

Sporadic autosomal dominant mutation is proposed as the mode of inheritance for progeria, an extremely rare disorder in which fewer than 80 patients have been reported since the turn of the century.

83. Khalifa MM: Hutchinson-Gilford syndrome: Report of a Libyan family and evidence of autosomal recessive inheritance. Clin. Genet. *35*:125–132, 1989.

A report of progeria affecting three children of two sisters provides strong support for an autosomal recessive pattern of inheritance in individuals with this disorder.

84. Carter DM, Gaynor A, McGuire J: Sister chromatid exchanges in dyskeratosis congenita after exposure to trimethyl psoralen and UV light. In Hanawalt PC, Friedberg EC, Fox CF (Eds.): DNA Repair Mechanisms. ICN-UCLA Symposium on Molecular and Cellular Biology, IX. Academic Press, Inc., New York, 1978, 671–674.

Studies suggest that dyskeratosis congenita is associated with a heritable defect in the repair of DNA cross-links.

85. Ling NF, Fenske NA, Julieus RL, et al.: Dyskeratosis congenita in a girl simulating chronic graft-vs-host disease. Arch. Dermatol. *121*:1424–1428, 1985.

Dyskeratosis congenita and graft-versus-host disease share several clinical and histologic features.

86. Goltz RW, Henderson RR, Hitch JM, et al.: Focal dermal hypoplasia syndrome, a review of the literature and report of two cases. Arch. Dermatol. *101*:1–11, 1970.

Report of two patients and a review of the distinguishing features of this disorder.

87. Christianson HB: Elastosis perforans serpiginosa: Association with congenital anomalies: Report of 2 cases. South. Med. J. *59*:15–19, 1966.

Two patients with elastosis perforans serpiginosa (one of whom had a congenital berry aneurysm of the circle of Willis), and review of 66 patients, of whom 44 per cent had associated congenital defects or anomalies.

88. Mehregan HM: Elastosis perforans serpiginosa: A review of the literature and report of 11 cases. Arch. Dermatol. *97*:381–393, 1968.

Pathologic changes of elastosis perforans serpiginosa, an attempt at transepidermal elimination of elastic tissue.

89. Feldman SR, Woosley JT: Use of Sedi-Stain for the diagnosis of elastosis perforans serpiginosa. J. Am. Acad. Dermatol. *20*:1137–1138, 1989.

A rapid Sedi-stain technique can avoid the need for biopsy for the diagnosis of patients with elastosis perforans serpiginosa.

90. Leeming JAL: Acquired linear nevus showing histologic features of keratosis follicularis. Br. J. Dermatol. *81*:128–131, 1969.

Linear and zosteriform configurations in Darier's disease.

91. Herndon JH Jr, Wilson JD: Acrokeratosis verruciformis (Hopf) and Darier's disease. Arch. Dermatol. *93*:305–310, 1966.

A review of 12 members of a single family with acrokeratosis verruciformis, Darier's disease, and minor disturbances of keratinization supports the thesis that Darier's disease and acrokeratosis verruciformis result from a single dominant defect.

92. Jegosathy BV, Humeniuk JM: Darier's disease: A partially immunodeficient state. J. Invest. Dermatol. *76*:129–132, 1981.

Studies of eight patients with Darier's disease suggest a

subtle defective cellular immunity in a subset of patients with this disorder.

93. Dicken CH, Bauer EA, Hazen PG, et al.: Isotretinoin treatment of Darier's disease. J. Am. Acad. Dermatol. 6:721–726, 1982.

A study of 104 patients revealed that treatment with isotretinoin, although helpful, failed to induce long-term remission in patients with Darier's disease.

94. Burge S, Wilkinson J, Miller JA: The efficacy of an aromatic retinoid, Tigason (etretinate), in the treatment of Darier's disease. Br. J. Dermatol. 104:675–679, 1981.

Etretinate, like isotretinoin, can be helpful for short-term management of patients with Darier's disease.

95. Caplan RM: Visceral involvement in lipoid proteinosis. Arch. Dermatol. 95:149–155, 1967.

Lipoid proteinosis in the intestine, pancreas, lung, kidney, lymph nodes, and striated muscle confirms the systemic nature of this disorder.

96. Hashimoto K, Klingmüller G, Rodermund OE: Hyalinosis cutis et mucosae. Acta Derm. Venereol. 52:179–195, 1972.

Electron microscopic studies show the hyalin infiltrate to be an abnormal product of fibroblasts.

97. Shore RN, Howard BV, Howard WJ, et al.: Lipoid proteinosis: Demonstration of normal lipid metabolism in cultured cells. Arch. Dermatol. 110:591–594, 1974.

An assay of fibroblast lipids from tissues from a cutaneous lesion of a woman with lipoid proteinosis revealed normal quantities of all lipid fractions, apparently confirming the fact that the accumulation of lipid in lesions of this disorder is a secondary phenomenon, probably due to the affinity between lipoproteins and glycoproteins.

98. Kainulainen K, Pulkkinen L, Savolainen A, et al.: Location on chromosome 15 of the gene defect causing Marfan syndrome. N. Engl. J. Med. 323:935–939, 1990.

Using linkage analyses with polymorphic markers of the human genone, the genetic defect of Marfan's syndrome was linked to chromosome 15.

99. Hollister DW, Godfrey M, Sakai LY, et al.: Immunohistologic abnormalities of the microfibrillar-fiber system in the Marfan syndrome. N. Engl. J. Med. 323:152–159, 1990.

Indirect immunofluorescence studies of skin and cultured dermal fibroblasts from patients with Marfan's syndrome suggest a deficiency of the microfibrillar-fiber system as the cause of the clinical manifestations of this disorder.

100. Gross DM, Robinson LK, Smith LT, et al.: Severe perinatal Marfan syndrome. Pediatrics 84:83–89, 1989.

Clinical, radiographic, and echocardiographic data in three patients with a severe perinatal form of Marfan's syndrome, a distinct subset in which patients suffer from severe cardiorespiratory problems and limited life expectancy.

101. Morse RP, Rockenmacher S, Pyeritz RE, et al.: Diagnosis and management of infantile Marfan syndrome. Pediatrics 86:888–895, 1990.

A report of 22 severely affected infants diagnosed as having Marfan's syndrome in the first 3 months of life and a review of the literature describing 32 additional infants with this variant of the disorder.

102. Gordon AM: Abraham Lincoln—a medical appraisal. J. Ky. Med. Assoc. 60:249–253, 1962.

Marfan's syndrome is believed to explain Abraham Lincoln's tall stature, loose-jointedness, kyphoscoliosis, dolichocephaly, and unusually long thin arms and legs.

103. Rosenberg E, Lang R, Boisseu V, et al.: Effect of long-term calcitonin therapy on the clinical course of osteogenesis imperfecta. J. Clin. Endocrinol. Metab. 44:346–355, 1977.

Calcitonin therapy appears to be helpful in the management of patients with osteogenesis imperfecta.

8

CUTANEOUS TUMORS IN CHILDHOOD

Because of their frequency and an increasing public awareness of skin cancer, physicians are continuously consulted regarding tumors or tumor-like lesions of the skin. In children the vast majority of cutaneous tumors are benign, and their importance lies predominantly in the cosmetic defect they may create or in their occasional association with systemic disease. Malignant lesions, however, despite their relative rarity, cannot be disregarded or ignored. Each lesion, in children as well as adults, must be assessed individually, with particular emphasis as to its cosmetic effect, its possible association with systemic disease, and its capacity for malignant degeneration.

Cutaneous tumors can be differentiated into those of the epidermal surface; those of epidermal appendages; those of fibrous, neural, vascular, fatty, muscular, and osseous tissues; those that are melanocytic; and those that are malignant. The term *nevus* has a broad meaning in dermatology. It refers to a circumscribed congenital abnormality of any cell type present at birth. When this term is used, therefore, it is appropriate to include a qualifying adjective (e.g., *epidermal, melanocytic, pigmented,* or *vascular*), thus specifying the particular cell of origin. Through common usage, however, this term is also used in a loose manner to refer to a benign tumor or pigment cells. In contrast to nevi, moles are pigmented cutaneous lesions *not* present at birth that are apparently hereditarily predetermined. Included in this group are pigmented nevocellular nevi and lentigines that develop after birth. In general, moles that appear during childhood and adolescence are flat or slightly elevated lesions. In adulthood they tend to be polypoid or dome-shaped, sessile, or papillomatous.

PIGMENTED MOLES AND NEVI

Pigmented moles and nevi are the most common neoplasms found in humans. Previous reviews suggest the incidence of moles and nevi to be 3 per cent in white and 16 per cent in black infants at birth. Although a study of 1,058 newborns younger than 72 hours of age noted pigmented lesions in 4 per cent of infants, cutaneous biopsies revealed only one third of these to be true melanocytic (nevus cell) nevi. This indicates that the incidence of melanocytic nevi in newborns is slightly more than 1 per cent.[1, 2] The incidence of melanocytic nevi increases throughout infancy and adulthood, reaching a peak at puberty and adolescence. The size and pigmentation of lesions also increase at puberty, during pregnancy, or following systemic estrogen or corticosteroid therapy. Acquired nevomelanocytic nevi are believed to appear after the first 6 to 12 months of life and enlarge with body growth. By 25 years of age most whites acquire their maximum number of lesions, usually 20 to 40 per person; in later life most lesions tend to fade and eventually disappear. In blacks, the over-all incidence of nevocellular nevi is lower and there tends to be a higher prevalence in those with lighter skin.

Pigmented nevi and tumors may be composed of melanocytes or nevus cells. The melanocyte is a dendritic cell that produces melanin and transfers it to the keratinocytes and hair cells, thus supplying all the normal brown pigment to skin and hair. Both melanocytes and nevus cells are of neural origin. Melanocytes originate in the neural crest and early in fetal life migrate from there with the nerves to the skin. After birth melanocytes will occasionally remain in the dermis of certain races (Asians, Native Americans, blacks, and individuals from the Mediterranean area), where they usually appear as mongolian spots. Blue nevi and the nevi of Ota and Ito also represent examples of melanocytic migration in which the melanoblasts remain in the dermis.

For many years there were two popular theories on the origin of pigment cell tumors. According to the most popular concept, nevus cells have a dual derivation and develop from the melanocytes in the epidermis and Schwann cells of the neural sheath.[3] Schwann cells line the peripheral nerves and appear to form a pathway between the central nervous system and the skin. As peripheral nerves branch into cutaneous nerve twigs, Schwann cells migrate into the dermis and give rise to a number of dermal tumors. Nevus cells, therefore, may locate at the dermal-epidermal junction (where they appear clinically as junction nevi), within the dermis (as intradermal nevi), or as a combination of both (compound nevi).

The contrasting theory suggests that nevus cells arise from a bipotential precursor cell (nevoblast) capable of developing into a melanoblastic or schwannian nevoblast.[4] In this theory the nevoblasts develop into epidermal nevus cells that give rise to the junction nevus and compound nevus; the schwannian nevoblasts develop into neural nevus cells and the intradermal nevus.

Nevocellular Nevi

Lesions composed of nevus cells are termed *nevocellular* or *pigmented nevi*. Subdivided and described on the basis of the location of the nevus cells, they may be designated as *junctional, intradermal,* or *compound lesions*. Junctional nevi have nevus cell nests confined to the dermal-epidermal junction (above the basement membrane separating the epidermis from the dermis). Intradermal moles and nevi have these nests in the dermis alone, and compound nevi have nevus cells in both locations.

Pigmented moles and nevi have a wide range of clinical appearances. They may occur anywhere on the cutaneous or mucocutaneous surface and range from flat to slightly elevated or dome-shaped, nodular, verrucous, polypoid, or papillomatous. Those that are flat (macular) are generally junctional (Fig.

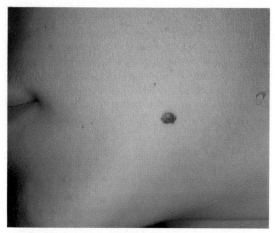

Figure 8–1. Junctional nevus. In contrast to a malignant melanoma, the skin surface is generally smooth and flat and skin furrows are preserved.

8–1). Lesions with only slight elevation are usually compound, and those that are nodular, dome-shaped, polypoid, or papillomatous tend to be intradermal (Fig. 8–2).

JUNCTIONAL NEVI

Junctional nevi are generally hairless, light to dark brown or brownish black macules. They range from 1 mm to 1 cm in diameter; their surface is smooth and flat; and skin furrows are preserved. Although most lesions are round, elliptical, or oval and show a relatively uniform pigmentation, some may be slightly irregular in configuration and color. Most junctional nevi represent a transient phase in the development of compound nevi and are found only in children. An exception to this rule, however, is seen on the palms, soles, and genitalia where the lesions generally retain their junctional appearance.

The nevus cell is the microscopic feature of all nevus cell nevi. In junctional nevi the cells are present as single cells or nests of nevus cells in the lower epidermis or immediately adjacent dermis. Those still in contact with the epidermis are said to be in the "dropping off" stage. Nevus cells are cuboidal, have a benign appearance without pleomorphism, and, when seen in nests, are characterized by an orderly arrangement and a central focus.

COMPOUND NEVI

Although more common in older children and adults, compound nevi may also be present at birth.[1, 2] Often similar in appearance to junctional nevi, they tend to be more elevated and accordingly vary from a slightly raised plaque to a lesion of a somewhat more papillomatous nature. They are flesh colored to brown, may have a smooth or warty surface, and, particularly when seen on the face, may have dark coarse hairs within the lesion (Fig. 8–3). In late childhood and adolescence, compound nevi frequently tend to increase in thickness and depth of pigmentation. It is at this stage that many children are brought to the physician for evaluation.

Compound nevi possess histologic features of both junctional and intradermal nevi. In this form, nevus cells are seen within the epidermis as well as in the dermis. The nevus cells in the lower part of the dermis frequently are spindle shaped and may extend around appendages and neurovascular bundles.

INTRADERMAL NEVI

Intradermal nevi are seen most frequently in adults. They are usually dome shaped, sessile (attached by a broad base), or pedunculated and range from a few millimeters to 1 cm or more in diameter. Often clinically indistinguishable from compound nevi, they vary from nonpigmented lesions to those of varying shades of brown to black

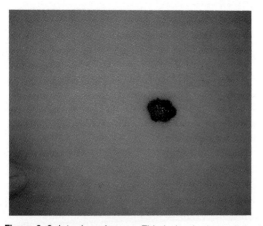

Figure 8–2. Intradermal nevus. This lesion is dome-shaped, slightly elevated, and irregularly pigmented.

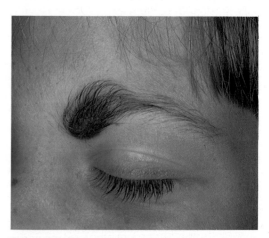

Figure 8–3. Compound nevus. Compound nevi tend to be more elevated, have a smooth or papillomatous surface, and, particularly when seen on the face, may contain dark coarse hairs.

(see Fig. 8–2). They may occur anywhere on the cutaneous surface and are frequently found on the head and neck; coarse hairs often are present. In older individuals intradermal nevi predominate. After the third decade of life, as maturation continues, there is often destruction and replacement of nevus cells by fibrous or fatty tissue, and by 70 years of age most individuals have few remaining moles or nevi.

On histopathologic examination, intradermal nevi reveal nests and cords of nevus cells, little to no junctional activity, and spindle-shaped nevus cells in the lower dermis. Multinucleated giant cells, with rosettes or clumping of small dark-staining nuclei, may be seen within the nests or theques. These giant cells occur only in mature nevi, are indicative of the benign nature of the lesion, and should not be confused with the more irregularly shaped giant cells seen in malignant melanomas or benign spindle cell tumors of Spitz.

For years it was presumed that malignant melanomas arise from preexisting junctional nevi. It is now conceded, however, that junctional moles are no more precancerous than other pigmented lesions and that malignant melanomas may originate from melanocytes in normal skin as well as those of pigmented nevi. The increased frequency of malignant change in moles appears to be related to an increased number of melanocytes in these lesions rather than to an inherent predisposition to malignant change on the part of melanocytes in pigmented lesions.

Treatment

The therapy for pigmented moles and nevi is usually related to their cosmetic appearance or the fear of potential malignant change. The majority of melanocytic lesions require no treatment; by careful clinical evaluation the patient can frequently be reassured as to their benign nature. Removal of nevi, when indicated, can be accomplished by shave excision techniques, shave excision and electrodesiccation, or complete elliptical extirpation (depending on the size, shape, and location of the lesion). Pedunculated tumors can be clipped off flush to the skin with scissors. Dome-shaped and other elevated nevi can be further elevated by injection of a local anesthetic beneath the lesion, and the elevated portion then may be shaved or sliced off level with the skin. Because of the mobility and muscularity of the upper arms, back, and shoulders, elliptical excision of moles in these areas often results in spreading of the scar and eventually a less cosmetically acceptable result.

Although some authorities suggest that simple shave excision with electrodesiccation of the underlying base may predispose to future malignant change, most lesions removed for cosmetic reasons or for reassurance can be shaved off with saucerization to include a portion of the underlying subcutaneous fat under local anesthesia. Such a procedure often yields a superior cosmetic result and frequently provides a specimen adequate for histopathologic examination. No matter which of these methods is used, careful histopathologic examination of all of the specimen is imperative.

After superficial removal of pigmented lesions a certain number will show a recurrence, often causing anxiety to the patient, parent, and, at times, the physician. This is not necessarily an indication of inadequate removal of malignancy but usually represents partial regrowth of nevus cells from the peripheral epidermis or hair root sheath.[5]

In the past, many authors advocated routine excision of pigmented lesions in certain anatomic locations (the palms, soles, and genitalia), owing to the belief that the likelihood of malignant transformation was greater in these areas. Allyn and his associates reviewed the incidence of malignancy of pigmented lesions on the palms and soles. On the basis of these and other studies it now appears that prophylactic removal of all pigmented lesions in these areas is neither warranted nor feasible.[6] The role that trauma plays as a cause of malignant transformation also remains to be proved. Removal of lesions in areas of trauma, therefore, is probably more a matter of convenience than a bona fide prophylactic measure.

Malignant Melanoma

The incidence of malignant melanoma in childhood is relatively low (approximately 2 per cent of malignant melanomas occur in children younger than 20 years of age).[7] Despite this rarity, the course of melanoma, when it does occur, bears the same prognosis as it does in adults. Many lesions previously thought to be melanomas of childhood are now recognized to be benign spindle cell tumors (Spitz nevi, benign juvenile melanomas). It now appears that malignant melanoma, when it occurs in childhood, is just as aggressive and potentially ominous as when it is found in adults.

Melanoma accounts for 1 to 2 per cent of fatal malignant disease in the United States and currently is associated with a mortality of 10 to 20 per cent. Of particular note is the fact that the incidence of melanoma is rising rapidly (doubling about every decade), and that its incidence is increasing in teenagers and young adults as well as in older individuals.[8, 9] Malignant melanomas most commonly affect patients with fair skin, blue eyes, and red or blond hair, particularly those of Celtic origin whose pigment cells have a limited capacity to synthesize melanin. Although melanomas may occur in blacks, the incidence, when compared with that of whites, is extremely low. In blacks, tumors usually arise in areas that are lightly pigmented, namely the mucous membranes (70 per cent), nail beds, or the sides of the palms and soles. Reports of familial cases have been documented, suggesting a genetic basis (at least in some patients) with perhaps an autosomal dominant trait with reduced penetrance.[10]

Although statistics vary, it has been estimated

that 60 to 70 per cent of malignant melanomas arise from preexisting nevi. In the average pigmented mole, however, neoplastic transformation rarely occurs, with estimates of malignant transformation of preexisting moles approaching 1 in 500,000 or 1 in 1 million lesions. The congenital pigmented nevus, however, is present in 1 per cent of all newborns. It appears to have a greater malignant potential than that seen in pigmented lesions appearing later in life,[11] and patients with a family history of melanoma and individuals with a large number of nevi appear to have a greater risk of developing cutaneous melanoma.[9]

Clinical Manifestations. Although nonpigmented (amelanotic) melanomas can occur, most malignant melanomas present as irregularly pigmented nodules with various shades of red and blue haphazardly intermingled with black, white, and brown. They often appear as deeply pigmented nodules with an irregular shape, nodules dotting the surface, absence of overlying skin markings, and occasionally surrounding erythema (Fig. 8–4). Benign pigmented lesions show order in color, symmetry or border, and uniform surface characteristics. Malignant lesions (usually but not necessarily greater than 6 mm in diameter) often lack regularity of these features; their overall color pattern is often nonhomogeneous, and their borders are frequently irregular or notched. Danger signals in pigmented nevi suggesting abnormal activity or malignant change include changes of any type, particularly rapid growth, crusting, ulceration, bleeding, change in pigmentation, the development of inflammation, satellite lesions, the loss of normal skin lines, or subjective symptoms such as tenderness, pain, or itching.

Extremely malignant, the melanoma may pro-

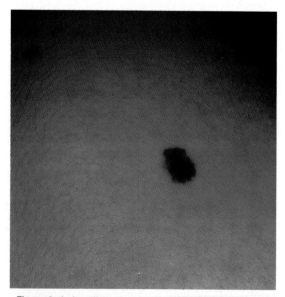

Figure 8–4. A malignant melanoma noted on the neck of a 19-year-old woman during a visit for the treatment of acne vulgaris reaffirms the need for constant vigilance for the possibility of cutaneous melanoma, even in this age group.

liferate locally, spread by satellite lesions, or extend through the lymphatics or bloodstream, from which it may eventually invade any organ of the body. Once it has begun to spread, response rates, in children as well as adults, have been low. Nodular melanomas, comprising 25 per cent of all pigment cell cancers, have the worst prognosis. They bypass the superficial spreading phase, immediately invade the dermis and subcutaneous fat, and soon metastasize to lymph nodes and distant sites. Survival rates with early diagnosis of patients with small superficial melanomas is materially higher (80 to 90 per cent) than those with large invasive lesions. The importance of early detection, therefore, is paramount.

The question of whether biopsy is advisable in a lesion suspected of being a malignant melanoma has been widely discussed. There has been widespread belief (particularly in Europe) that cutting into a melanoma, as in performing a cutaneous biopsy, may induce lymphatic or hematogenous spread or that incomplete removal can precipitate malignant degeneration in a premelanomatous junctional nevus. Many authors, however, refute this concept and believe that this procedure neither leads to spread nor alters the biologic behavior of the tumor.[12]

A melanoma that occurs beneath the nail fold is called a melanotic whitlow. The tumor begins as a brown or black discoloration, occasionally with mild deformity of the adjacent nail. Following the development of a pigmented band in the nail, granulation tissue may appear at the nail edge and the pigmented band frequently widens. *Hutchinson's sign* (pigmentation of the cuticle and dorsal skin proximal to the cuticle), however, although valuable, is not necessarily pathognomonic.[13, 14] If a melanoma is suspected, a biopsy (after a tourniquet has been placed on the finger) should be performed, frozen section should be carried out, and, if the diagnosis is confirmed, total amputation of the digit should generally be performed (Fig. 8–5).

Histopathologic examination of a typical malignant melanoma reveals irregular proliferations of melanoma cells from the dermal-epidermal junction into the dermis. These cells may vary considerably in appearance and mitotic activity. They may be cuboidal, with arrangement in irregular nests; loss of cohesiveness between cells may produce an alveolar appearance; or they may be composed primarily of spindle cells resembling those seen in fibrosarcoma.

In all malignant melanomas there is a direct correlation between the level of histologic invasion and prognosis. This can be determined either by the anatomic level of invasion of tumor within the skin (Clark's classification)[15] or by direct measurement of tumor thickness with an ocular micrometer (Breslow's classification).[16] In Clark's classification, level I refers to tumor confined above the basal lamina (in situ malignant melanoma). In level II the tumor has penetrated the basal lamina and extends into the papillary layer of the dermis, but not into the reticular dermis. In level III, the

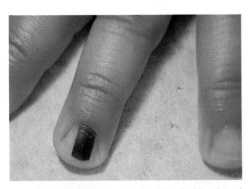

Figure 8–5. Intradermal nevus of nail bed with a broad pigmented band. Such lesions must be differentiated from melanotic whitlows. (Courtesy of Thomas Hansen, M.D.)

entire papillary region is occupied by neoplastic cells that impinge on, but do not invade, the epidermis. Invasion of the reticular dermis by neoplastic cells constitutes level IV; and in level V, the invasion has extended into the subcutaneous tissue.

Breslow's classification currently appears to be a more accurate and reproducible designation of tumor depth and prognosis. Using this classification, lesions with a thickness less than 0.76 mm have an excellent prognosis (96 to 99 per cent 5-year survival); those with a thickness of 0.76 to 1.50 mm have a 5-year survival of 87 to 94 per cent; those with a tumor thickness of 1.51 to 4.0 mm have a 66 to 77 per cent survival; and those with a thickness greater than 4 mm have an extremely poor prognosis (less than 50 per cent).[17] Other factors influencing survival include the anatomic site of the melanoma and the presence or absence of ulceration. In general, patients with lesions on the palms, soles, scalp, mid back, anterior chest, and genitalia have the poorest prognosis.[18]

Treatment. The treatment of choice of primary cutaneous melanoma is surgical excision. On the basis of current data, for melanoma in situ, excision of the lesion with a 0.5-cm border of clinically normal skin and subcutaneous tissue is usually sufficient; a 1-cm margin is usually adequate for melanomas less than 1.0 mm thick; for lesions greater than 1 mm thick, although surgical margins should be greater than 1.0 cm, no uniform standard exists. When clinically suspicious nodes are identified, except in patients with uncontrolled distant metastases or other medical contraindications, regional lymphadenectomy is recommended.[17] For metastatic disease, Dacarbazine is recommended as the most effective single drug. Therapy with cisplatin, vinblastine, cyclophosphamide, or dactinomycin and radiation therapy, regional limb perfusion chemotherapy, monoclonal antibodies, immunotherapy with interferon and interleukin-2, melanoma vaccines, and high-dose chemotherapy followed by autologous bone marrow transplantation have been used. Although advanced melanomas generally cannot be cured, adjuvant measures can often be used to relieve or prevent debilitating symptoms.[19]

Congenital Melanocytic Nevi

Congenital giant pigmented nevi represent a special group of melanocytic lesions with a predisposition to malignant melanoma. Although it has been suggested that the increased incidence of malignant melanoma in large garment-type nevi may be related to the increased number of cells in larger lesions, studies suggest that small congenital pigmented nevi also have an increased risk of malignant degeneration.[20–27]

Thus, small congenital pigmented nevi (Fig. 8–6), those that are less than 1.5 cm in diameter, which occur in 1 per cent of all newborns, have been estimated to have a lifetime risk of developing malignant melanoma of 2.6 to 4.9 per cent.[24] The risk of developing melanoma in medium-sized congenital nevi (those measuring 1.5 to 20 cm in diameter) (Figs. 8–7 and 8–8) is uncertain; and large or giant congenital pigmented nevi, those measuring greater than 20 cm in diameter, present in 1 in 20,000 newborns, are believed to have an estimated 6.3 per cent lifetime risk for developing malignant melanoma.[25, 26]

Most congenital nevi have a distinctive clinical appearance. Small and medium-sized congenital nevi usually present as flat, pale tan macules or papules (similar to café au lait spots) or as tan, well-circumscribed lesions with mottled freckling (see Figs. 8–6 through 8–8). With time they become elevated, and coarse dark brown hairs may or may not become prominent. Giant nevocellular nevi frequently lie in the distribution of a dermatome and vary in size to cover areas such as an arm, leg, or extensive areas of the trunk. Such lesions are frequently descriptively termed *coatsleeve, stocking, cape-like, bathing-trunk,* or *giant hairy nevi* (Figs. 8–9 through 8–11). These lesions are unevenly pigmented, their color ranges from dark brown to black, and over 95 per cent have a hairy component consisting of large coarse terminal hairs. Giant pigmented nevi have an uneven

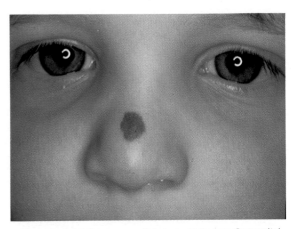

Figure 8–6. A 1.5-cm congenital pigmented nevus. Congenital nevi usually present as flat tan macules or papules with mottled freckling.

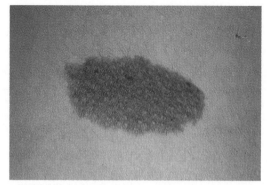

Figure 8–7. A 2.5-cm congenital pigmented nevus with a papular surface, uneven pigmentation, and irregular margin.

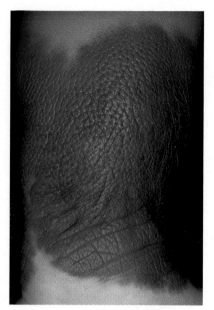

Figure 8–9. A garment-like (stocking type) congenital pigmented nevus on the skin of the ankle and lower aspect of the leg.

verrucous or papillomatous surface and irregular margin. Almost invariably satellite nevi appear at the periphery of the lesion, and numerous other pigmented nevi and café au lait spots coexist elsewhere on the body. As the infant grows the involved areas become thicker and frequently darker; the surface becomes rugose; and verrucous nodules frequently develop.

Giant hairy nevi, particularly those on the scalp and neck, may be associated with leptomeningeal melanocytosis and neurologic disorders such as epilepsy or other focal neurologic abnormality; those that overlie the vertebral column may be associated with spina bifida or meningomyelocele. Often seen in association with bathing-trunk nevi (particularly in the lumbosacral area) and, in a high proportion of patients, with multiple small or medium-sized congenital melanocytic nevi (especially on the scalp, face, or neck), most patients with this variant, termed *neurocutaneous melanosis* (see Fig. 8–11), present in the first 2 years of life and less frequently in the second or third decades with central nervous system manifestations of intracranial pressure or spinal cord compression, such as lethargy, irritability, headache, recurrent vomiting, generalized seizures, increased head circumference, bulging anterior fontanelle, photophobia, papilledema, neck stiffness, and occasionally nerve palsies, particularly of cranial nerves VI and VII. When confronted with patients with large or multiple nevi, particularly of the head, neck, or posterior midline, physicians should seek neurologic consultation; and when signs or symptoms of intracranial pressure appear, diagnostic procedures such as cerebrospinal cytology and magnetic resonance imaging with gadolinium contrast enhancement should be considered.[28]

On histopathologic examination the congenital nevus may appear as an intradermal or compound nevus. It is frequently characterized by nevus cells between the collagen bundles (as single cells or in

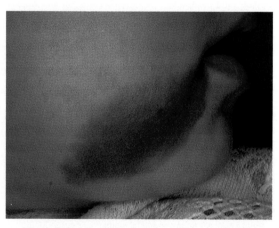

Figure 8–8. A 4- × 6-cm congenital pigmented nevus.

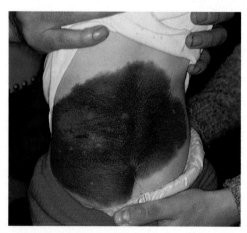

Figure 8–10. A bathing-trunk congenital pigmented nevus. (Courtesy of Marvin Arons, M.D.)

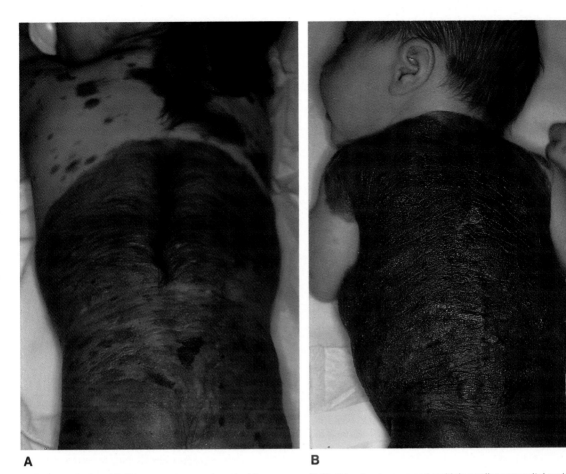

Figure 8–11. A and B. Neurocutaneous melanosis. A large congenital bathing-trunk nevus and multiple smaller congenital nevi are associated with leptomeningeal melanosis.

Indian file) in the lower two thirds of the dermis. In addition, the appendages, nerves, and vessels may also be invaded by nevus cells, and, at times, the melanocytic invasion may extend to involve subcutaneous tissue, fascia, lymphatic tissues, and underlying muscles or peritoneum.[29] Unfortunately, there is no consensus regarding the appropriate therapeutic approach to small and medium-sized congenital melanocytic nevi. Most authorities, however, agree that although individual circumstances must be taken into account, large congenital pigmented nevi should be removed whenever and as early as technically possible, with total excision, skin grafts when necessary, and careful examination of histology of such lesions.[30] There still remains considerable controversy, however, concerning the prophylactic removal of small and medium-sized congenital nevi. Since studies suggest that small congenital pigmented nevi that become malignant generally do so after the onset of adolescence or during adulthood,[24] it is generally agreed that small to medium-sized congenital pigmented nevi that are light colored and benign in appearance can generally be observed until the patient approaches adolescence, at which time the lesion can be easily removed with the use of local anesthesia. Potential danger signals include hemorrhage, crusting, erosion, friability, rapid growth, the development of satellite lesions, and focal hypopigmentation or hyperpigmentation. A congenital nevocellular nevus with a suspicious appearance or change suggestive of neoplastic growth, however, whether it be large or small, deserves consideration for excision at any age (Fig. 8–12). Patients with small to medium-sized congenital nevi that are light colored, benign in appearance, and located in an area where they can be observed may be offered an option of life-long follow-up, with removal only for cosmetic purposes or if clinical features suggest the possibility of neoplastic change.

Dermabrasion and Q-switched ruby laser therapy have been suggested for the removal of congenital nevi. Although these therapeutic approaches may give fairly favorable cosmetic results, they do not necessarily remove all pigment cells and, therefore, are not recommended.[31] In instances in which congenital pigmented nevi are large and difficult to remove, advances in soft tissue expansion techniques offer many technical and cosmetic advantages to the surgical approach.[32]

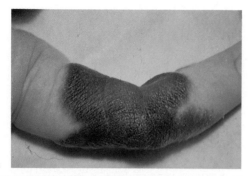

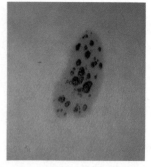

A   **B**

Figure 8–12. A. Malignant melanoma in a congenital pigmented nevus. (Courtesy of Department of Dermatology, Yale University School of Medicine.) B. Malignant melanoma in a congenital nevus overlying the scapular area of a 3½-month-old girl. Note the dark brown melanomas, which in this case appeared during the second week of life.

Dysplastic Nevi

Dysplastic nevi, also referred to as atypical or Clark's nevi, are acquired cutaneous melanocytic nevi regarded as markers and potential precursors for individuals with an increased risk for the development of melanoma. Described in 1978 under the designation of the B-K mole syndrome,[33] in addition to individuals with sporadic dysplastic nevi, a familial form of this disorder, termed the *familial dysplastic (familial atypical) nevus syndrome* or *familial atypical multiple mole-melanoma syndrome,* has also been recognized. Although the risk of malignant melanoma developing in patients with sporadic dysplastic nevi remains uncertain, such nevi are estimated to occur in 2 to 5 per cent of the white population (up to 4.6 million persons in the United States); the lifetime risk of developing a cutaneous melanoma of an individual with sporadic dysplastic nevi appears to be approximately 6 per cent (2 to 8 times greater than that of other individuals).[34] At the other end of the spectrum, for patients with dysplastic nevi who have two or more family members with dysplastic nevi and malignant melanoma, estimated to represent approximately 32,000 individuals in the United States, the lifetime risk of developing a cutaneous malignant melanoma approaches 100 per cent.

Thus a classification system of patients with dysplastic nevi and their risk factors has been suggested. Patients with sporadic dysplastic nevi, without melanoma and without family members with dysplastic nevi or melanoma, may be classified as type A (the lowest risk factor). In those with type B dysplastic nevus syndrome (DNS), dysplastic nevi are present in two or more family members, but there is no history of melanoma within the kindred. An individual with both dysplastic nevi and melanoma, but without either present in family members, represents type C DNS, and patients with type D DNS include kindreds in which both familial dysplastic nevi and familial melanoma are present. This group is further subdivided into type D-1, in which only one family member has had dysplastic nevi and mela-

noma, and type D-2, in which at least two family members have had both melanoma and dysplastic nevi.[34, 35] In individuals who are members of D-2 kindreds and thus at highest risk, the probability of melanoma developing between the ages of 20 and 59 years has been estimated to be approximately 56 per cent.[35]

Unlike ordinary acquired pigmented nevi, dysplastic nevi generally make their appearance during puberty, or at times in children as young as 5 to 6 years of age, and continue to appear throughout adult life. In contrast to ordinary acquired nevi, they have a variegated color ranging from shades of dark brown to tan and pink distributed irregularly throughout the lesions, have irregular or angulated borders, and often fade into the surrounding skin. Dysplastic nevi are frequently larger than common acquired nevi, generally measure 6 to 15 mm in diameter (common acquired nevi rarely exceed 5 mm in diameter), display marked lesion-to-lesion variability, and often have a cobblestone appearance or a small, dark, central papule surrounded by a lighter brown or tan macular periphery (described as a "fried egg" appearance) (Figs. 8–13 through 8–15). Individuals may occasionally have only a solitary or a few lesions or as many as 75 to 100 or more. Dysplastic nevi, although usually seen on sun-exposed areas of the trunk and extremities, with the back being the single site of the greatest number of dysplastic nevi, also have a predilection for apocrine areas such as the scalp (Fig. 8–16), groin, buttocks, and breasts.

Histologic criteria for the diagnosis of dysplastic nevi include architectural disorder with asymmetry, intraepidermal melanocytes extending singly or in nests beyond the main dermal component, lentiginous hyperplasia with elongation of the rete ridges (occasionally with fusing at their bases), spindle-shaped lentiginous or epithelioid melanocytes arranged into nests, fibrotic changes around the rete ridges, increased vascularity, and increased inflammation.

The management of patients with dysplastic nevi and dysplastic nevus syndrome should consist of a total body inspection (including the scalp, breasts, buttocks, and eyes) and evaluation of all

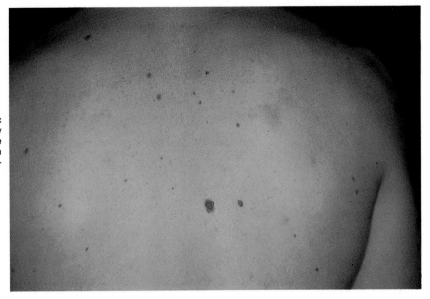

Figure 8–13. Multiple dysplastic nevi on the back of a 15-year-old boy with a melanoma noted on a routine visit for the treatment of acne again serve to emphasize the value of careful evaluation of cutaneous lesions.

first-degree relatives. A family history should be obtained with special attention to the location and number of unusual moles and whether or not the patient has a history of family members with skin cancer, especially melanoma. Although the physician should not create an atmosphere of cancer phobia, patients should be encouraged to minimize exposure to ultraviolet light by using effective sunscreens, wearing protective clothing, and limiting exposure to the sun. Optimal follow-up of patients includes photographs of the entire cutaneous surface and periodic re-examination at 6- to 12-month intervals if unusual or large numbers of atypical lesions are identified, or at yearly intervals

if only a few or mildly atypical nevi are noted. Wholesale removal of nevi is neither practical nor necessary, but lesions on the hairy scalp (since they are hard to follow) and ominous or changing lesions should be excised. Although the precise risk of dysplastic nevi is unresolved, awareness of their possible role as precursor lesions or potential markers of individuals with an increased risk of cutaneous melanoma, sun protective measures, regular follow-up examinations, and removal of ominous or malignant lesions at an early and curable stage are recommended in an effort to help reduce the incidence, morbidity, and mortality of cutaneous melanoma.

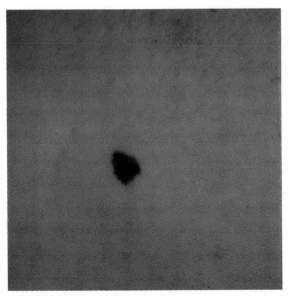

Figure 8–14. A dysplastic nevus with an irregular notched angular border and variegated color.

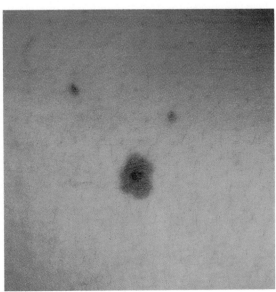

Figure 8–15. A dysplastic nevus with a central elevated papular "fried" or "sunny-side-up" egg-like appearance.

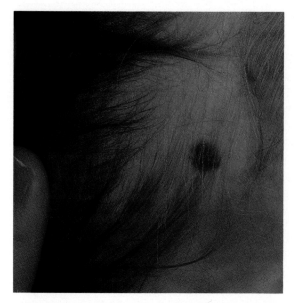

Figure 8–16. A dysplastic nevus on the right parietal scalp with severe atypia on histopathologic examination emphasizes the recommendation of prophylactic removal of dysplastic nevi in areas such as the hairy scalp that are difficult to monitor.

Spindle Cell Nevus (Spitz Nevus)

Prior to 1948 when Spitz clearly delineated the concept of benign juvenile melanoma (now termed *spindle cell nevus, spindle and epithelioid nevus,* or *Spitz nevus*), this lesion, which behaves in a benign fashion yet has certain histologic features resembling those of a malignant melanoma, was a great cause of concern to physicians and pathologists.[36] This tumor, a benign lesion of melanocytic origin, generally occurs on the face, usually the cheek, of children and adolescents (in about 15 per cent of cases) but may occur anywhere on the cutaneous surface. Spindle cell nevi on the uvea and iris have also been reported.[37]

The disorder usually presents as a smooth-surfaced, hairless, dome-shaped papule or nodule with a distinctive reddish brown color (Fig. 8–17). Usually solitary, multiple agminated (clustered) or widely disseminated lesions have also been described.[38] Seen most frequently in children in the 3- to 13-year-old age group, but also described in patients as young as 13 months and as old as 69 years,[37] spindle cell nevi may vary in size from a few millimeters to several centimeters, although most range from 0.6 to 1 cm in diameter. Surface telangiectasia may be a prominent feature, and the characteristic pink to reddish color, when present, is correlated with the vascularity of the tumor. In some lesions, particularly those on the extremities, the reddish color is replaced by a mottled brown to tan or black appearance, often with a verrucous surface and irregular margin. Clinically it is this type of lesion that is most easily confused with malignant melanoma (Fig. 8–18).

Spindle cell nevi must be differentiated from intradermal nevi, pyogenic granulomas, juvenile xanthogranulomas, mastocytomas, and malignant melanomas. When the diagnosis is uncertain, the rapid onset of the lesion and expression of its vascularity by diascopy with a glass slide or hand lens can assist in its clinical differentiation.

The histologic pattern of this disorder appears to be a variant of the compound nevus. The nevus cells are pleomorphic and generally consist of spindle-shaped and less frequently polygon-shaped epithelioid cells. Multinucleated giant cells and mitotic figures complete the histopathologic picture. This benign tumor can be differentiated from malignant melanoma by the presence of spindle and giant cells, an absence or sparsity of melanin, edema and telangiectasia of the stroma, and increased maturation of the tumor cells in the deeper aspect of the dermis. Important histopathologic aids to the diagnosis are recognition that the cells in Spitz nevi are larger than those of common melanocytic nevi and that coalescent eosinophilic globules resembling colloid bodies (Kamino bodies) are present in the basal layer above the tips of dermal papillae in 60 to 86 per cent of Spitz nevi.[39, 40]

After a period of initial growth (usually less than 1 year), untreated spindle cell nevi of Spitz may remain stable for years, may persist as such into adult life, or may develop into intradermal nevi. Once the diagnosis has been established, conservative management is advisable. Since incompletely removed lesions may recur and result in a histopathologic appearance that may be misinterpreted as malignant melanoma, conservative total surgical excision is frequently recommended. Biopsied lesions that leave a slight residual cellular or vascular component, or incompletely removed lesions in which the diagnosis has been firmly established, may be left alone or treated conservatively by cryosurgery with liquid nitrogen. This additional procedure may at times obvi-

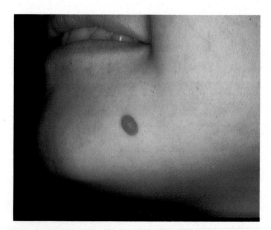

Figure 8–17. Spindle cell nevus (benign juvenile melanoma). A smooth-surfaced firm pink dome-shaped nodule is evident on the face of a young child.

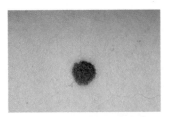

Figure 8–18. A mottled brownish black spindle cell nevus on the thigh. The reddish color may be replaced by a mottled brown, tan, or black appearance, often with a verrucous surface and irregular margin (this lesion may easily be confused with a malignant melanoma).

ate the need for further surgery and frequently will result in an excellent cosmetic result.

Halo Nevus

A halo nevus is a unique cutaneous lesion in which a centrally placed, usually pigmented skin tumor becomes surrounded by a 1- to 5-mm halo of depigmentation. Termed *Sutton's nevus* or *leukoderma acquisitum centrifugum*, this relatively common disorder occurs in both children and adults, generally between 3 and 45 years of age, with late adolescence as the average age at time of onset (Fig. 8–19).

The cause of the spontaneous depigmentation is unknown but appears to be related to an immunologic destruction of melanocytes and nevus cells. Adding support to this hypothesis is the fact that 30 per cent of patients with halo nevi have a tendency to vitiligo. Although compound or intradermal nevi are the tumors most frequently associated with this disorder, this phenomenon may also occur around blue nevi, neuromas, neurofibromas, melanomas, metastatic lesions of malignant melanoma, histiocytomas, seborrheic keratoses, angiomas, spindle

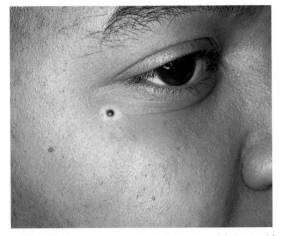

Figure 8–19. Halo nevus (leukoderma acquisitum centrifugum). A halo of depigmentation surrounds a spontaneously regressing nevus.

cell nevi, molluscum contagiosum, flat warts, and basal cell carcinomas; and giant congenital pigmented nevi have been sites of peripheral leukoderma with pigment regression and, at times, self-destruction.[41, 42] This phenomenon should not be confused with the *Cockarde nevus*, an unusual variant of the acquired nevomelanocytic nevus with a central nevus, an intervening nonpigmented zone, and a peripheral pigmented halo, which does not tend to self-destruct.

Halo nevi may appear on almost any cutaneous surface (except the palms, soles, nail beds, and mucous membranes), but the site of predilection for most halo nevi is the trunk, particularly the back. The course of halo nevi is variable, with a tendency toward spontaneous resolution, disappearance of the central lesion, and complete restitution of the site to normal-appearing skin (generally over a period of 5 months to 8 years) in about 50 per cent of affected lesions.

Histologic examination of halo nevi reveals reduction or absence of melanin and a dense inflammatory infiltrate composed primarily of lymphocytes with a few histiocytes and plasma cells around the central lesion. Electron microscopy may reveal complete absence of melanocytes and their replacement with Langerhans cells, ultrastructural findings identical to those seen in vitiligo.

Although the prognosis for benign halo nevi is excellent, attention must be focused on the rare instances in which a malignant melanoma can be the affected tumor or cases in which halo nevi develop when a primary malignant melanoma is located at a distant site. The management of halo nevi, therefore, is dependent on careful examination of the central pigmented tumor, its morphologic differentiation from malignant melanoma, and the exclusion of malignant melanoma on other parts of the cutaneous surface. If the central tumor has benign characteristics, the disorder need not be treated and the lesion may be observed at intervals until it has resolved. For lesions of unusual concern to the patient or physician, however, surgical excision, including the central tumor and its surrounding halo, with careful histologic examination is the method of choice.

Nevus Spilus

Nevus spilus (also termed *speckled lentiginous nevus*) is a solitary, nonhairy, flat, brown patch of melanization dotted by smaller dark brown to blackish brown freckle-like areas of pigmentation (Fig. 8–20). This relatively common disorder, although generally present at birth, may appear in infancy, in childhood, or at any age. Estimated to occur in 2 to 3 per cent of the adult population, it may vary from 1 to 20 cm in diameter and may appear on any area of the face, trunk, or extremities without relation to sun exposure.

Histologic examination reveals the presence of

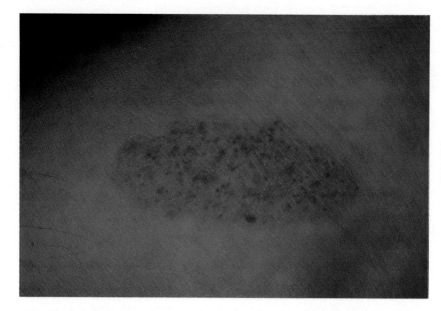

Figure 8–20. Nevus spilus. A solitary flat brown patch of melanization is dotted by smaller dark brown to blackish brown freckle-like areas of pigmentation.

nevus cells in a junctional or dermal location, basilar hyperpigmentation such as is present in café au lait spots, and elongation of the rete ridges. A nevus spilus, accordingly, should not be considered to be a lentigo or form of café au lait spot but should be considered to be a benign nevocellular nevus with the same potential for neoplastic change as any other pigmented nevus. Although there are reports of malignant melanoma developing within lesions of nevus spilus, this does not necessitate routine removal of uncomplicated lesions. For lesions of nevus spilus with melanocytic dysplasia or clearly documented congenital onset, routine clinical observation is indicated with cutaneous biopsy and surgical excision of any lesions suggested to be undergoing neoplastic change.[43–45]

EPIDERMAL MELANOCYTIC LESIONS

Becker's Nevus

In 1949 Becker described an irregular macular hyperpigmentation with hypertrichosis characteristically seen on the shoulders, anterior chest, or scapular region of adolescent males (Fig. 8–21).[46] This relatively common disorder, also known as pigmented hairy epidermal nevus or nevus spilus tardus, is classified as an epidermal rather than a melanocytic nevus.

Becker's nevus may begin in childhood, usually following exposure to sunlight in otherwise normal males (occasionally females), at or shortly after puberty. The first change generally appears as a grayish brown pigmentation on the chest, back, or

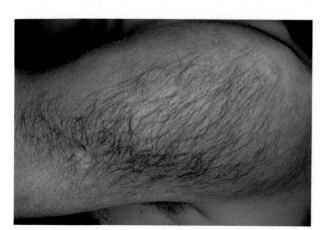

Figure 8–21. Becker's nevus (an irregular macular hyperpigmentation with hypertrichosis) on the shoulder of a 17-year-old boy.

upper arm that spreads in an irregular fashion until it reaches an area 10 to 15 cm in diameter (about the size of a hand or larger). The outline is sharply demarcated, irregular, and often surrounded by islands of blotchy pigmentation. Although characteristically seen unilaterally on the upper half of the trunk, especially around the shoulder, it has also been reported in other areas on the trunk, forehead, cheeks, supraclavicular region, abdomen, forearm, wrist, buttocks, and shins. After a period of time (often 1 or 2 years), coarse hairs appear in the region of, but not necessarily coinciding with, the pigmented area. The intensity of pigmentation may fade somewhat as the patient becomes older, but the hyperpigmentation and hypertrichosis tend to persist for life.

The etiology of Becker's nevus is unknown, but androgen receptor assays suggest that a localized increase in androgen sensitivity may help explain the clinical features seen in individuals with this disorder.[47] In addition, reports of familial cases raise the question of a genetic influence in some patients,[48] and the occasional association of smooth muscle hamartoma and Becker's nevi suggests that these disorders may perhaps represent two poles of the same hamartomatous change (Fig. 8–22).[49] Although most Becker's nevi occur without other pathologic findings, scattered reports of other associated abnormalities (such as unilateral breast and areolar hypoplasia, pectus carinatum, limb asymmetry, and spina bifida) suggest that Becker's melanosis may represent an organoid nevus and part of the spectrum of epidermal nevi and the epidermal nevus syndrome.[50, 51]

Histopathologic features reveal epidermal thickening, elongation of the rete ridges, and hyperpigmentation of the basal layer. There is no increase in the number of melanocytes, and since there are no nevus cells, malignant transformation does not occur. Treatment of this disorder, therefore, is purely cosmetic and consists of therapy with the Q-switched ruby laser or excision with split-thickness skin grafts. Unfortunately, these procedures are only partially satisfactory at best.

Freckles

Freckles (ephelides) are red or light brown well-circumscribed macules, usually less than 5 mm in diameter, which appear in childhood, especially on sun-exposed areas of the skin, and tend to fade during the winter and adult life (Fig. 8–23). They commonly arise in early childhood, generally between 2 and 4 years of age, but not in infancy, and appear to be inherited as an autosomal dominant trait linked with a tendency to fair skin and red or reddish-brown hair. Freckles are most common on the face (especially the nose), shoulders, and upper back. There is a seasonal variation in their appearance. They become darker and more confluent during the summer and are smaller, lighter, and fewer during the winter. They bear cosmetic but no systemic significance, except perhaps when they occur in brunette patients, are of early onset, or persist throughout the winter (a marker of xeroderma pigmentosum trait).

Ephelides must be differentiated from lentigines (Fig. 8–24), which are smooth, freckle-like pigmented macules that appear in childhood but may increase in number up to adult life. Lentigines are differentiated from freckles by their darker color, scattered distribution, comparative sparseness, and the fact that they do not darken or increase in number on sun exposure. Freckles become darker and more conspicuous after ultraviolet light exposure in the sunburn spectrum (290 to 320 nm) as well as in the long-wave ultraviolet range (320 to 400 nm). The long-wave spectrum is not blocked by window glass and sunscreen agents that filter out only the 290- to 320-nm sunburn spectrum.

Histopathologic features of ephelides include increased melanin pigmentation of the basal layer

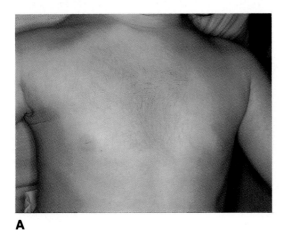

A

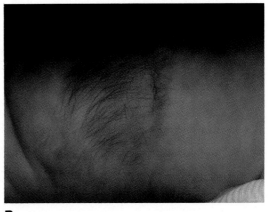

B

Figure 8–22. A. A localized patch of indurated skin with fine hairs and follicular papules (a congenital smooth muscle hamartoma) on the chest of a 19-month-old infant. B. A smooth muscle hamartoma with dark pigmented hairs on the left arm of a 2-month-old infant.

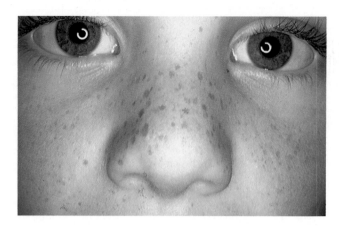

Figure 8–23. Freckles (ephelides). Red or light brown well-circumscribed macules appear in childhood on sun-exposed areas of the skin.

without an increase in the number of melanocytes. Ultrastructural studies reveal that the melanocytes in freckles produce increased numbers of large ellipsoid melanosomes, similar to those seen in blacks. The melanocytes are more highly arborized, react more intensely with dopa than those in normal adjacent skin, and contain more melanosomes in stages I through IV.

Treatment of freckles is best managed by avoidance of sun exposure and appropriate covering makeup. Although sunscreens do not prevent freckle formation, they do permit a more uniform tan in which freckling is less pronounced. When desired, although seldom necessary, gentle peeling with 50 per cent trichloroacetic acid or cryotherapy with carbon dioxide slush or liquid nitrogen may remove the superficial pigmentation and make many of the freckles less conspicuous. Monobenzyl ether of hydroquinone (Benoquin or Eldoquin) may also be partially effective. Unfortunately, the possibility of contact dermatitis and of occasional persistent hypopigmentation (leukoderma) suggests caution in the use of these physical or chemical methods.

Lentigines

Lentigines are small, tan, dark brown or black flat, oval, or circular lesions that usually appear in childhood and may increase in number up to adult life. They vary from 1 to 2 mm (occasionally up to 5 mm) in diameter and may occur on any cutaneous surface or, occasionally, on the mucous membrane or conjunctiva of the eyes. The pigmentation is uniform and darker than that seen in ephelides (freckles), and the color is unaffected by exposure to sunlight (see Fig. 8–24). Adult forms of this disorder, termed *senile lentigines,* or *"liver spots"* (due to their color and not their origin), are distinguished by their onset with advanced age and localization to the forearms, face, neck, and dorsal aspect of the hands.

Histopathologic features include elongated, often club-shaped rete ridges with small bud-like projections, an increase in the number of melanocytes just above the basal layer, and increased melanization of the keratinocytes of the basal layer.

Lentigines that appear early in life may fade or

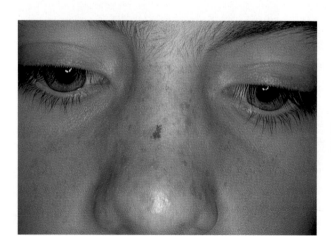

Figure 8–24. Lentigo. A smooth flat pigmented lesion is seen on the nose in a child who also has ephelides. Note the generally uniform dark pigment in the lentigo. This is unaffected by exposure to sunlight.

disappear; those appearing later in life tend to be permanent. Treatment other than for cosmetic purposes is ordinarily not indicated. When desired, however, excision by a small punch biopsy or by shaving, cryosurgery, Q-switched ruby laser, or electrodesiccation (after the diagnosis has been confirmed) may be beneficial.

Lentiginous Syndromes

PEUTZ-JEGHERS SYNDROME

The syndrome of mucocutaneous pigmentation and generalized intestinal polyposis constitutes a unique autosomal dominant disorder designated by the names of the authors, Peutz (Dutch) and Jeghers (American), who described it in 1921 and 1949, respectively.[52]

Characteristic bluish brown to black spots, often apparent at birth or in early childhood, represent the cutaneous marker of this syndrome. These flat pigmented lesions are irregularly oval and usually measure less than 5 mm in diameter. They are most commonly seen on the lips and buccal mucosa, nasal and periorbital regions, elbows, dorsal aspects of the fingers and toes, palms, soles, and periumbilical, perianal, or labial regions; occasionally the gums and hard palate, and, on rare occasions, even the tongue may be involved. The pigmented lesions on the skin and lips frequently tend to fade after puberty; those on the buccal mucosa, palate, and tongue, however, persist.

Although some authors tend to classify the pigmentary lesions of Peutz-Jeghers syndrome with freckles, histologic demonstration of increased melanocytes in the basal layer of the skin and mucous membranes suggest them to be either lentigines or a separate and distinct form of melanosis.[53]

The gastrointestinal polyps seen in this disorder may be found from the gastroesophageal junction down to the anal canal; the small bowel represents the most frequently involved portion of the intestinal tract (96 per cent of cases).[54] The polyps represent benign hamartomas and, contrary to previous descriptions, have a low malignant potential. The polyps may vary from minute pinhead lesions to those measuring several centimeters in diameter. They may occur in early childhood but frequently tend to develop during the second decade of life.

Symptoms in the pediatric patient frequently consist of abdominal pain, melena, or intussusception. The most common symptom, recurrent attacks of colicky abdominal pain, is believed to result from recurring transient episodes of incomplete intussusception. Hematemesis, although less common, may occur owing to involvement of the stomach, duodenum, or upper jejunum. Carcinoma rarely develops in the gross polyps of this disorder but has been associated with micropolyposis of the mucosa of the colon or gastroduodenal area.[53, 54]

Therapeutic management of polyposis in Peutz-Jeghers syndrome should be limited to relief of symptoms rather than radical multiple resections that may lead to malabsorption.[54–57] Multiple individual polypectomies are the treatment of choice when small bowel lesions become symptomatic and elective major resection of benign polyps is not indicated. After initial evaluation such patients can be followed by barium contrast studies, gastroscopy, and gastric cytology. When the colon or rectum is involved, however, the possibility of an independently developing malignancy suggests careful inspection and prophylactic resection, just as if the Peutz-Jeghers syndrome did not exist.[54]

MULTIPLE LENTIGINES SYNDROME (LEOPARD SYNDROME)

In 1969, Gorlin and his associates published a review of an autosomal dominant disorder with high penetrance and variable expressivity characterized by striking cutaneous pigmentation.[58] The various aspects of this syndrome are best remembered by the term LEOPARD syndrome, a mnemonic device derived from an acronym that encompasses many of the protean manifestations of this disorder: lentigines, electrocardiographic conduction defects, ocular hypertelorism, pulmonary stenosis, abnormalities of genitalia, retardation of growth, and deafness.[58]

The cutaneous marker heralding this syndrome consists of small, dark, 1- to 5-mm lentigines, which are usually congenital (but may appear soon after birth) and, with age, tend to increase in number, depth of color, and size (Fig. 8–25). Both light and electron microscopy confirm them to be lentigines with characteristic acanthosis, increase in melanocytes, and melanin deposition. The cutaneous lesions tend to be concentrated on the neck and upper trunk, but they may also appear on the skin of the face and scalp, arms, palms, soles, and

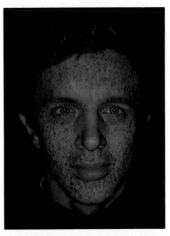

Figure 8–25. Multiple lentigines (LEOPARD) syndrome (Nordlund JJ, Lerner AB, Braverman IM, et al.: The multiple lentigines syndrome. Arch. Dermatol. *107*:259–261. 1973. Copyright © 1973, American Medical Association).

genitalia. Occasionally formes frustes of this disorder occur in which the characteristic lentigines are absent.[59]

Skeletal aberrations may include retardation of growth (below the 25th percentile), hypertelorism, pectus deformities (carinatum or excavatum), dorsal kyphosis, winged scapulae, and prognathism. Cardiac abnormalities, commonly seen in this disorder, may consist of valvular pulmonary stenosis, subaortic stenosis, or cardiac conduction defects. Endocrine disorders include gonadal hypoplasia, hypospadias, undescended testes, hypoplastic ovaries, and delayed puberty. Congenital neurosensory hearing loss, abnormal electroencephalograms, and slowed peripheral nerve conduction may complete the findings in this disorder.

In addition, a combination of cutaneous pigmented lesions and atrial myxomas have been reported in patients with the *NAME syndrome* (*n*evi, *a*trial myxomas, *m*yxoid neurofibromas, and *e*phelides) and the *LAMB syndrome* (*l*entigines, *a*trial myxomas, cutaneous papular *m*yxomas, and *b*lue nevi).[60, 61] Other disorders with lentiginous proliferation include *Moynahan's syndrome* (multiple symmetric lentigines, genital hypoplasia, dwarfism, congenital mitral stenosis, psychic infantilism, and mental deficiency); *inherited patterned lentiginosis in blacks*, a purely cutaneous disorder not associated with other abnormalities; *centrofacial neurodysraphic lentiginosis (Touraine's syndrome)*, an autosomal dominant disorder characterized by lentigines distributed across the center of the face (the nose and adjacent cheeks) without mucous membrane involvement, associated with mental retardation, congenital mitral valve stenosis, seizures, sacral hypertrichosis, coalescence of the eyebrows, high-arched palate, absent upper middle incisors, bony abnormalities, defective fusion of the neural tube (dysraphia), psychiatric disorders, dwarfism, and endocrine dysfunction; and *eruptive lentiginosis*, a disorder characterized by a widespread eruption of several hundred lentigines that may develop over a few months or years, usually in adolescents or young adults, without systemic manifestations.

Café au Lait Spots

Café au lait spots are large, round or oval, flat lesions of light brown pigmentation found in 10 to 20 per cent of normal individuals (Fig. 8–26). Frequently present at birth, or developing soon thereafter, they vary from 1.5 cm or less in their smallest diameter to much larger lesions that may measure up to 15 to 20 cm or more in diameter, often increase in number and size with age, and may occur anywhere on the body. Although most individuals with café au lait spots are normal, these pigmented macules may be a sign of neurofibromatosis and may be associated with other neurocutaneous disease.

They occur in 90 per cent of patients with neuro-

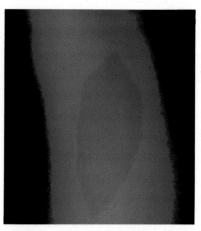

Figure 8–26. Café au lait spot. The presence of six or more café au lait macules with a diameter of 1.5 cm or more is diagnostic of neurofibromatosis. In prepubertal children six or more years old, café au lait spots 0.5 cm or greater in diameter may indicate the presence of neurofibromatosis.

fibromatosis (von Recklinghausen disease) and tend to be more numerous and often larger in individuals affected with this disorder. Crowe has shown that the presence of six or more café au lait spots greater than 1.5 cm in diameter is presumptive evidence of neurofibromatosis. This "six spot" criterion is particularly valuable in young children or adolescents before cutaneous neuromas make their appearance. In prepubertal children, however, six or more café au lait spots 0.5 cm or greater in diameter may indicate the presence of neurofibromatosis (see Chapter 23). Smaller café au lait spots (1 to 4 mm in diameter) in the axillae, termed *axillary freckling*, may also serve as a valuable early diagnostic sign of neurofibromatosis. Seen in 20 per cent of patients with this disease, axillary pigmentation (Crowe's sign), although highly characteristic, is not pathognomonic; it may also be seen in Watson's syndrome, an autosomal dominant disorder characterized by pulmonary stenosis, café au lait spots, low intelligence, and, in some instances, axillary freckling.[62]

In addition there is an increased incidence of café au lait spots in patients with tuberous sclerosis, similar lesions with a more irregular border occur in 50 per cent of individuals with polyostotic fibrous dysplasia (Albright's syndrome), and café au lait spots may also be found in association with the epidermal nevus syndrome, Bloom's syndrome, ataxia-telangiectasia, pulmonary stenosis, temporal lobe dysrhythmias, Silver's syndrome (a disorder of intrauterine growth retardation, hemihypertrophy, elevated gonadotropins giving rise to premature sexual development, inwardly curved fifth fingers, syndactylism of the toes, a triangular facies with turned-down corners of the mouth, and elongated arc or spike-shaped café au lait spots), basal cell nevus syndrome, Gaucher's disease, and Turner's syndrome (short stature, sexual infantilism, and congenital anomalies such as bicuspid aortic valve and coarctation of the aorta, webbed neck, and cubitus valgus of the elbows).

Histopathologic examination of the café au lait spots reveals an increase in pigment in the basal layer of the epidermis. Ultrastructural examination may reveal giant pigment granules in the keratinocytes and melanocytes in café au lait spots, particularly in those of individuals with neurofibromatosis. Giant pigment granules, however, have also been found in normal skin, pigmented macules of Albright's syndrome, melanocytic nevi, and nevus spilus and in patients with the LEOPARD syndrome. The lesions may occasionally be absent in café au lait spots in adults with neurofibromatosis and seem to be regularly absent in café au lait spots of children with neurofibromatosis.[63] The number of melanocytes per unit area in café au lait spots in patients with neurofibromatosis may be increased, decreased, or equal to the normal-appearing surrounding skin. In individuals without neurofibromatosis, however, the café au lait spots have fewer dopa-positive melanocytes per unit area than the normal surrounding skin.[64, 65] In addition, microscopic studies of café au lait spots suggest that the finding of more than 10 melanin macroglobules (macromelanosomes) per five high-power fields under light microscopy may be diagnostic of neurofibromatosis in individuals 15 years of age or older.[66]

Treatment of café au lait spots per se is unnecessary. They do not have an increased tendency to neoplastic change, depigmenting agents are of no value, and surgical excision is generally impractical and unnecessary. In cases in which therapy is desirable for cosmetic appearance, camouflage with appropriate cosmetics and removal of lesions with the Q-switched ruby laser may be considered.

McCune-Albright Syndrome

The McCune-Albright syndrome in its complete form is a triad characterized by café au lait spots, polyostotic fibrous dysplasia, and endocrine dysfunction, often manifesting as precocious puberty.[67, 68] When sexual precocity, generally seen in the female with menstruation prior to development of breasts or pubic hair, or in boys (as premature enlargement of the penis and testes accompanied by growth of pubic hair), is not present, the bone changes, seen radiographically as patchy areas of osteoporosis with a pseudocystic appearance (often with sclerosis, fractures, hyperostosis of the skull bones, and other skeletal deformities), can help establish the diagnosis. The pigmentary lesions, seen in approximately 50 per cent of patients, are frequently unilateral, stopping abruptly at the midline, and tend to follow a dermatomal distribution with a predilection for areas with most bony involvement (the forehead, nuchal area, face, neck, thorax, sacral areas, and buttocks). With their irregularly jagged or serrated borders (described as resembling the "coast of Maine," in contrast to café au lait spots, where the smooth borders are said to resemble the "coast of California"), the lesions are present early in life and frequently are the first sign of this disorder.[69]

DERMAL MELANOCYTIC LESIONS

Mongolian Spots

Mongolian spots are flat, deep brown to slate gray or blue-black, often poorly circumscribed, large macular lesions generally located over the lumbosacral areas, buttocks, and occasionally the lower limbs, back, flanks, and shoulders of normal infants (Fig. 8–27). Seen in over 90 per cent of black and Native American, 81 per cent of Asian, 70 per cent of Hispanic, and 9.6 per cent of white infants, this disorder develops in utero, is present at birth, and often fades somewhat during the first 1 or 2 years of life.[1] Occasionally, mongolian spots may persist into adulthood, but they usually disappear by 7 to 13 years of age.[70]

Mongolian spots may be single or multiple and vary from a few millimeters to 10 cm or more in diameter. They represent collections of spindle-shaped melanocytes located deep in the dermis, probably as the result of arrest during their embryonal migration from the neural crest to the epidermis. The slate blue to blue-black color depends on the Tyndall effect (a phenomenon in which light passing through a turbid medium such as the skin is scattered as it strikes particles of melanin). Long-wavelength light rays (red, orange, and yellow) tend to be less scattered and therefore con-

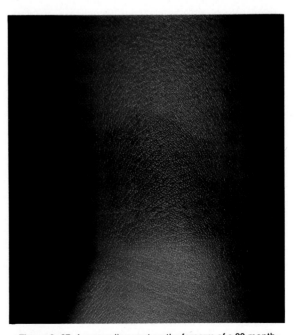

Figure 8–27. A mongolian spot on the forearm of a 22-month-old infant.

tinue to pass downward into the lower levels of the skin; colors of shorter wavelengths (blue, indigo, and violet) are scattered to the side and backward to the skin surface, thus creating the blue-black or slate gray discoloration.

The diagnosis is based on the clinical morphology and, when in doubt, is confirmed by histopathologic examination of lesions. Microscopic features of mongolian spots include collections of greatly elongated, slender, spindle-shaped, dopa-positive melanocytes that run parallel to the skin surface deep within the dermis or around the cutaneous appendages. Since this is a benign disorder, therapy is unnecessary.

Nevus of Ota and Nevus of Ito

The nevus of Ota (nevus fuscoceruleus ophthalmomaxillaris) represents a usually unilateral irregularly patchy bluish gray discoloration of the skin of the face supplied by the first and second divisions of the trigeminal nerve, particularly the periorbital region, the temple, the forehead, the malar area, and the nose (Fig. 8–28). About two thirds of patients with this disorder have a patchy bluish discoloration of the sclera of the ipsilateral eye, and occasionally the conjunctiva, the cornea, and the retina.[71] In about 5 per cent of cases the nevus of Ota is bilateral rather than unilateral, and, in rare instances, the lips, palate, pharynx, and nasal mucosa are similarly affected.

Most commonly seen in Asians, it has also been seen in blacks, and 80 per cent of the total number of cases appear in females. Unlike mongolian spots, which tend to disappear with time, the nevus of Ota generally persists (although some have been observed to fade during the course of years) and usually has a speckled rather than a uniform discoloration. Approximately 50 per cent of lesions are congenital; the remainder generally appear during the second decade of life. Rarely the onset

is later and may be associated with pregnancy. Nevus flammeus has been associated with this condition (this variant has been termed *phacomatosis pigmentovascularis*), and in a small percentage of cases, blotchy involvement (usually in association with persistent mongolian spots elsewhere) may be seen.

The nevus of Ito (nevus fuscoceruleus acromiodeltoideus) has the same features as the nevus of Ota except that the pigmentary changes tend to involve the shoulder, supraclavicular areas, sides of the neck, and upper arm, scapular, and deltoid regions. It may occur alone or may be seen in conjunction with the nevus of Ota.

Histopathologic features of the nevus of Ota and nevus of Ito show, similar to mongolian spots, elongated dendritic melanocytes scattered among the collagen bundles. The melanocytes, however, frequently appear to be situated somewhat higher in the dermis than those seen in ordinary mongolian spots.

Although these lesions do not disappear spontaneously, changes in color do occur. Darkening of lesions has been noted during menses, and intensification of pigmentation after the age of 11 is common. These disorders are generally benign. Malignant transformation (malignant melanoma) and sensorineural deafness, however, have been reported in association with the nevus of Ota.[72] Except for such cases, no treatment other than cryotherapy, laser ablation by the Q-switched ruby laser (or argon laser in patients in whom the pigmentation is sparse), or cosmetic cover-up is necessary.

Blue Nevi

Blue nevi consist of two distinct types: the common and the cellular. The common blue nevus is a small, round or oval, dark blue or bluish black, smooth-surfaced, sharply circumscribed, slightly elevated dome-shaped nodule or plaque (Fig. 8–29). Most common blue or plaque nevi range from 2 or 3 mm to 10 mm (less than 1 cm) in diameter. Although usually singular, they may be multiple. Lesions may be present at birth but may appear at any age, and women are usually affected at least twice as frequently as men. Although ordinary blue nevi may occur on any part of the body, areas of predilection include the buttocks, dorsal aspect of the hands and feet, and the extensor surfaces of the forearms. They also may occur on the face, bulbar conjunctiva, mucous membranes, and the hard and soft palates.

Once an ordinary blue nevus appears, it usually remains static and persists throughout life. Although fading of color and some degree of flattening may occur with time, malignant degeneration of this form of blue nevus is rare. When a diagnosis of malignant melanoma is considered, the common blue nevus can be differentiated from it by the presence of normal skin markings over the lesion,

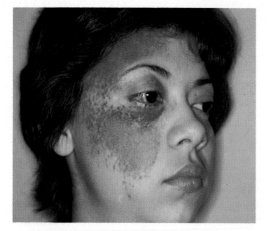

Figure 8–28. Nevus of Ota. (Courtesy of Department of Dermatology, Yale University School of Medicine.)

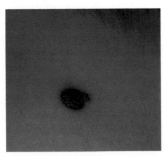

Figure 8–29. Blue nevus. The lesion is an oval bluish black smooth-surfaced, sharply circumscribed dome-shaped nodule.

in contrast to the loss of such marking in lesions of malignant melanoma.

Cellular blue nevi are considerably less common than ordinary blue nevi and differ in several respects. They tend to be larger and generally measure more than 1 cm in diameter, and they appear to have a relatively high incidence over the buttocks, sacrococcygeal areas, and occasionally the dorsal aspect of the hands and feet.

Although common blue nevi tend to remain benign, there is a low but distinct danger of malignant transformation in the cellular blue nevus.[73, 74] Malignant changes in cellular blue nevi are indicated by a sudden increase in size and, at times, an associated tendency toward ulceration. Malignant blue nevi are locally aggressive and, in about 5 per cent of individuals, produce regional lymph node metastases. Although this malignant tumor, except for local spread, is often relatively innocuous, as with malignant melanoma, patients may be asymptomatic for many years after the primary tumor excision, only to die of sudden development of widespread metastases.

Although the histogenesis of blue nevi has not been proved, it is assumed that the lesions represent hamartomas that result from the arrested embryonal migration of melanocytes bound for the dermal-epidermal junction. It would appear, therefore, that the blue nevus, mongolian spots, and the nevi of Ota and Ito are closely related and possibly represent different stages of the same physiologic process.

Histopathologic examination of common blue nevi reveals compactly and loosely arranged, greatly elongated spindle-shaped, bipolar, flattened or fusiform melanocytes. These cells have long, occasionally branching, dendritic processes, with their long axes parallel to the epidermis, and are grouped in irregular bundles, mainly in the middle and lower thirds of the dermis. The bundles of cells may be intimately mixed with the fibrous tissues of the upper reticular area of the dermis, or they may extend down into the subcutaneous layer. They often tend to aggregate about the adnexa, nerves, and blood vessels, and the normal dermal architecture (in contrast to that of mongolian spots) is frequently distorted.

In addition to spindle-shaped melanocytes,

cellular blue nevi also have nodular islands composed of densely packed, rather large, rounded or spindle-shaped cells with variously shaped nuclei and an abundant pale cytoplasm. Malignant cellular blue nevi, in addition, show mitotic figures, cellular pleomorphism, and evidence of invasion.

The treatment of choice for both types of blue nevus consists of conservative surgical excision with careful histologic examination of the lesion. Patients who have cellular blue nevi should be further examined for the presence of regional lymphadenopathy and, following surgery, should be studied at regular intervals for signs of recurrence or possible metastatic spread.[73, 74]

Other forms of blue nevi include eruptive blue nevi, a variant reported in a 14-year-old boy in whom a cluster of over 100 blue-brown papules appeared on the upper central chest, shoulders, and "V" of the neck following sunburn.[75] The Cockarde or target blue nevus is a benign clinical variant characterized by a concentric target-like appearance. Preferentially located on the back of the hands or feet, and occasionally on the back or anal rim, this variant may at times be mistaken for a malignant melanoma. In such instances, surgical removal and histopathologic examination can confirm the true nature of the disorder.[76]

TUMORS OF THE EPIDERMIS

Tumors of the epidermis range in severity from benign or nevoid lesions to those that are highly malignant. Benign tumors appear frequently; malignant tumors, less common in children, are often overlooked when they do occur.

Epidermal Nevi

Epidermal nevi represent a benign congenital disorder that is characterized by circumscribed hyperkeratosis and hypertrophy of the epidermis (Fig. 8–30). This disorder, usually apparent at birth or in early childhood, affects both sexes equally and is known by several descriptive names: nevus verrucosus, nevus unius lateris, and ichthyosis hystrix. The lesions may be deeply or slightly pigmented, have either a unilateral or a bilateral distribution, and often favor the extremities in what appears to be a dermatomal distribution, but may occur anywhere on the cutaneous surface and, at times, on the oral mucosa and ocular conjunctiva. Although single lesions may occur, the disorder generally consists of multiple lesions arranged in a linear distribution.

The localized form (nevus verrucosus) usually consists of a solitary lesion. Generally present at birth, it may also appear in infancy, early childhood, and occasionally in adult life. Lesions may be grayish to yellow-brown and velvety, granular, warty, or papillomatous. More often noted on the trunk or limb than on the head or neck, they may be

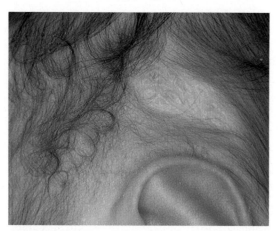

Figure 8–30. Epidermal nevus of the scalp in a newborn (this lesion must be differentiated from a nevus sebaceus of Jadassohn).

single or multiple and round or oval. They vary from 2 to 3 cm or more in diameter and, when seen on the limbs, frequently appear in a linear distribution.

The term *nevus unius lateris* is used when lesions are extensive and systematized. Nevus unius lateris may present as a single linear or spiral warty lesion or at times as an elaborate continuous or interrupted pattern affecting multiple sites, occasionally involving more than half of the body (Fig. 8–31). On the extremities lesions usually follow the long axis, and on the trunk or extremities they may be arranged in groups as spiral streaks (Fig. 8–32). On the trunk the lesions frequently tend to have a transverse orientation. If a large area of the body is affected, the term *systematized epidermal nevus* may be used. When the scalp, face, or neck is involved, adnexal tissues such as the sebaceous glands may be affected and become enlarged. For this form the term *linear nevus sebaceus* may be used. Linear nevus sebaceus should not be confused with nevus sebaceus (of Jadassohn), a distinct and unrelated disorder.

The term *ichthyosis hystrix* refers to widespread epidermal lesions that are usually bilateral and arranged in irregular geometric patterns. This variant frequently consists of feather-like or marbled patterns or sheets or whorls of hyperkeratosis (see Chapter 7, Fig. 7–16).

The predominant histologic features of epidermal nevi consist of hyperkeratosis, papillomatosis, and acanthosis. Nevus cells are absent, but in some cases an increase in melanin pigment in the basal layer may be present. Hyperkeratosis, vacuolization (ballooning) of the cells, and microvesicles, as seen in epidermolytic hyperkeratosis, may be seen in some lesions, particularly in the ichthyosis hystrix form of the disorder. In some patients both histologic patterns may be noted in a single lesion or in lesions from different areas of the same patient.

The occurrence of malignant degeneration of epidermal nevi is unusual. Although hemangiomas, lymphangiomas, apocrine cystadenomas, syringomas, and trichoepitheliomas may accompany the verrucose lesion, when malignant degeneration occurs, it usually consists of benign or low-grade malignant tumors such as Bowen's disease, keratoacanthoma, and basal or squamous cell carcinoma.[77, 78] Therapy, accordingly, depends on the site, the extent of the lesions, and the age of the patient. It is frequently wise, however, to delay surgery until the final extent of the process can be determined, since early excision may result in the appearance of new lesions in or adjacent to regions of previously treated areas. Excision by a plastic surgeon is the treatment of choice for lesions that are unsightly or uncomfortable, or when malignant change is suspected. Although cryosurgery (with liquid nitrogen), dermabrasion, or electrodesication and curettage may produce gratifying results initially, recurrences are common.

Inflammatory Linear Verrucous Epidermal Nevi

Inflammatory linear verrucous epidermal nevus (ILVEN) appears to be a special variant of epidermal nevus that presents as persistent, linear, pruritic eruptions composed of erythematous, slightly verrucous, scaling papules arranged in one or several linear plaques. Usually present at birth or appearing during early childhood, this disorder tends to run a chronic course and is generally resistant to

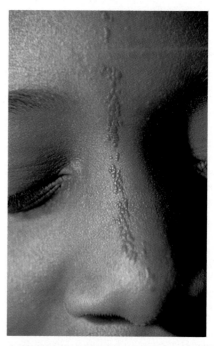

Figure 8–31. Linear epidermal nevus (nevus unius lateris). A linear arrangement of hypertrophic warty papules in an interrupted band was present since birth.

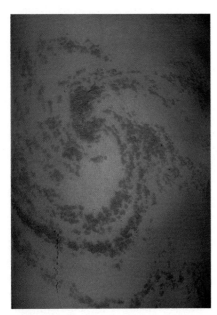

Figure 8–32. Nevus unius lateris in a whorled pattern (systematized epidermal nevus).

therapy.[79, 80] Frequently misdiagnosed as psoriasis, lichen simplex chronicus, or lichen striatus, the diagnosis can usually be established by the morphologic appearance of lesions, intense pruritus, resistance to therapy, and inflammatory and psoriasiform features that suggest the diagnosis of a nonspecific chronic dermatitis. Histopathologic features include hyperkeratosis with foci of parakeratosis, moderate acanthosis, elongation of rete ridges, occasional light spongiosis, and a chronic perivascular inflammatory infiltrate of lymphocytes and histiocytes.

Although topical and intralesional corticosteroids can reduce inflammation and produce a temporary remission, the disorder generally recurs. In such instances, surgical excision, deep-shave excision, or dermabrasion may be curative.

Epidermal Nevus Syndrome

Although there have been numerous isolated case reports of congenital anomalies associated with epidermal nevi, until recently little attention had been paid to them. The epidermal nevus syndrome is now delineated as a congenitally acquired syndrome consisting of deformities of the skin, the skeletal system, the central nervous system, and the cardiovascular system. Associated anomalies include cutaneous disorders (epidermal nevi, areas of hypopigmentation, other nevi, and café au lait spots), kyphoscoliosis, vertebral defects, hemihypertrophy, short limbs, phocomelia, angiomas of the skin, patent ductus arteriosus, coarctation and hypoplasia of the aorta, ocular abnormalities, and central nervous system involvement, with brain tumor, hydrocephaly, mental retarda-

tion, and convulsive disorders.[81, 82] In addition, affected individuals may also have increased susceptibility to a variety of tumors such as Wilms' tumor and other tumors of the urinary tract, astrocytoma, adenocarcinoma of the salivary glands, adenocarcinoma of the breast, ameloblastoma of the mandible, ganglioneuroblastoma, carcinoma of the esophagus and stomach, and metastatic squamous cell carcinoma.[83, 84] Although most cases of epidermal nevus syndrome occur sporadically, data suggest that, in some cases at least, an autosomal dominant transmission may be present.[81]

The nature of the verrucous lesions ranges from large unilateral hypertrophic deformities of the epidermis (nevus unius lateris) to whorled, brush stroke–like scaly lesions involving variable areas of the skin surface (ichthyosis hystrix) or large orange velvety changes of the scalp such as are seen in nevus sebaceus of Jadassohn. It now appears that the linear nevus sebaceus syndrome and epidermal nevus syndrome are probably the same entity, the only difference being that of topography. Biopsy specimens from patients with lesions in the sebaceous gland area (scalp, face, and ears) show sebaceous gland hyperplasia; those from patients with lesions on the arms, legs, and trunk (where a sebaceous component is not prominent) show histopathologic features of epidermal nevi (nevus unius lateris).

Patients with large epidermal nevi require a careful family history and thorough physical evaluation, with particular emphasis on the affected individual's developmental pattern and musculoskeletal, nervous, ocular, and cardiovascular systems; and although reports of individuals with epidermal nevi and malignancy may be coincidental, it is suggested that physicians remain alert to this possibility.

Basal Cell Carcinoma

Basal cell carcinoma (often termed *epithelioma*) is a slow-growing, usually nonmetastasizing but invasive malignant skin tumor with varying clinical patterns. This disorder arises from the basal cells of the epidermis or its appendages and is most commonly seen in persons of middle age. Although rarely seen in children, it can occur in childhood and must be considered even in the very young. Occurrence in young adults and children in association with xeroderma pigmentosum, nevus sebaceus of Jadassohn, and nevoid basal cell carcinoma is well recognized. The spontaneous occurrence of childhood forms of this disorder, however, also requires the consideration of basal cell carcinoma in the differential diagnosis of cutaneous lesions, even in the young.[85, 86]

The majority of basal cell epitheliomas occur on the head and neck, with a predilection for the upper central part of the face. Although basal cell tumors may arise without apparent cause, prolonged exposure to the sun is a predisposing factor, particularly in individuals with fair skin. The tumor, the least aggressive neoplasm among cutaneous cancers, is characterized by its capacity for local destruction. It should be noted, however, that congenital, metastatic, and invasive basal cell carcinomas, although rare, can indeed occur.[87–89] The regional lymph nodes, followed by the lung, bone, skin, liver, and pleura, are the most frequent sites of metastases, with an average of 9 years elapsing between the diagnosis of the primary tumor and the metastatic disease. Several clinical forms of basal cell epithelioma occur and are described below.

Noduloulcerative Type. The noduloulcerative type (by far the most common) begins as a small elevated translucent nodule with telangiectatic vessels on its surface. The nodule often increases in size, undergoes central necrosis, and results in an ulceration surrounded by a pearly rolled border. Although this form usually occurs as a single lesion, patients who develop this form of basal cell tumor frequently are likely to develop other such lesions. Basal cell epitheliomas enlarge more slowly than squamous cell carcinomas. In spite of the frequency of this disorder in adults, metastases are unusual and, when present, are usually associated with extremely aggressive primary lesions and repeated unsuccessful attempts at local treatment.

Pigmented Type. Pigmented basal cell carcinomas have all the features of the noduloulcerative type but also manifest an irregular dark pigmentation. The color may vary from light brown to dark black and often simulates the color of malignant melanoma.

Sclerosing Type. Sclerosing or morphea-like basal carcinomas usually present on the head and the neck as elevated, firm, yellowish waxy plaques with an ill-defined border and absence of the translucent rolled edge. Tumors of this type have been known to arise in early childhood and may grow for years before attracting medical attention.

Superficial Type. Superficial basal cell tumors appear as psoriasiform, erythematous, scaly, flat or slightly infiltrated patches with superficial ulceration, crusting, and a fine thread-like pearly border. Often multiple, these lesions generally occur on the trunk or extremities, expand slowly, and are easily mistaken for lesions of psoriasis or tinea corporis.

Histopathologic features of basal cell carcinoma generally correspond to the clinical manifestations of the lesion and are characterized by masses of basal cells with large oval or elongated nuclei and relatively little cytoplasm. The nuclei resemble those of basal cells in the epidermis, generally have a uniform rather than anaplastic appearance, and do not show abnormal mitoses or pronounced variations in size or intensity of stain.

No single method of therapy is applicable to all basal cell lesions. The goal, as with any skin tumor, is for permanent cure with the best functional and cosmetic result. Curettage and electrodesiccation is a simple office treatment most frequently used by dermatologists and has a cure rate of over 95 per cent. Although cure rates are calculated in 5-year periods, it is extremely rare to see recurrences 1 year or more after appropriate treatment. Large lesions are best treated by surgical excision, with grafting when necessary. Cryosurgery and Mohs' chemosurgery are particularly beneficial in recurrent basal cell carcinomas when other methods of therapy have proved unsatisfactory. Fractional doses of radiation therapy (used for large lesions in elderly patients in whom extensive surgical procedures are difficult) should be avoided whenever possible in the management of basal cell tumors in childhood. Although metastatic basal cell carcinoma is uncommon, with fewer than 200 cases recorded, once the tumor has metastasized beyond the regional lymph nodes it is usually fatal.[88, 89]

Basal Cell Nevus Syndrome

The basal cell nevus syndrome (multiple nevoid basal cell carcinoma syndrome, Gorlin's syndrome) is an autosomal dominant disorder with variable penetrance characterized by childhood onset of multiple basal cell epitheliomas associated with other abnormalities, such as odontogenic jaw cysts, bifid ribs, abnormalities of the vertebrae, and intracranial calcification.[90, 91] The most obvious feature of the syndrome is the appearance of multiple basal cell epitheliomas early in life. These basal cell epitheliomas are indistinguishable on histopathologic examination from ordinary basal cell carcinomas.

The skin lesions of basal cell nevus syndrome may appear as early as the second year of life, frequently develop at puberty, and generally occur between puberty and 35 years of age. They involve, in decreasing order of frequency, the face, neck, back, thorax, abdomen, and upper extremities. Lesions appear as flesh-colored to red or pale brown dome-shaped papules that measure 1 mm to 1 cm in diameter and tend to erupt in crops periodically throughout the lifetime of affected individuals (Fig. 8–33). Secondary changes such as ulceration, crusting, and bleeding rarely occur before puberty, but if left untreated, these lesions can become extremely destructive. Unlike ordinary basal cell carcinomas, basal cell nevi are not induced by prolonged exposure to sunlight.

In addition to nevoid basal cell carcinomas, affected individuals have a characteristic facies with sunken eyes, broad nasal root, true or apparent hypertelorism, and other cutaneous stigmata. These include small milia on the face, numerous comedonal lesions, large epidermal cysts of the limbs, lipomas, fibromas, café au lait pigmentation, multiple pigmented nevi, and ectopic calcium deposits in the skin. Shallow 2- to 3-mm palmar and plantar pits, a characteristic feature of the syndrome, are seen in 60 per cent of affected individuals. These defective areas of keratinization usu-

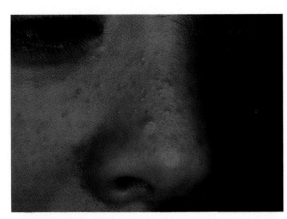

Figure 8–33. Basal cell nevus. A dome-shaped, skin-colored papule on the nose of a 13-year-old child with the basal cell nevus syndrome.

ally first appear during the second decade of life or later. Palmar and plantar pits also frequently tend to have an underlying area of erythema, which on casual observation appears as multiple small red spots on the palms and soles.

Musculoskeletal anomalies, present in 60 to 75 per cent of patients, consist of frontal and temporoparietal bossing, prognathism, mandibular and maxillary bone cysts, splayed or bifid ribs, kyphoscoliosis, cervical or upper thoracic vertebral fusion, spina bifida, a marfanoid build, pectus excavatum and carinatum, and shortened fourth metacarpals (seen in 10 per cent of affected persons).

Neurologic abnormalities include mental retardation, electroencephalographic abnormalities, agenesis of the corpus callosum, a peculiar calcification of the dura and falx cerebri, seizures, congenital communicating hydrocephalus, nerve deafness, and, in some patients, medulloblastomas, which generally appear during the first 2 years of life.

Cardiac tumors have been associated with this disorder,[92] and ophthalmic abnormalities, documented in approximately one third of patients, include hypertelorism and lateral displacement of the medial canthi (dystopia canthorum), congenital blindness due to corneal opacities, cataracts, strabismus, glaucoma, and colobomas of the retina and iris. Associated endocrine findings include ovarian fibromas and calcification, pseudohypoparathyroidism, hypogonadism, cryptorchidism or testicular agenesis, and adrenal cortical adenomas.

The relatively benign course of basal cell carcinomas in most individuals with the basal cell nevus syndrome suggests a nonradical therapeutic approach such as simple surgical excision, cryosurgery, or electrodesiccation and curettage. Radiation therapy, particularly in childhood, is not recommended. Mohs' fresh-tissue technique is helpful for the removal of deep or invasive tumors; and although systemic retinoids can produce recession of lesions, side effects limit their long-term

use in individuals with this disorder. Genetic counseling and periodic follow-up examinations are recommended and, except for the rare patients in whom medulloblastomas or aggressive deeply infiltrating destructive tumors occur, the prognosis in general is good.[93]

Squamous Cell Carcinoma

Squamous cell carcinoma (epidermoid carcinoma) is a malignant tumor of the epidermis rarely seen in children. Occasionally it may arise in normal skin, but generally it is seen in skin that has been injured by sunlight, trauma, thermal burn, or chronic irritation. In highly susceptible subjects, however, such as patients with xeroderma pigmentosum, squamous cell carcinoma may also occur in childhood or early adult life.

The most common sites for this tumor are the face (in particular the lower lip and pinna of the ear) and the dorsal aspect of the hands and forearms. Lesions are generally dull red, frequently contain telangiectasias, and appear as indurated plaque-like nodules with shallow, centrally crusted ulcerations surrounded by wide elevated and indurated borders. Lesions that arise de novo usually appear as solitary, slowly enlarging firm nodules with central crusting, underlying ulceration, and an indurated base.

Histopathologic examination of squamous cell carcinoma is characterized by irregular nests of epidermal cells that proliferate downward and invade the epidermis. The tumor masses are composed of varying proportions of differentiated squamous cells, keratinized cells, and anaplastic squamous cells. Of prognostic significance are the depth of the lesion and the histologic classification of squamous cell carcinomas into grades I to IV. In grade I, most cells are differentiated and the tumor has not penetrated beyond the level of the eccrine glands. In grade IV most of the cells are atypical and undifferentiated; the greater the number of atypical cells and depth of invasion, the higher the degree of malignancy.

The prognosis for squamous cell carcinoma of the skin is quite variable, ranging from easily cured small lesions arising in sun-damaged skin (which have a low propensity to metastasize) to lesions arising in burn scars, radiodermatitis, and chronic ulcers that are more aggressive and have reported incidences of metastases in the 20 to 30 per cent range and lesions on the lips where the metastatic risk is 10 to 20 per cent. Because of a tendency toward deep invasion of the tissues and the possibility of metastases, treatment by electrodesiccation may not be effective. This approach, however, may be of value for small lesions 1 cm or less in diameter, particularly when present on the head and neck or other areas where mutilating surgery is particularly undesirable. Excisional surgery may be used for lesions where primary closure or simple grafting is possible, and radiation therapy is often preferred for the treatment of large carcinomas. When properly executed, a 5-year cure rate of about 90 per cent can be attained for patients with this disorder. Other forms of therapy include Mohs' surgery, intralesional and intravenous bleomycin, interferon, and oral retinoids for the therapeutic and prophylactic management of patients with xeroderma pigmentosum.[94]

Keratoacanthoma

Keratoacanthomas are benign self-limiting epithelial tumors resembling squamous cell carcinoma in their gross appearance, histopathologic structure, and predilection to sun-exposed areas. Multiple keratoacanthomas characteristically have their onset in adolescence or early adult life. Although this tumor has been reported during childhood and even in infancy, it is rarely seen in individuals younger than 20 years of age. Solitary keratoacanthomas appear primarily in adults older than age 45, with approximately half of all such lesions occurring during the sixth and seventh decades of life.

The lesion consists of a firm dome-shaped nodule that generally measures 1 to 3 cm or more in diameter. The center contains a horny plug or is covered by a crust that conceals a central keratin-filled crater. The nodule generally reaches its full size within 2 to 8 weeks. Following a period of quiescence, which may last for 2 to 8 weeks, lesions heal spontaneously within a few months (frequently in less than 6 months) and resolve with only a slightly depressed, somewhat cribriform scar in the previously affected area.

The main problem in the diagnosis of this disorder is its differentiation from squamous cell carcinoma. In most cases the rapid evolution to a relatively large size and its crateriform shape with a keratotic plug help to establish the correct diagnosis. Inasmuch as the architecture of the lesion is as important as the cellular characteristics, elliptical excisional biopsy, including both edges and the center of the lesion, is important for proper histopathologic diagnosis of this disorder. The characteristic microscopic features include a central invagination of the epidermis from which strands protrude into the dermis. The central crater is filled with eosinophilic keratin, and a buttress or lip of epidermis overlaps the sides of the keratin-filled crater. Aside from the architecture, a high degree of keratinization, manifested by the eosinophilic glassy appearance of many cells, is an important diagnostic feature.

The treatment of keratoacanthomas is usually approached with a view toward its spontaneous resolution. Its close resemblance to squamous cell carcinoma, however, frequently dictates excisional biopsy. Treatment, when indicated, generally consists of surgical excision, electrodesiccation and curettage, topical application of 5-fluorouracil alone or under occlusion, intralesional methotrexate, and, at times, radiation therapy. Again, in treatment of children, radiation therapy is best avoided whenever possible.

TUMORS OF THE ORAL MUCOSA

White Sponge Nevus

White sponge nevus is an exuberant, extensive, and asymptomatic white spongy plaque on the oral and occasionally nasal, vaginal, labial, or anal mucosa that may be present at birth or may appear in early childhood; it usually does not reach maximal severity until adolescence or early adulthood. Both sexes are equally affected, and the condition is inherited as an autosomal dominant trait.

The lesions are symptomless, hence often discovered by accident. They appear as soft, gray-white, somewhat friable plaques with fissures, corrugations, and folds. The superficial keratin has a tendency to desquamate, at times leaving a raw mucosal surface. The disorder is differentiated from leukoplakia, pachyonychia congenita, and cheek biting by its history, diffuseness, and soft, spongy feel of the lesions. Histologic alterations are characterized by marked spongiosis of the epithelium, parakeratosis, and vacuolization of cells.

The disorder is benign, requires no specific therapy, and should not be confused with oral focal epithelial hypoplasia (Heck's disease), a rare disorder of the oral mucosa with the mucosa of the lower lip being most commonly involved. Oral focal epithelial hypoplasia, a human papillomavirus (HPV type 13) infection that usually occurs in children and tends to regress spontaneously after a few months, is characterized clinically by soft, white, asymptomatic 2- to 4-mm papules and histologically by acanthosis, thickening and elongation of the rete ridges, and vacuolization throughout the oral epithelium.

Leukoplakia

Leukoplakia (leukokeratosis) is a term used to describe a somewhat variable whitish thickening of the epithelium of the lower lip, oral mucosa, and the vulva of older women.

Usually seen in individuals older than age 40, it may also be seen in children in association with dyskeratosis congenita (see Fig. 7–30). When seen in older persons, it is frequently associated with chronic irritation (cheilitis, pipe-smoking, biting of the lips, dentures, tobacco, and, in vulvar leukoplakia, involutional atrophy of the mucosa after menopause).

The clinical appearance and extent of lesions are variable. They generally consist of well-demarcated and irregularly outlined white patches resembling drops of candle wax, extensive thick leathery plaques, or fine opalescent patches. The histopathologic features of leukoplakia include hyperkeratosis, individual cell dyskeratosis, and cellular atypism. Since 10 per cent of lesions of leukoplakia may eventuate in squamous cell carcinoma unless treated, therapy includes removal of the source of irritation,[95] improvement of dental hygiene, surgical removal in the form of "shaving" or "stripping" techniques, cryosurgery with liquid nitrogen, electrodesiccation and curettage, radiation therapy (in adults), surgical excision, and long-term follow-up examinations.

TUMORS OF THE EPIDERMAL APPENDAGES

Nevus Sebaceus

Nevus sebaceus of Jadassohn (also referred to as an organoid nevus because the entire organ, possibly with the exception of eccrine glands, takes part in its formation), is a well-circumscribed hairless plaque that is usually solitary. It is generally present at birth or in early childhood, but at times it may arise in adult life. Although rare familial forms have been reported, these nevi are generally not inherited and occur with equal frequency in males and females and in all races.[96] In young persons it is yellow or yellow-brown to orange or pink and has a flat, velvet-like appearance (Fig. 8–34). The lesion is generally solitary; is round, oval, or linear; and varies from a few millimeters to several centimeters in diameter. Lesions on the scalp are usually round or oval, those on the face are often linear, and, on occasion, multiple and extensive lesions have been reported. They often enlarge gradually, but have been known to grow rapidly.[97] With puberty, lesions of nevus sebaceus become raised, thickened, and nodular, with closely set papillomatous projections.

Of particular significance is the fact that secondary neoplastic changes occur in 10 to 15 per cent or more of lesions, generally during adolescence or adult life. On occasion this change has occurred in children younger than 5 years of age.[97] The most common neoplasm arising from this disorder is a

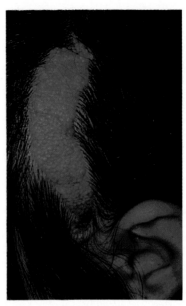

Figure 8–35. Nevus sebaceus with syringocystadenoma papilliferum.

basal cell carcinoma (epithelioma). Frequently the individual is a teenager or in the early 20s when the basal cell tumor appears. The second most common tumor is a *syringocystadenoma papilliferum* (a disorder derived from apocrine sweat glands) (Fig. 8–35). Ulceration or rapid enlargement of lesions of nevus sebaceus may indicate malignant change, usually the basal-cell type, but occasionally squamous cell carcinoma with metastasis. Other tumors arising from lesions of nevus sebaceous include keratoacanthoma, leiomyoma, piloleiomyoma, hidradenoma, apocrine cystadenoma, squamous cell carcinoma (2 per cent of cases), aggressive apocrine carcinoma, and malignant eccrine poroma, with at times widespread metastases and death.[98–100] Malignant degeneration, which is fortunately uncommon, is usually heralded by the appearance of a discrete nodule (often with superficial ulceration) on or within the lesion. At times the onset is insidious, and the clinical diagnosis of a carcinoma arising from a nevus sebaceus may be difficult.

On occasion, large lesions may be associated with ocular dermoids, major ophthalmic abnormalities, mental retardation, pigmentary and skeletal abnormalities, intracranial arteriovenous malformation, and seizure disorders. Although characterized by a predominance of sebaceous gland elements, this constellation of features, termed the *nevus sebaceus* (Schimmelpenning's) *syndrome,* probably represents a variant of the epidermal nevus syndrome.

Early in life, histopathologic examination of the sebaceous nevus reveals large numbers of immature sebaceous glands and incompletely formed hair follicles. At puberty papillomatous hyperplasia in association with hyperkeratosis and hyper-

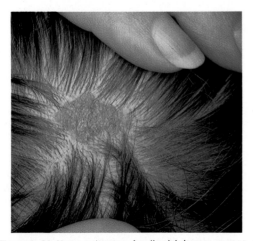

Figure 8–34. Nevus sebaceus. A yellowish brown, orange, or pink velvet-like plaque on the scalp.

granulosis takes place, and apocrine glands frequently are seen deep in the dermis beneath masses of sebaceous gland lobules.

The recognition of this lesion and its potential for neoplastic change is important. Local excision when the patient is prepubertal, preferably before enlargement of the sebaceous elements, is recommended, except perhaps for small facial lesions, which can easily be observed and do not present a cosmetic handicap. Since electrodesiccation and curettage may result in recurrences, deep-thickness surgical excision, preferably by a plastic surgeon, is generally recommended.

Nevus Comedonicus

The comedo nevus (nevus comedonicus) is a circumscribed or systematized disorder in which grouped hair follicles filled with horny plugs constitute a prominent and histologic feature. The disorder, a developmental or nevoid condition, is rarely reported. Believed by some to belong to the spectrum of epidermal nevi, it has been postulated that lesions of nevus comedonicus result from a failure in development of the mesodermal component of the pilosebaceous complex. There is no racial or sexual predisposition, and approximately half the cases are present at birth. In the remainder of the cases the lesions generally appear before 10 to 15 years of age.

The disorder is manifested by groups of closely set, slightly elevated papules that have in their center a dark, firm hyperkeratotic plug resembling a comedo (20 to 50 or more) in a linear or band-like distribution on any part of the body, with the face, neck, upper arm, chest, and abdomen as areas of predilection. The lesions tend to grow as the child matures, and large lesions extending above the surrounding cutaneous surface give a nutmeg grater–like feeling to the skin.

Histopathologic examination of lesions reveals a thickened epidermis with hyperkeratosis and acanthosis and large keratinous cysts with patulous openings extending into the cutaneous surface. Although lesions show little tendency to extension, secondary infection and abscess formation occasionally prove to be troublesome. Management includes appropriate antibiotics for secondary infection, when present, and topical retinoic acid (tretinoin) may at times be useful. When lesions are particularly troublesome, surgical excision is recommended.

Trichoepithelioma

Trichoepitheliomas may occur as a benign dominantly inherited disorder characterized by the presence of multiple small tumors, usually appearing on the face, or by a solitary nonhereditary tumor usually seen in early adult life, occasionally in childhood (Fig. 8–36). The terms *epithelioma*

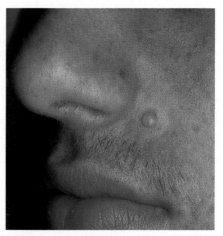

Figure 8–36. Trichoepithelioma (Brooke's tumor). A round translucent nodule with fine telangiectasia. Multiple trichoepitheliomas (epithelioma adenoides cysticum) is a disorder inherited as an autosomal dominant trait.

adenoides cysticum and *multiple benign cystic epithelioma* denote the hereditary disorder with a multiplicity of lesions, and the term *trichoepithelioma* may indicate either single or multiple lesions.

Multiple trichoepitheliomas (epithelioma adenoides cysticum) generally begin during early childhood or at puberty as small, firm, skin-colored papules and nodules on the face, particularly on the nasolabial folds and over the nose, forehead, upper lip, eyelids, and occasionally the scalp, neck, trunk, scrotum, and perianal area.[101] The lesions usually measure 2 to 5 mm in diameter, are firm, and have a translucent sheen. Occasionally, telangiectatic vessels are present over the rounded translucent surface of larger lesions. Trichoepitheliomas may enlarge slowly, reaching 5 mm in diameter on the face and ears and up to 2 to 3 cm in diameter in other sites; they often coalesce to form nodular aggregates and then remain static.

Desmoplastic trichoepithelioma is a usually solitary clinical variant of trichoepithelioma. Almost always located on the face, the lesion generally measures 3 to 8 mm in diameter, is markedly indurated, and often has a raised annular border and depressed nonulcerated center suggesting the clinical appearance of a granuloma annulare or basal cell epithelioma. Although most commonly seen in early adulthood, desmoplastic trichoepitheliomas are much more common in females, may be familial, and usually appear during the second decade of life.[102, 103]

Solitary nonhereditary trichoepitheliomas usually develop during the second or third decade of life and generally appear on the face. In 20 per cent of individuals they may be found on the scalp, neck, trunk, upper arms, or thighs. Solitary lesions usually appear as firm, flesh-colored tumors and generally reach 5 mm or slightly larger in diameter.

The gross and microscopic appearances of solitary trichoepithelioma and epithelioma adenoides cysticum are similar. Histologically these lesions are characterized by horn cysts surrounded by solid nests and lace-like strands of epithelial cells (basalioma cells). The latter show peripheral palisading of cells and, but for the characteristic horn cysts, are frequently indistinguishable from basal cell epitheliomas.

Simple surgical excision or electrodesiccation and curettage is the treatment of choice for solitary lesions. Surgical removal by electrodesiccation and curettage, dermabrasion, or cryosurgery with liquid nitrogen (for multiple trichoepitheliomas) frequently presents a problem, since attempts at removal are often followed by regrowth. Whatever the method of removal, microscopic examination to rule out the possibility of basal cell carcinoma is recommended.

Trichofolliculoma

Trichofolliculomas occur as benign solitary lesions. Usually seen on the face, scalp, ears, or neck of adults, they may occur at any age and occasionally can be seen in childhood. The lesion presents as a 0.2- to 1.0-cm slow-growing skin-colored or pearly papule or dome-shaped nodule with a smooth surface. Frequently there is a central pore with a protruding woolly or cotton-like tuft of hair (a highly diagnostic clinical feature). On occasion the protruding hairs may be so fine that a magnifying lens may be required to detect their presence.

Since this is an adnexal tumor of the hair follicle, histologic examination of lesions reveals large keratinous sinuses that contain horny material and fragments of birefringent hair shafts.

Treatment of trichofolliculoma by local surgical excision generally produces a good cosmetic result.

Pilomatricoma

Pilomatricoma (calcifying epithelioma of Malherbe),[104] a benign tumor of hair structures, usually develops before the age of 21 and manifests itself clinically as a solitary calcified deep-seated nodule on the face, neck, upper extremities, and at times perianal or genital area of children or young adults (Fig. 8–37). More than 50 per cent of lesions appear on the head and neck. The overlying skin may be normal or slightly discolored with a reddish blue tint, and although larger lesions may be encountered, the disorder generally measures 0.5 to 3 cm in diameter. Females are affected more often than males. Lesions are characterized by a stony-hard lobular consistency; and when the skin is stretched the disorder may show a "tent sign" with multiple facets and angles resembling a tent,

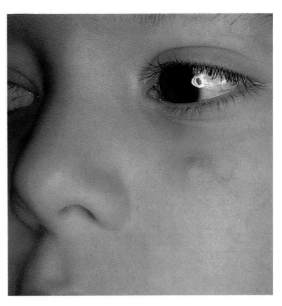

Figure 8–37. A pilomatricoma on the cheek of a young child.

a helpful clinical clue to the diagnosis of this disorder.

Although pilomatricomas as a rule are not hereditary, familial cases have been recognized and some familial forms have been associated with myotonic dystrophy (Steinert's disease), an uncommon autosomal dominant disorder characterized by hypotonia, muscle wasting, cataracts, hypogonadism, progressive mental retardation, and frontal baldness.[105] Other variants include a malignant form in which lesions arise suddenly, grow rapidly, and may have an aggressive malignant behavior[106]; cystic-appearing pilomatricomas in which hemorrhage may result in blue-red or purple translucent nodules with rapid enlargement; perforating pilomatricomas; and extruding pilomatricomas (draining lesions that spontaneously discharge a chalky material containing calcium).[107, 108]

Microscopic examination of lesions reveals sheets of epithelial cells with two patterns. Some sheets consist of compact basal cells resembling those seen in basal cell epithelioma. Adjacent cells devoid of basophilic material are seen as ghost cells or shadow cells, with transitional areas showing evolution of basaloid into shadow cells. A frequent but not constant feature, particularly in older lesions, is the presence of calcification within the areas of shadow cells, where it may occur either as fine granules within the cytoplasm of the shadow cells or as large sheets of calcification replacing these cells.

Lesions of pilomatricoma may be subject to periodic inflammation or granulomatous swelling, and treatment (usually for cosmetic purposes) consists of surgical excision by a plastic surgeon. Because of the possibility of malignant change, recurrent lesions, although uncommon, and those with rapid growth should be evaluated for this possibility.

Syringoma

Syringomas represent benign tumors of eccrine structures and are predominantly seen in females (2 : 1). The lesions occur at any age but frequently make their first appearance during puberty or adolescence as small, firm, usually multiple but occasionally solitary, translucent to skin-colored or somewhat yellowish 1- to 3-mm papules or nodules. In more than half the patients the lesions are located on the lower eyelids. Other common locations include the sides of the neck and upper thorax (especially the anterior aspect of the trunk) (Fig. 8–38), abdomen, back, upper arms, thighs, and genitalia.[109]

Children with Down's syndrome have an incidence of 19 to 37 per cent (30 times greater than that seen in other individuals).[110] In addition to their greater incidence in females and their tendency to proliferate at puberty, syringomas appear to be influenced by hormones, as evidenced by premenstrual swelling, enlargement in women on estrogenic hormones, and an increase in the size of lesions during pregnancy.

Histologic examination of lesions reveals dilated cystic eccrine ducts, some of which possess small comma-like tails of epithelial cells, with a resulting tadpole-like appearance.

Syringomas gradually enlarge until they attain their full size and then persist, with little tendency for spontaneous resolution. They are considered benign, and treatment, when desired for cosmetic reasons, consists of destruction by electrodesiccation, cryosurgery with liquid nitrogen, or local surgical excision. The disorder may sometimes regress spontaneously during adulthood; and because surgical and chemical destruction may produce unsightly scarring, laser therapy (primarily with the carbon dioxide laser) and reports of cosmetic improvement following oral administration of isotretinoin suggest alternative methods for the management of severe forms of this disorder.[111]

Eccrine Poroma

Eccrine poromas are benign cutaneous tumors that generally arise from the intraepidermal sweat duct unit. Generally seen in persons of middle age or older, they have also been noted to develop as early as 15 years of age. The disorder is manifested by firm, sometimes lobulated, asymptomatic, sessile or slightly pedunculated skin-colored to reddish nodules. Eccrine poromas generally appear as solitary lesions (2 to 12 mm in diameter) on the plantar surface of the foot and occasionally on other cutaneous surfaces such as the palms, fingers, neck, chest, or back. Although lesions tend to occur singly, multiple lesions may also occur. The disorder often has a vascular component, and the clinical appearance may, at times, suggest a pyogenic granuloma. A striking clinical feature is the frequent presence of a cup-shaped shallow depression from which the tumor grows and protrudes.

The histologic appearance of eccrine poromas is distinctive and consists of well-circumscribed, nonencapsulated tumor masses made up of broad anastomosing bands of basophilic epithelial cells that are connected by intracellular bridges and have a uniform cuboidal appearance with oval nuclei.

Since eccrine poromas may recur following incomplete removal and malignant variants have

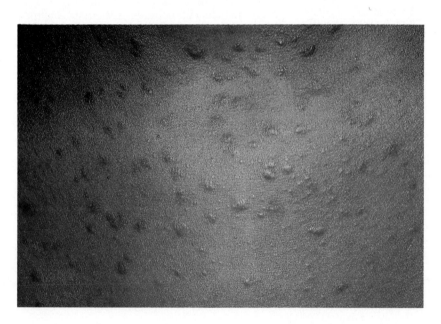

Figure 8–38. Multiple syringomas on the upper chest of a 19-year-old woman. Histopathologic evaluation of a skin biopsy specimen can help differentiate this disorder from steatocystoma multiplex.

been described,[112] surgical excision appears to be the treatment of choice for this tumor.

Cylindroma

Cylindromas (also known at times as turban or tomato tumors) are lesions of eccrine or apocrine origin characterized by spherical, firm, rubbery, pink to bluish nodules ranging from a few millimeters to several centimeters in diameter located primarily on the scalp and occasionally on the face, trunk, or extremities. Occurring in solitary or multiple forms, the solitary variant has no hereditary pattern and appears later in life; the dominantly inherited form manifests soon after puberty by numerous rounded, smooth, dome-shaped nodules resembling bunches of grapes or small tomatoes.

Cylindromas are characterized histologically by islands of epithelial cells surrounded and penetrated by thick bands of hyalin around and within the tumor lobules. Treatment consists of excision or electrosurgery, with skin grafting when necessary. Although lesions may recur if excision is incomplete and malignant degeneration has been reported, cylindromas almost invariably have a benign course.

DERMAL TUMORS

Angiofibroma

Angiofibromas may occur as isolated lesions or multiple lesions on the face. When seen as multiple lesions, they form an essential component (in 80 to 90 per cent) of the tuberous sclerosis complex. Angiofibromas (previously incorrectly termed *adenoma sebaceum*) represent hamartomas of fibrous and vascular tissue. They begin in childhood, only rarely are present at birth, generally appear between 2 and 5 years of age, and often do not occur until puberty.

Characteristically they are seen as small, 1- to 4-mm, firm, pink or flesh-colored dome-shaped tumors arranged in a symmetrical distribution in the nasolabial folds, on the cheeks or chin, and occasionally elsewhere on the face and scalp (Fig. 8–39 and, in Chapter 23, Fig. 23–5). They are rarely found on the upper lip except for the central area immediately below the nose. The lesions persist indefinitely and generally increase in size and number. Fully developed angiofibromas often appear as verrucous or polypoid growths, with or without the angiomatous hue (Fig. 8–40).

Histopathologic examination of angiofibromas reveals a proliferation of fibrous and vascular tissues. As the lesions mature, dermal fibrosis is more marked, plump spindle-shaped and stellate-shaped cells (some of which contain melanin) are loosely scattered in the areas of fibrosis, and the overlying epidermis reveals atrophy or acanthosis,

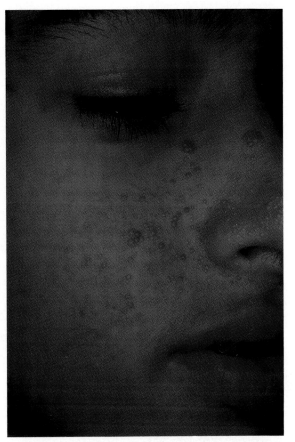

Figure 8–39. Angiofibromas (adenoma sebaceum). Multiple, firm, pink or flesh-colored dome-shaped tumors in a symmetrical distribution are evident on the face of a patient with tuberous sclerosis.

effacement of the rete ridges, and increased melanocytic activity.

These skin tumors require no treatment except for cosmetic reasons. Best results are seen following cryosurgery, electrodesiccation and curettage,

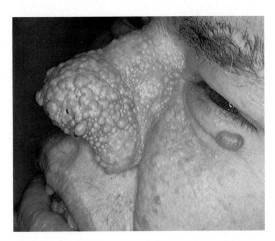

Figure 8–40. Florid adenoma sebaceum in an older person with tuberous sclerosis.

carbon dioxide or argon laser surgery, or dermabrasion, but some lesions tend to recur following superficial removal.[113]

Connective Tissue Nevi

Connective tissue nevi represent localized malformation of either or both dermal collagen and elastic fibers. These benign skin lesions, which are often hereditary, are usually seen in young children as firm, clustered, slightly raised, pea-sized, skin-colored oval lesions, distributed symmetrically over the abdomen, back, buttocks, arms, or thighs.

Early descriptions emphasized alterations in either elastic tissue (hence the term *nevus elasticus*, or juvenile elastoma) or collagen (*collagenoma*). More recently these distinctions have been obscured by a similarity in the appearance of all lesions and by the recognition of alteration of both collagen and elastic tissue. Microscopic examination of connective tissue nevi, accordingly, reveals disorganization of collagen fibers, elastic fibers, or both.

Connective tissue nevi may be familial and may sometimes be connected with other diseases. The collagenous plaques (shagreen patches of tuberous sclerosis) are flat, slightly elevated, flesh-colored lesions varying from 1 to 8 cm in diameter, with a wrinkled "pigskin" appearance, possibly due to indentation by the cutaneous appendages (Figs. 8–41 and 23–7).

Another form of connective tissue nevus, dermatofibrosis lenticularis disseminata, has been reported with osteopoikilosis (Albers-Schönberg disease, Buschke-Ollendorf syndrome), a rare hereditary dysplasia of bone affecting the long bones, pelvis, hands, and feet. The cutaneous changes usually appear in adult life, but their onset has also been reported as early as the first year of life or later in childhood. Histopathologic examination of lesions reveals a mixed pattern of increased abnormal distributed collagen and abnormal elastic fibers. The bony lesions are usually asymptomatic and found incidentally. Radiologically seen as focal sclerotic areas of bone dysplasia varying from 1 to 10 mm in diameter, bony lesions can be mistaken for metastatic disease and, if the true nature of the disorder is not recognized, may lead to unnecessary surgery and concern.

The management of connective tissue nevi consists of biopsy, when indicated, for diagnostic purposes. Surgical excision otherwise is unnecessary and, unless there is cosmetic deformity, generally not recommended.

Neurofibroma

Neurofibromas may appear as isolated, usually single, lesions in a healthy individual or as a cutaneous marker of dominantly inherited neurofibromatosis (von Recklinghausen's disease) (see Chapter 23). Tumors usually appear first in childhood or adolescence and gradually increase in size and, in neurofibromatosis, in number. The cutaneous tumors of neurofibromatosis generally appear in late childhood or adolescence, and their appearance is frequently associated with puberty. They may occur anywhere on the body, with no specific site of predilection other than that they usually avoid the palms and soles.

Solitary cutaneous neurofibromas are smooth, polypoid, and soft or firm. Although generally flesh colored, they tend to have a distinctive violaceous hue when small and, as they enlarge, they tend to become pink, blue, or pigmented. They may appear as superficial tumors, varying in size from 1 or 2 mm to several centimeters in diameter or as discrete beaded, nodular, elongated masses (plexiform neuromas) along the course of nerves, usually the trigeminal or upper cervical nerves. Small tumors may be deep-seated, sessile, or dome-shaped. As they become larger they become globular, pear-shaped, pedunculated, or pendulous. With moderate digital pressure the smaller lesions may be invaginated into an underlying dermal defect, an almost pathognomonic maneuver termed *buttonholing*.

In addition to solitary neurofibromas and the florid forms of neurofibromatosis, there are incomplete forms (formes frustes) of von Recklinghausen's disease in which only a few manifestations occur. The presence of café au lait spots, axillary freckling, scoliosis, and bilateral acoustic neuromas suggests formes frustes or minor manifestations of this disorder.

Histopathologic features consist of fine wavy fibrils of connective tissue and nerve fibers. The

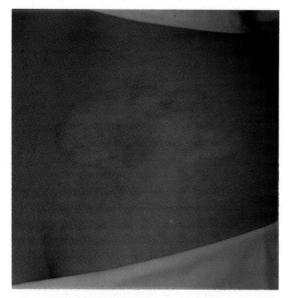

Figure 8–41. Connective tissue nevus. A slightly elevated, flesh-colored collagenous plaque (shagreen patch) on the lower back of a patient with tuberous sclerosis.

nuclei tend to parallel one another and at times may be arranged in whorl-like formations. Remnants of nerve bundles usually appear within the tumor. If nerve bundles are not seen, the distinction between neurofibroma and an ordinary fibroma may be difficult.

Treatment of cutaneous neurofibromas consists of surgical excision of tumors that are disfiguring, interfere with function, or are subject to irritation, trauma, or infection. Large plexiform neurofibromas have a small but definite incidence of fibrosarcoma in later life. Excision, accordingly, should be performed prophylactically when feasible. Although malignant degeneration of lesions is rare before age 40, complete surgical excision with histopathologic examination is required if cutaneous neurofibromas become painful or show signs of rapid enlargement.

Dermatofibroma

Dermatofibromas (histiocytoma cutis) are benign growths of connective tissue generally seen in adults; occasionally they are seen in children. They appear as small, well-defined dermal nodules, firmly fixed to the skin but freely movable over the subcutaneous fat. Nodules may be found on any part of the body and are common on the extremities, particularly on the anterior surface of the leg (Fig. 8–42).

Their size varies from 1 mm to 3 cm in diameter, and their color may range from a flesh color to red-brown, tan, or black. The majority of lesions are dome-shaped, but occasionally they will be depressed below the cutaneous surface. Usually lesions attain their maximum size and then remain stationary for years.

Generalized eruptive histiocytomas are characterized by symmetrical, discrete, flesh-colored or bluish red papules or papulonodules with no tendency to grouping. More closely related to juvenile xanthogranuloma (nevoxanthoendothelioma), histiocytosis X, and xanthoma disseminatum than to the classic solitary histiocytoma, these lesions tend to develop in crops and often involute spontaneously.

Dermatofibromas vary in their microscopic appearance. Some lesions show a well-circumscribed but encapsulated proliferation of fibroblasts and young collagen fibers, while in others histiocytes predominate. Lesions contain varying numbers of cells with small spindle-shaped nuclei that represent the fibroblasts. The collagen appears irregularly arranged in intertwining and anastomosing bands, and a significant acanthosis of the epidermis in the center of the lesion is of considerable diagnostic value. Histiocytic lesions are composed of histiocytes that show evidence of phagocytosis of lipid and hemosiderin. At times, multinucleated giant cells of the Touton type may be observed.

Although treatment of dermatofibromas or eruptive histiocytomas is unnecessary, surgical excision may be done for cosmetic or diagnostic purposes.

Dermatofibrosarcoma Protuberans

Dermatofibrosarcoma protuberans represents a slowly growing malignant tumor that, originating in the dermis, is locally invasive and, although it has a strong tendency to recur, rarely metastasizes.

Seen primarily in middle-aged adults (50 per cent are seen in individuals between 20 and 50 years of age), the disorder may also be seen at the time of birth, and about 10 per cent of cases arise in children younger than the age of 10.[114] It usually begins as an indurated plaque on which multiple red or purple nodules subsequently arise. As the nodules slowly increase in size, they may ulcerate. The trunk is the most frequent location, followed by the extremities, particularly their proximal regions; and the scalp, neck, and face are only rarely involved.

The histologic appearance of dermatofibrosarcoma protuberans is that of a subepidermal fibrotic lesion composed predominantly of cells with large spindle-shaped nuclei embedded in varying amounts of collagen. The cells are generally arranged in irregular, intertwining bands, resulting in a stariform (mat-like) pattern; and in some areas the cells radiate from a central hub of fibrous tissue in a whorl-like cartwheel fashion. Since the lesion is deeply invasive, metastases may be seen in 5 to 10 per cent of patients, and local recurrences are common, wide local excision and Mohs' micrographic surgical technique appear to be the treatments of choice.[114, 115]

Recurring Digital Fibroma of Childhood

Recurrent infantile digital fibroma (recurring digital fibroma of childhood) is a benign, asymptomatic fibrous tumor that appears on the distal phalanges during infancy or early childhood (Fig. 8–43). Eighty-six per cent of cases occur during the first year of life.[116] The fingers and toes are about equally affected in this disorder, but the thumb and great toe are spared. The tumor presents as a

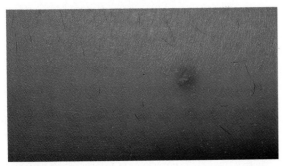

Figure 8–42. A dermatofibroma on the leg of a 17-year-old girl.

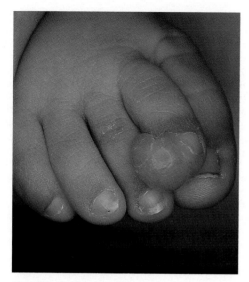

Figure 8–43. Recurring digital fibroma (of childhood).

smooth, dome-shaped, tense elevation up to 1 or 2 cm in diameter on the tips, sides, or dorsal aspect of affected digits. The overlying cutaneous surface is smooth, shiny, and erythematous.

The lesion affects both sexes equally and, although the etiology is unknown, the appearance of virus-like eosinophilic inclusion bodies in the dermis suggests a viral etiology. Electron microscopic examinations, however, are equivocal, and these cytoplasmic inclusions may actually represent degenerated organelles without viral causation.

Histopathologic features include interdigitating sheets of spindle-shaped fibroblasts, collagen fibers, and small, round, red perinuclear intracytoplasmic inclusion bodies in the proliferating fibroblasts (which are pathognomonic). Although nuclear atypia and the occasional presence of mitotic figures have been described, such features are not regularly present.

Despite the apparent benignity of this disorder, because of its high recurrence rate (60 per cent), either amputation of the digit or wide surgical excision with dissection down to the periosteum, with grafting when necessary, has been recommended. However, the fact that the tumor is benign and that, at least in some cases, spontaneous resolution has been reported suggests observation as a reasonable alternate to radical surgery once the diagnosis has been made. When functional impairment or deformity of the affected digit occurs, however, appropriate surgery appears to be warranted.[116, 117]

Infantile Myofibromatosis

Infantile myofibromatosis is a term used to describe two fibrous disorders (congenital multiple myofibromatosis and congenital generalized myofibromatosis), which actually represent two variants of the same disorder. In patients with *congeni-*

tal multiple myofibromatosis fibrous nodules composed of myofibroblasts are confined to the skin, subcutaneous tissue, skeletal muscle, and bone. There is no visceral involvement, and the nodules almost always regress spontaneously within 1 or 2 years. In patients with *congenital generalized myofibromatosis* visceral lesions are also present, and the disorder has a mortality as high as 80 per cent (generally within the first few months of life), usually as a result of obstruction of a vital organ (the lungs, gastrointestinal tract, or central nervous system), failure to thrive, debility, or intercurrent infection.[118, 119] In both disorders, 0.5- to 7.0-cm, firm, skin-colored to red or purple, ovoid or spherical dermal and subcutaneous nodules are usually present at birth or shortly thereafter. Although they may vary widely in distribution, they most commonly involve the trunk, head, and neck areas (Figs. 8–44 and 8–45). Skeletal lesions occur in more than one half of cases; and although any bone can be affected, the skull (Fig. 8–46), femur, tibia, spine, and ribs are the most commonly involved areas.

The histopathologic features consist of fibroblasts with oval to spindle-shaped nuclei arranged in interlacing bundles or a whorled pattern. Visceral lesions, when they occur, usually have a decreased cell density, less collagen and hyaline material, and greater vascularity. Since the cutaneous and subcutaneous nodules of infantile myofibromatosis tend to regress spontaneously, surgical excision is indicated only for diagnostic purposes, to alleviate obstruction or potential trauma, or to treat lesions in which the clinical course is prolonged and progressive. Surgery is recommended if vital structures are affected and chemotherapy with vincristine, actinomycin-D, and cyclophosphamide,

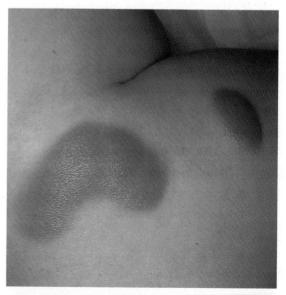

Figure 8–44. Infantile myofibromatosis. These firm rubbery nodules on the hip and upper thigh of an infant can be differentiated from lesions of granuloma gluteale infantum by histopathologic examination of a cutaneous punch biopsy.

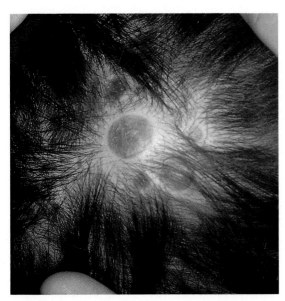

Figure 8–45. Infantile myofibromatosis on the scalp of a 13-month-old boy. The lesion also had involvement of the underlying bone and intracranial area.

with or without radiation, has been utilized for patients with recurrent or nonresectable tumors.

Epidermal Cysts

Epidermal cysts (epithelial, sebaceous, or pilar cysts) are discrete slow-growing, elevated, round, firm, slightly compressible 0.5- to 5.0-cm nodules that may appear at any time after puberty and most commonly occur on the face, scalp, nape of the neck, back, or scrotum. Although it has been well established that true sebaceous cysts do occur, most differentiate toward hair keratin and not sebaceous material. Accordingly, the term *sebaceous cyst* is frequently incorrectly applied to these common tumors.

Epidermal cysts are generally unilocular and result from the proliferation of surface epidermal cells situated within the dermis. Production of keratin and lack of communication with the surface are responsible for cyst formation. Most epidermal cysts arise from occluded pilosebaceous follicles. Some, however, arise from traumatic displacement of epidermal cells into the dermis, or from entrapment of epidermal cells along embryonic lines of closure (dermal cysts).

Milia (small multiple inclusion cysts within the dermis) differ from epidermal cysts only in size. They are multiple, 1- to 2-mm, whitish, hard globoid lesions that arise spontaneously on the face (Fig. 8–47). They occur as congenital lesions in newborns. In older persons, they also may arise as a result of trauma, such as may be seen following dermabrasion, or in the course of bullous disorders such as epidermolysis bullosa and porphyria.

Pilar cysts (wens) are epidermal cysts that occur on the scalp, and chalazions represent analogous cystic tumors of the eyelids that develop from meibomian glands. In Gardner's syndrome (a dominantly transmitted disorder characterized by premalignant colonic and rectal polyps and osseous and dental lesions) large disfiguring cysts may be found on the face, scalp, trunk, scrotum, or extremities. In Oldfield's syndrome, premalignant polyposis of the colon may also be seen in association with multiple sebaceous cysts.

Histopathologic examination of epidermal cysts reveals a wall of flattened or atrophic squamous and granular cells enclosing a keratin-filled cystic area. When the cyst ruptures and the contents are

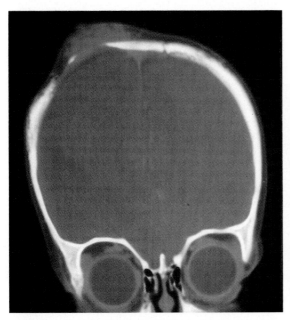

Figure 8–46. Infantile myofibromatosis. Computed tomography (CT scan) reveals bony and intracranial involvement in the patient in Figure 8–45.

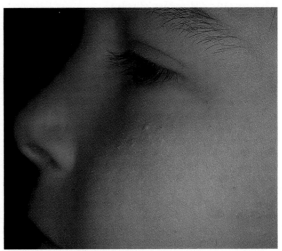

Figure 8–47. Milia. Small multiple inclusion cysts are noted on the cheek of an 8-year-old boy.

released into the dermis, a foreign body reaction with foreign-body giant cells may be noted.

Malignant degeneration (squamous cell or basal cell epithelioma) of epidermal and pilar cysts is rare. The treatment of epidermal cysts consists of local excision and suturing of the remaining cutaneous defect or a small puncture at the dome of the tumor with expression of the contents and removal of the cystic sac through the surgical opening. In treatment of epidermal cysts it is essential that the entire epidermal lining be removed or destroyed; otherwise small numbers of cells left behind may be responsible for recurrence.

Dermoid Cysts

Dermoid cysts are subcutaneous cysts of congenital origin seen chiefly along lines of embryonic fusion. Usually present at birth, they are most common on the head, mainly around the eyes, root of the nose, anterior aspect of the neck, scrotum, perineal raphe, and sacrum. Seen as painless firm tumors, they usually measure 1 to 4 cm in diameter and contain a highly characteristic, greasy, keratinous material and, at times, hair, bone, tooth, or nerve tissue. Since dermoid cysts may be attached to underlying structures and intracranial extension of nasal midline masses is common, biopsy, invasive techniques, or surgical intervention of any congenital midline mass should be avoided until intracranial connections are ruled out.[120] Untreated dermoid cysts persist and tend to grow as the child becomes older and, on rare occasions, carcinomatous degeneration may occur. Surgical excision is the treatment of choice and is curative if complete. Since dermoid cysts may be attached to underlying structures, particularly nasal dermoids in which there may be intracranial extension, prompt availability of a neurosurgical team and meticulous dissection are essential.

Mucoceles (Mucous Cysts)

Mucoceles (mucous cysts of the oral mucosa) are often seen as soft, white or bluish, solitary asymptomatic lesions, usually on the mucous surface of the lower lip and occasionally on the gums, tongue, or buccal mucosa. Generally less than 1 cm in diameter, lesions are dome shaped, are translucent, and contain a clear viscous fluid. The result of minor trauma causing rupture of a mucous duct and extravasation of sialomucin into the tissue, mucous cysts can be treated by surgical excision, incision and drainage followed by coagulation of the sac, carbon dioxide laser ablation, or cryosurgery.[121]

Digital Mucous Cysts

Digital mucous cysts (also known as myxoid or synovial cysts) are focal accumulations of mucin seen as soft, fluctuant white-to-pink dome-shaped nodules located on the dorsal aspect of the distal interphalangeal joint or proximal nail fold. Although controversy exists regarding their pathogenesis, they appear to represent a metabolic derangement of fibroblasts with increased production of hyaluronic acid in sites exposed to friction or minor trauma. As a result of degenerative joint changes, those located over the distal interphalangeal joints may result from herniation of an underlying tendon sheath or synovium (thus representing a ganglion) and may communicate with the underlying joint space. Digital mucous cysts may at times be misdiagnosed as a verruca or molluscum contagiosum and the true diagnosis may not be established until repeated unsuccessful attempts at therapy have been initiated. Although cryosurgery may at times be helpful in the treatment of mucoceles, they have limited success in the treatment of digital mucous cysts. Surgical excision is frequently effective, but recurrences are common and traditional surgical techniques can at times result in scarring and impairment of joint mobility. Carbon dioxide laser vaporization, therefore, has been suggested as a possible treatment of choice.[122]

Steatocystoma Multiplex

Steatocystoma multiplex is a disorder characterized by numerous small 2- to 4-mm, rounded, moderately firm, yellowish cutaneous cystic nodules located primarily on the chest and occasionally on the face, arms, and thighs of affected individuals. The disorder has a high familial tendency and is often dominantly inherited, and an occasional concomitant occurrence with pachyonychia congenita has been recognized.

Although lesions were formerly regarded as sebaceous or keratin-inclusion cysts, it now seems clear that they represent hamartomas and are a histologic variant of dermoid or vellus hair cysts. They usually appear or become larger at puberty. No punctum is apparent, and the more superficial lesions may have a yellowish color. On puncturing the cystic lesions, a syrup-like odorless liquid and, in some instances, small hairs may be noted.

On histopathologic examination the lesions have an intricately folded, thin, epidermal lining. The cyst wall incorporates abortive hair follicles and, at times, sebaceous, eccrine, or apocrine structures.

Because of the large number of lesions involved, treatment is generally not recommended. When desired, however, individual lesions can be excised, electrodesiccated, or incised and drained; on occasion, dermabrasion of multiple lesions of the face may be cosmetically acceptable. Isotretinoin has also been used for severe forms of this disorder. The possibility of exacerbation or worsening of the disorder in patients so treated, however, suggests caution when this modality is used.[123]

Keloids

Keloids represent an exaggerated connective tissue response to skin injury. Rare in infancy, their incidence increases throughout childhood, reaching a maximum between puberty and 30 years of age. Blacks and other deeply pigmented persons are more susceptible to keloids than individuals with fair skin, and the tendency often runs in families. Early growing lesions are pink, smooth, and rubbery and often tender, with surfaces extending beyond the area of the original wound (see Fig. 6–8). Hypertrophic scars, conversely, tend to stay within the margins of the lesion.

Microscopic examination of keloids reveals dense and sharply defined connective tissue in the dermis composed of whorl-like arrangements of hyalinized bundles of collagen. The superficial collagen bundles lie parallel to the epidermis, but those lower down interlace in all directions.

Elective cosmetic procedures in persons who have a tendency to form keloids should be avoided. Keloids less than 5 cm in diameter may respond to intralesional injections of long-acting corticosteroids (10 to 40 mg/ml of triamcinolone acetonide) with concomitant cryosurgery with liquid nitrogen. The use of intralesional steroid or radiation therapy in conjunction with careful plastic surgery is helpful for large lesions. Local or linear perilesional atrophy or hypopigmentation, however, may at times be seen as a complication following the use of intralesional corticosteroid injection. Fortunately, however, these usually disappear spontaneously, generally within several months to 1 year.[124]

TUMORS OF FAT, MUSCLES, AND BONE

Lipomas

A lipoma, one of the most common benign tumors, is composed of mature fat cells. It can be seen at any age but usually occurs from puberty on. Lesions may be present on any part of the body but predominantly appear in the subcutaneous tissues of the neck, shoulders, back, and abdominal wall. They may be single or multiple and of variable size, with a characteristic soft, often lobulated rubbery, putty-like consistency. Microscopic examination reveals encapsulated tumors composed of adipose tissue with essentially the same appearance as normal subcutaneous fat.

A rare nevoid variety, nevus lipomatosus superficialis of Hoffman-Zurhelle, is characterized by soft skin-colored to yellowish papules, nodules, or plaques located on the buttocks, sacrococcygeal areas, or thighs. A vascular variant, angiolipoma, is clinically indistinguishable except that the lesions are often tender or painful and have a greater tendency to be multiple.

Lipomas may be left untreated unless they become painful, increase in size, or are large enough to be objectionable. Malignant change is very rare except in lesions of 10 cm or more in diameter, particularly on the thighs. These should be investigated for malignancy, and surgical excision is the treatment of choice.

The Michelin-Tire Baby

The *Michelin-tire baby* is a term used to describe a rare disorder of newborns characterized by numerous, deep, conspicuous, cutaneous folds, apparently produced by excessive fat, some of which lie high in the dermis and result in a cutaneous appearance similar to that of the logo of the Michelin Tire Company. Although the cause of this disorder is uncertain, it appears to be associated with a lipomatous nevus, metaplasia of the dermis into adipose tissue, or an anomalous embryonic growth of fatty tissue. Abnormalities associated with this disorder include mental retardation, microcephaly, rocker-bottom feet, metatarsus abductus, hemiplegia, hemihypertrophy, chromosomal abnormalities, abnormal ears, and severe neurologic defects.[125]

Congenital Smooth Muscle Hamartoma

Congenital smooth muscle hamartoma is a benign disorder of the skin characterized by a proliferation of smooth muscles within the reticular dermis. Probably much more common than the literature suggests, the disorder is manifested by a localized patch or slightly elevated plaque of skin-colored or mildly hyperpigmented skin that generally measures several centimeters in diameter; there are multiple small follicular papules and at times fine hairs throughout the involved area (see Fig. 8–22).[126] Although usually present at birth, the disorder may not be noted until childhood or early adulthood and is seen as indurated areas of skin caused by hyperplasia of the smooth muscles in the dermis. This results in fasciculation of the skin (the pseudo-Darier sign) with a striking brief puckering or cobblestone appearance following stimulation of the arrector pili muscles by stroking, rubbing, or washing of the affected area.

Believed by many to be a part of the spectrum of Becker's nevus (see Fig. 8–21),[49, 50] the histopathologic features consist of thick well-defined bundles of smooth muscle fibers scattered throughout the dermis. In cases associated with hypertrichosis, the smooth muscle bundles frequently demonstrate connections with large hair follicles. Since this is a benign lesion, treatment is unnecessary.

Leiomyomas

Leiomyomas represent benign tumors principally derived from cutaneous smooth muscle. The majority of these lesions arise from arrector pili muscles, the media of blood vessels, or smooth muscle of the scrotum, labia majora, or nipples. Although found among all age groups, leiomyomas generally occur during the third decade of life and are relatively uncommon in childhood.

Cutaneous leiomymomas may be solitary or multiple and generally present as pink, red, or dusky brown, firm dermal nodules of varying size (Fig. 8–48). The lesions generally are subject to episodes of paroxysmal, often spontaneous, pain. Multiple cutaneous leiomyomas are reddish brown to blue, firm, elevated intradermal nodules, often with a translucent or waxy appearance. They tend to occur on the back, face, or extensor surfaces of the extremities and are usually arranged in groups.

Enlarging lesions often coalesce to form plaques with an arciform or linear configuration. Solitary leiomyomas have their onset at a later age than multiple lesions. They are generally somewhat larger but, although lesions as large as 10 cm in diameter have been described, seldom grow to more than 1.5 to 2 cm in diameter.

Leiomyomas may be classified as hereditary or nonhereditary types and are characterized by unencapsulated tumors of smooth muscle bundles and masses with an irregular arrangement. Although the smooth muscle cells of the tumor resemble normal smooth muscle, they are generally somewhat larger.

There are four types of leiomyomas of the skin: (1) multiple piloleiomyomas, by far the most common type; (2) solitary piloleiomyomas; (3) solitary genital or mamillary leiomyomas, derived from the smooth muscle of the nipple and genital regions (referred to as the dartoic type); and (4) angioleiomyomas, a variety of leiomyoma arising from the tunica media of the blood vessels and embryonic muscle rests. Most often found on the lower leg, they are made of smooth muscle bundles derived from the arrector pili muscles. Leiomyosarcomas seldom arise in the skin, but when they do they have the same general age distribution as leiomyomas but are more widely distributed and do not tend to favor the extensor surfaces. Clinically

they are larger than leiomyomas and present as nondescript subcutaneous masses. Metastases, when they occur, generally spread through the bloodstream and lymphatics, and lung involvement is a common complication. The microscopic appearance of leiomyosarcomas varies from a pattern closely resembling leiomyoma to a highly malignant appearance with an atypical cellular pattern and frequent mitotic figures.

Leiomyomas are benign but have a high incidence of recurrence (up to 50 per cent) following removal. Surgical excision is the treatment of choice with wide surgical excision and skin grafting, if necessary, for lesions of leiomyosarcoma. Cutaneous leiomyosarcomas, however, are extremely rare and when they do occur they probably did not arise from a preexisting leiomyoma. Hereditary leiomyomas are usually multiple and derived from piloarrector muscles, and reports of uterine leiomyomas in affected girls or women suggest evaluation for uterine involvement because of possible bleeding and leiomyosarcoma.

Calcinosis Cutis

Cutaneous calcification can be either focal or widespread and can be the consequence of cutaneous injury, secondary to metabolic alteration of calcium and phosphorus, or of unknown cause.

Solitary Nodular Calcification. Occasionally solitary small raised verrucous nodular calcifications of the skin may be seen in infants and small children (Fig. 8–49). Originally described as "solitary congenital nodular calcification of the skin," they are not always solitary, are frequently not congenital, and generally measure 3 to 11 mm in diameter. Cutaneous calcifications can also be seen as a consequence of diagnostic heel sticks in the newborn or as a result of calcium chloride used in electrode paste on abraded skin. Histologically, lesions of calcinosis cutis are characterized by a subepidermal mass of calcified material. Treatment, when desired, consists of surgical excision or gentle cryosurgery or electrodesiccation and curettage.

Calcinosis Universalis and Calcinosis Cutis Circumscripta. Calcinosis universalis and calcinosis cutis circumscripta may be idiopathic or secondary to tissue damage or connective tissue or metabolic disorders. They are characterized by papules, plaques, or tumors; are often purple-red; and are firm or stony to palpation.

Lesions of calcinosis circumscripta vary from 2 to 30 mm in diameter and occur chiefly on the upper extremities (particularly the fingers or the wrists) and have a tendency to be situated in locations subject to frequent motion or trauma, namely, the flexor tendons of the hands and the extensor tendons of the elbows and knees. Lesions consist of creamy material containing small gritty particles of calcium and are generally seen in patients with dermatomyositis or CRST syndrome (*calcinosis*

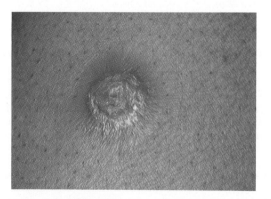

Figure 8–48. Solitary leiomyoma. An elevated, flesh-colored, pink, red, or dusky brown, firm dermal nodule is seen on the extensor aspect of the arm.

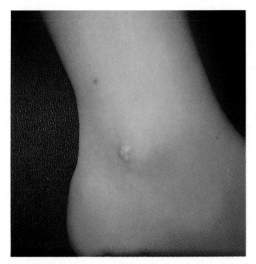

Figure 8–49. Cutaneous calcification (calcinosis cutis). Firm nodular flesh-colored deposition of calcium in the skin overlying the lateral malleolus of the ankle.

cutis, *R*aynaud's phenomenon, *s*cleroderma, and *t*elangiectasia).

Calcinosis universalis is a generalized disorder usually seen in girls. Although the etiology of this disorder is unknown, a local factor controlling calcification in the tissues is postulated. In this disorder, 0.5- to 5-cm nodules or plaques are distributed symmetrically over the extremities and, less commonly, the trunk.

Metastatic Calcinosis Cutis. This rare entity is characterized by metastatic calcifications to the skin, hyperphosphatemia, and elevated serum calcium. The cutaneous manifestations consist of small, firm, white papules 1 to 4 mm in diameter surrounded by slight edema. Occurring symmetrically in the popliteal fossae and over the iliac crests and posterior axillary lines, this type of calcinosis is seen in disorders such as parathyroid neoplasms, hypervitaminosis D, and diseases associated with excessive destruction of bone (severe osteomyelitis, Paget's disease, chronic renal disease, or metastatic carcinoma).

Treatment of calcinosis cutis consists of correction of the underlying disorder whenever possible, surgical removal of painful deposits, and, in some instances, administration of oral aluminum hydroxide antacids and a diet low in phosphorus and calcium.[127, 128]

Osteoma Cutis

Osseous formation in the skin may be primary or secondary. The term *osteoma cutis* generally refers to the primary type, which represents spontaneous new bone formation in the skin and is associated with Albright's hereditary osteodystrophy (pseudohypoparathyroidism and pseudopseudohypoparathyroidism)[129] or an isolated idiopathic occurrence. Secondary ossification occurs in areas of tissue degeneration caused by irritation, trauma, or various granulomatous disorders.

Cutaneous osteomas are usually multiple but may be solitary. Lesions may be present at birth or may arise at any age and occasionally have a familial pattern. Lesions generally occur over the face (especially the forehead, cheeks, and chin), are hard, raised, and sharply defined, and range from 1 to 5 mm in diameter. Lesions may be painful and tender, and the overlying skin may be normal, erythematous, pigmented, ulcerated, or atrophic.

Secondary osteomas of the skin can develop in pigmented nevi, fibromas, basal cell epitheliomas, tricholemmal cysts, lesions of acne vulgaris, folliculitis, scleroderma, and areas of scar tissue.

Histopathologic examination of lesions reveals proliferation of normal bone tissue in the dermis or subcutis. Osteoblasts and osteoclasts are also present on the periphery of these lesions.

Treatment, when necessary, consists of surgical excision of involved tissues.

Subungual Exostosis

Subungual exostosis is a solitary fibrous nodule on the terminal border of the distal phalanx of a finger or toe. Although the great toe reputedly has been described as the most commonly afflicted, this disorder may involve any of the toes and, on occasion, even a finger may be affected (Fig. 8–50).[130] When multiple lesions are noted, an autosomal dominant disorder (multiple exostoses syndrome) and possible involvement of the long bones (particularly the knees), the pelvis, scapulae, and ribs should be considered.

Although trauma has frequently been described as a precipitating factor, lesions commonly evolve spontaneously without a history of previous injury or trauma, usually develop in older children, ado-

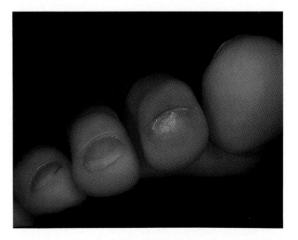

Figure 8–50. Subungual exostosis. A fibrous nodule on the distal phalanx of a toe may at times be misdiagnosed as a subungual wart.

lescents, or young adults between 12 and 30 years of age, and appear twice as often in females as in males.

The first appearance is a small pink or flesh-colored growth that develops beneath and projects slightly beyond the free edge of the nail. The portion of the nail overlying the lesion is lifted and becomes detached or may be removed by the patient or a parent in an effort to relieve the pain that frequently is associated with this disorder. The tumor then mushrooms upward, often above the nail as a mass of dense fibrous tissue, and generally attains 8 to 10 mm in diameter.

The differential diagnosis of subungual exostoses includes verrucae, pyogenic granuloma, glomus tumor, epidermoid carcinoma, or melanoma. When the diagnosis is in doubt, the firm, often stony nature of the disorder may suggest, and radiography generally will confirm, the diagnosis.

Once the diagnosis of subungual exostosis is established, total excision, preferably by an orthopedic surgeon under aseptic conditions, such as afforded by a hospital operating room, is the proper method of treatment. Complete excision with actual saucerization is generally required, since incomplete excision frequently results in recurrence of the disorder.

References

1. Jacobs AH, Walton RG: The incidence of birthmarks in the neonate. Pediatrics 58:218–222, 1976.

   A study of the various types of birthmarks in 1,058 newborns younger than 72 hours of age.

2. Walton RG, Jacobs AH, Cox AJ: Pigmented lesions in newborn infants. Br. J. Dermatol. 95:389–396, 1976.

   Clinical and pathologic evaluation of pigmented lesions in 1,058 newborns emphasizes the importance of pathologic examination to determine the true nature of various pigmented lesions.

3. Masson P: My conception of cellular nevi. Cancer 4:9–38, 1951.

   The neural theory of the origin of nevi.

4. Mishima Y: Macromolecular changes in pigmentary disorders. Arch. Dermatol. 91:519–557, 1965.

   Light microscopic, electron microscopic, and histochemical studies of various pigmentary disorders suggest a working hypothesis for the origin and pathogenesis of cellular nevi and melanotic tumors.

5. Schoenfeld RJ, Pinkus H: The recurrence of nevi after incomplete removal. Arch. Dermatol. 78:30–35, 1958.

   Recurrence of nevi by nevus cells from the periphery and hair root sheaths of the original lesion is common and does not imply malignant potential.

6. Allyn B, Kopf AW, Kahn M, et al.: Incidence of pigmented nevi. J.A.M.A. 186:890–893, 1963.

   Routine excision of pigmented nevi on palms and soles is unnecessary.

7. Roth ME, Grant-Kels JM, Kuhn K, et al.: Melanoma in children. J. Am. Acad. Dermatol. 22:265–274, 1990.

   A report of four children, all younger than the age of 17 years, with cutaneous melanomas. One, a 16-year-old girl with a history of frequent sun exposure, died of metastatic disease less than 1 year after the initial diagnosis was established.

8. Hurwitz S: The sun and sunscreen protection: Recommendations for children. J. Dermatol. Surg. Oncol. 14:657–660, 1988.

   The problem of sun exposure in childhood, its relationship to skin cancer, and recommendations for sun protection of children.

9. MacKie RM, Freudenburger T, Aitchison TC: Personal risk-factor chart for cutaneous melanoma. Lancet 2:487–490, 1989.

   An authoritative review of risk factors for malignant melanoma.

10. Anderson DE, Smith JL Jr, McBride CM: Hereditary aspects of malignant melanoma. J.A.M.A. 200:741–746, 1967.

    Data in 22 families, with particular emphasis on one kindred in whom malignant melanoma developed in a total of 15 individuals, demonstrates an autosomal genetic basis for some individuals with this disorder.

11. Rhodes AR, Melski JW: Small congenital nevocellular nevi and the risk of cutaneous melanoma. J. Pediatr. 100:219–224, 1982.

    Of 134 melanoma patients, 14.9 per cent recalled a history of a preexisting congenital pigmented lesion present at birth at the site of the tumor.

12. Lederman JS, Sober AJ: Does biopsy type influence survival in clinical stage I cutaneous melanoma? J. Am. Acad. Dermatol. 13:983–987, 1985.

    A study of 472 patients with clinical stage I melanoma offers further confirmation that the risk of tumor embolization after biopsy is more theoretical than real.

13. Mooney E, Bennett RG: Periungual hyperpigmentation mimicking Hutchinson's sign associated with minocycline administration. J. Dermatol. Surg. Oncol. 14:1011–1013, 1988.

    Periungual hyperpigmentation and pigmented nail streaks are not always pathognomonic of melanoma.

14. Baran R, Kechijian P: Longitudinal melanonychia (melanonychia striata): Diagnosis and management. J. Am. Acad. Dermatol. 21:1165–1175, 1989.

    A comprehensive review of longitudinal melanonychia and malignant melanoma of the nail, with clues to appropriate diagnosis and management.

15. Clark WH Jr, From L, Bernardino EA, et al.: The histogenesis and biologic behavior of primary human malignant melanomas of the skin. Cancer Res. 29:705–727, 1969.

    The relationship between prognosis and depth of invasion of primary malignant melanoma.

16. Breslow A: Prognostic factors in the treatment of cutaneous malignant melanoma. J. Cutan. Pathol. 6:208–212, 1979.

    Microscopic depths and their value in the prognosis and management of cutaneous malignant melanoma.

17. American Academy of Dermatology: Guidelines for Care of Malignant Melanoma. American Academy of Dermatology Bulletin, March 1991, 3–5.

    A current review of malignant melanoma, its diagnostic criteria and therapy.

18. Rigel DS, Rogers GS, Friedman RJ: Prognosis of malignant melanoma. Dermatol. Clin. 3:309–314, 1988.

    Although the depth of vertical invasion of the tumor appears to be the best prognostic factor, features such as the anatomic site of the lesion and ulceration also influence survival in patients with malignant melanoma.

19. Ho VC, Sober AJ: Therapy for cutaneous melanoma: An update. J. Am. Acad. Dermatol. 22:159–176, 1990.

An authoritative review of the diagnosis, staging, treatment, and follow-up of patients with cutaneous melanoma.

20. Greeley PW, Middleton AG, Curtin JW: Incidence of malignancy in giant pigmented nevi. Plast. Reconstr. Surg. 36:26–37, 1965.

The incidence of malignant change in giant pigmented nevi is greater than generally realized; although the majority of cases occur after puberty, malignant melanoma can occur in such lesions during infancy and early childhood.

21. Mark GJ, Mihm MC, Liteplo MG, et al.: Congenital melanocytic nevi of the small and garment type. Hum. Pathol. 4:395–418, 1973.

Small congenital nevi may share the same propensity for malignant degeneration as large garment nevi.

22. Trozak DJ, Rowland WD, Hu F: Metastatic malignant melanoma in prepubertal children. Pediatrics 55:191–203, 1975.

Review of 68 prepubertal cases of malignant melanoma with proven metastases suggest that there is no safe waiting period and suspicious cases should be removed as soon as technically feasible.

23. Arons MS, Hurwitz S: Congenital nevocellular nevi: Review of treatment controversy. Plast. Reconstr. Surg. 72:355–365, 1983.

An overview of the problem of congenital pigmented nevi, their risks and management.

24. Illig L, Weidner F, Hundeiker M, et al.: Congenital nevi ≤10 cm as precursors to melanoma. Arch. Dermatol. 121:1274–1281, 1985.

A review of 52 congenital melanocytic nevi supports the concept that even small congenital pigmented nevi (those equal or less than 10 cm in diameter) are potential precursors to melanoma. Although when giant congenital pigmented nevi become malignant this change generally occurs during the first 20 years of life, smaller lesions usually do not present a problem until after the onset of adolescence.

25. Hurwitz S: Pigmented nevi. Semin. Dermatol. 7:17–25, 1988.

An overview of pigmented nevi and their management in children.

26. Rhodes AR, Sober AJ, Day CL: The malignant potential of small congenital nevocellular nevi: An estimate based on histologic study of 234 primary cutaneous melanomas. J. Am. Acad. Dermatol. 6:230–241, 1982.

A review of small congenital nevocellular nevi and their role as precursors of cutaneous melanoma.

27. Quaba AA, Wallace AF: The incidence of malignant melanoma arising in large congenital naevi in the period 0–15 years. Plast. Reconstr. Surg. 78:174–179, 1986.

The authors believe that early prophylactic excision, due to the 8.5 per cent risk of malignant transformation and the invariably fatal course of this complication, be seriously considered for all patients with large congenital pigmented nevi.

28. Kadonga JN, Frieden I. Neurocutaneous melanosis: Definition and review of the literature. J. Am. Acad. Dermatol. 24:747–755, 1991.

A review of 39 reported cases of neurocutaneous melanosis, their clinical features and prognosis.

29. Stenn KS, Arons M, Hurwitz S: Patterns of congenital nevocellular nevi. J. Am. Acad. Dermatol. 9:388–393, 1983.

Only 14 (37 per cent) of 38 melanocytic nevi known to be congenital by history had nevus cell involvement of the lower third of the reticular dermis.

30. Jacobs AH, Hurwitz S, Prose NS, et al.: The management of congenital nevocytic nevi. Pediatr. Dermatol. 2:143–156, 1984.

Because of the continuous controversy regarding the appropriate management of congenital nevocellular nevi, this symposium highlights the views of various authorities (dermatologists and pediatric dermatologists) on this subject.

31. Johnson HA: Permanent removal of pigmentation from giant hairy naevi by dermabrasion in early life. Br. J. Plast. Surg. 30:321–323, 1977.

Although dermabrasion of congenital pigmented nevi can remove much of the discoloration of such lesions, it does not necessarily remove all pigment cells; this procedure is therefore not recommended as a treatment of choice for patients with congenital nevi.

32. Argenta LC, Marks MW, Pasyk KA: Advances in tissue expansion. Clin. Plast. Surg. 12:159–171, 1985.

A review of tissue expansion and its value in the management of patients with large cutaneous defects.

33. Clark WH Jr, Reimer RR, Greene M, et al.: Origin of familial malignant melanomas from heritable melanocytic lesions: The B-K mole syndrome. Arch. Dermatol. 114:732–738, 1978.

The association of familial melanoma in individuals with dysplastic (atypical) nevi is described under the designation of B-K mole syndrome.

34. Greene MH, Clark WH Jr, Tucker MA, et al.: Acquired precursors of cutaneous malignant melanoma: The familial dysplastic nevus syndrome. N. Engl. J. Med. 312:91–97, 1988.

A comprehensive review of dysplastic nevi, their risks and management.

35. Kraemer KH, Greene MH: Dysplastic nevus syndrome: Familial and sporadic precursors of cutaneous melanoma. Dermatol. Clin. 3:225–237, 1985.

The dysplastic nevus syndrome, its clinical features, melanoma risk, and management.

36. Spitz S: Melanomas of childhood. Am. J. Pathol. 24:591–602.

Clinical and histologic features of 13 patients (aged 18 months to 12 years) with benign juvenile melanoma.

37. Spielvogel RL: Spindle cell nevus (Spitz nevus). In Demis DJ (Ed.): Clinical Dermatology. J. B. Lippincott Co., Philadelphia, 1989, unit 11–51.

A review of the spindle cell nevus, its clinical and histologic features and management.

38. Smith SA, Day CL Jr, Van der Ploeg DE: Eruptive widespread Spitz nevi. J. Am. Acad. Dermatol. 15:1155–1159, 1986.

A report of a 12-year-old girl with numerous widespread spindle cell nevi of Spitz

39. Paniago-Pereira C, Maize JC, Ackerman AB: Nevus of large spindle and/or epithelioid cells (Spitz's nevus). Arch. Dermatol. 114:1811–1823, 1978.

Analysis and review of the histologic criteria for the diagnosis of the spindle cell nevus of Spitz.

40. Arbuckle S, Weedon D: Eosinophilic globules in the Spitz nevus. J. Am. Acad. Dermatol. 7:324–327, 1982.

Studies of 50 cases of malignant melanoma, Spitz nevi, and benign compound nevi confirm that the presence of coalescent eosinophilic globules can be helpful in the histopathologic differentiation of spindle cell nevi from malignant melanoma.

41. Frank SB, Cohen HJ: The halo nevus. Arch. Dermatol. 89:367–373, 1964.

Fourteen patients with a total of 34 halo nevi observed for periods of up to 17 years confirm previous reports of a self-destructive process that results in a patch of depigmentation, which itself may disappear over a period of 4 months to several years.

42. Zack LD, Stegmeier O, Solomon LM: Pigmentary regression in giant nevocellular nevus: A case report and a review of the subject. Pediatr. Dermatol. 5:178–183, 1988.

A report of a giant congenital nevocellular nevus that underwent pigmentary regression and clinical involution without apparent destruction of the nevus cells in the dermis and a discussion of possible mechanisms responsible for this phenomenon.

43. Cohen HJ, Minkin W, Frank SB: Nevus spilus. Arch. Dermatol. 102:433–437, 1970.

Review of 17 patients with nevus spilus suggests its classification as a nevus cell nevus.

44. Rhodes AR, Mihm MC Jr: Origin of cutaneous melanoma in a congenital dysplastic nevus spilus. Arch. Dermatol. 126:500–505, 1990.

For nevus spilus associated with elements of melanocytic dysplasia or clearly documented congenital onset, it appears to be prudent to recommend prophylactic surgical excision (if feasible) or periodic examination to detect the earliest possible malignant change.

45. Wagner RF, Cottel WI: In situ malignant melanoma arising in a speckled lentiginous nevus. J. Am. Acad. Dermatol. 20:125–126, 1989.

The development of a malignant melanoma in a nevus spilus suggests that patients with nevus spilus should be followed, just as patients with any other pigmented nevus, for the possibility of cutaneous malignant melanoma.

46. Becker SW: Concurrent melanosis and hypertrichosis in the distribution of nevus unius lateris. Arch. Dermatol. Syph. 60:155–160, 1949.

The original description of a unique epidermal hairy nevus (Becker's nevus).

47. Person JR, Longcope C: Becker's nevus: An androgen-mediated hyperplasia with increased androgen receptors. J. Am. Acad. Dermatol. 10:235–238, 1984.

Androgen receptor assays in a patient with a Becker's nevus suggests that a localized increase in androgen sensitivity may help explain the clinical features seen in individuals with this disorder.

48. Fretzin DF, Whitney D: Familial Becker's nevus. J. Am. Acad. Dermatol. 12:589–590, 1985.

A report of two brothers with Becker's nevi and reports of familial cases in the European literature suggest the possibility of a familial form of Becker's nevus in some patients.

49. Slifman NR, Harrist TJ, Rhodes AR: Congenital arrector pili hamartoma: A case report and review of the spectrum of Becker's melanosis and pilar smooth-muscle hamartoma. Arch. Dermatol. 121:1034–1037, 1987.

A report of an infant with smooth muscle hamartoma and a review of the controversy regarding its possible relationship with Becker's melanosis.

50. Glinick SE, Alper JC, Bogaars H, et al.: Becker's melanosis: Associated abnormalities. J. Am. Acad. Dermatol. 9:509–514, 1980.

A report of two patients and review of the world literature of patients with Becker's nevi and associated abnormalities.

51. Lucky AW, Saruk M, Lerner AB: Becker's nevus associated with limb asymmetry. Arch. Dermatol. 117:243, 1981.

A report of a 12-year-old girl with Becker's nevus and hypertrophy of the foot suggests that Becker's nevi may be part of the spectrum of epidermal nevi and the epidermal nevus syndrome.

52. Jeghers H, McKusick VA, Katz KH: Localized intestinal polyposis and melanin spots of the oral mucosa, lips and digits. N. Engl. J. Med. 241:993–1005, 1031–1033, 1949.

The classic description of a syndrome of intestinal polyposis and perioral pigmentation.

53. Dormandy TL: Peutz-Jeghers syndrome. N. Engl. J. Med. 256:1093–1102, 1141–1146, 1186–1190, 1957.

Although true malignant transformation in polyps of the small intestine rarely occurs, 4 of 21 patients with this disorder died of rectal or colonic cancer.

54. McKittrick JE, Lewis WM, Doane WA, et al.: The Peutz-Jeghers syndrome. Arch. Surg. 103:57–62, 1971.

When polyps are symptomatic, individual polypectomies are preferable to resection in Peutz-Jeghers syndrome.

55. Beck AR, Jewett TC.: Surgical implications of the Peutz-Jeghers syndrome. Ann. Surg. 165:299–302, 1967.

Surgical intervention in the Peutz-Jeghers syndrome should be limited to relief of intestinal obstruction or resection of polyps of the stomach, duodenum, or colon.

56. Wenzl JE, Bartholomew LG, Hallenbeck GA, et al.: Gastrointestinal polyposis with mucocutaneous pigmentation in children (Peutz-Jeghers syndrome). Pediatrics 28:655–661, 1961.

In order to avoid unnecessary loss of intestine and possible malabsorption states, conservative surgical treatment of Peutz-Jeghers syndrome is advocated.

57. Tovar JA, Eizaguirre A, Albert A, et al.: Peutz-Jeghers syndrome in children: Report of two cases and review of the literature. J. Pediatr. Surg. 18:1–6, 1983.

A report of two children with Peutz-Jeghers syndrome and a review of 70 patients with this disorder.

58. Gorlin RJ, Anderson RC, Blaw M: Multiple lentigines syndrome. Am. J. Dis. Child. 117:652–662, 1969.

Six family members with this syndrome demonstrate autosomal dominant inheritance with variable expressivity of the gene.

59. Nordlund JJ, Lerner AB, Braverman IM, et al.: The multiple lentigines syndrome. Arch. Dermatol. 107:259–261, 1973.

The basic genetic defect appears to be neuroectodermal in origin with associated changes in organs derived from mesoderm.

60. Atherton DJ, Pitcher DW, Wells RS, et al.: A syndrome of various pigmented lesions, myxoid neurofibroma and atrial myxoma: The NAME syndrome. Br. J. Dermatol. 103:421–429, 1980.

A report of a 10-year-old boy with generalized brown macules, multiple blue nevi, congenital pigmented nevi, myxoid tumors of the skin, and bilateral atrial myxomas.

61. Rhodes AR, Silverman RA, Harrist TJ, et al.: Mucocutaneous lentigines, cardiomucocutaneous myxomas, and multiple blue nevi: the "LAMB" syndrome. J. Am. Acad. Dermatol. 10:72–82, 1984.

The report of a young girl in whom mucocutaneous lentiginous macules and blue nevi were associated with cardiac and mucocutaneous myxomas.

62. Watson GH: Pulmonary stenosis, café au lait spots and dull intelligence. Arch. Dis. Child. 42:303–307, 1967.

A report of a patient with what appeared to be an incomplete form of the LEOPARD syndrome.

63. Benedict PH, Szabo G, Fitzpatrick TB, et al.: Melanotic macules in Albright's syndrome and in neurofibromatosis. J.A.M.A. 25:618–626, 1968.

Studies of 27 patients with Albright's syndrome and of 19 patients with neurofibromatosis revealed that melanocytes in café au lait spots have distinctive giant melanocytic granules not present in the pigmented lesions of patients with Albright's syndrome.

64. Jimbow K, Szabo C, Fitzpatrick TB: Ultrastructure of giant pigment granules (macromelanosomes) in cutaneous pigmented macules of neurofibromatosis. J. Invest. Dermatol. 61:300–309, 1973.

Giant pigment granules in melanocytes and keratinocytes in café au lait spots of patients with neurofibromatosis not found in café au lait macules of normal individuals.

65. Johnson BL, Charneco DR: Café au lait spots in neurofibromatosis and in normal individuals. Arch. Dermatol. *102*:442–446, 1970.

Giant melanin granules and increased numbers of melanocytes in café au lait spots and axillary freckles diagnostic of neurofibromatosis.

66. Martuza RL, Phillipe I, Fitzpatrick TB, et al.: Melanin macroglobules as a cellular marker for neurofibromatosis: A quantitative study. J. Invest. Dermatol. *85*:347–350, 1985.

A study of café au lait spots in patients with neurofibromatosis, in patients with bilateral acoustic neuromas, and in control subjects suggests that more than 10 macromelanosomes per 5 high-powered light microscopic fields may be a reliable marker for the diagnosis of von Recklinghausen's neurofibromatosis in individuals older than the age of 15 years. This finding has not yet been substantiated in children.

67. McCune DJ: Osteitis fibrosa cystica: The case of a 9-year-old girl who also exhibits precocious puberty, multiple pigmentation of the skin and hyperthyroidism. Am. J. Dis. Child. *52*:743–744, 1936.

Although the delineation of this syndrome has been attributed to Albright, McCunes' published report antedated that of Albright by several months.

68. Albright I, Butler AM, Hampton AO, et al.: Syndrome characterized by osteitis fibrosa disseminata, areas of pigmentation, and endocrine dysfunction, with precocious puberty in females. N. Engl. J. Med. *216*:727–746, 1937.

A review of five patients and 13 cases from the literature with peculiar pigmentation, multiple bone cysts, and precocious puberty in females.

69. Roth JG, Esterly NB: McCune-Albright syndrome with multiple café au lait spots. Pediatr. Dermatol. *8*:35–39, 1991.

A report of a 7-week-old infant with sharply marginated angular café au lait macules who, at the age of 15 months, developed a limp and radiologic evidence of fibrous bony dysplasia consistent with the diagnosis of the McCune-Albright syndrome.

70. Cole HN Jr, Hubler WR, Lund HZ: Persistent, aberrant mongolian spots. Arch. Dermatol. Syph. *61*:244–260, 1950.

Four patients with dermal and ocular melanosis (hypermelanosis of the nevi of Ota and Ito).

71. Kopf AW, Weidman AI: Nevus of Ota. Arch. Dermatol. *85*:195–208, 1962.

Clinical and histologic features of the nevus of Ota suggest a variant of the mongolian spot–blue nevus complex.

72. Jay B: Malignant melanoma of the orbit in a case of oculodermal melanocytosis (nevus of Ota). Br. J. Ophthalmol. *49*:359–363, 1965.

A 64-year-old woman with melanoma of the orbit associated with the nevus of Ota.

73. Silverberg GD, Kadin ME, Dorfman RF, et al.: Invasion of the brain by a cellular nevus of the scalp. Cancer *27*:349–355, 1971.

A 3-year-old boy with a large cellular blue nevus of the left frontoparietal scalp with focal invasion of the underlying skull, meninges, and brain.

74. Goldenhersh MA, Savin RC, Barnhill RL, et al.: Malignant blue nevus: Case report and literature review. J. Am. Acad. Dermatol. *19*:712–722, 1988.

A report of a woman with a dime-sized blue lesion on her scalp which, first noted at the age of 13, progressed to become a malignant lesion when she was approximately 70 years of age.

75. Hendricks WM: Eruptive blue nevi. J. Am. Acad. Dermatol. *4*:50–53, 1981.

A 14-year-old boy developed a cluster of blue nevi after a severe sunburn.

76. Bondi EE, Elder D, Gurray DP IV, et al.: Target blue nevus. Arch. Dermatol. *119*:919–920, 1983.

A report of two patients with blue nevi with a distinctive target-like configuration that on clinical examination suggested a diagnosis of malignant melanoma.

77. Braunstein BL, Mackel SE, Cooper PH: Keratoacanthoma arising in a linear epidermal nevus. Arch. Dermatol. *118*:362–363, 1982.

This article describing a keratoacanthoma in a linear epidermal nevus appears to be the first report of this association.

78. Horn MS, Sousker WF, Pierson DL: Basal cell epithelioma arising in a linear epidermal nevus. Arch. Dermatol. *117*:247, 1981.

A report of a basal cell carcinoma in a zosteriform verrucous nevus.

79. Golitz LE, Weston WL: Inflammatory linear verrucous epidermal nevus. Arch. Dermatol. *115*:1208–1209, 1979.

A report of an infant with skeletal anomalies and an inflammatory epidermal nevus suggests that this disorder may at times represent a variant of the epidermal nevus syndrome.

80. Morag C, Metzker A: Inflammatory linear verrucous epidermal nevus: Report of seven new cases and review of the literature. Pediatr. Dermatol. *3*:15–18, 1985.

A review of seven children with inflammatory linear verrucous epidermal nevus.

81. Solomon LM, Fretzin DF, Dewald RL: The epidermal nevus syndrome. Arch. Dermatol. *97*:273–285, 1968.

Review of the literature and report of findings in 23 patients with the epidermal nevus syndrome.

82. Rogers M, McCrossin I, Commens C: Epidermal nevi and the epidermal nevus syndrome. J. Am. Acad. Dermatol. *20*:476–488, 1989.

A review of 131 patients with epidermal nevi suggests that a high percentage of patients with this disorder are at risk of having associated abnormalities.

83. Goldberg LH, Collins SAB, Siegel DM: The epidermal nevus syndrome: Case report and review. Pediatr. Dermatol. *4*:27–33, 1987.

A report of a woman with multiple basal cell carcinomas complicating a large unilateral nevus sebaceus who also had signs of skeletal, neurologic, and vascular involvement.

84. Rosenthal D, Fretzin DF: Epidermal nevus syndrome: Report of an association with transitional cell carcinoma of the bladder. Pediatr. Dermatol. *3*:455–458, 1986.

A report of a 16-year-old boy with an extensive epidermal nevus, mild scoliosis and a transitional cell carcinoma of the bladder.

85. Milstone EB, Helwig EB: Basal cell carcinoma in children. Arch. Dermatol. *108*:523–527, 1973.

Clinical and pathologic features of 22 children with basal cell carcinoma and review of 25 previously cited cases in the literature.

86. Comstock J, Hansen RC, Korc A: Basal cell carcinoma in a 12-year-old boy. Pediatrics *86*:460–463, 1990.

A 12-year-old boy with a 1.1 × 1.0-cm basal cell carcinoma on the nose required Mohs' surgery followed by surgical reconstruction to remove this lesion.

87. Ledwig PA, Paller AS: Congenital basal cell carcinoma. Arch. Dermatol. *127*:1066–1067, 1991.

A report of a biopsy-proven basal cell carcinoma that apparently had been present from birth.

88. Mikhail GR, Boulos RS, Knighton RS, et al.: Cranial invasion by basal cell carcinoma. J. Dermatol. Surg. Oncol. 12:459–464, 1986.

A report of four patients with basal cell carcinoma with invasion of the cranial bone.

89. Bason MM, Grant-Kels JM, Govil M: Metastatic basal cell carcinoma: Response to chemotherapy. J. Am. Acad. Dermatol. 22:905–908, 1990.

A report of a patient with a basal cell carcinoma with extensive spread who exhibited a brief response to a combination of cisplastin, bleomycin, methotrexate, and 5-fluorouracil.

90. Howell JB, Caro MR: Basal-cell nevus: Its relationship to multiple cutaneous cancers and associated anomalies of development. Arch. Dermatol. 79:67–80, 1959.

Diagnosis, treatment, and review of four patients with basal cell nevus syndrome.

91. Gorlin RJ, Goltz RW: Multiple nevoid basal-cell epithelioma, jaw cysts, and bifid rib syndrome. N. Engl. J. Med. 262:908–912, 1960.

Case reports of two patients and review of the literature.

92. Cotton JL, Kavey RW, Palmer CE, et al.: Cardiac tumors and the nevoid basal cell carcinoma syndrome. Pediatrics 87:725–728, 1991.

Although often overlooked, cardiac tumors may also be associated with the nevoid basal cell carcinoma syndrome.

93. Pratt MD, Jackson R: Nevoid basal cell carcinoma syndrome: A 15-year follow-up of cases in Ottawa and the Ottawa valley. J. Am. Acad. Dermatol. 16:964–970, 1987.

A 15-year study of 12 patients with nevoid basal cell carcinoma syndrome (one patient had a highly destructive lesion requiring seven plastic surgical procedures).

94. Kraemer KH, DiGiovanna JJ, Moshell AN, et al.: Prevention of skin cancer in xeroderma pigmentosum with the use of oral isotretinoin. N. Engl. J. Med. 318:1633–1637, 1988.

A 3-year controlled study of five patients with xeroderma pigmentosum and multiple basal cell or squamous cell carcinomas treated with oral isotretinoin.

95. Roed-Petersen B: Effect on oral leukoplakia of reducing or ceasing tobacco smoking. Acta. Derm. Venerol. 62:164–167, 1982.

In a study of 138 patients with leukoplakia, in those who either reduced or stopped smoking, 56 per cent of lesions disappeared or regressed over a 3-month period and 78 per cent regressed or completely disappeared after 1 year of total smoking abstinence.

96. Sahl WJ Jr: Familial nevus sebaceus of Jadassohn: Occurrence in three generations. J. Am. Acad. Dermatol. 22:853–854, 1990.

This report, the second of a patient with inherited nevus sebaceus, reviews three generations of patients with this disorder.

97. Constant E, David DG: The premalignant nature of the sebaceous nevus of Jadassohn. Plast. Reconstr. Surg. 50:257–259, 1972.

Report of two patients with nevus sebaceus, one of whom had rapid growth of the lesion during the fourth and fifth months of life.

98. Burden PA, Gentry RH, Fitzpatrick JE: Piloleiomyoma arising in an organoid nevus: A case report and review of the literature. J. Dermatol. Surg. Oncol. 13:1213–1217, 1987.

In a report of a woman with a nevus sebaceus of the scalp with an unusual array of secondary tumors, including piloleiomyoma, the authors discuss reasons for replacing the term *nevus sebaceus* with the more inclusive designation of organoid nevus.

99. Domingo J, Helwig EB: Malignant neoplasms associated with nevus sebaceus of Jadassohn. J. Am. Acad. Dermatol. 1:545–556, 1979.

A report of 9 patients with nevus sebaceus who developed aggressive neoplasms in their lesions. Four patients had apocrine carcinomas (two of which metastasized), three had adnexal carcinomas, and of two patients who developed squamous cell carcinomas, one died of general metastases and the other had a large recurrent carcinoma that invaded the skull.

100. Tarkham II, Domingo J: Metastasizing eccrine porocarcinoma developing in a sebaceus nevus of Jadassohn: Report of a case. Arch. Dermatol. 121:413–415, 1985.

A 45-year-old man with an eccrine porocarcinoma in a nevus sebaceus that progressed to an extensive infiltrative metastatic tumor 6 months after wide surgical excision of the primary lesion.

101. Beck S, Cotton DWK: Recurrent solitary giant trichoepithelioma located in the perianal area: A case report. Br. J. Dermatol. 118:563–566, 1988.

A 31-year-old man developed a 3-cm trichoepithelioma in an excision scar on the scrotum 17 years after the original lesion had apparently been completely excised.

102. Brownstein MH, Shapiro L: Desmoplastic trichoepithelioma. Arch. Dermatol. 112:1782, 1976.

The first description of a variant of trichoepithelioma with an annular configuration and sclerotic consistency resembling granuloma annulare.

103. Shapiro PE, Kopf AW: Familial multiple desmoplastic trichoepitheliomas. Arch. Dermatol. 127:83–87, 1991.

A report of a kindred with familial mutiple desmoplastic trichoepitheliomas and a review of the clinical features, nosologic status, and treatment options for patients with this disorder.

104. Arnold HL Jr: Pilomatricoma. Arch. Dermatol. 113:1303, 1977.

Despite the term *pilomatrixoma* frequently seen in articles and textbooks, *pilomatricoma* is the correct spelling for this disorder.

105. Schwartz BK, Peraza JE: Pilomatricomas associated with muscular dystrophy. J. Am. Acad. Dermatol. 16:887–889, 1987.

A report of a 48-year-old man with a pilomatricoma and myotonic dystrophy (the patient's son and a distant maternal cousin also had myotonic dystrophy).

106. Green DE, Sanusi ID, Fowler MR: Pilomatrix carcinoma. J. Am. Acad. Dermatol. 17:264–270, 1987.

A report of a patient with a 13-cm ulcerated pilomatrix carcinoma and a review of 16 previous cases of pilomatricoma with malignant behavior.

107. Arnold M, McGuire LJ: Perforating pilomatricoma: Difficulty in diagnosis. J. Am. Acad. Dermatol. 18:754–755, 1988.

A report of a progressively enlarging and ulcerating pilomatricoma in a 17-year-old woman.

108. Brichta RF, Norvell SS Jr: Pilomatricoma: A case highlighting its variable presentation. J. Assoc. Milit. Dermatol. 14:14–16, 1988.

A report of a pilomatricoma presenting as a translucent nodule that appeared rapidly on the face prompted a review of the variable presentations of this disorder.

109. Scherbenske JM, Lupton GP, James WD, et al.: Vulvar syringoma occurring in a 9-year-old child. J. Am. Acad. Dermatol. 19:575–577, 1988.

A report of a preadolescent girl with a 4-year history of syringomas on the lower eyelids, neck, vulva, and perigenital skin.

110. Butterworth T, Strean LP, Beerman H, et al.: Syringoma and mongolism. Arch. Dermatol. 90:483–487, 1964.

Of 200 patients with Down's syndrome, 37 percent had syringomas.

111. Mainitz M, Schmidt JB, Gebhart W: Response of multiple syringomas to isotretinoin. Acta Derm. Venereol. *60*:51–55, 1986.

A 6-month regimen of isotretinoin was helpful for two women who had cosmetically objectional syringomas.

112. Kantor GR, Bergfeld WR, Pomeranz JR: Enlarging ulcerative tumor on the back. Arch. Dermatol. *122*:585–590, 1986.

A 25-year-old woman with a 4-year history of a slowly enlarging tumor on the back died of widespread metastases from an eccrine gland carcinoma.

113. Janniger CK, Goldberg DJ: Angiofibromas in tuberous sclerosis: Comparison of treatment by carbon dioxide and argon laser. J. Dermatol. Surg. Oncol. *16*:317–320, 1990.

In a comparison study of carbon dioxide and argon laser beam treatment of angiofibromas on the nose of a 12-year-old Hispanic boy with tuberous sclerosis, the carbon dioxide laser–treated sites seemed to have a better cosmetic result.

114. Goldberg DJ, Maso M: Dermatofibrosarcoma protuberans in a 9-year-old child: Treatment by Mohs micrographic surgery. Pediatr. Dermatol. 7:57–59, 1990.

A dermatofibrosarcoma protuberans in a child successfully treated by Mohs' surgery.

115. Robinson JK: Dermatofibrosarcoma protuberans resected by Mohs' surgery (chemosurgery): A five-year prospective study. J. Am. Acad. Dermatol. *12*:1093–1098, 1985.

Mohs' surgery in a patient with dermatofibrosarcoma protuberans suggests that this form of therapy may be ideal for this invasive, frequently recurrent disorder.

116. Beckett JH, Jacobs AH: Recurring digital fibrous tumors of childhood: A review. Pediatrics 59:401–406, 1977.

Review of the literature and two new cases reveal a tendency toward local recurrence in 61 per cent of patients with digital fibroma of childhood.

117. Ishii N, Matsui I, Ichiyama S, et al.: A case of infantile digital fibromatosis showing spontaneous regression. Br. J. Dermatol. *121*:129–133, 1989.

On the basis of a report of spontaneous regression of infantile digital fibromatosis in a 3-year-old girl and five previous cases, the authors recommend conservative management of patients with this disorder.

118. Spraker MK, Stack C, Esterly NB: Congenital generalized fibromatosis: A review of the literature and report of a case associated with porencephaly, hemiatrophy, and cutis marmorata telangiectatica congenita. J. Am. Acad. Dermatol. *10*:365–371, 1984.

A report of a 6-week-old infant with congenital fibromatosis, an unusual constellation of associated features, and a comprehensive review of the literature.

119. Goldberg NS, Bauer BS, Kraus H, et al.: Infantile myofibromatosis: A review of clinicopathology with perspectives on new treatment choices. Pediatr. Dermatol. 5:37–47, 1988.

A report of a 6-month-old infant with infantile myofibromatosis treated by surgery following the use of tissue expanders and a review of the fibromatoses of childhood and their management.

120. Paller AS, Pensler JM, Tomita T: Nasal midline masses in infants and children. Arch. Dermatol. *127*:362–366, 1991.

A review of 46 children with nasal dermoids, gliomas, and encephaloceles.

121. Böhler Sommeregger K, Kutchera-Henert G: Cryosurgical management of myxoid cysts. J. Dermatol. Surg. Oncol. *14*:1405–1408, 1988.

In a report of 18 patients with digital mucoid cysts and 31 with myxoid cysts of the oral mucosa treated by cryosurgery, those with digital mucoid cysts had a high recurrence rate.

122. Huerter CH, Wheeland RG, Bailin PL, et al.: Treatment of digital myxoid cysts with carbon dioxide laser vaporization. J. Dermatol. Surg. Oncol. *13*:723–727, 1987.

Ten patients with digital myxoid cysts were treated with carbon dioxide laser vaporization with good results.

123. Rosen BL, Brodkin RH: Isotretinoin in the treatment of steatocystoma multiplex: A possible adverse reaction. Cutis *37*:115, 120, 1986.

A 30-year-old black woman with severe steatocystoma multiplex developed exacerbation and worsening of her condition while receiving isotretinoin for her disorder.

124. Friedman SJ, Butler DF, Pittelkow MR: Perilesional linear atrophy and hypopigmentation after intralesional corticosteroid therapy: Report of two cases and review of the literature. J. Am. Acad. Dermatol. *19*:537–541, 1988.

Perilesional hypopigmentation and atrophy after intralesional corticosteroid injections for the treatment of keloids resolved spontaneously within a period of 10 to 12 weeks.

125. Gardner EW, Miller HM, Lowney ED: Folded skin associated with underlying nevus lipomatosus. Arch. Dermatol. *115*:978–979, 1979.

A report of a mentally retarded child with marked folding of the skin and multiple congenital defects suggests that the Michelin-tire baby syndrome may be part of a syndrome of cutaneous and systemic abnormalities.

126. Zvulunov A, Rotem A, Merlob P, et al.: Congenital smooth muscle hamartoma. Am. J. Dis. Child. *144*:782–784, 1990.

A report of 15 children with congenital smooth muscle hamartoma suggests that this condition is probably much more common than the literature indicates.

127. Nassim JR, Connolly CK: Treatment of calcinosis universalis with aluminum hydroxide. Arch. Dis. Child. *45*:118–121, 1970.

Calcinosis universalis (due to dermatomyositis in a 9-year-old boy) successfully treated with oral administration of aluminum hydroxide, 15 ml of Aludrox (Wyeth) four times a day.

128. Mozzafarian G, Lafferty FW, Pearson OH: Treatment of tumoral calcinosis with phosphorus deprivation. Ann. Intern. Med. 77:741–745, 1972.

A 16-year-old boy with a 7-year history of calcinosis of the hips and scapulae was successfully treated with aluminum hydroxide suspension.

129. Prendiville JS, Lucky AW, Mallory SB, et al.: Osteoma cutis as a presenting sign of pseudohypoparathyroidism. Pediatr. Dermatol. 9:11–18, 1992.

A report of four unrelated children with osteoma cutis and Albright's hereditary osteodystrophy.

130. Zimmerman EH: Subungual exostosis. Cutis *19*:185–188, 1977.

Subungual tumors should not be confused with subungual verrucae.

9

VASCULAR DISORDERS OF INFANCY AND CHILDHOOD

VASCULAR NEVI

Vascular lesions occur in up to 40 per cent of newborns and accordingly comprise the largest single group of neoplasms in infancy and childhood. These disorders are of developmental origin and are currently divided into three groups: hemangio-mas, salmon patches, and vascular malformations.

Hemangiomas are benign neoplasms composed of proliferating vascular endothelium that enlarge by cell proliferation rapidly during infancy, stabilize, and then undergo a slow period of involution characterized by fibrosis and diminished vascularity. Although this process is not completely understood, studies have shown that angiogenesis is influenced by hormonal factors (elevated estradiol levels and estrogen receptors) and mast cells and their product heparin, which binds to endothelium and enhances endothelial migration. This appears to explain, at least in part, the effect of corticosteroid therapy in the treatment of selected hemangiomas.

Vascular malformations, which are inborn errors of vascular morphogenesis, are hamartomas composed of mature endothelial cells that neither proliferate nor involute. They are true structural abnormalities that are present although not necessarily detected at birth and exhibit a normal rate of endothelial cell turnover throughout their natural history. Malformations grow commensurately with the child and may be subdivided into capillary, venous, arterial, and lymphatic abnormalities.[1-5]

Salmon patches represent a physiologic vascular phenomenon composed of distended dermal capillaries that, with the exception of some of those in the nuchal region, tend to fade, generally within the first year of life.

Strawberry Hemangiomas

The term *capillary hemangioma* has been used for both strawberry hemangiomas and port-wine stains (nevus flammeus). This term, however, is not entirely satisfactory since cavernous spaces may also be present in strawberry hemangiomas.

Although strawberry hemangiomas have been observed in several members of a family, there is no evidence of genetic predisposition. These lesions are present in approximately 2.6 per cent of all newborns and 8 to 12 per cent of white infants by 1 year of age; there is a higher frequency in girls (60 to 70 per cent) than in boys, and they appear to be somewhat more common in premature infants born before 30 weeks' gestation or who have birth weights less than 1500 g (Table 9–1).[6] Deep strawberry hemangiomas (cavernous hemangiomas), one tenth as common as superficial strawberry hemangiomas, are noted in 1 to 2 per cent of infants.

Strawberry hemangiomas (circumscribed capillary hemangiomas) may be present at birth but generally develop during the first few postnatal weeks. Although the majority are not seen at birth, 90 per cent are detected during the first month of life. Most reports of the onset of strawberry marks "at birth" as described by many authors are based on the statements of mothers, and most evidence suggests that the majority of these lesions make their appearance between the third and fifth weeks of life.[7] Eighty per cent are seen as single lesions, 20 per cent of individuals have more than one, and, in exceptional cases, there may be many hundreds. Strawberry hemangiomas may occur on any area of the body but are most commonly seen on the head and neck (38 per cent) and trunk (29 per cent) of affected individuals.[8]

Strawberry nevi initially appear as small, well-demarcated, telangiectatic macules or papules, as clusters of closely packed pinhead lesions, as telangiectatic patches, or as bright punctate stippling or fine thread-like telangiectases surrounded by an area of localized pallor (Fig. 9–1).[7] During the first 5 weeks of life these lesions become vascularized and grow to present as strawberry-type lesions. The classic strawberry hemangioma is a raised bright or purplish red lobulated tumor (Fig. 9–2) with well-defined borders and minute capillaries protruding from its surface, hence its "strawberry"-like appearance. Although it is compressible, it seldom blanches completely on pressure. It is important to recognize that it may at times be difficult to determine the exact nature of a vascular birthmark during the first few weeks of life. In such instances an accurate history and careful physical examination will determine the true nature of the cutaneous lesions and the physician can reassure the parents that another visit, in perhaps 2 or 3 months, can help establish a more definitive diagnosis.[1]

Cavernous Hemangiomas

Most cavernous hemangiomas (those that involute), seen in 1 to 2 per cent of infants, represent deep-seated strawberry hemangiomas with little

Table 9–1. INCIDENCE OF VASCULAR NEVI

1. Salmon patches (30–40%)
2. Strawberry hemangiomas
   a. Approximately 2.6% at birth
   b. Eight to 12% of white infants
   c. Somewhat more common in premature infants
   d. More common in girls than in boys (60–70%)
3. Cavernous hemangiomas (1–2% of infants)
4. Nevus flammeus (0.3%)

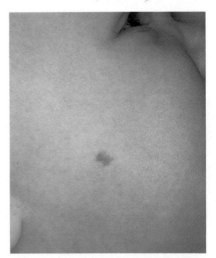

Figure 9–1. Early hemangioma. A well-demarcated vascular lesion is surrounded by an area of pallor. During the first few weeks of life this area becomes vascularized and progresses to the classic strawberry hemangioma.

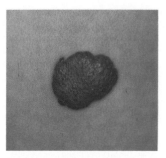

Figure 9–2. Strawberry hemangioma. This purplish red, raised, lobulated vascular tumor has well-defined borders and minute capillaries that protrude from its surface (hence its strawberry-like appearance).

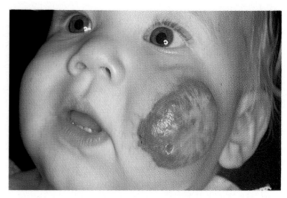

Figure 9–4. Mixed strawberry-cavernous hemangioma. A strawberry nevus with a deep cavernous component.

penetration of the overlying skin and therefore represent the same basic pathologic process as for strawberry nevi but are composed of larger, mature vascular elements (primarily dilated, well-differentiated vessels or sinusoidal blood spaces lined by a single layer of endothelial cells) in a delicate fibrous stroma that involves the dermis and subcutaneous tissues. Individual lesions occur chiefly on the head and neck but are found in other regions as well. They are present at birth, grow in proportion to the growth of the individual, and are generally seen as bluish red masses with less distinct borders than in strawberry hemangiomas (Fig. 9–3). If the lesion is deeply situated, the overlying skin may appear normal or show only a blue discoloration. Occasionally a combination of strawberry and cavernous hemangioma may occur. In mixed forms the deep component may be visible or palpable beneath a typical strawberry nevus (Fig. 9–4), or the entire lesion may consist of an irregularly bluish red mass, sometimes lobulated, involving the subcutaneous tissue.

Course. Strawberry hemangiomas grow rapidly during the first 6 months of life. The majority reach their maximal growth by the first year of life and although most lesions average 2 to 5 cm in diameter, the ultimate size ranges from 2 to 3 mm to 20 cm or more in diameter. In a study of 340 lesions, 80 per cent showed maximal increase in size (less than double their original size) during the first 2 years of observation, less than 5 per cent tripled in size, and 2 per cent quadrupled in size.[9, 10] Following their initial growth phase, most strawberry angiomas remain stationary and do not grow after the infant reaches 12 months of age. This stationary phase is soon followed by a period of involution, generally during the subsequent 6- to 12-month period (Fig. 9–5). This involutional period is variable; many lesions show complete involution by the time the child is 2 or 3 years of age. Cavernous hemangiomas that never involute represent venous malformations.

During the first year of involution the strawberry hemangioma becomes dull red and small foci of gray appear on the surface. These foci increase and coalesce, and gradually the entire lesion becomes pink-gray or gray (Fig. 9–6).

At least 90 per cent of strawberry and cavernous angiomas undergo complete or partial resolution (Fig. 9–7). Superficial lesions generally resolve completely without trace or with only slight atrophy of the area of involvement. Cavernous and mixed angiomatous lesions with a deep component also resolve (Figs. 9–3, 9–4, and 9–8 through

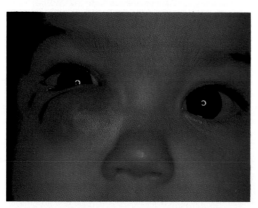

Figure 9–3. Cavernous-type strawberry hemangioma. Soft bluish red vascular tumor with a poorly circumscribed border.

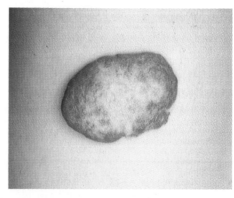

Figure 9–5. Strawberry hemangioma with focal areas of involution. Strawberry hemangiomas begin to show signs of involution in most children between the ages of 12 and 24 months.

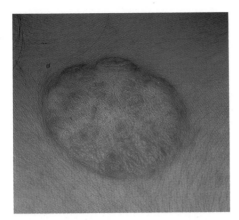

Figure 9–6. An involuting strawberry hemangioma in a 5-year-old child.

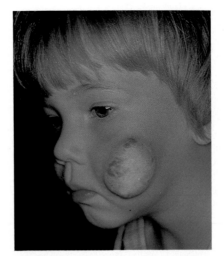

Figure 9–8. Partial resolution of a mixed strawberry-cavernous hemangioma at age 3 years (this is the same patient depicted in Figure 9–4).

9–11). Accordingly, fewer than 10 per cent of hemangiomas, whether they are strawberry, cavernous, or mixed, constitute any cosmetic handicap, and fewer than 2 per cent require active therapy.[8–11] In 50 per cent of cases the hemangiomas disappear by 5 years, in 70 per cent they disappear by 7 years, and in 90 per cent they disappear by age 9 years without leaving any scars or evidence that they ever existed.[12]

Cavernous-type hemangiomas generally tend to ·soften (and at times protrude as they soften) and, although little change occurs in their surface area, usually demonstrate a gradual decrease in thickness or volume during the second or third year of life. Although the natural history of cavernous hemangiomas parallels that of strawberry hemangiomas, cavernous lesions generally are less active. They have a lesser growth rate than strawberry hemangiomas, and although 90 per cent also improve by the time the child is 9 years of age,

regression of cavernous lesions is often not as complete but generally results in a satisfactory cosmetic appearance.

Management. Because of the tendency for the majority of strawberry and cavernous hemangiomas to regress completely, or almost completely, most cases require no therapy, and the final result in untreated lesions is generally far superior to that obtained from most forms of therapeutic intervention. In general, the end results of 7 years of observation of 210 children with 336 hemangiomas were cosmetically excellent and complications were uncommon (5 per cent). This was in sharp contrast to a 10-fold increase in complications (56 per cent) in the group that was actively treated.[9] Office management, accordingly, consists of judicious observation; avoidance, whenever possible, of active therapy; and constant reassurance to the parents of affected infants. For parents who find it difficult to accept the concept of conservative neglect, careful

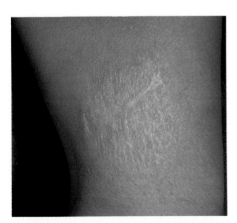

Figure 9–7. A completely resolved hemangioma with slight atrophy. In 90 per cent of cases the hemangioma (whether strawberry, cavernous, or mixed) will disappear by the age of 9 years without leaving any scar or cosmetic handicap; fewer than 2 per cent require therapy.

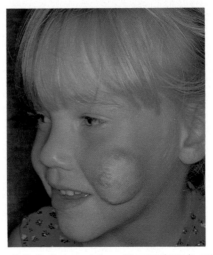

Figure 9–9. Further resolution of hemangioma in patient in Figure 9–8 at 5 years of age.

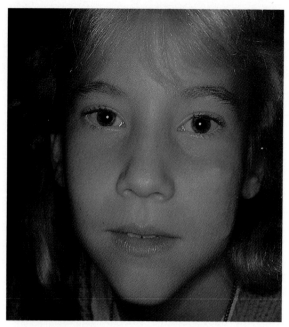

Figure 9–10. The same patient as in Figures 9–4, 9–8, and 9–9 at 10 years of age following almost complete spontaneous resolution of her lesion.

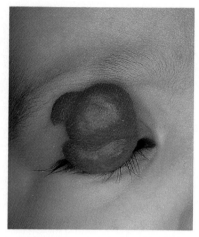

Figure 9–12. Strawberry hemangioma of the upper eyelid with obstruction of vision.

measurement and serial photographs of lesions, photographs of other typical cases, and discussion with parents of children who had similar lesions will usually help gain their confidence and cooperation.[9]

Hemangiomas that require intervention are those that by their size and growth compromise vital structures such as the eyes (Figs. 9–12 through 9–15, nares, auditory canals, pharynx, or larynx; those that have an alarming rate of growth,

tripling or quadrupling in size within a period of a few weeks; large, usually cavernous lesions that have an associated thrombocytopenia (Kasabach-Merritt syndrome); or lesions that by their size or location are particularly susceptible to trauma, hemorrhage, or secondary infection (Fig. 9–16). Unfortunately, no method of treatment is entirely satisfactory, and all forms of therapy may present complications.

In general, the cosmetic result is far better for lesions permitted to undergo spontaneous resolution than for those treated by sclerosing agents, radiation, or surgery. Light applications of liquid nitrogen or dry ice, grenz ray therapy, or tunable pulse dye laser therapy may be beneficial, particularly in small or early lesions.[13] If done too vigorously, however, cryosurgery may at times result in scarring or atrophy. Radiation therapy is not advisable and, other than grenz ray therapy, may have serious sequelae. If the location of the hemangioma is suitable, however, compression with a

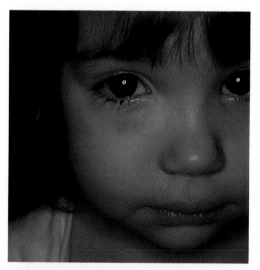

Figure 9–11. Spontaneous resolution of the cavernous hemangioma of the lower eyelid at the age of 2 years in the patient in Figure 9–3.

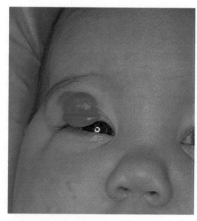

Figure 9–13. Partial resolution of hemangioma in patient in Figure 9–12 following 7 weeks of systemic corticosteroid therapy.

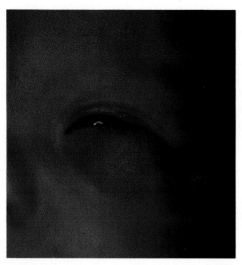

Figure 9–14. A cavernous hemangioma of the lower eyelid of a 3-month-old infant.

pressure dressing and frequent massage may help hasten its involution.[8]

Complications during spontaneous involution (ulceration, bleeding, or infection) fortunately are relatively infrequent. Therapy for ulceration and infection consists of open wet compresses, gentle cleansing with an antibacterial soap, and application of topical antibacterial agents. Bleeding and ulceration frequently hasten spontaneous involution, and residual scarring after complete involution is uncommon and rarely unsightly. Pulsed

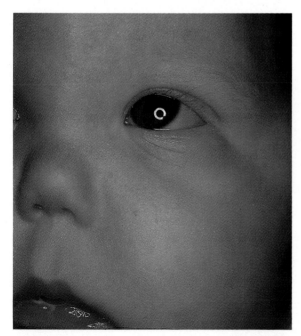

Figure 9–15. The child with the cavernous hemangioma of the eyelid shown in Figure 9–14, 1 month after the initiation of oral prednisone therapy.

tunable dye laser therapy can help heal ulcerated hemangiomas,[14] and most oozing and crusting lesions do better when left open to the air. When topical dressings are required, however, topical antibacterial agents and sterile Telfa dressings are preferable to gauze or occlusive adhesive bandages.

When intervention is required, oral corticosteroids or intralesional injection of sterile triamcinolone acetonide suspension, in a dosage of 1 to 3 mg/kg two or three times at 2- to 3-week intervals, may result in involution within several months (Figs. 9–16 and 9–17)[15]; or a course of oral prednisone may be used in a dosage of 2 to 4 mg/kg/day (or its equivalent) for 4 weeks, followed by alternate-day therapy using the same or doubled dosage for periods of 4 to 6 weeks, with gradual tapering of the dosage as the condition warrants (see Figs. 9–12 through 9–15). Involution usually begins about the second or third week and continues during the second month. If rebound occurs, a second or third course may be necessary.[16, 17]

Salmon Patches

The salmon patch (nevus simplex, telangiectatic nevus) is the most common vascular lesion of infancy. It occurs in 30 to 40 per cent of newborns and appears as a flat, dull pink, macular lesion (often with telangiectasia) on the nape of the neck, glabella, forehead (Fig. 9–18), upper eyelids, and nasolabial regions. When seen on the nape of the neck, it is frequently referred to as a "stork bite" (Fig. 9–19). Twenty-two per cent of infants have salmon patches only on the nape of the neck, 5 per cent have them either on the eyelids or on the glabella, and almost 20 per cent have them on both the glabella and the eyelids.

Histopathologic examination of salmon patches reveals distended dermal capillaries that represent the persistence of fetal circulation rather than newly formed capillaries. No treatment is necessary, since 95 per cent of salmon patches (with the exception of those on the nuchal region) fade, generally within the first year of life (unlike the true nevus flammeus, which is permanent). It should be noted, however, that a slight erythematous color may be more persistent or may reappear in salmon patches of fair-skinned children during episodes of crying, breath holding, or physical exertion. Those on the nuchal region (known as nuchal or Unna's nevus) persist in up to 50 per cent of individuals (see Fig. 9–19B). Since they are usually covered by hair, nuchal lesions do not generally present a cosmetic problem.

Nevus Flammeus

Macular stains, commonly known as port-wine stains (nevus flammeus) represent congenital vascular malformations composed of dilated capillary-

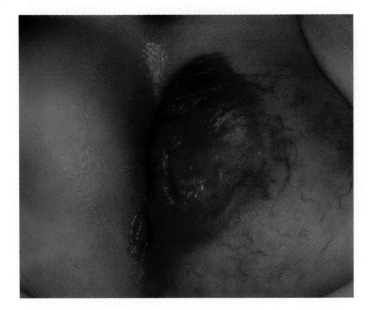

Figure 9–16. A large strawberry hemangioma with ulceration obstructing the perianal area of a 4-month-old infant.

like vessels. Often incorrectly referred to as capillary hemangiomas, such lesions are generally present at birth, persist throughout life, and usually do not grow out of proportion to the growth of the child (Fig. 9–20). Because this lesion is a congenital defect composed of mature dermal vessels, current studies suggest that a weakness in the capillary wall and a decrease in neural elements are responsible for the dilatation (ectasia) of the superficial capillary-like vessels seen in individuals with this disorder.[18, 19] Port-wine stains occur in 0.3 to 0.5 per cent of all newborns, and 5 to 8 per cent of patients with facial port-wine stains in a trigeminal (V_1) location within the ophthalmic area (above the palpebral fissure) or extending into the maxillary and mandibular regions are at risk for having ocular or intracranial vascular anomalies (see Sturge-Weber Syndrome).[20]

On histopathologic examination port-wine stains reveal numerous dilated capillary-like vessels without endothelial proliferation. Lesions are reddish purple, are flat or barely elevated above the surface of the surrounding skin, do not fade appreciatively with age, and, although benign, may be asociated with other syndromes. Their color ranges from pale pink to bright red or bluish purple, and, although initially flat, as the patient grows the areas may develop angiomatous papules and overgrowth of tissue. Port-wine stains are generally, but not necessarily, unilateral. Although

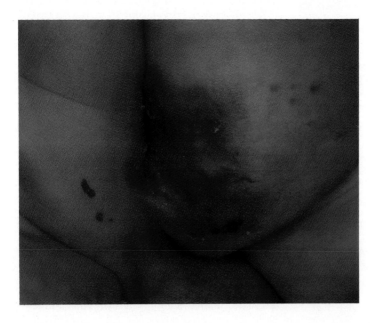

Figure 9–17. Involution of the strawberry hemangioma shown in Figure 9–16 two months later, after three treatments with intralesional triamcinolone.

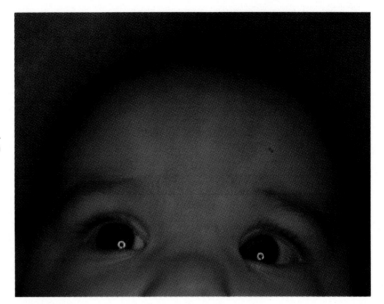

Figure 9–18. Salmon patch (nevus simplex). A dull pink macular lesion is seen on the forehead of a 5-month-old infant.

they most commonly involve the face, they may occur on any cutaneous surface.

Lesions of nevus flammeus show little tendency toward involution, and, until the recent introduction of laser therapy, treatment other than tinted opaque waterproof cosmetics (such as Covermark or Dermablend) was generally unsatisfactory. Argon laser beam therapy, introduced in the late 1970s, was the first major advance in therapy for port-wine stains (the word "laser" is an acronym for *l*ight *a*mplification by *s*timulated *e*mission *r*adiation). Although helpful, argon laser beam therapy produced cosmetically unacceptable scars in up to 40 per cent of children (generally those who were treated when younger than the age of 18 years).[21, 22] Pulsed tunable dye lasers, however, which emit light energy at 577 to 585 nm and penetrate to a

depth of 0.75 mm, allow the operator to target short bursts of energy at intravascular hemoglobin within the skin, while sparing other tissue components, thus allowing precise treatment—an ideal approach to the treatment of port-wine stains.[23] The pulse duration of 360 μsec, which closely matches the thermal relaxation time for dermal vessels, avoids diffuse thermal necrosis and subsequent scarring to adjacent skin and thus allows the successful treatment of up to 94 per cent of young children, even during infancy. This is accomplished with a minimum of discomfort and can do much to alleviate the severe psychological handicap of affected children and their families. In the United States, information relative to port-wine stains and their management can be obtained from the National Congenital Port-Wine Stain

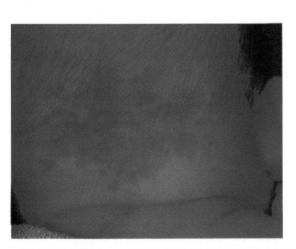
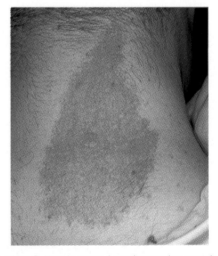

Figure 9–19. A. Salmon patch on the nape of the neck in a 3-month-old infant. B. Unna's nevus. A persistent salmon patch on the nucha (nape of the neck) of an adult.

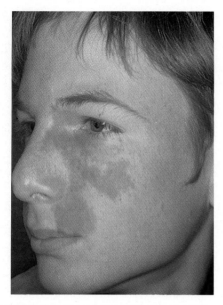

Figure 9–20. Port-wine stain (nevus flammeus), ectatic vessels within the upper dermis on the left side of the face of a 16-year-old boy.

Foundation, 125 East 63rd Street, New York, NY 10021 (212-755-3820).

Clinical Variants and Associated Syndromes

Hemangiomas and port-wine stains in special locations can often be a cause for complications, associated abnormalities, and concern. Ophthalmic sequelae, the most common complication of periorbital hemangiomas, occur in up to 80 per cent of patients with strawberry and cavernous hemangiomas and include amblyopia, astigmatism, myopia, strabismus, ptosis, retrobulbar involvement, orbital and palpebral asymmetry, keratitis,

and optic nerve atrophy (see Figs. 9–12, 9–14, 9–21, and 9–22).[24] Intralesional corticosteroid injections, currently advocated by many ophthalmologists, use local corticosteroid concentrations (up to 40 to 80 mg of triamcinolone acetonide in combination with 6 to 12 mg of betamethasone).[25, 26] This procedure, frequently done with the patient under general anesthesia, carries significant additional risks, including eyelid necrosis, localized lipoatrophy, retrobulbar or intracranial extension, and, as a result of corticosteroid embolization, at times retinal artery occlusion, resulting in visual loss or blindness.[27, 28] Most pediatric dermatologists, because of the potential side effects of local infiltration, the necessity of repeated injections, and the administration of general anesthesia, prefer to use oral corticosteroids for this purpose.

Infants with extensive facial hemangiomas have an increased risk of extension into retrobulbar, intracranial, paratracheal, intracervical, or intrathoracic spaces and, at times, neurologic malformations. Although aggressive facial hemangiomas may initially appear to represent less ominous-appearing port-wine stains or strawberry hemangiomas, careful follow-up visits can usually identify their ominous and aggressive features (see Fig. 9–21). Computed tomography (CT scans) and magnetic resonance imaging (MRI), with or without contrast enhancement, are recommended for patients with large, potentially aggressive facial hemangiomas (see Fig. 9–22). Although the treatment of aggressive hemangiomas is difficult, systemic corticosteroids and interferon can be beneficial.[29–33]

Like their cutaneous counterparts, when subglottic capillary hemangiomas occur, they usually develop during the first few months of life. The natural course of subglottic hemangiomas is one of gradual enlargement and spontaneous involution beginning at 9 or 10 months of age. Any infant with cutaneous hemangiomas with persistent inspiratory and expiratory laryngeal stridor, therefore, should be evaluated for possible laryngeal heman-

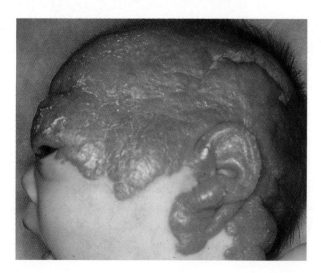

Figure 9–21. A large aggressive facial hemangioma in a 3-month-old infant.

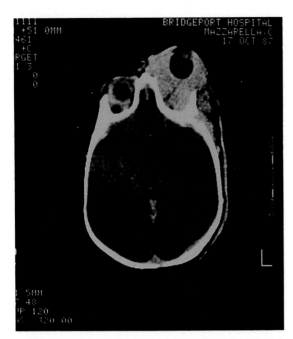

Figure 9–22. Computed tomographic study of the patient in Figure 9–21 showing retrobulbar extension of the hemangioma.

gioma. Tracheostomy is frequently required to secure an adequate airway in individuals with this disorder, and although therapeutic approaches such as irradiation, systemic corticosteroids, and surgical excision may at times be beneficial, carbon dioxide laser therapy (particularly during the time when natural involution begins) has been recommended.[34, 35]

Hepatic hemangiomas may be isolated or discovered in association with disseminated neonatal hemangiomatosis. They often tend to have a high mortality rate; and death, if it occurs, may be caused by high-output congestive heart failure, portal obstruction, or the Kasabach-Merritt syndrome. Although corticosteroids in dosages up to 5 mg/kg/day of prednisone (or its equivalent), interferon, cyclophosphamide, or surgical therapy may at times be lifesaving, no approach has met with uniform success. Obstruction of the external auditory canal by hemangiomatous involvement of the parotid regions or auditory canal may, at times, also be a cause for concern. Although the possibility of hearing loss must be considered when this occurs, it generally does not prove to be a problem unless it is bilateral and obstruction persists beyond the age of 1 year (when auditory conduction is necessary for the development of normal speech).[1] Lumbosacral hemangiomas or port-wine stains, like other cutaneous lesions centered over the midline, may be associated with underlying abnormalities such as spina bifida, spinal dysraphism, meningomyelocele, tethered cord syndrome, and other congenital abnormalities such as imperforate anus, rectoscrotal, rectoperineal, or rectovaginal fistulas, skin tags, leg

deformities, and neurologic, gastrointestinal, genitourinary, and skeletal anomalies.[36]

Nasal tip lesions (the "Cyrano nose" deformity) (Fig. 9–23) are notoriously slow to evidence regression, often leave behind extra fibrofatty tissue, and, because of their location, frequently result in extreme concern on the part of the family. Surgical correction, particularly when the child approaches school age, is therefore often considered. In such instances one should be certain that the lesion has reached its maximal growth and that there is no evidence of further spontaneous resolution before surgery is considered.[1, 37]

Usually becoming apparent in later childhood or during adult life (before the age of 30), cavernous hemangiomas of the skeletal muscle (skeletal muscle hemangiomas) may at times present as deep soft tissue masses with a predilection for the lower limbs. When seen in association with an overlying cutaneous purpuric discoloration, dilated veins, or a pulsatile mass with a bruit, they usually are easily diagnosed. Since most skeletal muscle hemangiomas do not present these associated features, however, they are often overlooked or misdiagnosed.[38] Computed tomography, nuclear scanning, magnetic resonance imaging, and angiography can help identify such lesions.

KASABACH-MERRITT SYNDROME

The Kasabach-Merritt syndrome (a variant of disseminated intravascular coagulopathy in which thrombocytopenia is reputedly caused by platelet sequestration in giant cavernous hemangiomas) is a vascular malformation that generally affects infants 3 months of age or younger. Although most cavernous hemangiomas associated with thrombocytopenia are exceedingly large, excessive size or extensive hemangiomatosis is not necessarily a prerequisite for diagnosis of this disorder. Patients with lesions as small as 5 or 6 cm in diameter have

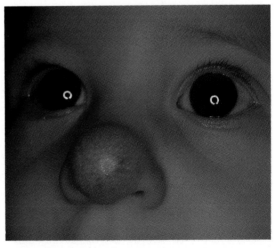

Figure 9–23. A cavernous hemangioma on the tip of the nose (the "Cyrano nose" deformity).

had confirmed thrombocytopenia, and this disorder has been reported in association with visceral hemangiomas, disseminated hemangiomatosis, and the Klippel-Trenaunay syndrome. Thrombocytopenia, frequently with blood platelet levels as low as 2,000 to 40,000/mm^3, anemia, decreased fibrinogen levels, and increased prothrombin and partial thromboplastin times may be detected during the first few weeks of life. Children with rapidly expanding cavernous lesions (with or without petechiae or ecchymoses), particularly during the early postnatal period, accordingly should be checked for platelet entrapment and incipient thrombocytopenia.[39]

The danger of the Kasabach-Merritt syndrome is the development of acute hemorrhage or possible compression of vital structures during a period of rapid growth. Nearly one fourth of reported infants with this complication died of bleeding disorders, respiratory distress, infection, or malignant transformation. Hence, infants with large cavernous hemangiomas and thrombocytopenia should be hospitalized and promptly treated.

Treatment consists of fresh whole-blood or platelet transfusions as needed, replacement of coagulation factors with fresh frozen plasma and cryoprecipitate, compression bandages over the hemangioma site whenever possible, a short intensive course of systemic corticosteroids, in dosages equivalent to the 2 to 5 mg/kg/day of prednisone, high-dose intravenous methylprednisolone, cautious use of anticoagulants in the presence of disseminated intravascular coagulopathy, aminocaproic acid (Amicar) alone or with cryoprecipitate, tranexamic acid (Cyclokapron), cyclophosphamide, a combination of aspirin (20 mg/kg/day) with dipyridamole (Persantine) 1 to 5 mg/kg/day, transcatheter embolization with magnesium seed foils, magnesium wire or intravenous Gelfoam pellets pentoxifylline, interferon, and surgical removal of the hemangiomatous lesions if and when feasible.[33, 39–42] It should be noted, however, that the disorder eventually resolves, that patients will recover if bleeding is prevented, and that surgery is relatively safe if fresh whole-blood transfusions are used and the surgeon is experienced in the management of patients with this disorder.

STURGE-WEBER SYNDROME

The Sturge-Weber syndrome (encephalofacial or encephalotrigeminal angiomatosis) is a syndrome characterized by a nevus flammeus (port-wine stain) in the distribution of the first branch of the trigeminal nerve associated with a vascular malformation of the ipsilateral meninges and cerebral cortex (Table 9–2 and Fig. 9–24). Although there have been reports of Sturge-Weber syndrome in the absence of a facial nevus, these cases do not fulfill the criteria for Sturge-Weber syndrome and are termed *meningeal angiomatosis*.[43–45]

Although the origin of the disorder is unclear,

Table 9–2. STURGE-WEBER SYNDROME

1. First branch of trigeminal nerve (V_1): 5–8% of patients with facial port-wine stains involving the upper eyelid or forehead
2. Ipsilateral meninges and cerebral cortex
3. Must involve area above palpebral fissure
4. Seizures (80%), retardation (60%), hemiplegia (30%)
5. Forty-five per cent associated with glaucoma (if both ophthalmic and maxillary divisions of trigeminal are involved); if only one branch is involved, glaucoma does not occur.

dysmorphogenesis of the cephalic neuroectoderm resulting in abnormality of the upper facial, choroid, and pia arachnoid vasculature, blood stagnation, and neuronal hypoxia of the underlying cortex appears to be, at least in part, responsible for the neurologic deficits associated with this congenital defect. Alexander and Norman, in their survey of 787 cases, showed part of the facial nevus involving the forehead and upper eyelid to some extent. When the nevus occurred exclusively below the palpebral fissure, the cerebral angiomatosis was not found.[46] From this observation it may be inferred that if the vascular nevus does not involve the upper eyelid or forehead, one generally need not worry about the possible association of central nervous system involvement.

The oral mucous membranes may show telangiectatic hypertrophy and studies suggest that if the vascular nevus involves both the ophthalmic and the maxillary divisions of the sensory branch of the trigeminal nerve, childhood glaucoma appears in 45 per cent of patients; involvement of one branch alone does not seem to be associated with glaucoma.[1, 47] When glaucoma occurs, it appears to be secondary to involvement of the filtration angle, resulting in increased venous pressure and subsequent elevated intraocular pressure.

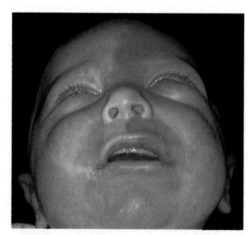

Figure 9–24. Sturge-Weber syndrome. Nevus flammeus in the distribution of the fifth cranial (trigeminal) nerve. It should be noted that Sturge-Weber syndrome is unlikely when the vascular nevus occurs exclusively below the palpebral fissure.

In 50 per cent of patients, the earliest symptoms of the intracranial lesions of Sturge-Weber syndrome develop during the first year. Although extensive meningeal lesions may remain silent throughout life, onset of symptoms after age 20 is unusual. Seizures, reported in 80 per cent of affected persons, often as early as 3 months of age, frequently present as the initial symptom of this disorder. Hemiplegia has been reported in up to 30 per cent, and mental retardation may be seen in 60 per cent of affected persons. *Phakomatosis pigmentovascularis*, a hereditary disorder with features of Sturge-Weber syndrome and ocular and cutaneous pigmentation suggestive of nevus of Ota and mongolian spots, although similar in some ways to the Sturge-Weber syndrome, is considered to have enough specific clinical as well as histopathologic features to be considered a distinct entity.[48]

Occurring in 5 to 8 per cent of patients with facial port-wine stains involving the upper eyelid or forehead, the association of a nevus flammeus in the region of the ophthalmic division (the upper eyelid and/or supraorbital area) of the trigeminal nerve (V_1) with epilepsy or hemiplegia is presumptive of a diagnosis of Sturge-Weber syndrome. Electroencephalography shows unilateral depression of cortical activity with or without spike discharges. Radiography of the skull reveals characteristic calcifications in two thirds of patients. These calcifications follow the convolutions of the cerebral cortex and are characterized by sinuous double-contoured parallel streaks of calcification (called "tram lines"). Although intracranial calcifications can be detected by radiographic examination or CT scan[45] in infants as young as 4 months of age, they often do not appear until after the first or second year of life and become more extensive up to the second decade, after which time they remain stable. Since CT scans and particularly MRI are more sensitive than standard radiography in the detection of intracranial calcifications, they often are recommended as the diagnostic procedures of choice.

Surgical treatment of the intracranial lesion is occasionally successful. Accordingly, neurosurgical consultation should be sought as soon as the diagnosis has been established, preferably, if possible, before the onset of seizures. Regular supervision by an ophthalmologist and control of glaucoma by goniotomy are important aspects of therapy. Parents of children with Sturge-Weber syndrome can obtain medical information from the Sturge-Weber Foundation, P.O. Box 460931, Aurora, CO 80046.

KLIPPEL-TRENAUNAY AND PARKES WEBER SYNDROMES

The Klippel-Trenaunay syndrome (nevus vasculosus hypertrophicus) is a vascular malformation characterized by extensive nevus flammeus (usually of a limb), underlying venous varicosities, and overgrowth of bone and soft tissue hypertrophy of the affected area. In 95 per cent of cases, the lower limb is the site of the malformations. The hypertrophy involves the length as well as the circumference of the extremity, males and females are about equally affected, and local hyperemia and augmented arterial flow due to the vascular abnormality and venous stasis are believed to account for the bony and soft tissue hypertrophy (Fig. 9–25). Although the syndrome was originally described in 1900 by Klippel and Trenaunay, in 1907 Frederick Parkes Weber described a similar syndrome with the additional finding of arteriovenous fistulas. Thus, when there are no arteriovenous fistulas the disorder is more correctly termed the *Klippel-Trenaunay syndrome*, and when the arteriovenous fistulas are the major vascular lesions *Parkes Weber syndrome* is the appropriate designation. The Parkes Weber syndrome is substantially less common, and although it generally affects the lower limb it is more likely to affect the upper limb than the Klippel-Trenaunay syndrome.[1]

Additional complicating features described in patients with the Klippel-Trenaunay and Parkes Weber syndromes include strawberry and cavern-

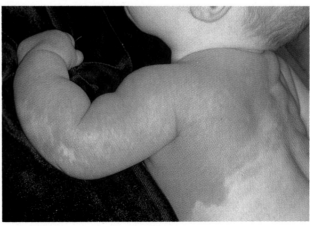

Figure 9–25. Klippel-Trenaunay syndrome. Local hypertrophy of the bone and soft tissue is associated with a port-wine stain in a 3-month-old infant.

ous hemangiomas, congenital varicosities, and combinations of these, with or without arteriovenous shunts, lymphangiomatous anomalies, varicosities, thrombophlebitis, cellulitis, lymphedema of the affected limb, congestive cardiac failure, limb disparity, compensatory vertebral scoliosis, stasis dermatitis, ulcerations, phleboliths, decalcification of involved bones, hyperhidrosis of the affected area, pulmonary hypertension, paresthesias, spina bifida, rectal bleeding, hematuria, and rarely Kasabach-Merritt syndrome. Although treatment is generally unsatisfactory, compression of dilated veins by support bandages has some merit, and surgery may be effective in the prevention of severe limb hypertrophy in occasional patients.[49] Surgery is not indicated for superficial venous varicosities resulting from hypoplasia or atresia of the deep venous system, however, and can produce disastrous results. Appropriate radiographic studies, therefore, are advisable prior to any attempts at surgical correction.

MAFFUCCI'S SYNDROME

Maffucci's syndrome (dyschondroplasia with hemangiomas) is a rare disorder characterized by vascular hamartomas (hemangiomas, phlebectasias, and lymphangiomas) and dyschondroplasia. Two thirds of reported patients have been male, up to 25 per cent of patients may be affected at birth or in the first year of life, and approximately 50 per cent will have recognizable disease by the age of 6 years. During the prepubertal years the multiple hemangiomas, usually manifested by hard or cauliflower-like nodules on the fingers or toes, followed by other nodular lesions elsewhere on the extremities, and dyschondroplasia become apparent. Subsequently, other progressive skeletal abnormalities due to defects of ossification (marked bony deformities complicated by pathologic fractures) and neurologic deficits from cerebral encroachment of enchondromas of the skull may be seen.

The vascular lesions consist of dilated veins and soft bluish cavernous hemangiomas, which occur on the affected limb or elsewhere. The distribution of vascular lesions does not necessarily correspond to that of the skeletal lesions. Of particular significance is the fact that 30 per cent of patients with this disorder develop some type of associated malignant disease (chondrosarcoma, fibrosarcoma, angiosarcoma, pancreatic adenosarcoma, glioma, or teratoma). The management of this disorder, accordingly, consists of surgery, when indicated, and periodic evaluation to detect and extirpate any lesions suggestive of neoplastic degeneration.

BLUE RUBBER BLEB NEVUS SYNDROME

The blue rubber bleb nevus is a variant of a cavernous hemangioma that presents as a soft, compressible, blue to purple, rubbery protuberance of the dermis and subcutaneous tissue (Fig. 9–26). Although most cases are sporadic, dominant inheritance of this syndrome through as many as five generations has been described.[50] Some lesions may be spontaneously painful and tender to palpation. In this syndrome the vascular lesions are sometimes present at birth and, with time, frequently tend to increase in size or number. The importance of this type of lesion lies in its frequent association with angiomas of the gastrointestinal tract. The gastrointestinal hemangiomas most frequently are found in the small intestine or colon but may occur anywhere throughout the gastrointestinal tract. They tend to bleed readily, frequently causing anemia.

The cutaneous lesions are blue and raised, their surfaces are wrinkled, and they vary from 0.1 to 5.0 cm in diameter. They may present as large cavernous hemangiomas, blood sacs resembling nipple-like blebs (blue rubber blebs), or irregular blue marks on the cutaneous surface. They may be solitary or may number in the hundreds and can occur anywhere on the cutaneous surface (usually the trunk or arms) or the mucous membranes of the nose and mouth. One of the diagnostic features is the fact that blood can be expressed from the lesions with pressure, leaving an empty wrinkled sac that then refills rapidly. Oral corticosteroids are of no value, and treatment is mainly symptomatic with excision of individual lesions for cosmetic purposes and bowel resection, when indicated, to control excessive bleeding and anemia.

DIFFUSE NEONATAL HEMANGIOMATOSIS

A number of infants have been reported with multiple hemangiomas of the visceral organs, the gastrointestinal tract, liver, central nervous system, and lungs. Although on occasion such infants have no cutaneous involvement, most affected children display widely disseminated small, red to bluish black papular cutaneous hemangiomas (usually present at birth or developing during the first few weeks of life), often numbering in the hundreds (diffuse neonatal hemangiomatosis, multinodular hemangiomatosis) (Figs. 9–27 and 9–28).

Hepatic hemangiomas, when present, may be delineated by liver and spleen scan, hepatic angiography, or both. Recognition of the cutaneous component, which may be minimal in some infants, will permit correct early diagnosis and help prevent confusion with cardiac failure seen in association with congenital heart disease. Patients with multiple cutaneous hemangiomas, therefore, should be observed for the possibility of systemic involvement, and those with clinical features of visceral involvement should have periodic physical examinations with auscultation for possible bruits; ophthalmologic examination to rule out ocular complications; hematocrit and hemoglobin

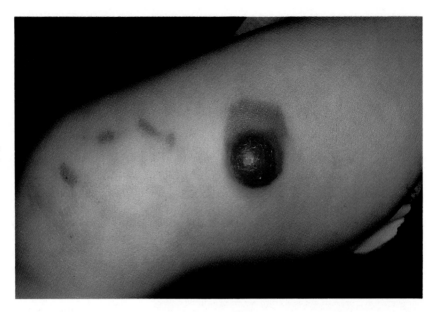

Figure 9–26. A blue rubber bleb nevus on the thigh of a 4½-month-old infant.

determinations to detect anemia secondary to bleeding; blood platelet counts to check for thrombocytopenia; ultrasound, computed tomography, or radiographic evaluation of suspicious areas; periodic examination of urine and stools for occult blood; echocardiography or electrocardiography if cardiac failure is suspected; careful neurologic examination; computed tomography if involvement of the central nervous system seems likely; and liver function tests if there is evidence of hepatic involvement.[51]

Affected infants may occasionally die of high-output cardiac failure, hepatic complications, gastrointestinal hemorrhage, respiratory tract obstruction, or severe neurologic deficit due to compression of neural tissue. When seen in association with multinodular hemangiomatosis, cardiac failure is believed to be the result of arteriovenous shunts in hepatic hemangiomas, which ultimately lead to increased venous return and increased cardiac output. When present, this complication occurs early in life (usually at 2 to 9 weeks of age). Surgical management of this complication by lobectomy or selective ligation of hepatic vessels can frequently be avoided by high-dose (5 mg/kg of prednisone or its equivalent) systemic corticosteroids and, if there is no response, interferon, and digitalis (particularly when initiated early).

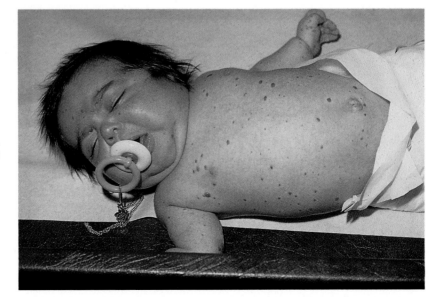

Figure 9–27. Multiple neonatal hemangiomatosis. (Courtesy of Robert Herzlinger, M.D.)

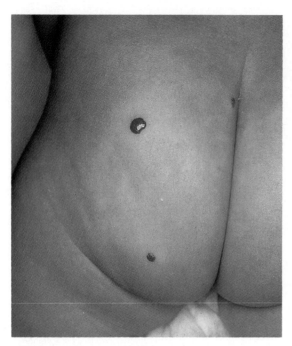

Figure 9–28. Neonatal hemangiomatoses on the buttock of a 4-month-old infant.

Although diffuse neonatal hemangiomatosis is frequently complicated by visceral involvement, some infants may have multiple cutaneous hemangiomas without visceral complications. This disorder has been termed *benign neonatal hemangiomatosis.*[52] Since there is no definitive way to distinguish the benign from the more serious cases, careful examination and follow-up for possible systemic involvement is necessary for all infants with cutaneous lesions suggestive of diffuse neonatal hemangiomatosis.

GORHAM'S SYNDROME

Gorham's syndrome (disappearing bones, vanishing bone disease, angiomatous nevi with osteolysis) is an extremely uncommon disorder that consists of cutaneous hemangiomas in association with massive osteolysis and complete or partial replacement of bone by extensive fibrosis. The skin and soft tissue involvement in this disorder is usually confined to areas near the bony lesions. Although the cause of increased bone resorption is not known, it has been theorized that this phenomenon may be due to localized hyperemia associated with the hemangiomas.

Usually a disorder of young children, involving single or multiple bones, Gorham's disease is believed to be a slowly developing, probably self-limiting condition and does not progress to neoplastic formation. Numerous methods of therapy have been employed, but not one has proved of value. The only reported deaths associated with this disorder are those that resulted from hemorrhage into serous cavities.[53, 54]

RILEY-SMITH SYNDROME

The Riley-Smith syndrome (macrocephaly with unusual cutaneous angiomatosis) is an autosomal dominant disorder characterized by multiple cavernous hemangiomas, macrocephaly, and pseudopapillomas. This disorder has been expanded to include persons with the Klippel-Trenaunay and Parkes Weber syndromes, a combination of the Sturge-Weber and Klippel-Trenaunay syndromes, cutis marmorata telangiectatica congenita, and macrocephaly with multiple lipomas and hemangiomas (Fig. 9–29).[55, 56] Because normal central nervous system function is frequently seen in association with this syndrome, awareness of the possible benign nature of the macrocephaly should help avoid unnecessary concern or intervention, except in patients who also manifest signs of increased intracranial pressure or central nervous system dysfunction.

COBB SYNDROME

Cobb syndrome (cutaneomeningospinal angiomatosis) consists of a cutaneous vascular nevus (angiolipoma, cavernous hemangioma, port-wine stain, or angiokeratoma) and an associated angioma in the spinal cord corresponding within a segment or two of the involved dermatome.[57] The cutaneous lesion, although initially macular, often develops a deep cavernous hemangiomatous component and an overlying verruciform hyperkeratotic surface. Symptoms of anoxia and compression include pain in the areas supplied by the involved segment of the spinal cord, weakness and atrophy of the limb muscles, loss of sensation, and distal flaccid monoplegia or paraplegia. Males slightly outnumber females in most series, and in the majority of patients the neurologic problems occur during childhood or adolescence. Angiomas of vertebrae or the retina may be found, kyphoscoliosis is common, and, in most patients, lateral thoracic and lumbar spine radiographs may show early bone erosion.

Treatment, as well as diagnosis, may be aided by spinal angiography. Spinal angiomas fed by the posterior spinal artery are often juxtamedullary and can be extirpated surgically without appreciable damage to the spinal cord. Those fed by the anterior spinal artery, however, are often intramedullary and supply critical motor pathways and neurons. Surgical removal of such lesions, therefore, is frequently technically impossible.

VASCULAR TUMORS

Verrucous Hemangioma

A verrucous hemangioma is an uncommon variant of a capillary, cavernous, or mixed hemangioma that develops secondary proliferative epidermal change. Easily mistaken for verrucae, pigmented tumors, or angiokeratomas, they are

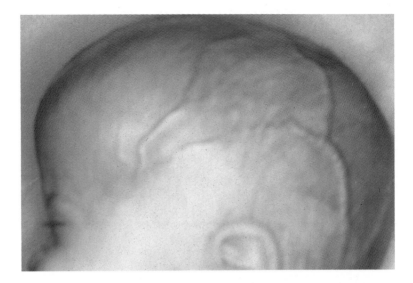

Figure 9–29. A port-wine nevus in a child with hydrocephalus (the Riley-Smith deformity).

vascular lesions that occur generally on the lower extremities and occasionally on the chest and forearms. Most are present at birth or appear during early childhood. Initially they are soft, bluish red, and well demarcated and range from 4 mm to as much as 5 to 7 cm in diameter. As the patient grows the lesions enlarge and frequently develop a brown or bluish black color with keratotic and verrucous features, which tend to obscure the true vascular nature of this disorder. When the diagnosis remains in doubt, histopathologic examination will reveal a capillary or cavernous hemangioma with overlying epidermal hyperkeratosis, irregular acanthosis, and papillomatosis.

Since verrucous hemangiomas do not regress spontaneously and tend to enlarge in proportion to the growth of the body, early excision generally is advisable. Smaller lesions (1 to 2 cm in diameter) are frequently amenable to local excision or electrocautery. Larger lesions, however, often extend into the subcutaneous fat and tend to recur (particularly when subjected to secondary infection or trauma). Such lesions are probably best treated by wide excision and subsequent skin graft.[58]

Pyogenic Granuloma

Pyogenic granuloma (granuloma pyogenicum, granuloma telangiectaticum) is a common vascular lesion, which in most instances consists of a bright red to reddish brown, soft or moderately firm, raised, usually slightly pedunculated nodule (Fig. 9–30). The mechanism that brings about the formation of pyogenic granuloma is unknown. It is believed to represent a true benign neoplasm or perhaps a reactive proliferative vascular process, possibly associated with trauma and the presence of pyogenic bacteria. Although there may indeed be an association with bacteria, pyogenic granuloma does not appear to be an infectious process. Affecting individuals of all ages, it occurs fre-

quently in children and young adults and may at times occur in patients receiving isotretinoin or etretinate.

Pyogenic granulomas develop rapidly and usually arise as solitary lesions. Some rare cases of multiple disseminated pyogenic granuloma have been reported, however, and removal or destruction of lesions has at times been followed by the development of recurrent or satellite lesions at or near the site of a previously treated lesion.[59, 60] Although they may occur on any cutaneous surface, they most commonly appear in areas subject to trauma, namely the hands (particularly the fingers), the forearms, the face, and occasionally the mucosal surfaces of the mouth. Pyogenic granulomas are vascular, range from 5 mm to 1 or 2 cm in diameter, and bleed easily, even on the slightest trauma. In most cases the history and clinical appearance are highly characteristic, and the correct diagnosis is easily established. The histologic picture is similar to that of a well-circumscribed capillary hemangi-

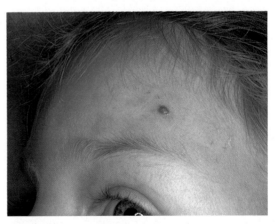

Figure 9–30. Pyogenic granuloma. A benign bright red elevated vascular nodule is evident on the forehead of a young child.

oma embedded in a loose edematous stroma and covered by a flattened epidermis.

Treatment consists of laser surgery or destruction of the lesion by electrodesiccation and curettage with coagulation of the base. A number of pyogenic granulomas recur after such treatment, however, because the proliferating vessels in the base extend in a conical manner into the deeper dermis. In such instances repeat electrodesiccation, cryosurgery with liquid nitrogen, carbon dioxide laser surgery, or surgical excision is generally effective.

Tufted Angioma

Acquired tufted angioma (angioblastoma) is a rare condition that occurs primarily on the upper trunk and neck in young persons. It may be present at birth and in up to 50 per cent of cases develops in the first five years of life. The disorder is characterized by single or multiple, slowly spreading erythematous macules and plaques, often with a deep nodular component. Occasionally clinically suggesting a diagnosis of pyogenic granuloma or Kaposi's sarcoma, the lesions tend to spread and in some patients eventually affect a large part of the trunk and neck. Histologically there are circumscribed angiomatous aggregates of closely packed capillaries, some of which are small and elongated (referred to as tufts) and others that consist of large round or irregularly shaped lobules. Despite the progressive spread of the angiomas, malignant change has not been encountered.[61]

Bacillary Angiomatosis

Bacillary angiomatosis, also called epithelioid angiomatosis, is a newly described visceral or cutaneous infection caused by a gram-negative *Rickettsia*-like organism of the *Rochalimaea* species or closely resembling that seen in cat-scratch disease with features of bartonellosis, occurring in immunosuppressed individuals infected with human immunodeficiency virus (HIV) and, at times, immunocompetent individuals. Cutaneous lesions are firm, nontender, red, purple, dusky, or skin-colored papules or nodules resembling angiomas up to 2 to 3 cm in diameter. Although they can be seen at any site, they tend to spare the palms, soles, and oral cavity.

Characterized histologically by lobular capillary proliferation surrounded by edematous and fibrotic stroma, neutrophils, and leukocytoclasis ("nuclear dust"), identification of the organism on Warthin-Starry stain can help establish the diagnosis. The possibility of HIV infection should be investigated in all individuals with this disorder; and, since death may result from visceral and mucosal involvement, treatment should be initiated as soon as possible.[62] The disorder usually responds to antibiotic therapy with erythromycin, doxycycline, trimethoprim-sulfamethoxazole, isoniazid, or rifampin.

Glomus Tumor

Glomus tumors are relatively uncommon hamartomas of the glomus body, a special temperature-regulating arteriovenous shunt that bypasses the usual capillary bed of the dermis. Rarely seen in infants, the lesions may be solitary or multiple and occur in children as well as adults.

Solitary glomus tumors, the more common form of this disorder, do not appear to have a familial tendency. They usually occur as bluish red cutaneous nodules that vary from 1 mm to several centimeters in diameter. Lesions usually appear on the upper extremities, particularly the nail beds, and occasionally on the lower extremities, head, neck, or penis. They are extremely tender and frequently give rise to paroxysms of pain. Although the etiology is unknown, some lesions appear to be associated with previous trauma to the involved area.

In contrast to the solitary type, multiple glomus tumors are dominantly transmitted, may be painful or painless, and vary from a few lesions to several hundred (Fig. 9–31). They are relatively more common in children than adults, and the majority of lesions involve the lower extremities and only sometimes the upper extremities. The face, neck, and subungual areas are generally spared. Multiple glomus tumors appear as flesh-colored to bluish red, flat to dome-shaped papules that vary from a few millimeters to several centimeters in diameter and blanch completely on diascopy. When grouped in one area, glomus tumors may resemble a blue rubber bleb nevus.

Solitary glomus tumors must be differentiated from neurofibromas, dermatofibromas, melanomas, blue nevi, and leiomyomas; multiple lesions must be differentiated from leiomyomas and cavernous hemangiomas. When the diagnosis remains

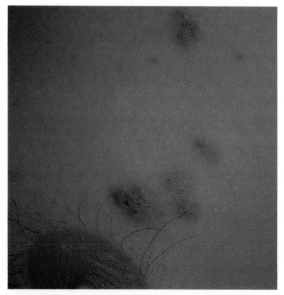

Figure 9–31. Multiple glomus tumors on the chest of a 19-year-old man.

in doubt, the true nature of the disorder may be verified by cutaneous biopsy.

On histopathologic examination solitary glomus tumors are surrounded by a fibrous capsule and contain numerous small vascular lumina lined by a single layer of glomus cells that have a faintly eosinophilic cytoplasm and a large, oval, or cuboidal pale nucleus. Multiple glomus tumors possess no capsules and are much more vascular than the solitary type. They are lined by a single layer of flat endothelial cells, and glomus cells are seen peripheral to the endothelial cells as a narrow rim of only one to three layers.

Glomus tumors are not radiosensitive, and electrocoagulation is frequently followed by recurrence. Surgical excision is the best method of treatment, but recurrences, particularly in the subungual region, are common, and sclerotherapy with care to avoid the risk of injection of arterial lesions of the distal extremities can be utilized for individuals with multiple, unsightly, or discomforting lesions.

Hemangiopericytoma

Hemangiopericytomas are very rare tumors of the skin, subcutaneous, and muscular tissues and may appear on any part of the body. Derived from pericytes (smooth muscle cells that surround small blood vessels), these usually solitary, firm nodules have been reported in individuals from birth to 93 years of age but usually appear shortly after birth, during early childhood, or in middle life.[63] Their clinical appearance is not distinctive, and their course is highly variable. Lesions are painless, are often well circumscribed, vary from 1 to 8 cm or more in diameter, and are flesh colored to reddish blue. Some lesions are benign and remain quiescent. Others show rapid growth and an incidence of neoplastic change estimated at 20 per cent, with a predilection for the musculoskeletal system. In children, those that are superficial or located in the subcutis generally tend to remain benign, however.

Histologically, hemangiopericytomas often resemble glomus tumors and may indeed be related to them. They are characterized by branching capillaries surrounded by closely packed cells with oval or spindle-shaped nuclei (pericytes) embedded in a network of reticulum fibers.

Since the histologic behavior of hemangiopericytomas is unpredictable and there is a high incidence of neoplastic change (generally during the second or third decade of life), wide local excision is the treatment of choice.

Cellular Angioma of Infancy

Angioendotheliomas (epithelioid or spindle cell hemangioendotheliomas, cellular angioma of infancy), despite their invasiveness, are benign vascular tumors that clinically and histologically represent an intermediate classification between hemangiomas and hemangiosarcomas. Cutaneous lesions are characterized by erythematous to reddish brown to bluish purple, usually firm patches, plaques, or nodules, petechiae, ecchymoses, telangiectasia, necrosis, ulceration, and poikiloderma vasculare atrophicans–like changes that occur most commonly on the trunk. Despite its local invasiveness and mitotic activity, in contrast with angiosarcoma of adults, it is benign; therefore, radical surgical excision is unnecessary.[64]

Angiolymphoid Hyperplasia With Eosinophilia (Kimura's Disease)

Angiolymphoid hyperplasia with eosinophilia is an uncommon vascular disorder occurring most commonly in young adults and, at times, in children, characterized by solitary or more commonly multiple, purplish red, intradermal or subcutaneous nodules of angiolymphoid hyperplasia. Its etiology is unknown, but the disorder appears to represent an inflammatory reactive process following trauma, infection, or humoral imbalance rather than a neoplastic process. It is usually seen as smooth, dome-shaped, bright or dusky red papules, nodules, or plaques in the dermis or subcutaneous tissue of the head and neck region, particularly in and around the ears. Although the dermal lesions generally measure less than 1 cm in diameter, the subcutaneous lesions may attain a size of 5 to 10 cm.

Histologically the lesion has a vascular and a cellular component. The vascular component consists primarily of irregularly shaped capillaries with greatly swollen pleomorphic cells with nuclei protruding into the lumen. The cellular component consists of an extensive inflammatory infiltrate with eosinophils, lymphocytes, histiocytes, and mast cells. Although this disorder and Kimura's disease are often considered to be part of the same spectrum, Kimura's disease may represent a separate entity.

The duration of lesions may vary from 3 weeks to several years; in approximately 5 per cent of patients lesions may persist for periods of 5 years or more. Deep-seated lesions, particularly those located in bones and soft tissue, often tend to run a more aggressive course. Although lesions can at times be locally destructive, malignant change does not occur; and in most instances, although recurrences are common, surgical excision results in a definitive cure. In addition, intralesional corticosteroids and carbon dioxide laser beam therapy have been helpful, and, in cases of long duration, oral corticosteroids and vinblastine have also been show to be effective.[65–68]

ANGIOKERATOMAS

The term *angiokeratoma* is applied to a group of disorders characterized by ectasia (dilatation of the superficial vessels of the dermis) and hyperkeratosis of the overlying epidermis. All have in common the presence of asymptomatic vascular lesions, seen as firm dark red to black papules that measure from 1 to 10 mm in diameter, with varying degrees of secondary hyperkeratosis (Figs. 9–32 and 9–33).

At least six forms of angiokeratoma have been recognized. Four represent cosmetic problems only. These include solitary or multiple angiokeratomas, angiokeratoma circumscriptum, angiokeratoma of Mibelli, and angiokeratoma of Fordyce. The fifth and sixth forms are diffuse diseases of systemic significance. They are known as angiokeratoma corporis diffusum or Fabry's disease (a sex-linked disorder characterized by storage of a neutral glycolipid, ceramide trihexoside, in many types of cells in the body) and fucosidosis (an autosomal recessive disease characterized by the abnormal intracellular accumulation of a fucose-containing glycosphingolipid).

Solitary or Multiple Angiokeratomas

Solitary or multiple angiokeratomas represent a group of individual lesions generally seen on the lower extremities. They appear to follow trauma and begin as an area of telangiectasia followed by hyperkeratosis and angiokeratoma formation. Although they may be seen in childhood, these lesions are not congenital but appear to be acquired as a result of injury to the papillary vessels, with resultant dilatation and impaired contractility of the capillary wall. Single angiokeratomas may be mistaken for nevi or malignant melanoma but can be differentiated on the basis of histopathologic examination.[69]

Microscopic features include groups of dilated papillary blood vessels, acanthosis and hyperkeratosis of the epidermis, and elongation of the rete ridges, which often tend to enclose the underlying capillary spaces. Treatment of asymptomatic angiokeratomas is usually unnecessary. When desired, however, because of trauma or for cosmetic purposes, argon or carbon dioxide laser beam surgery, local excision, or electrodesiccation generally produces good cosmetic results.

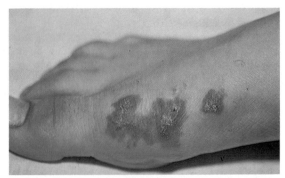

Figure 9–33. Angiokeratoma of Mibelli. Hyperkeratotic vascular lesions occur over the bony prominences of the foot. (Courtesy of Hillard H. Pearlstein, M.D.)

Angiokeratoma Circumscriptum

Angiokeratoma circumscriptum, the only form of angiokeratoma that is likely to be present at birth, is usually seen as a solitary large hyperkeratotic plaque or nodule. In half of the reported cases the lesion begins in infancy or early childhood, with females reportedly affected three times as frequently as males. Usually deep red or blue-black, lesions are seen as localized unilateral papules, nodules, or plaques, often arranged in streaks or bands, with an uneven verrucous surface. Although they may occur on the back, forearm, or penis, the thighs, lower legs, and buttocks are the more typical areas of involvement. Lesions usually increase only in proportion to general body growth but may go on to enlarge during adolescence or early adult life; and in several instances, extensive lesions covering as much as one fourth of the body have been reported.

Angiokeratoma circumscriptum does not show a tendency to spontaneous involution. Small lesions may be removed by electrodesiccation and curettage or laser beam surgery; in larger lesions extensive surgical excision appears to be the treatment of choice.

Angiokeratoma of Mibelli

Angiokeratoma of Mibelli is a rare disorder first described by Mibelli in 1989. It is characterized by hyperkeratotic vascular lesions that occur over the bony prominences of the extremities of children, usually girls, during late childhood or early adolescence. Since it has been described in siblings and children with an affected parent, a dominant mode of inheritance with variable penetrance has been suggested[70, 71]

Lesions usually occur over the dorsal and lateral aspects of the fingers and toes but may also involve the ears, knees, ankles, elbows, palms, soles, and backs of the hands and feet. This distribution and the frequent association of lesions with acrocya-

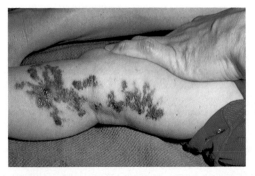

Figure 9–32. Angiokeratoma circumscriptum on the leg of a 15-month-old child. (Courtesy of Department of Dermatology, Yale University School of Medicine.)

nosis, chilblains, and frostbite suggest cold sensitivity as the precipitating factor in this disorder.

Early lesions are minute reddish to purple macules or soft papules. With time they increase to 5 to 8 mm or more in diameter and become elevated, verrucous, and darker. Although often numerous and disfiguring, lesions are generally asymptomatic. They do, however, bleed easily and, at times, may involute spontaneously following trauma. In patients with associated acrocyanosis and chilblains there may be abnormalities of immunoglobulin levels, with elevations of IgG, IgA, and IgM. One patient, an 11-year-old mentally retarded spastic girl, also had oral ulcerations and bony and soft tissue necrosis of the fingertips.[72]

Treatment of this disorder consists of cryosurgery with solid carbon dioxide or liquid nitrogen, electrocautery, or surgical excision.

Angiokeratoma of Fordyce

Angiokeratoma of the scrotum is a relatively common disorder first described by Fordyce in 1896. It occasionally appears in adolescents but most commonly occurs in males older than the age of 30, with an increasing incidence with age.[73] Clinically and histologically similar lesions may also appear on the labia of older women.

Lesions are distributed along the superficial vessels of the scrotum in a linear configuration, generally perpendicular to the scrotal raphe. Occasionally they may appear on the glans or shaft of the penis, and rarely they may be noted on the upper thigh or inguinal area.

Scrotal angiokeratomas are seen as multiple, small, 1- to 4-mm, reddish purple to black, dome-shaped vascular-appearing papules (Fig. 9–34). With increase in the age of the patient they become larger, darker, more numerous, nodular, and keratotic. The cause of these papules is unknown. Some investigators believe them to be neoplastic. Others consider them to be venous telangiectases,

possibly associated with venous obstruction. In support of the latter hypothesis is a frequent associated finding of varicocele, hernia, prostatitis, tumors of the bladder or epididymis, lymphogranuloma venereum, or thrombophlebitis in patients with this disorder.

Although angiokeratomas of the scrotum generally tend to be asymptomatic, they may become pruritic and tend to bleed when traumatized. Treatment, when desired, consists of electrocoagulation or cryosurgery with solid carbon dioxide or liquid nitrogen.

Angiokeratoma Corporis Diffusum

In 1898, Fabry, in Germany, and Anderson, in England, independently described a form of angiokeratoma now known as angiokeratoma corporis diffusum or Fabry's syndrome. The disorder appears to be an X-linked recessive disease with complete penetrance and variable clinical expressivity in homozygous males and occasional mild penetrance in heterozygous females.[74, 75] The disorder is characterized by systemic intracellular accumulation of glycosphingolipid (ceramide trihexoside) in the skin and viscera, particularly in the cardiovascular-renal system. The primary metabolic defect is the deficient activity of a specific α-galactosidase (ceramide trihexosidase), which normally catabolizes the accumulated glycosphingolipid.

The cutaneous vascular lesions characteristic of this disorder are telangiectases. They usually appear before puberty, often between 5 and 13 years of age. Occasionally they may occur during infancy. The lesions generally appear as clusters of individual punctate macular or papular dark-red angiectases that do not blanch with pressure. The eruption is usually symmetrical, and the lesions generally increase progressively in size and number with age. Despite their name, they generally show little to no hyperkeratosis.

Angiokeratomas of Fabry usually appear in the area between the umbilicus and knees. They may number into the thousands and tend to cluster in the iliosacral areas, about the umbilicus, and over the scrotum, buttocks, posterior thorax, and thighs. The first lesions frequently appear in the scrotum and must be differentiated from angiokeratoma of Fordyce. Lesions seldom occur on the hands or feet, have not been reported on the scalp, ears, or face, except for a small area on the chin, and are permanent unless they become thrombosed, after which they may disappear (which is rare). A majority of patients have pinpoint macular purplish spots on the lips, particularly near the vermilion border of the lower lip. These lesions are smaller than those on the skin. The tongue is not affected, but hemoptysis and epistaxis have been reported with involvement of the buccal and nasal mucosae. In addition to the typical cutaneous lesions, fine telangiectases have been described in the axillae

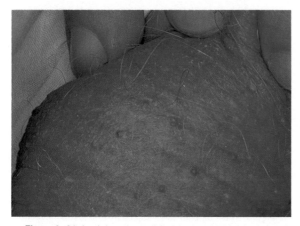

Figure 9–34. Angiokeratoma of the scrotum (angiokeratoma of Fordyce).

on the upper chest. In heterozygous females angiomas appear in only 20 per cent of cases and, when present, are less numerous and more limited in extent than in males.[76]

In childhood, recurrent episodes of fever, agonizing attacks of pain, and paresthesias of the hands and feet often accompany the eruption. Although often spontaneous or elicited by exertion, they are apparently associated with vasomotor disturbances and usually occur subsequent to temperature changes. Paralyses, scant body hair, and hypohidrosis are often present; and pedal and ankle edema are common and may result in stasis ulcers. Edema, when present, is presumably due to increased vascular permeability and is more prominent in summer than winter.

Patients with angiokeratoma corporis diffusum are often hypertensive and, with advancing age, are particularly susceptible to cerebrovascular accidents, coronary artery disease, and renal disease. Neurologic complications are common and include aphasia, paresis, tremors, paralyses, loss of consciousness, and psychotic disturbances. Other systemic manifestations include diarrhea, colitis, proctitis, an unusual arthritis of the distal interphalangeal joints with some loss of motion, cataracts, corneal opacities, and tortuosity of the conjunctival blood vessels with characteristic sausage-like constriction and dilatation.

The corneal opacities are usually present during childhood; they are found in all affected males as well as most (80 to 90 per cent) of the heterozygous female carriers with this disorder. Of particular diagnostic importance is the fact that the posterior capsular cataracts have a characteristic spoke-like appearance, which is pathognomonic for this disorder.

Most men with angiokeratoma of Fabry die in their 30s as a result of renal failure with uremia and hypertension. Others succumb to cerebrovascular accidents and congestive heart failure.

The course in female heterozygotes is more benign. Afflicted women have skin lesions (in 20 per cent of cases), cataracts, and relatively normal longevity. Although the disorder is generally asymptomatic in women, some have hypohidrosis, attacks of pain in the extremities, arthritis, urinary tract infection, and renal failure.

The diagnosis of angiokeratoma corporis diffusum is made by the presence of cutaneous angiomas, a positive family history, corneal opacities on slit lamp examination, and the presence of ceramide trihexoside, also referred to as trihexosyl ceramide, in the urine, plasma, or cultured fibroblasts. Hemizygotes and heterozygotes may also be diagnosed by hair root analysis.[77] Early in the course of the disease, casts, erythrocytes, fat-laden epithelial cells (mulberry cells), and lipid inclusions with characteristic birefringent "Maltese crosses" appear in the urinary sediment. Proteinuria, gradual deterioration of renal function, and azotemia occur in the second to fourth decades of life. Biopsy of the skin or kidney is confirmatory if intracellular birefringent lipoid deposits can be demonstrated, and prenatal detection can be accomplished by the demonstration of deficient α-galactosidase activity in cultured fetal cells obtained by amniocentesis.[78]

Unfortunately, there is no specific therapy to correct the biochemical defect of Fabry's disease. Treatment, therefore, is generally supportive. Replacement transfusion and periodic infusion with normal plasma have been suggested in an attempt to provide ceramide trihexosidase to patients with this inherited metabolic disease.[79]

Fucosidosis

Disseminated angiokeratomas may also be seen in patients with fucosidosis, an autosomal recessive disease characterized by absence or deficiency of the lysosomal enzyme α-L-fucosidase (Figs. 9–35 and 9–36). This disorder, first described by Durand in 1966, is associated with tissue accumulation of polysaccharides, mucopolysaccharides, and glycolipids and is characterized by mental retardation, weakness, spasticity, and retardation, with or without angiokeratomas.[80, 81]

Three variants of fucosidosis have been described, but only one is associated with angiokeratomatous lesions. Fucosidosis type I occurs in infancy and is characterized by progressive neurologic degeneration, mental retardation, weakness, spasticity, marked growth retardation, enlarged heart, repeated respiratory tract infec-

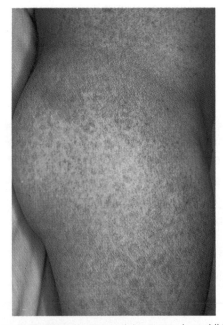

Figure 9–35. Disseminated angiokeratomas in a child with fucosidosis. (Courtesy of Benjamin K. Fisher, M.D.)

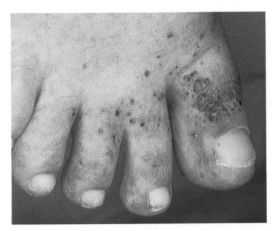

Figure 9–36. Angiokeratoma diffusum of the foot in a patient with fucosidosis. (Courtesy of Benjamin K. Fisher, M.D.)

DISORDERS ASSOCIATED WITH VASCULAR DILATATION

Livedo Reticularis

Livedo reticularis is a mottled or reticulated, bluish red discoloration of the skin that occurs chiefly on the trunk, legs, and forearms of both children and adults. The etiology of livedo reticularis is not completely understood, but exposure to cold usually intensifies the vascular pattern of this disorder. Most investigators attribute its reticulated appearance to vasospasm of the arterioles in response to cold, with subsequent hypoxia and dilatation of capillaries and venules. This results in sluggish blood flow through the subpapillary venous plexuses and a mottled livid or cyanotic appearance to the involved areas.

The blotchy pattern of livedo reticularis, in contrast to that of cutis marmorata, persists even when the skin is rewarmed. Livedo is usually benign when it affects the trunk or limbs of girls and young women in a continuous or persistent pattern. When livedo reticularis develops in a blotchy or interrupted asymmetrical distribution, it often represents an early sign of systemic disease, such as rheumatoid arthritis, rheumatic fever, lupus erythematosus, idiopathic thrombocytopenia, thrombotic thrombocytopenic purpura, leukemia, neurologic disorders (cerebrovascular accidents), adverse effects of drugs, vasculitis, infection, metabolic disorders, neoplasms, hematologic diseases, pancreatitis, or cryoglobulinemia.[84] In rare cases, recurrent small ulcerations may develop on the lower legs and feet in adults with idiopathic livedo reticularis (this disorder has been termed *livedo vasculitis, livedoid vasculitis,* or *livedo reticularis with summer ulceration*).[85] Mild hypertension and edema of the skin of the ankles, feet, and legs have been described in such cases. A variant of this disorder (atrophie blanche) characterized by whitish atrophic areas, hyperpigmentation, and ulcerations with telangiectatic vessels at their periphery, usually on the ankles and dorsal aspect of the feet, may be seen in young to middle-aged women. In addition, Sneddon's syndrome, characterized by multiple cerebrovascular accidents, may also be seen in adult patients with endarteritis obliterans and livedo reticularis.[86] Although there is no specific treatment for livedo reticularis, vasodilating (pentoxifylline [Trental]) and anticoagulant drugs have been used with moderate success in patients with severe ulceration.

Flushing and the Auriculotemporal Syndrome

Flushing, a transient diffuse erythema of the blush areas (the face, neck, and/or adjacent trunk), is caused by dilatation of superficial cutaneous blood vessels mediated by neural mechanisms or

tion, hypoplastic lumbar vertebrae, and death generally within the first few years of life. Cutaneous signs of this variant include hyperhidrosis and thickening of the skin.

Fucosidosis type II, a milder form of fucosidosis described in 1971, is referred to as lysosomal bone disease. This unusual form is associated with normal intelligence, moderate growth retardation, and spondyloepiphyseal dysplasia.

The third type, fucosidosis type III, is compatible with life, at least until adolescence. It is associated with central nervous system involvement (mental retardation, weakness, spasticity, and at times, seizures), coarse facies, mild spondyloepiphyseal dysplasia, retardation of growth, frequent respiratory tract infection, decreased sweating, purple nail bands in some patients, and cutaneous lesions practically indistinguishable from those seen in angiokeratoma circumscriptum or angiokeratoma corporis diffusum.[82, 83]

Patients with all three types of fucosidosis have markedly decreased or absent α-L-fucosidase activity, which results in increased levels of fucose-containing compounds in all tissues. Asymptomatic carriers of this autosomal recessive trait have also been found to have abnormally low α-L-fucosidase activity in cells and serum. Patients with Fabry's disease may be confused with those with the third variant of fucosidosis. Those with fucosidosis, however, do not have hypertensive cardiovascular disease, cerebral hemorrhage, or renal failure; and fat stains of histologic material from patients with fucosidosis do not show lipids, as seen in the cytoplasmic inclusions of Fabry's disease.

There is no effective form of therapy for fucosidosis. Efforts at enzyme replacement, as in other lysosomal diseases, however, show promise.

the direct action of a vasodilator substance on vascular smooth muscles. Flushing can be caused by emotion; the ingestion of alcoholic or hot beverages, or food additives such as sulfites, nitrites, and monosodium glutamate (MSG) in what has been described as the "Chinese restaurant syndrome"; calcium channel blockers such as nifedipine (Procardia); disulfiram (Antabuse); the carcinoid syndrome (a disorder of adults caused by malignant carcinoid neoplasms in which large amounts of serotonin and bradykinin are released into the circulation, diagnosed by the finding of high levels of 5-hydroxyindoleacetic acid in the urine); and other tumors that produce catecholamines such as neuroblastoma, renal cell carcinoma, or ganglioneuroma.

The *auriculotemporal syndrome (Frey's syndrome)* is a relatively common phenomenon characterized by hyperhidrosis and unilateral or bilateral flushing, which usually occurs on the face over the cutaneous distribution of the auriculotemporal nerve but may occur on other parts of the body in otherwise normal persons and is generally triggered by olfactory or gustatory stimuli. The disorder is believed to be the result of increased irritability of the cholinergic fibers resulting at times from infection or injury to the parotid area. Although there is no known treatment for this disorder, spontaneous resolution may occur after a period of time and patients with excessive sweating in the affected area may achieve some relief by the use of a β-adrenergic receptor-blocking agent such as nadolol (Corgard) or topical application of aluminum chloride formulations (e.g., Xerac-AC or Drysol). Attempts to suppress the flushing by the use of atropine or antihistamines have been unsuccessful; and upper dorsal sympathectomy and surgical section of the auriculotemporal nerve, although temporarily successful, tend to result in recurrence of the disorder, frequently within a few months.[87, 88]

Erythermalgia (Erythromelalgia)

Erythermalgia (also known as erythralgia or erythromelalgia) is characterized by paroxysmal burning pain, redness, tingling or itching, and warmth of one or more extremities (the feet, lower legs, and occasionally the hands) precipitated by heat, exercise, or dependency of the affected extremity. The disorder, attributed to vasodilatation with concomitant increased blood flow in the affected area, may appear as a primary or idiopathic syndrome in otherwise healthy persons, primarily children, or as a secondary disorder, seen usually in adults, associated with the taking of ergot derivatives or calcium channel antagonists or myeloproliferative disorders such as polycythemia vera, thrombocythemia, thrombocytopenic purpura, systemic lupus erythematosus, peripheral vascular disease, diabetes, or hypertension.[89, 90] Although

the pathogenesis remains speculative, mild heat in the range of 89.6° to 96.8°F (32° to 36°C) appears to provoke burning pain in a predisposed individual.

Generally characterized by attacks of burning pain associated with erythema and warmth of the affected extremity, lasting from a few minutes to 2 or 3 hours, acute attacks can be relieved by elevation of the affected area, cold applications, nonsteroidal anti-inflammatory drugs, methysergide maleate (alone or in combination with ephedrine) presumably due to its antiserotinin properties, and, in patients in whom thrombocythemia is present, busulfan (Myleran).

Cutis Marmorata Telangiectatica Congenita

Cutis marmorata telangiectatica congenita (congenital generalized phlebectasia) is a disorder of infants and children characterized by a serpiginous, reticulated, bluish mottling of the skin that resembles an exaggerated form of cutis marmorata. Seen in boys as well as girls, the disorder is characterized by dilated reticulated venous and capillary channels measuring 3 to 4 mm or more in diameter (Fig. 9–37). Usually present at birth, the vascular pattern generally extends somewhat during the first few weeks of life and, in most patients, eventually improves substantially during childhood. In some cases the cutaneous marbling pattern persists into adulthood.[91–93] In most patients the vascular pattern of cutis marmorata telangiectatica congenita is distributed in a generalized manner over the trunk and extremities, and at times the face (Fig. 9–38). In some, however, the involvement may be segmental or localized to one extremity or a limited portion of the trunk.

The etiology is unknown, but the disorder appears to represent a developmental ectasia involving both capillaries and veins; and, although spo-

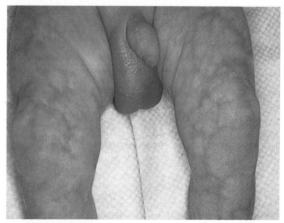

Figure 9–37. Congenital generalized phlebectasia (cutis marmorata telangiectatica congenita). This disorder must be differentiated from cutis marmorata.

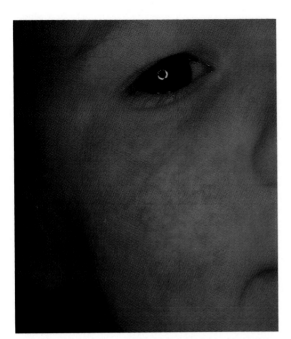

Figure 9–38. Cutis marmorata telangiectatica congenita on the cheek of a 2-year-old girl.

radic in most instances, an autosomal dominant inheritance pattern with low penetrance has been proposed for some individuals with this disorder. In some patients little or no histopathologic abnormality can be seen. In others, however, microscopic examination of a cutaneous biopsy specimen may reveal dilated capillaries, capillary and venous lakes, and large dilated veins in all layers of the dermis and subcutaneous tissue. Since histopathologic features are variable, diagnosis is best made on clinical criteria.

Ulcerations over the reticulated vascular pattern have been seen in a few patients with this disorder. In general, however, cutis marmorata telangiectatica congenita has a benign course and requires no specific therapy. Other defects in association with this disorder have been reported. These include hemangiomatous abnormalities and varicosities, telangiectatic capillary nevi, patent ductus arteriosus, cleft palate, skeletal demineralization, short fingers, acral cyanosis, congenital fibromatosis, scoliosis, spina bifida, high-arched palate, dystrophic teeth, syndactyly of the toes, short stature, congenital glaucoma with mental retardation, Sturge-Weber syndrome, macrocephaly or asymmetric skull, micrognathia, triangular facies, scaphoid scapulae, branchial cleft cysts, imperforate anus, rectovaginal and urethrovaginal fistulas, absent clitoris, aplasia cutis, and atrophy or hypertrophy of soft tissue or bone suggesting a possible defect of the mesoderm. Although studies suggest an association with other congenital anomalies in a high percentage (as high as 27 to 52 per cent) of patients with this disorder, patients without associated defects are often not reported and severe congenital malformations are probably not as common as the literature suggests.

Diffuse Phlebectasia

Diffuse phlebectasia (Brockenheimer's syndrome) is a rare hamartomatous malformation involving the deeper venous channels of a limb or part of a limb. This disorder is characterized by gradual onset during infancy, childhood, adolescence, or early adult life. It consists of multiple spongy, irregular venous sinusoids and dilated veins that assume bizarre patterns, with tumor-like vascular swelling of the involved area. The overlying skin may be atrophic, and secondary complications consisting of thromboses and phleboliths, with resultant bleeding, ulceration, or infection of the affected limb, may occur. The name *congenital phlebectasia* had been used as synonym for *cutis marmorata telangiectatic congenita*. Although the latter is more cumbersome, it is probably more accurate and helps avoid confusion between the congenital and diffuse forms of phlebectasia.

TELANGIECTASES

Telangiectases are permanent dilatations of capillaries, venules, or arterioles in the skin that may or may not disappear on diascopy (gentle pressure with a microscope slide or hand lens). Many processes affecting the blood vessel endothelium and its supporting structure can lead to the development of this common vascular lesion. Some of these are primary disorders of the blood vessels themselves for which the cause is unknown. Others are secondary and are related to some other known disturbances, such as aging, light exposure, radiation, or systemic disorders for which they may serve as useful diagnostic clues. Although the disorder is usually a solitary finding without associated underlying abnormalities, a benign hereditary form has also been described.[94] Medical intervention is usually unnecessary, but electrocoagulation or laser beam therapy may be considered if desired for cosmetic purposes.

Spider Angioma

The spider angioma (nevus araneus) is the best-known type of telangiectasia. It is characterized by a central, occasionally elevated, vascular punctum with symmetrically radiating thin branches (legs). Spider angiomas appear most commonly on exposed areas of the face, upper trunk, arms, hands, and fingers, and occasionally on the mucous membranes of the lip and nose. The central body is an arteriole (which at times can be shown to pulsate by gentle diascopy) (Fig. 9–39).

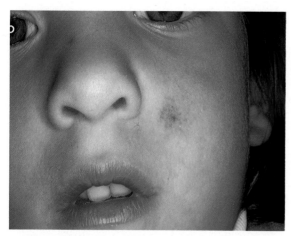

Figure 9–39. Spider angioma (nevus araneus). The lesion has a central vascular body with radiating vascular legs and a surrounding flush. Diagnosis can be confirmed by blanching the legs and demonstration of pulsations of the central vessel by gentle pressure with a glass slide (diascopy).

Although spider angiomas can be associated with liver disease, pregnancy, and estrogen therapy, they are frequently idiopathic and occur in 15 per cent or more of normal children and young adults. A small proportion of spider nevi regress spontaneously. The majority of such lesions, particularly in children, however, tend to persist indefinitely.

Diagnosis of spider angioma depends on recognition of the typical morphology of the lesion, demonstration of the central pulsating vessel, and blanching of the surrounding legs with diascopy of the central body. Therapy, when desired, consists of gentle electrodesiccation, electrocoagulation, laser therapy, or cryosurgery with solid carbon dioxide or liquid nitrogen and usually has a good cosmetic result.

Angioma Serpiginosum

Angioma serpiginosum is a rare nevoid disorder of the small vessels of the dermis that occurs predominantly in females (90 per cent) and usually has its onset during childhood. Lesions may affect any part of the body but generally are seen on the lower limbs and buttocks of affected individuals. They are characterized by minute copper-colored to red or purple angiomatous puncta with a background of diffuse erythema, which often measures 1 cm or more in diameter. The condition generally begins as one or more small lesions and characteristically extends slowly over a period of months or years. Individual puncta often disappear, and although complete clearing of lesions may occur at times, the prognosis for complete spontaneous resolution is generally poor.

Histopathologic characteristics include dilated and tortuous capillaries (ectasia), acanthosis, scattered parakeratosis and hyperkeratosis, occasional

atrophy of the epidermis, and varying degrees of liquefaction necrosis of the basal layer.

Although electrocoagulation and electrodesiccation of individual puncta may give partial resolution, treatment of this disorder is unsatisfactory and generally not recommended.

Hereditary Hemorrhagic Telangiectasia

Hereditary hemorrhagic telangiectasia (Osler's disease, Osler-Rendu-Weber disease) is an autosomal dominant disorder characterized by the presence of numerous telangiectases on the skin and mucous membranes of the nose and mouth, recurrent nosebleeds, and a family history of the disorder (Fig. 9–40). Recurrent epistaxis, the usual presenting symptom of this disorder, may begin in early childhood (generally at about 8 or 10 years), or early in infancy, but more commonly does not begin until puberty or adult life. The characteristic mucocutaneous lesions, however, are rarely observed in children and generally do not become evident until the third decade of life, or later.

True lesions of this disorder tend to be slightly elevated with an ill-defined border and one or more legs radiating from an eccentrically placed punctum.[84] They develop primarily on the lips, tongue, palate, nasal mucosa, conjunctiva, ears, and palms; under the nails; on the plantar surfaces of the feet; and occasionally on the trunk and toes. Similar lesions may also occur in the pharynx, larynx, bronchi, liver, brain, retina, urinary bladder, and gastrointestinal tract. Hemorrhages may occur from any site, and their severity and frequency determine the clinical manifestations and course of the disorder. Pulmonary arteriovenous fistulas are present in some cases and tend to occur in certain families but are rare in children. When such fis-

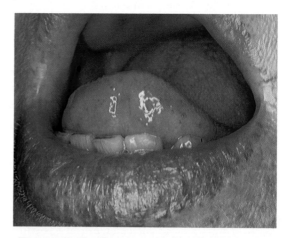

Figure 9–40. Hereditary hemorrhagic telangiectasia (Osler's disease, Osler-Weber-Rendu disease). Cutaneous manifestations usually appear after puberty and are characterized by 1- to 4-mm, slightly elevated, bright red to purple telangiectatic vessels with one or more legs radiating from an eccentrically placed punctum.

tulas are present, associated signs and symptoms include dyspnea, cyanosis, polycythemia, and clubbing of the fingers and toes in adolescence.

Diagnosis depends on the history and morphologic configuration of individual telangiectatic lesions. Microscopic examination reveals a subepidermal tortuous mass of dilated vessels with a markedly thin wall composed almost entirely of a single layer of endothelium.

Treatment of mild cases is not necessary. Individual lesions may be cauterized, and iron supplements may help control secondary anemia. In severe disorders, systemic estrogens have been advocated but when used in small dosages (as in contraceptive pills) actually may aggravate the disorder. Resection of pulmonary arteriovenous shunts and involved segments of the gastrointestinal tract may be necessary; and for severe epistaxis, dermoplasty may be beneficial for some individuals.

Ataxia-Telangiectasia

Ataxia-telangiectasia (Louis-Bar syndrome) is an autosomal recessive multifaceted syndrome characterized by progressive cerebellar ataxia, oculocutaneous telangiectasia, and frequent severe respiratory tract infections. The frequency of this disorder has been estimated to be approximately 1 in 40,000 births. A disorder of defective thymic development, generalized lymphoreticular abnormalities, immunologic deficiency, and susceptibility to lymphoreticular malignancy 1,200 times that of otherwise normal individuals, it is estimated that 1 per cent of the unaffected population are heterozygous for this disorder and are carriers of the trait, having a higher incidence of malignant disease, particularly breast cancer in women.[95, 96]

Ataxia-telangiectasia usually develops between the ages of 3 and 5 years (occasionally as early as the second year of life). Fine, symmetrical, bright red telangiectases are generally first noted in the temporal and nasal areas of the bulbar conjunctiva, and subsequently the cutaneous telangiectases appear on the ears, eyelids, butterfly areas of the cheeks, the neck, and the "V" area of the upper chest (areas receiving the greatest sun exposure). With time they extend to the popliteal and antecubital fossae and the dorsal aspect of the hands and feet. With continued sun exposure and aging, the skin tends to become sclerodermatous, with a mottled pattern of hyperpigmentation and hypopigmentation. Other cutaneous findings include café au lait spots, diffuse graying of the scalp hair, seborrheic dermatitis, follicular hyperkeratosis, excessive dryness of the skin and hair, eczema (in 40 to 60 per cent of patients), and hirsutism of the arms and legs. Patients who reach the second decade of life may also have sclerodermoid features with generalized loss of subcutaneous fat, hidebound skin, decreased mobility across the joints, peripheral neuropathy, and progressive spinal muscular atrophy.

Children are usually small for age and appear to be normal until the ataxia and clumsiness become apparent during the second year of life. In association with the ataxia, affected persons develop choreoathetosis, drooling, peculiar ocular movements, a sad mask-like facies, and a stooped posture with drooping shoulders and the head sunk forward and tilted to one side. About 30 per cent of affected individuals also have a mild to moderate intellectual deficit, and those who survive beyond adolescence frequently develop peripheral neuropathy and progressive spinal muscular atrophy, with, by the age of 12, the ataxia becoming so severe that patients are frequently confined to wheelchairs and unable to walk without assistance.

Recurrent sinopulmonary infections varying from acute rhinitis with infections of the ears to chronic bronchitis, recurrent pneumonia, and bronchiectasis occur in 75 to 80 per cent of affected patients. Death, when it occurs, is generally associated with bronchiectasis, pulmonary insufficiency, and pneumonia. Among the immunologic defects seen in association with this disorder are deficiencies of IgA and IgE, structural anomalies of the thymus and lymph nodes, impaired lymphocyte transformation, and lymphopenia. Of those individuals who survive to the late teens, about 10 per cent develop lymphoreticular malignancy (lymphosarcoma, Hodgkin's disease, reticular cell sarcoma, or leukemia). Other neoplastic disorders include ovarian dysgerminoma, medulloblastoma, glioma, adenocarcinoma, and primary carcinoma of the stomach, liver, ovary, salivary glands, breast, or pancreas.

A rapid diagnostic test for ataxia-telangiectasia consists of a 2-day culture of peripheral lymphocytes grown in phytohemagglutinin, which can distinguish normal cells from ataxia-telangiectasia cells by their sensitivity to radiation. Although this test can be used for prenatal diagnosis on amniotic fluid cells of affected infants, it does not detect carriers of the disorder.[97]

Generalized Essential Telangiectasia

Generalized essential telangiectasia is a benign cutaneous disorder generally seen in females (2:1), which frequently has its onset in late childhood or early adult life but most often develops in the fourth and fifth decades. The etiology of this disorder is unknown.

Essential telangiectasia may be generalized or segmented and usually begins on the legs and slowly spreads to involve the thighs, lower abdomen, and occasionally the arms or face (Fig. 9–41). Two varieties of telangiectases are present: (1) large venous stars consisting of superficial varicosities and (2) bright red blotchy erythema produced by many fine wiry vessels. Although the disorder is usually slowly progressive and asymptomatic for many years, it can subside spontaneously. Regression of lesions, however, except on the face of

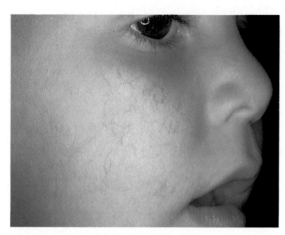

Figure 9–41. Essential telangiectasia on the face in a 3-year-old girl.

young children is rare and this basically cosmetic defect is not associated with any systemic disorder.

There is no effective treatment for this condition. If lesions are cosmetically significant, however, cover makeups, tunable dye laser therapy, or electrodesiccation or electrocoagulation may help to a limited degree.

PIGMENTED PURPURIC ERUPTIONS

The pigmented purpuric eruptions consist of a group of related benign dermatoses of unknown etiology characterized by increased capillary fragility or permeability. The primary lesion, related to a lymphocytic vasculitis, results in pinhead-sized reddish puncta occurring in irregularly shaped, dusky red or yellowish brown patches of purpura, with secondary pigmentation from hemosiderin deposition. Five dermatoses are included in this group of disorders. Whether they are separate entities or expressions of the same pathologic process remains controversial. These include progressive pigmentary dermatosis of Schamberg, itching purpura (eczematid-like purpura of Doucas and Kapetanakis), pigmented purpuric lichenoid dermatitis of Gougerot and Blum, purpura annularis telangiectodes (Majocchi's purpura), and lichen aureus.

Schamberg's disease (progressive pigmented purpuric dermatosis) is an uncommon asymptomatic disorder of the lower extremities that may occur in childhood (Fig. 9–42) but is generally seen in adolescent and young adult males. Typical lesions are discrete brown or yellow patches with red or reddish brown pinpoint-sized spots representing freshly extravasated erythrocytes and hemosiderin deposition (cayenne pepper spots) in the center or on the periphery of the lesions. This disorder begins on the lower legs (generally the shins, ankles, and dorsa of the feet and toes), may at times be unilateral, and only occasionally involves the trunk or upper limbs. Its course is chronic and the condition may persist for years. Although the cause is unknown, ingestion of drugs such as aspirin, acetaminophen, carbromals, thiamine, and meprobamate has been associated with the disease, and immunohistologic studies suggest that a cellular immune reaction in lesional skin may play a role in the pathogenesis of this disorder.[98–100] In addition, a report of three males with eruptions resembling Schamberg's disease, which progressed into cutaneous T-cell lymphoma (mycosis fungoides), suggests that some cases may represent a subset of mycosis fungoides with an early age at onset and male predominance.[101]

The histopathologic picture of Schamberg's disease, as with other pigmented purpuric eruptions, consists of a lymphocytic vasculitis with extravasation of erythrocytes and hemosiderin deposition.

Itching purpura appears to represent a generalized form of Schamberg's disease except that the disorder is extremely pruritic and occasionally lichenified owing to persistent scratching. The histopathologic picture consists of spongiosis and inflammation of the epidermis in association with the usual vasculitic pattern. *Eczematid-like purpura of Doucas and Kapetanakis,* seen primarily in adult males, probably represents the same condition. Itching purpura is generally localized to the legs, with dissemination to the thighs, trunk, and upper extremities and is more pronounced at the sites of friction. The disorder persists for months with marked fluctuations and episodic recurrences and may remit spontaneously or with the use of topical corticosteroids.

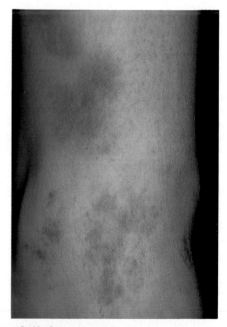

Figure 9–42. Schamberg's disease (progressive pigmented purpuric dermatosis). Discrete reddish-brown patches with pinpoint-sized cayenne pepper spots are seen on the lower leg and ankle of an 11-year-old girl.

Pigmented purpuric lichenoid dermatosis of Gougerot and Blum and purpura annularis telangiectodes (Majocchi's disease) also probably represent variants of the same disorder. The former, however, favors older men (between 40 and 60 years of age). Majocchi's disease generally occurs in adolescents and young adults of either sex but may occur at any age. The eruption generally begins symmetrically on the lower extremities and may extend to the trunk and arms. Lesions may be few or numerous and consist of small plaques 1 to 3 cm in diameter that are usually annular, often with clearing or atrophy in the center of some lesions. Treatment is generally ineffective, and the eruption usually persists for months to years.

Although the etiology of lichen aureus is not well understood, it has been described as a further variant within the spectrum of pigmented purpuric eruptions. Seen in children as well as adults, the disorder is characterized by distinctive rust-yellow patches, 2 to 10 cm in diameter, most commonly located on the lower legs and thighs.[102, 103] Its histologic picture is characterized by a dense band of lymphocytes and histiocytes (the latter often containing hemosiderin granules) separated from the epidermis by a band of normal connective tissue. The course of this disorder is generally protracted; lesions develop suddenly and usually remain unchanged for years; and various therapies, including ascorbic acid, antihistamines, topical corticosteroids, and support stockings, as with the other benign pigmented purpuric eruptions, have been largely ineffective. Although systemic corticosteroids may sometimes produce beneficial effects, because of the benign nature of these disorders, such therapy is generally not recommended.

PURPURA FULMINANS (DISSEMINATED INTRAVASCULAR COAGULATION)

Purpura fulminans and disseminated intravascular coagulation are terms used to describe a form of nonthrombocytic purpura characterized by an acute, severe, often rapidly fatal hemorrhagic infarction and necrosis of the skin. Usually occurring in children, the disease is triggered by a preceding infectious process such as scarlet fever or other streptococcal infection, meningococcal and other septicemias, chickenpox, measles, vaccinia, or rickettsial disorders such as Rocky Mountain spotted fever (Fig. 9–43). In addition, acquired or congenital protein C and protein S deficiencies have been shown to cause neonatal purpura fulminans, and transient lowering of protein C and protein S levels has been documented in infection-associated purpura fulminans.[104–107]

Although the etiology of purpura fulminans has not been firmly established, it usually has its onset within 3 to 30 days after a resolving infection. The cause appears to represent a nonimmunologic hypersensitivity reaction similar to that of an induced Schwartzman phenomenon. The primary pathol-

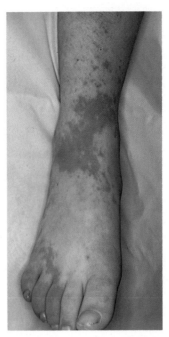

Figure 9–43. Purpura fulminans in a 4-year-old boy with Rocky Mountain spotted fever.

ogy is a consumptive coagulopathy (disseminated intravascular coagulation) characterized by intravascular consumption of plasma coagulation factors (fibrinogen and factors, II, V, and VIII), with low-normal to severely reduced platelet counts, hypofibrinogenemia, and hypoprothrombinemia associated with microthrombosis and a hemorrhagic diathesis.

The disorder is characterized by symmetrically distributed localized cutaneous ecchymoses, often with sharp irregular borders on the extremities, particularly in the areas of pressure. Lesions are tender, enlarge rapidly, coalesce, and develop central necrosis, with hemorrhagic blebs and a raised edge with surrounding erythema. They spread to the trunk and occasionally may involve the lips, ears, and nose. Chills, fever, tachycardia, anemia, and prostration are common. Visceral involvement with hematuria or gastrointestinal bleeding may occur; and shock and coma eventuating in death frequently develop. When hemorrhage and necrosis of the adrenal glands are present the designation Waterhouse-Friderichsen syndrome has been applied to this disorder.

Since current studies support the concept that purpura fulminans is usually the result of disseminated intravascular coagulation, the presence of a consumptive coagulopathy should be confirmed prior to the institution of therapy. Although the outlook is grave and death frequently occurs within 48 to 72 hours (until recently the mortality was over 90 per cent), prompt initiation of therapy improves the prognosis for most patients. Thus, with good supportive care and treatment of the underlying disease, mortality currently appears to be in the range of 18 per cent. Treatment consists of early recognition of the disorder, prompt identification and therapy for associated infection, correction of clotting factor deficiencies due to intravascular coagulation, and general supportive measures.

GARDNER-DIAMOND SYNDROME

The Gardner-Diamond syndrome (autoerythrocyte sensitization syndrome, painful bruising syndrome) is a relatively uncommon purpuric disorder of uncertain etiology. Although 95 per cent of patients are adolescent girls or women, the disorder has also been reported in male patients and children. Characterized by crops of painful, warm, red, slightly edematous patches that become ecchymotic over the course of several hours to one day, this disorder has probably engendered more debate over whether it is an organic disease or psychiatric syndrome than any other comparable disorder in medicine.[84, 108] The lower extremities and trunk are the usual sites of involvement, but lesions may also present on the face or any part of the cutaneous surface (Fig. 9–44). Emotional upsets frequently represent precipitating factors, and some patients can actually predict the appearance of new lesions by tingling or burning sensations at future eruptive sites.

Many cases cannot be discerned from factitial purpura, particularly since psychological disturbance is often a prominent feature of both disorders. Affected patients frequently tend to have a self-centered and demanding nature and often have a history of masochistic or hysterical characteristics (hallucinations, aphonia, paresthesia, paralyses, or hysterical convulsions). Bleeding from internal organs and neurologic symptoms may occur, and approximately half of the affected patients have gastrointestinal manifestations such as upper abdominal pain, nausea, vomiting, diarrhea, gastrointestinal bleeding, hemarthroses, hematuria, and epistaxis. Histologic features include vasculitis, dermal edema, a lymphocytic and monocytic perivascular infiltrate, and extravasation of erythrocytes; and whether the disorder has an organic or a factitial origin continues to be a source of considerable debate. In favor of the organic basis is the fact that typical bruises, in some patients at least, can be induced by intradermal injection of their own erythrocytes or phosphatidyl-L-serine derived from their own erythrocyte membranes. In favor of a factitial origin are the findings that intradermal injections of autologous erythrocytes do not necessarily produce the lesions and that patients in whom lesions were believed to have been reproduced by autologous injections or erythrocytes were not always clinically observed to exclude the possibility of factitial intervention by the patient.

The prognosis of this disorder is highly variable; and although the course of the disorder may last for years, it frequently becomes less active and eventually disappears, occasionally after a period of months and sometimes longer. Patients should be carefully evaluated to rule out other possible causes of purpura and, once the diagnosis has been established, treatment is usually unsuccessful. Although psychological evaluation and psychotherapy directed at emotional problems has helped in some cases, the disease, possibly exacerbated by emotional stress or physical injury, frequently follows an irregularly intermittent course.

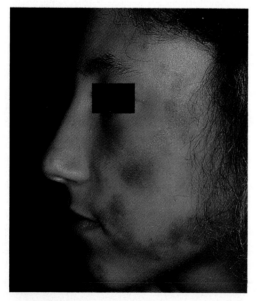

Figure 9–44. Gardner-Diamond syndrome (autoerythrocyte sensitization syndrome) in a 17-year-old girl.

SCURVY

Vitamin C deficiency (scurvy) is characterized by capillary hemorrhages surrounding hyperkeratotic follicular papules, swollen bleeding gums, petechiae, ecchymoses, weakness and tenderness of the lower extremities, hemorrhages into joints and splinter hemorrhage in the nail beds, and broken-off corkscrew hairs (hairs curled within hair follicles) capped by keratotic plugs. A disorder that occurs for the most part when nutrition is poor, scurvy can also be seen in individuals with behavioral or psychiatric problems, feeding disorders, or alcoholism, those with unusual dietary habits (food faddists),[109] patients with underlying medical problems resulting in malnutrition and ascorbic acid deficiency, and individuals taking medications such as aspirin, phenylbutazone, and anticonvulsant drugs known to reduce ascorbic acid levels.

DISORDERS OF LYMPHATIC VESSELS

Tumors of lymphatic origin are classified as hamartomas of the lymphatic system. They consist of dilated lymph channels lined by normal flat or cuboidal lymphatic endothelium. They may be superficial or subcutaneous and, at times, may extend into the underlying muscle tissue. Lymphangiomas are generally slow growing, and their clinical appearance depends on their size, depth, and location. Four major forms of lymphangioma (lymphangioma simplex, lymphangioma circumscriptum, cavernous lymphangioma, and cystic hygroma) have been described. Of these, 70 to 90 per cent are present at birth or develop within the first 2 years of life. They rarely appear after the age of 5 years.

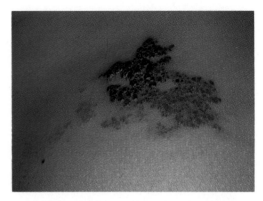

Figure 9–45. Hemangiolymphangioma (lymphangioma circumscriptum with a hemangiomatous component).

Lymphangioma Simplex

Simple lymphangiomas appear in infancy as solitary, well-circumscribed, flesh-colored dermal or subcutaneous tumors. They may occur anywhere on the subcutaneous or mucosal surface and are most often seen on the neck, upper trunk, proximal extremities, and tongue. Their surface is generally smooth, but on occasion they may be verruciform in character. Simple lymphangiomas either remain stable or grow quickly. Uncomplicated tumors can be removed easily by simple excision. For those that are more widespread, however, simple excision is not always satisfactory.

Lymphangioma Circumscriptum

This is the most common form of lymphangioma. Present at birth or appearing in early childhood, it is characterized by groups of deep-seated thick-walled vesicles that have the appearance of frog spawn. Common sites of involvement include the proximal limbs, shoulders, neck, axillae and adjacent chest wall, perineum, tongue, and mucous membranes; and although treatment by surgical excision, fulguration, or coagulation is often unsatisfactory because of recurrences, carbon dioxide laser ablation has been successful in selected cases.[110] Frequently there is also a hemangiomatous component (hemangiolymphoma) so that some of the vesicles are filled with fresh or altered blood (Figs. 9–45 and 9–46). Mixed lesions may increase rather suddenly because of bleeding into the lymphatic spaces. Although usually localized, these lesions may be quite extensive. If therapy is desired, such lesions require deep and extensive surgery (down to the fascial plane), and recurrences are common.

Cavernous Lymphangloma

Cavernous lymphangiomas consist of diffuse soft tissue masses of large cystic dilatations of lymphatic vessels in the dermis, subcutaneous tissue, and intermuscular septa. These lesions are ill defined and frequently involve large areas of the face, trunk, and extremities. They may appear in childhood or adult life. Surgical excision may be effective for local lesions, but extensive cavernous lesions require full-thickness skin grafts, and recurrences are common.

Cystic Hygroma

Cystic hygromas are benign, unilocular or multilocular lymphatic tumors (Fig. 9–47). These lesions are often found in the neck region (hygroma colli) and occasionally are seen in the axillae, groin, or popliteal fossae. Cystic hygromas may on rare occasion undergo spontaneous regression. The majority, however, tend to grow and frequently infiltrate adjacent vessels and nerves. In

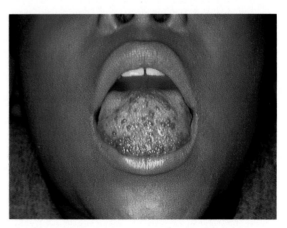

Figure 9–46. Hemangiolymphangioma of the tongue.

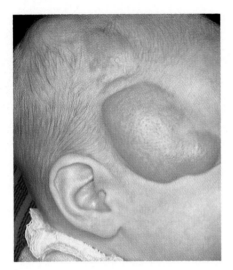

Figure 9–47. Cystic hygroma on the scalp and face of a 2-month-old infant.

general, when surgery is considered, the earlier the lesions can be removed the better the clinical result. In contrast to cavernous lymphangiomas, however, recurrences following surgical removal of cystic hygromas are uncommon.

Lymphedema

Lymphedema is a term used to describe a diffuse soft tissue swelling caused by increased accumulation of lymph due to inadequate lymphatic drainage. It may be divided into primary and secondary forms.

Primary lymphedema may be subdivided into congenital (13 per cent of patients), lymphedema praecox (that appearing after birth and before age 35), and lymphedema tarda (that appearing after age 35).

Secondary lymphedema is due to obstruction of lymphatic pathways by some pathologic process (following surgery, from recurrent lymphangitis or cellulitis, or from filariasis) or by some extralymphatic process, such as compression by direct invasion of lymphatics or lymph nodes by neoplasms or by fibrosis resulting from radiation therapy and scar formation. Secondary lymphedema is generally a disorder of adults and is relatively uncommon in childhood.

In congenital lymphedema the involved area is swollen at birth. The swelling is firm and is characterized by pitting on pressure. In lymphedema praecox, females are primarily affected, and the swelling appears spontaneously, generally between the ages of 9 and 25 years.

The term *Milroy's disease* refers to a familial disorder with autosomal dominant transmission in which the edema is almost always confined to the legs and feet. This disorder may be present at birth but usually appears during adolescence or the early 20s. The age at onset and severity tend to be similar in affected members in a family. Hot weather, menses, and pregnancy may accentuate the edema, and serum protein levels and results of hepatic, cardiac, and renal function studies are normal. In some affected individuals, aldosterone levels have been found to be abnormal.

The pathogenesis of Milroy's disease is unknown. Treatment consisting of trial on a low-sodium diet, elastic stockings or bandages, a variety of pneumatic compression devices such as the Jobst and the Wright linear pumps,[49, 111] and systemic diuretics may be helpful but is not curative. In children with moderate to severe lymphedema praecox, subcutaneous lymphangiectomy may be performed. This reduces the swelling of the extremity but, unfortunately, generally results in unsightly scars.

References

1. Mulliken JB, Young AE: Vascular Birthmarks: Hemangiomas and Malformations. W.B. Saunders Co., Philadelphia, 1988.

   A comprehensive update on vascular birthmarks and their pathogenesis and management.

2. Glowacki J, Mulliken JB: Mast cells in hemangiomas and vascular malformations. Pediatrics 70:48–51, 1982.

   A high incidence of mast cells in proliferating hemangiomas, but not in involuting lesions, suggsts that mast cells and heparin may play a major role in angiogenesis.

3. Folkman J: Toward a new understanding of vascular proliferative disease in children. J. Pediatr. 74:850–856, 1984.

   An illuminating review of angiogenesis offers new insight into the pathogenesis of vascular disorders of childhood.

4. Sasaki GH, Pang CY, Witliff JL: Pathogenesis and treatment of infant strawberry hemangiomas: Clinical and in vitro studies of hormonal effects. Plast. Reconst. Surg. 73:359–370, 1984.

   The finding of 17β-estradiol in sera of children with capillary hemangiomas at a level four times that found in controls suggests a hormonal influence in the pathogenesis of strawberry hemangiomas.

5. Silverman RA: Hemangiomas and vascular malformations. Pediatr. Clin. North Am. 38:811–834, 1991.

   An overview of hemangiomas, vascular malformations, their classification, pathogenesis, and management.

6. Jacobs AH, Walton RG: The incidence of birthmarks in the neonate. Pediatrics 58:218–222, 1976.

   A statistical study of birthmarks in 1,058 infants younger than 72 hours of age.

7. Hidano A, Nakajima S: Earliest features of the strawberry mark in the newborn. Br. J. Dermatol. 87:138–144, 1972.

   The majority of strawberry angiomas are not detectable at birth, but many are apparent as telangiectatic lesions surrounded by a pale halo during the first week of life.

8. Margileth AM: Hemangiomas: A before-and-after look. Contemp. Pediatr. 3:14–31, 1986.

   A comprehensive review of vascular lesions confirms the fact that even large hemangiomas often tend to disappear by the time the child reaches the age of 10 years, often with good cosmetic results.

9. Margileth AM, Museles, M: Cutaneous hemangiomas in children. J.A.M.A. 194:523–526, 1965.

Evaluation of the course of 366 hemangiomas in 210 patients reveals that conservative management results in spontaneous involution in the majority of lesions.

10. Margileth AM, Museles M: Current concepts in diagnosis and management of congenital cutaneous hemangiomas. Pediatrics 36:410–416, 1965.

Observations in over 200 children confirm previous studies in which over 90 per cent of congenital cutaneous hemangiomas involute spontaneously.

11. Illingworth RS: Thoughts on treatment of strawberry naevi. Arch. Dis. Child. 51:138–140, 1976.

A review of several studies discussing the clinical course of strawberry hemangiomas reveals that fewer than 2 per cent require active treatment.

12. Bowers RE, Graham EA, Tomlinson KM: The natural history of the strawberry nevus: Arch. Dermatol. 82:667–680, 1960.

A study of 169 untreated cases of strawberry nevi: 50 per cent had complete resolution by age 5, 70 per cent by age 7, and, of those that did not resolve, only 6 per cent had a cosmetic handicap.

13. Edwards EK Jr, Edwards EK Sr: Grenz ray therapy. Int. J. Dermatol. 29:17–18, 1990.

This article serves to remind us that grenz rays can be used as a safe, rapid, and painless form of therapy for selected disorders.

14. Morelli JG, Tan OT, Weston WL: Treatment of ulcerated hemangiomas with pulsed tunable dye laser. Am. J. Dis. Child. 145:1062–1064, 1991.

Healing of ulcerated hemangiomas can be enhanced, usually within two to three treatments, by vascular specific (585-nm) 450-μsec pulsed tunable dye laser therapy.

15. Moschella S: Capillary and cavernous hemangioma. Transactions of the Philadelphia Dermatologic Society (discussion). Arch. Dermatol. 113:1308, 1977.

Intralesional corticosteroids in five patients with hemangiomas.

16. Fost NC, Esterly NB: Successful treatment of juvenile hemangiomas with prednisone. J. Pediatr. 72:351–357, 1968.

Of six children with extensive hemangiomas treated with oral prednisone, all except one showed dramatic regression of the lesion within 2 weeks of therapy.

17. Zarem, HA, Edgerton MT: Cavernous hemangiomas and prednisolone therapy. Plast. Reconstr. Surg. 39:76–83, 1976.

Both cavernous and strawberry hemangiomas treated with oral prednisolone (20 mg/day with gradual reduction to 2.5 mg/day) resulted in rapid cessation of growth in four patients, and partial cessation in three, within 2 weeks of the start of therapy.

18. Barsky SH, Rosen S, Geer DE, et al.: The nature and evolution of port wine stains: A computer-assisted study. J. Invest. Dermatol. 74:154–157, 1980.

Studies suggest that collagen degeneration of dermal structures supporting blood vessels may be associated with the progressive ectasia of the cutaneous vasculature in individuals with port-wine stains.

19. Smoller BR, Rosen S: Port-wine stains: A disease of altered neural modulation of blood vessels? Arch. Dermatol. 122:177–179, 1986.

In biopsy specimens of port-wine stains, hemangiomas, and benign lesions stained for S100 protein, a deficiency in the number of perivascular nerves in lesions of nevus flammeus suggested a lack of neural modulation of vascular tone as a factor in the pathogenesis of the disorder.

20. Tallman B, Tan OT, Morelli JG, et al.: Location of port-wine stains and the likelihood of ophthalmic and/or central nervous system complications. Pediatrics 87:323–327, 1991.

A study of 310 patients with port-wine stains and their locations and associated complications.

21. Noe JM, Barsky SH, Geer DE, et al.: Port wine stains and the response to argon laser therapy; successful treatment and the predictive role of color, age, and biopsy. Plast. Reconstr. Surg. 65:130–136, 1980.

A comprehensive review of argon laser beam therapy and its results related to the depth and color of lesions and the age of patients treated with this modality.

22. Landthaler M, Haina D, Waidelich W, et al.: A three-year experience with argon laser dermatotherapy. J. Dermatol. Surg. Oncol. 10:456–461, 1984.

Of 337 patients with vascular lesions, argon laser therapy gave good results in 70 per cent of adult patients but was disappointing when used for the treatment of patients younger than 18 years.

23. Garden JM, Polla LL, Tan OT: The treatment of port-wine stains by the pulsed dye laser: Analysis of pulse duration in long-term therapy. Arch. Dermatol. 124:889–896, 1988.

Evaluations of 52 patients with port-wine stains treated by the pulsed dye laser revealed a good response, even after multiple treatment sessions to the same area, regardless of the anatomic location, color of the lesion, or age of the patient.

24. Robb RM: Refractive errors associated with hemangiomas of the eyelids and orbit in infancy. Am. J. Ophthalmol. 83:52–58, 1977.

Astigmatic and myopic errors in 46 per cent of 37 patients who had hemangiomas with extensive involvement of the upper eyelids.

25. Nelson LB, Melick JE, Hurley RD: Intralesional corticosteroid injection for infantile hemangiomas of the eyelid. Pediatrics 74:241–245, 1985.

Two cases of strawberry hemangiomas of the eyelids treated with intralesional corticosteroids.

26. Kushner BJ: The treatment of periorbital infantile hemangioma with intralesional corticosteroid. Plast. Reconstr. Surg. 76:517–524, 1985.

This report details the use of intralesional corticosteroid injections for the treatment of periorbital hemangiomas in 25 patients.

27. Schorr N, Seiff SR: Central retinal artery occlusion associated with periocular corticosteroid injection for juvenile hemangioma. Ophthalmic Surg. 17:229–231, 1986.

Retrograde blood flow resulted in retinal artery occlusion in a patient with a periorbital hemangioma treated by intralesional steroids.

28. Sutula FC, Glover AT: Eyelid necrosis following intralesional corticosteroid injection for capillary hemangioma. Ophthalmic Surg. 18:103–105, 1987.

The treatment of periorbital hemangiomas with intralesional corticosteroid injections carries an additional risk of rapid involution and necrosis.

29. Rizzo R, Micali G, Incorpora G, et al.: A very aggressive form of facial hemangioma. Pediatr. Dermatol. 5:263–265, 1988.

A 3-month-old girl with a particularly aggressive mixed hemangioma of the face with severe ulcerations of the earlobe and nasal septum, and cerebral anomalies.

30. Pascual-Castroviejo I: Vascular and nonvascular intracranial malformations associated with external capillary hemangiomas. Neuroradiology 16:82–84, 1978.

A 3-year-old girl with a left-sided facial hemangioma, ipsilateral cerebellar hypoplasia, and angiomatous malformation of the left carotid and hypothalmic area.

31. Mizuno Y, Kurokawa T, Numaguchi Y, et al.: Facial hemangioma with cerebrovascular anomalies and cerebellar hypoplasia. Brain Dev. *4*:376–378, 1982.

A 5-year-old girl with a strawberry hemangioma of the left side of the face, ipsilateral optic atrophy and ipsilateral cerebellar hypoplasia, and cerebrovascular anomalies.

32. White CW, Wolf SJ, Korones DN, et al.: Treatment of childhood angiomatous diseases with recombinant interferon alfa-2a. J. Pediatr. *118*:59–66, 1991.

In this multicentered uncontrolled study the authors treated five patients with progressive invasive angiomatous diseases with interferon, thus offering another mode of therapy for progressive hemangiomatous disease unresponsive to other forms of therapy.

33. Ezekowitz RAB, Mulliken JB, Folkman J: Interferon α-2a for therapy of life-threatening hemangiomas of infancy. N. Engl. J. Med. *326*:1456–1463, 1992.

A study of 20 infants with life-threatening or vision-threatening hemangiomas treated with daily subcutaneous injections of interferon alfa-2a (1 to 3 million units/m² of body surface for at least 6 months).

34. Healy G, McGill T, Friedman EM: Carbon dioxide laser in subglottic hemangioma: An update. Ann. Otol. Rhinol.Laryngol. *93*:370–373, 1984.

A review of 31 cases indicated that early treatment (at 1 or 2 months) with carbon dioxide laser therapy could prevent the need for a tracheostomy and would lead to few recurrences.

35. Cleland WJD, Riding K: Subglottic hemangiomas in infants. J. Otolaryngol. *15*:119–123, 1986.

A review of carbon dioxide laser treatment of children with subglottic hemangiomas suggests that early treatment can lead to a high recurrence rate and that the age of 9 months (when natural involution begins) would be an appropriate age for the treatment of infants with this disorder.

36. Goldberg NS, Hebert AA, Esterly NB: Sacral hemangiomas and multiple congenital abnormalities. Arch. Dermatol. *122*:684–687, 1986.

A report of five infants with sacral hemangiomas with associated neurologic, gastrointestinal, urologic, and skeletal abnormalities.

37. Thomson HG, Lanigan M: The Cyrano nose: A clinical review of hemangioma of the nasal tip. Plast. Reconstr. Surg. *63*:155–160, 1979.

Special problems associated with cavernous hemangiomas of the nasal tip (the "Cyrano nose" deformity).

38. Weisberg AL, Haller JO, Wood BP: Radiological case of the month: Hemangioma of the thigh. Am. J. Dis. Child. *143*:379–380, 1989.

A report of a 10-year-old girl with a deep, solid, tender, skeletal muscle hemangioma of the left thigh.

39. Esterly NB: Kasabach-Merritt syndrome in infants. J. Am. Acad. Dermatol. *8*:504–513, 1983.

A report of four patients with Kasabach-Merritt syndrome and a comprehensive overview of the disorder and its pathogenesis, clinical manifestations, and management.

40. Warrell RP Jr, Kempin SJ: Treatment of severe coagulopathy in the Kasabach-Merritt syndrome with aminocaproic acid and cryoprecipitate. N. Engl. J. Med. *313*:309–312, 1985.

A report of a 45-year-old woman with intrathoracic hemangiomas refractory to treatment with estrogens, pyridamole, indomethacin, aspirin, radiation, and heparin successfully treated with aminocaproic acid and cryoprecipitate.

41. Martins AG: Hemangioma and thrombocytopenia. J. Pediatr. Surg. *5*:641–648, 1970.

In a review of 19 of 94 patients with Kasabach-Merritt syndrome who died, 10 deaths were unavoidable and 4 were from unnecessarily aggressive therapy.

42. Larsen EC, Zinkham WH, Eggleston JC, et al.: Kasabach-Merritt syndrome: Therapeutic considerations. Pediatrics *79*:971–980, 1987.

A review of six children with Kasabach-Merritt syndrome and an analysis of possible pathologic mechanisms and therapeutic approaches for individuals with this disorder.

43. Jacobs AH: Response to a letter. Sturge-Weber syndrome without port-wine nevus. Pediatrics *60*:785, 1977.

Sturge-Weber syndrome consists of a combination of facial port-wine nevus and vascular malformations of the meninges and cerebral cortex; those without facial nevus represent cases of meningeal angiomatosis.

44. Taly AB, Nagaraja D, Das S, et al.: Sturge-Weber-Dimitri disease without facial nevus. Neurology *37*:1063–1064, 1987.

A patient with intractable seizures, progressive intellectual deterioration, bilateral calcification in a parieto-occipital gyral pattern, and extensive calcification of vessel walls in parieto-occipital cortices without port-wine nevus.

45. Ambrosetta P, Ambrosetta G, Michelucci R, et al.: Sturge-Weber without port-wine facial nevus: Report of 2 cases studied by CT. Child's Brain *10*:387–392, 1983.

In a report of 2 patients with Sturge-Weber syndrome without facial nevus the importance of computer-assisted tomography (CT) as a diagnostic procedure for this disorder is emphasized.

46. Alexander GL, Norman RM: The Sturge-Weber Syndrome. John Wright and Sons, Ltd., Bristol, 1960.

An extensive monograph on the problem of Sturge-Weber syndrome and report of seven cases in detail; in all of 257 cases at least part of the facial nevus involved the forehead and upper eyelids.

47. Stevenson RF, Thomson HG, Marin JD: Unrecognized ocular problems associated with port-wine stain of the face in children. Can. Med. Assoc. J. *111*:953–954, 1974.

Of 50 children with port-wine stains, glaucoma was present in 45 per cent of those with vascular lesions involving areas of skin supplied by *both* ophthalmic and maxillary divisions of the sensory branch of the trigeminal nerve. Those with involvement of only one area of involvement did not manifest glaucoma.

48. Ruiz-Maldonado R, Tamayo L, Laterza AM, et al.: Phacomatosis pigmentovascularis: A new syndrome? Pediatr. Dermatol. *4*:189–196, 1987.

A report of four patients with extensive nevus flammeus, oculocutaneous pigmentation, and severe neurologic alterations.

49. Alexander MA, Wright ES, Wright JB, et al.: Lymphedema treated with a linear pump: Pediatric case report. Arch. Phys. Med. Rehabil. *64*:132–133, 1983.

Report of the successful use of a custom-made programmable intermittent pressure pump (the Wright Linear Pump). Those interested in information regarding compression therapy with the Wright Linear Pump can call 1-800-631-9535.

50. Oranje AP: Blue rubber bleb nevus syndrome. Pediatr. Dermatol. *3*:304–310, 1986.

A review of 22 patients with the blue rubber bleb nevus syndrome and their clinical features, complications, and management.

51. Esterly NB, Margileth AM, Kahn G, et al.: Special symposia: The management of disseminated eruptive hemangiomata in infants. Pediatr. Dermatol. *4*:312–317, 1984.

A comprehensive review of the management of diffuse neonatal hemangiomatosis.

52. Stern JK, Wolfe JE Jr, Jarratt M: Benign neonatal hemangiomatosis. J. Am. Acad. Dermatol. *4*:442–445, 1981.

A review of diffuse neonatal hemangiomatosis suggests that all infants with this disorder need not have visceral involvement.

53. Frost JI, Caplan RM: Cutaneous hemangiomas and disappearing bones with a review of cutaneo-visceral hemangiomatosis. Arch. Dermatol. *92*:501–508, 1965.

A 15-year-old boy with multiple hemangiomas, massive osteolysis of the left side of the pelvis, osteolysis of lumbar vertebrae, "soap-bubble" osteolysis of the skull and humerus, and massive osteolysis of the bones of the left lower extremity, necessitating partial amputation of the left lower extremity because of multiple recurrent fractures.

54. Gellis SS, Feingold M: Picture of the month. Contributed by Ryan ME, Spahr RC: Hemangioma with osteolysis (Gorham's disease, vanishing bone disease). Am. J. Dis. Child. *132*:715–716, 1978.

A patient with hemangiomas involving mainly the skin of the back and left femur with osteolytic areas of the left pelvis and femur.

55. Stephan MJ, Hall BD, Smith DW, et al.: Macrocephaly in association with unusual cutaneous angiomatosis. J. Pediatr. *87*:353–359, 1975.

Ten patients with macrocephaly, unusual angiomatosis, and limb asymmetry.

56. Zonana J, Rimoin DL, David DC: Macrocephaly with multiple lipomas and hemangiomas. J. Pediatr. *89*:600–603, 1976.

A family of three individuals with an apparent autosomal dominant disorder consisting of macrocephaly with multiple hemangiomas and lipomas.

57. Jessen RT, Thompson S, Smith EB: Cobb syndrome. Arch. Dermatol. *113*:1587–1590, 1977.

The combination of a cutaneous angioma in a dermatomal distribution and spinal cord angioma comprises a rare but potentially crippling or fatal syndrome.

58. Imperial R, Helwig EB: Verrucous hemangioma—a clinicopathologic study of 21 cases. Arch. Dermatol. *96*:247–253, 1967.

Verrucous hemangiomas (variants of capillary or cavernous hemangiomas with secondary epidermal change) often misdiagnosed as nevi, pigmented tumors, verrucae, or angiokeratomas.

59. Dillman AM, Miller RC, Hansen RC: Multiple pyogenic granulomata in childhood. Pediatr. Dermatol. *8*:28–31, 1991.

A report of two young boys with numerous pyogenic granulomas at areas remote from the original lesion and a review of the literature on multiple, recurrent, or disseminated pyogenic granulomas.

60. Blickenstaff RD, Roenigk RK, Peters MS, et al.: Recurrent pyogenic granulomas with satellitosis. J. Am. Acad. Dermatol. *21*:1241–1244, 1989.

Recurrence of a pyogenic granuloma with satellite lesions following carbon dioxide laser treatment of a previously treated recurrent lesion.

61. Wilson Jones E, Orkin M: Tufted angioma (angioblastoma): A benign progressive angioma, not to be confused with Kaposi's sarcoma or low-grade angiosarcoma. J. Am. Acad. Dermatol. *20*:214–225, 1989.

A report of 20 patients with small circumscribed angiomatous tufts and lobules sometimes resembling pyogenic granulomas and Kaposi's sarcomas.

62. Cockerell CJ, LeBoit PE: Bacillary hemangiomatosis: A newly characterized pseudoneoplastic infectious cutaneous vascular disorder. J. Am. Acad. Dermatol. *22*:501–512, 1990.

A review of a newly described vascular or proliferative disorder seen primarily, but not necessarily, in individuals with HIV infection.

63. Kaufman SL, Stout AP: Hemangiopericytoma in children. Cancer *13*:695–710, 1960.

Thirty-one children with hemangiopericytoma.

64. Kobayashi H, Furukawa M, Fukai K, et al.: Cellular angioma of infancy with dermal melanocytosis. Int. J. Dermatol. *27*:40–42, 1988.

A report of a 7-month-old Japanese boy with a dark pedunculated vascular growth over a dome-shaped nodule on the left parietal region of the scalp.

65. Olsen TG, Helwig EB: Angiolymphoid hyperplasia with eosinophilia: A clinical pathologic study of 116 patients. J. Am. Acad. Dermatol. *12*:781–796, 1985.

A review of 116 patients with angiolymphoid hyperplasia with eosinophilia.

66. Nelson DA, Jarratt M: Angiolymphoid hyperplasia with eosinophilia. Pediatr. Dermatol. *1*:210–214, 1984.

A 12-year-old girl with angiolyphoid hyperplasia with eosinophilia and a review of the literature.

67. Massa MC, Fretzin DF, Chowdhury L, et al.: Angiolymphoid hyperplasia demonstrating extensive skin and mucosal lesions controlled with vinblastine therapy. J. Am. Acad. Dermatol. *11*:333–339, 1984.

A 28-year-old male with angiolymphoid hyperplasia with a wide range of clinical features controlled by vinblastine therapy.

68. Hobbs ER, Bailin PL, Ratz JL, et al.: Treatment of angiolymphoid hyperplasia of the external ear with carbon dioxide laser. J. Am. Acad. Dermatol. *19*:345–349, 1988.

A report of two patients with long histories of angiolymphoid hyperplasia successfully treated with carbon dioxide laser.

69. Imperial R, Helwig EB: Angiokeratoma. Arch. Dermatol. *95*:166–175, 1967.

Analyses of 116 examples of angiokeratoma support the concept of solitary and multiple angiokeratomas.

70. Pringle JJ: Four cases of angiokeratoma from one family. Br. J. Dermatol. *25*:40–53, 1913.

An early description of angiokeratoma.

71. Smith RBW, Prior IAM, Park RG: Angiokeratoma of Mibelli: A family with nodular lesions of the legs. Aust. J. Dermatol. *9*:329–334, 1968.

Four sisters and a female cousin with angiokeratomas confirm a genetic basis for this disorder.

72. Dave VK, Main RA: Angiokeratoma of Mibelli with necrosis of the fingertips. Arch. Dermatol. *106*:726–728, 1972.

A case of angiokeratoma of Mibelli in an 11-year-old girl with elevated IgG, IgA, and IgM, oral ulcerations, and necrosis of the fingertips.

73. Imperial R, Helwig EB: Angiokeratoma of the scrotum (Fordyce type). J. Urol. *95*:379–387, 1967.

One hundred thirty-five patients with angiokeratoma of the scrotum.

74. Danehower CC, Moyer DGM: Angiokeratoma corporis diffusum. Arch. Dermatol. *94*:628–631, 1966.

Diagnosis prior to onset of the rash can be aided by demonstration of mulberry cells on urinalysis and ophthalmologic examination.

75. von Gemmingen G, Kierland RR, Opitz JM: Angiokeratoma corporis diffusum (Fabry's disease). Arch. Dermatol. *91*:206–218, 1965.

A description of a pedigree that includes five males and one female with clinical evidence of Fabry's disease.

76. Burda CD, Winder PR: Angiokeratoma corporis diffusum universale (Fabry's disease) in female subjects. Am. J. Med. 42:293–301, 1967.

A report of a case of Fabry's disease in a 47-year-old woman with review of 12 living women with manifestations of the disease, and six women, including the propositus, who died of the disease.

77. Beaudet AL, Caskey CT: Detection of Fabry's disease heterozygotes by hair root analysis. Clin. Genet. 13:251–258, 1978.

Measurement of enzyme ratios in individual hair roots appears to be an accurate technique for the detection of carriers of this disorder.

78. Brady RO: Fabry's disease. Science 172:174–175, 1971.

Enzyme assays performed on extracts of cells obtained by transabdominal amniocentesis confirmed the diagnosis of a hemizygous male with Fabry disease in a fetus during the 17th week of pregnancy.

79. Mapes CA, Anderson RL, Sweeley CC: Enzyme replacement in Fabry's disease, an inborn error of metabolism. Science 169:987–989, 1970.

Studies describe the treatment of Fabry's disease by infusion with normal human plasma.

80. Durand P, Borrone C, Della Cella G: A new mucopolysaccharide lipid-storage disease? Lancet 2:1313–1314, 1966.

Clinical, histochemical, and microscopic findings in two brothers suggest a distinct autosomal recessive mucopolysaccharide/lipid complex disease.

81. Smith EB, Graham JL, Ledman JA, et al.: Fucosidosis. Cutis 19:195–198, 1977.

Three children with mental retardation, retarded growth, corneal opacities, dilated and tortuous conjunctival and retinal vessels, and angiokeratomas with low or absent α-L-fucosidase activity.

82. Dvoretzky I, Fisher BK: Fucosidosis. Int. J. Dermatol. 18:213–216, 1979.

A comprehensive review of fucosidosis and its variants.

83. Epinette WW, Norins AL, Drew AL, et al.: Angiokeratoma corporis diffusum with α-L-fucosidase deficiency. Arch. Dermatol. 107:755–757, 1973.

Report of a case of a 21-year-old mentally and physically retarded man who first developed angiokeratoma corporis diffusum at the age of 4 years, with normal α-galactosidase activity and reduced α-L-fucosidase activity (α-fucosidosis).

84. Braverman IM: Blood vessels. In Braverman IM: Skin Signs of Systemic Disease, 2nd ed. W.B. Saunders Co., Philadelphia, 1981, 532–565.

The value of skin lesions in the recognition of systemic disease.

85. Feldaker M, Hines EA Jr, Kierland RR: Livedo reticularis with summer ulcerations. Arch. Dermatol. 72:31–42, 1955.

Twelve patients with a syndrome of edema and ulcerations of the legs and feet.

86. Quimby SR, Perry HO: Livedo reticularis and cerebrovascular accidents. J. Am. Acad. Dermatol. 3:377–383, 1980.

A report of a 52-year-old man with generalized livedo reticularis, endarteritis obliterans, and cerebrovascular accidents that began at a relatively young age.

87. Davis RS, Strunk RC: Auriculotemporal syndrome in childhood. Am. J. Dis. Child. 135:832–833, 1981.

A report of three children with auriculotemporal syndrome, suggesting that this disorder is not as rare as most textbooks imply.

88. Harper KE, Spielvogel RL: Delayed onset of Frey's syndrome following trauma. J. Assoc. Milit. Dermatol. 9:32–34, 1983.

A 52-year-old white man with a 6-month history of sweating over his right temple while eating subsequent to multiple lacerations of the right side of the face suffered in an automobile accident 30 years earlier.

89. Mandell F, Folkman J, Matsumoto S: Erythromelalgia. Pediatrics 59:45–48, 1977.

A report of an 11-year-old Japanese girl incapacitated by erythromelalgia in whom symptoms began at the age of 3 years.

90. Michiels JJ, von Joost T: Erythromelalgia and thrombocythemia: A causal relation. J. Am. Acad. Dermatol. 22:107–111, 1990.

Studies of erythromelalgia suggest that platelet-mediated arteriolar inflammation, thrombosis, and platelet-derived growth factors and prostaglandins have a causal relationship in the etiology of this disorder.

91. Picascia DD, Esterly NB: Cutis marmorata telangiectatica congenita: Report of 22 cases. J. Am. Acad. Dermatol. 20:1098–1104, 1989.

A report of 22 cases of cutis marmorata telangiectatica congenita (8 male and 14 female infants): 4 had focal cutaneous atrophy, 8 had ulcerations of involved skin, and 6 had other associated anomalies.

92. Powell ST, Su WPD: Cutis marmorata telangiectatica congenita: Report of nine cases and review of the literature. Cutis 34:305–312, 1984.

A report of nine patients and a comprehensive review of the literature.

93. Delgiudice SM, Nydorf ED: Cutis marmorata telangiectatica congenita with multiple congenital anomalies. Arch. Dermatol. 122:1060–1061, 1986.

A report of a newborn with cutis marmorata telangiectatica congenita and multiple congenital anomalies (imperforate anus, rectovaginal and urethrovaginal fistulas, and absence of the clitoris).

94. Gold MH, Eramo L, Prendiville JS: Hereditary benign telangiectasia. Pediatr. Dermatol. 6:194–197, 1989.

A report of a father and two daughters with hereditary benign telangiectasia and a discussion of the differentiation of this entity from other primary disorders of telangiectasia.

95. Smith LL, Conerly SL: Ataxia-telangiectasia or Louis-Bar syndrome. J. Am. Acad. Dermatol. 12:681–694, 1985.

A report of two sisters with ataxia-telangiectasia and a comprehensive review of the clinical features of the disorder.

96. Swift M, Reinauer PJ, Morrell D, et al.: Breast and other cancers in families with ataxia-telangiectasia. N. Engl. J. Med. 316:1289–1294, 1987.

A retrospective review of 110 adult blood relatives with ataxia-telangiectasia suggests that heterozygous carriers of the gene for ataxia-telangiectasia have increased risk of cancer, particularly breast cancer in women.

97. Sheaham M, Voss R, Becker Y, et al.: Prenatal diagnosis of ataxia-telangiectasia. J. Pediatr. 100:134–137, 1982.

A report of a prenatal test for ataxia-telangiectasia based on a factor in the amniotic fluid that can induce chromosome breakage in lymphocytic cultures from normal donors.

98. Hersh CS, Shwayder TA: Unilateral progressive pigmentary purpura (Schamberg's disease) in a 15-year-old boy. J. Am. Acad. Dermatol. 24:651, 1991.

A report of a patient with unilateral Schamberg's disease on the left leg, apparently a unique variant of this disorder.

99. Draelos ZK, Hansen RC: Schamberg's purpura in children: Case study and literature review. Clin. Pediatr. 26:659–661, 1987.

A report of 2 girls and a literature review of Schamberg's purpura.

100. Aiba S, Tagami H: Immunohistologic studies in Schamberg's disease: Evidence for cellular immune reaction in lesional skin. Arch. Dermatol. *124*:1058–1062, 1988.

Monoclonal antibody studies of eight patients with Schamberg's disease suggest that the progressive pigmentary purpuras may represent an immunologic disorder of the skin.

101. Barnhill RL, Braverman IM: Progression of pigmented purpura-like eruptions to mycosis fungoides. J. Am. Acad. Dermatol. *19*:25–31, 1988.

Report of three relatively young males with pigmented purpuric eruptions characterized by petechial patches with varying degrees of scale, pigmentation and lichenification and brownish pigmentation from hemosiderin accumulation which progressed to mycosis fungoides.

102. Khana M, Levy A, Shewach-Millett M, et al.: Lichen aureus occurring in childhood. Int. J. Dermatol. *10*:666–667, 1985.

An 8-year-old girl with lichen aureus characterized by scattered bruise-like patches on the posterior left thigh.

103. Shelley WB, Swaminathan R, Shelley ED: Lichen aureus: A hemosiderin tattoo associated with perforator vein incompetence. J. Am. Acad. Dermatol. *11*:260–264, 1984.

A report of 4 patients with lichen aureus suggest that the disorder may be caused by venous insufficiency and that a local venous incompetence may be associated with the pathogenesis of this disorder.

104. Woods WG, Corman Lubin NL, Hilgartner MG, et al.: Disseminated intravascular coagulation in the newborn. Am. J. Dis. Child. *133*:44–46, 1979.

Disseminated intravascular coagulation in newborns is frequently more difficult to diagnose because of normal prolonged coagulation values in premature infants.

105. Auletta MJ, Headington JT: Purpura fulminans: A cutaneous manifestation of severe protein C deficiency. Arch. Dermatol. *124*:1387–1391, 1988.

A report of 5-day-old infant with congenital protein C deficiency and neonatal purpura fulminans and a review of the disorder.

106. Yuen Cheung A, Ju Lin H, et al.: Purpura fulminans in a Chinese boy with congenital protein C deficiency. Pediatrics 77:670–676, 1986.

Severe recurrent purpura fulminans associated with disseminated intravascular coagulation in a Chinese boy that began at 1 day of age.

107. Israels SJ, Seshia SS: Childhood stroke associated with protein C or S deficiency. J. Pediatr. *111*:562–564, 1987.

A report of 2 children with acute hemiplegia as a result of protein C or its cofactor protein S deficiency as a reminder that protein C or S deficiency can be a primary or contributing cause of cerebrovascular accident in childhood.

108. Gardner FH, Diamond LK: Autoerythrocyte sensitization: A form of purpura producing painful bruising following autosensitization to red blood cells in certain women. Blood *10*:675–690, 1955.

A report of four women with unusual bruising following autosensitivity to their own erythrocytes.

109. Ellis CN, Vanderven EE, Rasmussen JE: Scurvy: A case caused by peculiar dietary habits. Arch. Dermatol *120*:1212–1214, 1984.

A 9-year-old girl with a 2-week history of petechial rash, lethargy, friable gums with gingival erosions, bone tenderness, follicular hyperkeratosis, and perifollicular hemorrhages as a result of a 1-year diet of tuna fish sandwiches without lettuce, vitamins, or other foods.

110. Bailin P, Kantor G, Wheeland R: Carbon dioxide laser vaporization of lymphangioma circumscription. J. Am. Acad. Dermatol. *14*:257–262, 1986.

Successful treatment of six children and one adult with lymphangioma circumscriptum with carbon dioxide laser.

111. Bastien MR, Goldstein BG, Lesher JL Jr, et al.: Treatment of lymphedema with a multicompartmental pneumatic compression device. J. Am. Acad. Dermatol. *2*:853–854, 1989.

A report of a 14-year-old girl with congenital lymphedema treated with a pneumatic compression device.

10

BACTERIAL AND PROTOZOAL INFECTIONS OF THE SKIN

The normal skin of healthy infants and children is resistant to invasion by most bacteria because the cutaneous surface provides a dry mechanical barrier from which contaminating organisms are constantly removed by desquamation. Under normal conditions the skin is sterile at delivery and for a short period thereafter. During the process of vaginal birth it picks up organisms from the birth canal, which gradually increase in number during the first 10 days of life. If the newborn is delivered by cesarean section, however, the cutaneous surface remains sterile until after delivery but soon becomes exposed to bacteria from human contactants and fomites.

Almost any organism may live on the cutaneous surface under appropriate conditions. A complete list of transient organisms accordingly would include virtually all microorganisms found in the human environment. The number of species comprising the resident flora, however, is relatively small. It consists predominantly of gram-positive organisms and a few gram-negative species and includes *Propionibacterium acnes* (normally found in high concentrations about the pilosebaceous follicles of the face and less commonly in areas such as the axillae and forearms), aerobic diphtheroids (*Corynebacterium minutissimum* and *C. tenuis*), *Staphylococcus epidermidis* (formerly termed *S. epidermidis albus*), micrococci, anaerobic gram-positive cocci, and gram-negative bacilli found uncommonly on normal skin except about the moist intertriginous areas of the groin, axillae, and toe webs (*Escherichia coli, Proteus, Enterobacter, Alcaligenes, Pseudomonas, Acinetobacter calcoaceticus, A. lwoffi*), and *Staphylococcus aureus*. The organisms of *S. aureus*, a common pathogen, appear to be seeded from a carrier state in the anterior nares.

Since the cutaneous surface is continuously exposed to microorganisms, it is most helpful to be able to distinguish between transient, resident, and pathogenic flora. The transient flora consists of a multiplicity of organisms that are deposited on the skin from the environment, presumably do not proliferate, and are removed easily by washing or scrubbing of the affected area. The resident flora consists of a smaller number of organisms that are found more or less regularly in appreciable numbers on the skin of normal individuals, multiply on the skin, form stable communities on the cutaneous surface, and are not easily dislodged. Pathogenic bacteria, not ordinarily a regular part of this flora, persist on the skin if there is continuous replacement from some internal or external source, or if the integrity of the skin is disrupted by injury or disease. It should be noted that the mere presence of potentially pathogenic bacteria in a cutaneous lesion does not necessarily prove the demonstrable organism to be a cause of bacterial infection.

In the past it was believed that a low pH on the cutaneous surface limited proliferation of skin flora. This "acid mantle" theory, however, has currently fallen into disrepute. It now appears that the relative dryness, rather than the pH, constitutes the major factor in the retardation of growth of gram-negative bacteria with high moisture requirements.[1] Accordingly, it is not the acidity or fatty acids that protect the skin. It is a combination of normal epidermal shedding, the dryness of the cutaneous surface, the virulence of the organisms, the presence of normal flora, which contributes to host defenses, and the host response that determines the clinical picture.

Children have a more varied cutaneous flora than adults and often harbor soil bacteria on their skin. Prepubertal children lack sebum and accordingly have less diphtheroid organisms than adults. It is estimated that 20 per cent of individuals are persistent nasal carriers of *S. aureus*, that 60 per cent are intermittent carriers, and that 20 per cent of individuals are resistant to nasal colonization. Coagulase-positive staphylococci (*S. aureus*) are not considered part of the normal cutaneous flora of glabrous skin in adults but are frequent transients acquired from carrier sites such as the anterior nares and perineum.

Many individuals carry *S. aureus* in the nose without skin colonization, and, with certain virulent strains, colonization of staphylococci of the axilla and groin, in addition to the nose, is common.

Colonization with staphylococci, therefore, may not necessarily be related to a process of seeding from a carrier state but may be due to the acquisition of an outside organism that, once acquired, persists in a tenacious manner.

Pathogenic streptococci are usually not found on the skin of normal persons, and impetigo occurs in a high percentage of patients after cutaneous contamination. This is particularly important as a source of disease in children in warm moist climates where the infection rate during the summer may exceed 50 per cent, with the streptococci invading damaged skin with resultant pyoderma. The nasopharynx is probably contaminated from this site, and isolation of streptococci from this mucous membrane area is common even though clinical pharyngitis does not occur.

The introduction of a vast array of specific antibiotics and chemotherapeutic agents has affected striking changes in the management of bacterial infection. With the availability of these agents the focus of attention is directed to determination of the specific bacterial cause and its sensitivity, when indicated, so that a proper choice of antibacterial agents can be made. In purulent infections of the skin it is easy to obtain adequate specimens for microscopic examination and culture. When the lesion is dry or crusted, however, the superficial area must be cleansed with an antiseptic solution (alcohol, povidone-iodine [Betadine], or chlorhexidine gluconate) to prevent contamination of the specimen. The crusted lesion is then gently lifted off and cultures are obtained from the moist underlying surface. In nonpurulent infections (erysipelas or cellulitis) a diagnostic specimen may be obtained by aspiration of the most active area (not the surrounding area of erythema) with a 25-gauge needle attached to a syringe containing 2.0 ml of sterile saline without added preservatives. A drop of this specimen may be Gram stained for microscopic examination, and the remainder may be cultured in blood agar and thioglycollate broth.

BACTERIAL INFECTIONS

Impetigo

The primary bacterial infections of the skin are impetigo and folliculitis. Impetigo is a contagious superficial infection of the skin caused by streptococci, staphylococci, or both. Although seen in all age groups, the disease is most common in infants and children. Lesions may involve any body surface but occur most frequently on the exposed parts of the body, especially the face, hands, neck, and extremities.

Clinical Manifestations. The disease begins with 1- or 2-mm erythematous macules, which soon develop into thin-roofed vesicles or bullae surrounded by narrow areolae of erythema. The vesicles rupture easily, with release of a thin cloudy yellow fluid. The serous discharge subsequently dries, with formation of thick, soft honey-colored crusts, the hallmark of impetigo (Fig. 10–1). Crusts can be removed easily, leaving a smooth, red, weeping surface, which rapidly becomes encrusted again (Fig. 10–2). The exudate is easily spread by autoinoculation by fingers, towels, or clothing, with resultant satellite lesions to adjacent areas or other parts of the body. Individual lesions sometimes extend peripherally, with central clearing, and frequently eventuate in annular, circinate, or gyrate lesions (Figs. 10–3 and 10–4).

Impetigo is seen in two forms: (1) a bullous impetigo associated with phage group II staphylococci (Fig. 10–5) and (2) a vesiculopustular form with resulting thick crusted lesions due to β-hemolytic streptococci (alone or in combination with staphylococci). Lesions of impetigo due to *S. aureus* generally affect the face, trunk, and extremities; do not appear to have a seasonal predilection; and consist of superficial blisters that rupture and leave a "scalded skin"–like appearance. Fever and lymphadenopathy appear late in the course of the disorder. Lesions due to streptococci tend to occur on traumatized skin, frequently affect the lower extremities, appear in the hot, muggy summer months, and often consist of punched-out ulcers on the legs with superimposed crusts. Fever and lymphadenopathy are early prominent features of this disorder.

Current information suggests that the reservoir for staphylococci is the upper respiratory tract (particularly the nose) of asymptomatic persons. These carriers spread the agent to the skin of infants, probably with their hands. The reservoir for streptococci responsible for cutaneous infection appears to be cutaneous lesions of other individuals, not the respiratory tract of affected or asymptomatic persons. The presence of streptococci on normal skin does not seem to be the only factor responsible for cutaneous infection. Factors such as trauma and insect bites probably contribute to the pathogenesis of this disorder. Staphylococci, when

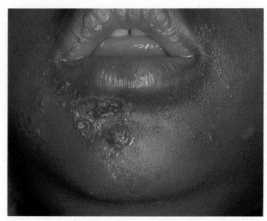

Figure 10–2. Impetigo. Red weeping surface has overlying encrustation.

seen, are late colonists and accordingly play no role in the pathogenesis of streptococcal pyoderma.

Treatment. Although appropriate management of impetigo is generally prompt and highly effective, untreated impetigo may last for 2 to 3 weeks, with continuous spread and development of new lesions. In severe neglected cases there may be large crusted vegetations with deep extension and ulcerative lesions. Simple uncomplicated lesions, however, ordinarily do not produce ulceration or deep infiltration and heal without scarring or atrophy. Gentle washing of lesions, removal of crusts, and drainage of blisters and pustules help prevent local spread and reaccumulation of crusts. If crusts

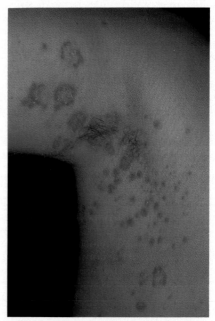

Figure 10–3. Autoinoculation of lesions of impetigo in the axillary region with multiple gyrate and circinate lesions due to peripheral extension and central clearing.

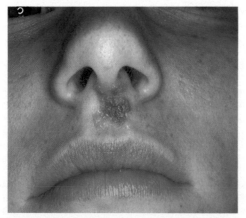

Figure 10–1. Impetigo. Moist, thin-roofed vesicles and honey-colored crusts surrounded by an areola of erythema.

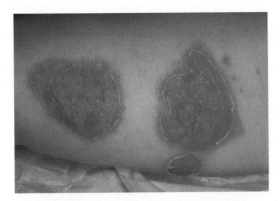

Figure 10–4. Large impetiginous lesions with smooth, red, weeping surfaces.

are firmly adherent, warm soaks or compresses are useful. Topical antibiotics, if used properly, are frequently highly effective in the treatment of early superficial pyoderma due to S. aureus. In cutaneous infection due to β-hemolytic streptococci or persistent staphylococcal infection, however, systemic antibiotics produce a swifter response and fewer failures.

Owing to changing patterns and increasing resistance to penicillin, penicillin G is generally not recommended for the treatment of S. aureus infection. Patients with impetigo caused by S. aureus may be treated with erythromycin, 30 to 50 mg/kg/day (up to 250 mg four times day) for 7 to 10 days. For those acutely ill or with severe forms of bullous impetigo, however, an alternate drug such as dicloxacillin should be administered (12.5 to 25 mg/kg/day given at 6-hour intervals) for 7 to 10 days. Other effective drugs include cloxacillin, the cephalosporins, clindamycin, or a combination of amoxicillin and clavulanic acid (Augmentin). Clin-

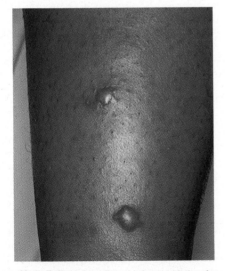

Figure 10–5. Bullous impetigo, a characteristic of group II staphylococcal infection.

damycin can be prescribed for individuals who cannot take penicillin or erythromycin. Because of the risk of pseudomembranous ulcerative colitis, however, long-term use of clindamycin is not recommended.

Bacitracin, polymyxin, gramicidin, and erythromycin are effective topical agents and are relatively nonallergenic. Although a high incidence of allergenicity has been attributed to the topical use of neomycin, this has probably been exaggerated. The majority of contact allergies to this agent follow prolonged use on chronically inflamed skin. When that group is excluded, the incidence of neomycin allergy falls drastically, with an estimated incidence of 1 in 100,000 usages.[2] In addition, mupirocin (pseudomonic acid A, Bactroban) exerts a high level of bactericidal activity against a broad spectrum of gram-positive organisms and has little or no potential for irritation, side effects, cross-reaction with other antibiotics, or systemic problems, even in infants with damaged skin, thus making it particularly safe and effective for the treatment of primary and secondary cutaneous infections. Although findings are not conclusive and the possibility of bacterial resistance exists, topical mupirocin ointment has been said to be as effective as oral erythromycin or cloxacillin and, because of its efficacy and excellent safety and tolerance profiles, currently appears to be a helpful topical agent for the treatment of superficial skin infections.[3–5]

Lesions of impetigo caused by group A β-hemolytic streptococci are shallow and usually heal well, and there are no recorded instances of rheumatic fever following streptococcal skin infection. In contrast, however, acute glomerulonephritis and scarlet fever can follow cutaneous streptococcal infection. Of these, acute glomerulonephritis is the most significant. As in the case of nephritis following streptococcal infection of the throat, only certain serologic types, different from those producing nephritis as a sequel of streptococcal pharyngitis, appear to result in this complication of cutaneous infection.[6] Clinical glomerulonephritis secondary to impetigo is uncommon, except for certain epidemics due to nephritogenic strains of streptococci. The risk of developing nephritis following skin infection with a nephritogenic strain of streptococcus, however, is high (12 to 28 per cent).[7] It must be emphasized that although systemic antibiotics help eliminate cutaneous streptococci, they do not appear to prevent glomerulonephritis due to streptococcal impetigo.[8] In areas where nephritogenic M strains of streptococci are endemic, urinalysis should be performed and patients should be watched for signs of glomerulonephritis for at least 7 weeks after the cutaneous streptococcal infection. In general, however, with our changing bacteriology, and the fact that staphylococci are becoming more important in the etiology of impetigo, concerns of cutaneous streptococcal-induced glomerulonephritis have been greatly reduced.

Folliculitis

The term *folliculitis* refers to a superficial or deep infection of hair follicles. The clinical appearance varies according to the location and depth of follicular involvement. Superficial folliculitis (Bockhart's impetigo), an infection of the follicular ostium, begins with superficial, small, dome-shaped, thin-walled yellow pustules, often with a narrow red areola and a hair shaft in the center of the lesion. The disorder occurs most commonly in children and usually is seen on the scalp, face, buttocks, and extremities. Most lesions are painless, occur in crops, and generally heal in 7 to 10 days. Coagulase-positive *S. aureus* is the most common pathogen; occasionally other organisms (*Streptocuccus, Proteus, Pseudomonas,* or coliform bacilli) may be responsible for the infection. Superficial folliculitis is not always primarily or exclusively infectious. Occupational contact with oil, occupational or therapeutic contact with tar and tar products, and occlusive dressings with polyethylene or adhesive may cause obstruction of pilosebaceous follicles, resulting in follicular plugging and inflammation. Although those lesions are usually sterile, *S. epidermidis* may occasionally be isolated from them.

Superficial folliculitis usually responds to gentle cleansing and the application of topical antibiotics. Occasionally, systemic antibiotics (a penicillinase-resistant synthetic penicillin or erythromycin) may be required for persistent or recurrent folliculitis. In such instances, bacterial culture should be obtained prior to the initiation of systemic therapy.

FOLLICULITIS BARBAE

Folliculitis barbae (sycosis barbae) is a term used to describe a deep-seated folliculitis of the bearded area involving the entire depth of the follicle and perifollicular region (Fig. 10–6). A pruritic follicular or perifollicular infection is usually the initial lesion, with the process spreading from one follicle to another by trauma from scratching, shaving, or impetiginization. The disorder is characterized by follicular papules and pustules and, as the condition progresses, by erythema, crusting, and boggy infiltration of the skin. Although occasionally other bacteria may be isolated, the infection is usually staphylococcal. Care in the technique of shaving should be taken, and the use of an electric rather than a safety razor is sometimes helpful in the prevention and treatment of this disorder. Although relapses are common, warm compresses and topical antibiotics are often sufficient to control minor forms of sycosis barbae. If the condition is chronic, severe, or recurrent, however, several weeks of systemic antibiotics are often required.

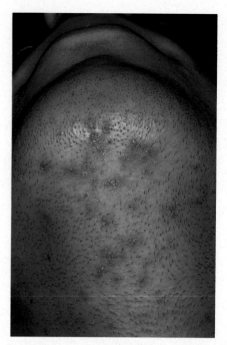

Figure 10–6. Folliculitis barbae of the submental area and upper aspect of the anterior neck. Follicular papules, pustules, boggy erythema, and crusting with spread from one follicle to another are due to shaving and impetiginization.

PSEUDOFOLLICULITIS BARBAE

Pseudofolliculitis barbae is a common and troublesome inflammatory disorder of the pilosebaceous follicles of the beard caused by shaved hairs that curve inward with resultant repenetration of the skin, seen particularly in blacks and in persons with curly hair. On reentry into the epidermis, the hairs grow in a curved or arcuate path, with the creation of an inflammatory foreign body reaction. Although cocci, particularly *S. epidermidis,* can be cultured from lesions at times, pathogenic bacteria seem to play little role in this type of folliculitis. Mild cases may be managed by careful shaving and occasionally by changing from a safety razor to an electric razor, or vice versa. Since close shaving promotes oblique penetration of hairs into the skin, this should be avoided whenever possible. A chemical depilatory alternating with careful shaving will often help control this disorder to a moderate degree, and the topical use of vitamin A acid (Retin-A), as in the treatment of acne vulgaris, is often helpful in the prevention of this disorder. When all else fails, individuals with moderate or severe pseudofolliculitis should avoid shaving for approximately 1 month. Thus, although many hair tips will reenter the skin, as their growth continues the hair segments that have not reentered the skin will act like springs and pull the ingrown hair tips out and hairs that remain buried can be gently lifted manually (not plucked) from the epidermis. Following this, in an effort to avoid recurrences, patients should be advised to shave gently (not too closely) with a sharp blade, should not pull the skin taut or shave repeatedly over the same area, and, since secondary bacterial infection is often associated with this disorder, should use a topical antibacterial agent whenever necessary.

FOLLICULITIS KELOIDALIS NUCHAE

Folliculitis keloidalis nuchae (acne keloidalis) represents a chronic perifollicular infection of the nape of the neck seen in men. Early cases are characterized by follicular papules, pustules, and occasionally abscesses. The lesions are gradually replaced by fibrous nodules and, in some individuals, by keloidal scarring, The condition usually occurs in males after puberty and is most commonly seen between the ages of 15 and 25, especially in blacks. Seen most frequently, but not exclusively, in those with a tendency toward acne vulgaris, the condition is extremely chronic and new lesions may continue to form at intervals for years.

The bacteriology varies from case to case and at different time intervals. Although pathogenic staphylococci are often found, they appear to be secondary invaders. Treatment consists of long-term antibiotic therapy, as in the treatment of severe acne and chronic folliculitis, with intralesional triamcinolone in an effort to minimize keloid formation, and with incision and drainage of lesions. In severe cases, excision and plastic surgical repair may be necessary.

EOSINOPHILIC PUSTULAR FOLLICULITIS

Eosinophilic pustular folliculitis (Ofuji's syndrome) is a dermatosis of unknown cause characterized by erythematous patches with largely follicular papules and pustules, often in an annular or serpiginous arrangement, with at times eosinophilia and leukocytosis of the peripheral blood.[9] Although not of bacterial origin, this disorder, seen on the face, trunk, and extremities, including the palms and soles, is included in this section as a form of folliculitis that occurs in children as well as adults. Whereas adults tend to have annular, serpiginous, or polycyclic lesions, prominent scalp involvement and failure to form annular rings appear to distinguish the infantile form from that of adults.[10] Histopathologic features include eosinophilic exocytosis of the epidermis, eosinophilic intradermal abscesses involving the hair follicles and sebaceous glands, and a perivascular or perifollicular infiltrate with mononuclear cells, neutrophils, and eosinophils.[11]

This chronic cutaneous condition has intermittent recurrences and a marked (4.8 : 1) male predominance. Although oral erythromycin, sulfapyridine, dapsone (alone or in combination with systemic corticosteroids), oral and topical indomethacin, and oral and topical corticosteroids have been used for the treatment of this disorder with varying degrees of efficacy, the typical course is one of spontaneous remission and exacerbation.[12, 13]

PSEUDOMONAS FOLLICULITIS (HOT TUB DERMATITIS)

Since the mid 1970s cutaneous infections caused by *Pseudomonas aeruginosa* have been linked to the use of whirlpools, hot tubs, and, less commonly, community swimming pools and water slides.[14, 15] Referred to as whirlpool dermatitis, *Pseudomonas* folliculitis, or hot tub dermatitis, the disorder is characterized by discrete pruritic papules and erythematous papulopustular lesions that develop, usually within 1 to 2 days after exposure, with greatest density on areas of the body covered by bathing suits (Fig. 10–7). Although spontaneous drainage or regression usually occurs within 5 to 14 days, recurrences have been reported in up to 24 per cent of affected individuals for up to 3 months after the original exposure. Although most patients are otherwise asymptomatic and well, many individuals manifest malaise, fever, headache, vomiting, conjunctivitis, upper respiratory tract infections, pneumonia, axillary adenopathy, and mastitis, at times obscuring the true nature of the disorder.[16, 17]

Since most cases of *Pseudomonas* folliculitis resolve spontaneously without serious complications, therapy other than mild symptomatic treatment is generally unnecessary. It should be noted, however, that persistent purulent otitis externa, *Pseudomonas* pneumonia, and urinary tract infections have been reported in individuals with this

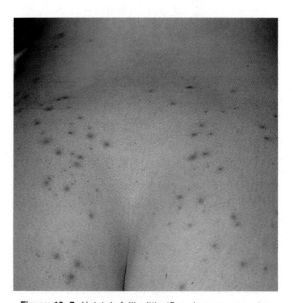

Figure 10–7. Hot tub folliculitis (*Pseudomonas aeruginosa* folliculitis). (Courtesy of Kenneth Greer, M.D.)

disorder. Preventive measures include the maintenance of a free chlorine level of 1.0 to 1.5 ppm (3 to 5 mg/liter) and pH between 7.2 and 7.8, frequent changing of the water, and thorough scrubbing of whirlpool baths and hot tubs with each water change.

Ecthyma

Ecthyma is a deep or ulcerative type of pyoderma commonly seen on the lower extremities and buttocks of children. It may occur as either a small punched-out ulcer (ecthyma minor) or a deep spreading ulcerative process (ecthyma major). The disorder begins in the same manner as impetigo, often following infected insect bites or minor trauma, but penetrates through the epidermis to produce a shallow ulcer. The initial lesion is a vesicle or vesiculopustule with an erythematous base, surrounding halo, and firmly adherent crust. Removal of the crust reveals a deeper lesion than that seen in impetigo, with an underlying saucer-shaped ulcer and raised margin (Fig. 10–8). Lesions are painful, slow growing, and chronic; healing occurs after a few weeks, often with scar formation. Scratching and a lack of appropriate hygienic measures may lead to progression and autoinoculation of the disease. Lesions are usually initiated by β-hemolytic streptococci, although in later stages other organisms are frequently isolated. Treatment, as in impetigo, consists of warm compresses with gentle removal of crusts, bacterial cultures, and appropriate systemic antibiotics.

Furuncles and Carbuncles

Furuncles or boils are painful circumscribed perifollicular staphylococcal abscesses that have a tendency to central necrosis and suppuration. Seen most frequently in older children and adults, they usually develop from a preceding folliculitis

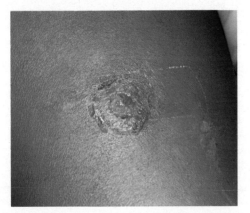

Figure 10–8. Ecthyma. A deep form of pyoderma with a saucer-shaped erythematous ulcer and raised margin associated with occlusion of the infection by an adhesive dressing.

with deeper extension into the dermis and subcutaneous tissue. They generally occur in areas of the skin that are unusually hairy and subject to friction and maceration, particularly the face, back of the neck, scalp, axillae, breasts, thighs, buttocks, and perineum. Clinically they appear as red tender nodules, which enlarge to a diameter of 1 to 5 cm. They gradually become boggy and fluctuant and, if untreated, often suppurate with a release of a purulent blood-tinged discharge. There is a high rate of contagion in patients with deep angry boils, and group I phage type 80-81 and certain other group I and II strains are reemerging as the cause of small epidemics of furunculosis.

The treatment of boils depends largely on the extent and location of lesions. Simple furunculosis may respond to warm moist compresses. Severe or persistent infections require systemic antibiotics, with incision and drainage after they have softened and become fluctuant. Since penicillin-resistant staphylococci are commonly seen as pathogens, cultures and sensitivity tests should be performed. Oral β-lactamase–resistant antibiotics such as dicloxacillin, cloxacillin, nafcillin, or cephalexin are usually the antibiotics of choice. If the patient is allergic to penicillin or its derivatives, erythromycin or clindamycin may be administered.

Carbuncles may be considered as large deep-seated staphylococcal abscesses composed of aggregates of interconnected furuncles that drain at multiple points on the cutaneous surface. Usually seen in men on the back of the neck, shoulders, buttocks, and outer aspect of the hip joints and thighs, they extend into the deeper dermis and subcutaneous tissues, reach a larger size than furuncles (3 to 10 cm in diameter), and undergo necrosis and suppuration more slowly than furuncles (usually 7 to 14 days are required before fluctuation becomes apparent). Because of the delay in suppuration and the larger size of lesions, patients may present with extreme pain and consitutional symptoms (fever, chills, malaise, and, in extreme situations, even prostration).

Carbuncles should be treated with appropriate antibiotics and incision and drainage of large lesions, preferably after appropriate antibiotics have been initiated and lesions have become fluctuant.

Cellulitis

Cellulitis is an acute suppurative inflammation of the skin, particularly the deeper subcutaneous tissues. It is characterized by erythema, swelling, and tenderness of the affected area. The borders of cellulitis are not elevated or sharply defined. This is in contrast to erysipelas, a more superficial form of cellulitis with a well-demarcated border, which is due to group A (or uncommonly group G) streptococci (Fig. 10–9).

Cellulitis usually occurs as a complication of a wound or trauma, which is followed within a day or two by markedly red, tender, warm swelling with

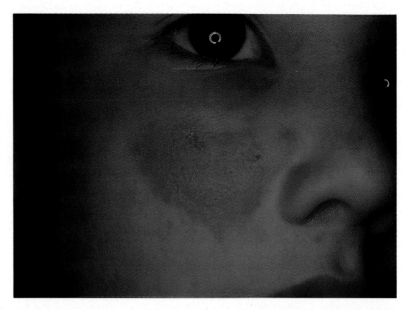

Figure 10–9. Erysipelas. Superficial streptococcal cellulitis has a distinct and well-marginated border.

an edematous infiltrated appearance. Although group A β-hemolytic streptococci and *Staphylococcus aureus* are the most common etiologic agents, occasionally other bacteria may be implicated. In young children, however, particularly those younger than 2 years of age, *Hemophilus influenzae* should be considered as a cause of cellulitis (in young children this agent is probably more common than either *Streptococcus* or *Staphylococcus*). Children with *H. influenzae* cellulitis may be extremely ill and toxic, often with accompanying upper repiratory tract symptoms and an associated bacteremia or septicemia.[18] In approximately 50 per cent of instances of *H. influenzae* cellulitis, the lesion has a peculiar dusky red, bluish, or purplish red discoloration. It should be noted, however, that bluish purple discoloration can also occur with cellulitis due to other organisms, such as *Streptococcus pneumoniae*.[19]

The treatment of cellulitis depends on identification of the affecting organisms whenever possible and use of appropriate antibiotics. Most cases of cellulitis should be aspirated with a needle to obtain a sample for Gram stain and bacterial culture. Patients with cellulitis due to *H. influenzae* can be treated with ampicillin (ampicillin and chloramphenicol for severe cases), methicillin, cefaclor, an amoxicillin–clavulanic acid combination (Augmentin), or cefuroxime or cefixime for ampicillin-resistant orgnaisms; penicillinase-resistant penicillins should be used for patients with cellulitis due to staphylococci; and penicillin should be used for those individuals with streptococcal cellulitis. For patients in whom needle aspiration and bacterial culture do not reveal the organism, therapy with both a penicillinase-resistant penicillin and ampicillin is recommended (a one-drug alternative is cefazolin). For those allergic to penicillin, erythromycin or clin-

damycin is indicated; for patients with penicillin-resistant staphylococci, a semisynthetic penicillinase-resistant penicillin (methicillin, nafcillin, oxacillin, dicloxacillin, cephalothin, or cefazolin) will generally result in a rapid clinical response. The dosage of ampicillin is 200 mg/kg/day and that of chloramphenicol is 100 mg/kg/day. Aplastic anemia, however, must be considered as a possible complication of chloramphenicol administration.

Facial, orbital, and periorbital cellulitis requires special attention because of the high rate of serious complication and the fact that unique bacterial infections and conjunctivitis may at times mimic orbital cellulitis. Treatment of orbital cellulitis requires hospitalization and a full 10-day course of therapy and when associated with paranasal cellulitis should be managed with the assistance of an ophthalmologist and an otolaryngologist.

Erysipelas

Erysipelas occurs most frequently in infants, very young children, and older adults as a superficial cellulitis of the skin, with marked lymphatic vessel involvement, due to group A β-streptococci. In most cases the organism gains access by direct inoculation through a break in the skin, but occasionally hematogenous infection may occur. After an incubation period of 2 to 5 days, the initial lesion begins as a small area of redness that gradually enlarges to reveal a characteristic tense, hot, painful, shiny bright-red, brawny infiltrated plaque with a distinct and well-marginated border (see Fig. 10–9). The periphery of the lesion may appear irregular because of projections of the inflammatory process. Although the face and scalp are favorite sites of involvement, the infection may appear anywhere on the cutaneous surface. The most common location of erysipelas, however, is the face, with involvement of the bridge of the nose and one or both cheeks.

Penicillin is the drug of choice for the treatment of erysipelas. For individuals allergic to penicillin, erythromycin or clindamycin is recommended. Penicillin-resistant staphylococci often coexist in chronic or persistent cases. For such individuals a semisynthetic penicillinase-resistant penicillin, such as methicillin, nafcillin, oxacillin, cephalothin, or cefazolin, is recommended.

Perianal Streptococcal Cellulitis

A frequently overlooked cutaneous manifestation of group A β-hemolytic streptococcal disease, perianal streptococcal cellulitis is characterized by a persistent, bright red, usually tender perianal eruption sharply demarcated from the adjacent normal skin with perianal itching, and at times rectal pain, painful defecation, fissures in the anal canal, streaks of blood on the stool, proctocolitis, and fecal hoarding (Fig. 10–10). Since signs of true cellulitis are not present, the term *streptococcal perianal disease* has been suggested as a more ap-

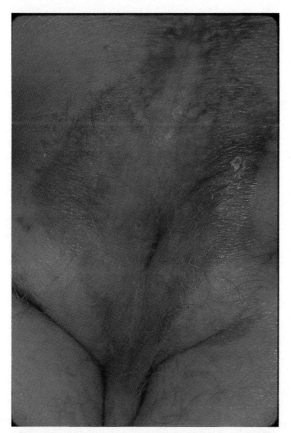

Figure 10–10. Streptococcal perianal disease. A persistent bright red, usually tender, perianal eruption sharply demarcated from the adjacent normal skin. (Courtesy of Department of Dermatology, Yale University School of Medicine.)

propriate designation for this disorder.[20–22] Often misdiagnosed as psoriasis, chronic perianal fissures, candidiasis, a behavior disturbance such as psychogenic stool holding, a manifestation of inflammatory bowel disease, pinworm infestation, or sexual abuse, the diagnosis can be confirmed by bacterial culture with a perianal swab. Treatment with oral penicillin V (25 to 50 mg/kg/day) for 10 to 14 days or with a single 1.2 million unit intramuscular injection of long-acting benzathine penicillin is usually curative. The disorder, however, has a high (up to 39 per cent) relapse rate and may at times be found as a source of streptococcal infection in individuals with guttate psoriasis and recurrent exacerbations of psoriasis.[23]

Blistering Distal Dactylitis

Blistering distal dactylitis is a unique bullous manifestation of a β-hemolytic streptococcal and, at times, *Staphylococcus aureus* infection in children, and occasionally adults, characterized by tender, dusky, fluid-filled tense blisters with surrounding erythema overlying the distal volar fat pads of the fingers or toes (Fig. 10–11).[24–27] Occasionally accompanied by systemic manifestations and fever, cutaneous lesions of blistering distal dactylitis can be differentiated from those of staphylococcal bullous impetigo, herpetic whitlow, and friction blisters by identification of the offending organism by Gram stain, bacterial culture of a fluid-filled blister, and their rapid response to treatment by incision and drainage and oral or intramuscular administration of penicillin or other appropriate antibacterial therapy.

Necrotizing Fasciitis

Necrotizing fasciitis is a rapidly progressive, acute, necrotizing infection of the skin and subcutaneous tissue frequently associated with severe systemic toxicity. Unless promptly recognized and treated aggressively, it is rapidly fatal. The disorder, which is generally found in individuals with decreased local resistance and general debilitation following surgery or perforating trauma, has been designated by a variety of terms (*hospital gangrene, acute infective gangrene, streptococcal gangrene, gangrenous erysipelas, necrotizing erysipelas, suppurative fasciitis,* and *Meleney's ulcer*). Frequently ascribed to a hemolytic streptococcal etiology, the disorder has also been associated with anaerobic streptococci, *Staphylococcus aureus, Proteus vulgaris, Bacteroides, Hemophilus,* and a variety of mixed aerobic and anaerobic flora. Characterized by a rapid fulminant course and rapid development of fascial necrosis, necrotizing fasciitis usually presents as an area of cellulitis with fever, redness, pain, and edema that quickly progresses to central patches of bluish discoloration, with or without serosanguineous blis-

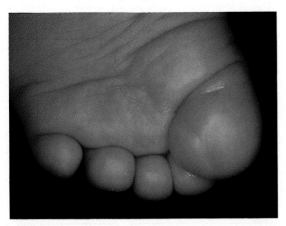

Figure 10–11. Blistering distal dactylitis. Tender, cloudy or dusky fluid–filled blisters with surrounding erythema overlie the distal volar fat pad, a frequently overlooked manifestation of a β-hemolytic streptococcal and at times staphylococcal infection.

ters, followed by ulceration, gangrene, and systemic toxicity (Fig. 10–12).

Rapid diagnosis and prompt surgical debridement of necrotic tissue are of prime importance in the management of patients with this disorder. Even in the best circumstances, however, there may be a relatively high (20 to 30 per cent) mortality. Treatment, therefore, should include early surgical debridement, intravenously administered antibiotics (penicillin, semisynthetic penicillin, gram-negative spectrum antibiotics, and a drug to treat anaerobic organisms, with later adjustment depending on culture results and sensitivities), and careful supportive care.[28, 29]

Noma

Noma (cancrum oris) is a rare progressive destructive infection usually involving the face and buccal mucosa. Caused by the invasion of buccal tissues by fusospirochetal organisms and other bacteria in children whose resistance has been lowered by concurrent disease or nutritional deficiency, the disorder is characterized by a gangrenous ulcerative infection of the gums, buccal mucosa, and eventually the cheeks and jaw. In newborns, fatal cases involving the perioral tissues, nasal areas, eyelids, and anal regions have been reported. Although mortality prior to the antibiotic era was 75 to 90 per cent, with the introduction of antibiotics and vigorous supportive care it has been lowered to closer to 10 per cent.[30]

Meningococcemia

During meningococcemia or meningococcal meningitis approximately two thirds of patients will develop skin lesions. Acute meningococcemia may present as an influenza-like illness associated with fever, malaise, myalgia, and arthralgias, followed by macular, morbilliform, urticarial, petechial, or purpuric lesions and profound hypotension. The petechiae are usually small and somewhat irregular, measure 1 to 2 mm in diameter, have a smudged appearance, and may have a slightly raised, pale grayish vesicular or pustular center. The trunk and lower extremities are the most common sites, but lesions may also appear on the face, palms, and soles, and the conjunctivae and other mucous membranes may have similar petechiae. More extensive hemorrhagic lesions are

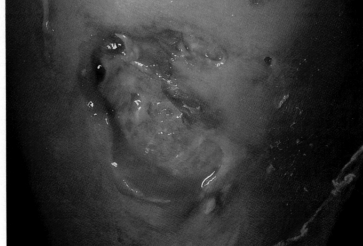

Figure 10–12. Necrotizing fasciitis. (Courtesy of Department of Dermatology, Yale University School of Medicine.)

seen in fulminant meningococcal infections, and a progressive increase on all areas of the body may be followed by coalescence of lesions to form large ecchymotic areas with sharply marginated borders. In overwhelming disease, necrotic bullae may advance to ischemic necrosis with sloughing, and the skin frequently becomes gangrenous in areas of extensive involvement (Fig. 10–13).

Chronic meningococcemia is rare in children. When it occurs, it is characterized by showers of erythematous macules and papules in association with fever, joint pain, and myalgia. Cutaneous lesions, seen in more than 90 per cent of cases, appear in crops coincident with or after a rise in fever. Lesions vary in character and size and are usually distributed on the trunk or the extremities, about one or more painful joints, or on areas of pressure. They generally appear as red macules and may evolve into tender papules or nodules with bluish or purpuric centers, often with ulceration.

Meningococcemia must be differentiated from gonococcemia, Henoch-Schönlein purpura, typhoid fever, rickettsial disease, erythema multiforme, purpura fulminans, and other bacterial septicemias. The cutaneous and visceral lesions in acute meningococcemia result from direct damage to capillaries and postcapillary venules; the purpura is caused by an acute vasculitis.

Diagnosis is suggested by a careful history and physical examination and can be confirmed by culture of the blood and cerebrospinal fluid. Isolation of meningococci from the nasopharynx is presumptive but not diagnostic. Petechial lesions can be smeared and examined for the presence of gramnegative diplococci and may be cultured for organisms. On histopathologic examination the walls of vessels may show necrosis; endothelial cells are swollen; lumina are often occluded by thrombi composed of platelets, erythrocytes, and fibrin;

and meningococcal organisms may be demonstrated in the lumina of vessels, within thrombi, in neutrophils, in perivascular spaces, and in the cytoplasm of endothelial cells.

The course of meningococcal infection is variable. In untreated cases the temperature is erratic, the symptoms of infection are persistent, and death nearly always occurs. Crystalline sodium penicillin G, in dosages of 100,000 to 400,000 units/kg/day administered intravenously in six divided doses is the treatment of choice. Chloramphenicol (100 mg/kg/24 hr given every 6 hours intravenously, with a maximum dose of 4 g/day) is an adequate alternative if the patient is allergic to penicillin; and a cephalosporin such as cefuroxime, cefotaxime, or ceftriaxone may be used if the patient's hypersensitivity is not anaphylactoid.

Gonococcemia

Gonococcemia is associated with lesions similar to those of meningococcemia and appears with bouts of fever, chills, arthralgia, and myalgia in patients with gonococcal septicemia. Skin lesions usually develop within 3 to 21 days of contact, are located principally on joints of the distal portions of the extremities, and usually appear as small erythematous or hemorrhagic papules, petechiae, or vesicopustules on a hemorrhagic and, at times, necrotic base (Fig. 10–14). Lesions usually heal spontaneously in 4 to 6 days.

The causative agent, *Neisseria gonorrhoeae*, may be demonstrated by smear or culture of early skin lesions, by specific immunofluorescent staining of vesiculopustular lesions, or by culture of the blood, genitourinary tract, or joint fluid on Thayer-Martin medium (chocolate agar with the addition

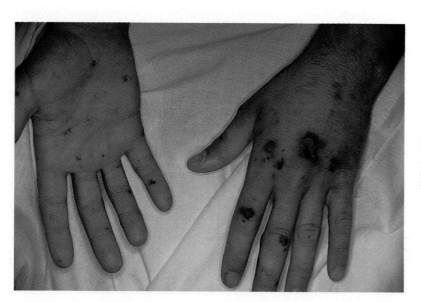

Figure 10–13. Purpuric lesions with sharply marginated borders on the hands of a patient with meningococcemia. (Courtesy of Department of Dermatology, Yale University School of Medicine.)

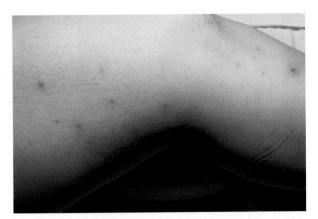

Figure 10–14. Gonococcemia. Small erythematous papules and vesiculopustules occur on a hemorrhagic base. (Courtesy of Department of Dermatology, Yale University School of Medicine.)

of antibiotics to inhibit normal flora and nonpathogenic neisserial organisms).

The treatment of choice is parenteral penicillin G in high doses (150,000 units/kg/day up to 10 million units of aqueous penicillin G daily) for 10 days. For patients sensitive to penicillin, the alternate drug of choice is tetracycline, 0.5 g every 6 hours for at least 7 days. Spectinomycin (Trobicin), the treatment of choice for individuals with gonorrhea who fail to respond to treatment with other antibiotics, is not recommended for the treatment of bacteremia due to this organism.

Staphylococcal Scalded Skin Syndrome

Staphylococcal scalded skin syndrome, previously known as Ritter's disease or pemphigus neonatorum, is a distinctive dermatosis caused by an epidermolytic toxin produced by certain strains of staphylococci (Figs. 10–15 and 10–16). In the United States, the majority of toxin-producing strains belong to phage group II staphylococci, usually phage types 3A, 3B, 3C, 55, or 71; in Japan, strains of other phage groups such as group 1 type 57 appear to be more prevalent.[31–33] Not to be confused with toxic epidermal necrolysis (Lyell's disease), when staphylococcal scalded skin syndrome is seen in adults it generally occurs in individuals with immunosuppression, renal impairment, or both.[34, 35] The reason for the increased incidence of staphylococcal scalded skin syndrome in infants and young children as opposed to adults appears to be related to the fact that most adults and 85 per cent of children older than 10 years of age have specific staphylococcal antibody, metabolic differences, or greater ability to localize, metabolize, and excrete the toxin, thus allowing the development of localized staphylococcal bullous impetigo (see Fig. 10–5) but limiting widespread bloodstream dissemination of the toxin.

Although cases of congenital and neonatal staphylococcal scalded skin syndrome have been reported,[36] the disorder usually begins in children, particularly in those younger than 5 years of age,

with malaise, fever, irritability, a generalized macular erythema, and a fine, stippled, sandpaper or nutmeg-like appearance that quickly progresses to a tender scarlatiniform phase over 1 or 2 days (Table 10–1). From the intertriginous and periorificial areas and trunk, the erythema and tenderness spread over the entire body, usually sparing the hairy parts. Affected children are extremely irritable, uncomfortable, and difficult to hold because of the extreme tenderness of the skin.

The exfoliative phase is heralded by exudation and crusting around the mouth and sometimes the orbits. Large fragments of crust often become separated, leaving radial fissures surrounding the mouth that give the disorder its characteristic and diagnostic appearance (see Figs. 10–15 and 10–16). Within 2 or 3 days, frequently over a period of a few hours, the upper layer of the epidermis may become wrinkled or may be removed by light stroking (often peeling off like wet tissue paper)—the characteristic Nikolsky sign (Fig. 10–17). Shortly thereafter, the patient develops flaccid bullae and eventual exfoliation of the skin (the desquamative phase). Unless further infection or

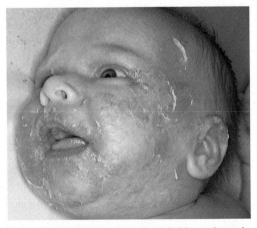

Figure 10–15. Staphylococcal scalded skin syndrome in an infant due to infection with coagulase-positive group II phage-type 71 staphylococci.

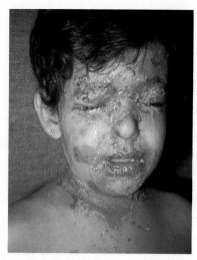

Figure 10–16. Scalded skin syndrome. Note characteristic facies with crusting about the eyes, nose, and mouth.

other skin irritation supervenes, the entire skin heals without scarring within 14 days of the onset of the process.

Diagnosis of staphylococcal scalded skin syndrome can be verified by isolation of coagulase-positive *Staphylococcus aureus*. In patients with this disorder the exfoliative (epidermolytic) toxin is disseminated from a primary infection site, usually in the nose or around the eyes. The organism may be recovered from pyogenic foci on the skin, conjunctivae, ala nasi, nasopharynx, stools, and occasionally the blood; the organism is not recovered from blisters or areas of exfoliation. When the diagnosis is indeterminate, differentiation from drug-induced toxic epidermal necrolysis and other bullous diseases can be made by a Tzanck preparation of scrapings from a blister base, examination of frozen sections of desquamating skin, or a cutaneous biopsy. In staphylococcal scalded skin syndrome, cleavage occurs in the epidermis, usually at the level of the granular layer; in toxic epidermal

Table 10–1. STAPHYLOCOCCAL SCALDED
SKIN SYNDROME

1. Generally in children younger than 5 years of age
2. Caused by an exfoliative (epidermolytic) toxin
   a. Usually group II staphylococci (phage types 3A, 3B, 3C, 55, or 71)
   b. Occasionally group I type 52 (in Japan)
3. Clinical features:
   a. Fever; tender erythematous skin
   b. Exfoliation with exudation and crusting around mouth, eyes, and paranasal areas
   c. Positive Nikolsky sign
4. Diagnosis
   a. Tzanck test—cleavage in the epidermis (usually at the level of the granular layer)
   b. Bacterial cultures positive for staphylococci (from skin, conjunctivae, ala nasi, nasopharynx, stools, or blood—*not* from blisters or areas of exfoliation)

necrolysis the split occurs in the upper dermis (below the dermal-epidermal junction).

Staphylococcal scalded skin syndrome has a mortality of slightly less than 4 per cent in children, with most fatalities occurring in newborns with generalized involvement. In adults, however, the mortality rate exceeds 50 per cent and is usually associated with coexistent disease or immunosuppressive therapy.[35] Treatment should be directed at the eradication of staphylococci from the focus of infection, thus terminating the production of toxin. Topical antibiotics are ineffective, and, since most of the organisms are resistant to penicillin and some are resistant to erythromycin, a penicillinase-resistant antistaphylococcal agent such as dicloxacillin is preferred. Dicloxacillin, 12.5 to 25 mg/kg/day in four equal doses, can be given to children weighing less than 40 kg (88 lb); for adults and children weighing 40 kg or more, 250 mg every 6 hours is usually an adequate dose. Although oral therapy is generally sufficient for limited bullous impetigo and in patients without evidence of sepsis or systemic involvement, parenteral antibiotics should be given to those who are severely ill or have extensive skin disease.

Toxic Shock Syndrome

Toxic shock syndrome, an acute febrile illness with multisystemic involvement, is a severe disorder characterized by myalgia, vomiting, diarrhea, pharyngitis, high fever, mucous membrane and conjunctival hyperemia, hypotension, a scarlatiniform rash, and, in severe cases, shock. Described by Todd and associates in 1978,[37] it appears that similar illnesses referred to as "staphylococcal scarlet fever" were reported as early as 1927.[38] Toxic shock syndrome, generally seen in female adolescents and young women, but also at times in men and young children, appears to be mediated by a blood-borne toxin (or toxins) produced by *S. aureus* at a focal site of infection. These include a phage group I *Staphylococcus aureus* (toxic shock syndrome toxin-1 [TSST-1]) in most patients and other toxins or toxin combinations such as enterotoxins A through C, epidermal toxin, yet unidentified toxins, and at times *Staphylococcus hyicus;* and a toxic shock–like syndrome has been described following infection by toxin-producing strains of group A streptococci (*S. pyogenes*).[39–41]

Although most case reports of toxic shock syndrome have been in women during the reproductive years of life, and 95 per cent of affected individuals have been women who used highly absorbent brands of tampons during the time of their menses, approximately 15 per cent of cases are not related to menstruation or tampon use. These include surgical wound infections; infections following submucous resection, sinusitis, rhinoplasty, and the use of nasal packings; ear-piercing; deep or superficial abscesses; infected

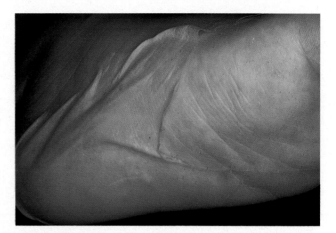

Figure 10–17. Tissue paper–like exfoliation on the foot of a child with staphylococcal scalded skin syndrome.

burns, abrasions, or insect bites; herpes zoster cellulitis; adenitis; bursitis; empyema; tracheitis; fasciitis; septic abortion; osteomyelitis; and infections in women during their postpartum period with mastitis or vaginal infection after cesarean section as well as vaginal delivery.[42, 43] In spite of much national publicity over the association of toxic shock syndrome with the use of highly absorbent brands of tampons, data regarding this linkage are poor, and it is still uncertain as to what roles tampons play in the pathogenesis of this disorder.[44]

Toxic shock syndrome is characterized by high fever, myalgia, vomiting, diarrhea, hypotension, severe prolonged shock, muscular or abdominal pain, mucous membrane and conjunctival hyperemia (Fig. 10–18), redness and swelling of the palms and soles (Fig. 10–19), and a diffuse scarlatiniform erythroderma that desquamates. The nails may be shed, and telogen effluvium may occur approximately 2 months later. The creatine phos-

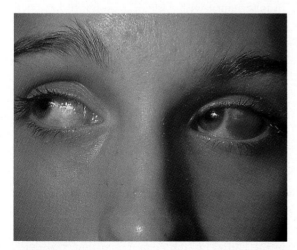

Figure 10–18. Conjunctival hemorrhage in a 13-year-old girl with toxic shock syndrome. This finding should not be confused with the bulbar conjunctival infection seen in patients with Kawasaki disease. (Courtesy of Andrew Margileth, M.D.)

phokinase level is often elevated (occasionally to extremely high levels), and some patients have been noted to have myoglobinuria. When tampons are found in place, they frequently emit a foul odor. Diffuse myalgia is almost always present, and many patients complain of exquisite skin or muscle tenderness when they are touched or moved.

Flaccid bullae with subepidermal blister formation have been seen in some infants with toxic shock syndrome, but subepidermal blisters per se are not histologic features of this disorder. Although it is well recognized that mild cases of toxic shock syndrome occur, case definition established by the Centers for Disease Control is based on specific criteria (Table 10–2). When the diagnosis is suspected a thorough search for a possible site of infection should be made and cultures should be obtained from a variety of sites (vagina, throat, nares, conjunctiva, blood, or stool, and any cutaneous or subcutaneous lesions, no matter how benign they appear).

The histopathology of skin lesions of toxic shock syndrome, although not always specific, is characterized by a superficial and interstitial mixed-cell infiltrate containing neutrophils, by foci of spongiosis containing neutrophils, and by scattered clusters of necrotic keratinocytes in the epidermis.

Because of the high morbidity and mortality rate, the treatment of patients with staphylococcal toxic shock syndrome should be aggressive with early initiation of antistaphylococcal antibiotics. Although the reported case fatality is still significant, with appropriate treatment the mortality has fallen from 15 per cent to 3 to 5 per cent. In severe cases, aggressive fluid replacement is essential and vasopressors to maintain normal blood pressure and other supportive measures such as respiratory assistance or dialysis should be used when necessary. If a tampon is present, it should be removed and vaginal irrigation with sterile water, saline, or povidone-iodine should be performed in an effort to remove organisms, toxins, and possible retained pieces of tampon. Because of a high (18 to 68 per

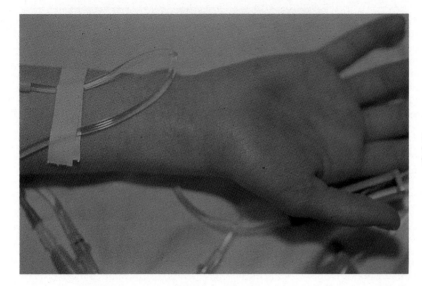

Figure 10–19. Swelling of the palm in a patient with toxic shock syndrome. (Courtesy of Andrew Margileth, M.D.)

cent) risk for recurrence, women with a history of toxic shock syndrome should avoid the use of tampons during subsequent menstrual periods, and those who prefer to continue to use tampons should have at least two negative cultures of the anterior nares and vagina before they resume this practice.[45]

Table 10–2. CRITERIA FOR THE DIAGNOSIS OF TOXIC SHOCK SYNDROME

1. Fever (temperature 102°F [38.9°C] or higher)
2. Rash (diffuse macular erythroderma)
3. Desquamation, particularly of the palms and soles (1–2 weeks after onset of illness)
4. Hypotension (a systolic blood pressure of 90 mm Hg or less for adults, and below the fifth percentile for children younger than 16 years); an orthostatic drop in diastolic blood pressure of 15 mm Hg or more with a change from lying to sitting; orthostatic syncope; or dizziness
5. Involvement of three or more of the following organ systems:
   a. Gastrointestinal (vomiting and diarrhea)
   b. Muscular (severe myalgia or elevated creatine phosphokinase levels)
   c. Mucous membranes (vaginal, conjunctival, or oropharyngeal)
   d. Renal
   e. Hepatic
   f. Hematologic (thrombocytopenia)
   g. Central nervous systems (disorientation or alterations in consciousness)
6. Negative results of following studies:
   a. Cultures of blood or cerebrospinal fluid
   b. Serologic tests for Rocky Mountain spotted fever, leptospirosis, and measles

Note: Toxic shock syndrome is probable when four or more major criteria, one of which is desquamation, or five criteria other than desquamation are fulfilled.

Chronic Granulomatous Disease of Childhood

Chronic granulomatous disease of childhood is an uncommon inherited disorder primarily affecting young males during the first year of life characterized by severe granulomatous reactions to a number of common bacteria that require phagocytic production of hydrogen peroxide to kill intracellular bacteria.[46–48] As many as nine different defects have been recognized. Six are inherited by X-linked transmission, and the remaining forms, in which females are also affected, are probably inherited by autosomal recessive transmission; in at least one family an autosomal dominant mode of inheritance with variable penetrance has been described.[49] Male patients seem to be more severely affected and outnumber females by approximately 7:1.

The earliest characteristic feature of chronic granulomatous disease is an eczematous eruption in infancy. Patients often have infectious eczematoid dermatitis, purulent miliaria, frequent pustules, paronychia, small indolent papules about the margins of the eyelids and lips, and apple-jelly granulomatous nodules about the face, particularly about the nares, the postauricular and periorbital areas, the scalp, the axillae, and the inguinal regions. Other clinical manifestations include pyoderma, stomatitis, conjunctivitis, osteomyelitis, chronic draining lymphadenitis (particularly in the cervical and inguinal regions), meningitis, pneumonia, peritonitis, septicemia, and abscesses or interstitial infiltrative granulomatous processes of the lungs, bone marrow, pericardium, and gastrointestinal tract; gastric outlet obstruction may at times be seen as the first clinical manifestation of the disorder.[50] The bacterial organisms usually associated with this disease are *Staphylococcus aureus, Klebsiella, Pseudomonas, Escherichia coli, Enterobacter aerogenes, Salmonella,* and *Serratia.* Fungal infections seen in patients with this disorder include those caused by *Candida, Aspergillus, Cryptococcus,* and *Nocardia* (Fig. 10–20).

The primary abnormality in chronic granulomatous disease (formally termed *fatal granulomatous disease of childhood*) is a defect in the ability of peripheral leukocytes (both neutrophils and monocytes) to kill bacteria. This defect is not a failure of the cells to phagocytize organisms but an abnormality in the intracellular killing process of the phagocytic cells. The leukocyte defect is detectable by the nitro-blue tetrazolium slide test. Whereas leukocytes from normal individuals reduce nitro-blue tetrazolium dye during phagocytosis, cells from patients with this disorder have an inability or marked decrease in the ability to reduce the dye from a colorless to a deep blue state during phagocytosis. Since some female carriers of the disorder, generally spared from severe infection, have been found to develop discoid lupus erythematosus, it is suggested that females with cutaneous lupus erythematosus with recurrent suppurative infections, or a family history of early childhood deaths or recurrent infections, have a nitro-blue tetrazolium test to rule out the possiblity of this disorder.[51]

Although treatment of chronic granulomatous disease in the past has been frustrating, aggressive diagnostic measures coupled with immediate and vigorous therapy have improved the prognosis of patients with this disorder. Genetic counseling, including carrier states in sisters of affected males, is recommended in all cases, and although the value of prophylactic antibiotics remains questionable, treatment with a bactericidal antibiotic specific for the patient's infecting organism and interferon gamma, alone or preferably in conjunction with antibiotics, appears to have a role in the prophylaxis and management of patients with this disorder.[52]

Erythrasma

Erythrasma is a superficial bacterial infection of the skin caused by *Corynebacterium minutissimum.* It is characterized by well-demarcated, reddish brown, slightly scaly to smooth shiny patches in the groin or axillae, or by maceration and scaling in the interdigital spaces of the toes. Fifteen percent of cases occur in children between 5 and 14 years of age. The incidence, however, increases with age and is noted most frequently during adolescence and adulthood.[53, 54] The most common sites of involvement are the genitocrural region and interdigital spaces, where the disorder may coexist with tinea cruris and tinea pedis. The disorder can also be found in intertriginous areas and, particularly in institutionalized individuals or diabetics, may be widely disseminated.[53]

Although erythrasma is frequently confused with a dermatophyte infection, with which it may coexist, it does not elicit an inflammatory response and does not progress to vesiculation. Erythrasma can often be differentiated from tinea infection by a characteristic coral red fluorescence under Wood's light (due to the production of porphyrins by the corynebacteria organisms in the stratum corneum). Since erythrasma may coexist with or may precede candidiasis, particularly in intertriginous regions, examination of the lesions for fungi is important.

Without treatment the disorder tends to persist indefinitely. Antibacterial soaps may help prevent recurrences of this disorder, and less restrictive clothing or other means to reduce friction and sweating may be helpful, particularly in the groin. Although tetracycline is frequently effective, the treatment of choice is oral erythromycin, 250 mg four times a day for 7 to 14 days (30 to 50 mg/kg/day in equally divided doses for young children).

Trichomycosis Axillaris

Trichomycosis axillaris is a relatively innocuous superficial infection of the axillary and, less commonly, pubic hairs that results in adherent white or yellow (occasionally red or black) concretions distributed irregularly along the hair shafts (Fig. 10–21). A diphtheroid organism (*Corynebacterium tenuis*) is believed to be the causative agent for this condition. The name trichomycosis axil-

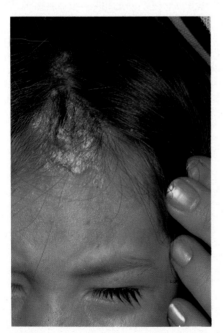

Figure 10–20. Chronic granulomatous disease with recurrent candidal granuloma of upper forehead and scalp.

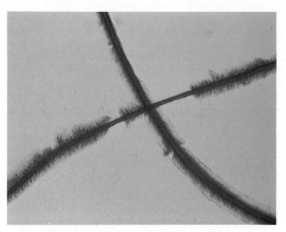

Figure 10–21. Trichomycosis axillaris with adherent concretions irregularly distributed along the hair shaft. (Courtesy of Joseph McGuire, M.D.)

laris, which implies a fungal etiology, accordingly is actually a misnomer.[55]

The disorder occurs only after puberty, owing to its association with axillary and pubic hair, but then occurs with equal frequency in all postpubertal age groups. It is common in adult males, but owing to the female practice of shaving axillary hair, is relatively uncommon in females. The most frequent sign of trichomycosis axillaris is the presence of red-stained perspiration on the clothing, and individuals with hyperhidrosis frequently complain of a particularly offensive axillary odor. The nodules of trichomycosis axillaris consist of bacterial elements embedded in an amorphous matrix and, except for the red form, produce a yellow or blue-white fluorescence under Wood's light examination.

Treatment consists of shaving the hairs of the affected areas, using deodorants (which decrease hyperhidrosis and growth of gram-positive bacterial flora), frequent washing with germicidal soaps, and the use of topical antibiotic formulations such as topical clindamycin or erythromycin used in the treatment of acne.[56]

Pitted Keratolysis

Pitted keratolysis is a superficial bacterial infection of the soles, lateral aspects of the toes, and at times the palms, characterized by violaceous or erythematous plaques, shallow asymptomatic round pits, crateriform depressions, or ulcerations. The causative organisms of this disorder are believed to be species of *Corynebacterium*, *Actinomyces*, *Micrococcus*, and *Dermatophilus congolensis*, or perhaps *Micrococcus sedentarius* or *C. minutissimum* alone or in combination with a *Corynebacterium* species.[57, 58] The disorder has worldwide distribution and occurs most commonly in hot tropical and semitropical climates where

hyperhidrosis, occlusive shoes or work boots, and prolonged immersion of the feet in water are predisposing factors.

Based on its distinctive appearance, diagnosis is usually not difficult and the disorder frequently resolves spontaneously after the affected area is removed from its moist environment. Patients with this disorder, therefore, should try to keep their feet as dry as possible, and the disorder generally responds to topical benzoyl peroxide or topical antibiotic agents (such as erythromycin or clindamycin), 40 per cent formalin ointment, Whitfield's ointment, or Castellani's paint, a combination of boric acid, phenol, resorcinol, fuchsin, and acetone in water currently available in a colorless formulation (Derma Cas Gel [Hill Dermaceuticals]).

Erysipeloid

Erysipeloid is an occupational infection of traumatized skin, particularly the fingers, hands, or arms of individuals who handle meat, raw saltwater fish, shellfish, or poultry, caused by *Erysipelothrix rhusiopathiae* (*E. insidiosa*), a gram-positive bacillus that can survive for months in soil or decomposed organic material. After an incubation period of 1 to 7 days, the disorder is usually seen as a localized cutaneous infection characterized by painful, violaceous, sharply demarcated, raised areas of cellulitis on the hands. In addition, a diffuse or generalized eruption in regions remote from the site of infection or regional lymphadenopathy and hemorrhagic vesicles may occur; and on rare occasions septicemia, purpura, endocarditis, septic arthritis, cerebral infarct, osseous necrosis, or pulmonary effusion may be seen as complications of this disorder.

The diagnosis of localized forms is best made by culture of biopsy specimens of cutaneous lesions, and blood culture will help confirm the diagnosis in patients with systemic forms of the disorder. Although the vast majority of patients with untreated localized erysipeloid tend to recover spontaneously within 3 weeks, antibiotics such as penicillin, orally or intramuscularly, in dosages of 2 to 3 million units daily, or erythromycin while awaiting sensitivity studies are recommended.[59]

Atypical Mycobacterial Infections

Abrasions from swimming pools or fish tanks, and at times cuts sustained from cleaning fish, may become infected with atypical mycobacteria (*Mycobacterium marinum*, formerly known as *M. balnei*) and possibly other unclassified mycobacteria. Most lesions are seen as solitary (occasionally multiple) subcutaneous nodules, ulcers, or abscesses at points of trauma, usually on the elbows (in 70 to 88 per cent of cases), knees, hands, feet, and, sometimes, the nose.

The classic clinical picture is characterized by

the appearance of reddish papules or pustules at a point of trauma that grow to be the size of a pea in about 3 weeks and tend to break down to form a crusted ulcer, dusky red or reddish brown papules, hyperkeratotic nodules, plaques, or suppurative ulcerations. Lesions tend to be solitary (multiple lesions are infrequent). They may remain in groups at the site of the abrasion or may ascend proximally from the point of trauma. Although they may at times resemble a sporotrichoid infection, lymphangitis and lymphadenitis do not appear. Healing usually occurs spontaneously in a few months, and although exceptional cases may persist for many years, almost all cases heal spontaneously within 1 or 2 years.

Mycobacterium marinum is an acid-fast nonmotile bacillus that often has transverse bands and is longer and wider than *M. tuberculosis*. The differential diagnosis of this disorder (often termed *swimming pool* or *fish-tank granuloma*) includes cellulitis, sporotrichosis, syphilis, cutaneous leishmaniasis, tularemia, foreign body reactions, cat-scratch disease, neoplastic skin tumors, and deep mycotic infections. The histologic changes resemble those of tuberculous granulation tissue, with a diffuse epithelioid cell reaction, tubercle formation without caseation, and, at times, scattered giant cells of the Langhans type. Cultures on Löwenstein-Jensen medium can help clarify the diagnosis; the greatest yield of positive cultures is obtained by direct inoculation of freshly biopsied material.

In all cases, a careful epidemiologic study should be performed to locate and eliminate the source of infection. Although there is no completely satisfactory treatment for this disorder, tetracycline, minocycline, doxycycline, and sulfamethoxazole-trimethoprim (Bactrim/Septra) or rifampin, alone or in combination with ethambutol, for periods of 6 weeks or more have been used with varying degrees of success. The use of hot soaks to the affected area twice daily for 30 minutes is also helpful.[60, 61] Electrodesiccation and curettage, cryosurgery with liquid nitrogen, or surgical excision may be satisfactory for early or small lesions, but recurrences are common. Studies suggest, however, that surgery is generally unnecessary, and since it may activate trivial lesions or cause extension of the infection into deeper tissues it may actually be contraindicated. Although rare cases of atypical myocbacterial infection have persisted for as long as 17 years, most lesions fortunately tend to heal spontaneously without scarring within 1 to 3 years.

Tuberculosis of the Skin

The incidence of cutaneous tuberculosis, until recently, has been declining the world over owing to the availability of effective antitubercular drugs, elimination of infected herds of cows that give milk, improvement in living standards, and vigorous preventive and therapeutic programs. However, it still occurs in some countries, and over the past several years the incidence of tuberculosis has shown an upward trend, presumably related to the human immunodeficiency virus epidemic, homelessness, and immigration.

Primary Tuberculous Complex. Primary tuberculous complex (tuberculous chancre) develops as a result of inoculation of *Mycobacterium tuberculosis* into the skin (occasionally into the mucosa) of an individual who has not previously been infected or who has not acquired natural or artificial immunity to the tubercle bacillus. Since tubercle bacilli cannot penetrate intact skin, this disorder occurs on exposed surfaces (the hands, most often the radial border of the dorsal aspect, the fingers, and, particularly in children, the lower extremities) through a small abrasion, insect bite, or cutaneous infection. After the bacteria have gained entry into the tissue, they remain at the site of infection, multiply, and, after 2 to 4 weeks produce cutaneous lesions.

The earliest lesion is a brownish red papule that develops into an indurated plaque that may ulcerate or scab over and is frequently associated with prominent regional lymphadenopathy.[62, 63] The ulcer may be quite insignificant or may enlarge to a diameter of up to 5 cm or more. The ragged reddish blue edges are undermined, and as they become older, they become more indurated. Thick adherent crusts and "apple jelly" nodules (lesions that on gentle pressure with a glass slide or hand lens [diascopy] result in a yellowish brown or "apple-jelly" color) may arise at the periphery of lesions. Healing generally takes place within a period of several weeks, with the regional lymphadenopathy remaining as the only indication of previous infection. This regional lymphadenopathy develops 3 to 8 weeks after the infection. The glands enlarge slowly and harden, are usually painless, and, after weeks or months, may soften and form "cold" abscesses, which form sinuses and perforate to the overlying cutaneous surfaces. With healing, scars may mark the sites of previous sinuses.

The histologic picture of tuberculous chancre (primary cutaneous tuberculosis) is that of an acute inflammatory reaction with numerous bacilli, epithelioid cells, and areas of necrosis and ulceration. After 3 to 6 weeks a more specific histologic picture, with caseation necrosis, epithelioid cells, lymphocytes, and Langhans giant cells, appears. During this stage the number of tubercle bacilli decreases, and organisms may no longer be demonstrable.

Lupus Vulgaris. Lupus vulgaris is the most common form of cutaneous tuberculosis. An extremely chronic, serious, and progressive disorder, it usually occurs in individuals with a high degree of sensitivity. Earlier studies suggested that it was essentially a disorder of childhood, but this predisposition has been overemphasized.

Although lupus vulgaris can arise at the site of a

primary inoculation, in the scar of scrofuloderma, or at the site of a vaccination with bacillus Calmette-Guérin (BCG), it generally appears in previously normal areas of skin. The disorder may affect any cutaneous surface, but over 90 per cent of lesions appear on the head and neck, usually originating on the nose or cheek as tiny brownish red papules with a soft consistency. As the disorder progresses, larger patches are formed by peripheral enlargement and coalescence of papules, with elevation of lesions and intensification of their brownish color (Fig. 10–22). As in tuberculous chancre, the infiltrate exhibits a characteristic apple-jelly color on diascopy.

The course of lupus vulgaris is slow, and lesions frequently remain limited to small areas for years, occasionally decades. Areas of involvement often tend to ulcerate, frequently healing by atrophic or hypertrophic scarring with gross disfigurement. This is especially prominent when nasal cartilages or eyelids are involved; the destruction of soft tissues, cartilage, and subsequent cicatricial changes frequently result in a "parrot-beaked" or "werewolf" appearance.

Lesions of lupus vulgaris must be differentiated from those of sarcoidosis, lymphocytoma cutis, lupus erythematosus, halogenoderma, leishmaniasis, leprosy, blastomycosis, coccidioidomycosis, and cutaneous malignancy. The histopathologic features consist of tubercles with epithelioid cells, Langhans giant cells, and a peripheral zone of lymphocytes. Caseation necrosis may be slight or absent, and tubercle bacilli are present, but in such small numbers that their demonstration is frequently difficult or impossible.

Scrofuloderma. The terms *scrofuloderma* and *scrofula* refer to tuberculous involvement of the skin by direct extension from underlying tuberculous lymph nodes or bones. A disorder of children and young adults infected from drinking milk containing tubercle bacilli, it has become exceedingly rare as a result of the routine pasteurization of milk

in the United States and Western Europe. Although scrofula from *M. tuberculosis* is rare today, draining lesions from atypical mycobacteria are not that uncommon.

Tuberculous scrofuloderma is seen most frequently over cervical lymph nodes, bones, and joints. Clinical manifestations include painless swelling in the parotid, submandibular, subclavicular, and lateral regions of the neck (Fig. 10–23). On the extremities and trunk the lesions may represent hematogenous spread or they may accompany tuberculous disease of the phalanges, joints, sternum, and ribs. The overlying skin is stretched, purplish, and depressed because of fixation to infected nodes, and, with time, ulcerations and draining fistulous sinuses develop. Untreated lesions of scrofuloderma may persist with little change for years, and when healing occurs, cordlike cicatricial bands overlying ulcerated regions or areas of otherwise normal-appearing skin may appear.

The histologic features of scrofuloderma consist of ulceration or abscess formation and tubercles, with caseation necrosis at the periphery and massive necrosis and abscess formation in the center of lesions. Plasma cells may be quite numerous in the surrounding inflammatory infiltrate, and tubercle bacilli may be detected by Ziehl-Neelsen stain.

Tuberculosis Verrucosa Cutis. Tuberculosis verrucosa cutis (warty tuberculosis) is an externally acquired, relatively uncommon inoculation type of tuberculosis in individuals who have had previous contact with *M. tuberculosis* and have thus acquired a degree of immunity and cutaneous hypersensitivity. The inoculation of tubercle bacilli occurs at sites of minor wounds or abrasions and generally appears in young or middle-aged persons whose occupations require the handling of tuberculous patients or tissues (physicians, laboratory attendants, veterinarians, medical students, nurses, butchers, or farmers) or by autoinoculation from sputum of a patient with active tuberculosis.

Lesions usually occur on the dorsal surfaces of the hands, on the fingers, and, in children, on the buttocks or lower extremities. Asymptomatic, they begin as small papules or papulopustules with a purple inflammatory halo. With time, they tend to become hyperkeratotic and wart-like and, with slow extension and growth, form a single verrucous plaque with an inflammatory border, papillomatous horny surface, and areas of pustule formation and suppuration. Multiple lesions may occur, but most areas of tuberculosis verrucosa are solitary; and although uncommon, tuberculous involvement of regional glands has been described.

The histologic picture shows acanthosis, hyperkeratosis, pseudoepitheliomatous hyperplasia of the epidermis, dense inflammatory dermal infiltrates, and abscesses consisting of polymorphonuclear leukocytes and lymphocytes. Epithelioid cells and giant cells are found in the dermis, but typical tubercle formation and caseation are un-

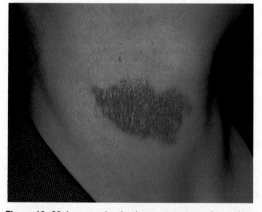

Figure 10–22. Lupus vulgaris, the most common form of cutaneous tuberculosis. An elevated brownish-red plaque is formed by coalescence of papular lesions. (Courtesy of Department of Dermatology, Yale University School of Medicine.)

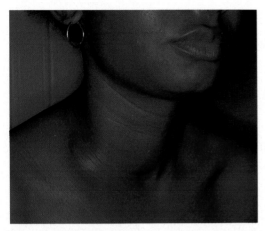

Figure 10–23. Scrofula (scrofuloderma). This painless tuberculous swelling is due to breakdown of tuberculous cervical nodes in the neck. (Courtesy of Department of Dermatology, Yale University School of Medicine.)

common. Although tubercle bacilli are not commonly found, they are more numerous than in lupus vulgaris and, occasionally, can be demonstrated.

Orificial Tuberculosis. Orificial tuberculosis (tuberculosis cutis orificialis) is a tuberculous disorder of the mucocutaneous junctions of the orifices (the nose, mouth, anus, urinary meatus, and genital orifices) due to autoinoculation of tubercle bacilli from tuberculosis of internal organs. A rare disorder, it affects males more frequently than females, and although it may occur in practically all age groups, it is relatively rare in childhood and most commonly seen in debilitated middle-aged or elderly individuals.

Lesions appear as shallow, oval, painful ulcers with a granulating base and undermined edges, with swelling, edema, and inflammation of the surrounding mucosa. Lesions are particularly painful, spontaneous healing is rare, and lesions often extend from the mucous membranes into contiguous cutaneous surfaces.

Painful ulcers of the mouth or other mucosal membranes in patients with visceral tuberculosis should arouse suspicion of this disorder. The histopathologic picture is not diagnostic and may merely reveal an ulcer surrounded by a nonspecific inflammatory infiltrate. The demonstration of tuberculous bacilli in cultures or histopathologic examination of material taken from clinically active mucosal ulcers is diagnostic.

Miliary Tuberculosis. Miliary tuberculosis (disseminated tuberculosis, tuberculosis cutis miliaris disseminata) is an extremely rare manifestation of fulminating pulmonary or meningeal tuberculosis. Cutaneous lesions are uncommon in infants and younger children and are seen even less frequently in adults. When present, the eruption is due to hematogenous spread in gravely ill individuals and is characterized by minute, symmetrically distributed, erythematous, ulcerated reddish brown macules, papules, vesiculopustules, or purpuric lesions. Children usually run a progressively downhill course, and the prognosis of this disorder is poor.

In miliary tuberculosis, the tuberculin test is usually negative, either because it is administered too early in the disease or because overwhelming infection prevents a positive reaction. Early histologic changes are nonspecific and often consist of necrosis, inflammation, and extravasation of erythrocytes. Numerous acid-fast bacilli are present; and if the patient survives, classic tuberculoid architecture with caseation eventually becomes apparent.

Treatment. The treatment of all forms of cutaneous tuberculosis is similar to that used for active pulmonary tuberculosis. Chemotherapy, to be adequate, must be continued without interruption for a minimum of 1 year or more depending on the bacteriologic and clinical findings. Isoniazid, p-aminosalicylic acid, streptomycin, ethambutol, ethionamide, pyrazinamide (an analogue of nicotinamide), and rifampin are the most effective antituberculous agents. All of the therapeutic agents, however, can be responsible for major toxic effects; and rifampin, when administered in excessive dosages, can result in striking reddish orange discoloration of the skin, red tears, red urine, histamine-related facial or periorbital edema, nausea, vomiting, and pruritus (the "red-man" syndrome).[64]

The Tuberculid Disorders

The term *tuberculid* is used to describe a group of recurrent cutaneous eruptions of unknown etiology. Originally considered to be related to toxins or possibly to an allergic response to tubercle bacilli, they are currently believed to be the result of hematogenous dissemination of mycobacteria from an internal focus into the skin, where they are destroyed by cutaneous defense mechanisms. Although the existence and pathogenesis of tuberculids is presently uncertain, most textbooks describe the following three "tuberculid" disorders: erythema induratum, papulonecrotic tuberculid, and lichen scrofulosorum. Lupus miliaris disseminatus faciei (formally described as a tuberculid) is probably more aptly described as a granulomatous disorder of the pilosebaceous units (see Chapter 6).

Erythema Induratum. Erythema induratum (Bazin's disease) is a chronic benign tuberculous vasculitis that typically occurs on the calves and occasionally thighs or heels of girls and young women. Although many authorities have contested the tuberculous origin of this condition, clinical and histopathologic features, and its response to antituberculosis therapy, seem to support a tuberculous cause.[65, 66] Lesions consist of symmetrical, chronic, painless but tender, deep-seated subcutaneous infiltrations that begin as subcutaneous plaques and nodules that eventuate in red or purple, tender, indurated masses that tend to ulcerate. The ulcers are irregular and shallow, have a bluish margin, rarely exceed 3 to 4 cm, and heal with an atrophic scar. The disease is chronic and recurrent; and in the majority of patients, a personal or family history of tuberculosis is reported. Patients have a positive tuberculin skin test, but mycobacteria are seldom recovered from lesions and there is no clinical or radiologic evidence of tuberculosis. The disease typically persists for years, with slow progression, relapses, and remissions.

Recurring bilaterally symmetrical nodules and ulcerations on the lower legs of young women are characteristic of this disorder. Histologic features include a tuberculoid infiltrate, inflammation of arteries and veins, and areas of caseation necrosis. Vascular changes consist of endothelial swelling, edema, hypertrophy of the vessel wall, occlusion of the lumen, fibrinoid necrosis, and vasculitis.

Many eruptions of erythema induratum undergo involution over a period of years simply as the result of supportive therapy, rest, careful bandaging, and elevation of the involved limbs. In cases in which active tuberculosis is considered present, chemotherapy should be carried out in the same manner as for other forms of tuberculosis.

Papulonecrotic Tuberculid. Papulonecrotic tuberculid, an eruption primarily seen in children and young adults, is characterized by symmetric crops of indolent, dusky-red, pea-sized papules and small nodules with central necrosis that heal spontaneously, with superficially depressed scars. Sites of predilection are the extensor aspects of the extremities, particularly the knees and elbows, the buttocks, and the lower trunk.

The histologic findings consist of small areas of necrosis in the upper dermis with extension into the epidermis. The inflammatory infiltrate surrounding the necrotic areas may be nonspecific but usually exhibits tuberculoid features. As a rule, bacteria cannot be demonstrated in the lesions. Epithelioid cells and occasional Langhans giant cells are present, and obliterative endarteritis and endophlebitis leading to thrombosis and occlusion of the vascular channels complete the picture.

The response of this disorder to antituberculous therapy appears to support a tuberculid nature.

Lichen Scrofulosorum. Lichen scrofulosorum is a disorder characterized by clusters of lichenoid papules on the trunk of children or young adults, with caseous tuberculous lymph nodes or bone or joint tuberculosis. Lesions are firm, pinhead-sized 1 to 5 mm or smaller, and skin colored or reddish brown. They are flat-topped follicular lichenoid papules. Asymptomatic, they are arranged in nummular groups, usually on the trunk, where they persist for months and slowly undergo spontaneous involution. Histopathologic examination reveals small tubercles that may show caseation, just below the epidermis, usually in relation to hair

follicles or eccrine ducts. Since sensitivity to tuberculin is often extreme, tuberculin tests should be performed only with high dilutions.

Spontaneous healing is the rule for this disorder.

Leprosy

Leprosy (Hansen's disease) is a chronic infectious disorder of worldwide distribution in which the acid-fast bacillus *Mycobacterium leprae* has a special predilection for the skin and nervous system. Although there is no universal agreement on the classification of leprosy, the disorder is currently divided into five or six types depending on the patient's degree of immunity to *M. leprae* (Table 10–3). At one end of the spectrum is the lepromatous (LL) form of the disorder, the disfiguring disease most familiar to the public. In this variant there is absence of cell-mediated immunity, the disorder is widely disseminated, and many bacilli are present in the tissues. Nodules or diffuse infiltrates, especially on the eyebrows, hands, and ears, produce a characteristic leonine facies, and patients are usually more infectious than those with other forms of the disorder.[67] At the opposite pole is tuberculoid leprosy (TT), a form that occurs only in patients with a very high degree of immunity. In this variant patients have only a single or occasionally a few large well-defined macules that show hypopigmentation and loss of sensation. The pe-

Table 10–3. CLASSIFICATION OF LEPROSY (IN ORDER OF DECREASING HOST RESISTANCE)

Group	Clinical Features
Tuberculoid (TT) (Mildest, high resistance)	A single or few localized anesthetic macules or plaques; few if any organisms; peripheral nerve involvement common
Borderline tuberculoid (BT)	Lesions similar to TT but more numerous; satellite lesions around larger lesions (at times); peripheral nerve involvement common
Borderline borderline (BB) (Intermediate dimorphous)	Features of both TT and LL; more lesions than BT; borders more vague; nerve involvement and satellite lesions common; many bacilli usually present
Borderline lepromatous (BL)	Multiple nonanesthetic symmetrically distributed lesions; late neural lesions; leonine facies
Lepromatous (LL) (most severe, low, or no resistance)	Generalized involvement (skin, mucous membranes, upper respiratory tract, the reticuloendothelial system, adrenal glands, and testes); no neural lesions until late; many bacilli in tissue

Note: The three intermediate forms (BT, BB, and BL) are clinically unstable and may pass from milder to more severe states and vice versa. Some authorities classify leprosy into six groups by subdividing the lepromatous (LL) form into polar (LLP) and subpolar (LLS) types.

ripheral nerves are thickened and palpable and as in the lepromatous type, anesthesia, trophic disturbances, and paralyses occur. In between, borderline forms of the disorder are seen (Fig. 10–24; Table 10–3).

Leprosy affects children as well as adults. The incubation period is typically very long (2 to 6 years), and incubation periods up to 40 years have been reported.[67] Early childhood forms reveal solitary lesions, which may occur on any exposed area of the skin. They appear as small, slightly raised hyperemic macules or groups of tiny papules surrounded by a blanched halo. Lesions are asymptomatic, tend to heal spontaneously after a period of 18 to 24 months, and leave a thin wrinkled hypopigmented scar. This is followed by a period of quiescence until puberty or early life when the condition may erupt into the more easily recognized forms of the disorder.

Leprosy should be suspected whenever a patient from a leprosy-endemic area presents with chronic skin lesions, skin anesthesia, thickened nerves, or eye complaints. The diagnosis is confirmed by the finding of acid-fast bacilli in skin smears or biopsy material.[67, 68] The histologic picture of leprosy features a granulomatous infiltrate containing large foamy histiocytes (lepra cells) in the epidermis. Acid-fast strains reveal the presence of the lepra bacilli, which frequently lie in bundles (like packs of cigars).

Sulfones are the treatment of choice for leprosy if there is no deficiency of glucose-6-phosphate dehydrogenase. Dapsone (4,4'-diaminodiphenylsulfone, Avlosulfon, DDS) is given in dosages of 50 to 100 mg/day for adults; for children, dosages of 1 mg/kg/day are recommended. Patients should be started on small doses and increased slowly in an effort to reduce possible reactions that might aggravate existing damage to vital areas such as motor nerves, eyes, or testes. Because resistance of *M. leprae* to dapsone has been reported, dapsone should not be used as monotherapy. Thus, rifampin (for adults, 600 mg/day; and for children, 10 mg/kg/day, not to exceed 600 mg/day) should be given with dapsone for 6 months for indeterminate, tuberculoid, and borderline tuberculoid disease, with close follow-up to detect relapses. Clofazimine, 50 mg/day for adults and 1 mg/kg/day for children (available from the National Hansen's Disease Control Center, Carville, Louisiana) should be added to the combination of dapsone plus rifampin for borderline, borderline lepromatous, and lepromatous disease and continued for at least 2 years and until skin smears are negative.[69]

Anthrax

Anthrax, an infectious disease caused by *Bacillus anthracis*, is occasionally transmitted to humans through exposure to infected animals or their byproducts. Although pulmonary, gastrointestinal, and oropharyngeal forms may occur, the cutaneous form (malignant pustule) is responsible for 95 per cent of the cases in the United States.[70, 71] Following an incubation period of 1 to 7 days, cutaneous anthrax is characterized by a painless lesion at the site of inoculation that progresses from a papule to a vesicle surrounded by a brawny, gelatinous, nonpitting edema (and at times small satellite vesicles or pustules), a feature that is practically pathognomonic of the disorder; necrosis occurs, and eventually a black eschar forms. Although some patients have no systemic manifestations, most develop headache, malaise, nausea, and low-grade fever during the course of the illness.

The diagnosis of anthrax can be made by (1) microscopic visualization of the causative organism on direct Gram-stained smear and cultures on blood agar of lesions or discharges; (2) detection of antibody to *B. anthracis* toxin by immunoblot; (3) a fourfold or greater titer rise in serum antibody between acute and convalescent sera by enzyme-linked immunosorbent assay (ELISA); (4) fluorescent antibody identification of the organisms in vesicle fluid, cultures, or tissue sections; or (5) histopathologic examination of a cutaneous punch biopsy specimen. The histopathologic features of cutaneous anthrax include epidermal necrosis, marked edema of the dermis, dilatation of blood vessels, diffuse degenerative changes of blood vessel walls, and identification of the anthrax bacillus with Gram stain, particularly in the necrotic tissue at the surface of the ulcer but also in the dermis.

Prior to the introduction of penicillin, cutaneous anthrax was fatal in approximately 20 per cent of patients. With effective treatment, however, mortality has been reduced to less than 1 per cent. In pulmonary and gastrointestinal anthrax and patients with septicemia and meningitis, the prog-

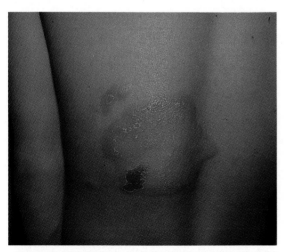

Figure 10–24. Infiltrated plaques on the back of a patient with lepromatous leprosy. (Courtesy of Department of Dermatology, Yale University School of Medicine.)

nosis is still poor (fatality rates range from 50 to 100 per cent for gastrointestinal anthrax to virtually 100 per cent for inhalation anthrax). Penicillin, the antibiotic of choice, administered by the oral route in a dosage of 50,000 units/kg/24 hr for 7 to 10 days is generally adequate for mild cutaneous anthrax. For systemic infection and cutaneous infection with signs of systemic toxicity, lesions on the head and neck, or patients with extensive edema, penicillin should be administered intravenously in a dosage of 300,000 to 400,000 units/kg/24 hr for at least 14 days. A combination of penicillin and streptomycin should be used for the treatment of meningitis or inhalation anthrax; and for individuals sensitive to penicillin and its derivatives, erythromycin, tetracycline (in individuals older than 8 years of age), or chloramphenicol can be used.

Cat-Scratch Disease

Cat-scratch disease is an acute, self-limiting infectious disorder of children and young adults caused by a pleomorphic gram-negative bacillus (*Afipia felis*). The disorder, characterized by a small edematous papule with central necrosis and regional lymphadenopathy, is generally transmitted to humans by cutaneous inoculation by a cat, in most instances a kitten younger than 6 months of age. Evidence of a cat scratch is present in about two thirds of patients, and a history of contact with a cat is present in more than 90 per cent of patients. Occasionally, the disorder has also been associated with dogs, rabbits, monkeys, fish hooks, fish bones, pins, wooden splinters, rose thorns, cactus spines, and porcupine quills.[72–74]

After an incubation period ranging from 3 to 30 days, usually between 7 and 12 days, one or more red papules measuring from 2 to 5 mm in diameter develop at the site of cutaneous inoculation (Fig. 10–25). Although often overlooked, with careful search, primary lesions can be found in over 90 per cent of patients and chronic lymphadenitis and regional lymphadenopathy (the hallmark of the disease) generally follow within 1 to 4 weeks (Fig. 10–26). Affected nodes are usually tender and the

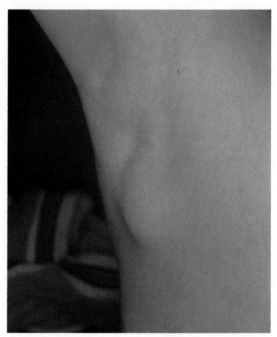

Figure 10–26. Axillary lymphadenopathy in the patient with cat-scratch disease shown in Figure 10–25.

overlying skin becomes warm, red, and indurated. Varying in size from 1 to 8 cm and persisting for 4 to 6 weeks (and up to 12 months in exceptional cases), 40 per cent of affected nodes eventually suppurate, occasionally with formation of a sinus tract to the skin surface. Additional features that may be seen at times with this disorder include Parinaud's oculoglandular syndrome (unilateral conjunctivitis with involvement of the homolateral preauricular lymph node), thrombocytopenic purpura, osteolytic lesions, pneumonitis, central nervous system involvement, and, in approximately 5 per cent of patients, dermatologic manifestations such as an erythematous nonpruritic maculopapular exanthem, erythema multiforme, erythema marginatum, erythema nodosum, or erythema annulare.[75, 76]

Diagnosis of cat-scratch disease is established by the combination of regional adenopathy, a history of a recent cat scratch, and identification of the organism by Warthin-Starry stain. A cat-scratch antigen skin test, which is prepared from suppurative lymph nodes of patients, although used by some investigators is not a licensed produce and is not available commercially[72] The histologic features of primary cutaneous lesions consist of acellular areas of necrosis in the dermis surrounded by histiocytic and epithelioid cells, giant cells, and eosinophils and identification of the gram-negative bacillus by Warthin-Starry silver stain.

The disease has an excellent prognosis and usually resolves spontaneously in 2 to 4 months. Tender, fluctuant nodes may be aspirated or drained with a 16- or 18-gauge needle (since the overlying skin is

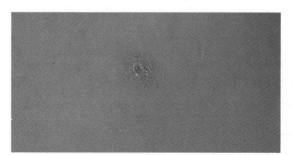

Figure 10–25. Cat-scratch disease. An erythematous crusted vesicular lesion is seen at the primary inoculation site on the chest of a 2-year-old boy.

usually too thin to permit injection of a local anesthetic, this can be done following the use of a local refrigerant spray such as ethyl chloride). Surgical removal of lymph nodes is not indicated, except in rare patients in whom the diagnosis is in doubt or repeated aspirations fail to relieve pain or resolution of the inflammatory process. Although antibiotics have generally not been shown to be effective in altering the course of cat-scratch disease, cefotaxime, intramuscular gentamicin, amikacin, tobramycin, rifampin, trimethoprim-sulfamethoxazole, erythromycin, netilmicin, mezlocillin, and ciprofloxacin (the latter is not recommended for the treatment of children) may at times be helpful, particularly if administered in the early stages of the disorder.[76, 77] Since animals believed to have transmitted the disease are not ill and the period of disease transmission appears to be transient, disposal or declawing of a cat or kitten believed to have been the source of the disease is unnecessary and not recommended.

Disorders Due to Fungus-like Bacteria

Actinomycosis and nocardiosis are disorders caused by actinomycetes, which are gram-positive organisms once thought to be closely related to fungi because of their tendency to grow in branches or mycelia in culture and infected tissue. Although these disorders can occur at any age and have been seen as early as the first month of life, most reported cases are seen in adults. Primary cutaneous infection is rare, and involvement of the skin and subcutaneous tissues is generally a result of contiguous spread from other sites or of secondary infection of injured skin and subcutaneous tissue, particularly in individuals who are debilitated or immunodeficient.

ACTINOMYCOSIS

Actinomycosis (lumpy jaw) is a chronic granulomatous disorder caused by *Actinomyces israelii*, an anaerobic gram-positive saprophyte of the tonsillar crypts or carious teeth, and rarely by *Actinomyces bovis* or other species. It is characterized by suppuration, painful induration, and the formation of multiple draining sinuses.

The disorder generally occurs at three sites: the cervicofacial area, the lungs, and the intestinal tract; two thirds of all human cases occur in the cervicofacial area. Cervicofacial actinomycosis, generally seen in individuals with poor oral hygiene and carious teeth, begins when the infecting organism invades a traumatized mucous membrane in the oral cavity. The primary lesion commonly develops as a swelling over the mandibular area and increases to form a brawny, erythematous lesion that breaks down to discharge serosanguineous or purulent material through multiple sinus tracts, from which the characteristic sulfuryellow granules consisting of masses of actino-

mycetes can be demonstrated. Destruction of bone, with periostitis and osteomyelitis, is common, and absence of regional lymph node involvement is characteristic.

Aspiration of the organism causes pulmonary infection, which progresses through the pleura, causing draining sinus tracts of the chest wall. The abdominal form develops in a similar fashion from the ileum, cecum, or appendix (through the gastrointestinal tract) and is seen as draining sinuses, tracts, or subcutaneous abscesses, extending to either the abdominal wall or the perineum. As in the skin and lungs, the disease progresses slowly, producing localized, granulomatous lesions, which may spread to involve adjacent soft tissue and bone, eventually presenting on the abdominal wall as a brawny erythematous mass with draining sinuses, from which the organism can be recovered.

Primary infection of other body sites may affect the urinary tract, central nervous system, bones, and joints. A localized form, known as mycetoma, occurs most frequently on the feet or ankles of individuals who walk around barefoot (see Chapter 13).

The diagnosis of actinomycosis is established by isolation and identification of the causative organism by strict anaerobic culture from tissue exudate of lesions. The diagnosis may also be confirmed by observation of the highly characteristic "sulfur" granules (groups of delicate filaments, frequently with club-shaped ends) in purulent or biopsied materials.

The course of the disease is prolonged, indolent, and characterized by closure of one sinus tract and the opening of another. Treatment consists of surgical incision and drainage of abscesses; excision of chronic, fibrotic, and avascular tissue; and chemotherapy, primarily with aqueous penicillin G, 150,000 to 300,000 units/kg/day, administered intravenously for 2 to 4 weeks, followed by oral penicillin for periods of 6 months or longer. Alternate antibiotics for patients who are allergic to penicillin include tetracycline or its derivatives minocycline or doxycycline (which should not be given to children younger than 9 years old), sulfonamides, erythromycin, clindamycin, streptomycin, a cephalosporin, and chloramphenicol.

NOCARDIOSIS

Nocardiosis is a severe acute or subacute, frequently fatal, primary pulmonary infection caused by an aerobic gram-positive, partially acid-fast, fungus-like organism, *Nocardia asteroides*. Acquired by the respiratory route with a focal infection in the lungs and frequent hematogenous dissemination, nocardiosis may be found in any organ of the body. Worldwide in distribution, the organism infects men more frequently than women (in a ratio of 3 : 1). The disease generally appears in individuals between 20 and 50 years of age, and although uncommon, it has been increasingly recognized in infants and children and is no longer considered a rarity.

Nocardiosis generally occurs through inhalation of contaminated dust, and the clinical picture is usually that of a primary pulmonary disease that resembles tuberculosis in its clinical and radiographic findings. In those instances in which the skin is involved (less than 15 per cent of cases) the most common lesions are abscesses of the chest wall with granulomatous lesions surrounding draining sinuses.[78] Although the disease is respiratory in origin, there may be dissemination to the brain, heart, spleen, and other organs; and lymphocutaneous infection with a typical chancriform syndrome, although relatively uncommon, has been described at the site of injury by a thorn or splinter.

Nocardiosis should be considered in obscure pulmonary and meningeal syndromes and chronic suppurative disorders of the bones or skin. The diagnosis is established by the presence of organisms in smears or cultures of sputum, aspirated material collected from lesions, or biopsied material. Unfortunately, the diagnosis is seldom established until the disease is far advanced. Accordingly, the prognosis is generally poor and mortality remains high.

Treatment consists of surgical incision and drainage of abscesses, excision and debridement of localized tissue, and sulfanomide therapy, up to 4 to 6 g/day in older children and adults (with blood levels maintained at 15 to 20 mg/dl), or trimethoprim-sulfamethoxazole (Bactrim/Septra), for 3 to 6 months. Immunocompromised patients or those with systemic disease should be treated for 6 to 12 months. If there is no response, erythromycin, ampicillin, streptomycin, tobramycin, cycloserine (Seromycin), amikacin, tetracycline, or minocycline (except in children younger than the age of 9 years, unless the benefits of therapy clearly outweigh the risk of dental staining) may be added. Even today, despite therapy, perhaps as a result of a delay in diagnosis and the debilitated state of patients with severely compromised host defenses, the overall mortality rate is approximately 50 per cent.

TREPONEMAL INFECTIONS

Syphilis

Syphilis is a contagious disease caused by the spirochetal organism *Treponema pallidum*. Transmitted principally through intimate contact with infectious lesions of the skin or mucous membranes, *T. pallidum* enters the body by the penetration of intact mucous membranes or minute abrasions of the stratum corneum. In congenital infection (prenatal syphilis) the fetus is infected by way of placental transmission from an untreated mother generally after the 16th week of pregnancy (for a discussion of neonatal syphilis, see Chapter

2). After a steady decline in the number of cases of syphilis in the early 1970s the incidence of syphilis is once again increasing, and the disorder continues to be an important health problem throughout the world.[79] Untreated acquired syphilis consists of the following five stages: (1) an incubation period of 3 to 4 weeks (outside limits 9 to 90 days); (2) a primary stage at the site of penetration by the treponemes, usually manifested by an initial syphilitic lesion or chancre, which lasts for 1 to 6 weeks; (3) a secondary stage 2 to 10 weeks later manifested by widespread cutaneous lesions and systemic symptoms, which last for 2 to 10 weeks; (4) a subclinical latent stage, with no symptoms or signs of the disease, that follows the disappearance of the eruption of the secondary stage, lasts for 1 to 40 years or more, and is diagnosable only by the presence of a reactive serologic test for syphilis; and (5) a tertiary or late stage (seen in about one third of cases) characterized by mucocutaneous, osseous, visceral, cardiovascular, and central nervous system lesions with, at times, debilitation and death.

Early syphilis (primary, secondary, and the first 2 to 4 years of latent syphilis) is infectious, tends to relapse, and seldom leads to scarring. The late latent (after the first 2 to 4 years of latent syphilis) and late stages, conversely, are considered noninfectious, rarely relapse, and often tend to be destructive and scarring.

Primary Syphilis. The initial lesion of syphilis appears at the site of penetration of the treponemes after an incubation period of 3 to 4 weeks following infection. The primary syphilitic lesion or chancre begins as a small red papule or crusted erosion, which in the course of a few weeks becomes round or oval and firm and indurated and develops a button-like papule or plaque a few millimeters to 1 or 2 cm in diameter with an erosive rather than ulcerative surface that is raw and exudes a serous fluid (Fig. 10–27). Since 95 per cent of all cases of syphilis are transmitted sexually, most syphilitic chancres appear on the genitalia. They are painless if free of secondary infection. They may occasionally be multiple but traditionally have been described as solitary lesions. In women, genital chan-

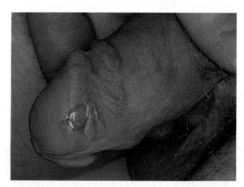

Figure 10–27. A chancriform plaque with an erosive surface as seen in primary syphilis.

cres are less commonly observed, because of their painless nature and frequent location on the cervix, and are generally detected only on intravaginal speculum examination.

Extragenital chancres may occur on any region of the body but most commonly occur about the anus or mouth, in the axillae or rectum, and on the lips, tongue, tonsils, eyelids, breasts, umbilicus, fingers, and toes. These may be single or multiple; and in the male homosexual, any anal lesion, even the smallest fissure or ulceration, must be viewed with suspicion. Regional lymphadenopathy usually accompanies primary syphilis. This may be unilateral or bilateral and is characterized by discrete, nonsuppurative, firm, freely movable painless nodes without overlying cutaneous change.

If left untreated, healing of the chancre generally occurs, and the lesion tends to disappear spontaneously after an interval of 3 to 6 weeks. The diagnosis of primary syphilis depends on the clinical picture, identification of *T. pallidum* by darkfield microscopy of serum from the lesion or fluid from an aspirated lymph node, by immunofluorescent staining of *T. pallidum* in serum from the lesion, by blood serologic tests, or by findings on cutaneous biopsy.

Serologic tests, which provide only indirect evidence of infection, are divided into nontreponemal and treponemal categories. The nontreponemal tests are flocculation tests (using cardiolipin, lecithin, and cholesterol as antigens) and include the Venereal Disease Reference Laboratory (VDRL) slide test, rapid plasma reagin card test (RPR), and the automated reagin test (ART). These tests provide quantitative results that are helpful as indicators of disease activity and useful for follow-up after treatment but may be falsely negative (nonreactive) in early primary, late acquired, and late congenital syphilis. Treponemal tests include the fluorescent treponemal antibody absorption (FTA-ABS) test, the microhemagglutination test for *T. pallidum* (MHA-TP), and the *T. pallidum* immobilization (TPI) test. Although the TPI test has been the standard against which all subsequent tests have been compared, since it is difficult, expensive, and only available in a few laboratories, it is rarely used today. The fluorescein-labeled antihuman antibody (IgM-FTA-ABS) test and its counterpart, the FTA-ABS double-staining (DS) test, are the most sensitive. Since the FTA-ABS test is expensive and time consuming, it is not recommended for general screening but for confirmation of positive nontreponemal tests and diagnosis of later stages of syphilis in which nontreponemal tests may be falsely negative. In summary, the nontreponemal antibody tests (VDRL, RPR, and ART) are useful for screening, the treponemal tests (FTA-ABS, MHA-TP) are used to substantiate the diagnosis, and quantitative nontreponemal antibody tests are used to assess the adequacy of therapy and detect reinfection or relapse.

Secondary Syphilis. Manifestations of secondary syphilis generally appear 6 to 8 weeks (occa-sionally up to 6 months) after the appearance of the primary lesion and, in almost one third of patients, the primary lesion is still present when the secondary eruption appears. The exanthem of secondary syphilis extends rapidly, and it is usually pronounced a few days after onset. It may be evanescent, lasting only a few hours or days, or, at times, it may persist for several months.

This stage is characterized by a generalized cutaneous eruption usually composed of brownish dull-red macules or papules (in dark-skinned individuals the lesions tend to be hyperpigmented). Lesions vary from a few millimeters to 1 cm in diameter; they are generally discrete and symmetrically distributed, and, particularly over the trunk, they tend to follow the lines of cleavage, often suggesting a diagnosis of pityriasis rosea. Papular lesions over the palms and soles which, because of the thickness of the stratum corneum, appear as macular or hyperkeratotic reddish brown hyperpigmented lesions, are often of help in the differentiation of these two disorders (Fig. 10–28). Papular lesions occasionally spread peripherally with central clearing to form ringed or arciform papulosquamous eruptions. These so-called annular syphilids are commonly seen on the face of darkskinned individuals (Fig. 10–29).

Of particular diagnostic significance is the presence of constitutional symptoms, namely general tiredness, a grippe-like syndrome consisting of headaches that are characteristically worse at night, sore throat, nasal discharge, lacrimation, arthralgia, generalized lymphadenopathy, and an associated anemia, leukocytosis with relative lymphocytosis, an increased sedimentation rate, and, at times, elevated alkaline phosphatase levels (with little to no jaundice). Particularly significant is swelling of lymph nodes that are otherwise seldom swollen, namely those of the posterior triangle of the neck and the occipital, auricular, paramammary, axillary, and supratrochlear nodes.

Other features of secondary syphilis include a patchy "motheaten" type of alopecia and mucous membrane lesions (mucous patches) that appear as slightly raised grayish white round or oval 5- to 10-mm plaques with central erosions and dull-red areolae. Mucous patches are painless and may occur on the buccal, labial, and lingual mucosae, the palate and tonsils, cervical and vaginal mucosae, labia minora, and the glans and corona of the penis. On the tongue the lesions are usually not eroded but appear as reddish flat papules with surfaces devoid of lingual papillae.

Condylomata lata are cutaneous lesions of secondary syphilis that occur in moist areas of the body, the folds of the genitalia, gluteal cleft, and medial thighs. They are highly infectious and must be differentiated from venereal warts (condylomata acuminata) that occur around mucocutaneous junctions and intertriginous areas. Syphilitic condylomata lata are highly infectious. They appear as smooth, moist, grayish pink 1- to 3-cm round or oval wide-based, often mushroom-like or

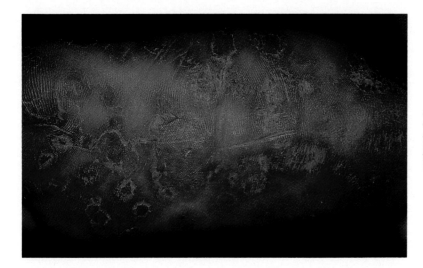

Figure 10–28. Reddish-brown crusted and hyperpigmented lesions on the plantar surface of the foot of a patient with secondary syphilis. (Courtesy of Department of Dermatology, Yale University School of Medicine.)

lobulated, papules, or nodules and, unlike condylomata acuminata, are never covered by digitate vegetations.

Cutaneous lesions of secondary syphilis usually heal without scarring, whether treated or not, within 2 to 10 weeks. Residual hyperpigmentation or hypopigmentation at sites of healed lesions may occur. Residual hypopigmentation on the skin of the neck has been termed *the necklace of Venus* (leukoderma colli).

The cutaneous manifestations of secondary

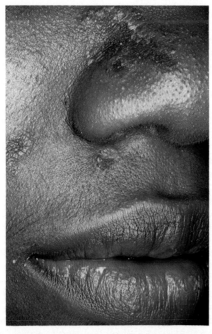

Figure 10–29. Arciform papulosquamous eruption (annular syphilids) as seen on the face of dark-skinned patients with secondary syphilis. (Courtesy of Department of Dermatology, Yale University School of Medicine.)

syphilis must be differentiated from pityriasis rosea, drug eruption, lichen planus, acute exanthemata, tinea versicolor, sarcoidosis, infectious mononucleosis, scabies, Mucha-Habermann disease (pityriasis lichenoides), urticaria pigmentosa, leprosy, and psoriasis.

Treponema pallidum is present in large numbers in the cutaneous and mucous membrane lesions of secondary syphilis. Early diagnosis and treatment, accordingly, is important to prevent progression of the disease and infection of contacts.

Latent Syphilis. Latent syphilis is that stage of the disease during which there are no clinical signs or symptoms of the disease or during which there are mild but generally unrecognized symptoms such as malaise, anorexia, headache, sore throat, arthralgia, and low-grade fever. A diagnosis of latent syphilis is usually established on the basis of a positive serologic test after other stages of syphilis have been ruled out by physical and cerebrospinal fluid examination.

Late Tertiary Syphilis. Late syphilis is divided into benign tertiary syphilis (gumma), neurosyphilis, and cardiovascular syphilis. It appears after a latent period of 3 to 12 years (often much longer) and is seen primarily in older individuals rather than children.

The cutaneous lesions of tertiary syphilis may appear as superficial nodules or deep granulomatous lesions that break down to form punched-out ulcers. Cutaneous nodular lesions can occur anywhere on the body but tend to favor the extensor surfaces of the arms, the face, and the back of the trunk. Characteristically they are asymptomatic and slow growing and consist of rounded, red to flesh-colored nodules that tend to be grouped in a rounded or polycyclic arrangement. These lesions may ulcerate, producing noduloulcerative lesions; and after the lesions heal, hyperpigmentation and atrophic scars may persist. Ulcerative lesions appear primarily on the face, scalp, arms, and presternal region. They begin as painless subcutaneous tumors, which may be single or multiple; and as the lesions increase in size, they eventuate in dull red lesions with punched-out ulcers.

Gummas may appear anywhere on the skin but most commonly appear on the scalp, the face (particularly the forehead, nose, and lips), the skin over the sternum, the thick portion of the calves, and the sternoclavicular joints. They usually develop at points of trauma, are almost always painless, and begin as soft cutaneous or subcutaneous swellings that tend to necrose at the center, forming one or more punched-out ulcers with a granulomatous base. When the hard or soft palate or nasal mucosa is affected, destruction is often pronounced and may lead to perforation of the affected areas. Large gummas may have several perforations and, as the intervening bridges of skin break down and necrose, lesions tend to produce arched or scalloped margins with arciform and geographic patterns.

Diagnosis. The diagnosis of syphilis depends on the history, clinical features, histopathologic findings, serologic studies, and, in primary and secondary lesions, darkfield examination. The fundamental histopathologic change consists of a predominantly perivascular infiltrate composed of lymphocytes and many plasma cells with endarteritis and endophlebitis. On special staining of primary lesions with Levaditi's stain, spirochetes can usually be found in the dermis and in and around the walls of capillaries and lymphatics. In secondary syphilis, the number of spirochetes varies with the type of lesions. In papular and condylomatous lesions they are almost always present in sufficient numbers to be found in the dermis and usually between epidermal cells. In macular lesions, spirochetes are few and generally cannot be found. In cutaneous lesions of tertiary syphilis, spirochetes may be demonstrated in early nodules or ulcerations but usually cannot be found in older gummatous lesions.

Treatment. The treatment of choice for all forms of syphilis (except congenital syphilis or neurosyphilis) is benzathine penicillin, 2.4 million units (1.2 million units in each buttock) intramuscularly, repeated in 1 week for a total of 4.8 million units, or aqueous procaine penicillin G, 600,000 units by intramuscular injection daily for 8 days (for a total of 4.8 million units). For patients allergic to penicillin, erythromycin (2 g/day for 15 days), tetracycline hydrochloride (2 g/day for 15 days), or minocycline (200 mg/day for 12 to 15 days) may be prescribed. Because of potential side effects, erythromycin estolate should not be used for syphilitic infection in pregnant women and tetracycline and minocycline should not be given to children younger than 9 years of age or to pregnant women.

Patients with early syphilis and congenital syphilis should have repeat quantitative, nontreponemal tests 3, 6, and 12 months after treatment. Patients with syphilis of more than 1 year's duration should also have a serologic test 24 months after therapy has been completed.

Pregnant women not allergic to penicillin should be treated with penicillin in dosages similar to those of nonpregnant patients appropriate to the stage of the disease, and erythromycin should be reserved for individuals with documented evidence of penicillin allergy (by skin tests or history of anaphylaxis) who are not candidates for penicillin desensitization. Infants born to women who have been treated for syphilis should be treated at birth if maternal treatment was inadequate, was indeterminate, or consisted of agents other than penicillin or if adequate follow-up of the infant cannot be assured. (Treatment of congenital syphilis is discussed in Chapter 2.)

Pinta

Pinta, a nonvenereal treponemal infection caused by *Treponema carateum*, occurs almost exclusively among the dark-skinned population of Central and South America and Cuba. It is transmitted by direct contact and is frequently seen in children of parents afflicted with this disorder. Although transmission by insects is possible, this mode of exposure is considered to be exceedingly rare.

There are three basic forms of this disease, termed *primary*, *secondary*, and *late*. The primary stage, seen on uncovered areas such as the face, arms, and legs, begins 7 to 10 days after inoculation as red papules, which, by proliferal extension, grow into oval or rounded erythematous squamous patches that measure up to 10 cm or more in diameter. Small papules frequently tend to become surrounded by satellite macules or papules that coalesce to form configurate patterns.

After a lapse of months or even years, secondary lesions appear. Clinically these lesions are hypochromic, pigmented, and erythematosquamous. In this secondary stage disseminated lesions appear. They, too, show proliferative enlargement, may coalesce, and are often covered with scales, frequently suggesting a diagnosis of psoriasis, eczema, tinea corporis, syphilis, or leprosy. The lesions always retain their tendency to merge and eventually become hypochromic, thus leading to the third or late phase of this disorder.

The late phase takes 2 to 5 years to develop and is characterized by irregular pigmentation with a range of different shades according to the site of deposition of melanin in the dermis. The pigmentary changes present a spotted and highly characteristic appearance. These lesions have an insidious onset, usually during adolescence or young adulthood. After a period of years hyperpigmented lesions become more widespread and are replaced by depigmented spots resembling vitiligo. The hypopigmented patches of pinta are located chiefly on the face, waist, and areas close to bony protuberances such as elbows, knees, malleoli, wrists, and backs of hands. Hyperkeratosis frequently develops on the legs, forearms, elbows, knees, and ankles, and the skin becomes thick and often scaly. Atrophy is the final stage of this disorder and is generally localized in the vicinity of the large joints.

Histopathologic lesions of the primary form of pinta show migration of lymphocytes through an edematous and slightly acanthotic epidermis. The basal layer shows loss of melanin and liquefactive degeneration. Numerous melanophores are found in the upper dermis, and a moderately dense infiltrate of plasma cells, lymphocytes, and some histiocytes and neutrophils are seen in the dermis. On silver staining, the causative organism can be seen between the cells of the epidermis. In the secondary stage, lesions show essentially the same histopathologic changes, and in the tertiary stage the hyperpigmented areas show atrophy of the epidermis with absence of melanin in the basal layer; the dermis presents accumulations of melanophages intermingled with a moderate number of lymphocytes. *Treponema* organisms are present in considerable numbers among the cells of the epidermis, and the depigmented lesions show atrophy of the epidermis, complete absence of melanin, no inflammatory infiltrate, and no *Treponema* organisms.

Diagnosis of this disorder is made by isolation of *T. carateum* by darkfield examination and serologic testing. In the late dyschromic stage of pinta, strongly positive serology is present in almost all patients with this disorder. The disease runs a progressive course and penicillin (a single injection of 1.2 million units of benzathine penicillin G) remains the treatment of choice for children older than 8 years of age; for children younger than 8 years of age, a dosage of 600,000 units is recommended.

Yaws

Yaws, caused by *Treponema pertenue*, is a nonvenereal treponemal disease endemic in many tropical regions that typically begins in childhood (usually before puberty) as a primary papule or group of papules. The initial lesion becomes larger (up to 2 to 5 cm in diameter and referred to as a "mother yaw") and undergoes ulceration, which persists for a period of a few months to as long as 3 years, after which healing occurs, leaving a residual hypopigmented scar. Weeks to months after the primary lesion, secondary yaws, relapsing frambesiform (raspberry-like) oozing papulomas that heal with little or no scarring, occurs. Hyperkeratotic involvement of the palms and soles is common, and painful fissuring of the palms and soles frequently develops. The latter may cause patients to walk on the sides of their feet, producing a characteristic gait known as "crab yaws."

Although the disorder generally terminates with the secondary stage, 10 per cent of patients develop a late tertiary stage in which gummatous lesions occur. Characteristically a disorder of children 10 years of age or older, late-stage lesions are usually solitary, ulcerated, and destructive and involve the skin, subcutaneous tissue, bone, and/or cartilage. Unlike the tertiary stage of syphilis, the central nervous and cardiovascular systems are not affected.

The diagnosis of yaws can be made on clinical manifestations in patients from endemic areas, darkfield demonstration of spirochetes from cutaneous lesions, and, since yaws like other treponemal disorders shares positive serologic tests for syphilis, a reactive serologic test for syphilis. Histopathologic examination of primary and secondary lesions reveals acanthosis and papillomatosis, pronounced edema of the epidermis, and neutrophils in the epidermis which lead to the formation of intraepidermal microabscesses; the dermis shows a dense dermal infiltrate composed primarily of plasma and mast cells and also neutrophils, lymphoid cells, histiocytes, fibroblasts, and eosinophils. The causative organism can be demonstrated in lesions during the first two stages of the disease by darkfield examination, and large numbers of organisms can be seen between the epidermal cells on silver impregnation. In late yaws, the ulcerative changes generally resemble those seen in late syphilis.

As in pinta, the treatment of choice is benzathine penicillin; tetracycline is the antibiotic of choice for penicillin-allergic patients older than 8 years of age and for women who are not pregnant. Although studies to determine the efficacy of erythromycin have not been reported, this may be an appropriate alternative for children younger than 9 years of age.

Lyme Disease

Lyme disease, first recognized in southeastern Connecticut in 1975 and named for the town where the first cases were identified, is an immune-mediated multisystemic disorder caused by the spirochete *Borrelia burgdorferi* and transmitted by *Ixodes* ticks. Initially called Lyme arthritis, the disorder begins in 60 to 83 per cent of cases with a cutaneous eruption (erythema migrans, erythema chronicum migrans) and may be followed several weeks to months later by cardiac, neurologic, or joint abnormalities, alone or in combination.[80, 81] Lyme disease is recognized throughout the United States, except for the states of Hawaii, Alaska, and Montana, and on all continents except South America and Antarctica.[82] In Europe, the disorder is usually manifested by erythema migrans and neurologic features; arthritis and carditis as well as neurologic features and erythema chronicum migrans (erythema migrans) are more common in the United States. In addition, linear morphea, lichen sclerosis et atrophicus, and lymphocytoma cutis have also been linked to the *Borrelia* spirochete; and in Europe *B. burgdorferi* has been associated with Bannworth's syndrome (focal radicular pains, lymphocytic meningitis, and cranial nerve *Borrelia* paralysis), lymphocytoma (usually during the second stage of the disorder), anetoderma, atrophoderma of Pasini and Pierini, eosinophilic fasciitis, progressive facial hemiatrophy, acrodermatitis chronica atrophicans (a late-stage disorder characterized by diffuse atrophic reddish or bluish red paper-thin skin on the backs of the hands and feet, forearms, and lower extremities seen almost exclusively in older individuals), and focal neuralgias near cutaneous lesions.[83–85]

The spirochete is borne by the tick vectors *Ixodes dammini* in the northeastern and midwestern United States, *I. pacificus* and *I. scapularis* in the western United States, *I. scapularis* in Georgia, and *I. ricinus* in Europe. In addition, the recognition of isolated cases over a wide distribution, including Australia where none of the currently recognized vectors are known to exist, suggest an even broader range of vectors and that *Amblyomma americanum* ticks may also be potential vectors of the disorder.[86] In the United States the white-tailed deer (*Odocoileus virginianus*) is the preferred host of the adult stage of the tick, and the white-footed mouse (*Peromyscus leucopus*) is the host for the larval and nymph stages. Other hosts include small mammals, rabbits, horses, chipmunks, raccoons, dogs, and birds. The finding of *B. burgdorferi* in deerflies, horseflies, and mosquitoes, coupled with the finding of deer ticks on 30 species of insects and birds, suggests that insects and birds may be temporary hosts and that avian and mammalian hosts may be responsible for the transmission of the disorder to previously unaffected areas.[87]

Lyme disease was originally described as having three clinical stages. However, since staging is somewhat arbitrary and stages may overlap or be skipped, the terms *early* (localized and early disseminated) and *late* (persistent) infection are currently used. The acute illness is characterized by malaise and easy fatigability (90 per cent of cases), fever and flu-like sensations (80 per cent), and cutaneous lesions of erythema migrans in approximately 75 per cent (60 to 83 per cent) of patients. Erythema migrans (*erythema chronicum migrans*), originally described by Afzelius in Sweden in 1909 and first reported in the United States in 1970,[88] usually begins 3 to 32 days after the tick bite as a red macule or papule that becomes annular and rapidly enlarges, often reaching a diameter of 20 to 68 cm, with an average diameter of 15 cm. It then usually disappears, generally within 2 months (Figs. 10–30 through 10–33). Because of the small pencil-point size of the *Ixodes* tick (see Chapter 14, Fig. 14–16), only about 30 per cent of patients recall having a tick bite. The annular border of erythema migrans is 1 to 3 cm wide, slightly edematous or flat, pink or red, and without epidermal change; occasionally smaller rings within the original lesion may suggest a diagnosis of erythema multiforme. Secondary rings are also commonly noted on other areas of the body (Fig.

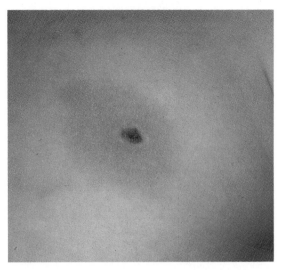

Figure 10–30. Erythema chronicum migrans (erythema migrans) with a central eschar at the site of a tick bite on the chest of a child with Lyme disease.

10–34). These lesions, seen in 25 to 50 per cent of cases, are smaller than the primary ring, lack indurated centers, wax and wane over shorter periods (independent of the initial lesion), and probably represent spirochetemia or lymphatic spread. Although erythema migrans may occur anywhere on the cutaneous surface, the thighs, groins, and axillae are particularly common sites of involvement. Lesions are usually asymptomatic but may be hot to touch, itch, sting, or burn; and evanescent flares may occur during subsequent attacks of arthritis.

Except for lethargy and fatigue, which may be constant and at times incapacitating, the early signs and symptoms of Lyme disease usually fade within 3 to 4 weeks (range, 1 day to 14 months)

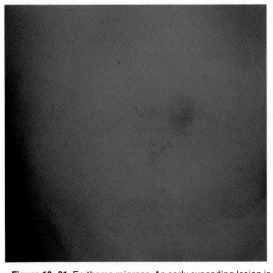

Figure 10–31. Erythema migrans. An early expanding lesion is seen on the chest of a child with early Lyme disease.

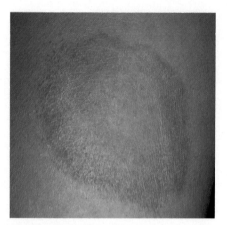

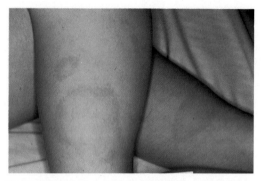

Figure 10–34. Multiple lesions of erythema migrans in a child with Lyme disease. (Courtesy of Steere AC, Malawista SE, Hardin JA, et al.: Ann. Intern. Med. 86:685, 1977.)

Figure 10–32. Erythema chronicum migrans (erythema migrans). An expanding ringed lesion with central clearing is caused by an *Ixodes* tick bite in a patient with Lyme disease.

even without therapy. Appropriate antibiotic therapy at the onset of Lyme disease, however, can shorten the duration of erythema migrans and associated symptoms and prevent the development of later stages of the illness (during this stage the disease can be cured in approximately 90 per cent of patients).

After several weeks to months, approximately 15 per cent of untreated patients in the United States manifest neurologic abnormalities, 5 to 8 per cent develop cardiac involvement, 50 per cent develop frank arthritis (single or intermittent attacks of joint swelling lasting from several days to 1 year) and about 10 per cent of the latter group develop chronic arthritis at times associated with permanent bone destruction.

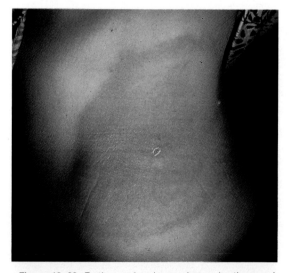

Figure 10–33. Erythema chronicum migrans (erythema migrans) with the area of the tick bite still visible in the center of the lesion. (Courtesy of William Burrows, M.D., reprinted from J. Assoc. Milit. Dermatologists 8:18–21, 1982.)

Symptoms suggestive of meningeal irritation frequently occur early in the illness (when erythema migrans is present) and, after several weeks to months, about 15 per cent of patients may develop frank neurologic abnormalities such as meningitis, cranial neuropathy (particularly Bell's palsy), and peripheral neuropathy, alone or in combination. Later neurologic abnormalities, which generally develop about 4 weeks after the onset of the acute illness, include encephalitis, chorea, cerebellar ataxia, peripheral neuritis, myelitis, Guillain-Barré syndrome, photophobia, blurred or double vision, lethargy, somnolence, emotional lability, depression, poor memory and/or concentration, dizziness, ataxia, sensory loss, oculomotor or limb weakness, involuntary movements, decreased hearing, and positive Babinski and/or Brudzinski signs. Neurologic complications generally have a favorable prognosis, and although most patients improve within a period of 2 weeks to 8 months without treatment, a few continue to manifest nerve palsy, eyelid weakness, poor memory, or behavioral changes for longer periods of time.

In 5 to 8 per cent of patients, cardiac abnormalities develop 3 to 21 weeks (generally about 5 weeks) after the tick bite. Complications are usually brief, last several days to 6 weeks, and rarely recur. The most common clue to cardiac involvement is tachycardia or bradycardia, with clinical features of myopericarditis, varying degrees of atrioventricular block (first-degree, Wenckebach, or complete heart block), and/or cardiomegaly with left ventricular dysfunction. Although the cardiac manifestations of Lyme disease often resemble those of rheumatic fever, complete heart block appears to be more common, myopericardial involvement tends to be milder, and the heart valves do not seem to be affected in individuals with Lyme disease.

When joint involvement develops it generally occurs within a few (4 to 6) weeks after the tick bite, while acute symptoms are still present, or up to 2 years after the onset of the disorder. If joint involvement occurs early in the illness, the typical pattern is one of migratory musculoskeletal pain, often with joint swelling; frank arthritis, however, generally does not begin until months after the onset of Lyme disease. In order of prevalence, the knee, shoulder, temporomandibular joint, ankle, hip, wrist, and small joints of the fingers are the most frequently involved. Affected joints are often hot (but rarely red), and they generally are much more swollen than painful. Joint fluid leukocyte counts range from 500 to 110,000 cells/mm^3 and consist predominantly of polymorphonuclear leukocytes. In about 10 per cent of patients with arthritis, joint involvement may become chronic with erosion of cartilage and bone.

Diagnosis. Although the diagnosis of Lyme disease is frequently difficult in nonepidemic areas, a history of erythema migrans followed within weeks to months by recurrent arthritis and/or neurologic and cardiac abnormalities is highly suggestive. Skin lesions of erythema migrans can be differentiated from those of tinea corporis and erythema annulare centrifugum by rapid peripheral expansion, lack of vesiculation and scaling along the peripheral border, microscopic examination of skin scrapings, and fungal culture. Histopathologic features of initial lesions are consistent with an arthropod bite and reveal edema of the papillary dermis and a heavy mononuclear infiltration, primarily lymphocytic, with plasma cells and eosinophils around the dermal blood vessels and cutaneous appendages (Fig. 10–35). Confirmation by serologic findings, although useful, is not yet standardized, and results often vary between different laboratories. Specific IgM titers peak between the third and sixth weeks following disease onset. Antibody titers of 200 or greater determined by ELISA, an indirect immunofluorescence assay (IFA) titer of 256 or greater, or a fourfold rise in titer is generally considered positive. Since sero-

logic response may be aborted by early antibiotic therapy and may be absent in patients with early disease, a negative result does not exclude the diagnosis. Polymerase chain reaction assay for detection of borrelial DNA holds promise as a more specific diagnostic technique, and, although diagnostic, culture of the organism from the skin, blood, or cerebrospinal fluid is difficult and generally impractical. The Western blot assay is more sensitive and specific than the ELISA test for detecting early Lyme disease, but its specificity in patients with late-stage disease or diffuse musculoskeletal complications is less clear. A combination of the two, however, can often help establish the diagnosis.[89]

Treatment. The most effective way to prevent Lyme disease, of course, is the development of an effective vaccine (currently under investigation) and to avoid exposure to *Ixodes* ticks and their habitats (tall grass, bushes, and woods, particularly from the months of April to October) in endemic areas. Individuals in possibly tick-infested areas should wear light-colored clothing, long-sleeved shirts with snug collars, socks pulled up over long pants, and closed shoes or boots. Tick repellents containing N,N-diethyl-m-toluamide (DEET) are effective but require repeated application every 2 hours, and spraying of clothing with permethrin-based repellents, currently available in lawn and garden centers or sports stores in the United States as Permanone Tick Repellent, is helpful. It should be noted, however, that DEET applied to the skin can be absorbed and that toxic and allergic reactions, including toxic encephalopathy, may occur following excessive or prolonged use, particularly in infants and children.[90] It is recommended, therefore, that this agent be used sparingly, only to exposed skin (but not on children's hands or faces), and washed off as soon as individuals come indoors. Since the *Ixodes* tick must be attached to the skin for at least 24 to 48 hours before infection is transmitted, daily inspection should be performed on individuals following exposure to potentially infested areas, and prompt tick removal, preferably be grasping the tick with a forceps, tweezers, or gloved fingers, within 18 to 48 hours of attachment will help prevent transmission of the disease.[91] Prophylactic antibiotic use is not recommended for individuals living in or traveling to potentially infested areas, and antimicrobial prophylaxis after a tick bite, even in endemic areas, is not warranted. Early treatment with tetracycline, doxycycline, penicillin, amoxicillin, or erythromycin, however, can shorten the duration of erythema migrans and its associated symptoms and can prevent or ameliorate subsequent arthritis and major complications.[92, 93] The current recommended treatment for early Lyme disease in children older than 8 years of age, nonpregnant women, and other adults is tetracycline (250 mg four times a day), doxycycline (100 mg twice daily), or amoxicillin (500 mg three times daily) for 10 to 30 days. For younger children, penicillin V or amoxicillin (25 to

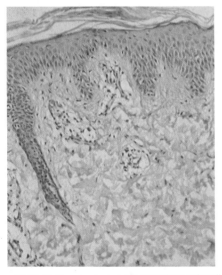

Figure 10-35. Erythema migrans. Mononuclear, primarily lymphocytic, perivascular infiltration (occasional eosinophils may also be noted).

50 mg/kg/day, with a maximum of 1 to 2 g/day), in three divided doses, is recommended. Although less effective, erythromycin (30 mg/kg/day, in divided doses up to 250 mg three times a day) for the young penicillin-allergic patient may be used as an alternative (Table 10–4). Occasional patients, generally those with severe disease, may develop intensification of symptoms during the first 24 hours after initiation of treatment. This Jarisch-Herxheimer–like reaction appears to occur more often with penicillin, amoxicillin, tetracycline, or doxycycline therapy than with erythromycin, presumably because of faster killing of larger numbers of organisms by these agents.[94] Although physicians should be aware of this reaction and forewarn patients that it can occur, the Jarisch-Herxheimer reaction usually disappears in 1 or more days and is not a reason to discontinue therapy.

Furthermore, since an association between Lyme disease in pregnant women and fetal malformations (cortical blindness, cardiac abnormalities, premature births, intrauterine deaths, neonatal rash, and perhaps syndactyly) have been noted,[95, 96] although *B. burgdorferi* could not be specifically linked to any of the adverse outcomes, this possibility warrants further surveillance. Pregnant women with Lyme disease or suggested Lyme disease should be treated with high doses of penicillin (penicillin V, 250 to 500 mg four times a day, or amoxicillin, 250 to 500 mg three times a day) for 10 days (or if penicillin allergy is suspected, erythromycin). Although there may be a role for intravenous penicillin in stage I Lyme disease in pregnant women with relatively severe symptoms, this approach requires further study and evaluation.

PROTOZOAL DISORDERS

Leishmaniasis

The term *leishmaniasis* refers to three different diseases caused by the protozoan parasite of the genus *Leishmania:* (1) cutaneous leishmaniasis (oriental sore, Delhi boil, Jericho sore) caused by *Leishmania tropica,* prevalent throughout tropical and subtropical zones of the world; (2) mucocutaneous (American) leishmaniasis, a somewhat similar disease caused by *L. braziliensis;* and (3) visceral leishmaniasis (kala-azar), caused by *L. donovani.* This terminology represents an oversimplification of the conditions but is maintained for descriptive purposes. Primarily a parasite of wild and domestic animals, for which humans are only accidental hosts, it is transmitted by various species of the *Phlebotomus* sandfly which harbor the flagellated form of the parasite in their gut.

Cutaneous Leishmaniasis. There are an estimated 12 million cases of leishmaniasis worldwide with approximately 400,000 new cases reported each year. Believed to be second only to malaria in world public health significance, as with so many other tropical disorders, increase in travel to endemic areas of South and Central America (and the Mideast as in Operation Desert Storm in 1991) has led to an increase in the number of cases of cutaneous leishmaniasis diagnosed in the United States.[97] In endemic regions, visceral leishmaniasis is seen in children more frequently than adults. The disease has an average incubation period of about 2 months, but this may vary from 2 weeks to more than a year and is seen primarily on an exposed area (generally the face). There are four clinically distinct forms of cutaneous leishmaniasis: (1) a moist or rural type, (2) a dry urban type, (3) a tuberculoid type, and (4) a lepromatoid type.

The moist or rural type first appears as a maculopapule that tends to enlarge slowly over a period of a few months to form a nodule, finally becomes ulcerated and crusted, and, after a period varying from several months to a year or longer, spontaneously resolves, leaving a depressed pigmented scar. The dry, urban, or later ulcerative form appears as a small brownish nodule, develops more slowly, and forms a slowly extending plaque 1 to 2 cm in diameter over a period of approximately 6 months (Fig. 10–36).[98] At this stage, a shallow ulceration appears in the center. It develops a closely adherent crust. Multiple secondary nodules may

---

Table 10–4. TREATMENT OF LYME DISEASE

Nonpregnant women, other adults, children older than 8 years:
  Tetracycline, 250 mg qid, *or* doxycycline, 100 mg bid, for 10 days to 3 weeks
Children younger than 8 years:
  Penicillin V, 250–500 mg qid (*or* 50 mg/kg/day) *or* amoxicillin, 250 mg tid (or 20 mg/kg/day)
For those allergic to tetracycline or penicillin:
  Erythromycin, 250 mg qid (or 30 mg/kg/day)
Late manifestations:
  Ceftriaxone, 2 g/day IV for 14 days
Neurologic complications:
  Penicillin, 200,000–300,000 units/kg, IV up to 20 million units/day for 14 days. Patients with mild neurologic symptoms can be treated in a manner similar to that given for early Lyme disease for up to 31 days
Lyme arthritis:
  Benzathine penicillin, 2.4 million units/wk for 3 weeks IM *or* penicillin G, 20 million units/day IV for 2 to 3 weeks. Adults with mild disease may be treated with oral doxycycline, 100 mg twice daily, *or* amoxicillin, 500 mg four times daily with probenecid, 500 mg four times a day, for 31 days
Cardiac disease with severe atrioventricular block:
  Penicillin G, 10 million units/day IV *or* ceftriaxone (2 g/day) for 10 days

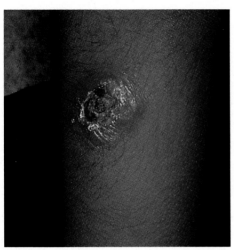

Figure 10–36. Cutaneous leishmaniasis. An erythematous crusted ulcerative plaque is evident on the arm of a 4-year-old child. (Courtesy of William Burrows, M.D.)

occur (much less frequently than in the moist form), and after a period of 8 to 12 months, the lesion begins to regress and the ulcer heals, leaving a scar. The average time from nodule to scar is about a year (twice that of the moist form). Disseminated cutaneous lesions that evolve into diffuse infiltrations and peripheral nerve involvement with anesthetic or hypoanesthetic skin lesions can also be seen in patients with cutaneous leishmaniasis. These are of particular significance since cutaneous leishmaniasis often exists in areas where leprosy is common and thus may prove to be a source of confusion or misdiagnosis.[99–101]

Chronic lupoid leishmaniasis (leishmaniasis recidivans), the result of a peculiar host reaction, is manifested by red to yellowish brown papules that appear in or close to a scar of an old lesion of cutaneous leishmaniasis, or in distant normal skin. Lesions coalesce to form a ring or plaque and spread peripherally on a common erythematous base, often resembling lupus vulgaris with apple-jelly nodules (the lupoid type). Leishmaniasis recidivans is exceedingly chronic and the nodules frequently reach considerable size.

A fourth, nonulcerating generalized form, the lepromatoid type, is characterized by papillomatous nodules over the entire body. Lesions resembling lepromatous leprosy occur chiefly on the face and ears. Patients with this form of the disorder present a public health hazard, since the skin is heavily infested and may act as a reservoir for transmission by the *Phlebotomus* fly.

Mucocutaneous (American) Leishmaniasis. Mucocutaneous (American) leishmaniasis, due to *L. braziliensis,* is an endemic and rural disease of damp forested country of Central and South America, generally seen in young men who work as foresters or as tea or cocoa plantation workers. The disorder is characterized by fungating oral and nasopharyngeal lesions that develop along with nodules and ulcers resembling those of the cutaneous form. The disease differs from the cutaneous form by its predisposition to involve mucocutaneous lesions, as the result of spread of the original cutaneous lesion (the uta form), or as a particularly mutilating form that develops several months after healing of the primary site (the espundia form). Lesions may heal without treatment in a period of 6 to 15 months. Secondary infection with regional adenitis and lymphangitis is common, and in some cases, nodular and vegetative (rather than ulerative) lesions may occur. Secondary mucous membrane lesions occasionally attack the nasal septum and nasopharynx. In this form the disorder may be characterized by erosions and necrotic ulcers, which if untreated, may erode soft tissue and cartilage, with resulting deformities of the nose, lips, and palate.

Visceral Leishmaniasis. Visceral leishmaniasis (kala-azar, dum-dum fever), caused by *L. donovani,* is endemic in Asia, along the Mediterranean coast, and in Africa and South America. In India the disease is transmitted from human to human; in some endemic areas of China, the Mediterranean countries, and Brazil, dogs represent an animal reservoir, their cutaneous lesions allowing the *Phlebotomus* fly direct access to the infected macrophages.

The diagnosis of leishmaniasis is based on the demonstration of nonflagellated (amastigote) intrahistiocytic forms (Leishman-Donovan bodies) in the stained smears of material scraped or aspirated from cutaneous lesions, lymph nodes, bone marrow, spleen, or cerebrospinal fluid; in stained tissue; by the Leishman skin test; or by culture of the organism on Nicolle-Novy-MacNeal (NNM) media. The *Leishmania* organisms appear as round or oval bodies 2 to 4 μm in diameter. Although visible in routine stains, they are best seen when stained with Giemsa's, Wright's, or Feulgen's stain. They have no capsules, but within the body there is a relatively large, peripherally placed round nucleus with a small rod-like paranucleus (the kinetoplast) tangential to the nucleus.

Delayed skin test reactions (the Montenegro or leishmania intradermal test) become reactive 3 months after infection and are positive in 95 per cent of cases of cutaneous leishmaniasis. The test is performed with a suspension of leptomonad antigen, 0.1 to 0.2 ml injected intradermally and read 48 to 72 hours later. The reaction reaches its maximum at 48 hours, appears as a papule or nodule formation with an erythematous halo, and disappears in 4 to 5 days. Although the Montenegro antigen is not available commercially in the United States, it is available from Instituto Adolfo Lutz, São Paulo, Brazil, and from Burroughs Wellcome, Barkhempstead, England.

Tissue may be cultured at room temperature on Schneider's *Drosophilia* medium, with various modifications, and on NNM media. In the fluorescent antibody test the patient's serum is layered on promastigote forms of *Leishmania* obtained from cultures on NNM media and counterstained with fluorescein-labeled antihuman γ-globulin. Unfortunately this test lacks sensitivity and gives a substantial number of false-negative results. Walton and associates have described a fluorescent antibody test for South American leishmaniasis. In this test the antigen used is the amastigote form of *L. braziliensis* obtained by osmotic lysis of cultured monkey kidney cells infected with *Leishmania* organisms. Since the amastigote form is the only one found in infected human tissue, it provides a more specific antigenic assay in serologic tests. Other tests include indirect hemagglutination, gel diffusion tests, ELISA, and identification of the amastigotes (Leishman-Donovan bodies) in tissue smears, touch smears, or skin biopsy specimens or as promastigotes in a parasite culture. When the touch preparation is done, samples should be taken from the edge of the active lesion, as far away from the crusting, ulceration, and secondary infection as possible.[102]

Amphotericin B is a highly effective leishmanicidal agent, but its toxicity has limited its use to cases resistant to antimony compounds. Antimony sodium stibogluconate (Solustibosan, Pentostam) (10 mg/kg, with a maximum 600 mg) administered intramuscularly into the buttocks for 6 to 10 days is effective for all forms of visceral leishmaniasis, and pyrimethamine is effective in cutaneous and mucocutaneous forms of the disorder. Pentostam is available in the United States from the Drug Service of the Centers for Disease Control. Also reported to be effective are electrosurgery; cryosurgery; surgical excision; topical antimony potassium tartrate; topical 15 per cent paromycin sulfate and 12 per cent methylbenzethonium chloride in white soft paraffin; oral ketoconazole; rifampin (300 to 600 mg/day for 3 to 15 weeks, alone or with isoniazid); metronidazole; allopurinol, alone or in combinatin with meglumine antimoniate; and pyrimethamine (Daraprim), a folic acid antagonist, although it is not listed as an antileishmaniasis agent in the manufacturer's instructions.[103–105]

References

1. Kligman AM, Leyden JJ, McGinley KJ: Bacteriology. J. Invest. Dermatol. *67*:161–168, 1976.

   Microflora of the skin, their ecology and role in disease.

2. Leyden JJ, Kligman AM: The case for topical antibiotics. Prog. Dermatol. *7*:11–14, 1973.

   Topical antibiotics are helpful in the therapy for superficial staphylococcal pyodermas. Although effective in the great majority of cases of streptococcal pyoderma, systemic antibiotics produce a swifter clinical response with fewer failures.

3. Leyden JJ: Mupirocin: A new topical antibiotic. J. Am. Acad. Dermatol. *22*:879–883, 1990.

   In a study of experimental infections in human volunteers, topical therapy with 2 per cent mupirocin was found to be more effective than oral erythromycin in suppression of both *Staphylococcus aureus* and *Streptococcus pyogenes*.

4. Dux PH, Fields L, Pollack D: 2% topical mupirocin versus systemic erythromycin and cloxacillin in primary and secondary skin infections. Curr. Ther. Res. *40*:933–940, 1986.

   Clinical trials demonstrate topical mupirocin to be more effective than erythromycin and cloxacillin in achieving clinical cure and improvement of primary skin infections.

5. May JA, Caldwell-Brown D, Lin AN, et al.: Mupirocin-resistant *Staphylococcus aureus* after long-term treatment of patients with epidermolysis bullosa. J. Am. Acad. Dermatol. *22*:893–895, 1990.

   Although topical mupirocin ointment has been shown to be especially useful in the treatment of epidermolysis bullosa by decreasing bacterial infection and promoting wound healing, the possibility of bacterial resistance must be considered.

6. Wannamaker LW: Medical progress: Differences between streptococcal infections of the throat and skin. N. Engl. J. Med. *282*:23–31, 78–85, 1970.

   The prevention of nephritis by penicillin preceding respiratory infection of streptococcal etiology is only partially successful; it is even more difficult and generally is unsuccessful in patients with streptococcal impetigo.

7. Anthony FB, Kaplan EL, Wannamaker LW, et al.: Attack rates of acute nephritis after type 49 streptococcal infection of the skin and respiratory tract. J. Clin. Invest. *48*:1697–1704, 1969.

   In study among children at the Red Lake Indian Reservation in Minnesota acute nephritis or unexplained hematuria developed in 28.8 per cent of children with type 49 streptococcal skin infection.

8. Lasch EE, Frankel V, Vardy PA, et al.: Epidemic glomerulonephritis in Israel. J. Infect. Dis. *124*:141–147, 1971.

   Penicillin treatment of streptococcal pyoderma, given early and adequately, succeeded in eradicating most of the streptococci, but did not prevent the appearance of glomerulonephritis nor have any effect on the course and severity of the nephritic process.

9. Ofuji S, Ogino A, Horio T, et al.: Eosinophilic pustular folliculitis. Acta. Derm. Venereol. *50*:195–203, 1970.

   A report of three Japanese young males with an eosinophilic pustular folliculitis on the face, chest, back, and extensor surfaces of the upper arm that extended to form annular lesions with a tendency toward central clearing and residual hyperpigmentation.

10. Lucky AW, Esterly NB, Heskel N, et al.: Eosinophilic pustular folliculitis in infancy. Pediatr. Dermatol. *1*:202–206, 1984.

    A report of five infants with recurrent crops of pruritic papulopustules of the scalp similar to those of adult patients with eosinophilic pustular folliculitis.

11. Jaliman HD, Phelps RG, Fleischmajer R: Eosinophilic pustular folliculitis. J. Am. Acad. Dermatol. *14*:479–482, 1986.

    A report of a 33-year-old American male with a 6-year history of eosinophilic pustular folliculitis and a review of the histopathologic features and management of the disorder.

12. Nishimaru M: Eosinophilic pustular folliculitis effectively controlled with topical indomethacin. Int. J. Dermatol. *28*:206, 1989.

    A report of a 36-year-old man with a 6-year history of eosinophilic pustular folliculitis in which a combination of oral and topical indomethacin was suggested as the treatment of choice for individuals with this disorder.

13. Colton AS, Schachner L, Kowalczyk AP: Eosinophilic pustular folliculitis. J. Am. Acad. Dermatol. *14*:469–474, 1986.

    A report of a 39-year-old Brazilian man with eosinophilic pustular folliculitis and a review of 23 cases in the literature.

14. Rasmussen JE, Graves WH III: *Pseudomonas aeruginosa*, hot tubs and skin infections. Am. J. Dis. Child. *136*:553–554, 1982.

In a report of eight teenage girls with *P. aeruginosa* folliculitis, the disorder developed within 24 to 48 hours after an all-night slumber party in which 1 to 3 hours were spent lounging in a hot tub.

15. Perrott DM, Johns RE, Jr., Jacobson J, et al.: An outbreak of *Pseudomonas* folliculitis associated with a waterslide—Utah. J.A.M.A. *250:*1259, 1983.

A report of 265 cases of *Pseudomonas* folliculitis following the use of a waterslide by 650 persons.

16. Salmen P, Dwyer DM, Vorse H, et al.: Whirlpool-associated *Pseudomonas aeruginosa* urinary tract infection. J.A.M.A. *250:*2025–2032, 1983.

A report of three previously healthy adults who developed *Pseudomonas aeruginosa* urinary tract infections within 2 days after whirlpool bath exposures.

17. Rose HD, Franson TR, Shem NK, et al.: *Pseudomonas* pneumonia associated with use of a home whirlpool spa. J.A.M.A. *250:*2027–2029, 1983.

A report of a 47-year-old man who developed *Pseudomonas aeruginosa* pneumonia following use of an inadequately sanitized whirlpool spa.

18. Green M, Fousek MD: *Hemophilus influenzae* type b cellulitis. Pediatrics *19:*80–83, 1957.

Six cases of cellulitis due to *Hemophilus influenzae* type b suggest a characteristic picture of tender, dusky bluish red discoloration in individuals with this disorder.

19. Thirumoorthi MC, Asmar BJ, Dajani AS: Violaceous discoloration in pneumococcal cellulitis. Pediatrics *62:*492–493, 1978.

Bluish red discoloration also can occur with cellulitis due to organisms other than *H. influenzae*, and *H. influenzae* cellulitis may occur in the absence of violaceous discoloration of the involved skin.

20. Amren DR, Anderson AS, Wannamaker LW: Perianal cellulitis associated with group A streptococci. Am. J. Dis. Child. *112:*546–552, 1966.

In a report of 10 children with perianal streptococcal infection, although none had clinically apparent pharyngitis, four of eight children who had throat cultures were found to be positive for *β*-hemolytic streptococci.

21. Spear RM, Ruthman RJ, Keating JP, et al.: Perianal streptococcal cellulitis. J. Pediatr. *107:*557–559, 1985.

In a report of 14 children with perianal streptococcal disease, signs and symptoms were present for an average of 6 months before the diagnosis was established.

22. Kokx MP, Comstack JA, Facklam RR: Streptococcal perianal disease in children. Pediatrics *80:*659–663, 1987.

In a study of 31 children, since the authors note that perianal streptococcal cellulitis is not truly a cellulitis, the term perianal streptococcal disease was suggested as a more appropriate name for this disorder.

23. Honig PJ: Guttate psoriasis associated with streptococcal perianal disease. J. Pediatr. *113:*1037–1039, 1988.

A report of four children with psoriasiform eruptions associated with group A *β*-hemolytic streptococcal infection of the perianal area suggests that physicians inspect the perianal area as well as the pharynx for possible streptococcal infection in children with psoriasis.

24. Hays GC, Mullard JE: Blistering distal dactylitis: A clinically recognizable streptococcal infection. Pediatrics *56:*129–131, 1975.

A report of 13 patients with blistering distal dactylitis, a *β*-streptococcal infection of the anterior fat pads of the distal portion of the fingers or thumbs.

25. McCray MK, Esterly NB: Blistering distal dactylitis. J. Am. Acad. Dermatol. *5:*592–594, 1981.

A report of two children with bullous *β*-hemolytic streptococcal infections of the volar fat pad of a distal phalanx.

26. Schneider JA, Parlette HL: Blistering distal dactylitis: A manifestation of group A *β*-hemolytic streptococcal infection. Arch. Dermatol. *118:*879–880, 1983.

In a report of blistering distal dactylitis the authors state that this disorder is probably much more common than generally recognized.

27. Parras F, Ezpeleta C, Romero J, et al.: Blistering distal dactylitis in an adult. Cutis *41:*127–128, 1988.

A report of a 23-year-old woman with blistering distal dactylitis serves as a reminder that this disorder can be seen in adults as well as children.

28. Umbert IJ, Winkelmann RK, Oliver GF, et al.: Necrotizing fasciitis: A clinical, microbiological, and histopathologic study of 14 patients. J. Am. Acad. Dermatol. *220:*774–781, 1989.

A comprehensive review of necrotizing fasciitis, its bacterial, clinical and histopathologic features.

29. Goldberg GN, Hansen RC, Lynch PJ: Necrotizing fasciitis in infancy: Reports of three cases and review of the literature. Pediatr. Dermatol. *2:*55–63, 1984.

A report of three infants with necrotizing fasciitis, its clinical features and management.

30. Lieberman J, Lynfield Y, Rosen P: Noma. Cutis *39:*501–502, 1987.

A report of an adult with noma and a review of the disorder.

31. Melish ME, Glasgow LA: The staphylococcal scalded skin syndrome—development of an experimental model. N. Engl. J. Med. *282:*1114–1119, 1970.

Seventeen children with exfoliative dermatitis associated with phage group II staphylococci.

32. Melish ME, Glasgow LA: Staphylococcal scalded skin syndrome: The expanded clinical syndrome. J. Pediatr. *78:*958–967, 1971.

Twenty-eight patients with dermatologic disease associated with phage group II *Staphylococcus* (staphylococcal scalded skin syndrome).

33. Sarai Y, Nakahara H, Ishikawa T, et al.: Bacteriological study on children with staphylococcal toxic epidermal necrolysis in Japan. Dematologica *154:*161–167, 1977.

Bacteriologic study of 21 infants and children with typical staphylococcal toxic epidermal necrolysis revealed that exfoliatin production is not necessarily restricted to staphylococcal phage group II.

34. Lyell A: Toxic epidermal necrolysis (scalded skin syndrome): A reappraisal. Br. J. Dermatol. *100:*69–86, 1979.

A review of toxic epidermal necrolysis and scalded skin syndrome confirms the fact that these two disorders are indeed distinctive and unrelated.

35. Ridgway HB, Lowe NJ: Staphylococcal scalded skin syndrome in an adult with Hodgkin's disease. Arch. Dermatol. *115:*589–590, 1979.

A report of staphylococcal scalded skin syndrome in a 68-year-old man with Hodgkin's disease who was receiving multiple drug chemotherapy.

36. Loughead JL: Congenital staphylococcal scalded skin syndrome: Report of a case. Pediatr. Infect. Dis. J. *11:*413–414, 1992.

A report of staphylococcal scalded skin syndrome in the first 24 hours of life in an infant born to a mother whose pregnancy was complicated by uterine infection, puerperal sepsis, and chorioamnionitis at the time of delivery.

37. Todd J, Fishaut N, Kapral F, et al.: Toxic-shock syndrome associated with phage-group-I staphylococci. Lancet *2:*1116–1118, 1978.

A report of a distinctive staphylococcal infection with multisystemic involvement in seven patients 8 to 17 years of age.

38. Stevens FA: The occurrence of *Staphylococcus aureus* in-

fection with a scarlatiniform rash. J.A.M.A. *88*:1957–1958, 1927.

Staphylococcal as well as streptococcal infections can be manifested by a scarlatiniform rash.

39. Todd JK: Toxic shock syndrome. Clin. Microbiol. Rev. *1*:432–446, 1988.

A comprehensive review of toxic shock syndrome, its epidemiology, pathology and clinical features.

40. Bartter T, Dascal A, Carroll K, et al.: Toxic strep syndrome: A manifestation of group A streptococcal infection. Arch. Intern. Med. *148*:1421–1424, 1988.

Although staphylococcal infection is recognized in the vast majority of patients with toxic shock syndrome, a similar clinical picture may be induced by streptococcal infection.

41. Rizkallah MF, Tolaymat A, Martinez JS, et al.: Toxic shock syndrome caused by a strain of *Staphylococcus aureus* that produces enterotoxin C but not toxic shock syndrome toxin-1. Am. J. Dis. Child. *143*:848–849, 1989.

A report of an 8-month-old infant with pneumonia and pleural effusion associated with clinical manifestations of toxic shock syndrome in whom the *Staphylococcus aureus* strain isolated from the pleural fluid produced enterotoxin C.

42. Green SL, La Peter KS: Evidence for postpartum toxic-shock syndrome in a mother–infant pair. Am. J. Med. *72*:169–172, 1982.

A report of a mother with postpartum toxic shock syndrome who was delivered of an infant with clinical features of toxic shock syndrome.

43. Rheingold AC: Nonmenstrual toxic shock syndrome: The growing picture. J.A.M.A. *249*:932, 1983.

A review of patients with toxic shock syndrome not related to menstruation and tampon usage.

44. Todd JK: Toxic shock syndrome: A perspective through the looking glass. Ann. Intern. Med. *96*:839–842, 1982.

Public opinion, press reports and attention to a disorder by the lay press (such as that which appeared to incriminate super-absorbent tampons in the etiology of toxic shock syndrome) should not divert scientific investigative processes and critical review.

45. Davis JP, Chesney PJ, Wand PJ, et al.: Toxic-shock syndrome: Epidemiologic features, recurrence, risk factors, and prevention. N. Engl. J. Med. *303*:1429–1435, 1980.

Ten of 38 patients with toxic shock syndrome had one or more recurrent episodes of the disorder during subsequent menstrual periods.

46. Berendes H, Bridges RA, Good RA: A fatal granulomatosis of childhood. Minn. Med. *40*:309–312, 1957.

The first definitive description of chronic granulomatous disease of childhood.

47. Bridges RA, Berendes H, Good RA: A fatal granulomatous disease of childhood: The clinical, pathological, and laboratory features of a new syndrome. Am. J. Dis. Child. *97*:387–408, 1959.

A description of four male children suffering from a previously unreported syndrome consisting of chronic suppurative lymphadenitis, hepatosplenomegaly, pulmonary infiltrations, and eczematoid dermatitis of characteristic distribution.

48. Quie PG, Kaplan EL, Page AR, et al.: Defective polymorphonuclear-leukocyte function and chronic granulomatous disease in two female children. N. Engl. J. Med. *278*:976–980, 1968.

Although chronic granulomatous disease in males is X-linked, studies of leukocyte function in two girls demonstrate that defective bactericidal function and metabolic abnormalities of polymorphonuclear leukocytes associated with chronic granulomatous disease are not necessarily familial and are not limited to male patients with X-linked hereditary disease.

49. Hitzig WH, Seger RA: Chronic granulomatous disease: A heterogeneous syndrome. Hum. Genet. *64*:207–215, 1983.

A review of chronic granulomatous disease of childhood and its variants with subdivisions on the basis of defective initiation of oxidative metabolism, defective NADPH, and genetic linkage.

50. Dickerman JD, Colletti RB, Tampas JP: Gastric outlet obstruction in chronic granulomatous disease of childhood. Am. J. Dis. Child. *140*:567–570, 1986.

In a review of 17 patients with chronic granulomatous disease of childhood, 23 per cent were found to have gastric outlet obstruction as the first clinical manifestation of the disorder.

51. Barton LL, Johnson CR: Discoid lupus erythematosus and X-linked chronic granulomatous disease. Pediatr. Dermatol. *3*:376–379, 1986.

In a review of three generations of a large kindred, three patients with evidence of chronic granulomatous disease and discoid lupus erythematosus led the authors to suggest an NBT test for females with discoid lupus erythematosus with a personal history of recurrent suppurative infections, a family history of early childhood deaths, or recurrent infections.

52. International Chronic Granulomatous Disease Cooperative Study Group: A controlled trial of interferon gamma to prevent infection in chronic granulomatous disease. N. Engl. J. Med. *324*:509–516, 1991.

In a randomized double-blind placebo-controlled study of 128 patients, interferon gamma was shown to be safe and effective as a prophylactic and therapeutic agent for patients with chronic granulomatous disease.

53. Somerville, DA: Erythrasma in normal young adults. J. Med. Microbiol. *3*:57–64, 1970.

A diphtheroid organism that fluoresced when grown in tissue culture media was demonstrated in 42 per cent of students with erythrasma of the toe webs.

54. Munro-Ashman D, Wells RS, Clayton YM: Erythrasma in adolescence. Br. J. Dermatol. *75*:401–404, 1963.

Coral-red fluorescence was detected in 17 per cent and *Corynebacterium minutissimum* was cultured from 14 per cent of individuals during an epidemic of erythrasma at a boys' boarding school.

55. Freeman RG, McBride ME, Dunkin WC, et al.: Pathogenesis of trichomycosis axillaris. South. Med. J. *62*:78–80, 1969.

Studies in seven patients with trichomycosis axillaris suggest corynebacterial infection of the hair cuticle (with rare involvement of the cortex or medulla) as the etiology of this disorder.

56. Bergman H: Trichomycosis of the scrotal hair. Arch. Dermatol. *120*:299–300, 1984.

Twice-daily applications of topical clindamycin lotion produced a cure of trichomycosis in 2 weeks.

57. Zaias N: Pitted and ringed keratolysis. J. Am. Acad. Dermatol. *7*:787–791, 1982.

An authoritative review of pitted keratolysis, its etiology, clinical features, and management.

58. Nordstrum KM, McGinley KH, Cappiello L, et al.: Pitted keratolysis: The role of *Micrococcus sedentarius*. Arch. Dermatol. *123*:1320–1325, 1987.

Studies of eight patients suggest that pitted keratolysis may result from *Micrococcus sedentarius*, a *Corynebacterium* species, or a combination of the two.

59. Barrett JH, Estes SA, Wirman JA, et al.: Erysipeloid. J. Am. Acad. Dermatol. *9*:116–123, 1983.

In a report of a 62-year-old man with erysipeloid (which developed following trauma to his hand while removing spoiled meat, fowl and fish from a refrigerator after a power failure), the authors recommended erythromycin as the drug of choice for the treatment of this disorder.

60. Loria PR: Minocycline hydrochloride treatment for atypical acid-fast infection. Arch. Dermatol. *112*:517–519, 1976.

    Three patients with swimming pool granulomas with an excellent response to minocycline hydrochloride within a period of 2 weeks.

61. Huminer D, Pitlik SD, Block C, et al.: Aquarium-borne *Mycobacterium marinum* skin infection: Report of a case and review of the literature. Arch. Dermatol. *122*:698–703, 1986.

    A report of a fish fancier with atypical mycobacterial infection and a review of 30 previous reports involving 44 cases acquired from aquariums in which sulfamethaxazole-trimethoprim or ethambutol hydrochloride plus rifampin appeared to be drugs of choice for treatment of this disorder.

62. Fisher I, Orkin M: Primary tuberculosis of the skin. J.A.M.A. *195*:314–316, 1966.

    A review of four childhood cases of primary inoculation type tuberculous chancre.

63. Kakahel KU, Fritsch P: Cutaneous tuberculosis. Int. J. Dermatol. *28*:355–362, 1989.

    An update on cutaneous tuberculosis, its clinical manifestations, diagnosis, and therapy.

64. Bolan G, Laurie RE, Broome CV: Red man syndrome: Inadvertent administration of an excessive dose of rifampin to children in a day-care center. Pediatrics *77*:633–635, 1986.

    A striking, glowing, red discoloration of the skin, facial or periorbital edema, nausea, vomiting, and pruritus of the head were found to be markers of rifampin toxicity in 19 children who inadvertently received five times the normal dose of rifampin for chemoprophylaxis of *Hemophilus influenzae.*

65. Rademaker M, Lowe DG, Munro DD: Erythema induratum (Bazin's disease). J. Am. Acad. Dermatol. *21*:740–745, 1989.

    A study of 26 patients helps support the hypothesis that erythema induratum is a true tuberculid.

66. Kuramoto Y, Aiba S, Tagamin H: Erythema induratum of Bazin as a type of tuberculid. J. Am. Acad. Dermatol. *22*:612–616, 1990.

    Three patients with erythema induratum who showed extreme tuberculin hypersensitivity reactions and a good therapeutic response to isoniazid.

67. Lauer BA, Lilla JA, Golitz LE: Experience and reason: Leprosy in a Vietnamese adoptee. Pediatrics *65*:335–337, 1980.

    This report of a 10-year-old Vietnamese adoptee with lepromatous leprosy serves to remind us that leprosy is a common infection among Vietnamese and, because of its long incubation period, may not become manifest for several years.

68. Sehgal VN, Sehgal S: Leprosy in young urban children. Int. J. Dermatol. *27*:112–114, 1988.

    A review of 1,460 cases of leprosy in children from infancy to 14 years of age.

69. Report of the Committee on Infectious Diseases: The Red Book, 22nd ed. American Academy of Pediatrics, Elk Grove, IL, 1991.

    Current recommendations for the control of infectious diseases in childhood.

70. Leads from the Morbidity and Mortality Weekly Reports: Human cutaneous anthrax—North Carolina. J.A.M.A. *260*:616, 1988.

    A report of cutaneous anthrax contracted in a North Carolina textile mill.

71. Kutluk MT, Sesmeer G, Kanra G, et al.: Cutaneous anthrax. Cutis *40*:117–118, 1987.

    Cutaneous anthrax on the face of a 9-year-old boy in Turkey who presumably developed the disorder following contact with an infected cow.

72. Margileth AM, Wear DJ, Hatfield TL, et al.: Cat scratch disease: Bacteria in the skin at the primary inoculation site. J.A.M.A. *252*:928–931, 1984.

    Small gram-negative pleomorphic bacilli in the inoculation site and lymph nodes of patients with cat-scratch disease suggest that the skin is the primary site of bacterial infection and proliferation.

73. Carithers HA: Cat scratch disease: An overview based on a study of 1,200 patients. Am. J. Dis. Child. *139*:1124–1133, 1985.

    An authoritative review of the clinical spectrum of cat-scratch disease.

74. English CK, Wear DJ, Margileth AM, et al.: Cat-scratch disease: Isolation and culture of the bacterial agent. J.A.M.A. *259*:1347–1352, 1988.

    A gram-negative bacterium isolated from lymph nodes and an increase in antibody titers in patients with cat-scratch disease help fulfill Koch's postulates confirming this bacterium's role in the etiology and pathogenesis of this disorder.

75. Margileth AM: Dermatologic manifestations and update of cat scratch disease. Pediatr. Dermatol. *5*:1–9, 1989.

    A review of the cutaneous manifestations of cat-scratch disease.

76. Shinall EA: Cat-scratch disease: A review of the literature. Pediatr. Dermatol. *7*:11–18, 1990.

    A comprehensive overview of cat scratch disease, its clinical features and management.

77. Margileth AM: Antibiotic therapy for cat-scratch disease. Pediatr. Infect. Dis. J. *11*:474–478, 1992.

    Although conservative symptomatic treatment is recommended for the majority of patients with mild or moderate cat-scratch disease, rifampin, ciprofloxacin, trimethoprim-sulfamethoxazole, and gentamicin may be considered for patients with severe disease.

78. Beaman BL, Burnside J, Edwards B, et al.: Nocardial infections of the United States, 1972–1974. J. Infect. Dis. *134*:286–289, 1976.

    A survey of members of the Infectious Diseases Society of America indicates that nocardial infections are not rare and that probably 500 to 1,000 cases are recognized in the United States each year.

79. Rolfs RT, Nakashima AK: Epidemiology of primary and secondary syphilis in the United States, 1981 through 1989. J.A.M.A. *264*:1432–1437, 1990.

    Statistics from the Centers for Disease Control revealed a 34 per cent increase in the incidence of syphilis in the United States between 1981 and 1989.

80. Steere AC, Malawista SE, Syndam DR, et al.: Lyme arthritis, an epidemic of oligoarticular arthritis in children and adults in three Connecticut communities. Arthritis Rheum. *20*:7–17, 1977.

    The first report of Lyme disease (initially termed Lyme arthritis), a previously unrecognized entity named for the community along the Connecticut River where the disorder was first studied and identified.

81. Burgdorfer W, Barbour AG, Hays SF, et al.: Lyme disease: A tick-borne spirochetosis? Science *216*:1317–1319, 1982.

    A comprehensive review of Lyme disease and evidence suggesting a spirochete as its etiologic agent.

82. Schmid GP: The global distribution of Lyme disease. Rev. Infect. Dis. *7*:41–50, 1988.

    As of 1985, Lyme disease had been described in the United States, Europe, North Africa, the Middle East, Turkey, Egypt, and Australia.

83. Asbrink E, Hovmark A, Hederstedt B: The spirochetal etiology of acrodermatitis chronica atrophicans Herxheimer. Acta. Derm. Venereol. *64*:506–512, 1984.

A borrelial spirochete similar to that seen in patients with Lyme disease appears to be the etiologic agent in some individuals with acrodermatitis chronica atrophicans.

84. Hovmark A, Asbrink E, Olsson I: The spirochetal etiology of lymphadenosis benigna cutis solitaria. Acta. Derm. Venereol. 66:479–484, 1986.

Clinical findings, serologic tests, and spirochetal cultures suggest that *Ixodes ricinus*–transmitted *Borrelia* spirochetal infection may be related to the etiology in some patients with lymphadenosis benigna cutis.

85. Aberer E, Kollegger H, Kristoferitsch W, et al.: Neuroborreliosis in morphea and lichen sclerosus et atrophicus. J. Am. Acad. Dermatol. 19:820–825, 1988.

Studies of nine patients with morphea and two with lichen sclerosus et atrophicus suggest that *Borrelia burgdorferi* may also be linked to morphea, lichen sclerosus et atrophicus, and acrodermatitis chronica atrophicans.

86. Schulze TR, Bowen SG, Bosler EM, et al.: *Amblyomma americanum*: A potential vector of Lyme disease in New Jersey. Science 224:601–603, 1984.

The tick *Amblyomma americanum* is incriminated as a possible vector of Lyme disease.

87. Anderson JF, Magnarelli LA: Avian and mammalian hosts for spirochete-infected ticks and insects in a Lyme disease focus in Connecticut. Yale J. Biol. Med. 57:627–641, 1984.

Epidemologic investigations reveal that birds and rodents may also be hosts for spirochete-infected ticks responsible for Lyme disease.

88. Scrimenti RJ; Erythema chronicum migrans. Arch. Dermatol. 102:104–105, 1970.

A migratory erythematous ring following a tick bite in a physician in Milwaukee appears to be the first recorded case of erythema chronicum migrans in the United States.

89. Rose CD, Fawcett PT, Singsen BH, et al.: Use of Western blot and enzyme-linked immunosorbent assays to assist in the diagnosis of Lyme disease. Pediatrics 88:465–479, 1991.

The combination of a positive ELISA and a positive Western blot is strongly associated with the presence of Lyme disease.

90. Gryboski J, Weinstein D, Ordway NK: Toxic encephalopathy apparently related to the use of an insect repellent. N. Engl. J. Med. 264:289, 1961.

A report of a child who developed encephalopathy as a result of prolonged and excessive use of DEET as an insect repellent.

91. Piesman J, Mather TN, Sinsky RJ, et al.: Duration of tick attachment and *Borrelia burgdorferi* transmission. J. Clin. Microbiol. 25:557–558, 1987.

Studies on hamsters and white-footed mice exposed to infected *Ixodes* ticks revealed that the proportion of hosts infected by *Borrelia burgdorferi* is correlated with the duration of tick attachment and that removal of the tick within 18 hours of attachment can prevent transmission of this infection.

92. Mast WE, Burrows WM Jr: Erythema chronicum migrans and "Lyme arthritis" (letter). J.A.M.A. 236:2392, 1976.

Clinical studies suggest that oral antibiotics can help in the treatment of patients with erythema chronicum migrans and Lyme disease.

93. Steere AC, Hutchinson J, Rahn DW, et al.: Treatment of early manifestations of Lyme disease. Ann. Intern. Med. 99:22–26, 1983.

A comprehensive evaluation of antibiotics and their efficacy in the early management of patients with Lyme disease.

94. Moore JA: Jarisch-Herxheimer reaction in Lyme disease. Cutis 39:397–398, 1987.

Although more commonly associated with the treatment of

syphilis, this report of a 22-year-old man with Jarisch-Herxheimer reaction serves as a reminder that this phenomenon can also occur as a side effect in individuals treated for the spirochetosis of Lyme disease.

95. Schlesinger PA, Duray PH, Burke BA, et al.: Maternal-fetal transmission of the Lyme disease spirochete, *Borrelia burgdorferi*. Ann. Intern. Med. 103:67–68, 1985.

An infant born to a mother who developed Lyme disease during the first trimester of pregnancy died at 39 hours of age; the infant had multiple cardiovascular malformations and postmortem evidence of spirochetal infection in the spleen, kidneys, and bone marrow.

96. Markowitz LI, Steere AC, Benach JL, et al.: Lyme disease during pregnancy. J.A.M.A. 255:3394–3396, 1986.

A review of 19 cases of Lyme disease in pregnancy with five adverse outcomes, including syndactyly, cortical blindness, intrauterine fetal death, prematurity, and rash in the newborn. Subsequent studies suggest that the syndactyly may have been an incidental finding rather than a consequence of spirochetal infection.

97. Furner BF: Cutaneous leishmaniasis in Texas: Report of a case and review of the literature. J. Am. Acad. Dermatol. 23:368–371, 1990.

A report of a patient with cutaneous leishmaniasis and a review of eight other cases of leishmaniasis acquired in Texas.

98. Kubba R, Al-Gindan Y, El-Hassan AM, et al.: Clinical diagnosis of cutaneous leishmaniasis (oriental sore). J. Am. Acad. Dermatol. 16:1183–1189, 1987.

A review of the clinical features of leishmaniasis, their frequency and diagnostic value.

99. Nelson DA, Gustafson TL, Spielvogel RL: Clinical aspects of leishmaniasis acquired in Texas. J. Am. Acad. Dermatol. 12:985–992, 1985.

A report of five patients with cutaneous leishmaniasis in which two patients showed spontaneous healing; one was cured by lesion excision, another by the use of topical antimony potassium tartrate 10 per cent cream, and one by two courses of intravenous sodium stibogluconate.

100. Satti MB, El-Hassan AM, Al-Gindany, et al.: Peripheral nerve involvement in cutaneous leishmaniasis: A pathologic study of human and experimental lesions. Int. J. Dermatol. 28:243–247, 1989.

Studies of a 37-year-old man with hyperesthetic lesions of cutaneous leishmaniasis and neural involvement in 13 mice following subcutaneous injection of *Leishmania major* promastigotes help clarify the pathogenesis of neural lesions in individuals with this disorder.

101. Sharma VK, Kaur S, Mahajan RC, et al.: Disseminated cutaneous leishmaniasis. Int. J. Dermatol. 28:261–262, 1989.

A report of a 50-year-old mason with disseminated cutaneous lesions of leishmaniasis on the upper abdomen, chest, thighs, arms, and back.

102. Berger RS, Perez-Figaredo RA, Spielvogel RL: Leishmaniasis: the touch preparation as a rapid means of diagnosis. J. Am. Acad. Dermatol. 16:1096–1105, 1987.

A report of a patient with leishmaniasis and the value of the touch preparation as a rapid means of diagnosis.

103. Livshin R, Weinraugh L, Even-Paz Z, et al.: Efficacy of rifampin and isoniazid in cutaneous leishmaniasis. Int. J. Dermatol. 26:55–59, 1987.

A study of 39 patients with leishmaniasis comparing treatment with rifampin alone versus rifampin in combination with isoniazid revealed no significant difference in efficacy with either regimen.

104. El On J, Livshin R, Even-Paz Z, et al.: Topical treatment of cutaneous leishmaniasis. J. Invest. Dermatol. 87:284–288, 1986.

Twice-daily topical applications of 15 per cent paromomycin sulfate and 12 per cent methylbenzethonium chloride in white soft paraffin cleared cutaneous lesions of leishmaniasis in 87 per cent of 67 patients within 10 to 30 days.

105. Martinez S, Marr JJ: Allopurinol in the treatment of American cutaneous leishmaniasis. N. Engl. J. Med. 326:741–744, 1992.

Allopurinol alone appears to be as effective as the combination of allopurinol and meglumine antimoniate (Glucantime) for the treatment of American cutaneous leishmaniasis.

11

VIRAL DISEASES OF THE SKIN

Viruses are ultramicroscopic organisms that grow only within living cells. The antigenic material responsible for viral immunologic reactions is present in the outer protein membrane (capsid) of the virus. The nucleoprotein core is composed of either deoxyribonucleic acid (DNA) or ribonucleic acid (RNA), but not both. Lacking ribosomes, viruses depend on the use of the host cells' enzyme systems. Here they blend with metabolic material of the host cell and frequently remain undetected until some stimulus incites the production of new viral particles.

Viral infections of the skin vary in their morphologic appearance from inflammatory changes (macules, papules, vesicles, or pustules) to localized growths or tumors composed of virus-laden cells and their products (warts, molluscum contagiosum, milkers' nodules). The following discussion will describe the common cutaneous viral disorders of childhood (warts, herpes simplex, herpes zoster, molluscum contagiosum), viral-like disorders of the oral mucosa, milkers' nodules, orf, and the acquired immunodeficiency syndrome.

HERPES SIMPLEX VIRUS INFECTION

The herpesvirus family includes the herpes simplex virus, Epstein-Barr virus, cytomegalovirus,

human herpesvirus-6 (HHV-6, the virus recently recognized as the etiologic agent of roseola), and the varicella-zoster virus. Herpes simplex, one of the most common viral infections of humans, is caused by *Herpesvirus hominus*, a relatively large (175 nm) DNA virus. There are two major antigenic types of *H. hominus*. Type 1 herpes simplex virus (HSV-1) has traditionally been associated with oral herpes (herpes labialis) and other nongenital infections, and herpes simplex virus type 2 (HSV-2) has been associated with genital infection. However, oral type 2 and genital type 1 infections have become increasingly common, probably as a result of increased orogenital sexual activity and promiscuity. Both HSV-1 and HSV-2 produce primary and recurrent infections. Although infections due to HSV-1 and HSV-2 are clinically indistinguishable, differentiation of the two types can be made by differences in growth in chick embryo cells, microneutralization tests, and immunofluorescent techniques.

Infections with herpesvirus are classified as primary or recurrent. Primary infections occur in exposed individuals without circulating antibodies. Following an incubation period of 1 to 26 days, with a median of 6 to 8 days, they may appear as subclincal or inapparent infections, characterized only by the development of antibodies to the virus, as a localized or generalized eruption, or as a serious systemic infection with encephalitis, hepatosplenomegaly, high fever, and, at times, serious sequelae.[1]

Recurrent herpes simplex infection occurs only in individuals who have been previously infected, either clinically or subclinically. It is characterized by repeated infections manifested by repeated eruptions of vesicles on an erythematous base at or close to one particular affected site. Cultures of herpes simplex virus in spinal ganglia of mice and humans suggest that the viruses are maintained in a quiescent state from which they may be reactivated, thus producing overt disease.[2, 3]

PRIMARY HERPES SIMPLEX VIRUS INFECTION

Herpetic Gingivostomatitis

The most common clinical presentation of primary herpesvirus-induced type 1 infection in children is gingivostomatitis. It may occur at any age, but its peak incidence is in children between the ages of 10 months and 5 years. The clinical presentation is frequently associated with fever, malaise, myalgias, inability to eat, restlessness, irritability, cervical adenopathy, and sudden high fever. After a brief incubation period of a few days (usually 2 to 12 days), vesicular lesions appear in the oral cavity (on and around the lips, along the gingiva, on the anterior tongue, and hard palate) and soon become eroded and ulcerated, appearing as 1- to 3-mm shallow gray ulcers on an erythematous base. The gums become mildly swollen, red, and ulcerated and bleed easily. Salivation may be present, there may be a foul odor to the breath, soreness and dysphagia may interfere with intake of food or fluids, and marked cervical lymphadenopathy is common. The fever generally subsides in 3 to 5 days, but the oral manifestations usually persist for 10 days to 2 weeks.

Although herpetic gingivostomatitis is often falsely diagnosed as Vincent's infection, hand-foot-and-mouth disease, aphthous stomatitis, erythema multiforme, or Behçet's disease, the diagnosis can be confirmed by the Tzanck test and viral cultures. Therapy consists of acetaminophen; lidocaine (Xylocaine 2 per cent viscous solution) to decrease pain and allow intake of fluids; avoidance of citrus fruits, juices, or spicy foods; intravenous fluids for individuals (generally infants or small children) who become dehydrated as a result of poor fluid intake; and, in severely affected or immunosuppressed patients, acyclovir or vidarabine.

Herpetic Keratoconjunctivitis

Primary herpetic infection of the eye often causes a severe purulent conjunctivitis characterized by edema, erythema, and vesicles, with opacity and superficial erosion or ulceration of the cornea. Marked pain, photophobia, lacrimation, and discharge from the eye is common, and the eyelids may be discolored or inflamed. Although uncomfortable and alarming in appearance, most cases of primary herpetic keratoconjunctivitis generally heal within a period of 2 weeks, without residual corneal damage. Occasionally, however, secondary infection and ulceration may persist and, in severe cases, may cause serious impairment of sight.

Herpetic keratoconjunctivitis should be treated by an ophthalmologist. Cortisone therapy, either topical or systemic, should be avoided, since it appears to facilitate increased dissemination of virus, with subsequent scarring and, in some cases, perforation. The treatment of herpetic keratoconjunctivitis has been facilitated by the use of idoxuridine, available as Herplex Liquifilm ophthalmic solution or Stoxil ophthalmic solution or ointment; trifluridine (Viroptic Ophthalmic Solution); acyclovir ophthalmic ointment; or vidarabine (Vira-A ophthalmic ointment). Although systemic antiviral therapy is usually not necessary for superficial herpetic keratitis, severe ophthalmic herpesvirus infections warrant systemic therapy with intravenous vidarabine or oral or intravenous acyclovir.[4]

Genital Herpes

Genital herpes, (herpetic vulvovaginitis and herpes progenitalis) currently the most common sexually transmitted disease in the United States, is increasing at an alarming rate in the adolescent and young adult population. With estimates of new cases approximating 500,000 to 750,000 a year, primary herpetic infection of the genitalia generally appears 2 to 8 days following contact with an infected individual.

Herpetic Vulvovaginitis. Although herpetic vulvovaginitis in young women and adolescent girls is usually caused by HSV-2 and associated with sexual contact, it may also occur with HSV-1 infection and in young children without sexual contact. Its presence in a young child, however, as with any disease that can be sexually transmitted, should raise the question of possible sexual molestation. The disorder is usually seen on the external genitalia and on the mucosa of the vulva, vagina, and cervix. Primary illness may be accompanied by fever, malaise, and regional lymphadenopathy and is characterized by burning vaginal pain, vesicles (often with a yellowish gray membrane), superficial ulcerations and extensive erosions on the vaginal mucosa, erythema, and edema of the mons pubis, perineum, labia majora and minora, and vagina, accompanied by intense soft tissue edema and exquisite pain. The vesicles generally measure 2 to 4 mm in diameter, but coalescence frequently results in the formation of larger ulcerations on the affected mucosal and cutaneous surfaces.

Treatment consists of warm sitz baths, topical anesthetics, topical antibacterial ointment to prevent secondary infection, and oral analgesics. The fever and constitutional symptoms subside within 5 to 7 days, lesions crust over and tend to resolve within 10 to 14 days, and healing is generally complete within 2 to 4 weeks. Although topical acyclovir (Zovirax ointment 5 per cent) applied five times a day for 5 to 10 days may be helpful in the treatment of primary genital herpes infection, it offers little benefit for patients with recurrent infection. For severe, persistent, or discomforting forms of the disorder, oral acyclovir (Zovirax), 200 mg five times a day for 5 to 10 days, can accelerate healing and shorten the duration of symptoms and viral shedding.[5]

Herpes Progenitalis. Although rare in young children, herpes progenitalis has also become increasingly common in male adolescents and young adults. Usually but not necessarily associated with HSV-2, herpes progenitalis most commonly involves the penile shaft and less frequently the glans, urethra, or scrotum. It is manifested by single or multiple painful vesicular eruptions that are transformed to painful shallow ulcers covered with exudate (Fig. 11–1). Urethral discharge is uncommon. When it occurs, it should suggest the possibility of another etiology, such as a gonococcal or chlamydial infection. In addition, genital, anal, and rectal lesions are especially common among homosexual men; and when genital or perianal lesions are present in young children, one should always consider the possibility of sexual abuse.

The severity of herpes progenitalis depends on the patient's previous history. If it is a primary infection, systemic symptoms can be severe and the duration is close to 2 or 3 weeks; in recurrent infections the disorder usually runs its course in about 8 days.

Treatment consists of topical analgesics, open

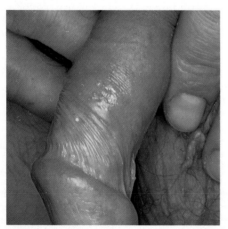

Figure 11–1. Herpes progenitalis. Multiple painful vesicles and ulcerations on the penile shaft, usually but not necessarily associated with herpes simplex type 2 infection.

wet compresses with Burow's solution or tap water, and topical antibiotics to help prevent secondary infection. Topical acyclovir (Zovirax ointment) may be helpful in the treatment of primary genital herpes but is of little value in recurrent disease; and, as in herpetic vulvovaginitis, oral acyclovir can shorten the duration and ease symptoms during a recurrent or primary infection and may be used prophylactically for patients with frequent recurrent genital HSV infection.[5–8]

Neonatal Herpes

Neonatal herpes usually develops when infants are born vaginally to mothers who have genital herpes. Like other herpetic infections this disease varies considerably in severity, with a wide spectrum of illness ranging from death or recovery with severe central nervous system involvement or ocular damage to a mild or asymptomatic infection with complete recovery (see Chapter 2, Figs. 2–22 and 2–23).

Kaposi's Varicelliform Eruption

Kaposi's varicelliform eruption is generally seen as a form of HSV infection in infants with atopic dermatitis but may also be seen in patients with Darier's disease. It is characterized by the sudden appearance of umbilicated vesicles distributed principally in the areas of the dermatitis (see Chapter 3, Figs. 3–17 and 3–18). The treatment of eczema herpeticum requires maintenance of adequate hydration, control of fever, and prevention of bacterial superinfection. Lesions frequently resemble an extensive burn. Topical application of silver sulfadiazine is beneficial, and in patients with severe viral infection, the systemic administration of vidarabine or oral or intravenous acyclovir should be considered (see Chapter 3).

Herpetic Whitlow

Primary cutaneous herpes may be found anywhere on the cutaneous surface. Herpetic whitlow is a special type of cutaneous inoculation herpes. Seen primarily in physicians, dentists, dental hygienists, and nurses who work in the mouth or genital regions of patients with herpetic lesions, the virus is inoculated into the skin of one or more fingers, causing a superficial vesiculopustular or extremely painful deep vesicular eruption that forms a honey-combed, bullous, whitish blue swelling (Fig. 11–2).[9] The pain usually subsides in 10 days, but the disorder takes about 3 weeks to resolve.

Diagnosis is assisted by Tzanck test preparations of vesicular lesions and viral culture. Systemic antibiotics and surgical drainage are ineffective. Analgesics may be prescribed as needed. Drilling of the nail to relieve pressure followed by com-

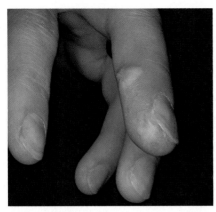

Figure 11–2. Primary cutaneous inoculation herpes (herpetic whitlow). A bullous swelling on the finger of a house staff physician was acquired from a patient with herpes simplex infection.

presses helps reduce inflammation, and exposure to the air; topical applications of ether or of Castellani's paint, and/or topical antibiotics may help prevent scarring, secondary bacterial infection, and loss of the overlying nail. In severe cases, a 5- to 10-day course of oral acyclovir (200 mg five times a day) can relieve symptomatology and hasten healing.[10]

Herpes Gladiatorum

Herpes gladiatorum is a term used to describe a widespread primary inoculation HSV infection occurring in contact sports enthusiasts, such as wrestlers or rugby players, who abrade their skin and come into contact with active HSV lesions on the skin or mucocutaneous surface of their opponents. Patients often present with systemic manifestations such as fever, malaise, anorexia, weight loss, and regional lymphadenopathy. The disorder, usually seen on the head, trunk, or extremities, is manifested by scattered groups of vesicular lesions on an erythematous base (sometimes associated with edema and pain) and regional lymphadenopathy. In addition to the treatment of individuals with this disorder, it is necessary to educate wrestlers, parents, and coaches and to increase their awareness of herpes gladiatorum as a potential health risk.[11]

RECURRENT HERPES SIMPLEX VIRUS INFECTION

Clinical Manifestations. Recurrent HSV infection appears in previously infected individuals in whom the herpesvirus remains latent. On reactivation, a recurrent infection ensues. Triggering mechanisms believed to be responsible for reactivation include febrile illness, menstruation, emotional disturbances, gastrointestinal upset, sun-

burn, or local trauma. It is not clear where the virus resides during the latency period between attacks, but it appears to be the regional nerve ganglion. From here it is activated or triggered by any of the above factors and spreads distally to the skin.[2]

Recurrent infections differ from primary infections in the smaller size of vesicles, their close grouping, and the usual absence of constitutional symptoms. They occur most commonly on the lips, perioral region, cheeks, or chin but may occur in any cutaneous area (Figs. 11–3 through 11–8). Grouped herpetic vesicles generally appear at or near previous areas of involvement; and, in some instances, patients may develop an associated herpes simplex lymphangitis. Following an initial period of itching, stinging, or burning (a few hours to 2 or 3 days prior to the eruption), the area becomes tender, swollen, and red; and soon thereafter several closely set, thick-walled tense vesicles containing yellowish serous fluid appear.

The individual vesicles are small at their onset, do not coalesce, and overlie an erythematous base. They persist for varying short periods, ordinarily 2 or 3 days. The lesions then become purulent and form scabs that eventually fall off. Before the skin lesions appear, satellite lymph nodes may enlarge and become tender, remaining inflamed during the infection and regressing slowly after the lesions heal. An individual attack of recurrent herpes simplex may last for 4 or 5 days (small lesions) or for as long as 2, and sometimes 3, weeks.

Recurrent Genital Herpes. The genital region is an increasingly common site for HSV infection. Usually associated with HSV-2 infection, the changes in sexual mores and the concomitant increase in orogenital sexual exposures make herpes progenitalis a common venereally induced disorder, with an associated increase in the incidence of HSV-1 infection in this area. In males, lesions appear on the prepuce, glans, or sulcus, and occasionally on the penile shaft or in the urethra. Frequent sites in the female are the labia, vulva, clitoris, and cervix. The disorder is manifested by single or clustered vesicles that rupture, generally within a

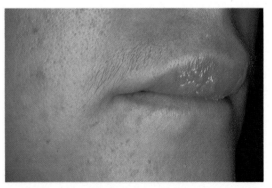

Figure 11–3. Herpes labialis. Recurrent herpes simplex infection with grouped vesicles on the upper lip. Generally caused by herpes simplex type 1 infection, this disorder usually follows an acute febrile illness or intense sun exposure.

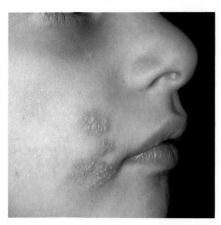

Figure 11–4. Recurrent herpes simplex infection. Grouped vesicular lesions appear on a tender red swollen area at or near previous areas of involvement.

few days, to form erosions and ulcers. Lymphadenopathy, although uncommon, may also be present at times. Symptoms include pain, burning, and dysuria, and, occasionally, malaise, headache, and anorexia may accompany the cutaneous lesions. The infection runs its course in about 8 days, and healing does not produce scarring (see Fig. 11–1).

Recurrent Ocular Herpes. The most important type of recurrent HSV infection is that which affects the eye. Presenting as a recurrent marginal keratitis or dendritic corneal ulcer, vesicles may be noted on the eyelids and palpebral conjunctivae as well as on the surrounding skin. Prevention of bacterial infection is of utmost importance, and broad-spectrum ophthalmic antibiotics are valuable in the management of this disorder. If keratitis is severe or if uveitis appears, tonometric examination is important, and mydriatic and anti-inflammatory therapy, preferably under the management of an experienced ophthalmologist, is recommended. Although topical corticosteroids are contraindicated in suspected HSV conjunctivitis, ophthalmologists may at times use these agents in conjunction with antiviral agents for deep-seated lesions.

Recurrent HSV lesions must be differentiated from lesions of impetigo, herpes zoster, primary syphilitic chancre, and contact dermatitis. Although mixed viral and bacterial infections are not unusual, the history of itching or burning prior to the eruption and clear or straw-colored, serous, fluid-filled vesicles on an erythematous base is characteristic of recurrent herpetic infection.

Diagnosis. When the true nature of the disorder is not apparent, rapid diagnosis can be confirmed by demonstration of multinucleated giant cells, balloon cells, and, on rare occasion, intranuclear inclusions on a Giemsa-, Papanicolaou-, or Wright-stained smear of the scraping of the base or roof of a vesicle (the Tzanck test) (see Fig. 2–24) or by tissue culture of vesicular fluid or crusts, indirect fluorescent antibody studies using the fluid

scraped from the base of the vesicles, complement fixation or viral neutralization tests, the enzyme-linked immunosorbent assay (ELISA), the polymerase chain reaction technique, or cutaneous biopsy for light or electron microscopy. It should be noted, however, that the cytologic appearance of a scraping of herpes simplex cannot be differentiated from that of varicella and that complement fixation and viral neutralizing antibody tests are not helpful in the diagnosis of recurrent herpes infections, since viral antibody titers are usually high at the time of the eruption. To distinguish between primary and recurrent infections, it is necessary to demonstrate a rising antibody titer in acute and convalescent sera.

The characteristic histopathologic features of a herpetic infection consist of an intradermal vesicle produced by degeneration of epidermal cells, marked acantholysis, reticular degeneration, ballooning degeneration, and, as in varicella and herpes zoster infection, inclusion bodies located within the nucleus. This is in contrast to lesions of variola in which the inclusion bodies lie predominantly in the cytoplasm.

Traditional methods of diagnosing herpes simplex infection, although generally successful, may at times be inconclusive; and a rapid accurate diagnosis is often required. In such instances, identification of HSV DNA by polymerase chain reaction, which permits the isolation and repetitive duplication of specific DNA fragments, is extremely helpful.[12]

Treatment. Except for oral or intravenous acyclovir, or intravenous vidarabine, there is no single therapeutic modality that is fully effective in decreasing the duration or recurrence rate of cutaneous HSV infection. The evidence that herpesvirus persists in nerve cells, specifically within the nuclei of the cells found in the sensory ganglia, should suggest the limited effectiveness of any

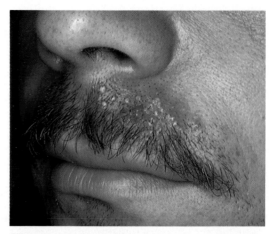

Figure 11–5. Herpes simplex. Vesicles and vesicopustules are grouped on the mustache area. The period from the appearance of vesicles to complete healing generally lasts 8 to 10 days, occasionally longer.

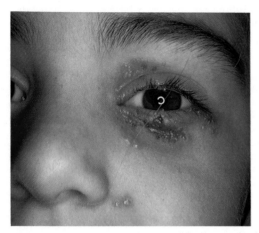

Figure 11–6. Herpes simplex of the eyelids. Herpes simplex infection around the eye requires a search for the possibility of herpetic keratitis.

topical approach to the treatment of herpesvirus infections of the skin. Although agents that interfere with viral reproduction and the resulting damage to cells may possibly abort the infection and lead to somewhat more rapid healing, if used early in the course of recurrent cutaneous herpes infection, in controlled studies none of the currently recommended therapeutic regimens has proved to be consistently beneficial.

The key to management of recurrent herpetic infections of the skin appears to be early treatment. Once the virus has stopped spreading and no more tissue damage is occurring (usually within 1 or 2 days of the appearance of lesions), the goal is to aid the healing of damaged tissue and to prevent secondary bacterial infection.

When vesicles first appear, merely opening the lesions and treating them with any liquid preparation will result in the dilution of viral particles and help to shorten the course of infection. There is theoretical justification, therefore, for the use of 70 per cent alcohol or ether, which destroys the lipoprotein particles and renders them noninfectious. Ethyl ether is a topical anesthetic agent and lipid solvent that dissolves the capsule of the herpesvirus particle. Although reports of clinical results are controversial,[13] topical applications of ether with a cotton swab or moistened pledget until the skin blanches and local anesthesia is produced, three or four times a day to *early* recurrent lesions, has been recommended in an effort to obtain symptomatic relief and help decrease the duration of lesions. Since ether is highly flammable, topical application of 70 per cent alcohol is recommended as a safer alternative.

Thymol is also available as a topical anesthetic and antiviral agent that interferes with protein synthesis. Topical application of 4 per cent thymol in chloroform (also a lipid solvent capable of dissolving the herpesvirus capsule) twice daily at the earliest sign of a new lesion can also produce

symptomatic relief and possibly decrease the duration of lesions. A light freeze with liquid nitrogen on a cotton applicator to a very early recurrent lesion may also help prevent further progression of the herpetic infection.

Ophthalmic preparations of 0.1 per cent idoxuridine in solution or ointment base (Stoxil, Herplex, or Dendrid) and 3 per cent vidarabine (Vira-A), although beneficial in the treatment of herpetic keratoconjunctivitis, appear to be ineffective in recurrent disease such as herpes labialis, herpes genitalis, and herpetic whitlow.

Double-blind studies of repeated smallpox vaccinations for the management of recurrent HSV infection indicate that repeated smallpox vaccination is not effective in the prevention or management of recurrent HSV infection. Since this approach is also potentially hazardous, it is not recommended for the management of this disorder.[14]

Since patients with recurrent HSV infections have high circulating humoral antibody titers to herpesvirus, there is good reason to suspect that a herpesvirus vaccine might not prove effective in the therapy for recurrent diseases. Animal model evidence suggests that herpesvirus vaccines and circulating anti-herpesvirus IgG may interact with the cell-mediated immune system and enhance resistance against HSV infection. This approach, however, is controversial and studies have not confirmed a beneficial response to the use of HSV vaccines in the treatment of this disorder.

Another recommendation for the management of cutaneous HSV infections has been the oral administration of the amino acid lysine monohydrochloride (Enisyl). A daily dose of 800 to 1,000 mg during overt infection has been suggested for the reduction of pain during acute infection, the prevention of new vesicles, and more rapid resolution of new lesions. In addition, a maintenance dose of 500 mg of lysine given daily between infec-

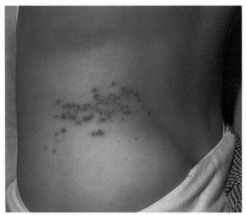

Figure 11–7. Herpes simplex simulating herpes zoster on the lateral aspect of the trunk of an immunosuppressed child with leukemia.

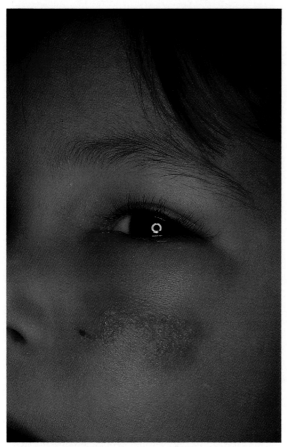

Figure 11–8. Herpes simplex on the cheek of a 3-year-old girl with localized edema and lymphangitis.

tions has been suggested as a means of preventing recurrences of this disorder. Since arginine appears to encourage and lysine appears to antagonize herpesvirus replication and cytopathogenicity, intake of foods high in arginine (nuts, seeds, chocolate) is discouraged with this form of therapy. Although lysine treatment of cutaneous herpesvirus lesions is benign, further carefully controlled double-blind studies are necessary before oral lysine can be accepted as an effective cure for cutaneous HSV infection.[15, 16]

Topical administration of acyclovir (5 per cent Zovirax ointment) is helpful in the treatment of primary herpes genitalis and in non–life-threatening mucocutaneous HSV infections. Its effect, however, is less evident in the treatment of recurrent infection; and since its polyethylene glycol base may cause vaginal erythema, acyclovir ointment is not approved for intravaginal use. Primary herpetic whitlow responds to oral acyclovir, and intravenous vidarabine and acyclovir can be used for potentially serious or severe HSV infections, neonatal herpes, ophthalmic herpes, immunocompromised patients, and patients with

disseminated disease or encephalitis. The administration of acyclovir, orally (25 to 30 mg/kg/day up to 200 mg five times a day) or intravenously, can produce dramatic results for patients with herpetic Kaposi's varicelliform eruption (eczema herpeticum). Patients with frequent recurrences of herpetic infection (six or more per year) can also benefit from chronic suppressive therapy (oral acyclovir, 400 mg twice daily for a 6- to 12-month course). Although acyclovir has not been shown to be teratogenic, its potential for causing chromosome breakage must be taken into consideration when treating women who are pregnant. This modality, therefore, is not recommended during pregnancy unless its potential benefit justifies the potential risk to the fetus.[17]

HERPES ZOSTER

Herpes zoster (shingles) is an acute vesiculobullous infection of the skin caused by the varicella-zoster virus (herpesvirus varicellae), the same virus that produces chickenpox (Figs. 11–9 through 11–12). As in herpesvirus infections, after an initial varicella infection, the varicella-zoster virus remains dormant in cells of the dorsal root ganglia or cranial nerve ganglia, inapparent and nonreplicating until reactivation and subsequent propagation of the virus along the nerve to the skin where infection of the dermis gives rise to the grouped vesicular eruption characteristic of this disorder. Reactivation, although not fully defined, may result from a reexposure to varicella, physical trauma to the spinal column, radiation therapy, immunosuppressant drugs, cancer, leukemia, or Hodgkin's disease. Acting as a trigger mechanism, any of these may release the virus from the dorsal root ganglia (a situation perhaps analogous to recurrent HSV infection).

Although herpes zoster is chiefly a disease of adults, the disorder has been noted as early as the first week of life, presumably in infants born to a mother who contracted varicella during pregnancy.[18–20] It has been suggested that the infrequent occurrence of this disorder in infants and young children (see Fig. 11–10) might be due to the relatively low incidence of previous varicella (chickenpox) infection in this age group. Since 50 per cent of children have varicella by age 5 years and 80 to 90 per cent by age 15 years, a more likely hypothesis suggests that a long latent period is required after primary infection (a period during which various aspects of immunity presumably decrease, thus allowing herpes zoster to develop on reexposure to varicella virus).

Clinical Manifestations. Herpes zoster is characterized by a segmental papulovesicular eruption on an inflammatory base arranged in a continuous or interrupted band along the dermatomes of the skin supplied by the affected sensory nerves or extramedullary cranial nerves, usually with a degree of hyperesthesia, pain, and tenderness. The

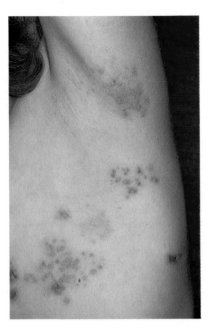

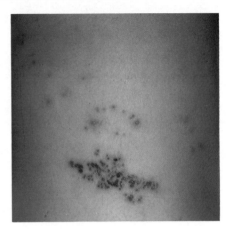

Figure 11–9. A and B. Herpes zoster. Typical segmental papulovesicular eruptions on an inflammatory base occur in an interrupted band with dermatomal distribution.

most frequently affected dermatomes are those innervated by the second dorsal to second lumbar nerves (C2 to L2) and the fifth and seventh cranial nerves.

Patients typically develop pain of variable severity in a dermatomal distribution 4 to 5 days (occasionally 1 to 10 days) before the eruption appears. Herpes zoster generally tends to appear first at a point nearest the central nervous system and extends peripherally along the course of the nerve, thus producing its characteristic band-like distribution of lesions. Generally the eruption is unilateral but may cross the midline and, at times, may involve (to a lesser degree) the contralateral side. Successive crops continue to appear for about 7 days. They extend along the course of the nerve

and eventually dry out and crust over in the course of another 5 to 10 days. In 90 per cent of individuals younger than the age of 20 the disorder resolves in 7 to 14 days. Occasionally, however, particularly in older individuals, the process may persist for 1 to 5 weeks. During this time, mild constitutional symptoms, low-grade fever, and/or regional lymphadenopathy may be present. It is not unusual to see a few randomly scattered vesicular lesions beyond the primary dermatomal involvement. Such scattered lesions do not constitute disseminated zoster.

Infection associated with the ophthalmic branch of the fifth (trigeminal) nerve may involve the cornea with keratitis and uveitis and may lead to permanent damage. This disorder (zoster ophthal-

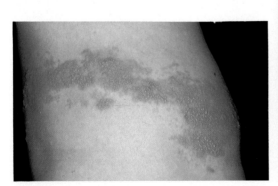

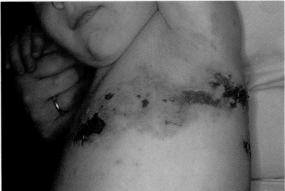

Figure 11–10. A. Herpes zoster on the trunk of a 7½-month-old infant following exposure to varicella. (The infant's mother had chickenpox during the eighth month of pregnancy.) B. Herpes zoster with severe crusting and ulceration on the left hemithorax of a young child who had chickenpox at the age of 3 months.

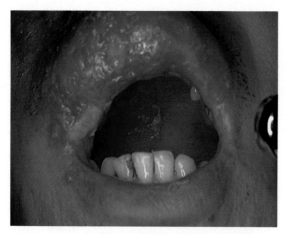

Figure 11–11. Herpes zoster with vesiculation of the lips and hard palate.

micus) appears when the nasociliary branch is involved and, accordingly, is present in those individuals who manifest cutaneous involvement of the nose (Hutchinson's sign).

Zoster of the maxillary division of the trigeminal nerve produces vesiculation of the palate, uvula, and tonsillar area (see Fig. 11–11). Involvement of the mandibular division produces vesicular involvement of the anterior aspects of the tongue, floor of the mouth, lips, and buccal mucous membranes. Involvement of the geniculate ganglion produces lesions on the tongue, the ear, and the skin of the auditory canal. When accompanied by Bell's palsy and disturbances of hearing and equilibrium, it is part of the Ramsay Hunt syndrome.

Herpes zoster in prepubertal children is usually a mild disease, and it is unusual to see a prolonged course. Neuralgia, so common to adults (particularly those older than 65 years of age), is unusual but occasionally may be seen in adolescents. Hematogenous dissemination of herpes with viremia and resulting spread of the eruption may occur in approximately 2 per cent of cases. Such patients initially present with the usual zosteriform eruption, which progresses, becomes generalized, and assumes a varicella-like distribution. The majority of patients with this complication have a serious underlying disease, usually a malignancy of the reticuloendothelial system. Generalized zoster is a serious disorder and occurs mainly in immunosuppressed individuals, patients with Hodgkin's disease, lymphoma, or leukemia, or those on immunosuppressive medications.[21] Although children with cancer have an increased risk of childhood zoster, the presence of herpes zoster in an otherwise apparently healthy child should not be taken as a marker of malignancy.[22, 23] Children or adults with disseminated herpes zoster infection, however, should be investigated for the possibility of malignancy, immunodeficiency, or acquired immunodeficiency syndrome (AIDS)-related complex.[24]

Diagnosis. The diagnosis of herpes zoster is based on the presence of a painful, unilateral, grouped vesicular eruption along the course of a sensory nerve. The Tzanck test may demonstrate multinuclear giant cells, viral culture of vesicular fluid or, demonstration of an increase in paired varicella antibody titers, and polymerase chain reaction studies can confirm the diagnosis. The characteristic histologic picture is similar to that of HSV infection and varicella.

Management. The management of herpes zoster is limited to symptomatic treatment and prevention of secondary infection. Uncomplicated cases may be treated with local applications of heat, open wet compresses, topical application of drying lotions such as calamine lotion (plain or with 1 per cent phenol), or ethyl chloride spray. When present, intractable pain and post-herpetic neuralgia, seldom a problem in preadolescent children, can frequently be controlled with analgesics.

Patients with severe involvement or ophthalmic infection and individuals older than 60 years of age (in the absence of contraindication) may be given systemic corticosteroids, preferably administered

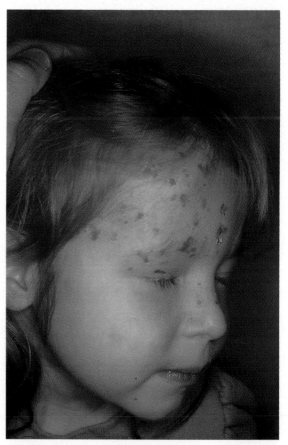

Figure 11–12. A child with severe herpes zoster on the left forehead, nose, and ophthalmic area that was treated successfully with high oral doses of acyclovir.

early in the course of the disorder. Administration of prednisone (or its equivalent), if given early in the course of the disease, in a dosage of up to 40 to 60 mg/day for 1 week, 30 mg/day for 1 week, and then 15 mg/day for 1 week, frequently decreases the severity of the illness and, particularly in those older than age 50, appears to decrease the incidence as well as the duration of post-herpetic neuralgia.[25] Topical applications of capsaicin (Zostrix)[26] three to four times daily and subcutaneous sublesional injection of 15 ml of triamcinolone acetonide and procaine have also been helpful in the treatment of postherpetic neuralgia.[27, 28]

Lesions of the tip of the nose indicate involvement of the nasociliary nerve and possible ocular involvement. In ophthalmic zoster, ocular complications occur in about 50 per cent of cases. The conjunctiva is red and swollen, and superficial or deep keratitis may develop. Although fortunately relatively uncommon, uveitis, when it occurs, may be intense and prolonged and may produce keratic precipitates, secondary glaucoma, and, in severe cases, permanent loss of vision. Patients with herpes zoster ophthalmicus, accordingly, should be referred to an ophthalmologist early in the course of the disease.

Patients with ophthalmic or disseminated herpes zoster (see Fig. 11–12) may be treated with intravenous vidarabine or intravenous or oral acyclovir. Since the varicella-zoster virus is less sensitive to acyclovir than HSV, levels two to eight times greater than those required for the treatment of HSV infection are required for the treatment of herpes zoster. Thus, since gastrointestinal absorption is somewhat erratic, with only about 20 per cent of the drug being absorbed, 20 mg/kg orally four times a day, with a maximum of 400 to 800 mg orally five times daily, for 7 to 10 days is recommended if there is evidence of viremia or systemic complications. Intravenous vidarabine (10 to 20 mg/kg/day) or acyclovir (7.5 mg/kg three times a day) and hyperimmune convalescent zoster serum or zoster immune globulin (ZIG) may be used, preferably within 48 to 72 hours of exposure, for the treatment of immunocompromised individuals and patients with disseminated herpes zoster.[29–33]

VIRAL-LIKE DISORDERS OF THE ORAL MUCOSA

Aphthous Stomatitis

Recurrent aphthous stomatitis is a common disorder characterized by recurrent single or multiple ulcerations (canker sores) that appear on the inner cheeks, lips, gums, tongue, palate, and pharynx (Fig. 11–13). Previously believed to represent a manifestation of herpes simplex, attempts to isolate a virus have been uniformly unsuccessful, and mounting evidence currently favors an autoimmune phenomenon as the basis of this disorder.[34]

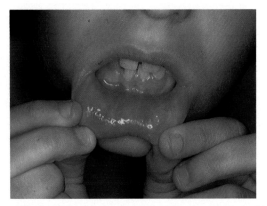

Figure 11–13. Aphthous stomatitis. Tiny superficial grayish white erosions and ulcerations are surrounded by sharp borders and narrow, slightly elevated, bright red areolae.

Aphthous stomatitis occurs in individuals of all ages but is relatively uncommon in children. Before puberty the sexes are affected equally; in adult life, however, the disorder appears somewhat more frequently in women, with a peak incidence during the third decade of life.

Prior to the clinical appearance of lesions the patient is frequently aware of their impending development by a tingling or stinging sensation. Twenty-four to 48 hours later a focal erythema develops, and soon thereafter tiny, superficial, grayish white erosions appear. Usually there are one to three lesions, and the area of erosion increases and evolves into one or more sharply defined shallow ulcers covered by gray membranes and surrounded by sharp borders and narrow, slightly elevated, bright red areolae. Lesions measure 3 to 6 mm in diameter and, if left untreated, generally persist for 8 to 12 days (sometimes longer) and heal without scarring.

Studies suggest that emotional stress, trauma, and hormonal changes such as in menstruation appear to play an important role in the precipitation of attacks. Commonly, one to three ulcers develop at irregular intervals of weeks or months, and many patients are almost continually afflicted.

Aphthous stomatitis must be differentiated from herpetic stomatitis, Vincent's angina, candidiasis, traumatic ulcers, mucous patches of early syphilis, erythema multiforme, pemphigus, Behçet's syndrome, and Reiter's disease.

In general there is no one specific treatment for aphthous stomatitis. The most effective topical therapy appears to be the use of tetracycline suspension (250 mg/5 ml), held in or swished around in the mouth for 2 minutes and then swallowed, four times a day for 5 to 7 days, or application of a tetracycline compress of cotton soaked in a suspension of 250 mg of tetracycline in 30 ml of water placed directly on the ulcers for 20 minutes four to six times a day. Although the mechanism is not known, the presence of the L-form of *Streptococcus sanguis* in lesions may explain the apparent shortening of the course of aphthous stomatitis by tetracycline.

Other useful modalities include topical anesthetic agents such as lidocaine (Xylocaine 2 per cent viscous solution), dyclonine (Dyclone), 0.5 per cent, swirled around the mouth for several minutes or applied directly to the lesions, clobetasol (Temovate) ointment applied about six times a day for several days, or a mixture of equal parts of elixir of diphenhydramine (Benadryl) and Kaopectate or Maalox held in the mouth for 5 minutes prior to meals. Early lesions are frequently helped by topical applications of silver nitrate or by the topical use of triamcinolone acetonide (Kenalog, 0.1 per cent, in Orabase) applied four times daily to nonulcerated lesions. Large painful ulcers frequently respond dramatically to intralesional injections of 0.1 to 0.5 ml of triamcinolone acetonide (10 mg/ml) into the base of lesions. In addition, although not available in the United States, thalidomide, 100 to 300 mg/day for 3 months, has been used for the treatment of severe, persistent, or recurrent aphthae.[35]

Acute Necrotizing Gingivitis

Acute necrotizing gingivitis (trench mouth, Vincent's stomatitis, Vincent's angina) is a painful ulcerative disorder that chiefly affects adolescents and young adults. Although formerly common in schools and military establishments, the disorder, perhaps owing to improved oral and dental care, is rare in the United States and Western Hemisphere.

The pathogenesis remains uncertain, but *Fusobacterium fusiforme* and *Borrelia vincentii* organisms usually predominate in smears from infected tissues. Clinical findings consist of painful gingivae that bleed easily and an inflamed oropharynx with eroded hemorrhagic appearance and ulcerations at both the gingival margins and interdental papillae. The ulcerations are covered by a grayish white slough or pseudomembrane that can be removed, leaving a raw, bleeding surface. Single or multiple papillae may be involved, and the necrotizing ulceration can be very extensive. As a result of tissue necrosis and suppuration there is bleeding of the gums, discomfort, and a characteristic fetid odor. Systemic involvement consists of varying degrees of malaise, lymphadenopathy, and fever, depending on the severity of the disease.

The clinical manifestations are characteristic, and diagnosis generally can be made on the basis of clinical evidence alone. Smears of the lesions usually reveal spirochetes, fusobacteria, cocci, vibrios, and filamentous organisms. Since these organisms can also be found in smears from normal mouths, such findings are not specific for the disease.

It must be emphasized that Vincent's stomatitis does not usually occur in healthy persons with normal tissue resistance. The possibility of underlying systemic disease or other predisposing factors, therefore, must be considered.

The course of necrotizing gingivitis is indefinite, and the disease, if untreated, may progress into a serious and, at times, even potentially fatal complication referred to as *noma*. Extremely uncommon in the United States, this complication is seen in individuals with severe nutritional deficiency or debilitating diseases such as terminal cancer, kala-azar, or kwashiorkor.

Treatment of Vincent's stomatitis consists of antibiotic therapy (penicillin, erythromycin, or tetracycline) for 5 to 7 days, detection and relief of any underlying disorders, and the use of sodium perborate or 3 per cent hydrogen peroxide (diluted one half to one third with warm water) mouth washes every 2 to 3 hours. After the acute phase has passed, oral hygienic measures (brushing, flossing, scaling of the teeth, and removal of gingival irritants) are beneficial. Occasionally gingivectomy may be necessary to correct the deep ulcerations that may have developed between the teeth.

WARTS

Warts (verrucae) and molluscum contagiosum are common viral disorders of the skin caused by DNA viruses.

Warts are intraepidermal tumors caused by infection with the human papillomavirus (HPV) of the papova group. The word "papova" is an acronym derived from the first two letters of the first three oncogenic viruses discovered: *pa*pilloma (wart), *po*lyoma (mouse tumors), and *va*cuolating (simian virus 40). There are four basic types of verrucae: verruca vulgaris, verruca plana, verruca plantaris, and condyloma acuminatum. Seen in 7 to 10 per cent of the population, they are among the most common skin disorders of childhood. Although rarely a serious health problem, verrucae are often responsible for cosmetic problems to those who have them and therapeutic problems for those who attempt to treat them.

Seen in patients of all ages, warts generally occur during childhood and adolescence, with the highest incidence in individuals between 10 and 19 years of age. Their incubation period varies from 1 to 6 months or more, and although their course is totally unpredictable, the range of duration of lesions varies from a few months to 5 years or more, with 25 per cent disappearing spontaneously within 3 to 6 months and 65 per cent disappearing spontaneously within 2 years.[36] Warts are inoculable from one location to another and from one person to another, through direct or indirect contact. Since local trauma promotes inoculation by the virus, most warts are seen on the fingers, hands, and elbows, along the perionychial folds (often in a linear configuration due to biting or picking of the involved areas), in areas of trauma (the Koebner phenomenon), or on the plantar surfaces of the feet (plantar warts) (Figs. 11–14 through 11–18).

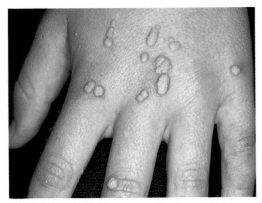

Figure 11–14. Multiple common warts (verrucae vulgaris) with Koebner's phenomenon.

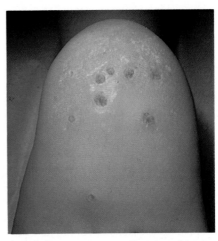

Figure 11–16. Plantar warts (verrucae plantaris) generally occur on weight-bearing areas of the heels, toes, and midtarsal areas.

Nearly 70 distinct types of HPV have been characterized, and various HPV types have been associated with a wide spectrum of cutaneous and mucosal lesions. Although the same DNA virus can be responsible for various types of warts, their morphologic and clinical characteristics appear to represent a manifestation of individual cutaneous or mucous membrane response to the localized viral infection. Thus, HPV types 1, 2, 4, and 7 are most frequently responsible for common warts (verrucae vulgaris); deep painful palmar and plantar warts are generally associated with HPV type 1; mosaic plantar warts are caused by HPV type 2; flat warts (verrucae plana) are associated with HPV types 3, 10, and, at times, 26, 27, and 28; laryngeal papillomatosis is caused by HPV types 6 and 11; epidermodysplasia verruciformis is associated with HPV types 5 and 8; HPV types 6 and 11, 16, and 18 commonly infect the genital tract; and HPV types 6 and 11 have a predilection for the external anogenital skin. In addition, cutaneous and genital malignancies have been associated with HPV infection, particularly in immunosuppressed individuals. Potentially oncogenic HPV types associated with cervical carcinomas include HPV types 16 and 18 (the most prevalent viruses associated with cervical cancers found to date) and types 31,

33, and 35. HPV types 5, 8, and 14 are associated with malignancy in patients with epidermodysplasia verruciformis.[37–40]

Verrucae Vulgaris

Verrucae vulgaris (common warts) appear predominantly on the dorsal surface of the hands or periungual regions but may be seen anywhere (see Figs. 11–14 and 11–17). Occasionally they may also occur on the oral mucosa. They may vary from a solitary isolated lesion to vast numbers in any given individual. Early verrucae are usually round, discrete, flesh colored, and pinpoint. With time usually within a period of a few weeks to months, they grow to larger yellowish tan, grayish black or brown lesions that measure anywhere from several

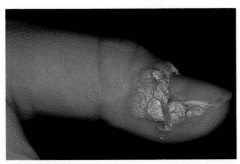

Figure 11–15. Periungual warts. These warts are frequently seen on the fingers of cuticle pickers or nail biters.

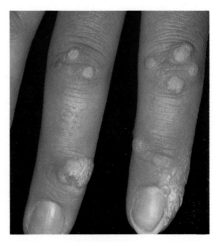

Figure 11–17. Common warts (verrucae vulgaris) on the dorsal aspect and periungual region of the fingers.

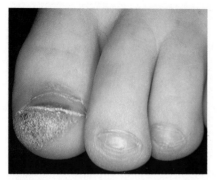

Figure 11–18. Subungual verruca with thrombosed capillaries.

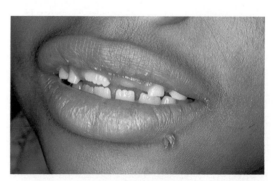

Figure 11–20. Multiple warts on the left nostril.

millimeters to 1 cm or more in diameter. Repeated irritation will often cause a wart to continue to enlarge and, with time, the surface generally takes on a roughened finely papillomatous (verruciform) surface.

Periungual warts and subungual verrucae occur around and beneath nail beds, particularly on the fingers of cuticle-pickers or nail biters (Figs. 11–15 and 11–17). These lesions, because of their location and susceptibility to trauma, frequently become irritated, infected, or tender and are often more persistent and resistant to therapy. Satellite lesions often grow around warts, particularly those that have been irritated, manipulated, or incompletely or inadequately treated. When the diagnosis is in doubt, gentle paring with a 15-gauge scalpel blade will reveal characteristic minute black dots due to the presence of thrombosed capillaries that tend to bleed when the surface is removed (Figs. 11–16 and 11–18).

Digitate warts, commonly seen on the cheeks, chin, neck, or scalp, are broad-based, finger-like projections with a horny surface. They usually occur on the face and neck and are particularly common on the eyelids or about the ala nasi (Figs. 11–19 and 11–20). Filiform warts are seen as thread-like digitate projections with a narrow base and delicate cornified tips (Fig. 11–21). The trauma of shaving plays a common role in the dissemination of filiform or digitate warts.

Verrucae Plana

Verrucae plana (flat warts) occur primarily on the face, neck, arms, and legs. They are usually seen as smooth, flesh-colored to slightly tan or brown, slightly elevated papules, 2 to 5 mm in diameter, with a round or polygonal base (Fig. 11–22). They vary from only two or three to several hundred in any given individual. In the bearded areas of men, and on the legs of women, irritation from shaving tends to cause flat warts to spread. Contiguous warts often coalesce to form firm, papular, plaque-like lesions. Again linear slightly elevated lesions in areas of scratch marks (the Koebner effect) are characteristic of this disorder (Fig. 11–23).

Verrucae Plantaris

Verrucae plantaris (plantar warts) occur on the plantar surfaces of the feet and are perhaps the most uncomfortable and therapeutically challenging form of this disorder. They generally occur on the weight-bearing areas of the heels, toes, and

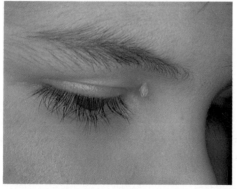

Figure 11–19. Digitate wart on medial aspect of upper eyelid.

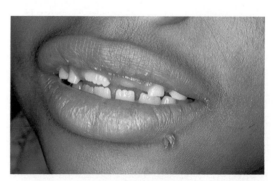

Figure 11–21. Digitate wart with bifid filiform tips.

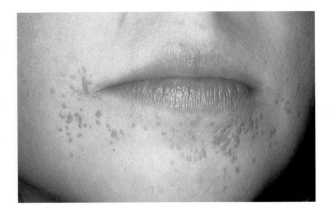

Figure 11–22. Verrucae plana (flat warts) on the chin of a 6-year-old girl.

mid-metatarsal areas (see Figs. 11–16 and 11–24). Pressed inward by walking, they frequently become deep, painful, and tender. Often there are several lesions on one foot. At times a cluster of small satellite warts, often pinhead sized with a grape-like vesicular appearance, may develop around a wart or group of warts. Thick keratotic plaques of closely grouped coalescent verrucae are termed *mosaic warts* (Fig. 11–24).

At times it may be difficult to differentiate plantar warts from corns, calluses, or scars (Fig. 11–25). Corns are localized hyperkeratoses that form over interphalangeal joints as the result of intermittent pressure and friction. Penetrating corns often appear at the base of the second or third metatarsal phalangeal joint. They can be distinguished from plantar warts by a lack of thrombosed capillaries, by a characteristic hard semiopaque core, and by the fact that, in contrast to verrucae plantaris, they are more painful on direct rather than lateral pressure. *Soft corns* are macerated hyperkeratotic lesions that persist at points of friction and pressure in intertriginous areas. They are usually seen on the lateral aspect of the toes, or in the webs between the fourth and fifth toes.

Black heel ("talon noir") is a common condition frequently confused with plantar warts (Fig. 11–26). In this disorder, papillary capillaries are ruptured by the shearing action associated with sudden stops in athletic individuals, usually tennis, handball, or basketball players.[41] Clinically this is characterized by clusters of brown or bluish black, pinpoint petechial hemorrhages in the horny layer along the backs or sides of the heels or lateral edges of the feet. Gentle paring of the surface of suspected lesions with a 15-gauge scalpel blade can help differentiate this condition from malignant melanoma, calluses, corns, scars, and plantar warts.

Condylomata Acuminata

Condylomata acuminata (genital warts) are fleshy verrucae that occur around mucocutaneous junctions and intertriginous areas (the glans penis, the mucosal surface of the female genitalia, and

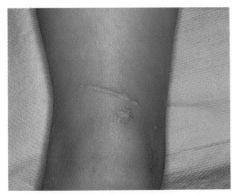

Figure 11–23. Verrucae with the Koebner effect in the line of a scratch on the leg.

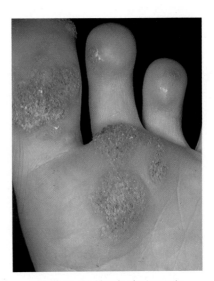

Figure 11–24. Mosaic plantar warts.

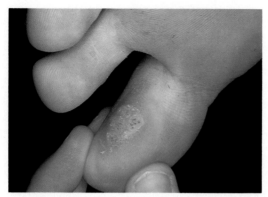

Figure 11–25. Verrucae on the medial aspect of the great toe. The presence of thrombosed capillaries helps differentiate them from soft corns.

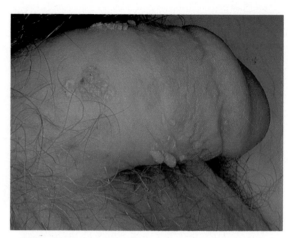

Figure 11–27. Condylomata acuminata (genital warts) on the penile shaft in a 16-year-old boy.

around the anus) as soft, flesh-colored, elongated, sometimes pedunculated or polypoid nodules (Figs. 11–27 through 11–29). In some patients, particularly young women, these lesions multiply and coalesce into large cauliflower-like masses (Figs. 11–30 and 11–31). Condylomata acuminata may be transmitted by sexual contact (the so-called venereal warts) or may be associated with verrucae on other parts of the body. Condylomata acuminata must be differentiated from the moist, wide-based, 1- to 3-cm, papular or nodular lesions of secondary syphilis (condylomata lata) that occur in the same regions. In rare instances, condylomata acuminata may attain considerable size, particularly on the penis of noncircumcised males. Known as giant condylomata acuminata of Buschke and Lowenstein, they frequently resemble squamous cell carcinomas (Fig. 11–32).

Anogenital warts are also being reported with increasing frequency in children, and in young children the route of transmission becomes one of paramount concern (see Fig. 11–29).[42] Although the transmission of genital warts to children is often venereal, nonvenereal transmission should be considered when the child is younger than 3 years

of age, when there is no evidence of child abuse, when lesions are somewhat distant from the anus or introitus, when warts are present in close contacts (particularly genital warts in mothers), and when the child is younger than 9 months of age when the lesions first appear.[43–45] Although the precise role of HPV and its possible oncogenetic potential have not been fully defined, it is recommended that adolescents and adults with genital warts, particularly HPV types 16 and 18, be examined carefully and periodically for the possibility of new lesions and possible neoplastic transformation.[46]

Epidermodysplasia Verruciformis

Epidermodysplasia verruciformis is a rare, lifelong disorder characterized by persistent disseminated, flat, wart-like lesions and erythematous, hyperpigmented, or hypopigmented macules (Figs. 11–33 and 11–34). First described by Lewandowsky and Lutz in 1922, the eruption usually starts in childhood and may be familial, suggesting a recessive inheritance pattern. In one kindred in which only male members were affected, an X-linked recessive form of the disorder has been de-

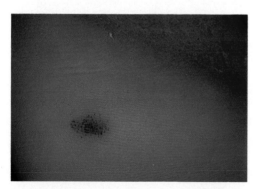

Figure 11–26. "Talon noir" (black heel). This common condition is caused by rupture of papillary capillaries due to shearing action associated with sudden stops by tennis, handball, or basketball players.

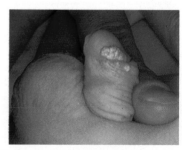

Figure 11–28. Verrucae on the glans penis and corona in an 8-month-old infant.

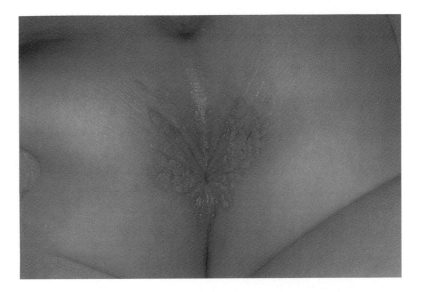

Figure 11–29. Condylomata acuminata in the perianal area of a 4-year-old girl. The presence of condylomata in the perianal or perigenital areas should arouse the suspicion of sexual abuse.

scribed.[47] Although at least 15 HPV types have been isolated in cutaneous lesions of patients with epidermodysplasia verruciformis, malignant changes appear to be limited to those infected with certain HPV types, primarily HPV types 5, 8, and 14. In a high percentage (30 to 80 per cent) of patients, lesions in sun-exposed areas may degenerate (usually within 2 or 3 decades) into bowenoid carcinomas and progress to squamous cell carcinomas. When malignant degeneration occurs, it generally develops on sun-exposed areas of the skin (especially the face, most often the forehead, the presternal areas, and backs of the hands). Lesions almost never regress spontaneously and are almost always refractory to therapy. Treatment of this disorder, therefore, consists of prompt detection and surgical excision of tumors, genetic counseling, and sun protection.

Laryngeal Papillomatosis

Laryngeal papillomas, HPV-associated tumors of the larynx, and at times the tracheal, bronchial, and pulmonary epithelium, are common tumors that, although primarily seen in infants, may occur at any age. HPV types 6 and 11 have been frequently found in this condition, and although a correlation between mothers and condylomata acuminata and infants with laryngeal papillomas has been shown, reports of newborns who developed laryngeal papillomatosis after delivery by cesarean section suggest an intrauterine source of infection. Thus, the value of prophylactic cesarean section for pregnant women with genital condylomata remains unclear.[38] Diagnosis of the disorder can be made by direct laryngoscopy; and although recurrences are common, most cases eventually resolve spontaneously. Treatment consists of forceps removal of individual lesions, with

care taken not to damage normal tissue. Cryosurgery and laser surgery may at times be beneficial.

Diagnosis

Common warts and plantar warts are characterized histologically by sharply demarcated localized hyperplasia of the epidermis with marked acanthosis, papillomatosis, and hyperkeratosis with interspersed areas of parakeratosis. The rete ridges are elongated and at the periphery of individual verrucae are frequently bent inward so that they appear to point radially toward the center of the lesion. The characteristic feature that distinguishes verrucae vulgaris from other papillomas is the presence of large vacuolated cells in the upper stratum malpighii and granular layer. The dermal papillae are thin and elongated and contain blood vessels that project high into the wart itself. These vessels appear as punctate dark spots when thrombosed and bleed when the wart is pared down or

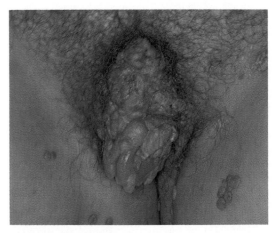

Figure 11–30. A large cauliflower-like mass of warts (giant condylomata acuminata).

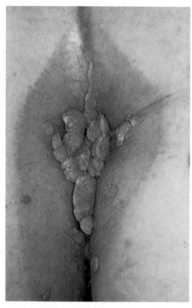

Figure 11–31. Condylomata acuminata of the perianal region.

traumatized. Verrucae plana show hyperkeratosis, acanthosis, and slight elongation of the rete ridges. In contrast to lesions of verrucae vulgaris, they have no papillomatosis and no areas of parakeratosis. The histologic picture of verrucae plantaris resembles that of verrucae vulgaris. The stratum corneum, however, is much thicker and frequently shows more extensive parakeratosis. In condyloma acuminatum the stratum corneum is only slightly thickened and is composed, as is usual on mucosal surfaces, of parakeratotic cells. The stratum malpighii shows papillomatosis, considerable acanthosis, and thickening and elongation of the rete ridges.

Treatment

There is no single effective treatment for warts. They are capricious (unpredictable), are occasionally highly resistant to therapy, and have a recurrence rate that varies from 5 to 10 per cent no matter what the therapeutic approach. Although these recurrences may at times be related to incomplete removal of individual lesions, latent HPV infection in apparently normal squamous epithelium beyond the areas of treatment appears to correlate with the high risk of recurrences.[48] Particularly in the treatment of flat or anogenital warts, barely perceptible or clinically inapparent warts may escape detection. In such instances, light application of liquid nitrogen on a cotton-tipped applicator or 3- to 5-minute soaking of suspicious areas with a 3 to 5 per cent solution of acetic acid can highlight the area and reveal small white verrucous papules or plaques. Vinegar can be used as a substitute for acetic acid, but the slightly more offensive odor of commercial vinegar may prove to be a deterrent to its use for this purpose.[49]

Whether warts should be treated depends entirely on the patient's and the patient's parents' desires. Only those with verrucae that are painful, spreading, enlarging, subject to trauma, or cosmetically objectionable need be treated. If treatment is to be given, the cardinal principle is that it shall not be harmful. It should be emphasized that some modalities employed for the treatment of warts in adults are neither feasible nor desirable for the treatment of warts in children. The choice of therapy, therefore, depends on the age and personality of the patient and the number, size, and location of the lesions. Whatever method the physician may select, he or she should be guided by conservatism if excessive trauma and scarring are to be avoided.

To be effective, any treatment must remove the entire wart and eradicate all virus; otherwise, recurrences are common. The simplest topical agents are keratolytic preparations. These include lactic acid and salicylic acid (in concentrations of 5 to 20 per cent in flexible collodion) or commercially available salicylic acid preparations such as Duofilm, Occlusal, Occlusal HP, or Duoplant, salicylic acid in a karaya gum patch (Trans-Ver-Sal or Trans-Plantar [Tsumara Medical]), and 40 per cent salicylic acid adhesive plasters (Mediplast).[50] The latter preparations are especially effective for the treatment of mosaic warts. Although clinically visible improvement will normally appear during the first 2 to 4 weeks of treatment, maximum resolution usually occurs after 6 to 12 weeks of continual application. Care should be exercised, however, to ensure that the adjacent normal tissues are not inadvertently treated, with resulting irritation. If irritation or discomfort occurs, 2-day intervals can be allowed between periods of application. This method can be used for flat warts (verrucae plana) if salicylic and lactic acids are kept at relatively low (5 per cent) concentrations.

Suggestion. The power of suggestion, or "charming of warts," is simple, nontraumatic, and in susceptible individuals (usually young children

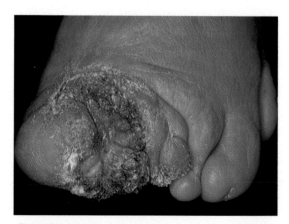

Figure 11–32. Giant verrucae (may at times resemble a squamous cell carcinoma).

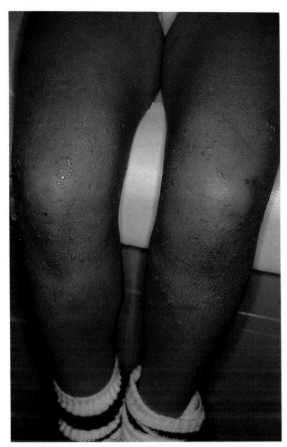

Figure 11–33. Epidermodysplasia verruciformis on the legs of a 10-year-old boy. (Courtesy of Israel Dvoretzky, M.D.)

5 to 10 years of age) may cure warts within a few days, leaving no trace of the previous lesion. How this works is unknown; however, it may explain the multiple spontaneous cures attributed to various inert preparations such as cod liver oil, lime juice, bits of hamburger, potato, garlic, and so on. Although at times parents may wonder about the credibility of the physician prescribing such therapy, it is harmless, is nontraumatic, and, when it works, can save many a child, parent, and physician from embarking on a long-term or more traumatic therapeutic approach. It is advisable to enlighten the parents to what the limits of the "power of suggestion" are and to have an alternate therapeutic plan available for those patients for whom this simple, but unfortunately not always reliable, approach fails. Most of the innumerable folk remedies for warts depend on the tendency of warts to spontaneously resolve and possibly the influence of suggestion.

An ointment containing ascorbic and pantothenic acids in a bland starch base, available in the past as Vergo (Daywell Laboratories), is safe and reputedly effective for the treatment of some patients with verrucae vulgaris or plantaris.[51] Although I personally have not been impressed with the results of this preparation, the ease of administration and its cosmetic acceptibility make it a benign agent that can be attempted by physicians, perhaps for its "power of suggestion" if not its clinical effect.

Cantharidin. Cantharidin, a potent blistering agent, is the purified active ingredient of cantharides, the dried, powdered, blister beetle (Spanish fly). A 0.7 per cent solution of cantharidin in acetone and flexible collodion, previously available as Cantharone, but currently unavailable in the United States, is easy to use and frequently effective, particularly in the management of periungual and plantar warts. At times it can be used for the treatment of other verrucae, particularly in children for whom other modalities may be painful, frightening, or traumatic. The disadvantage to the use of this agent, however, is the fact that occasionally a ring of satellite warts may develop at the periphery of the blister (Fig. 11–35).[52] Cantharidin should not be dispensed to the patient but should be applied carefully by the physician with a toothpick, cotton-tipped applicator, or glass adapter; allowed to dry; and occluded by a strip of adhesive tape. After 12 to 24 hours, or less if the

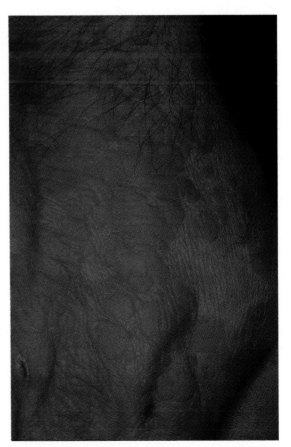

Figure 11–34. Confluent reddish verrucae on the dorsal aspect of the wrist and hand of an adult with epidermodysplasia verruciformis.

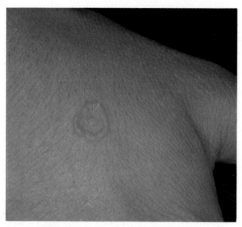

Figure 11–35. Annular satellite lesions in a "doughnut" formation following cantharidin treatment of a wart on the dorsal aspect of the hand.

area begins to sting or hurt, the adhesive covering should be removed and the area washed off. Stronger formulations containing 1 per cent cantharidin, 30 per cent salicylic acid, and 2 to 5 per cent podophyllin, also previously available as Cantharone Plus (Seres Laboratories) or Verrusol (C & M Pharmacal, Inc.), but again currently unavailable in the United States, can be applied under occlusion for shorter periods of time (1 to 2 hours).

The cantharidin produces a blister that in approximately 10 days, dries and peels off, removing part of the wart and leaving no scar. Following gentle debridement of the remaining verrucous tissue, cantharidin may be reapplied at 1- to 4-week intervals until the wart completely disappears. Although most patients note little discomfort, some may experience tingling, itching, or burning within a few hours, and at times the area may become tender for several days. When there is discomfort, relief may be obtained by removing the tape, puncturing a blister if present, and soaking the area with cool water for an hour or more.

Formalin and Trichloroacetic Acid. Formalin may be used successfully for the treatment of recalcitrant warts by the topical application of formaldehyde (4 ml of 40 per cent formaldehyde in 15 g of Aquaphor), once daily for 3 or 4 weeks or until the warts disappear, or of a saturated solution of trichloroacetic acid (or formalin in concentrations of 10 to 20 per cent) in combination with topical occlusion with 40 per cent salicylic acid plaster, with periodic gentle paring until the warts improve.[53]

Cryosurgery. Cryosurgery with liquid nitrogen (−196°C), although at times somewhat uncomfortable, is frequently a highly effective therapeutic approach to the treatment of individuals with multiple warts. A cotton-tipped applicator is dipped into the liquid nitrogen and applied to the lesion for periods varying from 2 or 3 to 10 seconds for superficial lesions to longer periods for deeper le-

sions. The freezing induces blister formation just above the dermal-epidermal junction, thus removing the cells infected with the virus while leaving the basement membrane intact. Care must be taken, however, not to freeze the warts too vigorously, particularly on the first occasion in young children, since there is considerable variation in pain threshold and the resulting reaction. The lesion should be re-examined at 2- to 4-week intervals. Remaining warty tissue or debris can be gently pared, and liquid nitrogen can be reapplied at each visit until the wart is completely destroyed. Speed and the simplicity of this technique make this method particularly valuable, since little or no scarring occurs and local anesthesia is not required.

Cryosurgery may at times be uncomfortable, and some children will not accept this mode of therapy. Although liquid nitrogen may be used for the treatment of warts in all areas, it is particularly effective and well tolerated in the treatment of flat warts. If periungual lesions are treated, however, extreme discomfort may be produced.

One particularly undesirable complication, that of neuropathy, has been reported as the result of liquid nitrogen therapy over superficial nerves on the volar or lateral aspects of the proximal phalanges of the fingers and medial epicondyle of the humerus at the elbow, over the common peroneal nerve at the head of the fibula, and over the digital plantar nerves to the toes. In treatment of lesions on the dorsum of the hand, sliding the skin back and forth over the underlying fascia during treatment may minimize the freezing effects on nerves lying between the skin and fascia.[54]

An alternate use of cryosurgical technique is that of gentle curettage of the verrucous lesions while the area under treatment is numb and temporarily frozen to a semisolid state by topical application of liquid nitrogen. This modification of cryosurgery is easy, convenient, and frequently can be used without the use of local anesthetic injection.

Smallpox Vaccination. The use of smallpox vaccination has been suggested for the treatment of verrucae. Although direct inoculation of smallpox vaccine into the wart may provide a remission rate in 30 to 60 per cent of cases, the risk of a permanent scar at the site of treatment and the possible pain or severe systemic reaction or both make this method unsound. Smallpox vaccination, therefore, is *not* a recommended form of therapy in the management of verrucae.[55]

Podophyllum Resin. Podophyllum resin, often useful in the treatment of moist warts (condylomata acuminata) in concentrations of 20 to 25 per cent in tincture of benzoin, acts as a cytotoxic agent, arresting epidermal mitoses in metaphase, with cellular disruption of the hypoplastic tissue. To prevent excessive irritation, this preparation must be applied carefully (only to lesions, with care to avoid adjacent tissues) and must be washed off with soap and water within 4 to 6 hours. Sitting in a tub bath with gentle washing of the treated area for a period of 20 to 30 minutes is a simple and effective measure for removal of the podophyllum preparation. Treatment may be repeated at weekly to monthly intervals, but failure of response after several treatments requires a change in therapy, possibly to liquid nitrogen or electrodesiccation and curettage, carbon dixoide laser therapy, or perhaps interferon. The expense, inconvenience, and recurrence rates of interferon, however, limit its use at this time.[56] Formulations containing cantharidin, salicylic acid, and podophyllin, if used, must be applied carefully, with care to avoid adjacent tissues, and washed off with soap and water after a shorter period of time (1 to 2 hours).

When extensive verrucae are present at the perianal mucocutaneous junction, proctoscopic examination may reveal warts within the anal mucosa. These verrucae of the anal mucosae require treatment by a gastroenterologist if recurrences are to be avoided. It is important to note that podophyllum resin derivatives occasionally have been shown to produce toxic hematologic effects (leukopenia and thrombocytopenia) when administered orally. Therefore, the container must be clearly labeled, and, when using large quantities on mucous membranes, the preparation should be used with extreme care and caution and should not be prescribed for self-administration by the patient.[57] Less toxic formulations containing podofilox (formerly known as podophyllotoxin, currently available from Oclassen Pharmaceuticals) may be dispensed as Condylox 0.5 per cent topical solution for the treatment of genital warts in males and external genital warts in females. These formulations can be applied carefully by the patient twice daily for 3 consecutive days followed by a rest period of 4 consecutive days. Patient selection for reliability, however, is imperative, and these formulations should not be used for the treatment of perianal, cervical, or vaginal condylomata. If there is no response after 4 weeks of treatment, alternative forms of therapy should be considered.[58]

Radiation. Irradiation, although effective in the management of recalcitrant—particularly plantar—warts, is not recommended for use in children because of the possibility of injury to underlying epiphyseal centers and the fact that instances of annoying or serious sequelae may result from such therapy.

Surgical Excision. Since some surgical procedures may lead to scarring that can be more painful and ugly than the wart itself, the physician should be guided by conservatism in the therapeutic management of warts. Surgical excision is not recommended, since it is painful and produces a scar, with warts frequently tending to recur in the area of the scar.

Electrodesiccation and curettage, however, is highly effective and often the method of choice for individual large warts (especially in older chil-

dren). Since warts are entirely epidermal, electrodesiccation should be neither extensive nor deep. The top of the lesion may be gently seared until the wart softens. It can then be curetted easily with gentle electrodesiccation of bleeders. Excessive coagulation of the base of the lesion is undesirable and may produce slow healing and undue scarring without better results or decrease in recurrence rate. This procedure should also be used with extreme caution on weight-bearing areas of the foot because of the possibility of painful and extensive scarring.

Bleomycin. Intralesional bleomycin may at times be used as an alternative form of therapy for large persistent warts and warts unresponsive to other modes of therapy. A cytotoxic drug isolated from a strain of *Streptomyces verticillus*, the main mode of action of bleomycin on recalcitrant warts appears to be related to its inhibition of DNA synthesis and, when injected locally, microthrombosis and hemorrhagic necrosis of the affected area. Available as bleomycin sulfate (Blenoxane) in 15-unit ampules, which when reconstituted with 15 ml of sterile saline produces a 0.1 mg/ml concentration (1 unit/ml), this mixture will remain stable under refrigeration for 4 months; and when injected into persistent warts at 2- or 3-week intervals for a total of two or three injections, it will effect a cure in 76 to 95 per cent of recalcitrant warts.[59, 60] Since intralesional bleomycin therapy can be painful, further dilution of the mixture with 2 per cent lidocaine and injections of minute amounts (0.1 to 0.2 ml) superficially, with just enough material to cause a slight blanching of the treated area, or a multiple puncture technique using bifurcated vaccination needles (available from Allergy Laboratories of Ohio Inc., 623 E. 11th Avenue, Columbus, Ohio) offers a less painful approach to the use of this modality.[61] It should be noted, however, that injections of bleomycin into periungual or cuticular tissue may result in onychodystrophy or loss of nails (Fig. 11–36).[62]

Laser Surgery. Although not recommended as a first-line form of treatment, carbon dioxide laser beam therapy can also be used as an alternative form of treatment for recalcitrant warts when other modes of therapy have been unsuccessful. Carbon dioxide ablation of warts, however, is not a cure-all, and careful patient selection is recommended.[63, 64]

Interferon Therapy. Topical and intralesional interferon-alfa and interferon-beta have at times been used for the intralesional and topical treatment of persistent verrucae vulgaris, genital warts (including giant Buschke-Lowenstein condylomata acuminata), flat warts, and epidermodysplasia verruciformis. Although headache, chills, myalgia, fever, malaise, nausea, flu-like symptoms, and leukopenia may occur after interferon treatment, these side effects are usually brief and mild and generally do not prove to be a problem in the treat-

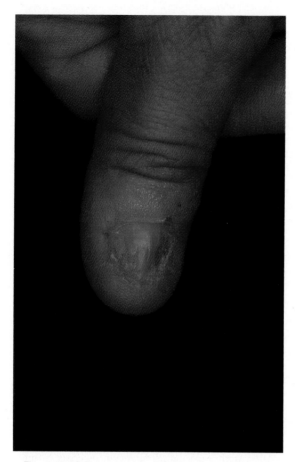

Figure 11–36. Permanent onychodystrophy on the thumb of a patient treated with intralesional bleomycin for periungual verrucae.

ment of affected individuals. Interferon therapy, however, is only suppressive. Thus, when treatment is discontinued, the papillomas often tend to return. If used, interferon should be administered cautiously in all patients, and particularly in those with debilitating medical conditions such as cardiovascular disease, pulmonary disease, diabetes mellitus prone to ketoacidosis, coagulation disorders, or severe myelosuppression.[56, 65, 66]

Summary. There is no single treatment for warts. All cases should be individually assessed, with the choice of therapy dependent on the age and personality of the patient and the number, size, and location of lesions. Whatever method the physician selects, he or she should be guided by conservatism if excessive trauma (psychological as well as physical) is to be avoided.

MOLLUSCUM CONTAGIOSUM

Molluscum contagiosum is a viral disorder of the skin and mucous membranes characterized by discrete single or multiple, flesh-colored, dome-shaped umbilicated papules (Figs. 11–37 through

11–39). Seen most frequently in childhood, molluscum lesions may appear at any age. The greatest incidence of this disorder appears in children between the ages of 3 and 16; the youngest reported case occurred in an infant whose lesions were noted during the first week of life.[67]

Both contagious and autoinoculable, lesions in children are generally located on the face, trunk, extremities (particularly in the axillae, antecubital, and crural regions), and sometimes on the mucous membranes of the lips, tongue, buccal mucosa, and conjunctiva. In adults, involvement of the pubic, genital, and perineal areas is common. The tendency for autoinoculation is supported by the presence of linear lesions in areas that are scratched. The contagious nature is suggested by the presence of lesions in areas of direct human contact, as is seen in wrestlers and masseurs, an increased incidence in swimmers (versus nonswimmers) who frequent swimming pools,[68] and the predominant genital distribution noted in sexually active individuals.[69] An epidemiologic study in Alaska revealed that multiple cases in families can occur (but are unusual), that males are more susceptible than females of similar age, and that the duration of lesions may vary from 2 weeks to 1½ years.[70]

The causative agent of molluscum contagiosum is a brick-shaped DNA virus of the pox virus group. Measuring 200 to 300 nm in diameter, it shares, with the viruses of psittacosis and lymphogranuloma venereum, the distinction of being one of the largest viruses known to infect humans. Although lesions are produced only rarely following experimental inoculations, most studies indicate incubation periods varying anywhere from 14 days to 6 months.[69] Reports of widespread lesions of molluscum contagiosum in individuals with atopic dermatitis, immunosuppressed individuals, and patients receiving prednisone and methotrexate support a correlation between depressed cellular immunity and the use of immunosuppressive

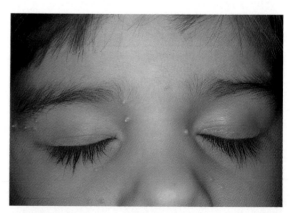

Figure 11–37. Discrete, flesh-colored, dome-shaped papules on the nasal area of a 3-year-old girl with molluscum contagiosum.

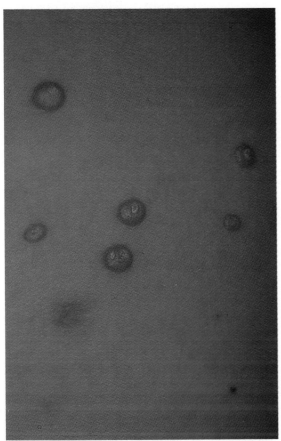

Figure 11–38. Multiple skin-colored, umbilicated, dome-shaped papules (molluscum contagiosum).

vitis of superficial punctate keratitis may complicate lesions located on the conjunctiva or eyelid margin. In such cases the dermatitis and conjunctivitis clear spontaneously after the molluscum lesions are treated.[74]

Diagnosis. The diagnosis of molluscum contagiosum is usually easily established by the appearance of distinctive flesh-colored papules with central umbilication. When the diagnosis remains in doubt, confirmation may be achieved by direct microscopic examination of the curd-like material extracted from lesions and, when necessary, by histopathologic examination of individual papules or nodules. The histopathologic changes of molluscum contagiosum are highly characteristic and consist of lobular proliferation of epidermal cells into the dermis. Individual epithelial cells contain large intracytoplasmic inclusion bodies (the so-called molluscum bodies), which give a unique and highly diagnostic histologic appearance to the lesions.

Treatment. Treatment generally depends on minor destructive techniques and should produce as little scarring or discomfort as possible. When treatment is deemed advisable, a topical cutaneous anesthetic such as fluorethyl ethylene chloride spray or a topical anesthetic cream containing 2.5 per cent lidocaine and 2.5 per cent prilocaine, available as EMLA cream (a *e*utectic *m*ixture of *l*ocal *a*nesthetics), applied under an occlusive semipermeable dressing for 45 to 60 minutes prior to treatment can help minimize discomfort.[75] It is important to inform the parent or patient at the first visit that, no matter which method is used, new

agents and increased susceptibility to viral disease (Figs. 11–40 and 11–41).[71, 72]

Clinical Manifestations. Most lesions of molluscum contagiosum are asymptomatic. They begin as small pinpoint elevations of the skin and gradually or rapidly increase, generally reaching 2 to 5 mm in diameter. Larger lesions measuring 10 to 15 mm in diameter are occasionally seen, and a giant molluscum lesion may even reach a diameter of 2 or 3 cm.[69] Papules of molluscum contagiosum are initially firm, solid, and flesh colored. With time they generally become soft and develop a waxy or pearly gray semitranslucent quality with a centrally located dimpled umbilication and a pulpy curd-like core, which can be expressed with a comedo extractor or a small sterile needle (Fig. 11–38). In some individuals an area of dermatitis may surround the molluscum lesions (Fig. 11–39). This inflammatory reaction, seen in up to 10 per cent of affected persons, may represent a delayed hypersensitivity to molluscum virus antigen and may vary from a mild reaction extending 5 mm around a discrete lesion to 10-cm areas of active dermatitis.[73] In some patients a chronic conjuncti-

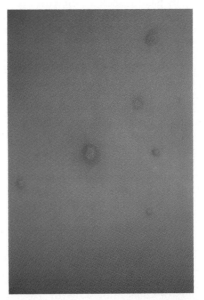

Figure 11–39. Molluscum contagiosum dermatitis. An umbilicated papule is surrounded by dermatitis. The inflammatory reaction may represent a delayed hypersensitivity reaction to the molluscum virus antigen.

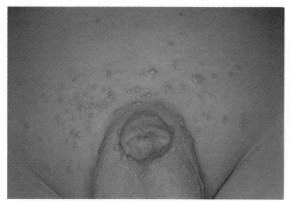

Figure 11–40. Molluscum contagiosum in the genital and suprapubic area of a 4½-year-old immunosuppressed child on chemotherapy for leukemia. Once the chemotherapy was discontinued the molluscum lesions resolved spontaneously.

lesions of microscopic size may be incubating and may possibly evolve within a period of several weeks. The easiest form of therapy is a light 2- to 3-second application of liquid nitrogen to each individual papule or nodule. This method is relatively painless and nonscarring and generally results in resolution of most lesions with two or three applications at intervals of 2 to 4 weeks.

Other methods include nightly scotch-tape or adhesive tape application followed, after a month or more, by gentle removal of individual lesions by a parent or physician; removal of individual lesions by gentle curettage (with or without cryosurgery), or piercing of each papule or nodule with a small needle and expression of the plug under aseptic technique; by light electrodesiccation; by touching the base of each lesion with silver nitrate, 7 to 9 per cent iodine, 1 per cent phenol, or 30 to 50 per cent trichloroacetic acid; or by the application of salicylic acid or cantharidin (as in the treatment of warts). Cantharidin, if available, although easily and painlessly applied in the office, may create a severe inflammatory reaction and, at times, a painful blister several hours later. Lesions on the eyelids and conjunctivae are probably best removed by light applications of liquid nitrogen or gentle curettage under local anesthesia (Fig. 11–42). No matter which method of therapy is used, since the disease is transmissible by autoinoculation, care must be taken to ensure that all molluscum lesions are destroyed.

MILKERS' NODULES

Milkers' nodule is a benign viral disease that generally consists of one or a few localized cutaneous nodules on the hand or forearm acquired from the udders of cows infected with pseudocowpox (paravaccinia virus), usually by dairy farmers, but occasionally by stock handlers, slaughterhouse employees, and, at times, children. The disorder is characterized by single or, at times, multiple 1- to 2-cm brownish red nodules usually confined to a finger, hand, or forearm. After an incubation period of 4 to 7 days the cutaneous lesions usually go through several stages, each lasting approximately 1 week. These usually start with a macule that progresses to a papular and then a vesicular stage and then a nodule; the histopathologic picture is consistent with that of a viral infection. During the maculopapular stage, lesions are characterized by vacuolization of cells and multilocular vesicles in the upper third of the stratum malpighii and, at times, eosinophilic inclusion bodies in the cytoplasm of the vacuolated epidermal cells.

Since the disorder is self-limiting and generally clears within about 6 weeks, only symptomatic treatment is generally indicated. Surgical removal of cutaneous lesions by razor blade transection, however, can often provide immediate relief, reduce the healing time, and minimize or eliminate the potential for complications such as lymphangitis, lymphadenopathy, secondary infection, or erythema multiforme.[76]

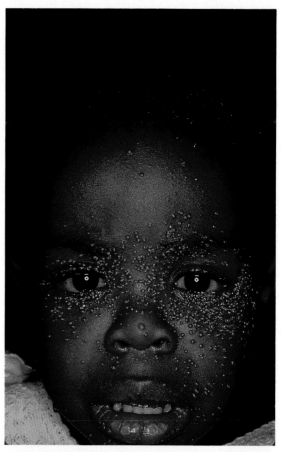

Figure 11–41. Multiple molluscum contagiosum in a 3-year-old child with acquired immunodeficiency syndrome. (Courtesy of Neal S. Penneys, M.D.)

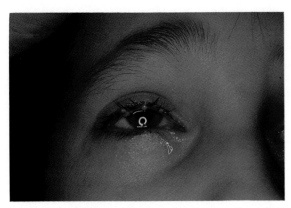

Figure 11–42. Multiple molluscum contagiosum on the eyelids of a 3-year-old child. These lesions were treated successfully with a light touch of liquid nitrogen and gentle curettage.

ORF

Orf, also known as contagious ecthyma (ecthyma contagiosum), is a parapox virus infection endemic among sheep and goats that can be transmitted to humans. In this self-limiting infection, which is generally manifested as nodules on the skin of individuals who raise or handle sheep, goats, or their byproducts, lesions appear after an incubation period of 3 to 6 days, and are characterized by single or multiple, 0.5- to 5.0-cm papules or nodules usually seen on the dorsal aspect of the right thumb or fingers of the right hand. Showing considerable clinical and histopathologic resemblance to milkers' nodules the disorder passes through similar stages, usually resolving spontaneously within 7 to 10 weeks. Although complications are rare, ocular involvement, erythema multiforme, papulovesicular or bullous rashes, extensive lesions in patients with atopic dermatitis, and superficial infection by bacterial organisms may be seen. Treatment is usually symptomatic and, as with milkers' nodules, superficial razor blade excision of lesions can reduce the healing time and minimize the complications.[76]

ACQUIRED IMMUNODEFICIENCY SYNDROME IN CHILDREN

First recognized as a clinical entity in 1981 when an unprecedented occurrence of Kaposi's sarcoma and severe opportunistic infections were reported in previously healthy persons, acquired immunodeficiency syndrome (AIDS) is a highly lethal viral infection caused by an RNA cytopathic human retrovirus, human immunodeficiency virus type 1 (HIV-1).[77] Children and adolescents as well as adults are affected, and it is estimated that as of 1991 there were 3,471 cases of AIDS in children younger than the age of 13 and 45,000 HIV-infected children in the United States. With 70 to 75 per cent of adult patients with AIDS presenting as male homosexuals in the third to fifth decades of life and with intravenous drug abusers accounting for 15 to 17 per cent of adults with this disorder, most children with AIDS (83 per cent) are born to mothers with HIV-1 infection, 10 per cent are recipients of blood transfusion or blood components contaminated with HIV, and an additional 5 per cent are hemophiliacs contaminated in the course of therapy for their disease.[78] Because of the variable and frequently long incubation period, ranging from months to years from the time of onset to the appearance of clinical manifestations, many of the young adults currently seen with this disorder appear to have been infected during their teenage years.[79, 80]

Currently accounting for 2 per cent of all reported cases in the United States, AIDS in children is manifested clinically by recurrent severe invasive bacterial infections caused by common bacteria (*Streptococcus pneumoniae, Hemophilus influenzae* type B, *Staphylococcus aureus,* and *Salmonella*), progressive neurologic disease, lymphoid interstitial pneumonitis, generalized lymphadenopathy and hepatosplenomegaly (often the earliest manifestations of pediatric AIDS), failure to thrive, developmental delay, recurrent diarrhea, parotitis, encephalopathy, hepatitis, cardiomyopathy, recurrent otitis media, thrush, diaper rash, nephropathy syndromes, clubbing of the nails, severe generalized atopic or seborrheic dermatitis, chronic varicella or severe herpes zoster infection, herpetic gingivostomatitis, condylomata acuminata, and widespread molluscum contagiosum (see Fig. 11–41). In addition there may be unusual vascular lesions clinically resembling Kaposi's sarcoma or pyogenic granuloma, recurrent widespread mucocutaneous candidiasis, oral hairy leukoplakia, an increased incidence of dermatophytosis, and low serum zinc levels (as a result of severe diarrhea) accompanied by the clinical features of acrodermatitis enteropathica.[78, 81–83] *Pneumocystis carinii* pneumonitis is the most common opportunistic infection of children with AIDS. Neoplasms, although commonly seen in adults, have been documented in only 2 per cent of children with AIDS. These include exceptionally rare reports of Kaposi's sarcoma (a common feature of HIV infection in homosexual men), non-Hodgkin's B-cell lymphomas of the Burkitt type, lymphomas of the central nervous system, fibrosarcoma of the liver, and multiple leiomyomas and leiomyosarcomas.[84] Cutaneous bacillary angiomatosis (see Chapter 10) and dark blue, purple-brown plaques or nodules characteristically seen on the skin of adults with AIDS (Fig. 11–43) have not been described in children.

Although craniofacial abnormalities in infants with prenatally acquired HIV infection have been reported, whether these represent other factors, such as maternal drug use, or genetic characteristics is controversial.[85, 86]

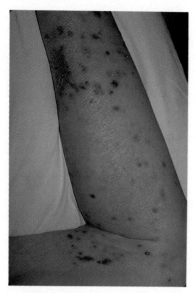

Figure 11–43. Multiple purple papules and nodules in a patient with acquired immunodeficiency syndrome (AIDS). (Courtesy of Department of Dermatology, Yale University School of Medicine.)

The diagnosis of HIV infection is based on clinical, immunologic, and serologic findings and the exclusion of other causes of immunodeficiency. A profound loss of T-cell immunity, particularly the T-helper (CD4) lymphocytes, with inversion of the normal T-helper to T-suppressor cell ratio to less than 1, is a nonspecific finding that also occurs in other acute viral infections such as those caused by cytomegalovirus or Epstein-Barr virus. Other helpful diagnostic tests include absent or delayed hypersensitivity skin tests to phytohemagglutinin or concanavalin A; anergy to skin test antigens such as mumps, *Candida*, *Trichophyton*, tetanus, and tuberculin purified protein derivative (PPD); abnormal lymphocyte responses to mitogens; and evidence of HIV infection by polymerase chain reaction and ELISA. Western blot and immunofluorescent antibody tests are used for confirmation of ELISA test results. Infants born to HIV-seropositive mothers are usually seropositive for up to 5 months due to passive transfer of maternal antibody. When an infant is suspected of having AIDS, therefore, sequential antibody tests should be used to determine whether the infant is truly infected.

The management of children, as well as adults, should be directed at prevention, nutritional support, and the treatment of individual manifestations of this syndrome. The controversy as to whether a child who has HIV infection may attend school, day care, or be placed in foster care should take into consideration the risks of the child acquiring secondary infection and the theoretical risk of transmission of HIV to other individuals. These decisions are best made by a team approach that includes the child's physician, public health personnel, the parents or guardians of the child, and personnel associated with the proposed care or educational setting. The benefit of monthly or biweekly administration of intravenous immune globulin for HIV-infected children is controversial. Early diagnosis and aggressive treatment of opportunistic infections such as *P. carinii* pneumonia will help prolong survival, and antiviral treatments such as ribavirin (Virazole) and zidovudine (formally called azidothymidine [AZT]) and studies of immunomodulators such as interferon and interleukin-2 are in progress.[87–90]

References

1. Corey L, Spear PG: Medical Progress: Infections with herpes simplex viruses. N. Engl. J. Med. *11*:686–691, 749–757, 1986.

   A comprehensive review of herpes simplex viruses, their epidemiology, pathogenesis, clinical features, and management.

2. Stevens JG, Cook ML: Latent herpes simplex in ganglia of mice. Science *173*:843–845, 1971.

   Cultures of herpesvirus obtained from spinal ganglia of mice suggest that these viruses are maintained in a "quiescent" state from which they may be reactivated, thus producing overt disease.

3. Baringer JR: Recovery of herpes simplex virus from human sacral ganglions. N. Engl. J. Med. *291*:828–830, 1974.

   Viral cultures of S3 and S4 ganglions of four patients suggest that virus residing in sacral sensory ganglions may serve as a source for recurrent genital infection.

4. Flowers FB, Araujo OE, Turner LA: Recent advances in antiherpetic drugs. Int. J. Dermatol. 27:612–616, 1988.

   An updated review of the newer antiviral drugs and their use in the treatment of herpesvirus infections.

5. Mertz GJ, Critchlow CW, Benedetti J, et al.: Double-blind placebo-controlled trial of oral acyclovir in first-episode genital herpes simplex virus infection. J.A.M.A. 252:1147–1151, 1984.

   In a study of 119 patients with primary and 31 patients with nonprimary genital herpes, oral acyclovir was shown to shorten the course and accelerate healing time in those who had primary genital herpes.

6. Straus SE, Takiff HE, Seidlin M, et al.: Suppression of frequently recurring genital herpes: A placebo-controlled double-blind trial of oral acyclovir. N. Engl. J. Med. *310*:1545–1550, 1984.

   In patients who had recurring genital herpes characterized by one or more episodes of the infection per month, a significant reduction in recurrences was demonstrated while patients were on suppressive acyclovir treatment.

7. Corey L, Nahmias AJ, Guinan ME, et al.: A trial of topical acyclovir in genital herpes simplex virus infections. N. Engl. J. Med. *306*:1313–1319, 1982.

   In a double-blind trial of 77 patients with primary genital herpes infection, the duration of viral shedding was reduced from 7.0 to 4.1 days and the healing time from 14.3 to 10.9 days (treatment of 111 patients with recurrent genital herpes showed equivocal results).

8. Kaplowitz LG, Baker D, Gelb L, et al.: Prolonged continuous acyclovir treatment of normal adults with frequently recurring genital herpes simplex virus infection. J.A.M.A. 265:747–751, 1991.

   A 3-year study of suppressive acyclovir for recurrent genital herpes confirms the efficacy and safety of oral acyclovir (400 mg twice daily) for periods of up to 3 years.

9. Feder HM Jr, Long S: Herpetic whitlow: Epidemiology, clinical characteristics, diagnosis and treatment. Am. J. Dis. Child. *137*:861–863, 1983.

A report of herpetic whitlow in four infants and young children, a 15-year-old girl, and two pediatric housestaff officers.

10. Tschen EH, Baack B: Treatment of herpetic whitlow in pregnancy with acyclovir. J. Am. Acad. Dermatol. *17*:1059–1060, 1987.

A report of a pregnant woman with a herpetic whitlow successfully treated with 10 days of oral erythromycin and a 5-day course of oral acyclovir without complication to mother or infant.

11. Belognia EA, Goodman JL, Holland EJ, et al.: An outbreak of herpes gladiatorum at a high-school wrestling camp. N. Engl. J. Med. *325*:906–910, 1991.

Herpes simplex was identified as a cause of cutaneous or ocular infection in 34 per cent (60 of 175) of high-school wrestlers attending a 4-week wrestling camp.

12. Penneys NS, Goldstein B, Nahass GT, et al.: Herpes simplex virus DNA in occult lesions: Demonstration by the polymerase chain reaction. J. Am. Acad. Dermatol. *24*:689–692, 1991.

A report of two patients in whom the clinical and histologic features were inconclusive and the polymerase chain reaction (PCR) was used to confirm the presence of herpes simplex virus DNA.

13. Guinan ME, MacCalman J, Kern ER, et al.: Topical ether and herpes labialis. J.A.M.A. *243*:1059–1061, 1980.

In a double-blind, placebo-controlled study of 51 patients with recurrent herpes simplex labialis there was no noteworthy difference between groups given ether or placebo in progression of lesions, healing time, duration or intensity of pain, and duration or quantity of virus excretion.

14. Neff JM, Lane JM: Vaccinia necrosum following smallpox vaccination for chronic herpetic ulcers. J.A.M.A. *213*:123–125, 1970.

Smallpox vaccination, a futile and potentially hazardous form of therapy for recurrent herpes simplex infection.

15. Griffith RS, Norins AL, Kagan C: Multicentered study of lysine therapy in herpes simplex infection. Dermatologica *156*:257–267, 1978.

In a study of 45 patients with frequently recurring herpes infection, L-lysine monohydrochloride in a daily dose of 800 to 1,000 mg during overt infection appeared to relieve pain, prevent appearance of new vesicles, and hasten resolution of lesions. Of further significance was an apparent prevention of recurrences by a maintenance dose of 500 g or more daily.

16. DiGiovanna JJ, Blank H: Failure of lysine in frequently recurrent herpes simplex infection: Treatment and prophylaxis. Arch. Dermatol. *120*:48–51, 1984.

A study of the use of lysine for recurrent herpes simplex infections showed no significant differences between the lysine- and placebo-treated groups.

17. Lagrew DC Jr, Furlow TG, Hager D, et al.: Disseminated herpes simplex virus infection in pregnancy: Successful treatment with acyclovir. J.A.M.A. *252*:2058–2059, 1989.

A 26-year-old pregnant woman with disseminated herpes simplex virus infection was successfully treated with intravenous acyclovir during her third trimester of pregnancy.

18. Feldman GV: Herpes zoster neonatorum. Arch. Dis. Child. *27*:126–127, 1952.

A case of herpes zoster in one of a pair of 4-day-old twins.

19. Baba K, Yabuuchi H, Takahashi M, et al.: Increased incidence of herpes zoster in normal children infected with varicella zoster virus during infancy: Community-based follow-up study. J. Pediatr. *108*:372–377, 1986.

A study of 849 infants and children who had clinical varicella during the first 4 years of life in which 9 subsequently developed herpes zoster at a significantly shorter interval in their life.

20. Helander I, Arstila P, Terho P: Herpes zoster in a 6-month-old infant. Acta. Derm. Venereol. *63*:180–181, 1983.

A report of herpes zoster in a 6-month-old infant whose mother had varicella during the second trimester of pregnancy.

21. Keiden SE, Mainwaring D: Association of herpes zoster with leukemia and lymphoma in children. Clin. Pediatr. *4*:13–17, 1965.

Five children, two with Hodgkin's disease and three with acute leukemia, with herpes zoster.

22. Guess HA, Broughton DD, Melton LJ III, et al.: Epidemiology of herpes zoster in children and adolescents: A population-based study. Pediatrics 76:512–517, 1985.

A review of 173 cases of herpes zoster in children younger than 20 years of age confirms previous concepts that the disorder is generally milder in children than it is in adults and that the risk of cancer in children with herpes zoster is no different than that of the general childhood population.

23. Wurzel CL, Kahan J, Heitler M, et al.: Prognosis of herpes zoster in healthy children. Am. J. Dis. Child. *140*:477–478, 1986.

In a review of 22 cases of childhood herpes zoster, the authors conclude that a detailed investigation for malignancy does not appear to be warranted for otherwise apparently normal children with herpes zoster.

24. Friedman-Kien AE, Lafleur FL, Gendler E, et al.: Herpes zoster: A possible early clinical sign for development of acquired immunodeficiency syndrome in high-risk individuals. J. Am. Acad. Dermatol. *14*:1023–1028, 1986.

A review of 300 patients with acquired immunodeficiency syndrome and Kaposi's sarcoma revealed a seven-times higher incidence of herpes zoster and a greater risk of disseminated disease in patients with AIDS than that of the general population.

25. Ashton H, Beveridge CW, Stevenson CJ: Management of herpes zoster. Br. J. Dermatol. *81*:874–876, 1976.

Systemic corticosteroids in disseminated herpes zoster and post-zoster neuralgia.

26. Bernstein JE, Korman NJ, Bickers DR, et al.: Topical capsaicin treatment of chronic postherpetic neuralgia. J. Am. Acad. Dermatol. *21*:265–270, 1989.

Local application of capsaicin, a phytochemical that results in depletion of substance P within the neuron, provided partial to complete relief from zoster-induced pain and pruritus in almost 80 per cent of patients with chronic intractable postherpetic neuralgia.

27. Epstein E: Treatment of herpes zoster and post zoster neuralgia by sublesional injection of triamcinolone and procaine. Acta Derm. Venereol. *50*:69–73, 1970.

The subcutaneous sublesional injection of triamcinolone-procaine solution appears to help control post-herpetic pain.

28. Epstein E: Treatment of herpes zoster and post-zoster neuralgia by subcutaneous injection of triamcinolone. Int. J. Dermatol. *20*:65–68, 1981.

Intralesional injections of triamcinolone acetonide solution helped control post-herpetic pain in 65 per cent of 272 patients with herpes zoster.

29. Serota FT, Starr SE, Bryan CK, et al.: Acyclovir treatment of herpes zoster infections: Use in children undergoing bone marrow transplantation. J.A.M.A. 247:2132–2135, 1982.

A report of three bone marrow recipient patients with herpes zoster treated with intravenous acyclovir with good results.

30. Huff JC: Antiviral treatment in chickenpox and herpes zoster. J. Am. Acad. Dermatol. *18*:204–206, 1988.

Intravenous acyclovir is effective for varicella and zoster infections in immunocompromised patients. Although oral acyclovir is also effective, its effect is less dramatic and the drug must be given early.

31. Whitley RJ, Chi'en LT, Dolin R, et al.: Early vidarabine therapy to control the complications of herpes zoster in immunosuppressed patients. N. Engl. J. Med. 307:971–975, 1982.

In a double-blind study of 121 patients, intravenous vidarabine (10 mg/kg over a period of 12 hours) for 5 days reduced the chance of disseminated lesions and post-herpetic neuralgia in immunocompromised patients with herpes zoster.

32. Groth KE, McCullough J, Marker SC, et al.: Evaluation of zoster immune plasma: Treatment of cutaneous disseminated zoster in immunocompromised patients. J.A.M.A. 239:1877–1879, 1978.

Since zoster immune plasma (ZIP) did not alter the clinical course of zoster, and because zoster patients produced high antibody titers without ZIP, it is suggested that ZIP is not useful for the treatment of cutaneous disseminated zoster and should be reseved for the prevention or modification of varicella in exposed susceptible immunocompromised patients.

33. Balfour HH Jr: Acyclovir therapy for herpes zoster: Advantages and adverse effects. J.A.M.A. 255:387–388, 1986.

A review of the use of intravenous acyclovir in immunocompromised patients, its side effects and recommendations for appropriate dosages and concentrations.

34. Rogers RS: Recurrent aphthous stomatitis: Clinical characteristics and evidence for an immunopathogenesis. J. Invest. Dermatol. 69:499–509, 1977.

A comprehensive review of aphthous stomatitis, its clinical features and etiology.

35. Grinspan D, Blanco GF, Agüero S: Treatment of aphthae with thalidomide. J. Am. Acad. Dermatol. 20:1060–1063, 1989.

In a report of 100 patients (44 with major and 56 with minor aphthae) treated with thalidomide (in dosages of 100 to 300 mg daily for 3 months), a cure was achieved in 34 per cent of cases and marked improvement was evident in the rest.

36. Massing AM, Epstein WL: Natural history of warts: A two year study. Arch. Dermatol. 87:301–310, 1963.

Observations on 1,000 institutionalized children revealed that two thirds of their warts resolved spontaneously within 2 years.

37. Lutzner MA: The human papillomaviruses: A review. Arch. Dermatol. 119:631–635, 1983.

A review of the human papillomaviruses, their subtypes, histologic patterns, and potential for oncogenicity.

38. Cobb MW: Human papillomavirus infection. J. Am. Acad. Dermatol. 22:547–566, 1990.

A comprehensive overview of the epidemiology, pathogenesis, clinical manifestations, and treatment of human papillomavirus infection.

39. Pfister H: Human papillomaviruses and impaired immunity vs. epidermodysplasia verruciformis. Arch. Dermatol. 123:1469–1470, 1987.

Although the vast majority of warts are benign, those associated with dysplasias of the uterine cervix, macules of epidermodysplasia verruciformis, and laryngeal papillomas in adults may progress to squamous cell carcinomas.

40. Beutner KR: Periodic synopsis: Human papillomavirus infection. J. Am. Acad. Dermatol. 20:114–123, 1989.

An authoritative review of the literature on human papillomavirus infection.

41. Crissey JT, Peachey JC: Calcaneal petechiae. Arch. Dermatol. 83:501, 1961.

The pigment in "talon noir" (black heel) appears to be hemoglobin that has extravasated from capillaries on the sides and backs of the heels and edges of the feet of athletes due to the shearing effect of sudden stopping on hard surfaces.

42. American Academy of Dermatology Task Force of Pediatric Dermatology: Genital warts and sexual abuse in children. J. Am. Acad. Dermatol. 11:529–530, 1984.

Sexual abuse must be considered when warts are noted in the anal and genital areas of children younger than 12 years of age, and, if there is reason to believe that abuse may have occurred, the case must be reported to the proper authorities.

43. Cohen BA, Honig P, Androphy E: Anogenital warts in children: Clinical and virologic evaluation for sexual abuse. Arch. Dermatol. 126:1575–1580, 1990.

Data from 73 children with anogenital warts examined for sexual abuse suggest that sexually transmitted anogenital warts are less common than the literature suggests, and when observed in children younger than the age of 3 years the disorder is unlikely to have been a result of sexual abuse.

44. Rock B, Naghashfar Z, Barnett N, et al.: Genital tract papillomavirus infection in children. Arch. Dermatol. 122:1129–1132, 1986.

A nonvenereal route should be sought when there is no evidence of sexual abuse, lesions are more than 1½ inches from the anus or introitus, and children are younger than 9 months of age at the time of onset of the disorder.

45. Obalek S, Jablonska S, Favre M, et al.: Condylomata acuminata in children: Frequent association with human papillomaviruses responsible for cutaneous warts. J. Am. Acad. Dermatol. 23:205–213, 1990.

A study of 32 children 10 months to 11 years of age with anogenital warts confirms nonsexual transmission and a high association with cutaneous warts transmitted perhaps by heteroinoculation or autoinoculation.

46. Chuang T-Y: Condylomata acuminata (genital warts): An epidemiologic view. J. Am. Acad. Dermatol. 16:376–384, 1987.

An overview of condylomata acuminata and a recommendation that patients with genital warts be examined carefully and periodically for the possibility of new lesions or neoplastic transformation of the cervical and other genital areas.

47. Androphy EJ, Dvoretzky I, Lowy D: X-linked inheritance of epidermodysplasia verruciformis. Arch. Dermatol. 121:864–868, 1985.

A report of a family with typical epidermodysplasia verruciformis in which only male members were affected suggests the presence of an X-linked recessive form of this disorder.

48. Ferenczy A, Mitao M, Nagai N, et al.: Latent papillomavirus and recurring genital warts. N. Engl. J. Med. 313:784–785, 1985.

The presence of papillomavirus in apparently normal squamous epithelium beyond treatment areas in patients with anogenital warts appears to correlate with the risk of recurrence in individuals with this disorder.

49. Rosenberg SK: Subclinical papilloma viral infection of male genitalia. Urology 26:554–557, 1985.

Inapparent genital warts were detected in 40 per cent of 154 male patients by the use of 3- to 5-minute soaks with 3 to 5 per cent acetic acid.

50. Bart BJ, Biglow J, Vance JC, et al.: Salicylic acid in karaya gum patch as a treatment for verruca vulgaris. J. Am. Acad. Dermatol. 20:74–76, 1989.

In a clinical study of 61 patients with verruca vulgaris on the hands, those using salicylic acid in karaya gum patches showed a significantly greater cure rate (68 per cent) than patients (28 per cent) treated with patches containing the same ingredients, with the exception of the salicylic acid, used as controls.

51. Linn E: Conservative management of warts. Clin. Med. 74:39–42, 1967.

Since untreated warts may undergo spontaneous resolution,

alone or by suggestion therapy, results associated with the use of an ointment containing ascorbic and pantothenic acid are difficult to assess.

52. Epstein WL, Kligman AM: Treatment of warts with cantharidin. Arch. Dermatol. 77:508–511, 1958.

Although cantharidin appears to be beneficial in the treatment of warts, patients should be forewarned of the possibility of recurrences in the surrounding blister margin.

53. Tromovitch TA, Kay DM: Plantar warts: Treatment with formalin and salicylic acid occlusion. Cutis 12:87–88, 1973.

A 94 per cent cure rate in 18 of 19 patients with plantar warts by formalin, salicylic acid plaster, and plastic tape occlusion.

54. Nix TE: Liquid-nitrogen neuropathy. Arch. Dermatol. 92:185–187, 1965.

In an effort to minimize the possibility of neuropathy, caution should be exercised in the use of liquid nitrogen on those sites where nerves are known to lie close to the skin surface.

55. Committee on Cutaneous Health and Cosmetics: Treatment of verrucae with smallpox vaccine. J.A.M.A. 206:117, 1968.

Even if vaccinia-induced inflammatory reactions may cause the resolution of verrucae, potential serious side effects associated with smallpox inoculation of warts makes this a medically unsound method of therapy.

56. Friedman-Kien AE, Eron LJ, Conant M, et al.: Natural interferon alfa for treatment of condylomata acuminata. J.A.M.A. 259:533–538, 1988.

In a randomized controlled study, treatment with interferon alfa injected intralesionally twice weekly for up to 8 weeks completely eliminated warts in 62 per cent of patients (as compared with only 21 per cent in placebo-treated patients).

57. Perez-Figaredo RA, Baden HP: The pharmacology of podophyllum. Prog. Dermatol. 10:1–4, 1976.

Podophyllum resin, the most frequently used drug in the treatment of genital warts, is cytotoxic and when used over large areas or in children should be used with appropriate precautions.

58. Beutner KR, von Krogh G: Current status of podophyllotoxin for the treatment of genital warts. Semin. Dermatol. 9:148–151, 1990.

An evolutionary process that began 50 years ago with a crude plant resin (podophyllum) has now been developed to the point where it appears that podophyllotoxin can be applied at home by patients for the treatment of their external genital warts.

59. Bunney MH, Nolan MW, Buxton PK, et al.: The treatment of resistant warts with intralesional bleomycin: A controlled clinical trial. Br. J. Dermatol. 111:197–207, 1984.

Treatment with intralesional bleomycin sulfate (up to 0.2 ml for a total of one to three treatments at 3-week intervals) resulted in a 76 per cent cure rate in patients with resistant warts.

60. Shumer SM, O'Keefe EJ: Bleomycin in the treatment of recalcitrant warts. J. Am. Acad. Dermatol. 9:91–96, 1983.

Intralesional bleomycin treatment of warts resulted in a high (81 per cent) cure rate with one to two biweekly injections of bleomycin (0.2 to 1.0 ml per wart) in concentrations of 1 unit/ml in normal saline.

61. Shelley WB, Shelley ED: Intralesional bleomycin sulfate therapy for warts: A novel bifurcated needle puncture technique. Arch. Dermatol. 127:234–236, 1991.

A multiple puncture technique using a bifurcated vaccination needle resulted in elimination of 92 per cent of a randomized series of warts after a single treatment.

62. González FU, del Carmen Cristobal Gil M, Martinez AA, et al.: Cutaneous toxicity of intralesional bleomycin in the treatment of periungual warts. Arch. Dermatol. 122:974–975, 1986.

A report of a patient with recalcitrant periungual warts treated with intralesional bleomycin who suffered finger nail loss in the involved fingers suggests caution in the use of this modality in the treatment of periungual warts.

63. McBurney EI, Rosen DA: Carbon dioxide laser treatment for verrucae vulgaris. J. Dermatol. Surg. Oncol. 10:45–48, 1984.

A cure rate of 81 per cent was achieved in recalcitrant warts on the hands and feet in 27 patients with a single CO_2 laser treatment; all others were cured following one or two additional treatments.

64. Garden JM, O'Banion K, Shelnitz LS, et al.: Papillomavirus in the vapor of carbon dioxide laser–treated verrucae. J.A.M.A. 259:1199–1202, 1988.

Since viral DNA is liberated into the air in the vapor of laser-treated verrucae, precautionary measures are recommended for all physicians who use CO_2 laser therapy in the treatment of viral infections or other viral-associated dermatologic disorders.

65. Olsen EA, Kelly FF, Vollmer RT, et al.: Comparative study of systemic interferon alfa-n1 and isotretinoin in the treatment of resistant condylomata acuminata. J. Am. Acad. Dermatol. 20:1023–1030, 1989.

Although side effects are common, subcutaneous interferon therapy appeared to be an effective alternative treatment for patients with refractory condylomata acuminata.

66. Schoenfeld A, Ovadia J, Stein L, et al.: Treatment of flat facial warts with interferon-beta cream. J. Dermatol. Surg. Oncol. 13:299–301, 1987.

A 20-year-old man with multiple verrucae plana was successfully treated, without side effects, by a topical formulation of human fibroblast interferon beta.

67. Mandel MJ, Lewis RJ: Molluscum cantagiosum of the newborn. Br. J. Dermatol. 84:370–372, 1970.

Molluscum contagiosum lesions noted during the first week of life.

68. Niizeki K, Karo O, Kondo Y: An epidemic study of molluscum contagiosum: Relationship to swimming. Dermatologica 169:197–198, 1984.

In a study of molluscum contagiosum, the incidence of this viral infection in swimmers was found to be twice that of children not permitted to swim in public pools.

69. Lynch PJ, Minkin W: Molluscum contagiosum of the adult: Probably venereal transmission. Arch. Dermatol. 98:141–143, 1969.

Lesions of molluscum contagiosum confined to the genital areas and inner thighs in 55 adult patients suggest a venereal transmission of the disorder in this group of military personnel.

70. Overfield TM, Brody JA: An epidemiologic study of molluscum contagiosum in Anchorage, Alaska. J. Pediatr. 69:640–642, 1966.

Proximity as a factor in 9 of 13 children (ages 10 months to 13 years) with molluscum contagiosum.

71. Paul CR, Artis WM, Jones HE: Atopic dermatitis, impaired cellular immunity and molluscum contagiosum. Arch. Dermatol. 114:391–393, 1978.

Patients with atopic dermatitis may have a functional defect or defects in cell-mediated immunity that may impair host defense and predispose to increased susceptibility to molluscum contagiosum.

72. Rosenberg EW, Yusk JW: Molluscum contagiosum, eruption following treatment with prednisone and methotrexate. Arch. Dermatol. 101:439–441, 1970.

Two patients under therapy with prednisone and methotrexate developed florid eruptions with hundreds of molluscum contagiosum lesions.

73. DeOrea GA, Johnson HH Jr, Binkley GW: An eczematous reaction associated with molluscum contagiosum. Arch. Dermatol. 74:344–348, 1956.

Patchy eczematoid eruptions around lesions of molluscum contagiosum.

74. Kipping HF: Letters to the editor: Molluscum dermatitis. Arch. Dermatol. *103*:106–107, 1971.

In 200 consecutive cases of molluscum contagiosum, 19 patients were observed to have a surrounding inflammatory dermatitis, which cleared after the molluscum lesions were treated.

75. Waard-van der Spek FB, Oranje AP, Lillieborg S, et al.: Treatment of molluscum contagiosum using a lidocaine/prilocaine cream (EMLA) for anesthesia. J. Am. Acad. Dermatol. *23*:685–688, 1990.

In a study of 83 children with molluscum contagiosum in which EMLA or a placebo cream was used, local redness, believed to be caused by the vasoactive properties of lidocaine and prilocaine, was the only observed adverse reaction to this agent.

76. Shelley WB, Shelley ED: Surgical treatment of farmyard pox: Orf, milker's nodules, bovine papular stomatitis pox. Cutis *31*:191–192, 1983.

Superficial razor excision of localized lesions can provide immediate relief and cure and, at the same time, eliminate the potential for secondary complications seen in individuals with the above disorders.

77. Friedman-Kien A: Disseminated Kaposi's sarcoma syndrome in young homosexual men. J. Am. Acad. Dermatol. *5*:468–471, 1981.

A report of an epidemic of a fulminant type of Kaposi's sarcoma in severely immunodeficient homosexual males.

78. Prose NS: Mucocutaneous disease in pediatric human immunodeficiency virus infections. Pediatr. Clin. North Am. *38*:977–990, 1991.

An overview of AIDS and its clinical manifestations in the childhood age group.

79. Manoff SB, Gayle HD, Mays MA, et al.: Acquired immunodefiency syndrome in adolescents: Epidemiology, prevention and public health issues. Pediatr. Infect. Dis. J. *8*:309–314, 1989.

Although little attention had been focused on AIDS in the adolescent, this article highlights the fact that the incidence of AIDS in adolescents has increased annually since 1986 and that many young adults with AIDS were actually infected during their teenage years.

80. Gayle HD, D'Angelo LJ: Epidemiology of acquired immunodeficiency syndrome and human immunodeficiency virus infection in adolescents. Pediatr. Infect. Dis. J. *10*:322–328, 1991.

A comprehensive overview of the epidemiology of AIDS in adolescents.

81. Pahwa S, Biron K, Lim W, et al.: Continuous varicella-zoster infection associated with acyclovir resistance in a child with AIDS. J.A.M.A. *260*:2879–2882, 1988.

A 4½-year-old girl congenitally infected with human immunodeficiency virus developed a continuous infection with varicella-zoster virus that persisted despite vigorous therapy with acyclovir and eventually resulted in her death.

82. Knobler EH, Silvers DN, Fine KC, et al.: Unique vascular lesions associated with human immunodeficiency virus. J.A.M.A. *260*:524–527, 1988.

A report of four patients with antibodies to human immunodeficiency syndrome, AIDS, or both, with unusual vascular lesions clinically resembling Kaposi's sarcoma or pyogenic granuloma.

83. Tong TK, Andrew LR, Albert A, et al.: Childhood acquired immunodeficiency syndrome manifesting as acrodermatitis enteropathica. J. Pediatr. *108*:426, 1986.

Severe diarrhea in children with AIDS can at times result in severe loss of zinc through the gastrointestinal canal and a syndrome manifesting as acrodermatitis enteropathica.

84. Chadwick EG, Conner EJ, Hanson CF, et al.: Tumors of smooth-muscle origin in HIV-infected children. J.A.M.A. *263*:3182–3184, 1990.

Multiple leiomyomas and leiomyosarcomas in three children with acquired immunodeficiency syndrome.

85. Marion RW, Wiznia AA, Hutcheon G, et al.: Human T-cell lymphotrophic virus type III (HTLV-III) embryopathy. Am. J. Dis. Child. *140*:638–640, 1986.

Although a review of 20 infants and children with positive serologic tests for the AIDS virus were noted to have similar features suggesting a dysmorphic syndrome, the presence of a distinctive craniofacial dysmorphism has not been validated by other observers.

86. Quazi QH, Sheikh TM, Fikrig S, et al.: Lack of evidence for craniofacial dysmorphism in perinatal human immunodeficiency virus infection. J. Pediatr. *112*:7–11, 1988.

A review of 30 children perinatally exposed to human immunodeficiency virus infection and 30 healthy controlled subjects matched for age, sex, and race failed to confirm the presence of a characteristic craniofacial dysmorphism in children exposed to perinatal human immunodeficiency virus infection.

87. Kaplan LD, Wolfsy C, Volberding PA: Treatment of patients with acquired immunodeficiency syndrome and associated manifestations. J.A.M.A. *257*:1367–1374, 1987.

A comprehensive review of the treatment of patients with AIDS and its complications.

88. Fischl MA, Richman DD, Causey DM, et al.: Prolonged zidovudine therapy in patients with AIDS and advanced AIDS-related complex. J.A.M.A. *262*:2405–2410, 1989.

Studies of 229 patients confirm the continued survival benefits of long-term zidovudine therapy in patients with AIDS and advanced AIDS-related complex.

89. Bartlett JA: Editorial: HIV therapeutics: An emerging science. J.A.M.A. *260*:3051–3052, 1988.

A review of therapy for patients with asymptomatic HIV infection, advanced AIDS-related complex, and AIDS.

90. Pizzo PA, Eddy J, Falloon J, et al.: Effect of continuous intravenous injection of zidovudine (AZT) in children with symptomatic HIV infection. N. Engl. J. Med. *319*:889–896, 1988.

Studies of intravenous AZT administration in children confirm its beneficial effect in children with symptomatic human immunodeficiency virus infection.

THE EXANTHEMATOUS DISEASES OF CHILDHOOD

Many viral and bacterial illnesses are accompanied by generalized erythematous eruptions called exanthems. These rashes, composed of macules, papules, vesicles, pustules, or petechiae, may be produced by many microorganisms. The classic exanthems of childhood include chickenpox, smallpox, measles, scarlet fever, rubella, erythema infectiosum, and roseola infantum. Other disorders added to this list of childhood exanthems include the exanthematous eruptions produced by echoviruses, coxsackieviruses, reoviruses, and the Epstein-Barr virus (infectious mononucleosis). Because of their exanthematous nature, the rickettsial diseases, caused by microorganisms that occupy an intermediate position between bacteria and viruses, are also included in this chapter.

VARICELLA (CHICKENPOX)

Varicella (chickenpox) is a highly contagious disease of childhood, and occasionally adulthood, caused by a primary infection with a complex herpes group DNA virus (herpesvirus varicellae), the varicella-zoster virus. Transmission of varicella is by close contact and droplet infection from individuals affected with the disorder and, since varicella and herpes zoster are caused by infection with the same virus, occasionally from contact with individuals with herpes zoster.

In normal children systemic symptoms are usually mild and serious complications are rare. In adults and children taking systemic corticosteroids or immunosuppressive drugs, or with deficiencies in cell-mediated immunity, the disorder is more likely to be characterized by an extensive eruption, severe constitutional symptoms, and, occasionally, varicella pneumonia with, at times, a potentially fatal outcome.

Because of its highly contagious nature this disorder is usually seen during childhood, but it may occur at any age, including the newborn period. Approximately 50 per cent of the cases occur prior to the fifth year of age and 80 to 90 per cent occur by the age of 15 years. The disorder occurs in epidemics with a peak incidence during late winter and spring and recurring high rates of incidence at intervals of 2 to 5 years.

Clinical Manifestations. Following an incubation period of 14 to 16 days (occasionally as early as 10 days or as late as 21 days) the disease begins with a low-grade fever, malaise, and the appearance of a highly characteristic vesicular exanthem manifested by delicate "teardrop" vesicles on an erythematous base (Fig. 12–1). In children the disease is characteristically a mild febrile disorder, occasionally preceded by a 24-hour prodrome of headache, malaise, and fever accompanied by successive crops of papulovesicles. Adults frequently exhibit a prodrome of 1 or 2 days, a more extensive rash, increased constitutional symptoms, and a predisposition to more severe complications.

A highly characteristic feature is the fact that all stages and sizes of lesions may be found at the same time and in the same vicinity. The eruption generally begins abruptly on the trunk, face, and scalp, with successive crops of pruritic lesions and

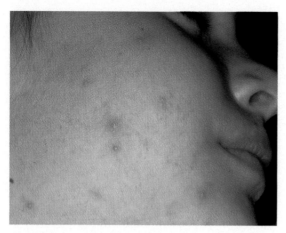

Figure 12–1. Varicella. Maculopapular lesions and "tear-drop" vesicles on an erythematous base are evident on the face of a 9-year-old girl.

minimal, if any, involvement of the distal aspect of the extremities. This centripetal distribution is in sharp contrast to the centrifugal distribution seen in variola (smallpox). Mucous membranes are characteristically involved, and ulcers may be present on the pharynx, palate, anterior tonsillar pillars, and occasionally on the larynx, the conjunctivae, vulva, and anal mucosa.

The average pock first appears as a small red macule, 2 or 3 mm in diameter, which, in the course of a few hours, becomes a papule. It then develops a small delicate vesicle of clear fluid (see Fig. 12–1). Although many of the lesions are surrounded by an irregularly shaped red areola, this may be entirely lacking, and occasionally a vesicle may appear directly on otherwise normal-appearing skin. The vesicle of chickenpox is usually rounded or pear shaped but may show a central depression or umbilicated appearance. Often, within 6 to 8 hours and usually within 24 hours, the rash of varicella progresses through maculopapular, vesicular, pustular, and crusted stages (Fig. 12–2). Except for secondarily infected lesions, the crusts fall off within 5 to 25 days, depending on the depth of involvement. Except for immunosuppressed individuals with severe varicella, unless deep excoriation or secondary infection occurs, lesions generally tend to heal without scar formation (Fig. 12–3).

Lesions of varicella appear in successive crops over a 3- to 5-day period, with all stages of development in the same anatomic area at the same time. The lesions may be modified by preexisting inflammation, such as may be seen in infants with diaper dermatitis, or by an increase in lesions in areas of sun exposure or sunburn. Although relatively little has been written about the accentuation of viral eruptions in areas of the body exposed to sunlight, photoexaggerated or photolocalized varicella, this phenomenon and the localization of varicella to areas of trauma or injection bear recognition.[1, 2]

The fever in individuals with chickenpox is vari-

able in severity and duration and roughly parallels the extent and severity of the rash. Successive lesions usually appear over a period of 3 days. Crusting of lesions occurs within 5 days in mild cases and within 10 days in severe cases. The disorder is considered to be contagious for approximately 24 hours preceding the rash and for 5 to 7 days afterward (when all vesicles have crusted). Infectivity, however, may persist much longer in patients with an altered immune response, as fresh moist lesions continue to appear. As in most other viral exanthems, although varicella generally confers lasting immunity, second attacks are rare but can occur.

Unusual forms of chickenpox may also occur. Varicella in an immunocompromised individual may be characterized by a hemorrhagic, progressive, and/or disseminated infection with severe viremia and a potentially fatal outcome.[3] Infants born to mothers who had varicella early in pregnancy may be born with multiple congenital anomalies (microphthalmia, cataracts, micrognathia, cutaneous scars, or atrophy of a limb), suggesting an intrauterine teratogenic potential to the varicella-zoster virus. Although transplacental IgG antibody passes from the mother to the infant in utero, the protection from this antibody is not as good as that of other viral disorders such as rubeola. Maternal varicella, accordingly, just prior to or at term may result in a severe or fatal disseminated disorder of the newborn (varicella neonatorum) characterized by hemorrhagic lesions and involvement of the lungs and liver. When an infant contracts the infection from its mother or through exposure to a sibling or other individual during the first 3 months of life, except when the onset is between the 5th and 10th days of life, the disorder is usually relatively mild and uncomplicated, except for the diaper area (where the eruption may be

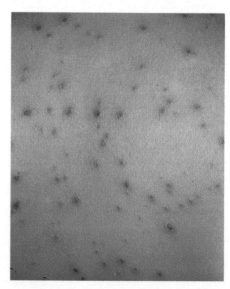

Figure 12–2. Varicella. Crusted lesions on the seventh day of illness.

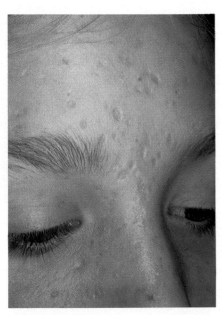

Figure 12–3. Post-varicella scars on the face of a young girl who developed chickenpox shortly after receiving systemic intramuscular corticosteroid for the treatment of poison ivy.

Diagnosis. The diagnosis of varicella can usually be made clinically, especially when one can elicit a history of contact with an infected sibling or playmate. When confirmation is required, examination of cells from scrapings of lesions for multinucleated giant cells containing intranuclear viral inclusions (the Tzanck smear), skin biopsy, viral cultures of vesicular lesions (particularly during the first 3 to 4 days of the eruption), immunofluorescent staining of vesicular scrapings, identification of viral particles by direct electron microscopic examination, the polymerase chain reaction technique, and serologic testing of acute and convalescent sera for varicella-zoster antibody can help establish the diagnosis.

Treatment. The treatment of chickenpox should be directed to alleviation of itching and prevention of secondary bacterial infection. Patients are believed to be contagious for 1 or 2 days before and possibly for as long as 5 days after the onset of the cutaneous eruption. Thus, children with uncomplicated chickenpox who have been excluded from school or day care may return on the sixth day after the onset of the rash. In mild cases with only a few lesions and rapid resolution, children may return sooner. Immunocompromised children, however, may have a more prolonged course and should be excluded for the entire period of eruption of new lesions. Pruritus may be decreased by starch baths or Aveeno baths, topical application of calamine lotion (to which 0.25 to 0.5 per cent menthol and 0.5 to 1.0 per cent phenol may be added), pramoxine-containing formulations such as Prax or PrameGel, or Sarna lotion (a combination of 0.5 per cent camphor and 0.5 per cent menthol). Acetaminophen (not aspirin) may be used to control fever, headache, or myalgia; and, when necessary, topical or systemic antibiotics can be used to control secondary bacterial infection.

Patients on systemic corticosteroids or other drugs that may depress immune response exposed to varicella should have the dosage reduced to physiologic levels or discontinued whenever possible. For immunologically depressed patients exposed to varicella, γ-globulin prophylaxis (1.3 ml/kg) or zoster immune globulin (ZIG) may be used to attenuate the subsequent clinical disease. [6–8] It is also recommended that seronegative pregnant women exposed to chickenpox receive varicella-zoster immune globulin (VZIG, 4 vials, each containing 125 units, one in each buttock and one in each thigh).[7] Since infants born to mothers with onset of varicella within 5 days before or within 48 hours after delivery and infants who develop varicella between the 5th and 10th days of life have a high risk of dissemination, fulminant infection, and mortality, ZIG or VZIG (125 units) should be administered to the infant as soon as possible after delivery. In addition, intravenous vidarabine and acyclovir, although not always successful, have been shown to inhibit cutaneous and visceral dissemination of the virus when given to immunocompromised patients and infants with varicella neonatorum.[9–11] Oral acyclovir, given

modified by diaper dermatitis or secondary infection).

When an adult contracts the disease, it generally appears in a more severe form, constitutional symptoms are more profound, and viral pneumonia is a common sequela. Although varicella pneumonia generally runs a fairly mild course, it may at times progress and result in death. Most such progression has been observed in patients on systemic corticosteroids or in individuals with neoplastic disease or on immunosuppressive drug therapy.[4] Bacterial infections of the skin due to excoriation are the most frequent complications. Other complications include appendicitis, orchitis, nephritis, cardiac and circulatory involvement, encephalitis, leukopenia, thrombocytopenia, arthritis, hepatitis, purpura fulminans, transverse myelitis, the Guillain-Barré syndrome, and, in 1 in 10,000 cases, Reye's syndrome, which is an acute disorder characterized by fatty degeneration of the liver, diffuse cerebral edema, vomiting, confusion, delirium, elevated serum ammonia, and coma. Since the administration of acetylsalicylic acid (aspirin) to children with varicella (and infections due to influenza B virus) appears to increase the risk of Reye's syndrome, it is recommended that, until the pathogenesis of this complication is better understood, children with varicella and influenza virus infection should not receive salicylates during the course of these illnesses.[5] Unlike other complications, encephalopathy (seen in 0.01 to 0.1 per cent of all cases of varicella) is not related to the severity of the primary disorder and the prognosis of varicella central nervous system disease is generally favorable.

four times a day in a dosage of 20 mg/kg per dose for children 2 to 12 years of age (up to 800 mg per dose), and 4 g/day to adults for 5 days, although not recommended for routine treatment of varicella, if started within 24 hours of the exanthem has been shown to shorten the duration and magnitude of fever, accelerate healing time, and reduce the number of skin lesions. This is particularly useful for patients with photoexaggerated lesions, patients who contract varicella while on systemic corticosteroid therapy, or immunocompromised children. It is also useful in otherwise healthy adults or children 13 or more years of age in whom severe varicella and the possibility of facial scarring may be a concern, and children with a chronic cutaneous or pulmonary disorder or those receiving chronic salicylate therapy whose clinical course may be adversely affected by varicella infection.[12] An attenuated live strain of varicella vaccine can also be used to prevent or modify varicella in sick or immunocompromised children with no history of chickenpox and no detectable complement-fixing antibody.[13–16]

RUBEOLA (MEASLES)

Prior to 1963 measles was the most common viral exanthem of childhood. It was not unusual to see a young child with high fever, cough, coryza, conjunctivitis, Koplik's spots, and a characteristic morbilliform rash, which involved the head, face, neck, trunk, and extremities and faded after 3 to 7 days. This disorder, unfortunately, produced a variety of complications, including otitis media, bronchopneumonia, subacute sclerosing panencephalitis, and encephalitis. The latter complication occurred in 1 of 1,000 affected individuals and proved fatal in 15 per cent of cases. Of those who survived, 45 per cent were left with permanent central nervous system damage, including hearing loss, mental retardation, or seizure disorders.

Clinical Manifestations. Transmitted by direct contact with droplets from infected persons, rubeola is caused by the measles virus (an RNA-containing paramyxovirus) with an incubation period of 10 to 14 days. The classic picture of unmodified measles begins with a prodromal period lasting 3 to 4 days, in occasional cases 1 to 6 days, manifested by systemic toxicity, with fever (101°F to 104°F [38.3°C to 40.0°C] or higher), chills, malaise, headache, perspiration, prostration, oculonasal catarrh, conjunctivitis, photophobia, coryza with mucopurulent discharge, and a persistent dry hacking cough refractory to most antitussive agents.

Approximately 2 days before the development of the characteristic morbilliform exanthem, Koplik's spots appear on the buccal mucous membranes opposite the first molar teeth and, as they become more numerous, all over the inside of the cheeks and, at times, on the mucous membranes of the

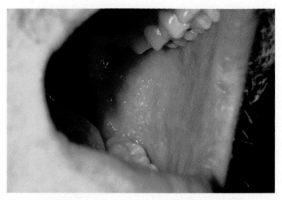

Figure 12–4. Koplik's spots. Pinpoint 1- to 3-mm white or bluish white elevations, resembling grains of sand, on the buccal mucosa of a patient with rubeola (measles).

gums and lips. When marked, these spots are characterized by many pinpoint 1- to 3-mm, white or bluish white elevations resembling grains of salt sprinkled on a bright erythematous background (Fig. 12–4). Koplik's spots are highly diagnostic of measles and usually disappear as the exanthem becomes full blown.

The exanthem of unmodified measles first makes its appearance 3 to 4 days after the onset of illness. It begins as an erythematous maculopapular eruption first on the scalp and hairline, the forehead, the area behind the ear lobes, and the upper part of the neck. It then spreads downward to involve the face, neck, upper extremities, and trunk and continues until it reaches the feet by the third day, the rash then fading in the same order as it appeared (Fig. 12–5). With the disappearance of the rash, a

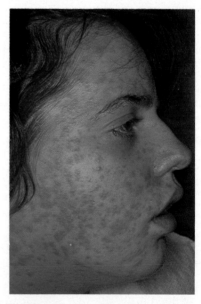

Figure 12–5. Rubeola. A purplish red maculopapular eruption is present on the face.

fine branny desquamation may be noted over the sites of the most extensive previous involvement.

The illness reaches its climax between the second and third days of the rash. At this time the temperature is at its peak, the eyes are puffy and red, the coryza is profuse, and the cough is most distressing. During this period the child feels miserable and looks "measly," but within the next 24 to 36 hours the temperature falls, the conjunctivitis and coryza clear, the cough decreases in severity, and within a few days, the child feels normal. Fever persisting beyond this point usually suggests a complication of the disorder.

Modified measles may develop in children who have been immunized with γ-globulin after exposure to the disease or in infants whose transplacental passive immunity has partially waned. The incubation period may be prolonged to 14 to 20 days; the usual prodromal period of 3 to 4 days may be absent or decreased to 1 or 2 days; there may be a low-grade fever or the temperature may be normal; and the cough, coryza, and conjunctivitis may be minimal or absent. Koplik's spots are absent or few and, if they develop, usually disappear within a day or less. The exanthem follows the same progressive pattern as regular measles but is much milder, and the characteristic confluence of the exanthem is generally absent, sparse, or so mild that it may be missed (Fig. 12–6).

The typical unmodified form of measles is usually easily recognizable. When the diagnosis is in doubt, it can be confirmed by a variety of serologic procedures such as complement-fixation or hemagglutination inhibition studies. Lesions of the skin and oral mucosa (Koplik's spots) share the following similar histologic features: parakeratosis, acanthosis, intercellular and intracellular edema, foci of multinucleate giant cells with pale-staining cytoplasm, and a sparse lymphohistiocytic inflammatory infiltrate around the dilated blood vessels in the dermis. Electron microscopy reveals viral microtubular aggregates within nuclei and cytoplasm of the syncytial giant cells. These microtubules are indistinguishable from those seen in tissue cultures infected with measles virus. These findings indicate that the measles virus initiates a similar pathologic process in lesions of the skin and oral mucosa.[17]

Management. In 1954 a breakthrough in the control of this disease occurred with the isolation of measles virus by Enders and Peebles, a milestone in the control of measles. Shortly thereafter two measles vaccines were developed and, following extensive trials, licensed in 1963: a "killed" formalin-inactivated alum-precipitated vaccine and an attenuated Edmonston-B type live vaccine. Between 1963 and 1967 an estimated 600,000 to 900,000 children were immunized with "killed" inactivated measles virus vaccine. Because febrile reactions caused by immunization with live Edmonston-B measles virus vaccines were common, many physicians preferred to use the killed measles virus vaccine, the live vaccine with a simultaneous injection of immune serum γ-globulin, or a combined killed and live measles virus regimen.

In 1965 an atypical form of measles following exposure to natural measles in children who had previously received killed vaccine was observed and, by 1967, it was apparent that the immunogenic and protective effects of inactivated measles virus vaccine were transient and that individuals with short-lived immunity were being seen with a bizarre new clinical syndrome termed *atypical measles.*

Atypical measles is manifested by extremely high fever, cough, headache, myalgia, abdominal pain, pneumonitis, pleural effusion, peripheral edema, and an unusual macular, vesicular, or petechial rash, principally involving the hands and feet, thus frequently suggesting a diagnosis of Rocky Mountain spotted fever (Fig. 12–7).[18]

There are two theories regarding the pathogenesis of atypical measles. In one, it has been suggested that this disorder represents a generalized Arthus reaction in an individual exposed to wild measles virus—an individual who has lost the protective antibody level but has been left with a persistent cell-mediated hypersensitivity to the virus. The second is that it is due to an imbalance

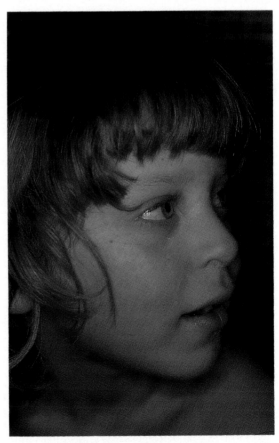

Figure 12–6. Modified measles.

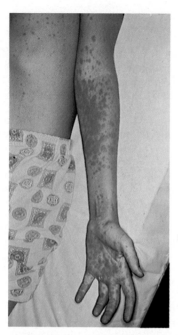

Figure 12–7. Purpuric rash on the trunk, forearm, and hand of a patient with the atypical measles syndrome. (Courtesy of William E. Lattanzi, M.D.)

between T-cell function and the lack of humoral antibody. Clinical and immunologic data currently favor this aberrant cell-mediated response.[19]

Although licensure of measles vaccine in the United States in 1963 dramatically altered the epidemiology of measles and the number of reported cases of measles (500,000 cases per year with 400 to 500 measles-associated deaths annually), despite the fact that measles vaccine is easily available and highly effective (95 per cent), the control of measles is not as yet completely resolved. Current data suggest that up to 20 per cent of immunized children remain susceptible to measles. This problem has been created primarily by the age at which vaccine was administered, the fact that many of those who apparently were properly immunized may have received vaccine that lost its potency because of exposure to heat or light, and the fact that many children still have not received measles vaccine.

In response to an increase in outbreaks of measles in the United States (from a low of 1,497 reported cases in 1983 to a provisional total of 27,672 cases and 89 suspected measles-associated deaths in 1990), the American Academy of Pediatrics has revised its policy for measles vaccination.[20, 21] It is currently recommended that live attenuated measles vaccine be administered as a combined measles, mumps, and rubella (MMR) vaccination at 15 months of age, with a second dose to be given at entry to middle school or junior high school (i.e., at age 11 or 12 years). Adolescents and adults should be considered susceptible unless they have docu-

mentation of physician-diagnosed measles, laboratory evidence of immunity, were born before 1957, or have documentation of two doses of measles vaccine at the appropriate time intervals. Although revaccination of children who previously received killed vaccine can result in mild local or severe general manifestations of hypersensitivity, most reactions are localized and the risk does not appear to be a deterrent to revaccination of such individuals.

Contraindications to live measles virus vaccine are pregnancy; leukemia, lymphoma, or other malignancy; diseases in which cell-mediated immunity is impaired; therapy that depresses resistance and immunity, such as corticosteroids, irradiation, antimetabolites, and alkylating agents; severe febrile illness; and untreated active tuberculosis. Few adverse effects have been seen in egg-sensitive children from administration of live measles vaccine grown in chick fibroblast culture, probably because egg albumin and yolk components of the egg are essentially absent from the culture, and data suggest that something other than egg sensitivity may trigger allergic reactions. Although it is recommended that skin testing with measles vaccine be performed for individuals with a history of anaphylactic reaction following egg ingestion, patients who have a history of minor reactions to egg white who merely develop a rash, abdominal pain, or other delayed manifestations and individuals with allergy to chickens or chicken feathers need not be skin tested prior to measles vaccine administration.[22] In addition, since measles vaccine contains trace elements of neomycin, persons who have experienced anaphylactic reactions to neomycin should not receive measles vaccine.

SCARLET FEVER

Scarlet fever (scarlatina), although of bacterial origin, is commonly considered in the differential diagnosis of viral exanthems. The diffuse punctate erythematous eruption of scarlet fever results from an erythrogenic toxin produced by group A streptococci, usually as the result of a pharyngeal infection, occasionally of a cutaneous infection (surgical scarlet). The disorder affects individuals of all ages and has its highest incidence in the late fall, winter, and early spring. The only difference between streptococcal tonsillitis or pharyngitis and scarlet fever is the fact that the latter disorder is accompanied by a cutaneous eruption. Although severe scarlet fever with systemic toxicity is now rare, milder forms of the disease still occur in association with certain strains of streptococci.

Clinical Manifestations. The clinical manifestations of streptococcal disease are governed by the portal of entry, the patient's age, and his or her immune status. The disease usually occurs in children, the maximal incidence being in the 1- to 10-year age group, and only rarely in adults. Although streptococcal infections are not uncommon in infants and very young children, scarlet fever is rarely seen in this age group.

The chief sources of pathogenic streptococci are discharges from the nose, thoat, ears, and skin of patients or carriers. After an incubation period of 2 to 5 days (with a range of 1 to 7 days), the disease is generally ushered in by the abrupt onset of fever, headache, vomiting, malaise, and sore throat. The enanthem includes lesions of the tonsils, pharynx, tongue, and palate. The oral mucous membranes are bright red, and there may be scattered petechiae and red punctate lesions on the soft palate. During the first few days the tongue is heavily coated. By the second or third day reddened and edematous papillae project through the white coating, producing the so-called white strawberry tongue. By the fourth or fifth day the coating peels off, leaving a red, glistening tongue studded with prominent papillae, thus presenting the appearance of a red strawberry.

Within 12 to 48 hours an erythematous punctate rash that blanches on pressure appears, first on the upper trunk, and then becomes generalized, rapidly within a period of a few hours or more gradually over 3 to 4 days (Fig. 12–8). The face is flushed but rarely shows a punctate erythematous rash, and there is a relative pallor from the triangle of the nose to the chin (circumoral pallor). The punctate lesions of scarlet fever give the skin a rough sandpaper-like texture. This is more intense in skin folds such as the axillae, antecubital, popliteal, and inguinal regions, and at sites of pressure such as the buttocks, the small of the back in bed-

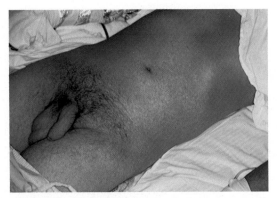

Figure 12–9. Scarlet fever with exaggeration of lesions (Pastia's sign) in the inguinal region.

fast patients, over the sternum, and between the scapulae. The lower legs generally are involved least and last. Capillary fragility is increased, and the eruption often exhibits transverse areas of hyperpigmentation with a petechial character in the antecubital fossae, axillary folds, and inguinal region (Pastia's lines) (Fig. 12–9). If the eruption is severe, minute vesicular lesions (sudamina) may be scattered over the abdomen, hands, and feet.

In mild cases the rash may be localized to the trunk and may be seen only as a faint erythema. In an effort to reassure anxious parents, this milder form, although actually the same disorder, is frequently referred to by physicians as scarlatina rather than scarlet fever. The eruption may become less pronounced when the circulation is poor or when the patient is cold, and generally may be brought out more strongly by wrapping the patient warmly in blankets. In dark-skinned individuals the exanthem often is visible only where pigmentation is less pronounced (on the palms and soles); in other areas the rash is frequently difficult to recognize and may consist only of punctate papular elevations resembling cutis anserina (goose flesh) (Fig. 12–10).

The exanthem lasts for 4 or 5 days, but in mild cases may be transient and short lived. As the exanthem fades it leaves a scale, which is branny in most areas but which may appear as large exfoliative lamellar scales on the hands, palms, soles, fingertips, elbows, knees, creases, and feet (Figs. 12–11 and 12–12). The extent and duration of the desquamation are directly proportional to the intensity of the rash. When present, this is a most characteristic feature of scarlet fever.

The diagnosis is usually made on the basis of clinical features of fever, pharyngotonsillitis, a characteristic enanthem, strawberry tongue, a punctate erythematous rash with circumoral pallor, postscarlatinal desquamation, isolation of group A streptococci from the pharynx, and a rising antistreptolysin-O titer.

The cutaneous histopathology consists of perivascular collections of polymorphonuclear leuko-

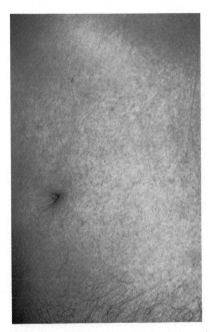

Figure 12–8. Fine punctate erythematous rash on the abdomen of a patient with scarlet fever.

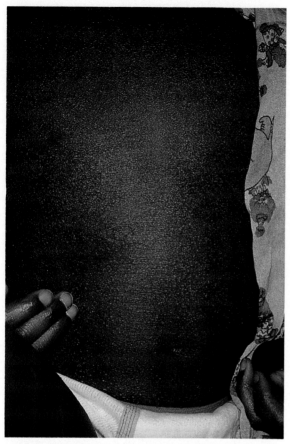

Figure 12–10. Scarlet fever. Since erythema is difficult to see on black skin, the exanthem of scarlet fever in blacks is often seen as punctate papular elevations (cutis anserina). (Courtesy of Mary Williams, M.D. and Steven Resnick, M.D.)

Scarlet fever–like rashes have also been associated with *Corynebacterium hemolyticum* infection, mercury intoxication (acrodynia, pink disease), and pseudoephedrine hydrochloride or codeine sensitivity.[23–25] The rash of *C. hemolyticum* has a fine diffuse macular and erythematous appearance, often with a fine papular component. It begins on the distal extremities 1 to 4 days after the onset of pharyngitis, spreads centrally during the next 2 to 3 days, sparing the face, palms, and soles, and persists longer than 48 hours. Pruritus is present in about half of the patients, and desquamation, when present, is mild. In contrast to streptococcal scarlet fever, neither palatal petechiae nor strawberry tongue is observed. Although streptococcal pharyngitis is primarily a disease of children, *C. hemolyticum* is most commonly seen in teenagers and young adults (particularly those in the 11- to 22-year-old age group).[23] Acrodynia (pink disease) is characterized by a pinkish color of the hands, feet, nose, fingers, and toes (with the cheeks and nose often acquiring a scarlet color), photophobia, profuse perspiration, swelling of the fingers and toes resulting from hyperplasia and hyperkeratosis of the skin in these areas, constant pruritus with excruciating pain in the hands and feet, darkening and occasional loss of nails, hypotonia, anorexia, and neurologic complications such as neuritis, mental apathy, and irritability. Once a common disorder (associated with ingestion or repeated contact with mercury in products such as house paints, wall papers, teething powders, diaper rinses, and the use of antihelminthics containing mercury), acrodynia may still occur as a result of accidental exposure but is rarely seen today.[24]

cytes and erythrocytes, dilated small blood vessels, and focal accumulations of exudate. The latter are responsible for the punctate erythematous eruption characteristic of this disorder.

Staphylococcal Scarlet Fever. A slightly similar syndrome caused by an exfoliative exotoxin produced by staphylococci of bacteriophage group II, types 3A, 3C, 55, 71, and 85, has also been documented. Staphylococcal scarlatiniform disease is characterized by generalized erythema with a sandpaper-like texture and diffuse tenderness of the skin. This disorder can be differentiated from streptococcal scarlet fever by the absence of streptococcal pharyngitis or palatal enanthem, negative bacterial cultures, the absence of elevated antistreptolysin titers, and a lack of the characteristic desquamation that frequently follows streptococcal scarlet fever. Many investigators currently believe that patients originally described as having staphylococcal scarlet fever may actually have represented individuals with abortive or mild forms of toxic shock syndrome or staphylococcal scalded skin syndrome.

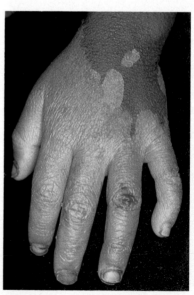

Figure 12–11. Post–scarlet fever exfoliation of the skin on the hand of a black child.

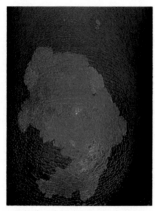

Figure 12–12. Post–scarlet fever exfoliation of the skin on the knee of a black child.

Treatment. The prognosis for adequately treated streptococcal infection is excellent. Early complications of inadequately treated scarlet fever include otitis media, bronchopneumonia, occasionally mastoiditis, septicemia, and osteomyelitis. Late complications include rheumatic fever and acute glomerulonephritis. Although their pathogenesis is unknown, poststreptococcal rheumatic fever and glomerulonephritis are thought to be due to a hypersensitivity to group A hemolytic streptococci or some of their byproducts.

The optimum treatment for streptococcal scarlet fever, as for other streptococcal disease, is penicillin. A single intramuscular injection of benzathine penicillin G is the most effective and secure mode of therapy (600,000 units for children weighing less than 60 pounds, and 1.2 million units for those weighing more than 60 pounds). If oral penicillin is prescribed, the patient should receive a full 10 days of therapy to eradicate the streptococci and help prevent rheumatic fever. Oral penicillin may be administered as 200,000 to 400,000 units of penicillin V three or four times a day for 10 days for children weighing less than 60 pounds and as 400,000 units three or four times a day for those weighing 60 pounds or more. Although adequate treatment appears to reduce the incidence of rheumatic fever, it is unclear if early treatment of pharyngitis can regularly prevent the development of acute glomerulonephritis. Erythromycin, 40 mg/kg/day in four divided doses (not to exceed a total of 1 g/day), is the drug of choice for patients with a history of penicillin allergy.

Follow-up cultures of patients are important, particularly for those individuals treated with oral therapy. Throat cultures should be obtained 7 to 10 days following a course of oral penicillin or 4 to 5 weeks after an injection of benzathine penicillin. If follow-up cultures are found to be positive, retreatment with intramuscular benzathine penicillin is recommended for those individuals not allergic to penicillin. For those with a history of penicillin allergy, a repeat course of therapy with erythromycin or with one of the cephalosporin group of antibiotics is advisable (see below).

Staphylococcal scarlatiniform eruptions should be treated by a semi-synthetic β-lactamase-resistant (penicillinase-resistant) penicillin (dicloxacillin, methicillin, nafcillin, or oxacillin). If there is a history of previous allergic reaction to penicillin, antistaphylococcal cephalosporins (cephalothin, cephapirin, or cephazolin) or clindamycin may be used. However, it should be noted that in 5 to 10 per cent of patients there is a cross-reactivity with penicillin and the cephalosporins and that, because of possible renal toxicity associated with cephaloridine, this agent should not be administered to individuals in the pediatric age group.

RUBELLA (GERMAN MEASLES)

Rubella is a common viral disease of children and young adults manifested by a generalized maculopapular rash and enlargement of the posterior occipitocervical lymph nodes. Before the widespread use of rubella vaccine, rubella was an epidemic disease, occurring in 6- to 9-year cycles, and most cases were reported in children. Currently, the incidence of rubella in the United States has declined more than 98 per cent from that seen before 1969, the year rubella vaccine was licensed; and in 1988, health departments in the United States reported an all-time low of 225 cases of rubella. Since 1989, however, as with measles, the number of reported cases of rubella has increased, and in 1990 a provisional total of 1,093 cases of rubella and 10 confirmed and 5 provisional cases of congenital rubella syndrome were reported.[26]

Clinical Manifestations. The portal of entry of the rubella virus is the respiratory mucosa, and the incubation period is 16 to 18 days, with a range of 14 to 21 days. The exanthem, usually the first evidence of the disorder, generally begins about the hairline and face and spreads rapidly to involve the neck, trunk, and extremities, generally within a period of 24 hours. The duration and extent of the rash may be variable. Although it generally lasts for about 3 days, it may be evanescent and may disappear in less than a day, or it may be prolonged and last for as long as 5 days.

The eruption is characterized by innumerable small, discrete, rose-pink maculopapules, which are generalized and discrete on the first day, fade on the face and coalesce over the trunk on the second day, and usually disappear by the third day (Fig. 12–13). The rash tends to fade as it spreads, and the face and shoulders may be fairly clear while the eruption remains prominent elsewhere on the body. The most notable feature of the exanthem is its rapid change in appearance, frequently over a few hours. The characteristic pink-red lesions of rubella differ from the more vivid purplish red lesions of measles and the fine punctate yellow-red lesions of scarlet fever. After

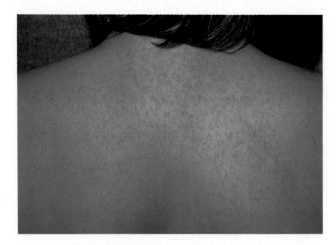

Figure 12–13. Rubella. Multiple, light reddish pink lesions on the back of a child with German measles.

severe rubella eruptions, a fine flaky desquamation may be observed in areas of maximum involvement. In contrast to measles, however, the eruption is not followed by a temporary period of hyperpigmentation.

In children, the temperature may be normal or slightly elevated and rarely persists beyond the first day of the exanthem. In adolescents and adults, however there may be a prodromal period. Lasting 1 to 5 days it consists of headache, malaise, anorexia, mild conjunctivitis, coryza, sore throat, and cough; and at times there is a low-grade fever during the prodromal period and first day of the rash. An enanthem termed *Forchheimer's sign* may be observed in up to 20 per cent of patients during the prodromal period or first day of the rash. Located on the soft palate, it is manifested by petechiae or reddish pinpoint or larger spots.

Besides the eruption, the other notable feature of rubella is the involvement of the lymph nodes in the back of the neck, particularly the suboccipital and postauricular nodes. This glandular involvement may precede the appearance of the rash by 1 to 5 days, ordinarily lasts for 2 to 7 days, and usually subsides quickly after the rash had disappeared. It is important to recognize the fact that, although highly characteristic, suboccipital, postauricular, or cervical lymphadenopathy is suggestive but not diagnostic of the disorder. They may also be associated with diseases such as measles, chickenpox, adenovirus infections, infectious mononucleosis, and others.

The clinical diagnosis is suggested by a maculopapular rash, which begins on the face, progresses rapidly downward to the trunk and extremities, and subsides, generally within a few days, accompanied by postoccipital and postauricular lymphadenopathy, which precedes the appearance of the rash, a low-grade fever or absence of fever, and absent or mild prodromal symptoms. When the diagnosis is indeterminate, rubella virus may be recovered from the pharynx as early as 7 days before and as late as 14 days after the onset of the rash. Since the introduction of the hemagglutination inhibition test in 1967, serologic studies have become increasingly important. The hemagglutination inhibition antibody test has the advantages of high sensitivity and speed with which results are obtained. A serologic diagnosis depends on acute and convalescent serum determinations. Ideally, the first blood sample should be drawn as soon as possible after the rash is noted, and a second blood test should be performed 2 to 4 weeks later. Evidence of a fourfold or greater rise in rubella titer is indicative of rubella infection.

Except for possible infection of the fetus during pregnancy, rubella is one of the most benign of all infectious diseases of childhood. A pregnant woman who contracts rubella in the first trimester of pregnancy has a high probability that intrauterine transmission will give rise to the congenital rubella syndrome. In the first few weeks of pregnancy the chance of transmission is 30 to 50 per cent, at 5 to 8 weeks it is 25 per cent, and from 9 to 12 weeks the risk is 8 per cent. (For a discussion of the congenital rubella syndrome, refer to the discussion in Chapter 2.)

In older children and adults arthritis may affect about 30 per cent of females and 5 per cent of males. The clinical picture is variable but characteristically involves the small joints of the hands and feet, occasionally the knees, elbows, shoulders, and spine. Occasionally the arthropathy lasts up to 2 weeks and has been associated with mild elevations of the erythrocyte sedimentation rate and false-positive latex fixation tests (the latter generally revert to normal within a period of 18 months). Other rare complications include thrombocytopenic or nonthrombocytopenic purpura, and in approximately 1 in 6,000 cases encephalitis has been reported. Most patients with purpura improve and become symptom free within 2 weeks. The clinical manifestations of encephalitis are similar to those observed in other types of postinfectious encephalitis and, although fatalities have been reported, complete recovery is generally the rule.

Present prophylactic recommendations for rubella include vaccination of all children with live attenuated rubella vaccine, either alone or in combination with measles and mumps vaccine, when a child is 15 months of age or older. As with measles prophylaxis, a second dose at 11 to 12 years of age is recommended. In addition, prenatal or antepartum screening for rubella susceptibility should be routinely undertaken. Since infection of the fetus with attenuated virus may take place in pregnant women, routine immunization of adolescent and adult females should be undertaken with caution, and rubella vaccine should not be administered to pregnant women or to women who might become pregnant within a period of 3 months.

DUKES' DISEASE

Historically the exanthems of childhood have been classified on a numerical basis (Table 12–1). This classification is no longer tenable and is included only for its historical significance.

The name Dukes' disease (fourth disease) is an antiquated term used to describe a group of exanthematous disorders described by Clement Dukes in 1900. Unfortunately, Dukes' descriptions were based on clinical and morphologic examination, before modern laboratory facilities were available to allow proper evaluation and classification. The disorder, or perhaps more correctly, disorders, as originally described were characterized by a mild prodromal period manifested by headache, anorexia, drowsiness, chills, and backache, followed by a diffuse, slightly red, raised eruption and a slight edema of the skin, which disappeared on the fourth or fifth days when a branny desquamation took place. In retrospect it now appears that Dukes described variants of rubella, rubeola, scarlet fever, exfoliative variants of *Staphylococcus aureus* infection, or viral exanthems of the Coxsackievirus-Echovirus group.

ERYTHEMA INFECTIOSUM

Erythema infectiosum (fifth disease), a viral infection caused by human parvovirus B19 infection, is a mildly contagious disease of childhood that tends to affect children from 3 to 12 years of age. Its incubation period has an estimated range of 6 to 14 days, and it is characterized by three stages: (1) an erythematous malar blush that suddenly develops in an asymptomatic child, giving the patient a "slapped cheek" or "sunburned" appearance (Fig. 12–14); (2) a second stage that begins the next day with an erythematous maculopapular eruption on the extensor surfaces of the extremities (Fig. 12–15), and less often the trunk and buttocks; and (3) a third stage that begins on or about the sixth day, when the rash fades, particularly on the proximal extremities, with areas of central clearing creating a reticulated or lacy marble-like pattern. The lesions of the second stage persist for several days to a week or more, after which they subside. The reticulated rash is the most characteristic finding of fifth disease. Its presence in a patient with few or no constitutional symptoms is highly pathognomonic.[27, 28]

The duration of the reticulated rash varies from 3 to 24 days, with an average of 9 to 11 days; and after the rash has seemed to subside, it frequently reappears, often several times, in response to friction, temperature changes, or sun exposure. There is no enanthem and rarely the disease may be accompanied by low-grade fever, malaise, fatigue, irritability, general aches and pains, and, at times, mild arthritis, arthralgia, and adenopathy. Joint manifestations, when present, are transient, self-limiting, and more common in adults than in children.

The diagnosis of erythema infectiosum is dependent on clinical and epidemiologic grounds and laboratory diagnosis can be made only by tests currently available in research laboratories. Although misdiagnosis often occurs, the characteris-

Table 12–1. THE NUMBERING OF EXANTHEMS*

First disease	Measles
Second disease	Scarlet fever
Third disease	Rubella
Fourth disease	Dukes' disease
Fifth disease	Erythema infectiosum
Sixth disease	Roseola infantum

* This classification is antiquated and included only because of historical significance.

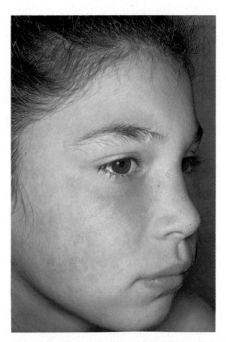

Figure 12–14. Erythema infectiosum ("fifth disease"). Note the "slapped-cheek" or sunburn-like malar flush.

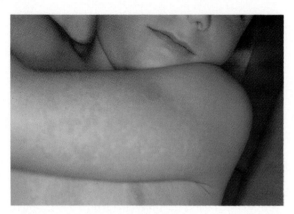

Figure 12–15. A maculopapular eruption on the arm (the second phase of erythema infectiosum).

tic "slapped-cheek" appearance and subsequent lacy marble-like pattern on the upper arms and thighs generally help establish the diagnosis.

Human parvovirus B19 is the same virus that induces aplastic crises in patients with sickle cell disease, hereditary spherocytosis, acquired and hereditary hemolytic anemia, chronic anemia in immunodeficient patients, and an arthritis similar to rheumatoid arthritis in adults. Because of its effect on erythrocyte precursor cells the possibility of parvovirus-induced hydrops fetalis and fetal death has become a growing concern among pregnant women exposed to children with erythema infectiosum.[29, 30] The risk of infection on exposure is approximately 8 per cent, and with maternal infection the risk of fetal death is 3 to 5 per cent; 60 per cent or more of adults have serologic evidence of past infection and probably are not susceptible to reinfection. Of particular concern is the risk to school teachers or nurses likely to be exposed to children with fifth disease. Since erythema infectiosum is only contagious during the first stage of the disease (the stage when children have symptoms such as headache, bodyache, sore throat, fever, or chills), children with erythema infectiosum are not contagious at the time that the rash is present and may attend day care or school.[31, 32]

ROSEOLA INFANTUM

Roseola infantum (exanthem subitum, sixth disease), the most common exanthem in children younger than 3 years of age, is characterized by a fever of 3 to 5 days' duration, rapid defervescence, and then the appearance of an erythematous or maculopapular rash that persists for a few hours to 1 or 2 days. Although roseola-like illnesses have been associated with other viral agents, such as parvovirus B19, echovirus 16, Coxsackievirus B5, other enteroviruses, and several adenoviruses, human herpesvirus-6 has now been implicated as the causal agent of roseola infantum.[33, 34]

The illness is of sporadic, nonseasonal occurrence without known contact, and the incubation period varies from 5 to 15 days. Although there are epidemics, communicability is quite low and one attack usually confers lasting immunity.[35] The disorder is characterized by constant or intermittent high fever that usually drops by crisis (occasionally by lysis). The appearance of a rash coincides with the subsidence of the fever, generally on the third or fourth day. Occasionally the rash may not be apparent until one day of normal temperature, and at times it may appear before the fever has subsided.

The eruption is characterized by discrete rose-pink macules or maculopapules, 2 to 3 mm in diameter, that fade on pressure, rarely coalesce, and are similar in appearance to those of rubella and modified measles. The rash characteristically first appears on the trunk and sometimes may spread to the neck, upper extremities, and lower extremities (Fig. 12–16). The duration of the eruption is usually 1 to 2 days; occasionally it may be evanescent, arising quickly and disappearing in a matter of hours (hence the name exanthem subitum). In spite of the elevated temperature the patient is frequently alert and playful and generally does not appear to be acutely ill. Periorbital edema is common and, when present in a febrile but otherwise apparently well child, is frequently a useful clue to diagnosis during the pre-exanthematous stage.

A diagnosis of exanthem subitum is made chiefly on the basis of the stiking contrast between the infant's general appearance and clinical course, periorbital edema (when present), and the appearance of the rash as the fever subsides. The leukocyte count is usually low (but may be slightly elevated during the first 2 days of the illness), and

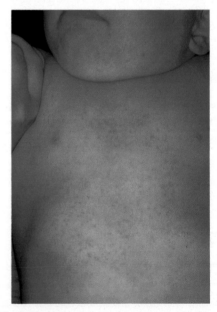

Figure 12–16. Roseola infantum (exanthem subitum).

leukopenia with relative lymphocytosis as a rule does not develop until the third day of the illness.

Febrile seizures, in all probability related to the abrupt rise of temperature, as in many other febrile disorders of childhood, are a common complication. Seen in less than 6 per cent of cases in private practice, seizures represent a common problem in children admitted to hospitals with this disorder.

There is no specific therapy for patients with exanthem subitum other than acetaminophen, fluids, and phenobarbital for those with a history of febrile seizures during either the current or a previous illness.

OTHER VIRAL EXANTHEMS

Recognition of a specific virus as the etiologic agent responsible for a particular exanthematous disorder is often difficult. During epidemics or localized outbreaks of similar cutaneous eruptions, an etiologic association may be established by the recovery of a particular viral agent or by serologic demonstration of an acute infection in a statistically greater number of ill patients than in a similar group of well subjects from the same community. Even in situations in which a specific etiologic agent cannot be identified, recognition of characteristic clinical findings or symptoms during epidemics will frequently suggest the association of specific etiologic agents with certain cutaneous eruptions.

Exanthems Due to Enteroviruses

Enteroviruses, a subgroup of the picornaviruses, are a common cause of exanthems. Although unknown 40 years ago, there now appear to be at least 30 types that have been associated with cutaneous eruptions. Polioviruses, coxsackieviruses, echoviruses, and reoviruses are grouped under this classification because of their many similarities and their habitat in the human enteric tract. These viruses, spread by contact from person to person, initiate infection first in the pharynx and shortly thereafter in the gastrointestinal tract.

The exanthems associated with coxsackievirus and echovirus infections are frequently morbilliform (Figs. 12–17 and 12–18). Cutaneous lesions are usually generalized, nonpruritic, and maculopapular but also have been described as scarlatiniform, vesicular, zosteriform, urticarial, petechial, or purpuric (Tables 12–2 and 12–3).[36, 37]

COXSACKIEVIRUS INFECTIONS

Eruptions associated with coxsackieviruses vary markedly (see Table 12–2). They may resemble maculopapular echovirus disorders, may be suggestive of roseola infantum, or may consist of urticarial lesions. In some cases lesions may resemble

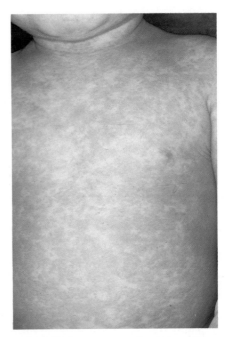

Figure 12–17. Erythematous maculopapular exanthem of the coxsackievirus-echovirus group.

varicella, but, unlike the latter, they heal rapidly without pustular formation, crusting, or scarring.

Hand-Foot-and-Mouth Disease. The most distinctive exanthem-enanthem complex of the "newer exanthems" is that caused by coxsackievirus A16 (occasionally A5, A9, A10, A16, B1, and B3) and appropriately called the hand, foot, and mouth syndrome. First described in the mid 1950s,

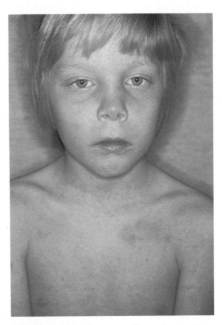

Figure 12–18. Erythematous maculopapular exanthem of the coxsackievirus-echovirus group.

Table 12–2. EXANTHEMS CAUSED BY COXSACKIEVIRUSES

Virus	Time	Distribution	Cutaneous Manifestations
Coxsackievirus A16	During fever	Hands, feet, buttocks	Maculopapules and vesicular lesions, ulcerations on tongue, soft palate, buccal mucosa, and gums
Coxsackievirus A9	During fever	Face, trunk, (occasionally palms and soles)	Erythematous maculopapules, vesicles, occasionally petechiae, purpura, or urticaria
Coxsackievirus A5	During fever	Hands, feet, occasionally legs, trunk, and buttocks	Maculopapules, vesicles, ulcers on tongue, soft palate, buccal mucosa, and gums
Coxsackievirus B5	During or after defervescence	Initially face and neck followed by spread to the trunk and extremities	Maculopapules, occasionally petechiae and urticaria

there have been repeated outbreaks of this disorder in the United States since 1963.[36] Infections are more common in late summer and fall. The disorder is highly contagious in a susceptible population and may occur as an isolated phenomenon or in epidemic form. During epidemics the virus is spread from child to child (horizontal spread) and then to adults (vertical spread) in various family groups.

The disorder is characterized by fever and a vesicular eruption that begins after a 3- to 6-day incubation period, occasionally with a brief prodrome of low-grade fever, anorexia, a sore mouth, malaise, and abdominal pain, which precedes the enanthem by 1 to 2 days; the exanthem occurs shortly after the enanthem. The fever lasts for 2 or 3 days, and temperatures average 101°F (38.3°C). The oral lesions begin as small red macules and evolve into small vesicles 1 to 3 mm to 2 cm in diameter on an erythematous base, which then ulcerate and last for 1 to 6 days. Similar lesions may also be seen on the soft palate, hard palate, buccal mucosa, gingivae, and tongue. The tongue is involved in 44 per cent of patients with this disorder, and lesions are suggestive of aphthous stomatitis. Involvement of the palate, uvula, and anterior tonsillar pillars (the classic herpangitic enanthem) is noted in about one third of cases.[36, 38]

One fourth to two thirds of affected patients also have highly characteristic vesicular lesions on the hands and feet, more commonly on the dorsal aspect, but also involving the lateral borders of the feet, the palms, soles, and buttocks, and occasionally the arms, legs, and face. The lesions on the skin are maculopapular at first, many later forming superficial gray vesicles on an erythematous base. The vesicles vary from 3 to 7 mm in diameter and are thin-walled, superficial, and nonloculated. They contain a clear fluid, sometimes coalesce to form bullae, and are only occasionally tender or pruritic. Vesicles are most frequently seen on the dorsal aspect of the fingers and toes as well as on the lateral borders of the feet and frequently have a characteristic elliptical football-shaped appearance (Figs. 12–19 and 12–20). Although the palms and soles are not involved as frequently, when affected they may show the greatest number of lesions. The vesicles, frequently surrounded by a red areola, usually clear by absorption of the fluid within 2 to 7 days; and on occasion, the vesicles may rupture, leaving a superficial scab.

The disorder tends to be more severe in infants and children than in adults but is usually mild, and the temperature falls after a few days. Some patients are afflicted with high fever, marked malaise, diarrhea, and occasionally joint pains. In 22

Table 12–3. EXANTHEMS CAUSED BY ECHOVIRUSES

Virus	Time	Distribution	Cutaneous Manifestations
Echovirus	With fever	Trunk, neck, and face	Pink to red papules, sometimes becoming coppery
Echovirus 4	With fever	Trunk, neck, and face	Macules, maculopapules, occasionally petechiae, rarely vesicles
Echovirus 5	After the onset of fever	Most marked on limbs and buttocks, also noted on trunk and face	A faint pink macular rash (a zosteriform eruption has also been noted)
Echovirus 9	Generally with but occasionally prior to fever	Face and neck, then trunk, extremities, and occasionally palms and soles	Rubelliform macules, maculopapules, occasionally petechiae, rarely vesicles
Echovirus 11		Trunk and extremities	Erythematous maculopapules, vesicles, urticarial lesions
Echovirus 16	During or after defervescence	Initially head and trunk, then generalized (occasionally palms and soles)	Macules, maculopapules, punched-out ulcers on soft palate and pillars

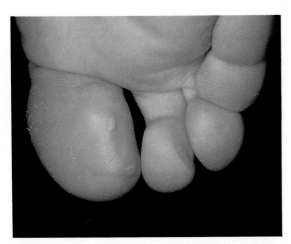

Figure 12–19. Hand-foot-and-mouth disease. A characteristic vesicular lesion is seen on the plantar surface of a great toe.

per cent of cases, marked cervical or submandibular adenopathy may be present. A few cases may recur at intervals for several months, and although the prognosis is generally excellent, rare cases of myocarditis, pneumonia, and meningoencephalitis have been reported.[38–40]

Other Exanthems Associated With Coxsackievirus Infection. Coxsackievirus A9, a common cause of aseptic meningitis, is also a common cause of exanthematous eruptions. The rash, which is most commonly erythematous and maculopapular, starts on the face and neck and spreads to the extremities. It is usually discrete and has been described as morbilliform, but urticarial and petechial or purpuric lesions simulating meningococcemia have been reported. The duration of the rash is from 1 to 7 days. Patients are usually febrile during the period of the rash and, except for those with aseptic meningitis, the majority of affected patients are generally not very ill.

In addition to the occasional association of hand-foot-and-mouth syndrome due to coxsackieviruses A5 and A10, coxsackievirus A5 has also been associated with scattered 4- to 5-mm yellow vesicles on the legs, which spread to the trunk; maculopapular lesions on the buttocks; and an enanthem consisting of 3- to 4-mm papules and vesicles on the soft palate. Coxsackievirus A10 has also been associated with an enanthem involving both the anterior and posterior oral cavities. Coxsackievirus B1 has been associated with a maculopapular rubelliform eruption with fever, headache, and aseptic meningitis and a roseola-like syndrome. Coxsackievirus B3 has been described in individuals with a maculopapular rash, fever, headache, diarrhea, splenomegaly and hepatomegaly, lesions typical of hand-foot-and-mouth disease, and, on occasion, petechial rashes suggesting a diagnosis of meningococcemia.[36]

Coxsackievirus B5, a frequent cause of human illness, may occasionally be associated with aseptic meningitis, encephalitis, paralytic disease, pleurodynia, myocarditis, pericarditis, peritonitis, vesicular pharyngitis, orchitis, and hepatitis. The exanthem occasionally described in association with coxsackievirus B5 infection varies considerably. Although maculopapular in the majority of instances, petechiae and urticaria have also been noted in isolated patients. The maculopapular exanthem associated with this infection appears first on the face and neck and spreads to the trunk and extremities in 4 to 24 hours. The head and neck have been described as most heavily involved. The cutaneous lesions associated with coxsackievirus B5 occur during or after defervescence and last about 36 hours.

Small outbreaks of enteroviral exanthems have also been associated with coxsackievirus A4 infection. Initial symptoms in affected patients consist of anorexia, drooling, sore throat, coryza, and fever; and a typical herpangitic enanthem lasting for 1 to 10 days has been described. The exanthem may begin with or after defervescence as 2- to 5-mm maculopapular lesions on the face and trunk. The lesions last 1 to 4 days and then disappear or become vesicular. The vesicular lesions have been described as occurring in crops and spreading to the extremities with exclusion of the palms and soles. Initially the vesicles tend to be yellowish, opaque, and 5 to 10 mm. Later they may become firm, may have a central punctum with a "bug-bite" appearance, persist for 1 to 2 weeks, and

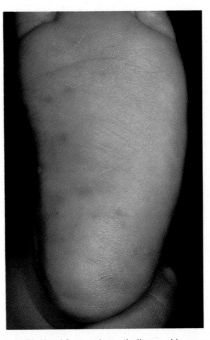

Figure 12–20. Hand-foot-and-mouth disease. Linear and crescentic vesicular lesions have a surrounding zone of erythema.

regress with brownish discoloration without crusting, pruritus, or desquamation.

ECHOVIRUS INFECTIONS

Except for the polioviruses, echovirus 9 infections are the best studied of all enterovirus infections. Exanthems have been noted in about 35 per cent of all echovirus 9 illnesses, but in young children the incidence is greater than 50 per cent. The rash most frequently occurs as a rubelliform eruption, but in addition, or as the sole manifestation, petechiae are occasionally noted. Lesions first appear on the face and neck and then spread rapidly to the trunk and extremities, including the palms and soles. Although the rash is usually discrete, on occasion confluence, particularly on the face, may be noted. The rash and fever usually occur simultaneously; but the rash has been noted to precede the fever by as much as 2 days, and, in most instances, the duration of the exanthem is 3 to 5 days. Of particular importance is the fact that disease due to enteroviruses (particularly those associated with echovirus 9 infection) with petechial exanthems and meningitis may closely mimic meningococcemia (see Table 12–3),[41] and, as in other viral exanthems, photoexaggeration (accentuation of the eruption in areas exposed to sunlight) is a common phenomenon (Fig. 12–21).

The "*Boston exanthem*" is an uncommon roseola-like infection caused by echovirus 16. Seen in large epidemics, summer outbreaks of this disease were first observed in Massachusetts in 1951 and then in Pittsburgh in 1954. After 22 years of relative absence, the demonstration of echovirus 16 in 10 states in 1974 suggested a general increase in the incidence of this disorder.[42]

Approximately one third of individuals with echovirus infection have a rubelliform eruption consisting of discrete pinkish red macules that are noted early in the course of the disease. Affecting first the face and neck, then the upper trunk and extremities, and only occasionally the palms and soles, the incubation period is usually 3 to 8 days, with fading of the lesions, usually within 4 or 5 days. Fifty per cent of cases show sparse yellow or grayish white lesions on the oral mucous membranes with, at times, lesions resembling Koplik's spots on the membranes opposite the molars. Fever, gastrointestinal symptoms (anorexia, nausea, vomiting, and colicky abdominal pain), respiratory symptoms, sore throat, cough, and conjunctivitis may be present. Characteristically the eruption in the Boston exanthem develops during or shortly after defervescence (this roseola-like feature sets echovirus 16 and coxsackievirus B5 infections apart from other enteroviruses). The exanthem consists of pink or salmon-colored discrete macular or maculopapular lesions measuring 0.5 to 1.5 cm in diameter, is centrifugal, and lasts for 1 to 2 days to about a week.

Other exanthems seen with echovirus infection include those associated with echovirus 2 infec-

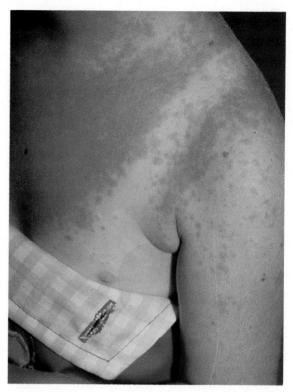

Figure 12–21. Photoexaggeration of the exanthem on the skin of a child with echovirus 9 infection. (Courtesy of Dr. Jonathan Schneider.)

tion, and a macular or rubelliform rash on the abdomen and back with spread, in some cases, to involve the chest, face, and neck. The cutaneous eruption has been noted to be coppery on the second day and persists for 2 to 7 days. Patients with this disorder have been noted to have rhinorrhea, pharyngitis, fever, cervical adenopathy, and, on occasion, aseptic meningitis and fatal paralytic infection. Echovirus 4 has been associated with aseptic meningitis, meningoencephalitis, and, in about 15 per cent of patients during epidemics, with a macular, nonpruritic erythematous rash, which has its onset 1 to 3 days after the onset of symptoms, lasts for 2 days, and begins on the trunk and occasionally the face, becomes semiconfluent, and spreads to the extremities.

An unusual epidemic of echovirus 5 has been described in newborns with fever, malaise, vomiting, diarrhea, and a faint pink macular rash that, most marked on the limbs and buttocks, was also noted on the trunk and face. The cutaneous eruption appeared 24 to 36 hours after the onset of fever and cleared after 2 days. In another child with echovirus 5 infection, fever, back pain, and an erythematous macular rash with a zosteriform distribution on the trunk has been noted.

Echovirus 6, a frequent cause of neurologic illness, has only sporadically been noted in association with an exanthem (usually a morbilliform eruption). It should be noted, however, that a zosteriform eruption has also been reported in association with this disorder.[37]

Exanthems associated with echovirus 11 infection have been described as urticarial and vesicular, and in echovirus 17 and echovirus 25 infections, transient erythematous, macular, maculopapular, and vesicular eruptions have been noted. In the latter, the rashes had their onset following 3 days of fever (during the period of defervescence), were most marked on the trunk, usually lasted 2 to 3 days, and then cleared without desquamation.

Other less common exanthems have, on occasion, been noted with other echoviruses. These include generalized erythematous maculopapular, morbilliform, and scarlatiniform eruptions and, as with many other enteroviral exanthems, do not appear to be particularly characteristic or diagnostic in appearance.[36] The various echovirus infections are self-limiting, the vast majority of patients recover completely, and there is no effective remedy for this group of disorders. Diagnosis is established on clinical grounds, on isolation of the affecting organism from the throat, rectum, or cerebrospinal fluid, and on serial antibody studies performed during the course of the illness and 2 weeks later.

REOVIRUS INFECTIONS

Reoviruses are common infectious agents of humans and lower animals. Despite their prevalence, human disease due to reoviruses has only occasionally been recognized (Table 12–4). Reovirus 2 infections were seen in seven children younger than the age of 10 years in Boston during the summer of 1960. Of these, one child was asymptomatic. Of the other six, five had maculopapular eruptions and one child had a vesicular eruption.[43] The eruption was mildly pruritic, persisted for 3 to 9 days, and then began to fade, first from the face and then from other affected areas. Other associated symptoms and signs included fever, which persisted for a total of 5 days, anorexia, and mild pharyngitis without exudate or cervical adenopathy.

Smallpox (Variola)

Smallpox (variola) is an acute, highly contagious, frequently deadly but preventable disease caused by poxvirus variolae, a specific virus immunologically related to vaccinia virus. Because of vigorous mass immunizations, skillful management, and sound epidemiologic principles, it appears that except for the possibility of laboratory accidents, with no natural instance of smallpox having oc-

curred since the last case was reported in Somalia in October 1977, a world free of smallpox has now become a reality.[44]

The smallpox virus (poxvirus variolae), a member of the genus *Orthopoxvirus*, probably first invades the upper respiratory tract where it multiplies locally in the mucosa and spreads to the regional lymph nodes from where it enters the bloodstream. The incubation period of classic smallpox, variola major, is 12 days, with a range of 8 to 16 days. The disease usually begins with chills, fever, headache, backache, severe malaise, delirium, and, particularly in children, seizures.

In some cases a transient eruption may develop during the prodromal period. It may be morbilliform, scarlatiniform, or petechial, with a characteristic bathing-trunk distribution. In most instances it disappears within 1 or 2 days. The duration of the prodromal period ranges between 2 and 4 days and, in most cases, it is terminated by the end of the third day.

The exanthem first appears on the face and forearms, spreads to the upper arms and trunk, particularly the back, and finally reaches the lower extremities. The eruption is characteristically more severe on the face and the distal parts of the arms and legs and least severe over the trunk and abdomen (this centrifugal distribution is distinct from that of varicella, which tends to be centripetal).

The initial lesions are macular. First detected on the third or fourth day of illness, they rapidly become papular (within a matter of hours), and by the end of the sixth day the papules develop into vesicles that measure up to 6 mm in diameter and are usually surrounded by red areolae. Between the seventh and ninth days the vesicles become pustular and measure up to 8 mm in diameter. During this stage the temperature again begins to rise and constitutional symptoms return, now aggravated by the intensely painful lesions. On the 10th day the pustules begin to rupture and dry and finally form crusts.

Lesions do not appear in crop-like fashion (a helpful point in diagnosis), and the mature pustular lesions are thick walled (in contrast to the thin-walled, dewdrop-like vesicles of varicella), discrete or confluent, umbilicated, and unilocular. Mucosal lesions are common and affect the mouth, nasopharynx, larynx, trachea, esophagus, and vagina as well as other areas and, among susceptible (previously unexposed or unvaccinated) populations, the fatality rate is high (up to 40 per cent).

The diagnosis is based on clinical manifestations, tissue culture, ultramicroscopic techniques, the Tzanck test, fluorescent antibody tests (a rapid diagnostic technique for the identification of ortho-

Table 12–4. EXANTHEMS CAUSED BY REOVIRUSES

Virus	Time	Distribution	Cutaneous Manifestions
Reovirus 2	With fever	Trunk, neck, and face (then occasionally the extremities)	Maculopapules

pox antigen), and hemagglutination and virus neutralization tests.

Smallpox vaccinations are no longer administered, except perhaps to laboratory workers and selected military personnel who may be exposed to smallpox virus, thus eliminating previously seen complications such as generalized vaccinia, accidental inoculation from contact with one's own or another individual's vaccination site (Fig. 12–22), vaccinia necrosum (a rare gangrenous form of vaccinia occurring primarily in immunocompetent individuals), Kaposi's varicelliform eruption (eczema vaccinatum), postvaccinial central nervous system disease, erythema multiforme or Stevens-Johnson disease, and primary malignancies such as squamous cell carcinoma, basal cell carcinoma, keratoacanthoma, or malignant melanoma that may develop in later life in smallpox vaccination sites.

Infectious Mononucleosis

Infectious mononucleosis is an acute infectious disease caused by the Epstein-Barr virus. Although infection with this virus is exceedingly common in young children, illness in this age group is frequently inapparent or so mild and atypical that the diagnosis is unrecognized. Infectious mononucleosis, therefore, generally described as a disorder primarily affecting adolescents and young adults between the ages of 15 and 25 years, occurs much more commonly in infants and young children than heretofore realized.[45, 46]

Transmitted by direct contact with a low degree of contagiousness, the incubation period of infectious mononucleosis is said to be between 33 and 49 days. The disorder begins insidiously with headache and malaise, and the early course is frequently marked by fevers of 101°F to 104°F (38.3°C to 40.0°C). Fever usually lasts 4 to 14 days, rarely up to 3 or 4 weeks. A sore throat commonly develops a few days after the onset of the illness, and an extensive membranous tonsillitis is characteristic. Lymphadenopathy begins early and is often generalized, and the cervical glands are usually most conspicuously affected. The spleen is moderately enlarged in one half to two thirds of cases, hepatomegaly is common, and icteric hepatitis is reported in 5 to 10 per cent of affected individuals.

An exanthem occurs in 10 to 15 per cent of cases, usually between the fourth and sixth days, and appears as a macular or maculopapular morbilliform eruption of the trunk or upper arms and occasionally the face, forearms, thighs, and legs (Fig. 12–23). The eruption may last for only a few days and may be followed by an urticarial or erythema multiforme–like eruption. Periorbital and eyelid edema, reported to occur in up to 50 per cent of patients with early infectious mononucleosis, may at times be the initial manifestation of the disorder (Fig. 12–24).[47] An enanthem appears in 25 per cent of cases on the palate between the 5th and 17th days of the illness. Manifested by discrete, bright red petechiae 0.5 to 1.0 mm in diameter, these lesions, seen at the junction of the hard and soft palates, are considered to be highly characteristic of the disorder and fade to a brownish hue in 2 days (Fig. 12–25).

In most cases spontaneous recovery occurs in 10 to 20 days, and virtually all patients return to their normal state of health and activity within 4 to 6 weeks after the onset of the illness. Deaths are extremely rare and, when reported, are generally associated with splenic rupture.

The spectrum of clinical manifestations in children may be mild and atypical, and young children frequently do not show the same hematologic antibody reactions as older individuals. Rashes and abdominal pain seem to be more common in children than adults, and children, particularly those younger than 4 years of age, are more likely to have significant neutropenia. Although failure to thrive, otitis media, episodes of recurrent tonsillopharyngitis, thrombocytopenia with hemorrhagic manifestations, airway obstruction, and neurologic problems appear to be more closely associated with childhood disease, jaundice appears to be less common in children than in adult patients with this disorder.[45, 46]

Since the 1930s a syndrome of chronic debilitating fatigue (the chronic fatigue syndrome) manifested by low-grade fever, sore throat, lymphadenopathy, myalgias, arthralgias, paresthesias, headache, depression, and cognitive deficits has at times been attributed to recurrent acute or chronic episodes of infectious mononucleosis. The status

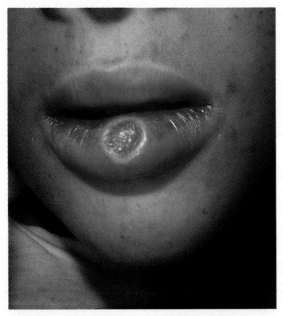

Figure 12–22. Accidental vaccination on the lip of an adult following exposure to an infant vaccinated for smallpox.

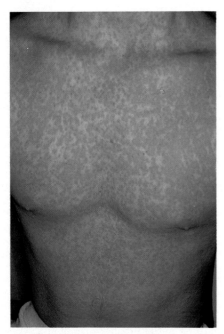

Figure 12–23. Infectious mononucleosis. An erythematous maculopapular eruption is seen in 10 to 15 per cent of patients with this disorder.

of "chronic infectious mononucleosis" is controversial, and although a small group of patients with recurrent symptoms have markedly abnormal serologic tests for Epstein-Barr virus, it appears that an insult to the immune system may at times be the cause of these recurrent symptoms.[48, 49]

The diagnosis of infectious mononucleosis is based on a triad of clinical, hematologic, and serologic findings. Hematologic features include a leukocyte count of 10,000 to 40,000/mm^3 with abnormally large basophilic-staining lymphocytes containing foamy cytoplasm. Heterophile antibody studies (agglutination of sheep erythrocytes by the Paul-Bunnell test) resulting in titers of 1 : 112 or higher are diagnostic, and the mono-spot test, a slide test using formalized horse cells, is a valuable presumptive test for rapid diagnosis. It should be noted, however, that multiple leukocyte counts and Paul-Bunnell heterophile tests may need to be repeated during the first 3 to 4 weeks of illness before diagnostic results are achieved. In addition, the rapid mono-spot test and Paul-Bunnell test are not as sensitive in children younger than 4 years of age[46] as they are in adults and a high proportion of false-negative tests occur in this age group. In cases in which the heterophile test is negative, multiple specific serologic antibody tests for IgA antibodies against the viral capsid antigen may be used to help identify the disorder.

The treatment of infectious mononucleosis is symptomatic. During the acute phase, rest is the most important aspect of treatment. In severe forms of the disorder corticosteroids have been shown to reduce the duration and severity of the illness, and 20 to 25 per cent of patients are reputed to have a concurrent β-hemolytic streptococcal infection. Penicillin or erythromycin is beneficial for those individuals with streptococcal disease, but ampicillin should be avoided, since 80 to 90 per cent of individuals with infectious mononucleosis have an unusual sensitivity to this drug characterized by a copper-colored maculopapular or generalized erythematous eruption that occurs 5 to 8 days after the initiation of therapy (Fig. 12–26). As stated previously, the frequency of cutaneous eruptions in patients with infectious mononucleosis is between 10 and 15 per cent. If penicillin is administered, this incidence increases to 44 per cent. This unusual cutaneous reaction to ampicillin and at times other antibiotics appears to be created by an altered immunologic state with abnormal lymphocytes and is part of a transient serologic abnormality involving a number of antigens during infection with this disease. Since this association is not permanent it is reassuring to know that on reexposure to ampicillin 1 to 17 months after the acute illness only 5 per cent of patients continue to display this cutaneous reaction.[50–52]

In patients with life-threatening upper airway obstruction, hospitalization, maintenance of hydration and a 4- to 7-day course of systemic corticosteroids (prednisone, 40 mg/kg/day, or its equivalent) can help relieve inflammation and soft tissue swelling. Although acyclovir has been shown to reduce the replication of Epstein-Barr virus in vitro and has been used in patients with severe clini-

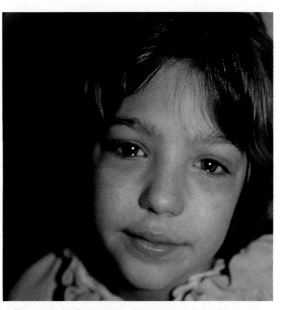

Figure 12–24. Edema of the eyelids in a patient with infectious mononucleosis. (Courtesy of Dr. Jonathan Schneider.)

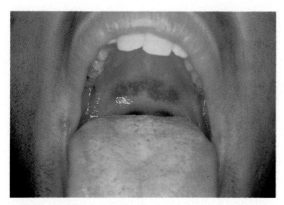

Figure 12–25. Petechial lesions at the junction of the hard and soft palate of a patient with infectious mononucleosis.

cal disease, results to date with this agent have not been striking.[53]

EXANTHEMS ASSOCIATED WITH *MYCOPLASMA PNEUMONIAE* INFECTION

For many years the agent (Eaton agent) of cold agglutinin–positive primary atypical pneumonia was thought to be a virus. In 1962 it was shown not to be a virus but a pleuropneumonia-like organism. Rashes, often of short duration and usually described as maculopapular or urticarial, have occurred in up to 16 per cent of cases. Other cutaneous eruptions associated with *M. pneumoniae* infection include erythema multiforme (and its severe bullous form, Stevens-Johnson syndrome), erythema nodosum (see Chapter 18), and, on rare occasions, pityriasis rosea and purpura.[36]

RICKETTSIAL DISEASES

Rickettsial infections are arthropod-borne diseases caused by microorganisms that occupy an intermediate position between bacteria and viruses. Spread by blood-sucking insects such as the body louse, the flea, tick, and mite, the various rickettsial diseases that occur in the United States include endemic or murine typhus, rickettsialpox, Rocky Mountain spotted fever, and Q fever.

Epidemic Typhus Fever. Epidemic typhus fever (louse-borne typhus) is an acute, severe, potentially fatal infectious disease caused by *Rickettsia prowazekii* and characterized clinically by high fever, headaches, general aches and pains, and a centripetal maculopapular eruption that, in severe cases, becomes hemorrhagic. The diagnosis can be established by the clinical picture, isolation of *R. prowazekii* from the blood, and the Weil-Felix agglutination reaction with *Proteus* OX-19.

Endemic Typhus Fever. Endemic typhus fever (flea-borne or murine typhus) is an acute, relatively mild infection caused by *Rickettsia mooseri* and

characterized chiefly by headache, fever, malaise, and a centripetal maculopapular eruption. Essentially a modified version of epidemic typhus, it is spread to humans by the rat flea *Xenopsylla cheopis* and is diagnosed on the basis of the clinical picture, isolation of the organism by inoculation of the patient's blood into guinea pigs and adult white mice, and a positive Weil-Felix agglutination reaction with *Proteus* OX-19.

Rickettsialpox. Rickettsialpox is an acute benign infectious disease caused by *Rickettsia akuri*, spread by the rodent mite *Allodermanyssus sanguineus* and ectoparasites of the mouse, *Mus musculus* (the reservoir of the infection). The disorder is characterized by an initial papule at the site of the bite, a grippe-like syndrome, and a papulovesicular eruption (papules surmounted by vesicles) with an irregular distribution. Diagnosis can be made on the basis of the clinical picture, isolation of the causative agent from the blood during the acute stage of the disease, negative Weil-Felix agglutinations, and a complement fixation test that shows a fourfold or greater rise in antibody titer in paired sera obtained early and late in the disease. It should be noted that because of cross-reactions, the Rocky Mountain spotted fever complement

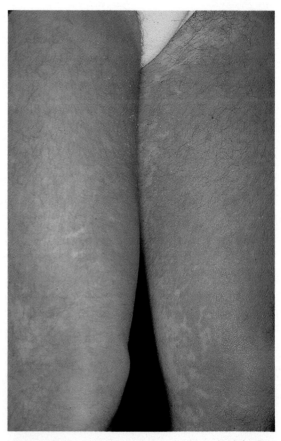

Figure 12–26. Ampicillin rash in a patient with infectious mononucleosis.

fixation test is positive and accordingly should not be misdiagnosed in patients with this disorder.

Q Fever. Q fever, a widespread infection affecting a wide variety of domestic farm animals, caused by the rickettsia *Coxiella burnetti*, can at times be transmitted to humans by inhalation of infected materials, tissues, and dust from infected animals on research facilities and farms. Following an incubation period of 9 to 20 days, the disorder is characterized by the abrupt onset of fever, chills, weakness, headache, anorexia, myalgia, and, at times, pneumonitis, hepatitis, a glandular fever-like syndrome, glomerulonephritis, myocarditis, or endocarditis. The disease is usually mild and generally lasts 1 to 4 weeks with a mortality less than 1 per cent. The mortality in patients with endocarditis, however, is 30 to 60 per cent. Although generally described as not having a cutaneous eruption, fine discrete macules lasting for 2 to 7 days may sometimes be seen (particularly on the trunk) and transient urticarial eruptions and palatal petechiae have been reported. The diagnosis can be established by immunofluorescent or complement-fixation antibody tests using paired serum specimens and specific enzyme-linked immunosorbent assay, complement fixation, or immunofluorescent studies. Tetracycline, which should not be given to children younger than 9 years of age unless the benefits are greater than the risk of dental staining, is the drug of choice.[54] Therapy should be continued until the patient is afebrile for 2 to 3 days. The organism, however, can remain latent in tissues for years, and relapses are not uncommon.

Rocky Mountain Spotted Fever. Rocky Mountain spotted fever is an acute febrile exanthematous illness caused by *Rickettsia rickettsii* and transmitted by the bite of a tick. Although for years a disorder primarily confined to the Rocky Mountain states, the disorder is also endemic in the South Atlantic states, and cases are now reported from all parts of the United States. In the western United States, *Dermacentor andersonii*, the wood tick, is the most important vector and the disease usually occurs in men who acquire a wood tick bite in wooded areas; in the eastern United States, *Dermacentor variabilis*, the dog tick, is the usual vector, and most patients are women and children. In the southwestern United States, the Lone Star tick (*Amblyomma americanum*) is the vector of the disease.[55–58]

The incubation period usually is 5 to 7 days. Most often the rash begins on the third or fourth day of illness as a maculopapular eruption on the extremities (the flexors of the wrists and ankles), spreads centrally to involve the back, chest, and abdomen, and within 2 days becomes generalized. At first the macules are erythematous and later become purpuric, and the palms and soles are usually involved. Occasionally the face is also affected. The lesions are at first discrete, macular, and maculopapular, blanching on pressure. Within 1 or 2 days the rash becomes hemorrhagic, and the severity and extent of the eruption are directly proportional to the severity of the disease (Fig. 12–27).

The history of a tick exposure in an individual with fever, headache, thread-like purpuric lesions on the palms and soles, a peripherally distributed hemorrhagic eruption, ecchymotic lesions following trauma (particularly on the ankles), conjunctivitis, and peripheral and periorbital edema suggest the possibility of Rocky Mountain spotted fever. Although serologic tests are unable to establish the diagnosis early in the course of illness, the demonstration of rickettsiae on direct immunofluorescence of a cutaneous punch biopsy can help establish the diagnosis and, when rapid diagnosis is desired, many commercial laboratories can provide a 24- to 48-hour turn-around time for immunofluorescent antibody testing.[59, 60] Diagnosis can usually be confirmed by Weil-Felix agglutinations positive with OX-19 and OX-2 strains by the second or third week of the infection and by complement fixation tests. Since the pathogenic organism cannot routinely be cultured and the Weil-Felix or complement fixation tests may be negative during the acute stages of the disorder, a high index of suspicion and careful epidemiologic history are important.

Rocky Mountain spotted fever is a curable but potentially fatal disease with a confirmed death rate of about 20 per cent, with a range of 13 to 40 per cent without treatment. Fatalities are more common in individuals older than age 40 and less common in children and young adults. With effective rapid therapy, however, mortality can be lowered to 5 per cent. The primary factor in patient survival is early diagnosis and therapy. Reduction

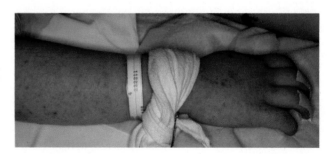

Figure 12–27. Maculopapular and hemorrhagic eruption on the forearm and hand (Rocky Mountain spotted fever).

of deaths from Rocky Mountain spotted fever, accordingly, requires that a presumptive diagnosis be made early enough for appropriate antibiotic therapy to be effective.

The tetracyclines and chloramphenicol are highly effective and usually curative when given early and in adequate dosages. Although tetracyclines are generally contraindicated for patients younger than 9 years of age, physicians must weigh the benefits and risks of each drug.[61] Tetracycline, the preferred drug, may be administered orally in a dosage of 30 to 40 mg/kg/day (in four equally divided doses) with a maximum of 2 g/day for 7 to 10 days (or until the patient is afebrile for at least 2 or 3 days). When administered intravenously, the dosage of tetracycline is 20 mg/kg/day. In the more severely ill, intravenous chloramphenicol (50 to 100 mg/kg/day, with a maximum of 2 to 4 g/day) may be used. When chloramphenicol is given, patients and their families should be advised of the potential toxicity of this preparation, complete blood cell counts should be done every 2 days (or daily if the leukocyte count is below 7,000/mm^3), and chloramphenicol should be replaced with tetracycline if the leukocyte count decreases to below 5,000/mm^3 or the polymorphonuclear cell count becomes less than 30 per cent.

All patients with Rocky Mountain spotted fever have vasculitis to a varying degree. The more severely ill patients may have edema involving the periorbital area, face, and extremities. Disseminated intravascular coagulation or purpura fulminans (see Fig. 9–43), myocarditis, and heart failure are common complications of patients severely ill with this disorder. Although rarely necessary, the platelet deficit may be lessened temporarily by platelet or whole blood transfusion and intravenous heparin (50 to 100 units/kg intravenously every 4 to 6 hours appears to decrease or stop the progression of the coagulopathy). Central nervous system vasculitis, when present, is manifested by delirium, confusion, stupor, and seizures. Phenobarbital sodium, intravenously, in a dose of 4 mg/kg will usually control the seizures. Widespread increase in capillary permeability and hyponatremia may be prominent abnormalities in patients with Rocky Mountain spotted fever. Accordingly, intravenous therapy with plasma and whole blood infusions followed by appropriate fluid and electrolyte replacement is frequently necessary.[59]

Mediterranean Spotted Fever. A number of other distinct but clinically similar tick-borne spotted-fever infections caused by rickettsiae have been recognized. *Mediterranean spotted fever* (boutenneuse fever, Kenya tick-bite fever, African tick typhus) is an acute febrile illness usually endemic in southern Europe and northern Africa caused by *Rickettsia cornorii*. Seen primarily in children living in or visiting that part of the world and transmitted by the dog tick, the disorder is characterized by a generalized maculapapular rash, often affecting the palms and soles; and, in three fourths of patients, an indurated papule (known as *tache noir*) that becomes a necrotic ulcer may be noted at the presumed site of the previous tick attachment. Like all rickettsial diseases, laboratory diagnosis of Mediterranean spotted fever is difficult. At onset, fewer than half of the patients have a positive reaction to one or more of the Weil-Felix antigens, but, as in Rocky Mountain spotted fever, a rapid diagnosis can be obtained by direct immunofluorescence staining of a cutaneous biopsy specimen. Almost always a benign disease, adenopathy, splenomegaly, and conjunctivitis are common; fatalities are rare. Although the choice of antibiotic and the duration of therapy have not been established, tetracyclines, chloramphenicol, and sulfamethoxazole-trimethoprim have been used with success.[62]

Human Ehrlichiosis. *Human ehrlichiosis,* currently the most common rickettsial disease in the United States, is an acute febrile illness clinically similar to Rocky Mountain spotted fever but with more frequent leukopenia and less frequent occurrence of a rash. Caused by a tick-borne rickettsia (*Ehrlichia canis,* or another closely related rickettsial species), and primarily a disorder of adult men but also reported in children,[63–65] the spectrum of illness ranges from subclinical infection to a severe multisystemic disorder manifested by fever, headache, anorexia, myalgias, and a variety of cutaneous (macular, petechial, scarlatiniform, maculopapular, or vasculitic) eruptions. The rash is variable in appearance and location, develops approximately 1 week after the onset of illness, and only occurs in approximately one half of reported cases. The diagnosis can be confirmed by demonstration of a fourfold or greater increase in antibody titer between acute and convalescent sera, preferably obtained 2 to 4 weeks apart using an indirect fluorescent antibody test with *E. canis,* with a minimum positive titer being 1:80. The disease typically lasts 1 to 2 weeks. Although recovery generally occurs without sequelae, reported complications include pulmonary infiltrates and respiratory and renal failure, and fatalities have been reported. Tetracycline appears to be effective, with a treatment dose and schedule similar to that used for the treatment of Rocky Mountain spotted fever. Limited data suggest that chloramphenicol may also be considered as an alternative form of therapy.

References

1. Cupoli JM: Photodistribution of viral exanthems (letter). Pediatrics 59:484, 1977.

   A profound photodistribution of viral exanthems as manifested in a brother and sister with varicella.

2. Gilchrest B, Baden H: Photodistribution of viral exanthems. Pediatrics 54:136–138, 1974.

   Two children with viral exanthems (echovirus 9 and varicella) with the eruption almost exclusively in sun-exposed areas.

3. Feldman S, Hughes WT, Daniel CB: Varicella in children with cancer: Seventy-seven cases. Pediatrics 56:388–397, 1975.

Of 77 children with cancer who contracted varicella, no complications were noted in the children not treated with corticosteroids or chemotherapeutic agents at the time of infection. In contrast, 32 per cent of 60 children receiving anticancer therapy had evidence of visceral dissemination and 7 per cent died of varicella pneumonia or encephalitis.

4. Kasper WJ, Howe PM: Fatal varicella after a single course of corticosteroids. Pediatr. Infect. Dis. J. 9:729–732, 1990.

The death of a 12-year-old boy from extensive dissemination of varicella following oral and intravenous corticosteroids for the treatment and exacerbation of asthma suggests the need for early acyclovir treatment in high doses in an effort to prevent dissemination of varicella in individuals receiving or who recently received corticosteroids during or prior to the onset of varicella.

5. Orlowski JP, Gillis J, Kilham HA: A catch in the Reye. Pediatrics 80:638–642, 1987.

A review of 26 patients with Reye's syndrome adds fuel to the controversy regarding the role of salicylates, if any, in the pathogenesis of this disorder.

6. Brunnell PA, Gershon AA, Hughes WT, et al.: Prevention of varicella in high risk children: A collaborative study. Pediatrics 50:718–722, 1972.

Zoster immune globulin (ZIG) in adequate dosage, administered within 48 hours of exposure, may be expected to prevent or modify varicella in high risk children.

7. Prober CG, Gershon AA, Grose C, et al.: Varicella-zoster infections in pregnancy and the perinatal period. Pediatr. Infect. Dis. J. 9:865–869, 1990.

An authoritative consensus opinion on the management of varicella-zoster in pregnant women and their offspring.

8. Oglivie MM, Stephen JRD, Larkin M: Letter to the editor: Chickenpox in pregnancy. Lancet 1:915–916, 1986.

The authors suggest a higher dose of VZIG (250 mg versus 100 mg) for infants born to mothers who develop varicella within 4 days before or after delivery.

9. Whitley R, Hilty M, Haynes R, et al.: Vidarabine therapy of varicella in immunosuppressed patients. J. Pediatr. 101:125–131, 1982.

Intravenous vidarabine (Ara-A) was shown to be beneficial in the treatment of immunosuppressed patients with varicella.

10. Pahwa S, Biron K, Lim W, et al.: Continuous varicella-zoster infection with acyclovir resistance in a child with AIDS. J.A.M.A. 260:2879–2882, 1988.

A report of a 4½ year-old girl congenitally infected with human immunodeficiency virus who developed a varicella-zoster viral infection that persisted over a 14-month period despite repeated acyclovir therapy.

11. Shepp DH, Dondliker PS, Myers JD: Treatment of varicella-zoster infection in severely immunocompromised patients: A randomized comparison of acyclovir and vidarabine. N. Engl. J. Med. 314:208–212, 1986.

In a study of varicella-zoster virus infection in severely immunocompromised patients, intravenous acyclovir appears to be more effective than intravenous vidarabine.

12. Balfour HH Jr, Kelly JM, Suarez CS, et al.: Acyclovir treatment of varicella in otherwise healthy children. J. Pediatr. 116:633–639, 1990.

Although not a panacea and not recommended for general use in children with varicella, oral acyclovir can hasten the healing and lessen the total number of cutaneous lesions and time of defervescence if given early (within the first 24 hours of the onset of the cutaneous eruption).

13. Gershon AA, Steinberg SP, Gelb L, et al.: Live attenuated varicella vaccine in immunocompromised children and adults. Pediatrics 78 (suppl):757–762, 1986.

Studies in 307 children with leukemia in remission who received live attenuated varicella vaccine showed varicella vaccination to be safe and effective in decreasing the attack rate of varicella in leukemic children.

14. Brunell PA, Geiser CF, Novelli V, et al.: Varicella-like illness caused by live varicella vaccine in children with acute lymphocytic leukemia. Pediatrics 79:922–927, 1987.

Although a varicella-like illness occurred in 52 children with acute lymphocytic leukemia following the administration of live varicella vaccine, the morbidity associated with vaccine administration was shown to be considerably less than that which would have occurred if the patients had not received prophylactic administration.

15. Brunell PA, Novelli VM, Lipton SV, et al.: Combined vaccine against measles, mumps, rubella and varicella. Pediatrics 88:779–784, 1988.

Although live varicella vaccine is not routinely recommended for chickenpox prophylaxis for children in the United States, the administration of varicella vaccine in combination with routine MMR vaccinations is recommended in this article.

16. White CJ, Kuter BJ, Hildebrand CS, et al.: Varicella vaccine (VARIVAX) in healthy children and adolescents: Results from clinical trials, 1987 to 1989. Pediatrics 87:604–610, 1989.

A study of 3,303 healthy children and adolescents confirmed findings of previous studies attesting to the efficacy and safety of varicella vaccine.

17. Suringa DWR, Bank LJ, Ackerman AB: Role of measles virus in skin lesions and Koplik's spots. N. Engl. J. Med. 283:1139–1142, 1970.

On the basis of histopathologic and electron microscopic features, measles virus appears to initiate a similar pathologic process in lesions of the skin and oral mucosa.

18. Cherry JD, Feigin RD, Lobes LA Jr, et al.: Atypical measles in children previously immunized with attenuated measles virus vaccines. Pediatrics 50:712–721, 1972.

Twelve children with clinical illnesses suggesting "atypical measles" during an epidemic of measles in the winter and spring of 1970 to 1971.

19. Krause PJ, Cherry JD, Naiditch MJ, et al.: Revaccination of previous recipients of killed measles vaccine: Clinical and immunologic studies. J. Pediatr. 93:565–571, 1978.

Clinical and immunologic studies suggest low serum antibody and increased measles specific lymphocyte reactivity as the cause of the atypical measles syndrome and severe local reactions following reimmunization with live measles vaccine.

20. Hutchins SS, Escolan J, Markowitz LE, et al.: Measles outbreak among unvaccinated preschool-aged children: Opportunities missed by health care providers to administer measles vaccine. Pediatrics 83:369–374, 1989.

An epidemic of measles among unvaccinated preschool children suggests that new immunization strategies are required in an effort to increase protective antibody levels in this susceptible age group.

21. Morbidity and Mortality Weekly Report: Measles—United States, 1990. J.A.M.A. 265:3227–3228, 1991.

Failure to vaccinate children at the appropriate age level was the major factor contributing to the resurgence of measles in the United States in 1989–1990.

22. Stiehm ER: Skin testing prior to measles vaccination for egg-sensitive patients. Am. J. Dis. Child. 144:32, 1990.

Although most egg-sensitive individuals do not require skin testing prior to measles vaccination, those with severe sensitivity (anaphylactic reaction following egg ingestion) should be tested with diluted vaccine prior to its administration.

23. Miller RA, Brancato F, Holmes KK: *Corynebacterium hemolyticum* as a cause of pharyngitis and scarlatiniform rash in young adults. Ann. Intern. Med. *105*:867–872, 1986.

In a retrospective study, 20 of 32 patients with cultures positive for *C. hemolyticum* had erythematous eruptions on the trunk and extremities similar to those seen in individuals with scarlet fever.

24. Dinehart SM, Dillard R, Raimer SS, et al.: Cutaneous manifestations of acrodynia (pink disease). Arch. Dermatol. *124*:107–109, 1988.

A report of a 14-month-old girl with acrodynia exposed to mercury when the parents inadvertently spilled a bottle of mercury in a room where she played.

25. Taylor BJ, Duffill MB: Recurrent pseudo-scarlatina and allergy to pseudoephedrine hydrochloride. Br. J. Dermatol. *118*:827–829, 1988.

A report of a 32-year-old woman with seven episodes of a scarlet fever–like eruption associated with the administration of pseudoephedrine hydrochloride. The authors also note that codeine can give a similar picture.

26. Morbidity and Mortality Weekly Report: Increase in rubella and congenital rubella syndrome—United States, 1988–1990. Arch. Dermatol. *127*:465–466, 1991.

Following a substantial decrease in rubella and congenital rubella in the 1980s, a moderate resurgence of rubella and a major increase in congenital rubella syndrome occurred in the United States in 1990. As in measles prevention programs, it is suggested that failure to vaccinate rather than vaccine failure was responsible for this increase.

27. Balfour HH Jr: Fifth disease: Full fathom five (marginal comments). Am. J. Dis. Child. *130*:239–240, 1976.

Erythema infectiosum, a mild evanescent disorder of childhood, is presumed to be a viral disorder, although the etiologic agent has not yet been established.

28. Hall CB, Horner FA: Encephalopathy with erythema infectiosum. Am. J. Dis. Child. *131*:65–67, 1977.

The second reported case of encephalitis following erythema infectiosum and apparently the first with permanent sequelae.

29. Anand A, Gray ES, Brown T, et al.: Human parvovirus infection in pregnancy and hydrops fetalis. N. Engl. J. Med. *316*:183–186, 1987.

Two of six women with serologic evidence of parvovirus infection had midtrimester abortions in which both fetuses were grossly hydropic and profoundly anemic.

30. Leads from the Morbidity and Mortality Weekly Report: Risks associated with human parvovirus B19 infection. J.A.M.A. *261*:1555–1563, 1989.

A comprehensive review of human parvovirus B19 infection in pregnant women and recommendations for the management of individuals when this complication occurs.

31. Centers for Disease Control: Risks associated with human parvovirus B19 infection. M.M.W.R. *38*:81–97, 1989.

A comprehensive report helpful to physicians and public health and health-care professionals regarding the concerns and management of individuals with human parvovirus B19 infection.

32. McDonald NE: School policies for children with erythema infectiosum. Pediatr. Infect. Dis. J. *8*:64–65, 1989.

Recommendations on the management of children with erythema infectiosum with emphasis on the contagiousness of this disorder and advice for the physician and health communities regarding school attendance of affected children.

33. Yamanishi K, Okuno T, Shiraki K, et al.: Identification of human herpesvirus-6 as a causal agent of exanthem subitum. Lancet *1*:1065–1067, 1988.

Human herpesvirus-6 obtained from peripheral blood lymphocytes of four infants with exanthem subitum provides evidence implicating this virus as the etiologic agent of this disorder.

34. Suga S, Yoshikawa T, Asano Y, et al.: Human herpesvirus-6 infection (exanthem subitum) without rash. Pediatrics *83*:1003–1006, 1989.

Human herpesvirus-6 was isolated from peripheral blood mononuclear cells in two patients with a 3-day febrile episode in whom exanthem subitum, without the typical roseola rash, was suspected.

35. Berenberg W, Wright S, Janeway CA: Roseola infantum (exanthem subitum). N. Engl. J. Med. *241*:253–259, 1949.

A review of the clinical and laboratory features of roseola infantum (exanthem subitum).

36. Cherry JD: Enteroviruses: Poliovirus (poliomyelitis), coxsackieviruses, echoviruses, and enteroviruses. In Feigin RD, Cherry JD (Eds.(: Textbook of Pediatric Infectious Diseases, 2nd ed. W.B. Saunders Co., Philadelphia, 1987, 1729–1790.

A comprehensive review of the various enteroviruses and their cutaneous manifestations.

37. Meade RH III, Chang T: Zoster-like eruption due to echovirus 6. Am. J. Dis. Child. *133*:283–284, 1979.

A 7-year-old boy with a unilateral vesiculobullous eruption, which on the basis of viral culture of fluid from several bullae and the development of high titers of serum neutralizing antibody appeared to be associated with echovirus type 6 infection.

38. Tindall JP, Miller GD: Hand, foot and mouth disease. Cutis *9*:457–463, 1972.

A review of hand-foot-and-mouth disease, its clinical and laboratory aspects.

39. Goldberg MF, McAdams AJ: Myocarditis possibly due to Coxsackie group A, type 16, virus. J. Pediatr. *62*:762–765, 1963.

A 10½-month-old girl with interstitial myocarditis, cardiac failure, and death presumably due to an infection with Coxsackievirus group A type 16 infection.

40. Wright HT Jr, Landing BH, Lennette EH, et al.: Fatal infection in an infant associated with Coxsackie virus Group A, type 16. N. Engl. J. Med. *268*:1041–1044, 1963.

A fatal case of hand-foot-and-mouth disease in a 7-week-old male infant with enteritis, interstitial myocarditis, lymphohistiocytic arachnoiditis, and what was interpreted as a nonspecific interstitial pneumonia.

41. Frothingham TE: ECHO virus type 9 associated with three cases simulating meningococcemia. N. Engl. J. Med. *259*:484–485, 1958.

Three patients with echovirus type 9 infection, aseptic meningitis, and a petechial rash.

42. Hale CB, Cherry JE, Hutch MH, et al.: The return of the Boston exanthem: Echovirus infections in 1974. Am. J. Dis. Child. *131*:323–328, 1977.

Ten children aged 1 week to 7 years with the Boston exanthem in Rochester and Los Angeles.

43. Lerner AM, Cherry JD, Klein JO, et al.: Infections with reoviruses. N. Engl. J. Med. *267*:947–952, 1962.

Seven children younger than age 10 years with reovirus 2 infection.

44. Wehrle PF: Smallpox eradication: A global appraisal. J.A.M.A. *240*:1977–1979, 1978.

Barring unforeseen problems, it appeared that a world free from smallpox was at hand in 1978.

45. Sumaya CV, Ench Y: Epstein-Barr virus infectious mononucleosis in children. I. Clinical and general laboratory findings. Pediatrics *75*:1003–1010, 1985.

A review of 113 children aged 6 months to 16 years with documented Epstein-Barr virus–induced infectious mononucleosis serves to expand our knowledge of this disease in children of all ages.

46. Sumaya CV, Ench Y: Epstein-Barr virus infectious mononucleosis in children: II. Heterophile antibody in viral specific responses: New perspectives on infectious mononucleosis. Pediatrics 75:1011–1019, 1985.

Advances in Epstein-Barr virus–specific testing show that infectious mononucleosis occurs much more frequently in young children than physicians have heretofore realized.

47. Decker GR, Berberian BJ, Sulica VI: Periorbital and eyelid edema: The initial manifestation of acute infectious mononucleosis. Cutis 47:323–324, 1991.

Periorbital and eyelid edema in an 18-year-old student occurring 1 week before the typical prodrome period presented as the initial manifestation of acute infectious mononucleosis.

48. Buchwald D, Sullivan JL, Komaroff AL: Frequency of chronic active Epstein-Barr virus infection in a general medical practice. J.A.M.A. 257:2303–2307, 1987.

Although 21 per cent of 500 patients found to be suffering from chronic fatigue syndrome had serologic evidence of Epstein-Barr virus infection, the frequency of this virus infection in general medical practice makes it difficult to prove that Epstein-Barr virus plays a causal role in the pathogenesis of the chronic fatigue syndrome.

49. Holmes GP, Kaplan JE, Stewart JA, et al.: A cluster of patients with a chronic mononucleosis-like syndrome: Epstein-Barr virus the cause? J.A.M.A. 257:2297–2302, 1987.

A study of 134 patients suggests that chronic Epstein-Barr virus infection or perhaps another insult to the immune system may be the cause of the "chronic fatigue syndrome."

50. Patel BM: Skin rash with infectious mononucleosis. Pediatrics 40:910–911, 1967.

A 100 per cent incidence of a copper-colored maculopapular rash in 13 patients with infectious mononucleosis treated with ampicillin.

51. Levene G, Baker H: Ampicillin and infectious mononucleosis. Br. J. Dermatol. 80:417–418, 1978.

Infectious mononucleosis appears to have a tendency to render patients sensitive to ampicillin.

52. Lund A, Bergan T: Temporary skin reactions to penicillins during acute stage of infectious mononucleosis. Scand. J. Dis. 7:21–28, 1975.

Studies in 19 patients with infectious mononucleosis allergic to penicillin and ampicillin during the acute stages of their illness with reversal of the reactivity after recovery from the disease.

53. Anderson J, Britton S, Ernberg I, et al.: Effect of acyclovir on infectious mononucleosis: A double-blind placebo-controlled study. J. Infect. Dis. 153:283–294, 1986.

In a randomized study of 31 patients with infectious mononucleosis, although intravenous acyclovir appeared to inhibit oropharyngeal shedding of virus, the virus was found to recur after treatment was discontinued.

54. Spelman DW: Q fever: A study of 111 consecutive cases. Med. J. Aust. 1:547, 1982.

An overview of 111 cases of Q fever confirming that, although unusual, patients with this disorder may at times display a cutaneous eruption.

55. Selgo MP, Telzak EE, Currie B, et al.: A focus of Rocky Mountain spotted fever within New York City. N. Engl. J. Med. 318:1345–1348, 1988.

A report of two children and two adults who acquired Rocky Mountain spotted fever in New York City.

56. Leads from the Morbidity and Mortality Report: Rocky Mountain spotted fever—United States, 1985. J.A.M.A. 255:2861–2867, 1986.

In 1985 a provisional total of 600 cases of Rocky Mountain spotted fever were reported in the United States. Of these, Oklahoma had the highest incidence, North Carolina reported the largest number of cases, and South Carolina and Kansas had incidence rates of 1/100,000 or higher.

57. Haynes RE, Sanders DY, Cramblett HG: Rocky Mountain spotted fever in children. J. Pediatr. 76:685–693, 1970.

A review of 78 children with Rocky Mountain spotted fever.

58. Bradford WD, Hawkins HK: Rocky Mountain spotted fever in childhood. Am. J. Dis. Child. 131:1228–1232, 1977.

Review of 138 cases of Rocky Mountain spotted fever indicates that the characteristic rash in combination with fever, tick bite, low serum sodium concentration, and thrombocytopenia is helpful in recognition of this serious and potentially lethal infectious disease.

59. Hattwick MAW, Retailliau H, O'Brien RJ, et al.: Fatal Rocky Mountain spotted fever. J.A.M.A. 240:1499–1503, 1978.

Comparison of 44 fatal and 50 nonfatal cases of Rocky Mountain spotted fever emphasizes the need for early diagnosis and therapy for this disorder.

60. Newby JG: Letter to the editor: The Weil-Felix test is archaic and misleading. J.A.M.A. 255:1020, 1986.

The indirect fluorescent antibody test is recommended as a more specific and reliable study for the diagnosis of Rocky Mountain spotted fever.

61. Abramson JS, Givner LB: Editorial: Should tetracycline be contraindicated for therapy of presumed Rocky Mountain spotted fever in children less than 9 years of age? Pediatrics 86:123–124, 1990.

Contraindications to the use of tetracycline in patients younger than 9 years of age do not seem warranted when treating children with Rocky Mountain spotted fever.

62. Treadwell TL, Phillips S, Jablonski WJ: Mediterranean spotted fever in children returning from France. Am. J. Dis. Child. 144:1037–1038, 1990.

A report of two children from New England found to have Mediterranean spotted fever on return from a school trip to Nice.

63. Barton LL, Foy LL: Ehrlichia canis infection in a child. Pediatrics 84:580–582, 1989.

A 4-year-old child with ehrlichiosis, although rare and not endemic in the United States, reaffirms the fact that this disorder should be considered in the differential diagnosis of Rocky Mountain spotted fever and other rickettsial disorders in the Mediterranean area and in individuals who travel to this part of the world.

64. Eng TR, Harkess JR, Fishbein DB, et al.: Epidemiologic, clinical, and laboratory findings of ehrlichiosis in the United States, 1988. J.A.M.A. 264:2251–2258, 1990.

A review of 40 patients with human ehrlichiosis identified by the Centers for Disease Control and the Oklahoma State Department of Health.

65. Malpass DG, Heiman HS, Sumaya CV: Childhood ehrlichiosis: A case report and review of the literature. Int. Pediatr. 6:354–358, 1991.

A report of human ehrlichiosis in an 8-year-old girl, a disorder reported to date in 16 different states, most in the southern half of this country, underscores the importance of early diagnosis and treatment, especially in the seriously ill and those with significant underlying medical conditions.

13

SKIN DISORDERS DUE TO FUNGI

Fungi are a group of simple plants that lack flowers, leaves, and chlorophyll and get their nourishment from dead or living organic matter, thus depending on plants, animals, and humans for their existence. Fungal infections that affect humans may be superficial, deep, or systemic, and sometimes fatal. Often regarded as trivial, diseases caused by fungi are no longer unimportant and remote problems in medicine and public health. Although they do not rank as pathogens with the bacteria or viruses, a number of species once thought to be ubiquitous and harmless have been implicated in various diseases, and with increasing use of broad-spectrum antibiotics, corticosteroids, and potent cytotoxic agents and the increasing incidence of acquired immune deficiency disease,

deep mycoses have become increasingly frequent and significant.

The pathogenic fungal diseases are divided into superficial and deep infections. The superficial infections are those that are limited to the epidermis, hair, nails, and mucous membranes. The deep fungal infections are those in which the organisms affect other organs of the body or invade the skin through direct extension or hematogenous spread.

SUPERFICIAL FUNGAL INFECTIONS

There are three common types of superficial fungus infection, the dermatophytoses, tinea versicolor, and candidiasis (moniliasis). Those caused by dermatophytes are termed *tinea, dermatophytosis*, or, because of the annular appearance of the lesions, *ringworm*. In addition, tinea nigra, a superficial infection of the stratum corneum caused by a yeast-like fungus (frequently misdiagnosed as a melanocytic lesion or silver nitrate or India ink stain), and piedra, an asymptomatic infection of the hair shaft, may also be noted in children as well as adults.

The dermatophytes are a group of related fungi that live in soil, on animals, or on humans, digest keratin, and invade the skin, hair, and nails, producing a diversity of clinical lesions. Depending on the involved site, the infection may be termed *tinea capitis, tinea barbae, tinea corporis, tinea manuum, tinea pedis, tinea cruris*, or *onychomycosis* (tinea of the nails). The diagnosis and management of fungal diseases of childhood have become easier in the past decade owing to the development of more effective diagnostic techniques and therapeutic agents.

Diagnosis of Fungal Infections

Tests for fungal infection are rewarding procedures readily available to all physicians, not merely to those trained in dermatology.[1, 2] Diagnosis of ringworm of the scalp can frequently be aided by the presence of fluorescence under a Wood's light, by direct microscopic examination of cutaneous scrapings or infected hairs, or by fungal culture. These tests can be performed simply, inexpensively, and rapidly, as an office procedure. With the ready availability of these tests, I believe that it is best not to treat a possible fungal disorder without fungal culture, just as it is best not to treat a possible streptococcal throat infection without bacterial culture.

WOOD'S LIGHT EXAMINATION

The discovery in 1925 that hair infected by certain dermatophytoses would fluoresce when exposed to ultraviolet light filtered by a Wood's filter led to a helpful but occasionally improperly used diagnostic tool. When Wood's light examination is performed, it must be remembered that infected hairs, not the skin, fluoresce when exposed to light rays emitted in the 356-nm range by this lamp. Although the nature and the source of the fluorescent substance in infected hairs are not fully understood, this phenomenon is believed to be the result of a substance, perhaps a pteridine, emitted when the fungus invades the hair (Fig. 13–1).

Optimally, a powerful Wood's lamp should be used in a completely darkened room. Under these conditions the majority of cases of tinea capitis will show fluorescence. Hairs infected by *Microsporum audouinii* and *M. canis* produce a brilliant green fluorescence, and those infected by *Trichophyton schoenleinii* produce a pale green fluo-

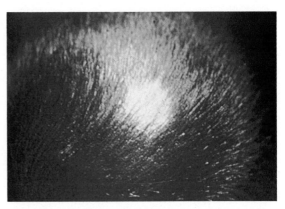

Figure 13–1. Tinea capitis. Fluorescence is evident with Wood's light (Courtesy of Alfred W. Kopf, M.D.)

rescence. It must be remembered, however, that infections due to *Trichophyton tonsurans* and *T. violaceum* do not fluoresce. Sources of error include Wood's light examination in an insufficiently darkened room; the bluish or purplish fluorescence produced by lint, scales, serum exudate, or ointments containing petrolatum; and failure to remember that it is the infected hair and not the skin that fluoresces.

POTASSIUM HYDROXIDE WET-MOUNT PREPARATIONS

Microscopic examination of scrapings of cutaneous fungal infection is an important but frequently overlooked aid in the diagnosis of suspected fungal infection of the skin or hair. This examination will yield rapid results but requires considerable experience, as a consequence of which, unfortunately, it has achieved wide use only by those trained in the dermatologic disciplines (Fig. 13–2).

Material for mycologic study should be taken by gently scraping outward from the active border of a suspected lesion with a dull scalpel blade. Cut hairs, nail scrapings, subungual debris, and material from the edge of the affected nail may also be used for wet-mount examination. Suspected material should be placed on a glass microscope slide with care and spread out flat and evenly in a single layer. A coverslip is applied, and one or two drops of 10 to 20 per cent potassium hydroxide are added at the side of the coverslip until the entire space between coverslip and slide is filled. This preparation should be heated slowly and gently (with care to prevent boiling of the potassium hydroxide, since this will cause crystallization) until the horny cells and debris are rendered translucent. If the potassium hydroxide solution contains dimethylsulfoxide (DMSO), the slide should not be heated, since heating a DMSO potassium hydroxide preparation will dissolve fungi as well as epidermal cells.[1]

After preparation of the specimen, gentle pres-

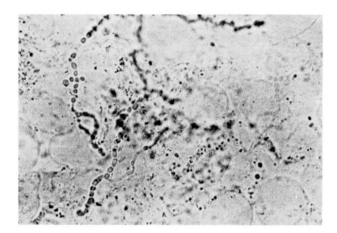

Figure 13–2. Fungal elements (hyphae) as seen on microscopic examination of a potassium hydroxide preparation. (Courtesy of Alfred W. Kopf, M.D.)

sure is applied to the coverslip. When the material has been softened, this will improve the preparation by forcing out trapped air and thinning the specimen, thus allowing better visualization of fungi. It is further recommended that the light of the microscope condenser be dimmed, to enhance contrast between branched hyphae and epidermal elements.

FUNGAL CULTURE

Although direct microscopic examination of skin scrapings will often confirm the suspicion of a fungal disorder, definitive identification of the responsible agent requires isolation of the fungus by culture. There are several types of fungal culture media, but those with Sabouraud's maltose peptone agar, selective for fungi because of an acid pH, are most popular. However, since nonpathogenic fungi grow as well and more rapidly than most pathogenic organisms, a simple modification includes chloramphenicol to inhibit bacterial growth and cycloheximide to discourage nonpathogenic fungi.

The formulation and introduction of Dermatophyte Test Medium (DTM) in 1969 brought a new dimension to the gross screening of pathogenic dermatophytes.[2, 3] Dermatophyte test medium has antibiotics (cycloheximide, gentamicin, and chlortetracycline), which inhibit saprophytic fungi and bacteria. Of particular significance is the fact that the medium also contains phenol red as a color indicator. Nonpathogenic fungi ferment the glucose in culture media with an acidic byproduct. Thus, when not inoculated by a pathogenic dermatophyte, the medium maintains its original yellow color. Dermatophytes, conversely, do not cause fermentation of glucose but use nitrogenous ingredients, resulting in the production of alkaline byproducts and a color change from yellow to red. Although not quite as reliable as standard Sabouraud's media, DTM (available from Acuderm, Inc., Fort Lauderdale, Florida [1-800-327-0015] and

Baker/Cummins, Miami, Florida [1-305-590-2282]) is 95 to 97 per cent accurate, thus making it particularly useful for physicians who lack detailed knowledge of fungus colony morphology.[2–4]

The Dermatophytoses

TINEA CAPITIS

Tinea capitis, the most common dermatophytosis of childhood, is a fungal infection of the scalp characterized by scaling and patchy alopecia. Generally a disease of prepubertal children, chiefly those between 2 and 10 years of age, it only rarely affects infants (Fig. 13–3). Dermatophytes have a short incubation period (generally 1 to 3 weeks and, at times, as brief as 2 to 4 days), boys are afflicted with tinea capitis five times more frequently than girls, and infection beyond the age of puberty (in adolescents and adults) may occur but is uncommon, and an asymptomatic carrier state can be present.[5–10] The cause of increased resistance to tinea capitis infection after puberty is unknown but has been attributed to a higher content of fungistatic fatty acids in the sebum of postpubertal individuals. Although this hypothesis has not been proved, it has widespread acceptance and support.[5]

Clinical Manifestations. Primary lesions of tinea capitis are characterized by the presence of broken-off hairs, 1 to 3 mm above the scalp, and partial alopecia. The infected areas are round or oval and sometimes irregular, and there may be coalescence of lesions, with formation of gyrate patterns. Individual patches generally measure 1 to 6 cm in diameter, and multiple patches are common (Figs. 13–3 through 13–5).

Although almost any species of dermatophyte can cause tinea capitis, it is usually produced by species of *Microsporum* and *Trichophyton*. Lesions can be classified clinically as inflammatory or noninflammatory. The latter type is exemplified by

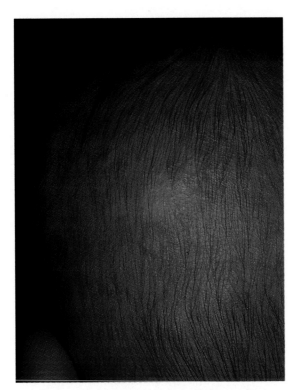

Figure 13–3. A 2-month-old infant with tinea capitis.

lesions of *Microsporum audouinii*. The designation *noninflammatory* is actually a misnomer. On histologic examination tinea capitis displays an inflammatory response and, with careful clinical examination, the presence of erythema and slight scaliness can be detected in most cases. However, the term *inflammatory* has gained wide acceptance and is useful in the description of lesions of tinea capitis associated with widespread pustulation, suppuration, or kerion formation. Tinea capitis due to *M. audouinii* is characteristically noninflammatory at the outset, and most cases remain so throughout the course of the disease. In the early phases the features of the lesions are similar to those of tinea infection of glabrous skin. The central areas show scaling, and the borders are active and slightly elevated. The disorder is characterized by sharply delineated, usually rounded areas of alopecia on the scalp, which is not devoid of hair but covered with short lusterless stubs of hair broken off at 1 to 3 mm of length. The term *gray patch ringworm* has been applied to this disorder. Although *M. audouinii* and *M. canis* in the past were the most common causes of tinea capitis in the United States, they have been replaced by *Trichophyton tonsurans*, the major cause of tinea capitis in Europe.[11, 12]

Any dermatophyte causing tinea capitis may at times produce a sharply demarcated, painful, inflammatory, indurated, boggy granulomatous tumefaction called a kerion (Fig. 13–6). The onset of this condition is acute, lesions usually remain localized to one spot, and the area of involvement is studded with vesicles and pustules. Elicited most often by *M. canis* and *T. tonsurans,* and in rural areas by *T. verrucosum,* an inflammatory kerion is believed to be associated with an intense allergic sensitization to the fungi. Although kerions often heal spontaneously, frequently over 4 to 6 weeks, when the inflammatory reaction is severe and diagnosis is delayed, scarring alopecia may result (Figs. 13–7 and 13–8).

"Black dot" ringworm is a form of tinea capitis caused by *T. tonsurans* and *T. violaceum* and characterized by multiple, small, circular patches of alopecia, with only a few involved hairs, which are broken off very close to the cutaneous surface, resulting in a polka dot–like appearance (Fig. 13–9). This type of involvement tends to produce a chronic diffuse alopecia. It should be noted that the "black dot" sign is probably overemphasized and, although present, is frequently relatively inconspicuous.

Favus, a severe chronic form of tinea capitis rarely seen in the United States (Fig. 13–10), is caused by the fungus *T. schoenleinii*. This disorder is characterized by scaly erythematous patches with honeycomb-yellow cup-like crusts that are termed *scutula.* A chronic disorder, with onset often in childhood, it begins as a yellowish or red papule surrounded by a circle of vesicles, which progress to form friable nummular crusts that are yellowish brown to greenish brown; they coalesce to form plaques and exudate with a characteristic mouse-like odor. Such infections frequently result in considerable scarring and permanent alopecia.[13]

Diagnosis. Tinea capitis may occasionally mimic other scalp conditions and may be confused with seborrheic dermatitis, psoriasis, alopecia areata, trichotillomania, folliculitis, impetigo, lupus erythematosus, folliculitis decalvans, and pseudopelade. When the diagnosis remains uncer-

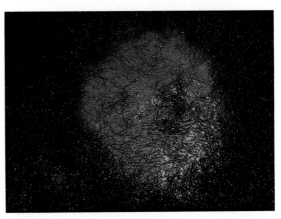

Figure 13–4. Tinea capitis. Broken hairs and scaling occur in a sharply circumscribed area of alopecia.

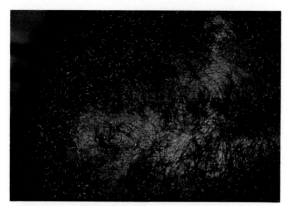

Figure 13–5. Inflammatory tinea capitis manifested by a diffuse circumscribed area of scaling and broken hairs.

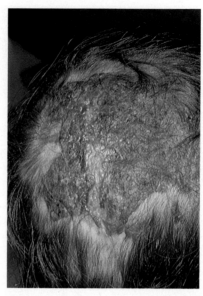

Figure 13–7. *T. tonsurans* infection of the scalp with kerion and alopecia.

tain, Wood's light examination, demonstration of the fungus by potassium hydroxide wet-mount preparations of loose hairs removed from suspected areas, and fungal culture will help confirm the diagnosis. It must be reemphasized, however, that hairs infected with *T. tonsurans* and *T. violaceum* do not fluoresce.

Microscopic examination of a potassium hydroxide preparation of an infected hair will reveal tiny arthrospores surrounding the hair shaft in *Microsporum* infection (ectothrix involvement) (Fig. 13–11) and chains of arthrospores within the hair shaft (endothrix type) in *T. tonsurans* and *T. violaceum* infections; favus is characterized by arthroconidia and hair spaces within the hair shaft. Final definitive diagnosis may be obtained by planting several of the infected hairs and epidermal scales on appropriate culture media (Sabou-

raud's glucose agar or Dermatophyte Test Medium [DTM]). A distinctive growth appears within 5 to 14 days on Sabouraud's agar. With DTM medium, a color change from yellow to red in the medium surrounding the fungus colony suggests the presence of a dermatophyte (Fig. 13–12).

The color change in DTM may begin within 24 to 48 hours for fast-growing dermatophytes and appears as a pinkish or red zone around the developing colony. The color will intensify as growth proceeds, with full color development for most cultures in 3 to 7 days. When DTM medium is used, however, the culture should not be evaluated for color after 10 days, since contaminant fungal growth may cause color change by this time, thus leading to false-positive results. It must be remem-

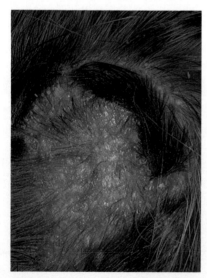

Figure 13–6. Kerion. This inflammatory boggy mass with pustules represents an exaggerated host response to a fungal infection.

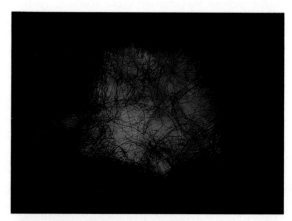

Figure 13–8. Permanent scarring alopecia on the scalp of a 12-year-old boy who had a kerion due to a *Trichophyton tonsurans* infection of the scalp 9 years earlier.

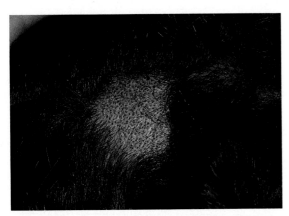

Figure 13–9. "Black dot" ringworm in a patient with *T. tonsurans* infection.

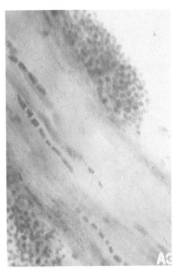

Figure 13–11. Tinea capitis: microscopic examination of a potassium hydroxide preparation. Endothrix infections (e.g., *T. tonsurans* and *T. violaceum*) show spores within the hair shaft; in ectothrix involvement (e.g., *Microsporum* infection), as in this illustration, the arthrospores surround the hair shaft. (Courtesy of Alfred W. Kopf, M.D.)

bered that fungi grow best at room temperature and require oxygen. Accordingly, the culture media should be left at room temperature, and the tops of the culture tubes or bottles should be left slightly unscrewed (or the tubes may be covered only with a cotton plug) to allow aeration of the preparation.

The most frequent errors in microscopic examination of potassium hydroxide preparations of patients with tinea capitis are the choosing of long hairs and looking for hyphae rather than arthrospores in the hair shafts. When fungal cultures are performed, one should culture affected hairs as well as the adjacent scaling. Fungal culture for suspected tinea capitis can be performed by the use of a dull No. 15 scalpel blade, a glass slide, a sterile toothbrush, or a cotton swab. Short broken hairs from the periphery of an affected area should be gently removed and placed on the media with part of the specimen being implanted into the agar.

Treatment. Currently available topical antifungal agents do not appear to reach the hair bulb

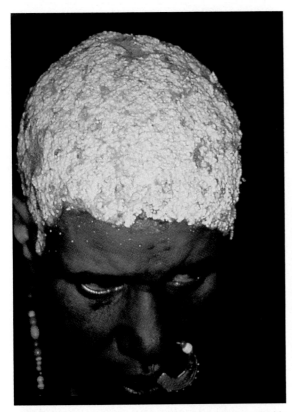

Figure 13–10. Favus, a severe chronic from of tinea capitis caused by *Trichophyton schoenleinii*. (Courtesy of Israel Dvoretzky, M.D., and Benjamin K. Fisher, M.D.)

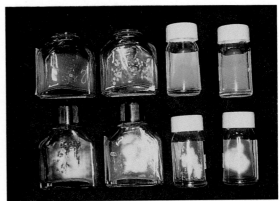

Figure 13–12. Fungal cultures on Sabouraud's agar (left) and dermatophyte test medium (right). A color change from yellow to red in the DTM medium helps establish the presence of a dermatophyte.

and therefore are ineffective in the treatment of tinea capitis. The introduction of griseofulvin (a metabolic product of several species of *Penicillium*) in 1958 marked the first effective systemic antidermatophytic agent, one that was curative for tinea capitis. The effect of griseofulvin appears to be related to its capacity to attach to newly formed keratin in skin, hair, and nails, where it exerts a fungistatic effect. Administered for 6 to 8 weeks or more, it is effective against all forms of tinea. The oral dose of microcrystalline griseofulvin is 10 to 20 mg/kg/day (generally 125 to 240 mg/day for children weighing 30 to 50 pounds and 250 to 500 mg/day for those weighing over 50 pounds). Although the dosage for children younger than the age of 2 years has not been specifically spelled out, I have used a dosage of 10 to 20 mg/kg/day for infants as young as 2 months of age (Fig. 13–3) without adverse effects. For children unable to swallow tablets, Grifulvin-V suspension, 125 mg per teaspoon (Ortho) may be recommended, or Grisactin capsules, 125 mg (Ayerst), can be pulled apart and the powder dispensed in milk or other suitable vehicles.

An ultramicrocrystalline griseofulvin dispersed in polyethylene glycol has allowed the dosage to be cut to one half of the recommended dose of microcrystalline forms. Although the manufacturer's recommended dosage of ultramicrosized griseofulvin (Gris-PEG) is not yet established for children 2 years of age or younger, 5 to 10 mg/kg/day (half the microcrystalline dose) is effective for most children. Thus children older than the age of 2 years who weigh 30 to 50 pounds should receive 62.5 to 125 mg/day; those weighing more than 50 pounds should receive 125 to 250 mg of Gris-PEG daily. It should be recognized, however, that except for enhanced bioavailability and lower dosage schedules, the ultramicrocrystalline preparation does not appear to offer any significant increase in efficacy or safety over other available microsized formulations.

Griseofulvin appears to be absorbed more rapidly after a fatty meal and therefore is probably best given after ingestion of a meal containing fats (milk or ice cream may be recommended for this purpose). Medication should be continued for 4 to 8 weeks (2 weeks after all clinical and laboratory examinations confirm absence of the fungus). Although a single 3- to 4-g dose of microcrystalline griseofulvin will result in cure of most children with tinea capitis (particularly those cases due to *Microsporum* species that fluoresce under Wood's light examination), the 6- to 8-week dosage regimen appears to have a higher curative rate with fewer recurrences.

Reported reactions to griseofulvin consist of hypersensitivity (morbilliform eruptions, urticaria, and angioneurotic edema), photosensitivity, gastrointestinal disturbances, mental confusion, dizziness, headaches (particularly in adults), insomnia, paresthesias of the hands and feet, albuminuria, reversible lymphocytosis, leukopenia,

and aplastic anemia. Although the administration of griseofulvin should be discontinued if granulocytopenia occurs, true agranulocytosis has not been encountered and most reported side effects are minor and probably have been exaggerated.[14]

Griseofulvin also has some effect on porphyrin metabolism, and there have been reports of precipitation of acute porphyria in patients receiving this antibiotic. It also has been shown to cause exacerbations of lupus erythematosus,[15] to inhibit the effect of rifampin and oral contraceptive pills, to increase the effect of cyclosporine, and to induce microsomal enzymes in the liver, thus decreasing the activity of warfarin-type anticoagulants. It is embryotoxic and teratogenic in rats, and evidence suggests hepatic carcinogenicity in male mice when given in amounts and duration comparable to dosages used in humans. More than 20 years of use, however, have revealed no evidence of hepatic carcinoma in humans. Griseofulvin, accordingly should be avoided in patients with porphyria or hepatocellular failure; and since barbiturates tend to depress griseofulvin activity, concomitant administration may necessitate raising the dosage of the antifungal agent. Griseofulvin has been shown to be embryotoxic and potentially teratogenic. Hence, unless the potential benefit justifies the potential risk, its administration is not recommended during pregnancy.

Griseofulvin should be reserved for ringworm infections of the scalp, for severe tinea infection of the nails, or for severe proven ringworm infections in other sites that have not responded to topical agents. Although griseofulvin is generally recognized as the treatment of choice for dermatophyte infections that require oral therapy, in cases in which griseofulvin is not tolerated or ineffective, ketoconazole (Nizoral), or the more recently introduced itraconazole (Sporanox), may be used. Ketoconazole is effective against a wide range of systemic fungal infections such as candidiasis, oral thrush, chronic mucocutaneous candidiasis, candiduria, blastomycosis, cryptococcosis, coccidioidomycosis, histoplasmosis, chromomycosis, paracoccidioidomycosis, and tinea versicolor but, since it penetrates poorly into the cerebrospinal fluid, it is not recommended for fungal meningitis.[16–19] Imidazole compounds such as ketoconazole and itraconazole also increase the anticoagulant effect of coumarin-like medications, increase blood levels of cyclosporin A, and may cause adverse cardiac effects in individuals taking terfenadine (Seldane) or astemizole (Hismanal). In addition, concomitant administration with rifampin and isoniazid appears to affect blood levels of ketoconazole, and its administration with phenytoin may alter the metabolism of one or both drugs. The usual adult dose of oral ketoconazole is 200 mg to 400 mg/day, and although the dosage has not yet been determined for children younger than age 2 years, 3.3 to 6.6 mg/kg/day has been used successfully in the treatment of young children with chronic mucocutaneous candidiasis.[20–22]

Approximately 10 per cent of patients treated with oral ketoconazole have had adverse reactions such as anorexia, nausea, vomiting, diarrhea, headache, dizziness, somnolence, nervousness, and pruritus. Other side effects include chills and fever, photophobia, cutaneous eruptions, myopathy, bulging fontanelles, leukopenia, thrombocytopenia, hemolytic anemia, gynecomastia, hypogonadism, decreased libido, impotence, and hypoadrenalism.[23, 24] The most serious adverse reaction is hepatic toxicity. Estimated to occur in 1 in 10,000 to 15,000 patients, the hepatic toxicity appears to be idiosyncratic and does not appear to be related to daily or cumulative dosage or duration of therapy. Although the mean duration of treatment at the time of onset of symptoms of this reaction is approximately 2 months, it has been reported as early as 3 to 10 days following the initiation of therapy. Monitoring of hepatic function, therefore, and discontinuation of ketoconazole on signs of hepatic toxicity are essential.

Oral griseofulvin and ketoconazole are both effective for the treatment of tinea capitis, but griseofulvin currently appears to be the drug of choice. Concomitant twice-weekly shampooing with 2.5 per cent selenium sulfide shampoo (Selsun, Exsel) will generally result in suppression of viable spores within 2 weeks and helps limit spread to adjacent areas and contacts.[25] Topical antifungal agents are not as effective for this purpose. Although further studies are required, itraconazole and terbinafine (which is not yet released for use in the United States) appear to be more potent than griseofulvin and less toxic than ketoconazole. Accordingly, they may eventually prove to be of even greater value for the treatment of tinea capitis and other mycotic infections.[26, 27]

If a kerion is present, remember that this deep boggy inflammation is caused by an allergic reaction to the fungus. In resistant cases, a combination of prednisone and griseofulvin generally will ensure rapid clearing and help keep atrophy and permanent hair loss to a minimum.[28, 29] The oral administration of saturated solution of potassium iodide has also been recommended for the treatment of patients with kerion. Although I have had no personal experience with this modality for the treatment of tinea infection, Dr. Richard L. Dobson reports good results with this agent and believes that this form of therapy can eliminate the need for systemic corticosteroid therapy for patients with resistant kerion formation.[30] The dosage of potassium iodide solution is discussed under the treatment of sporotrichosis in this chapter.

TINEA BARBAE

Tinea barbae is an uncommon fungal infection of the bearded area and surrounding skin of adolescent and adult males. Since the most common etiologic agents are zoophilic species of *T. mentagrophytes* and *T. verrucosum* (occasionally *T. violaceum* and *T. rubrum*), it occurs primarily among individuals from rural areas in close contact with cattle or other domestic animals.

The infection generally is solitary or confluent and confined to one side of the face. Its clinical appearance is dependent on the species of organism producing the infection. The majority of infections are characterized by highly inflammatory lesions with purulent follicles, inflammatory papules, pustules, exudate, crusts, and boggy nodules. The hairs in infected areas are loose or absent, and pus may be expressed through the follicular openings. Spontaneous resolution may occur, or the lesions may persist for months with resultant alopecia and scar formation.

Occasionally, a less inflammatory superficial variety may appear. This variant is characterized by mild pustular folliculitis, erythematous patches with or without broken-off hairs, and a raised vesiculopustular border and central clearing similar to that seen in lesions of tinea corporis.

Tinea barbae must be differentiated from bacterial folliculitis of the bearded area (sycosis barbae), contact dermatitis, herpes zoster, or severe herpes simplex. Sycosis barbae may be differentiated by the presence of papular and pustular lesions pierced in the center by a hair that is loose and easily extracted; herpes simplex or zoster frequently can be diagnosed by the presence of characteristic balloon cells on Tzanck smear preparations or viral culture. When the diagnosis remains indeterminate, microscopic examination of a potassium hydroxide wet-mount for fungal elements and fungal culture generally will establish the correct diagnosis.

Although superficial inflammatory cases of tinea barbae frequently resolve spontaneously, generally after a period of months, both forms of tinea barbae may result in scar formation and alopecia. Warm saline compresses frequently aid in the removal of crusts, and topical antibacterial agents may help to control secondary bacterial infection. As in patients with tinea capitis, oral microcrystalline griseofulvin is generally required and will produce clearing, frequently within 4 to 6 weeks.

TINEA CORPORIS

Superficial tinea infections of the nonhairy (glabrous) skin are termed *tinea corporis*. Sites of predilection include the nonhairy areas of the face (particularly in children), the trunk, and limbs, with exclusion of ringworm of the scalp (tinea capitis), bearded areas (tinea barbae), groin (tinea cruris), hands (tinea manuum), feet (tinea pedis, and nails (onychomycosis). Although frequently misdiagnosed or overlooked in infants and young children, with its short incubation period, tinea faciei has been reported in an infant as young as 2 days of age and a cutaneous fungal infection has been described (but not proved by culture) in an infant within 6 hours of birth.[31–35] Contact with other individuals, such as is seen in high school and college wrestlers (tinea corporis gladiatorum), and domestic animals, particularly young kittens and puppies, is a common cause of the affliction in children. The causative organism in young children frequently is *M. canis*, occasionally *M. audouinii* or *T. mentagrophytes*. In adults, *T. rubrum*, *T. verrucosum*, *T. mentagrophytes*, or *T. tonsurans* is more likely to be found. In children with infection caused by *T. rubrum* or *Epidermophyton floccosum*, parents with tinea infection are commonly noted to be the source of infection.

Tinea corporis tends to be asymmetrically distributed and is characterized by one or more annular, sharply circumscribed scaly patches with a clear center and scaly vesicular, papular, or pustular border (hence the term *ringworm*) (Figs. 13–13 and 13–14). When multiple lesions are present, they may join together, thus giving rise to bizarre polycyclic configurations. Although the infection may involve persons of all ages, the disorder is most commonly seen in children, in individuals in warm, humid climates, and at times in those with systemic diseases, such as diabetes mellitus, leukemia, or other debilitating illnesses.

Clinical Manifestations. Tinea corporis is frequently manifested as a classic ringworm with annular, oval, or circinate lesions. At times, however, the pattern can vary and may mimic a wide variety of other dermatoses. Lesions may be eczematous, vesicular, pustular, and, less often, granulomatous. Lesions may resemble the herald patch of pityriasis rosea, nummular eczema, psoriasis, contact dermatitis, seborrheic dermatitis, tinea versicolor, vitiligo, erythema migrans (erythema chronicum migrans), various granulomatous lesions (particularly granuloma annulare), fixed drug eruptions, and lupus erythematosus. The use of topical corticosteroids may further mask the diagnosis by amelioration of signs and symptoms while the infection persists (Figs. 13–15 and 13–16). The term *tinea incognito* has been suggested for this phenomenon.[36] Of further significance is the fact that individuals with certain immunologic abnormalities

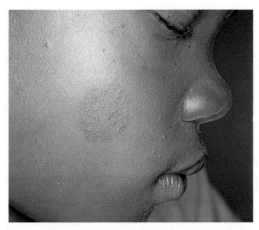

Figure 13–14. Resolving tinea corporis in same patient as in Figure 13–13 following 2 weeks of treatment with a topical antifungal preparation.

such as atopic dermatitis, presumably due to a decreased cell-mediated delayed sensitivity and an increase in humoral (IgE) response, are particularly prone to chronic and recurrent dermatophyte infections.[37]

Although granulomatous lesions are uncommon in children, a perifollicular granulomatous disorder (Majocchi's granuloma) may appear, especially on the limbs of young women who shave their legs closely. This distinctive variant of ringworm is essentially a granulomatous folliculitis and perifolliculitis caused by *T. rubrum* or *T. mentagrophytes*, the primary focus frequently being a diffuse *T. rubrum* infection of the feet. The nodular lesions in this disorder usually involve only one leg, rarely exceed 1 cm in diameter, and are flat or only slightly elevated (Fig. 13–17). If observed early, a hair may be noted in the center of the lesion. It is

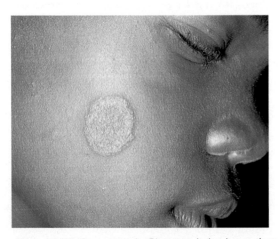

Figure 13–13. Tinea corporis. Ringworm lesion has a clear center and a circinate papulovesicular border.

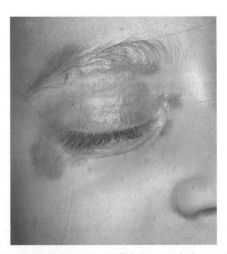

Figure 13–15. Tinea incognito. This is an atypical presentation of tinea corporis (the characteristic clinical features are masked owing to the use of topical corticosteroids).

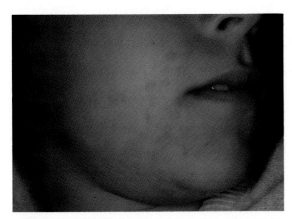

Figure 13–16. Tinea incognito on the cheek and chin of a 9-year-old girl originally thought to have atopic dermatitis.

this infected ingrown hair (secondary to close shaving) that presumably frequently incites the surrounding granulomatous skin infection.

The classic erythematous scaling with a sharply defined papulovesicular border is by no means the most common expression of this disorder, and any red scaly rash should be suspect for fungus until proved otherwise. Accordingly, a potassium hydroxide wet-mount examination and fungal cultures of appropriately collected cutaneous scrapings should be performed on any suspected lesions. As previously described, fluorescence under a Wood's light is not helpful in diagnosis of suspected lesions on glabrous (hairless) skin unless the lanugo hairs are infected. In this case, if the infection is associated with the *Microsporum* species, a light green fluorescence similar to that of *Microsporum*-induced tinea capitis may be observed. Infection of lanugo hairs, however, is extremely unusual. Accordingly, Wood's light examination of suspected tinea corporis generally is fruitless and unnecessary.

Management. Unfortunately there frequently is confusion among nondermatologists regarding the classification and management of cutaneous infection due to fungus. By definition, the term *fungus infection* incorporates disorders due to both tinea and *Candida* infection. It must be recognized, however, that dermatophytes and *Candida* are not synonymous, and that although nystatin is effective against candidal infection, it is inappropriate and ineffective in the treatment of tinea (dermatophyte) infection. Tolnaftate and undecylenic acid, although beneficial in the management of dermatophytoses such as tinea pedis, tinea cruris, and tinea corporis, are also ineffective against disorders due to candidal infection. Topical anticandidal agents include nystatin, amphotericin B (Fungizone), clioquinol (Vioform), and iodochlorhydroxyquin (Iodoquinol) in combination with hydrocortisone (Vytone). Since clioquinol and iodoquinol have limited topical antibacterial and antifungal activity and can be absorbed (particularly when used under occlusion in areas such as the diaper area of infants), these agents have largely been supplanted by other currently available formulations, such as ciclopirox (Loprox), clotrimazole (Lotrimin, Mycelex), econazole (Spectazole), haloprogin (Halotex), ketoconazole (Nizoral), miconazole (Micatin, Monistat-Derm), naftifine (Naftin), oxiconazole (Oxistat), and sulconazole (Exelderm), which can be used for the topical treatment of dermatophyte and candidal infections. Most patients with tinea corporis, tinea pedis, and tinea cruris, therefore, will respond to topical application of these agents and the recently introduced fungicidal allylamine derivative, terbinafine (Lamisil Cream, Sandoz), gently rubbed into the affected area and surrounding skin morning and evening; once-daily application of ketoconazole, oxiconazole, or sulconazole is also effective and may be used if desired. Even though clinical clearing and relief of pruritus is frequently seen within the first 7 to 10 days after initiation of therapy, treatment should be continued for a minimum period of 2 to 3 weeks after the affected area is clinically clear and fungal cultures are no longer positive. If a patient shows no clinical improvement after 4 weeks of therapy, the diagnosis should be reevaluated, and in unusually severe or extensive disease, a course of systemic therapy with an agent such as griseofulvin (as described for the treatment of tinea capitis) may be required.

Although a mild topical corticosteroid such as hydrocortisone may be used to reduce accom-

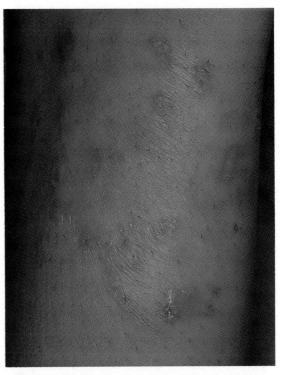

Figure 13–17. Majocchi's granuloma. A deep tinea infection manifested as a granulomatous folliculitis on the leg of a 16-year-old girl.

panying inflammation and pruritus, potent cortico-steroid formulations such as those containing betamethasone dipropionate (Diprosone, a Class 3 topical corticosteroid [see Chapter 3] in combination with clotrimazole [as in Lotrisone]) are not recommended.[38] For unusual cases such as severe tinea manuum or tinea pedis, however, clotrimazole in combination with betamethasone dipropionate may be used, but for periods of no longer than 2 to 4 weeks (Fig. 13–18); this combination should not be used in the diaper area or under occlusion, and it is not recommended in children younger than 12 years of age.

TINEA IMBRICATA

Tinea imbricata (tokelau), caused by *Trichophyton concentricum*, is a superficial fungal infection seen in tropical regions of the Far East, South Pacific, South and Central America, and parts of Africa. Like favus, tinea imbricata is probably contracted in early childhood and can persist for a lifetime. The disorder is characterized by concentric rings of scales forming extensive patches with polycyclic borders. With time, the lesions spread peripherally and form large plaques, which cover almost the entire cutaneous surface, with sparing, usually, of the scalp, axillae, palms, and soles. When fully developed, the concentrically arranged rings are seen as parallel lines of scales overlapping each other, often resembling tiles or shingles (*imbrex* means "shingle") on a roof. Diagnosis is based on the characteristic clinical presentation, microscopic demonstration of interlacing, septate, mycelial filaments that branch into two parts, and identification of the organism by fungal culture. Although treatment with griseofulvin, ketoconazole, or itraconazole for 6 weeks will usually clear the cutaneous eruption (within 2 to 4 weeks), there is a tendency for recurrence or reinfection when treatment is discontinued.

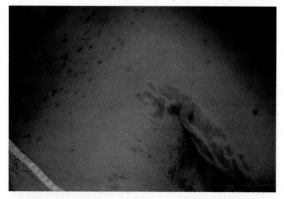

Figure 13–18. Striae in the axilla of a patient following long-term topical application of betamethasone dipropionate in combination with clotrimazole. (Courtesy of Leonard Milstone, M.D.)

TINEA CRURIS

Tinea cruris ("jock itch") is an extremely common superficial fungus disorder of the groin and upper thighs. Seen primarily in male adolescents and adults, it may occur but is less common in females. It is more symptomatic in hot, humid weather and is most frequently noted in obese individuals or persons subject to vigorous physical activity, chafing, and tight-fitting clothing such as athletic supporters, jockey shorts, wet bathing suits, panty hose, or tight-fitting slacks. *Epidermophyton floccosum* traditionally has been associated with this infection, but both *T. rubrum* and *T. mentagrophytes* frequently are responsible for this disorder, and it is commonly seen in association with tinea pedis.

The eruption is sharply marginated, is usually but not invariably bilaterally symmetrical, and involves the intertriginous folds near the scrotum, the upper inner thighs (Fig. 13–19), and occasionally the perianal regions, buttocks, and abdomen. The scrotum and labia are usually spared or only mildly involved, unless the eruption is caused by *Candida albicans*, overtreatment, or an associated neurodermatitis (Fig. 13–20). The margins are abrupt and frequently half-moon shaped, and the skin in the involved area is erythematous and scaly. The color may vary from red to brown, central clearing may be present, and an active vesiculopustular border, although uncommon, may be noted. In chronic infection the redness and scaling may be slight, the active margin may be subtle or ill defined, and lichenification may be present.

Tinea cruris must be differentiated from intertrigo, seborrheic dermatitis, psoriasis, primary irritant dermatitis or allergic contact dermatitis (generally due to therapy), or erythrasma (a fairly common chronic superficial dermatosis of the crural area caused by the diphtheroid *Corynebacterium minutissimum*). A characteristic coral-red fluorescence under Wood's light is helpful in diagnosis of the erythrasma (see Chapter 10). The presence of tinea cruris can be confirmed by potassium hydroxide microscopic examination of cutaneous scrapings and by fungal culture on appropriate media.

The treatment of tinea cruris consists of topical therapy, as described under the treatment of tinea corporis, for 3 to 4 weeks, reduction of excessive chafing and irritation by loose-fitting cotton underclothing, reduction of friction and perspiration by the use of a bland absorbent powder such as ZeaSorb-AF Medicated Powder (Stiefel), and, for dermatophyte-induced lesions that are resistant or recur frequently, oral griseofulvin for 4 or 5 weeks.

TINEA PEDIS

Tinea pedis, or athlete's foot, relatively uncommon in young children, is more common in adolescents and adults and represents the most prevalent

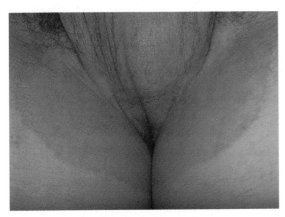

Figure 13–19. Tinea cruris.

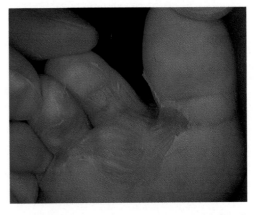

Figure 13–21. Tinea pedis in a 21-month-old child. This disorder (uncommon in prepubertal children) is characterized by fissuring, maceration, and scaling of the interdigital webs.

ringworm infection seen in adults. Although children are not completely immune, most instances of "athlete's foot" in prepubertal individuals actually represent misdiagnosed examples of foot eczema, shoe dermatitis, or some other dermatosis (Fig. 13–21).[39–41]

The etiologic agents usually responsible for tinea pedis are *T. rubrum and T. mentagrophytes,* and less often *E. floccosum.* The disorder may present clinically as an intertriginous inflammation, as a vesiculopustular eruption, or as a chronic scaling disorder with or without hyperkeratosis. Of these, interdigital lesions are the most common expression of the disorder and appear as fissuring, maceration, and interdigital scaling, generally in the web between the fourth and fifth toes, accompanied by maceration and peeling of the surrounding skin. In many instances the disorder remains localized to the interdigital webs and sides of the toes. In others, it may spread to affect the soles and, less often, other parts of the feet (Fig. 13–22). Contrary to the eruption seen in foot ec-

zema, the dorsal aspect of the toes and feet generally remains clear.

The inflammatory vesiculopustular lesions generally result from *T. mentagrophytes* infection. Lesions may involve all areas of the foot, including the dorsal surface, but usually are patchy in distribution, with a predisposition to the midanterior plantar surface or instep (Fig. 13–23). Lesions occur most often in summer, and allergy to fungal elements may be reflected by a vesicular eruption on the palms and sides of the fingers, and occasionally by an erythematous vesicular eruption on the extremities and trunk, the so-called dermatophytid ("id") response. Although the mechanism of this frequently described but relatively uncommon eruption is not completely understood, it appears to result from absorption of the fungus or fungal products and an associated reaction between circulating antigen originating from the primary infection site and skin-sensitizing antibodies.

Although vesicular dermatophytid reactions of the fingers and palms may appear as "id" reactions

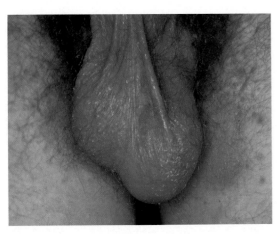

Figure 13–20. Scrotal infection caused by *Candida albicans.*

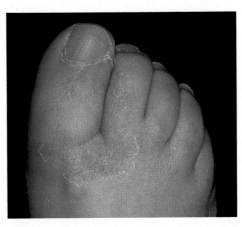

Figure 13–22. Tinea pedis with extension to the dorsal aspect of the foot.

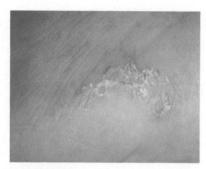

Figure 13-23. Tinea pedis. Scaly vesicular eruption is evident on the instep of the foot.

to tinea pedis, other causes of eczematous dermatitis or dyshidrotic eczema frequently are misinterpreted as true dermatophytid reactions in individuals with tinea pedis. The diagnosis of an "id" reaction accordingly is dependent on absence of fungus in the area of the id reaction, a demonstrable focus of pathogenic fungus (generally on the feet), and spontaneous disappearance of the rash when the focus of infection has been eradicated.

The scaly hyperkeratotic variety of tinea pedis is extremely chronic and resistant to treatment and may affect the soles, heels, and sides of the feet. In this form of tinea pedis, seen in adolescents and adults more frequently than children, the disorder is generally bilateral (occasionally unilateral) and is characterized by a dull red or skin-colored, diffuse, often bran-like scaling, relative lack of inflammation, and extreme chronicity (Fig. 13–24). When the process becomes diffuse over the entire plantar surface, the term *moccasin foot* is applied to this disorder.

The diagnosis of tinea pedis is dependent on the clinical picture, with corroboration by potassium hydroxide examination of cutaneous scrapings and fungal culture. Tinea pedis is often difficult to control because of the moist and warm environment of the feet. Efforts to keep the feet dry are helpful. These include thorough drying of the feet after bathing, avoidance of occlusive footwear, frequent airing of the affected areas, avoidance of nylon socks or other fabrics that interfere with dissipation of moisture, and the wearing of sandals or perforated shoes to permit drying of the affected areas. Absorbent powders containing undecylenic acid, miconazole, or tolnaftate may be used liberally once or twice a day, and 3 to 6 per cent salicylic acid in rubbing alcohol, aluminum chloride 20 per cent in anhydrous ethyl alcohol (available as Drysol [Persōn and Covey]), or aluminum chloride in a 30 per cent concentration aids in the management of the hyperhidrosis commonly associated with persistent or recurrent lesions.

Acute vesicular lesions should be treated with open wet compresses (Burow's solution 1 : 80) applied for 10 to 15 minutes three to four times a day for 3 to 5 days (see Chapter 3), bed rest if the disorder is severe, and topical antifungal prepara-

tions (as described for the treatment of tinea corporis) for at least 6 weeks, and in resistant cases or when recurrences are common for 6 months or more. In instances in which the diagnosis is indeterminate, a topical antifungal agent and a corticosteroid formulation may be used for a short period of time (up to 3 or 4 weeks), at which time a fungal culture performed at the initiation of therapy can generally establish the appropriate diagnosis, and if the diagnosis of tinea pedis is confirmed, the topical corticosteroid can be discontinued. Severe, chronic, and recalcitrant forms of tinea pedis that are uncontrollable by topical therapy may require treatment with systemic microsize griseofulvin (10 to 20 mg/kg/day) for up to 6 to 12 months. "Id" reactions, generally seen on the hands, when present, are best treated by open wet compresses, topical corticosteroids, and eradication of the primary source of infection.

TINEA MANUUM

Ringworm infections of the hand (tinea manus, tinea manuum) are uncommon in childhood and, when present, are generally seen on the palms in postpubertal individuals. The disorder is usually unilateral and has morphologic changes similar to those seen in individuals with chronic scaly dermatophytosis of the feet. Usually it is caused by the same fungi responsible for tinea pedis, *T. rubrum*, *T. mentagrophytes*, and *E. floccosum*, and may be seen in association with ringworm infection of the feet.

Clinical manifestations range from diffuse hyperkeratosis of the fingers and palm, accompanied by a fine branny adherent scale that is especially prominent in the flexural creases, to a less common patchy inflammatory vesicular reaction. Other clinical variants include discrete erythematous papular and follicular scaly patches or severe scaling and exfoliation (Fig. 13–25). Involvement of the fingernails frequently occurs in association with

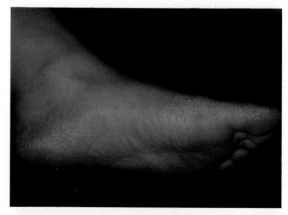

Figure 13-24. A chronic scaly hyperkeratotic form of tinea pedis on the foot of a 19-year-old young woman. The term *moccasin foot* has been applied to this disorder.

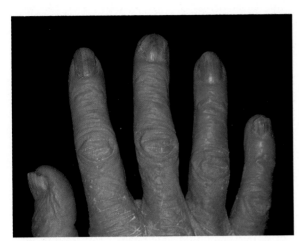

Figure 13–25. Onychomycosis. Tinea of the hand (tinea manuum) with nail involvement.

this disorder. When present, it is seldom that all the nails of the involved hand are infected. Total nail involvement, when seen, should make one suspect psoriasis and, less commonly, lichen planus.

Ringworm infections of the hand frequently masquerade as psoriasis, allergic contact or primary irritant dermatitis, dyshidrosis, and, less commonly, as a dermatophytid reaction. The fact that the infection is frequently unilateral is a clue to the diagnosis, which then can be corroborated by potassium hydroxide microscopic examination and fungal culture of cutaneous scrapings.

The management of tinea manuum is essentially the same as that recommended for tinea pedis, with the exception of the environmental measures outlined for the treatment of dermatophytosis of the feet. It must be remembered, however, that ringworm of the hand is often accompanied by tinea pedis and that when both sites are affected they should generally be treated simultaneously.

TINEA UNGUIUM (ONYCHOMYCOSIS)

Tinea unguium (onychomycosis) is a chronic fungal infection of the fingernails or toenails caused by *T. rubrum*, *T. mentagrophytes*, and *E. floccosum* (the dermatophytes that usually affect the hands and feet), and, at times, *Candida albicans*. Ordinarily a disease of adults and less common in chidren,[42] the disorder generally occurs in association with tinea pedis or tinea manuum but may occur as a primary infection or in association with other dermatophytoses (Figs. 13–25 through 13–27).

The disorder usually has its origin at the distal edge of the nail and first becomes evident at the lateral border of the distal tip of the nail. The onset is slow and insidious, and toenails are affected more frequently than fingernails. The disorder first begins as an opaque white or silvery, then yellow and later brown, patch at the sides and distal tip of the nail plate. Subungual debris collects and actual invasion of the nail plate then occurs, and the nail slowly becomes discolored, thickened, deformed, and friable, and, because of accumulation of subungual keratin, loosened from the nail plate.

In onychomycosis due to *C. albicans* there is often an associated paronychia (Fig. 13–28). The adjacent cuticle is pink, swollen, and tender, and on pressure, occasionally a small amount of pus may be expressed from the lateral border. In other instances the nail plate may show brown or gray discoloration at the lateral nail edge or white or gray spots without development of further dystrophy. In contrast to onychomycosis due to tinea infection, candidal onychomycosis almost exclusively affects the fingernails rather than toenails and is seen more commonly in individuals, usually women, who frequently have their hands in water (Fig. 13–29). Except in immunologically impaired patients, such as those with chronic mucocutaneous candidiasis, the nail plate is rarely invaded by these organisms.

Onychomycosis must be differentiated from psoriasis, dystrophy secondary to eczema or chronic paronychia, trauma, tetracycline-induced photo-onycholysis, pachyonychia congenita, lichen planus, nail-patella syndrome, and other nail dystrophies (see Chapter 17). It must be remembered that onychomycosis is seldom symmetrical and that it is common to find involvement of only one, two, or three nails of only one hand. In all suspected cases the feet should be examined with care, since infection is frequently found there, and if all ten fingernails are abnormal, some cause other than ringworm should be sought.

Accurate diagnosis depends on direct microscopic examination of potassium hydroxide preparations and identification of the organism by fungal culture. When collecting specimens it is essential to obtain samples from the ventral nail plate and subungual keratinous material rather than from the nail surface, and since the responsible organism in

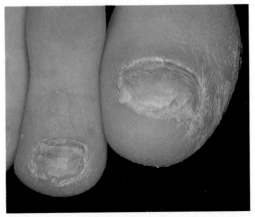

Figure 13–26. Onychomycosis. Thickening, discoloration, and crumbling of the nail plate in a 16-year-old boy.

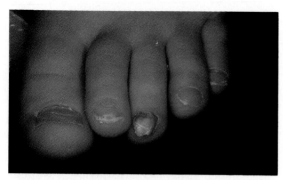

Figure 13–27. Onychomycosis (tinea unguium). A tinea infection of the nail on the toe of a 4½-year-old child. Although much less common in children than adults, the disorder may at times occur in children and generally is contracted from a parent with tinea pedis.

onychomycosis is difficult to demonstrate, repeated scrapings and cultures frequently may be necessary.

Despite recent advances in antifungal therapy, topical agents are generally ineffective and oral administration of griseofulvin (for periods of 6 months for fingernails, 12 to 18 months for toenails) for the treatment of onychomycosis is a long-term process, and patients should be advised that even prolonged therapy may not lead to cure and that recurrences are all too frequent.[43] Children with onychomycosis and patients with superficial white onychomycosis, however, will frequently respond to gentle mechanical curettage of the loose white material followed by topical application of appropriate antifungal agents.[44, 45] Itraconazole (and terbinafine, not yet released for use in the United States) and chemical nail removal with 40 per cent urea compounds and surgical avulsion of the nail, combined with topical agents and oral griseofulvin, may increase the cure rate. In general, however, unless the nail matrix is completely destroyed and the nail bed and lateral grooves carefully curetted, this mode of therapy is only moderately effective.[46, 47]

If the disorder proves to be associated with *Candida albicans*, topical applications of anticandidal agents to the periungual region can be beneficial. The treatment of candidal onycholysis (see Fig. 13–29), however, is not effective unless the affected digits (usually the fingers) are kept dry. Exposure to water should be kept to a minimum, and inexpensive cotton gloves should be worn under protective rubber or latex gloves when immersion in water cannot be avoided. Cotton-lined rubber gloves are of relatively little value, since the lining frequently becomes saturated with perspiration. A solution of 4 per cent thymol in chloroform applied under the nail folds two or three times daily and immediately following immersion in water frequently will help keep the area dry and may prove helpful in the management of persistent *Candida*-induced nail disorders. When *Candida*-induced

onycholysis persists, keeping the onycholytic area of the nail trimmed and as dry as possible and taking ketoconazole (Nizoral), 400 mg/day orally for 2 to 4 weeks is beneficial, but recurrences are common.

Tinea Versicolor

Tinea versicolor (pityriasis versicolor) is an extremely common superficial fungal disorder of the skin characterized by multiple scaling, oval, macular, and patchy lesions, usually distributed over the upper portions of the trunk, proximal arms, and occasionally the face or other areas (Figs. 13–30 and 13–31).[48] The lesions may be hypopigmented or hyperpigmented (fawn-colored or brown), depending on the patient's complexion and exposure to sunlight. This disorder is caused by the dimorphic fungus *Pityrosporum orbiculare* (originally called *Malassezia furfur*), which exists predominantly in the yeast phase on normal skin and causes clinical lesions only when substantial numbers of filamentous forms develop. The reason for proliferation of hyphal forms in lesions is unknown, but findings of glycogen granules in unusual amounts in the normal skin of patients with tinea versicolor suggests the presence of some underlying disorder such as malnutrition, poor general health, treatment with corticosteroids, or a genetic predisposition to the disorder.[49]

Usually seen as a disorder of adolescents and young adults 15 to 30 years of age, tinea versicolor has been found in senior citizens, prepubertal children, and, at times, even in infants.[50–52] Generally asymptomatic and extremely chronic, the lesions become more prominent during the summer months when the patient is exposed to sunlight and the involved areas fail to tan following sun exposure. Lesions accordingly become lighter

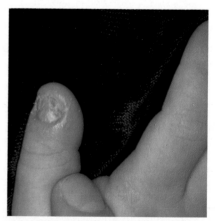

Figure 13–28. Onychomycosis due to *Candida albicans*. Candidal onychomycosis, in contrast to onychomycosis due to tinea infection, almost exclusively affects fingernails rather than toenails.

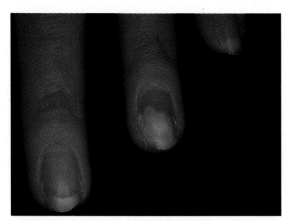

Figure 13–29. Candidal onycholysis. *Candida* infection of the nail involves lifting of the distal nail plate and a characteristic opaque white discoloration of the affected nail.

than the surrounding skin in summer and relatively darker during winter, hence the term *tinea versicolor*. In the past, the hypopigmentation was attributed to a sun-screening effect. However, closer observations do not support this hypothesis but suggest that the organism may suppress the formation of melanin or that an abnormal transfer of pigment from melanocytes to keratinocytes may be the cause of the pigmentary disturbance seen in this disorder.[53]

Diagnosis. The eruption in tinea versicolor is usually distinctive and the diagnosis can frequently be made on clinical grounds and confirmed by potassium hydroxide wet-mounts of cutaneous scrapings. Conditions most commonly confused with this disorder include pityriasis alba, postinflammatory hypopigmentation, vitiligo, melasma, seborrheic dermatitis, pityriasis rosea, and secondary syphilis. When the diagnosis is uncertain, demonstration of a yellow, coppery orange, bronze, or blue-white fluorescence under Wood's light (in a darkened room) or demonstration of highly characteristic fungal hyphae and spores in grape-like clusters (in a "spaghetti-and-meatballs" appearance) (Fig. 13–32) on microscopic examination of a potassium hydroxide slide preparation of scrapings from lesions generally will help confirm the diagnosis. Fungal cultures, however, are unsatisfactory, because the organisms are difficult to grow on culture media.

Treatment. Tinea versicolor generally responds readily to a variety of topical preparations. However, since the course of the disorder generally is chronic and the primary etiologic agent (*P. orbiculare*) is a normal saprophytic inhabitant of the skin, treatment generally must be thorough and recurrences are common. Wood's light fluorescence of lesions of tinea versicolor is valuable in the management of this disorder, since it helps to delineate distal areas of involvement not seen in ordinary light. Selenium sulfide shampoo (Exsel, Selsun) in a 2.5 per cent concentration is a conve-

nient, rapid, and highly effective mode of therapy for this disorder.[54] This is accomplished by application of a thin layer of the preparation to the affected area overnight, with care to see that the entire cutaneous surface is covered, once a week for 3 to 4 weeks, followed by monthly applications for 3 months (in an effort to help prevent recurrences of this disorder). The preparation is washed off in the morning by bath or shower, at which time the patient should be instructed to change all night clothes, bedding, and undergarments.

Response to therapy should be assessed by potassium hydroxide wet-mount microscopic examination of cutaneous scrapings. The patient should be advised that this is a benign, occasionally pruritic, but otherwise primarily cosmetic disorder; that the hypopigmentation will not return to normal until sun exposure allows remelanization of the affected areas; and that recurrences, especially during the hot and humid months, are common. Recurrences, when noted, should be treated early in an effort to prevent extensive cutaneous involvement. Alternate remedies include a 15 to 25 per cent solution of sodium hyposulfite or thiosulfate, 50 per cent propylene glycol in water, or sulfur–salicylic acid or zinc-pyrithione shampoos. Topical antifungal agents, although effective, are

Figure 13–30. Tinea versicolor (pityriasis versicolor). This disorder is frequently seen as yellowish or brownish patches on pale skin and hypopigmented macules on dark-skinned persons.

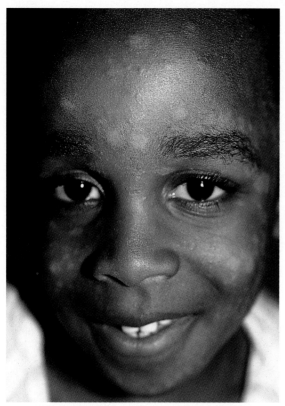

Figure 13–31. Tinea versicolor. Multiple hypopigmented macules with fine scaling are present on the face of a black child. (Courtesy of Kenneth Greer, M.D.)

United States, following a long incubation period (of up to 20 years or more),[59] the disorder is manifested by mottled greenish or brownish black sharply marginated macular areas on the palm or volar aspect of the fingers, and, less commonly, feet or other cutaneous areas.

Misdiagnosed at times as melanocytic lesions (junctional nevi or melanoma), or silver nitrate or India ink stains,[60] the disorder can be readily diagnosed by microscopic examination of potassium hydroxide–prepared scrapings from a lesion and identification of brownish or olive-colored hyphae and budding yeast cells, and fungal culture is confirmatory. Treatment of tinea nigra can be accomplished by the topical application of keratolytic agents such as salicylic acid, Whitfield's ointment (6 per cent benzoic acid and 3 per cent salicylic acid), tincture of iodine, undecylenic acid (Desenex), a 10 per cent solution of thiabendazole suspension (Mintezol),[61] and topical antifungal agents such as clotrimazole, econazole, ketoconazole, miconazole, or sulconazole (alone or in combination with topical retinoic acid), by Scotch tape stripping, or by gentle shaving of the infected stratum corneum with a scalpel blade.

more expensive and, except on small, localized, or facial lesions, do not offer any substantial advantage. For individuals with persistent, extensive, or recurrent lesions, a 200- to 400-mg daily dose of oral ketoconazole for 5 to 10 days, followed perhaps by 200 to 400 mg/day for 3 consecutive days once a month for 6 months, or oral itraconazole (200 mg/day for 5 to 7 days) may be considered. Since ketoconazole-induced hepatitis has been reported following even relatively short courses of oral ketoconazole, patients and physicians should be cognizant of this potential risk whenever oral ketoconazole is used.[55–58]

Tinea Nigra

Tinea nigra is an asymptomatic superficial fungal infection of the stratum corneum caused by the black somewhat yeast-like mold *Phaeoannellomyces werneckii* (formerly called *Cladosporium* or *Exophiala werneckii*). Most often found in warm humid areas of Central or South America, Africa, Asia, and at times the coastal areas of southern

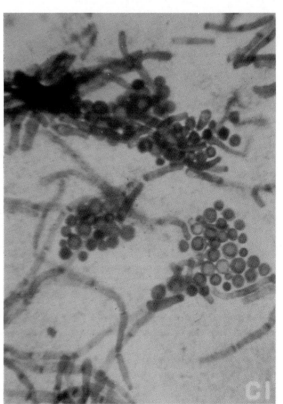

Figure 13–32. Blunt-ended hyphae and grape-like clusters of spores in a "spaghetti-and-meatball" pattern on a potassium hydroxide mount of a patient with tinea versicolor. (Courtesy of Alfred W. Kopf, M.D.)

Piedra

Piedra is an asymptomatic fungal infection of the hair shaft caused by *Piedraia hortae* (black piedra) and *Trichosporon beigelii*, occasionally called *T. cutaneum* (white piedra). Black piedra, seen commonly in tropical areas of South America, the Far East, and Pacific Islands and less frequently in Africa, Asia, and other tropical areas, is characterized by small, black, firmly attached, hard, brown-black nodules on the hair shafts of the scalp composed of honeycomb-like masses of brown fungus cells with hyaline loculi occupied by ovoid spores (asci). Fungal cultures can confirm the diagnosis, and removal of the hair by clipping or shaving is usually curative.

White piedra, seen in temperate climates of South America, Europe, Asia, Japan, Europe, Australia, and the southern United States, tends to affect the eyelashes, eyebrows, mustache, beard, and axillary or pubic hair and is more sporadic. Characterized by asymptomatic, soft, white to brown-black or green nodules on the hair shaft caused by the yeast-like fungus *T. beigelii* and other *Trichosporon* species, the diagnosis of white piedra can be established by microscopic examination of the nodules and the finding of hyphae that are perpendicular to the hair shaft (lacking the organized appearance of black piedra) and by fungal culture. Again, clipping or shaving the hair is usually curative.[62]

Candidiasis

Candidiasis (moniliasis) is an acute or chronic infection of the skin, mucous membranes, and occasionally the internal organs, caused by yeast-like fungi of the *Candida* genus. Although other candidal species can be responsible for human infection, *C. albicans* is the most frequent cause of this disorder.

C. albicans is not a saphrophyte of normal skin. It exists in the microflora of the oral cavity, gastrointestinal tract, and vagina and becomes a cutaneous pathogen when an alteration in the host defenses, either localized or generalized, allows the organism to become invasive.

Factors that predispose to candidiasis include endocrinologic disorders (diabetes mellitus, hypoparathyroidism, and Addison's disease), genetic disorders (Down's syndrome, acrodermatitis enteropathica, chronic mucocutaneous candidiasis, granulomatous disease of childhood), debilitating disorders such as leukemia or lymphoma, and the administration of systemic antibiotics, corticosteroids, anovulatory drugs, or immunosuppressive agents.

Newborns are physiologically susceptible to candidal infection, which may be manifested as oral candidiasis (thrush) or, less commonly, as a localized or generalized dermatitis. Candidiasis in the infant is traceable almost invariably to an infected mother who may be a vaginal or intestinal carrier of the organism. These infants invariably harbor *C. albicans* in the mouth or intestinal canal (see Figs. 2–30 through 2–32), and the infected saliva or stools constitute a focus for cutaneous infection.[63] See Chapter 2 for a more in-depth discussion of candidal diaper dermatitis.

ORAL CANDIDIASIS (THRUSH)

Oral candidiasis (thrush) is a painful inflammation of the tongue, soft and hard palates, and buccal and gingival mucosae characterized by whitish gray, often confluent, friable, cheesy pseudomembranous patches or plaques on a markedly reddened mucosa (see Fig. 2–31). Often not clinically apparent until 8 or 9 days of life, the disorder is acquired at the time of delivery during passage through the vaginal canal.

Occurrences of oral candidiasis in adults, infants, and children are clinically similar and can be diagnosed by gentle removal of the curd-like plaques, which, unlike milk particles, adhere to the underlying oral mucosa, by gently rubbing the area with a cotton applicator or tongue blade with a resulting underlying inflammatory mucosal erosion. The organism may be identified by potassium hydroxide wet-mount preparation or Gram-stained material removed from a plaque or by fungal culture. Lesions usually respond promptly to careful removal of the curd-like lesions after each feeding by a cotton-tipped applicator dipped into a mixture of one-fourth teaspoon of baking soda and one or two drops of liquid detergent mixed in a glass of warm water or to careful removal of lesions by a cotton-tipped applicator dipped into a nystatin suspension (Mycostatin Oral Suspension or Nilstat Oral Suspension). Persistent or recurrent lesions in infants and young children may be treated by oral administration of nystatin suspension (100,000 units/ml) 2 ml four times a day until 48 hours after the lesions have disappeared and cultures have been normal for 48 hours (generally a period of 7 to 14 days). Oral candidiasis in older individuals can be treated by Mycostatin Oral Tablets, one to three tablets (500,000 to 1 million units) three times daily, or by the use of clotrimazole troches (Mycelex) held in the mouth and allowed to dissolve five times a day for 14 consecutive days. Clotrimazole troches can also be used as prophylaxis in high-risk patients. However, since only limited data are available on their safety and effectiveness after prolonged administration, it is suggested that this form of therapy be limited to short-term use.[64–66] Although it has been suggested that clotrimazole or nystatin troches or suppositories be inserted into a slit in the tip of a pacifier or nipple for the treatment of infants with oral candidiasis, the possibility of aspiration must be considered when this form of therapy is used.[67] When treating infants with persistent or recurrent oral candidiasis, asymptomatic maternal vaginal candidiasis and candidal contamination of nipples or pacifiers should be considered as possible reservoirs for reinfection.[68]

CUTANEOUS CANDIDIASIS

Candidiasis may present a variety of cutaneous manifestations. The moist warm conditions found in intertriginous areas favor its development. Accordingly the disorder frequently affects the folds of the body (the groin, perineum, intergluteal, and, particularly in obese individuals, the inframammary folds). It also affects the interdigital spaces, particularly those of the third and fourth fingers; see Erosio Interdigitalis Blastomycetica later in this chapter.

Two types of candidiasis have been reported in the newborn period, a congenital form in which the skin lesions are present at birth or shortly thereafter and a neonatal form commonly seen after the first week of life.[69] In the congenital form the skin lesions involve the head, face, neck, trunk, and extremities. The diaper area is spared, but the intertriginous areas, posterior aspect of the trunk, and extensor surfaces of the extremities may be severely affected. Occasionally, the nails, palms, and soles may be involved. The rash begins with an intense erythema and small white papules that gradually increase in number and become pustular.[70]

The syndrome of *congenital cutaneous candidiasis* differs from the classic form of candidal dermatitis of the newborn. Whereas congenital cutaneous candidiasis represents an intrauterine infection, candidial dermatitis of the newborn is acquired by passage through an infected vagina, with onset of cutaneous lesions at a later date. The clinical features of congenital cutaneous candidiasis may resemble erythema toxicum, bacterial folliculitis, bullous impetigo, congenital herpes, varicella, or syphilis.[70] It is distinguished by a progressive but relatively benign course, absence of constitutional signs, and the recovery of *Candida* organisms by direct smear and fungal culture. Although the prognosis of congenital cutaneous candidiasis is usually good, with lesions generally progressing from erythema and pustular lesions to a drying exfoliative stage that clears spontaneously, systemic candidiasis can develop, particularly in infants who are premature or have other problems that may compromise their ability to ward off systemic infection. Since immunosuppressed infants and premature infants weighing less than 1500 g with cutaneous candidiasis may progress to disseminated disease and high mortality, it is recommended that such infants be carefully monitored and that prompt systemic therapy be initiated regardless of the presence or absence of evidence of systemic disease.[71]

In late-onset neonatal candidiasis, in contrast to congenital cutaneous candidiasis, early lesions radiate from the perianal area into the gluteal folds with satellite lesions and spread to the perineum, genitalia, suprapubic areas, buttocks, and inner thighs. The infection may be restricted in extent or may go on to involve the entire area. The typical vivid-red hue, glistening skin, and characteristic pustulovesicular border, when present, are the hallmarks of this disorder (see Fig. 2–30). It is highly significant that a majority of older infants with cutaneous candidiasis harbor C. *albicans* in the intestine, suggesting infected stools as the primary focus of candidiasis in the diaper area.

Occasionally a widespread cutaneous dermatitis may occur, either as a result of progression from an untreated localized area or by contamination of the skin from an infected maternal vagina during the process of delivery. In this variant, superficial vesiculopustules rupture, leaving a denuded surface. Lesions spread peripherally and form confluent plaques of dermatitis with generalized scaling. When the etiology of the dermatosis is not readily apparent, direct microscopic examination of cutaneous scrapings (particularly the white scale and the edge of lesions) and fungal culture will help establish the correct diagnosis (see Figs. 2–32 and 2–33).

The treatment of superficial infections of the skin caused by C. *albicans* consists of the use of topical anticandidal agents such as amphotericin B (Fungizone cream or lotion), ciclopirox, clotrimazole, econazole, haloprogin, ketonazole, miconazole, naftifine, nystatin, oxiconazole, or sulconazole. Although Mycolog and Lotrisone are effective for the treatment of topical candidiasis, because of the potent topical corticosteroids contained in these agents these preparations are not recommended for this purpose.

CANDIDAL VULVOVAGINITIS

C. *albicans* is a common inhabitant of the vaginal tract, but its incidence increases in diabetes and pregnancy and in females taking antibiotics or oral anovulatory preparations. When vulvovaginitis occurs, the labia become edematous and red, white patches appear on an erythematous mucosal surface, and leukorrhea develops, with painful itching, burning, and an associated discomfort on micturition. The infection may spread to the perineum, perianal region, gluteal folds, and upper inner aspects of the thigh.

Diagnosis is established by the clinical signs and symptoms and by demonstration of the fungus by potassium hydroxide microscopic examination and fungal culture. Treatment consists of nystatin vaginal tablets (available as Mycostatin Vaginal Tablets [Squibb], 100,000 units) deposited high in the vagina by means of an applicator twice daily for 7 to 14 days, or clotrimazole vaginal tablets (available as Gyne-Lotrimin Vaginal Tablets or Mycelex-G Vaginal Tablets, 100 mg per tablet) inserted intravaginally at bedtime for 7 consecutive days. A one-dose regimen using a 500-mg vaginal tablet of clotrimazole (Mycelex-G) has also been shown to be clinically effective when one-day therapy is deemed to be appropriate.[72] In patients with severe or persistent vulvovaginal candidiasis, however, the 7- to 14-day 100-mg tablet regimen appears to be preferable; and for resistant cases, 400 mg of oral ketoconazole (Nizoral), given daily for 1 week, can be used.

PERLÈCHE

Perlèche (angular cheilitis) is a common disorder characterized by fissuring and inflammation of the corners of the mouth, with associated maceration and softening of the adjacent cutaneous surface (Fig. 13–33). This condition is not due to vitamin B deficiency. It is associated with moisture collecting in the corners of the mouth. In adults it is generally due to ill-fitting dentures; in children it is seen in conjunction with overbite, overlapping, the wearing of braces, and poor closure of the mouth. This disorder is best managed by the use of petrolatum or corticosteroid ointments applied two or three times a day to the corners of the mouth, avoidance of the habit of lip-licking, and, when *Candida* or secondary bacterial infection is present, the application of topical antibiotics and topical anticandidal agents, alone or in combination.

EROSIO INTERDIGITALIS BLASTOMYCETICA

Erosio interdigitalis blastomycetica (derived from the Latin, meaning an erosion between digits caused by a budding fungus) is a red, itchy, and occasionally slightly painful, well-defined oval eruption of the webs between and extending to the sides of fingers (Fig. 13–34). Usually, but not necessarily, involving the area between the third and fourth fingers (occasionally the second and third or fourth and fifth fingers, and rarely a corresponding surface of the toes), the disorder is manifested by fissuring, maceration, and exfoliation of the affected region, with a characteristic scaly and occasionally vesicular or papulovesicular border. It appears to be associated with infection due to *C.*

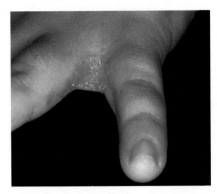

Figure 13–34. Erosio interdigitalis blastomycetica. This patient has cutaneous candidiasis of the interdigital web.

albicans and an associated, possibly syngergistic gram-negative infection, particularly in individuals who tend to perspire a great deal or who frequently have their hands immersed in water. Treatment of erosio interdigitalis blastomycetica consists of avoidance of moisture to the intertriginous webs and the use of topical antibacterial as well as topical anticandidal preparations.

BLACK HAIRY TONGUE

Black hairy tongue is a term used to describe a disorder of adults and occasionally adolescents characterized by hypertrophic elongated filiform papillae, which form a dense black, bluish black, or brown mat-like surface on the midportion of the dorsum of the tongue (Fig. 13–35). The etiology of this disorder is unknown, but it is frequently attributed to the prevalence of *C. albicans*, aspergillosis, or the filamentous mycelia of fungi that grow on the tongue's dorsal surface and is often associated with prolonged use of antibiotics.

The most effective treatment consists of discon-

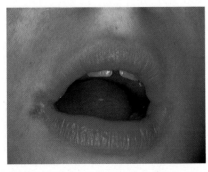

Figure 13–33. Perlèche. Maceration, erythema, and fissuring of the corners of the mouth associated with *Candida albicans*.

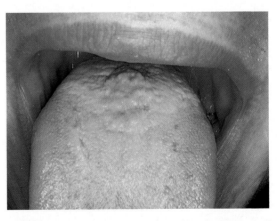

Figure 13–35. Black hairy tongue. Hypertrophic filiform papillae on the dorsal aspect of the tongue due to *Candida albicans* (a complication of long-term systemic tetracycline therapy for acne vulgaris).

tinuation of possible offending systemic antibiotics, clotrimazole (Mycelex) troches, and gentle brushing of the dorsum of the tongue with a soft toothbrush, alone or with a papain paste made up of a solution of four parts water and one part Adolph's Meat Tenderizer. This helps remove retained debris and generally results in clinical improvement of the disorder.

SYSTEMIC CANDIDIASIS

Although superficial skin and mucosal infections are common in the neonatal period, serious *Candida* infections are encountered much less frequently. Systemic candidiasis presents a major challenge to the clinician, since neither diagnostic nor therapeutic measures are entirely satisfactory. The disorder may affect the lungs, bronchial tree, meninges, kidneys, bladder, joints, and, less commonly, the liver, myocardium, endocardium, and eyes. Drug addition and indwelling intravenous catheters, as well as direct trauma during intracardiac surgery, have been implicated in this disorder.[73]

Although almost indistinguishable from corresponding bacterial, viral, or other fungal diseases, the disorder may be suspected in patients with intermittent, spiking, therapy-resistant fever, with cutaneous or unusual candidal lesions or cellulitis at the site of an intravenous catheter. The diagnosis is confirmed by isolation of *Candida* from blood, abscesses, urine, or other body fluids, by demonstration of the organism in cutaneous biopsy or other surgical specimens, and by the presence of hypergammaglobulinemia and precipitating antibodies to cytoplasmic antigens of *C. albicans*.

Treatment is directed toward removal of iatrogenic factors, treatment of the underlying illness, and specific antifungal therapy. Nystatin, 1 to 1.5 million units per day in infants or 3 to 6 million units per day in older children, may be administered as the oral suspension (for infants) or in tablet form (for older individuals). Amphotericin may be administered in dosages of 0.25 to 1 mg/kg intravenously daily, or 1.5 mg/kg every other day. The toxicity of amphotericin B (anemia, thrombocytopenia, and nephrotoxicity), however, requires caution with the use of this preparation. In such cases, oral clotrimazole (60 to 150 mg/kg/day) in three divided doses, oral itraconazole, flucytosine (100 mg/kg/day) divided into four doses, or intravenous miconazole (30 to 60 mg/kg/day), given at 8-hour intervals, may be administered.[74, 75] Although flucytosine may be given orally and is relatively safe, resistant strains of *Candida* often develop during therapy.[76] Except for chronic mucocutaneous candidiasis, intravenous drug addicts with cutaneous or ocular candidiasis, and selected patients with osteoarticular candidiasis who are unwilling to remain in the hospital for a course of intravenous amphotericin B, ketoconazole is not recommended as the drug of choice for systemic candidiasis. As an alternative, fluconazole (an antifungal azole derivative available as Diflucan [Roerig]) has been approved for the treatment of oropharyngeal, esophageal, and severe systemic candidiasis. Fluconazole, although very expensive, appears to be less toxic than amphotericin B or flucytosine and is better tolerated than ketoconazole. Like other azole antifungal agents, however, fluconazole should be discontinued in patients with progressive hepatic dysfunction. Although the efficacy of this drug has not been established in children, a small number of children between the ages of 3 and 13 years have been treated safely with dosages of 3 to 6 mg/kg/day.

CHRONIC MUCOCUTANEOUS CANDIDIASIS

Chronic mucocutaneous candidiasis is a progressive candidal infection that may be congenital or acquired and is usually associated with endocrinopathy (hypoadrenalism, hypothyroidism, diabetes, hypoparathyroidism), vitiligo, immunologic deficiency, and defects in the thymus-controlled lymphocyte defense system. Although the disorder may have its onset in the neonatal period, it usually manifests itself later in infancy or early childhood.

It may begin as an oral candidiasis (thrush), candidal diaper dermatitis, candidal intertrigo, or paronychia that is persistent and resistant to the usual modes of therapy. The disorder persists and spreads to involve the scalp, eyelids, nose, hands, and feet and may be characterized by intertrigo, pathognomonic satellite pustules, erythematous lesions covered with dry scaly patches, or thick macerated crusts (see Chapter 10, Fig. 10–20). Coalescence of individual lesions often leads to the formation of crusted granulomatous areas with verrucous surfaces and horn-like projections. Dystrophy of the nails, scarring, and loss of hair are common sequelae.

Although the disorder has been refractory to therapy, systemic candidiasis is uncommon. Death, when it occurs, is usually seen in individuals with immunodeficiency syndromes and associated severe and recurrent infections of various types. Although there are patients with chronic mucocutaneous candidiasis who also have extensive and persistent dermatophytosis, this is usually not found in association with this disorder.

Nystatin and amphotericin B in the past have been the treatments of choice for this disorder. Unfortunately, neither of these antifungal antibiotics is absorbed from the gastrointestinal tract sufficiently to be of value in the oral treatment of systemic infection. Although the intravenous or prolonged administration of amphotericin B may result in clearing of chronic mucocutaneous candidiasis, recurrence invariably occurs when treatment is discontinued, and nephrotoxicity precludes its continued use.

In addition, there have been reports of successful treatment of chronic mucocutaneous candidiasis with the newer antifungal agents. Clotrimazole (60 to 150 mg/kg/day taken in three divided doses) or intravenous miconazole (30 to 60 mg/kg/day, given at 8-hour intervals) may be administered. Clotrimazole can be given orally, and side effects are limited to gastrointestinal intolerance, leukopenia, and elevated liver enzyme levels, all of which are reversible. Because the drug induces hepatic microsomal enzymes that affect its metabolism, it has been recommended that it be given for 2-week courses, followed by a 2-week rest period.[77] Oral ketoconazole and itraconazole[78] have also been found to be effective. Unfortunately, since relapses are common and prolonged therapy may be necessary, owing to its potential for hepatotoxicity and the possible development of resistant yeast strains, oral ketoconazole therapy should be used intermittently and with caution in children as well as adults.

DEEP FUNGAL DISORDERS

In contrast to the superficial dermatophytes, which are confined to dead keratinous tissue, certain mycotic infections have the capacity for deep invasion of the skin or produce skin lesions secondary to systemic visceral infection, usually of the lungs and reticuloendothelial system.

Subcutaneous Mycoses

The subcutaneous mycoses are a group of disorders caused by a number of fungi that exist as soil saprophytes and are normally of low virulence. Although these infections (sporotrichosis, chromoblastomycosis, histoplasmosis, blastomycosis, coccidioidomycosis, and cryptococcosis) are found most often in adults with occupational exposure to soil and plants, all age groups are potentially susceptible.

SPOROTRICHOSIS

Sporotrichosis is a granulomatous fungal infection of the skin and subcutaneous tissues caused by *Sporotrichum schenkii,* a dimorphous fungus of worldwide distribution commonly isolated from soil and plants. It occurs in patients of all ages and is observed most commonly in adult males who,

because of their occupation or leisure-time activities, are likely to be exposed to contaminated soil or vegetation (farmers, florists, gardeners, forestry workers, miners, individuals who work with contaminated packing material, or children at play). In addition, multiple familial cases have also been reported. Although human transmission can occur in individuals caring for patients with suppurating wounds of sporotrichosis, the majority of familial cases appear to be related to simultaneous inoculation from the same recognized or unrecognized source.[79-82]

Lymphocutaneous sporotrichosis is the most common manifestation of the disease. Seen in 75 per cent of all reported cases, it follows a wound inflicted by an object, such as a splinter, thorn, straw, grain, rock, glass, cat bite, or cat scratch (cats are perhaps the only animals capable of transmitting this disorder) contaminated with the organism.[83] The initial lesion is characterized by a small, firm, painless dusky papule that develops at the site of trauma 1 to 12 weeks (frequently within 3 weeks) after inoculation, slowly enlarges, and eventually ulcerates; this papule is followed by a series of subcutaneous nodules with overlying erythema and occasional ulceration along the course of lymphatic drainage (Fig. 13–36). The disorder is almost always unilateral. A well-developed lesion appears as a 2- to 4-cm violaceous nodule with central ulceration, undermined edges, and considerable crusting. In adult cases most lesions occur on exposed surfaces of the arms and legs; in childhood cases, lesions on the face and trunk are fairly common as well.[79]

The second most common form of sporotrichosis is a fixed cutaneous form, which appears in endemic areas, in which infection in a previously sensitized person does not spread along lymphatic channels but remains localized at the site of entrance of the organism. Localized forms of this disorder range from scaly maculopapular lesions to verrucous and weeping ulcerations with or without satellite lesions. In other instances there may be primary chancriform lesions, with enlargement of the regional lymph nodes without intervening nodules along the lymphatic channels, and in some cases, mucous membrane involvement may give rise to suppurative ulcerating, vegetative, or granulomatous lesions. It has been hypothesized that

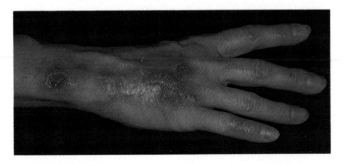

Figure 13–36. Sporotrichosis. Subcutaneous nodules, ulceration, and erythema occur along the course of lymphatic drainage.

children manifesting fixed cutaneous forms may possess host factors that limit the infection to the inoculation site, even if the strain is capable of producing the more classic lymphocutaneous form commonly seen in adults.[82, 84]

Disseminated sporotrichosis is an uncommon manifestation of this disorder seen in individuals with compromised immunologic capacity, such as those with sarcoidosis, malignant neoplasms, diabetes mellitus, or chronic alcoholism. In such cases the cutaneous lesions may be widespread and may be located on the extremities in a pattern suggestive of embolic spread. When disseminated cutaneous lesions occur, they originate as subcutaneous nodules similar to and following the same course as that seen in the lymphocutaneous form of the disorder and eventually end as chronic crusted ulcers. Seen in less than 1 per cent of infected patients, the disseminated form develops following hematogenous spread of the infection from a primary focus in the skin or an occult pulmonary focus (as a result of inhalation, ingestion, or laboratory complication) with spread to the skin, skeletal system, and at times the liver, spleen, pancreas, thyroid, myocardium, or central nervous system.[85]

Atypical mycobacterium infections, localized granulomatous lesions, bacterial infections, primary syphilis, cat-scratch disease, leishmaniasis, tuberculosis, anthrax, blastomycosis, tularemia, and occasionally nocardial infections can all cause lesions that mimic cutaneous sporotrichosis. When the diagnosis is uncertain, demonstration of the organism on fungal culture, preferably from ulcerative lesions or aspiration of unopened nodules, is confirmatory. Direct examination of smears or biopsy material is usually unrewarding, but a fluorescent antibody-staining technique may aid in rapid diagnosis of this disorder.

The treatment of choice for cutaneous sporotrichosis is orally administered saturated solution of potassium iodide, 1 to 2 drops per year of age three times a day and increased to a maximum of 90 to 120 drops/day or until signs of toxicity (increased lacrimation or salivation, swelling of the salivary glands, burning mouth, abdominal discomfort, diarrhea, headache, or gastric intolerance) appear. This is administered after meals and if necessary may be supplemented by intravenous sodium iodide. Treatment is continued for 4 to 6 weeks after resolution of lesions. The therapeutic effect of iodides is not due to a fungistatic activity but to some unknown influence on tissue reaction that increases the resistance of the host.

Amphotericin B, given by slow intravenous infusion (0.25 mg/kg to a maximum of 1.0 mg/kg) with appropriate precautions, is the method of choice for extracutaneous (disseminated) sporotrichosis, especially in the presence of a rising titer with agglutination or complement fixation tests. Itraconazole, recently approved for clinical use in the United States, and fluconazole (Diflucan) appear to be effective for patients with cutaneous and lymphangitic sporotrichosis.[86]

CHROMOBLASTOMYCOSIS

Chromoblastomycosis (chromomycosis) is an uncommon chronic cutaneous and subcutaneous fungal infection of the skin caused by several species of *Phialophora*, *Fonsecaea* or *Cladisporium*, all of which are common inhabitants of soil and decaying vegetation. Confined most frequently to one of the lower extremities, the disorder usually results from a puncture or splinter of wood and occurs most frequently among barefoot farm laborers in rural tropical or subtropical countries, but it has also been seen in North America, Northern Europe, and Australia, and has occurred in children as young as 3 years of age.

Chromoblastomycosis is characterized by the formation of small papular, verrucous nodules, plaques, and tumor masses, usually on the distal portion of one of the extremities (most frequently the foot, occasionally an upper extremity, rarely the face, neck, or trunk). Lesions have a dull reddish gray color, may be slightly scaly, and are usually painless unless secondary infection is present. In early stages of this disorder the appearance is not very distinctive and may resemble other granulomatous disorders. The occurrence of verrucous lesions is an outstanding feature of all cases of chromoblastomycosis, thus accounting for the name dermatitis verrucosa once given to this disorder. Eventually, after a period of months or years, the extremity may become edematous and swollen, enlarged masses may form with exudate, debris, and crusts, and lesions may become papillomatous, with masses of elevated, hard, brownish or reddish nodules surmounting the plaques, with a resultant cauliflower-like appearance.

Chromoblastomycosis can be diagnosed by recognition of the causative fungus in microscopic examination of potassium hydroxide preparations, in biopsy specimens from clinical lesions, or in fungal culture. When the foci of infection are localized and limited, the treatment of choice is surgical removal of the infected tissue by excision, electrodesiccation, or cryosurgery. In cases of long duration and extensive involvement, although the organism may be sensitive to amphotericin B, the required local concentration generally is too high for intravenous infusion to be effective. In such instances, the use of intralesional amphotericin B given in a concentration of 5 mg/ml in dextrose and water or in 2 per cent lidocaine may be curative.[87] Patients with localized chromoblastomycosis have been completely cured solely by prolonged topical application of heat obtained from the use of pocket warmers[88]; and flucytosine (Ancobon) (either alone or combined with amphotericin B), thiabendazole, ketoconazole, and itraconazole (which may prove to be the treatment of choice) have also been effective in the management of this disorder.[89]

MYCETOMA

Mycetoma, also termed *Madura foot* or *maduromycosis*, is a chronic localized granulomatous disorder of the subcutaneous tissues followed by marked invasion of the fascia, muscles, and bone, and, when an extremity is involved, enlargement of the affected area. Although the majority of lesions are seen on the foot or hand, lesions also may occur on the shoulder, buttocks, knees or other parts of the body; thus the term *Madura foot* actually is inappropriate for this disorder.

The infection may be caused by various species of true fungi (*Allescheria boydii, Madurella mycetomii, M. grisea, Phialophora jeanselmii, Cephalosporium recifei*), by aerobic fungus-like bacteria, and by actinomycetes (usually species of *Nocardia* and *Streptomyces*), which occur as saprophytes in soil or on vegetable matter. Uncommon in childhood and relatively rare in the United States, mycetoma occurs most commonly in young adults and workers in rural tropical and subtropical areas who walk barefoot and accordingly are more readily exposed to the fungi.

The infection begins as one or more, small, nondescript, firm painless papules that gradually evolve into subcutaneous nodules with sinus tracts, draining abscesses, edema, and, when an extremity is affected, enlargement of the area of involvement. The diagnostic features of mycetoma are distortion and enlargement of the involved area, draining sinus tracts, and bloody or purulent drainage with characteristic pinpoint-sized granules seen on microscopic examination of the suppurative fluid. Definitive diagnosis can be made by microscopic identification of the granules and their actinomycete or fungal nature, with confirmation by culture of the etiologic organism.

The treatment of mycetoma depends on early diagnosis and the nature of the infection. Disease due to actinomycetes frequently responds to sulfonamides, penicillin, tetracycline, or chloramphenicol (alone or in combination), or in some instances to amphotericin B, and that due to *Nocardia brasiliensis* to dapsone. Unfortunately, there is no single drug that can give consistently good results, and long-standing cases with extensive tissue destruction and fibrosis frequently are resistant to all forms of drug therapy. Surgery may be effective during the early stages. In more advanced cases, however, particularly when there is extensive sinus tract formation, except for amputation procedures, surgical treatment rarely is curative.

Systemic Mycoses

The systemic mycoses comprise a group of fungal disorders that arise from internal foci, usually the lungs or upper respiratory tract. When the skin lesions result from dissemination of the disease from one or more internal foci, the prognosis is generally poor. Disorders in this group include blastomycosis, coccidioidomycosis, cryptococcosus, histoplasmosis, rhinosporidiosis, and those due to opportunistic infection, aspergillosis, and mucormycosis. Actinomycosis and nocardiosis, although frequently included under the group of disorders due to true fungi, are actually caused by fungus-like gram-positive bacteria. Accordingly, they are described in the chapter on bacterial infections (see Chapter 10).

BLASTOMYCOSIS

Blastomycosis is seen in two forms, North American and South American. North American blastomycosis is caused by *Blastomyces dermatitidis*. It occurs in three forms, primary cutaneous inoculation blastomycosis, pulmonary blastomycosis, and disseminated (systemic) blastomycosis. South American blastomycosis is a chronic granulomatous disease caused by *B. brasiliensis*. It characteristically begins on the skin or mucosa about the mouth or nasal cavity, occasionally in the lungs, with dissemination by hematogenous spread to various internal organs, namely, the central nervous system, brain, bones, adrenal glands, spleen, and skin.

An infrequent disorder of childhood, North American blastomycosis is almost exclusively restricted to individuals on the North American continent from Canada to Mexico and Central America (usually men older than 50 years of age), with most cases occurring in the central eastern and midwestern United States.[90] Except for rare cases of primary cutaneous inoculation blastomycosis, which appears in physicians or laboratory workers who have accidentally inoculated themselves with *B. dermatitidis*, most cases of North American blastomycosis are pulmonary in origin. Those caused by inoculation show an indurated ulcerated chancriform lesion with lymphangitis and lymphadenitis of the affected limb. The primary lesion and affected nodes heal spontaneously, generally within 8 months, and, except for a resultant scar, the prognosis is excellent.

Pulmonary blastomyocosis may be asymptomatic or may produce mild to moderately severe acute pulmonary involvement characterized by low-grade fever, pleuritic chest pain, cough, and hemoptysis. The disorder may heal spontaneously, may cause chronic pulmonary disease with or without cavitation, or may disseminate, primarily to the skin, subcutaneous tissues, bones, and joints, and less frequently to the gastrointestinal tract, liver, spleen, and central nervous system. If untreated, pulmonary blastomycosis often progresses, eventuating in the patient's death.

Cutaneous lesions disseminated from a primary pulmonary focus are usually symmetrical and generally appear on the exposed areas of the body (the face, wrists, hands, and feet). They appear as papules or nodules, which subsequently ulcerate and discharge purulent material; as elevated verrucous crusted lesions, with active arciform or serpiginous borders and violaceous margins, and a tendency toward central healing with a thin depigmented atrophic scar; or as a raised, firm, subcutaneous nodule with multiple small pustules over its surface.

South American blastomycosis (paracoccidioidomycosis) occurs almost exclusively in all sections of South and Central America with the exception of Chile, Guyana, and French Guiana. The disorder is most frequently noted in Brazil and, as in North American blastomycosis is found more often in males than in females (in a proportion of 10 to 12 to one), with the highest incidence in inhabitants of rural areas, especially farmhands. The highest incidence occurs in individuals between 20 and 50 years of age, and it is uncommon in childhood. It is thought that the organism lives as a saprophyte on vegetation or in soil, and that the infection is acquired by direct implantation into the skin or mucous membranes, possibly through the practice of cleaning the teeth with small pieces of infected vegetation or, in pulmonary lesions, by direct inhalation of the organism.

The primary lesions usually appear on the lips or in the mouth, pharynx (extending to the larynx), or nasal cavity as infiltrated ulcerated lesions. The ulcers extend and ultimately progress to destroy the nose, lips, and facies. Hematogenous or lymphatic spread results in subcutaneous abscesses, and the lymph nodes draining the affected areas are palpable, painful, and adherent to the overlying skin, and occasionally progress to form chronic sinuses and suppurate.

The diagnosis of cutaneous blastomycosis is dependent on the demonstration of characteristic round budding organisms in potassium hydroxide mounts or stained smears of material from skin, ulcers, or purulent discharge, or by culture of organisms on Sabouraud's agar. Although a mild self-limiting form of pulmonary blastomycosis not requiring therapy has been reported, before the advent of chemotherapy blastomycosis was fatal in 90 per cent of cases. Despite the fact that amphotericin B has been the standard therapy for years and is currently the treatment of choice for meningeal forms of the disorder, many cases of blastomycosis can now be successfully managed by ketoconazole, fluconazole, or itraconazole.

COCCIDIOIDOMYCOSIS

Coccidioidomycosis is an acute, subacute, or chronic infectious disease caused by the fungus *Coccidioides immitis*, a soil saprophyte endemic in the hot, arid, desert areas of the southwestern United States (especially the San Joaquin Valley in California), Mexico, and parts of South America. Seen in infants as early as the first few months of life and in children as well as adults, it affects individuals of all ages, particularly men engaged in agricultural occupations, with a peak incidence of the acute infection among field workers during the hot months of autumn. The disease is not believed to be transmitted through the placenta, but cases of disseminated coccidioidomycosis have been reported beginning as early as 2 to 3 weeks of age.[91]

As in blastomycosis, coccidioidomycosis may also occur as a primary cutaneous inoculation, pulmonary, or systemic disorder. Primarily an airborne disease, the common pulmonary form is acquired by the inhalation of dust that contains arthrospores, and it varies in severity from a mild inapparent upper respiratory tract infection to an acute, disseminated fatal disease. The primary pulmonary disorder is the most common form of coccidioidomycosis. Following an incubation period of 10 days to several weeks, 60 per cent of cases are asymptomatic, and 40 per cent of affected individuals develop a respiratory infection consisting of a "flu-like" syndrome, with fever, malaise, cough, chest pain, chills, dyspnea, nodular densities, localized infiltrations in the lung, and hilar adenopathy. Ninety-five per cent of patients with clinically manifest coccidioidomycosis recover completely; 5 per cent develop pulmonary residua and complications consisting of persistent pulmonary granulomas or thin-walled cavities, pleural effusion, bronchiectasis, and pneumothorax; and 0.1 per cent progress to a disseminated disorder, with involvement of the skin, subcutaneous tissue, bone, lymph nodes, or central nervous system.

Cutaneous signs of primary pulmonary coccidioidomycosis include a generalized erythematous macular exanthem that appears within the first 1 or 2 days of illness (seen in up to 10 per cent of patients) or erythema multiforme or erythema nodosum (seen in up to 20 per cent of individuals with the acute pulmonary form, particularly females). Supraclavicular lymphadenopathy is frequently an early sign of dissemination, and the disseminated form consists of nondescript papules or pustules, granulomas or erosions, plaques, nodules, or abscesses with thick mucoid pus or chronic ulcers with, at times, superimposed verrucous or vegetative surfaces.

Primary cutaneous inoculation is relatively rare and occurs through injury by contaminated splinters or thorns or by accidental inoculation in laboratory or autopsy rooms. This form of coccidioidomycosis is characterized by a painless, indurated ulcerated lesion with lymphangitis and lymphadenopathy (similar to that seen in sporotrichosis or blastomycosis). Although healing usually takes place within a few months, at least one patient with primary cutaneous inoculation developed an associated coccidioidal meningitis.[92]

Diagnosis of coccidioidomycosis can be established by demonstration of the characteristic large (up to 60 to 100 μ) thick-walled globular spherules in potassium hydroxide mounts of sputum, purulent discharge, biopsy specimens, or cerebrospinal fluid or by isolation of the fungus by culture. Since *C. immitis* is highly infectious, special precautions are necessary to prevent laboratory accidents due to airborne spread of arthrospores. Serologic tests are also of value in the diagnosis and prognosis of this disorder. The coccidioidin skin test usually becomes positive in 3 to 4 weeks but may revert to negative or never become positive in overwhelming disease. A negative test result, therefore, may be misinterpreted or may indicate a poor prognosis. Complement fixation antibodies develop more slowly, increase with the severity of the disease, and diminish with clinical improvement. A high titer or complement fixation denotes severe extensive disease and poor prognosis; complement fixation antibodies in cerebrospinal fluid indicate the presence of central nervous system infection.

The majority of infections with coccidioidomycosis are self-limiting and do not require specific therapy. The illness of nondisseminated primary coccidioidomycosis commonly lasts 1 to 2 months, but the disseminated course may be fulminant or may persist for several years, and until the advent of amphotericin B therapy, disseminated forms were fatal in more than 50 per cent of cases. Although most patients with coccidioidomycosis do not require treatment, amphotericin B is currently recommended for severe pulmonary disease, disseminated infection, central nervous system infections, and immunocompromised patients; and oral ketoconazole has been shown to be effective for the management of primary pulmonary and nonpulmonary soft tissue infections. Although the optimum dose of oral ketoconazole for children has not been established, a single daily dose of 5 to 10 mg/kg has been used (with up to 20 mg/kg/day for severe infections, particularly those involving the central nervous and skeletal systems). Alternative agents include itraconazole and intravenous miconazole.[93] Reports of treatment failure in patients with coccidioidomycosis and other fungal infections, however, suggest that intravenous miconazole should be used for individuals who are unable to take ketoconazole or fail to respond to other modes of therapy.

CRYPTOCOCCOSIS (TORULOSIS)

Infection due to the encapsulated yeast *Cryptococcus neoformans* affects all age groups in a worldwide distribution and usually occurs as a systemic disease with the respiratory tract as the portal of entry. The organism has been found in various fruits, soil, pigeon excreta, and cow's milk; and, when it affects humans, there is marked predilection for the brain and meninges, although the lungs and occasionally the skin and other parts of the body may be involved. The disease usually occurs in individuals between 30 and 60 years of age and, although uncommon, does occur in children and has been seen in newborns. In some cases of neonatal cryptococcosis, symptoms begin so promptly after birth that the question of transplacental transmission must be considered. However, since *Cryptococcus* is an occasional in-

habitant of the female genital tract, it is believed that the infant acquires infection during passage through the birth canal.

Clinically apparent cryptococcosis may remain localized to the lungs, producing focal pneumonia, patchy infiltrates, solitary nodules, and, infrequently, abscesses and pleural effusion. Pulmonary symptoms may be absent or minimal and, although pulmonary involvement may progress and produce death, in most instances central nervous system manifestations predominate, and infection is detected only after dissemination to the central nervous system has occurred.

Central nervous system manifestations consist of occipital or frontal headaches, behavioral abnormalities, confusion, dizziness, vomiting, stiff neck, and with progression, cranial nerve palsy, seizure disorders, delirium, coma, and death. Although most patients have isolated meningeal involvement occasionally accompanied by pulmonary infiltrates, other organs, including the liver, spleen, kidney, bones, and lymph nodes, may be involved. Skin lesions, when present, may be related to trauma or extension from bony involvement but are usually due to hematogenous spread from a pulmonary focus. Approximately 30 per cent of cases of disseminated cryptococcosis are associated with some form of reticuloendothelial system malignancy (usually Hodgkin's disease). The presence of cutaneous involvement, therefore, suggests a search for a possible underlying malignant disorder.

Cutaneous lesions, seen in 10 to 15 per cent of cases, are located most commonly on the head and neck (including the scalp); less commonly they are found on the extremities or thorax. Lesions usually begin as painless, well-demarcated, firm, pink, red, or bluish purple papular, pustular, acneiform eruptions without surrounding inflammation. These lesions are especially characteristic of widespread infection and often occur around the nose and mouth. As the lesions enlarge they form infiltrated plaques and develop firm, rubbery, indolent tumors, subcutaneous abscesses, or ulcers, often with raised papillomatous borders.

The diagnosis of cryptococcosis depends on demonstration of the organism by examination of cerebrospinal fluid, pus from skin lesions, sputum, or tissue sections, by indirect immunofluorescence, or by culture on Sabouraud's dextrose agar. The organisms are oval or rounded, thick-walled spherules 5 to 20 μm in diameter. The organism is surrounded by a polysaccharide capsule, often with characteristic budding. This is best demonstrated by the addition of one drop of India ink to potassium hydroxide wet-mounts and cerebrospinal fluid preparations or by special staining with methylene blue, alcian blue, or mucicarmine.

Untreated cryptococcosis is fatal in 90 per cent of cases; intravenous and intrathecal amphotericin B, however, will result in cure in about 80 per cent of cases of disseminated forms of this disorder. Intravenous amphotericin B is administered in increasing increments, beginning with 0.1 to 0.3 mg/kg/ day (never exceeding a total daily dose of 1.5 mg/kg). Sterilization of foci of cryptococci is accomplished in 10 to 14 days, and treatment should be given daily, generally for a period of 2 months, with a total intravenous dose of 30 mg/kg. For patients with central nervous system involvement, intrathecal therapy in addition to intravenous therapy often produces a cure.

Oral flucytosine (Ancobon), an antifungal fluorinated pyrimidine chemically related to fluorouracil, 150 to 200 mg/kg administered daily in four divided doses, is effective. Since emergence of flucytosine-resistant strains has been a major cause of treatment failure, the combination of flucytosine with intravenous amphotericin B is now recommended to avert development of resistant strains and to avoid the potential toxic effects associated with high doses of amphotericin B. Intravenous miconazole, oral ketoconazole, and itraconazole and, although data on its use in children are limited, oral fluconazole (Diflucan) as an adjunct to amphotericin B have been shown to be effective in the management of patients with cryptococcal meningitis who fail to respond to other therapeutic modalities.

HISTOPLASMOSIS

Histoplasmosis is a common, highly infectious disorder affecting primarily the lungs caused by the fungus *Histoplasma capsulatum*. The disease is widely distributed throughout the world, is endemic in the Mississippi and Ohio valleys of the United States, and affects infants and children as well as adults. *H. capsulatum* exists as a saprophyte in the soil in endemic areas, most often in soil contaminated by chicken feathers or droppings. Infection is usually acquired by inhalation and is contracted more frequently in rural rather than urban areas. In children, who are more likely to have generalized histoplasmosis, the frequency of extensive ulcers along the gastrointestinal mucosa that give rise to diarrhea and other gastrointestinal disturbances suggests that organisms of histoplasmosis may be ingested rather than inhaled in these individuals. Approximately three fourths of infected individuals have asymptomatic benign, self-limiting pulmonary infections, which may leave calcified residua in the lungs. Twenty-five per cent develop a "flu-like" pulmonary infection, and less than 1 per cent progress to the disseminated form of the disease.

Many classifications of histoplasmosis have been recommended. The most recognized include an acute pulmonary form, a febrile disorder of varying severity in which there may be malaise, cough, chest pain, chills, dyspnea, and nodular densities or localized infiltration in the lung; chronic pulmonary forms often resembling tuberculosis clinically and radiographically; disseminated forms with fever, hepatosplenomegaly, anemia, and weight loss (more commonly seen in young children and individuals older than 50 years of age); and an extremely rare traumatic primary form (seen in laboratory or autopsy room workers) characterized by chancriform lesions at the site of inoculation accompanied by regional lymphadenopathy.

Cutaneous lesions are uncommon but may be seen in the disseminated form of histoplasmosis. Quite variable, they include lesions of erythema multiforme and erythema nodosum; purpura; papules; pustules; plaques; chronic abscesses; patches of impetiginized or exfoliative dermatitis; vegetative lesions; characteristic ulcerations of the nose, mouth, pharynx, genitalia, and perianal regions; and punched-out or circumscribed granulomatous ulcers.

The diagnosis of histoplasmosis consists of identification of the small intracellular yeast-like organisms in sputum or peripheral blood, smears from open or ulcerated tissue, biopsy specimens of cutaneous lesions, lymph nodes, liver, or bone marrow, and fungal culture on Sabouraud's dextrose agar. Since in endemic areas as many as 90 per cent of the population react positively, the skin test is not diagnostic. In infants a positive reaction probably indicates active infection, but in older children and adults it may signify past or present infection and accordingly is reliable only as a screening procedure. It must be remembered, however, that the histoplasmin skin test does not become positive for 2 or 3 weeks after infection and that it may be negative in extensive debilitating disease.

Serologic tests may be of value, but blood for serologic studies must be collected prior to skin testing, since the skin test itself may produce a rise in serologic titer. Serologic tests (agar gel precipitin test, yeast phase complement fixation, and collodion or latex particle agglutination) usually are positive except in chronically ill patients with severe disseminated lesions. Since low titers frequently are present in healthy persons living in endemic areas, titers less than 1:16 should be viewed with suspicion, and titers exceeding 1:32, although not conclusively diagnostic, are highly suggestive of histoplasmosis infection.

In more than 99 per cent of infections histoplasmosis has a benign self-limiting course. The disseminated forms, however, particularly in the very young and very old, have a high mortality. Amphotericin B, as in blastomycosis and coccidioidomycosis, and perhaps itraconazole, appear to be the treatments of choice for this disorder. Lesser infections may be treated with triple sulfa, but since there is considerable tendency to spontaneous resolution, controlled studies are lacking. Studies have shown ketoconazole to be as effective as amphotericin B in the treatment of histoplasmosis in the immunocompromised host, but potential hepatic and endocrinologic side effects suggest caution in its use in children with this disorder.

RHINOSPORIDIOSIS

Rhinosporidiosis is a rare chronic disorder caused by the fungus *Rhinosporidium seeberi*. Endemic in India and Sri Lanka (Ceylon), it occurs in other parts of the world, including the southern part of the United States. Males are infected most commonly (11:1), and the disease occurs at any age but is more common in children and young adults.

The disorder is characterized by papules, nodules, and pedunculated vascular polypoid growths on the mucous membranes of the nose, nasopharynx, and soft palate (in 75 per cent of cases) and in upper respiratory passages, conjunctivae, lacrimal sacs, skin, larynx, genitalia, or rectum. The surface of the growth has a raspberry-like appearance and is studded with tiny white or yellowish nodules containing the fungal spores.

The lesions become hyperplastic and may reach enormous size, and symptoms are associated with obstruction of the respiratory passages or esophagus. Typical lesions are recognizable by their pink to purple color, their friable consistency, and the presence of the white sporangia within the lesion itself. Diagnosis is confirmed by microscopic demonstration of typical sporangia on the surface of the polyps or in tissue section, and treatment consists of electrosurgical destruction and surgical removal of lesions when feasible.

Opportunistic Mycotic Infections

With the emergence of acquired immunodeficiency syndrome (AIDS) and the frequent use of broad-spectrum antibiotics and potent cytotoxic agents, fatal deep mycoses have become increasingly frequent. Opportunistic mycoses (e.g., aspergillosis, mucormycosis) are those that are very low in pathogenic potential but capable of causing infection when alteration or breakdown of host defenses occurs, thus permitting them to invade the host.

ASPERGILLOSIS

Aspergillosis is an uncommon opportunistic fungal disease of the respiratory tract and other sites caused by a variety of *Aspergillus* species. Although *A. fumigatus* is the most commonly identified pathogen, *A. niger* and an increasing number of species have been reported in recent years. There is no predilection for sex or race, and although a state of altered susceptibility is more common in adults, it also occurs in susceptible infants and children.

The fungi are ubiquitous, are normally nonpathogenic, and primarily affect debilitated individuals in the respiratory tract, although the skin, cornea, external auditory canal, gastrointestinal tract, nasopharynx, vagina, and urethra may also be affected. There are no features pathognomonic of aspergillosis, the clinical picture being related to the organs of involvement.

One of the most common characteristic manifestations of aspergillosis is the pulmonary intracavitary fungus ball. This is composed of colonies of *Aspergillus*, inflammatory exudate, cells, and fibrin in the form of a sphere, which may measure from 1 to 5 cm in diameter. Although it occasionally causes hemoptysis, most patients with fungus balls are asymptomatic.

In some patients, especially those with lymphoma or malignancy and those who are receiving systemic corticosteroids or other immunosuppressive therapy, the fungus may invade the tissues directly and spread hematogenously to other organs, characteristically the central nervous system, kidney, liver, spleen, gallbladder, heart, aorta, thyroid, bones, lymph nodes, uterus, and skin (Fig. 13–37). Less commonly, an opportunistic infection of the paranasal sinuses may result in mucopurulent or blood-tinged nasal discharge, headache, periorbital neuralgia, and rhinitis; and, with extension, the face may become erythematous, swollen, warm, and tender, suggesting a diagnosis of cellulitis or erysipelas. Cutaneous lesions are rare, but various species of *Aspergillus* have been recovered from the external auditory canal. Whether the fungus is a causative factor of otomycosis, however, remains controversial. In addition, palmar aspergillosis, characterized by erythematous papules, hemorrhagic bullae, and erythematous to violaceous plaques with central necrosis, has been seen in patients with aspergillosis receiving intravenous therapy. Since this complication appears to involve a hand previously secured to an intravenous armboard, it is hypothesized that this cutaneous manifestation may have been the result of localization of the organism in an area of stasis during a period of fungemia or direct contamination during the course of intravenous therapy.[94]

Although *Aspergillus* organisms may be identified on culture, clinical findings must be carefully

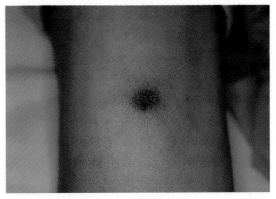

Figure 13–37. Cutaneous aspergillosis on the arm of an immunosuppressed patient with leukemia. (Courtesy of Department of Dermatology, Yale University School of Medicine.)

evaluated before a diagnosis of aspergillosis is established. Clinical material should be examined carefully for the presence of hyphae, and although culture of the organism is ideal, this is not always possible. Treatment consists of amphotericin B or oral flucytosine and surgical removal of pulmonary fungus balls, when present. As with cryptococcosis, amphotericin B and flucytosine in combination are recommended to avoid toxicity and development of resistant strains; and, as an alternative, itraconazole has been shown to be effective for the treatment of invasive osseous and chronic necrotizing pulmonary forms of aspergillosis.[95]

PHYCOMYCOSIS

Phycomycosis (mucormycosis) is an opportunistic infection that occurs in immunocompromised individuals, patients with a variety of debilitating diseases, such as diabetes, anemia, heart or liver disease, burns, leukemia, or other lymphomas, and in individuals receiving corticosteroids, cytotoxic agents, or immunosuppressive therapy. It may involve any organ of the body but most commonly affects the skin, lungs, meninges, gastrointestinal tract, and structures in the head and neck.

The causative fungi of mucormycosis belong to the class Phycomycetes and include species of *Mucor, Rhizopus, Absidia, Mortierella,* and *Cunninghamella,* the portal of entry varying with the site of the disease. The term *phycomycosis* refers to the subcutaneous form of the disorder. Caused by *Basidiobolus* and *Entomophthura* species, this form is characterized by inflammatory subcutaneous swellings that spread over the upper part of the chest, neck, or arms; involve the fat, muscle, and fascia; and heal spontaneously.

Cutaneous or subcutaneous infections are rare and occur most frequently in diabetics with recurrent acidosis or in patients with severe burns. They are characterized by papular lesions, chronic indolent ulcers, and slowly enlarging painless subcutaneous nodules. The initial lesion is usually a small area of macular discoloration or dusky erythema, which gradually enlarges and ulcerates. Necrosis may be marked, and there is usually a profuse foul-smelling purulent exudate and, in some cases, cutaneous infarction resembling ecthyma gangrenosum.[96, 97] Subcutaneous phycomycosis occurs most frequently in children and adolescents. It is characterized by localized subcutaneous nodular eosinophilic granulomas, usually with an intact but inflamed epidermis, multiple purulent ulcerations, and paronychia.

The cerebral form may be recognized by a suppurative necrotizing infection of the paranasal sinuses, orbital pain, swelling, edema, proptosis, ptosis, pupil fixation, and loss of vision. Acute inflammation, infarction, or necrosis in the lungs, gastrointestinal tract, orbits, and the central nervous system in a patient debilitated by disease or immunosuppressant therapy should suggest the possibility of mucormycosis.

Diagnosis depends on microscopic examination of the organism in clinical lesions and definitive fungal culture. Therapy requires treatment of the underlying disease process, discontinuation of predisposing therapeutic agents whenever possible, and, when necessary, the use of intravenous amphotericin B.

References

1. Zaias N, Taplin DM: Improved preparation for the diagnosis of mycologic diseases. Arch. Dermatol. 93:608–609, 1966.

   Microscopic demonstration of fungi in skin, nail, and hair scrapings can be facilitated by the use of 20 per cent potassium hydroxide in a solution of 60 per cent water and 40 per cent dimethyl sulfoxide (DMSO).

2. Rockoff AS: Fungus cultures in a pediatric outpatient clinic. Pediatrics 63:276–278, 1979.

   In a total of 76 fungal cultrues, of which 24 yielded dermatophytes, results on dermatophyte test medium (DTM), read by nonmycologists (pediatric house officers), compared favorably with those on standard media processed in a laboratory.

3. Taplin D, Zaias N, Rebell G, et al.: Isolation and recognition of dermatophytes on a new medium (DTM). Arch. Dermatol. 99:203–209, 1969.

   Dermatophyte test medium (DTM) contains a phenol red indicator, enabling the nonmyocologist to determine the presence of dermatophytic fungi by a change in the color of the agar from yellow to red.

4. Rosenthal SA, Furnari D: Efficacy of dermatophyte test media. Arch Dermatol. 104:486–489, 1971.

   Although not quite as reliable as Sabouraud's media, the distinctive color change in DTM is helpful in the evaluation of fungal cultures for those not proficient in dermatophyte colony morphology.

5. Kligman AM: Tinea capitis due to *M. audouinii* and *M. canis:* II. Dynamics of host-parasite relationship. Arch. Dermatol. 71:313–337, 1955.

   Clarification of the pathogenesis of tinea capitis through sectioned biopsy specimens taken from the scalps of experimental subjects inoculated with *M. audouinii* and *M. canis.*

6. Mangalani PR, Ramanan C, Durairaj P, et al.: *Trichophyton tonsurans* infection in a 9-day-old infant. Int. J. Dermatol. 27:128, 1988.

   A report of a 15-day-old infant with *Trichophyton tonsurans* infection on the scalp, forehead, and trunk that began 6 days earlier.

7. Barlow D, Saxe N: Tinea capitis in adults. Int. J. Dermatol. 27:388–390, 1988.

   In a study of 46 adults with scalp problems and 25 asymptomatic adult contacts of children with tinea capitis, adult forms of the disorder were found to be much more common than previously noted in the literature.

8. Babel DE, Baugmans A: Evaluation of the adult carrier stage in juvenile tinea capitis caused by *Trichophyton tonsurans.* J. Am. Acad. Dermatol. 21:1209–1212, 1989.

   This study of parents and grandparents of 50 children with *T. tonsurans* tinea capitis in which 14 of 46 fungal cultures of asymptomatic adults grew out *T. tonsurans* confirms the fact that asymptomatic adult carriers are common.

9. Hebert AA, Head ES, Macdonald EM: Tinea capitis caused by *Trichophyton tonsurans.* Pediatr. Dermatol. 2:219–223, 1985.

   A report of a 16-year-old black mother who, having harbored a subclinical tinea infection of the scalp for years, apparently transmitted tinea capitis to her mother, grandmother, two aunts, her daughter, and newborn son.

10. Sharma V, Hall JC, Knapp JF, et al.: Scalp colonization by *Trichophyton tonsurans* in an urban pediatric clinic. Arch. Dermatol. *124*:1511–1513, 1988.

A study in which random culturing of the scalp of 200 apparently healthy children revealed a 4 per cent incidence of positive cultures for *T. tonsurans* suggested the possibility that tight braiding and dressing of the hair with petrolatum or other oils might contribute to scalp colonization by this organism.

11. Laude TA, Shah BR: Tinea capitis in Brooklyn. Am. J. Dis. Child. *136*:1047–1050, 1982.

A study of 144 children with tinea capitis in Brooklyn, New York, in which 96 children had positive cultures and 89 per cent were associated with *T. tonsurans*.

12. Rippon JW, Lucky AW, Hebert AA, et al.: Tinea capitis: Current concepts. Pediatr. Dermatol. *2*:224–237, 1985.

A comprehensive review of tinea capitis, its epidemiology, diagnosis, and management.

13. Dvoretzky I, Fisher BK, Movshovitz M, et al.: Favus. Int. J. Dermatol. *19*:89–91, 1980.

A report of two patients and a comprehensive review of favus, its clinical features and management.

14. Sheretz EF: Are laboratory studies necessary for griseofulvin therapy? J. Am. Acad. Dermatol. *22*:1103, 1990.

An extensive review of patients who received griseofulvin on a long-term basis questions the need for routine laboratory monitoring of individuals receiving this preparation.

15. Miyagawa S, Okuchi T, Shiomi Y, et al.: Subacute cutaneous lupus erythematosus lesions precipitated by griseofulvin. J. Am. Acad. Dermatol. *21*:343–346, 1989.

A report of a patient with dermatomyositis in whom griseofulvin, given for the treatment of onychomycosis, was associated with eruptions similar to those of subacute cutaneous lupus erythematosus.

16. Tanz RR, Hebert AA, Esterly NB: Treating tinea capitis: Should ketoconazole replace griseofulvin? J. Pediatr. *112*:987–991, 1988.

In a 12-week study of patients with tinea capitis, 25 of 26 (95 per cent) patients who received griseofulvin were treated successfully and only 16 (73 per cent) of 22 patients treated with ketoconazole had a favorable response.

17. Robertson MH, Rich P, Parker F, et al.: Ketoconazole in griseofulvin-resistant dermatoses. J. Am. Acad. Dermatol. *6*:224–229, 1982.

The authors recommend griseofulvin over ketoconazole as the drug of choice for the treatment of dermatophytoses.

18. Lambert DR, Seigle RJ, Camisa C: Griseofulvin and ketoconazole in the treatment of dermatophyte infections. Int. J. Dermatol. *28*:300–304, 1989.

A review of griseofulvin and ketoconazole in the treatment of dermatophyte infections recommends griseofulvin as the drug of choice for dermatophyte infections that require systemic therapy and that ketoconazole be reserved for patients who do not respond to or cannot tolerate griseofulvin because of adverse effects.

19. Gan V, Petruska M, Ginsburg CM: Epidemiology and treatment of tinea capitis: Ketoconazole vs. griseofulvin. Pediatr. Infect. Dis. J. 6:46–49, 1987.

In a study in which tinea capitis was cured in 92 per cent of griseofulvin-treated (as compared with 59 per cent of ketoconazole-treated) patients, the authors suggest that recommended dosages of ketoconazole may be inadequate for the treatment of tinea capitis.

20. Lesher JL, Smith JG Jr: Antifungal agents in dermatology. J. Am. Acad. Dermatol. *17*:383–394, 1987.

A comprehensive review of currently available antifungal agents.

21. Lesher JL Jr, Smith JG Jr: Antifungal agents in dermatology (letter reply). J. Am. Acad. Dermatol. *18*:760–761, 1989.

The authors, commenting on the conflicting reports in the literature regarding the effect of food, if any, on the absorption of ketoconazole, conclude that there is no definitive answer on this question.

22. Sheretz EF: Pharmalocogy: II. Systemic drugs in dermatology. J. Am. Acad. Dermatol. *21*:298–305, 1989.

A review of the mechanism of action, metabolism, potential drug interactions and adverse effects of the major systemic agents used in clinical dermatology.

23. Sonino N: The use of ketoconazole as an inhibitor of steroid production. N. Engl. J. Med. *317*:812–818, 1988.

Ketoconazole, because of its action as a steroid inhibitor, can also be used as a therapeutic tool in the management of prostatic cancer, precocious puberty, Cushing's syndrome, and disorders of androgen excess.

24. Britton H, Shehab Z, Lightner E, et al.: Adrenal response in children receiving high doses of ketoconazole for systemic coccidiomycosis. J. Pediatr. *112*:488–492, 1988.

In a study of 10 children who received long-term (3 to 52 months) ketoconazole therapy the authors suggest that ketoconazole blocks aldosterone and cortisol at the 11-hydroxylase step of steroid biosynthesis.

25. Allen HB, Honig PJ, Leyden JJ, et al: Selenium sulfide: Adjunctive therapy for tinea capitis. Pediatrics 69:81–83, 1983.

In children with *Trichophyton tonsurans* scalp infection treated with oral griseofulvin, the addition of twice-a-week selenium sulfide shampooing resulted in negative hair cultures after 2 weeks. In patients who were treated with griseofulvin alone, or griseofulvin in combination with daily application of clotrimazole lotion, the cultures remained positive for up to 8 weeks.

26. Legendre R, Escola-Macre J: Itraconazole in the treatment of tinea capitis. J. Am. Acad. Dermatol. *23*:559–560, 1990.

Studies of 50 patients with tinea capitis revealed itraconazole to be safe and effective for the treatment of this disorder.

27. Hay RJ, Logan RA, Moore MK, et al.: A comparative study of terbinafine versus griseofulvin in "dry-type" dermatophyte infections. J. Am. Acad. Dermatol. *24*:243–246, 1991.

In a double-blind comparative study of chronic dermatophyte infections of the feet or hands, oral terbinafine showed a significantly better response after long-term follow-up than griseofulvin. Six months after treatment all nine patients whose skin had cleared with terbinafine therapy remained in remission versus only one of seven patients treated with griseofulvin.

28. Kahn G: Letters to the editor: Kerion treatment. Pediatrics *61*:501, 1978.

Prednisone with griseofulvin appears to be the most effective form of therapy for kerion.

29. Keipert JA: Beneficial effect of corticosteroid therapy in *Microsporum canis* kerion. Aust. J. Dermatol. *25*:127–130, 1984.

In a report of three children with microsporum kerion, the addition of systemic prednisolone to their therapy produced an extremely rapid decrease in the inflammatory changes associated with this disorder.

30. Dobson RL: Editorial comment. In: 1979 Year Book of Dermatology. Year Book Medical Publishers, Chicago, 1979, 124.

In a discussion of an article on children with tinea capitis, the editor suggests the use of oral saturated solution of potassium iodide for the treatment of kerion.

31. Yesudian P, Kamalam A: *Epidermophyton floccosum* infection in a three-week-old infant. Trans. St. John's Hosp. Dermatol. Soc. *59*:1, 66–67, 1973.

A 3-week-old infant with ringworm infection (*E. floccosum*) infection on the skin overlying the left hip.

32. Kramalam A, Thambiah AS: Tinea facei caused by *Microsporum gypseum* in a 2-day-old infant. Mykosen *24*:40–42, 1981.

A report of a tinea infection on the face of a 2-day-old infant.

33. Khare AK, Singh G, Pandey SS, et al.: Kerion, tinea faciei and tinea corporis in an infant. Indian J. Dermatol. Venereol. Lepro. *50*:271–272, 1984.

A report of *Trichophyton mentagrophytes* infection in a 3-day-old infant.

34. Jacobs AH, O'Connell BM: Tinea in tiny tots. Am. J. Dis. Child. *140*:1034–1038, 1986.

A review of tinea infections frequently overlooked and misdiagnosed in infants and young children.

35. Cavanaugh RM, Greeson JD: *Trichophyton rubrum* infection of the diaper area. Arch. Dermatol. *118*:446, 1982.

A report of a 9-month-old infant with a *T. rubrum* infection in the diaper area.

36. Ive FA, Marks R: Tinea incognito. Br. Med. J. *3*:149–152, 1968.

Fourteen patients with "Tinea incognito," an unusual presentation of tinea corporis due to topical application of corticosteroids.

37. Jones HE, Reinhardt JH, Rinaldi MB: A clinical, mycological, and immunological survey for dermatophytosis. Arch. Dermatol. *108*:61–65, 1973.

Data in a study of 180 subjects suggest that susceptibility to chronic tinea infection in atopic individuals appears to be related to a lack of delayed cell-mediated immunity coexistent with increase in antibody (presumably IgE).

38. Reynolds RD, Boiko S, Lucky AW: Exacerbation of tinea corporis during treatment with 1% clotrimazole/0.05% betamethasone dipropionate (Lotrisone). Am. J. Dis. Child. *145*:1224–1225, 1991.

Fluorinated topical corticosteroid/antifungal combinations should not be used for conditions in which a single topical antifungal agent would suffice.

39. Schwartz BK, Clendenning WE: Tinea pedis during childhood. Cutis *40*:477–478, 1987.

A report of a 4-year-old boy with a dermatophyte infection on the dorsal aspect of both feet reaffirms the fact that this disorder must be considered in the differential diagnosis of persistent cutaneous dermatoses of the feet, even in young children.

40. Kearse HL, Miller OF III: Tinea pedis in prepubertal children: Does it occur? J. Am. Acad. Dermatol. *19*:619–622, 1988.

Although tinea pedis is less common in prepubertal children, the authors were able to demonstrate dermatophyte infection in 8 of 15 consecutive prepubertal children with foot dermatitis.

41. Broberg A, Faergemann J: Scaly lesions on the feet in children: Tinea or eczema? Acta Paediatr. Scand. *79*:349–351, 1990.

A report of 20 children with juvenile plantar dermatosis, a common disorder of childhood often misdiagnosed as tinea pedis. (This disorder is discussed in Chapter 3.)

42. Philpot CM, Shuttleworth D: Dermatophyte onychomycosis in children. Clin. Exp. Dermatol. *14*:203–205, 1989.

Dermatophyte onychomycosis, although uncommon in children, should alert the physician to the possibility of parental tinea pedis as a source of infection.

43. Davies RR, Everall JD, Hamilton E: Mycological and clinical evaluation of griseofulvin for chronic onychomycosis. Br. Med. J. *3*:464–468, 1967.

Griseofulvin, even when given over a 2-year period, rarely cures dermatophyte infections of the toenails.

44. Quadripur SA, Horn G, Hohler T: On the local efficacy of ciclopiroxolamine in onychomycoses. Arzneimittelforschung *31*:1369–1372, 1981.

Topical applications of ciclopirox (Loprox) seem to be helpful for the treatment of some patients with dermatophytic onychomycosis.

45. Klaschka F: Treatment of onychomycosis with naftifine gel. Mykosen *30*(suppl 1):119–123, 1987.

In a study of 50 patients with onychomycosis, a cure was achieved in 42 per cent of those treated with twice-daily applications of naftifine gel for 6 months.

46. Baran R, Hay RJ: Partial surgical avulsion of the nail in onychomycosis. Clin. Exp. Dermatol. *10*:413–418, 1985.

Twenty patients with onychomycosis were treated successfully by a combination of systemic or topical fungal therapy in conjunction with surgical removal of the segment of the nail plate harboring the disease.

47. Farber EM, South DA: Urea ointment in the nonsurgical avulsion of nail dystrophies. Cutis *22*:689–692, 1978.

Topical application of a formulation containing 40 per cent urea, 20 per cent anhydrous lanolin, 5 per cent white wax, and 35 per cent white petrolatum applied to the nail plate under occlusion for a period of 7 to 10 days is recommended as a nonsurgical approach to the removal of nails.

48. Pontasch MJ, Kyanok ME, Brodell RT: Tinea versicolor of the face in black children in a temperate region. Cutis *43*:81–84, 1989.

The authors comment on the use of cocoa butter and its possible role in the production of tinea versicolor on the faces of two young black children.

49. McGinley KJ, Lantis LR, Marples RR: Microbiology of tinea versicolor. Arch. Dermatol. *102*:168–171, 1970.

Studies of normal and affected skin of patients with tinea versicolor support the dimorphous concept that *Pityrosporum orbiculare* becomes pathogenic when it changes from a *yeast* to a *filamentous* form.

50. Smith EB, Gellerman GL: Tinea versicolor in infancy. Arch. Dermatol. *93*:362–363, 1966.

Report of an 8-week-old infant with tinea versicolor and review of the subject of tinea versicolor in infancy.

51. Michalowski R, Rodziewizc H: Pityriasis versicolor in children. Br. J. Dermatol. *75*:397–400, 1963.

A study of 305 children between the ages of 4 months and 10 years with tinea versicolor.

52. Powell DA, Hayes J, Durrell DE, et al.: *Malassezia furfur* skin colonization of infants hospitalized in intensive care units. J. Pediatr. *111*:217–220, 1987.

Of 361 infants studied over 1 year, 36.8 per cent had at least one positive culture for *M. furfur;* the more premature the infant and the longer the hospitalization, the more apparent the risk of cutaneous colonization.

53. Charles RC, Sire DJ, Johnson BL, et al.: Hypopigmentation in tinea versicolor: A histochemical and electron microscopic study. Int. J. Dermatol. *12*:48–58, 1973.

Electron microscopic studies suggest an abnormal pigment transfer from melanocyte to keratinocyte as the cause of the pigmentary disturbance seen in lesions of tinea versicolor.

54. Albright SD, Hitch JM: Rapid treatment of tinea versicolor with selenium sulfide. Arch. Dermatol. *93*:460–462, 1966.

Selenium sulfide shampoo, applied to the skin of patients with tinea versicolor (dried and left on overnight) offers a convenient and effective therapeutic approach to the management of this disorder.

55. Alteras I, Sandbank M, Segal R: Two years of follow-up of oral ketoconazole therapy in 60 cases of pityriasis versicolor. Dermatologica *175*:142–144, 1987.

Despite excellent initial results, patients with tinea versicolor treated with 200 mg of ketoconazole daily for 21 days showed high recurrence rates.

56. Faergemann J, Djárv L: Tinea versicolor: Treatment and prophylaxis with ketoconazole. Cutis 30:542–545, 1982.

Ketoconazole (200 mg/day) cured 26 of 32 patients with tinea versicolor in 3 weeks (the remaining 6 patients were cured in 5 weeks). In 30 of the patients, subsequent doses of ketoconazole (200 mg/day) for 3 consecutive days each month for 6 months prevented recurrences in all but one.

57. Zaias N: Correspondence: Pityriasis versicolor with ketoconazole. J. Am. Acad. Dermatol. 20:703–704, 1989.

The author recommends a 5-day course of oral ketoconazole (200 mg/day) as the treatment of choice for pityriasis versicolor (a 5-day regimen appeared to be just as effective as a 10-day course of treatment).

58. Jones HE: Pityriasis versicolor with ketoconazole. J. Am. Acad. Dermatol. 20:704–705, 1989.

Since some patients appeared to require an additional treatment, a 400 mg dose of ketoconazole, repeated 7 to 10 days later, is recommended as an effective form of systemic therapy for patients with tinea versicolor.

59. Blank H: Tinea nigra: A twenty-year incubation period? J. Am. Acad. Dermatol. 1:49–51, 1979.

Twenty years after studying tinea nigra in two volunteers, Dr. Harvey Blank and one of his volunteers developed tinea nigra palmaris at the original infection sites.

60. Palmer SR, Bass JW, Mandojana R, et al.: Tinea palmaris and plantaris: A black fungus producing black spots on the palms and soles. Pediatr. Infect. Dis. J. 8:48–50, 1989.

A report of three children with tinea nigra, an uncommon fungal infection easily confused with other disorders such as pigmented junctional nevi or malignant melanoma.

61. Carr JF, Lewis CW: Tinea nigra palmaris: Treatment with thiabendazole topically. Arch. Dermatol. 111:904–905, 1975.

Tinea nigra palmaris, unresponsive to topical applications of tolnaftate or salicylic acid ointment, cleared following a 2-week course of topical thiabendazole (Mintezol, 100 mg/ml) suspension application.

62. Kalter DC, Tschen JA, Cernoch PL, et al.: Genital white piedra; Epidemiology, microbiology, and therapy. J. Am. Acad. Dermatol. 14:982–993, 1986.

A study in Houston, Texas, suggests that infection with Trichosporon beigelii is common in young patients with genital complaints, also occurs in female patients, and is endemic in Houston and perhaps other parts of the United States.

63. Kozinn PJ, Taschdjin CL, Dragutsky D, et al.: Cutaneous candidiasis in early infancy and childhood. Pediatrics 20:827–834, 1957.

In a study of 2175 infants, 100 per cent of neonates and 80 per cent of older infants and young children with candidal diaper rashes harbored C. albicans in the intestines.

64. Harris LJ, Pritzker HG, Laski B, et al.: Effect of nystatin (Mycostatin) on neonatal candidiasis (thrush). Method of eradicating thrush from hospital nurseries. Can. Med. Assoc. J. 79:891–896, 1958.

Although the prophylactic treatment of newborns with oral nystatin can reduce the incidence of thrush tenfold (from 4.0 to 0.4 per cent), the rarity of serious pathology due to Candida does not warrant oral nystatin prophylaxis in newborns.

65. Schechtman LB, Funaro L, Robin T, et al.: Clotrimazole treatment of oral candidiasis with neoplastic disease. Am. J. Med. 76:91–94, 1984.

Clotrimazole troches, dissolved in the mouth and then swallowed, cleared candidal esophagitis in five of six patients.

66. Gombert ME, DuBouchet L, Aulicinol TM, et al.: A comparative trial of clotrimazole troches and oral nystatin suspension

in recipients of renal transplants: Use in prophylaxis of oropharyngeal candidiasis. J.A.M.A. 258:2553–2555, 1987.

Clotrimazole troches and oral nystatin suspension three times a day for 60 days were found to be equally effective for the prevention of oropharyngeal candidiasis in renal transplant recipients.

67. Mansour A, Gelfond EW: A new approach to the treatment of infants with persistent oral candidiasis. J. Pediatr. 98:161–162, 1981.

Although two infants with persistent oral candidiasis were successfully treated with clotrimazole or nystatin suppositories or troches inserted into the tips of nipples or pacifiers, the possibility of aspiration must be considered when this form of therapy is used.

68. Abramovits W: Persistent oral candidiasis in an infant due to pacifier contamination. Clin. Pediatr. 20:393, 1981.

Persistent oral candidiasis in a 3-month-old infant, despite treatment with nystatin oral suspension, was traced to candidal contamination of the infant's pacifier (the infection cleared rapidly once the use of the contaminated pacifier was discontinued).

69. Kam LA, Giacoia GP: Congenital cutaneous candidiasis. Am. J. Dis. Child. 129:1215–1218, 1978.

Two cases of congenital cutaneous candidiasis and a summary of the clinical characteristics of this disorder and its differentiation from neonatal cutaneous candidiasis.

70. Rudolph N, Taria AA, Reale MR, et al.: Congenital cutaneous candidiasis. Arch. Dermatol. 113:1101–1103, 1977.

Macular, papular, vesiculopustular, and bullous lesions followed by desquamation are the cutaneous manifestations in three newborns with congenital cutaneous candidiasis.

71. Baley JE, Silverman RA: Systemic candidiasis: Cutaneous manifestations in low birth weight infants. Pediatrics 82:211–215, 1989.

A review of 18 infants treated for systemic candidiasis suggests that infants with birth weights less than 1500 g are at greater risk for systemic involvement and that premature infants suspected of having candidal infection should be treated with systemic therapy regardless of the presence or absence of positive systemic cultures.

72. Hughes D, Kriedman T: Treatment of vulvovaginal candidiasis with a 500-mg vaginal tablet of clotrimazole. Clin. Ther. 6:662–668, 1984.

In a prospective randomized double-blinded study of patients with clinically and mycologically proven vulvovaginal candidiasis, 9 of 10 patients treated with a one-dose, 500-mg vaginal clotrimazole tablet were shown to be clinically and mycologically clear of infection.

73. Keller MA, Sellers BB Jr, Melish ME, et al.: Systemic candidiasis in infants: A case presentation and literaturre review. Am. J. Dis. Child. 131:1260–1263, 1977.

A 4½-month-old infant with systemic candidiasis following exchange transfusion for hyperbilirubinemia and subsequent surgical repair of a patent ductus arteriosus at 20 days of age.

74. Rockoff AS: Chronic mucocutaneous candidiasis: Successful treatment with intermittent oral doses of clotrimazole. Arch. Dermatol. 115:322–323, 1979.

Report of a 9-year-old girl with chronic mucocutaneous candidiasis who achieved a prolonged remission following treatment with the imidazole antibiotic clotrimazole.

75. Fisher TJ, Klein RB, Kershnar HE, et al.: Miconazole in treatment of chronic mucocutaneous candidiasis: Preliminary report. J. Pediatr. 91:815–819, 1977.

Evaluation of intravenous miconazole in the treatment of five children with chronic mucocutaneous candidiasis.

76. Logan RI, Goldberg MJ: C. albicans resistance to 5-fluorocytosine. Br. Med. J. 3:531, 1972.

A 53-year-old man who developed a 5-fluorocytosine resistant *Candida albicans* infection of the throat and bloodstream while on treatment for endocarditis.

77. Leikin S, Parrott R, Randolph J: Clotrimazole treatment of chronic mucocutaneous candidiasis. J. Pediatr. *88*:864–866, 1976.

   Report of a beneficial response to oral clotrimazole in an 11-year-old girl with multiple immunologic defects and chronic mucocutaneous candidiasis.

78. Burke WA: Use of itraconazole in a patient with chronic mucocutaneous candidiasis. J. Am. Acad. Dermatol. *21*:1309–1310, 1989.

   Itraconazole was found to produce a dramatic clinical improvement in an 11-year-old patient with chronic refractory dermatophytosis and extensive *Candida* granulomas.

79. Lynch PJ, Botero F: Sporotrichosis in children. Am. J. Dis. Child. *122*:325–327, 1971.

   Nine of 11 childhood cases of sporotrichosis developed their initial lesion on an exposed area of the face, arms, or legs.

80. Orr ER, Riley HD Jr: Sporotrichosis in childhood. J. Pediatr. *78*:951–957, 1971.

   Ten children ages 3 to 16 with sporotrichosis.

81. Dahl BA, Silberfarb DM, Sgrosi GA, et al.: Sporotrichosis in children: Report of an epidemic. J.A.M.A. *215*:1980–1982, 1971.

   A report of sporotrichosis in nine children who had been playing among contaminated bales of prairie hay.

82. Frumkin A, Tisserand ME: Sporotrichosis in a father and son. J. Am. Acad. Dermatol. *20*:964–967, 1989.

   A report of two father-and-son pairs with sporotrichosis and a summary of published familial cases.

83. Dunstan RW, Langham RF, Reimann KA, et al.: Feline sporotrichosis: A report of five cases with transmission to humans. J. Am. Acad. Dermatol. *15*:37–45, 1986.

   A report of seven individuals with lymphocutaneous forms of sporotrichosis following bite wounds, a traumatic wound, or contact with infected cats.

84. Rafal ES, Rasmussen JE: An unusual presentation of fixed cutaneous sporotrichosis: A case report and review of the literature. J. Am. Acad. Dermatol. *25*:928–932, 1991.

   A report of an 84-day-old girl with fixed sporotrichosis, presumably transmitted by a cat; to the authors' knowledge this is the youngest reported patient with this disorder.

85. Smith PW, Loomis GW, Luksasen JL, et al.: Disseminated cutaneous sporotrichosis: Three illustrative cases. Arch. Dermatol. *117*:143–144, 1981.

   A report of three patients and a discussion of the pathogenesis, diagnosis, and treatment of disseminated sporotrichosis.

86. Restropo A, Reboldo J, Gomez I, et al.: Itraconazole therapy in lymphangitic and cutaneous sporotrichosis. Arch. Dermatol. *122*:413–417, 1986.

   Itraconazole, 100 mg/day for periods of 90 to 180 days, was shown to be a safe and effective form of therapy for sporotrichosis.

87. DeFeo CP, Harber LC: Chromoblastomycosis treated with local infiltration of amphotericin B solution: Report of a second case. J.A.M.A. *171*:1961–1963, 1959.

   Choromoblastomycosis of 22 years' duration caused by *Hormodendrum pedrosoi*—the second case of favorable response to amphotericin B injected locally in a 2 per cent procaine solution.

88. Tagami H, Ginoza M, Imaizumi S, et al.: Successful treatment of chromoblastomycosis with topical heat therapy. J. Am. Acad. Dermatol. *10*:615–619, 1984.

   Five patients with localized chromoblastomycosis were cured by topical heat therapy (pocket warmers) over a median period of 3 months.

89. Tuffanelli L, Milburn PB: Treatment of chromoblastomycosis. J. Am. Acad. Dermatol. *23*:728–732, 1990.

   A review of chromoblastomycosis and its treatment with emphasis on itraconazole as the possible drug of choice.

90. Klein BS, Vergeront JM, Weeks RJ, et al.: Isolation of *Blastomycoses dermatidis* in soil associated with a large outbreak of blastomycosis in Wisconsin. N. Engl. J. Med. *314*:529–534, 1986.

   An outbreak of blastomycosis in children and adults who visited a camp in Wisconsin suggests that *B. dermatidis* in the soil along ponds and river banks may be an important source of human blastomycosis infection.

91. Townsend TE, McKey RW: Coccidioidomycosis in infants. Am. J. Dis. Child. *86*:51–53, 1953.

   Although human transmission of coccidioidomycosis is extremely rare, a 3-week-old female infant, who did not live in an endemic area but was exposed to a father who lived in southwestern United States where coccidioidomycosis is endemic, had pneumonitis, meningoencephalitis, and positive cerebrospinal fluid cultures of *Coccidioides immitis*.

92. Winn WA: The treatment of coccidioidal meningitis: The use of amphotericin B in a group of 25 patients. Calif. Med. *101*:78–79, 1964.

   Intracisternal amphotericin B as an adjunct to intravenous and intraspinal therapy in the treatment of coccidioidal meningitis.

93. Tucker RM, Denning DW, Arathoon EG, et al.: Itraconazole therapy for nonmeningeal coccidioidomycosis: Clinical and laboratory observations. J. Am. Acad. Dermatol. *23*:593–601, 1990.

   Itraconazole, in dosages of 50 to 400 mg/day for a median of 10 months, showed impressive activity in a large series of patients with refractory disseminated coccidioidomycosis.

94. Barson WJ, Ruymann FB: Palmar aspergillosis in immunocompromised children. Pediatr. Infect. Dis. *5*:264–268, 1986.

   A report of five children with palmar aspergillosis, all of whom had an underlying hematologic or oncogenic disorder, were granulocytopenic and had received parenteral immunosuppressive therapy adjacent to the area of the palmar infection.

95. Dupont B: Itraconazole therapy in aspergillosis: Study in 49 patients. J. Am. Acad. Dermatol. *23*:607–614, 1990.

   Itraconazole, 200 to 400 mg orally, once a day at mealtime, was found to be useful as an alternative to amphotericin B for the treatment of patients with invasive osseous and pulmonary forms of aspergillosis.

96. Kramer BS, Hernandez AD, Reddick RL, et al.: Cutaneous infarction, manifestation of disseminated mucormycosis. Arch. Dermatol. *113*:1075–1076, 1978.

   Cutaneous infarction resembling ecthyma gangrenosum as a manifestation of mucormycosis.

97. Meyer RA, Kaplan MH, Ong M, et al.: Cutaneous lesions in disseminated mucormycosis. J.A.M.A. *225*:737–738, 1973.

   An 8-year-old boy with leukemia, widespread systemic mucormycosis, and cutaneous vasculitis as an unusual cutaneous manifestation.

INSECT BITES AND PARASITIC INFESTATIONS

Parasites are a fascinating and important cause of skin disease in children. They produce their effects in various ways: mechanical trauma of bites or stings, injection of pharmacologically active substances that induce local or systemic effects, allergic reactions in a previously sensitized host, persistent granulomatous reactions to retained mouth parts, direct invasion of the epidermis, or transmission of infectious disease by blood-sucking insects.

ARTHROPODS

Arthropods are elongated invertebrate animals with segmented bodies, true appendages, and a chitinous exoskeleton. Those of dermatologic significance are the eight-legged arachnids (mites, ticks, spiders, and scorpions), the six-legged insects (lice, flies, mosquitoes, fleas, bugs, bees, wasps, ants, beetles), caterpillars, and moths.

Arachnids

The term *mite* refers to a large number of tiny arachnids, many of which live at least part of their lives as parasites upon animals or plants or in prepared foods. Of greatest medical significance are itch mites (*Sarcoptes scabiei*), grain mites, and harvest mites (chiggers). They attack humans by burrowing under or attaching themselves to the skin where they inflict trivial bites and cause associated dermatitides.

ITCH MITES (SCABIES)

Scabies is a contagious disorder caused by an itch mite, *Sarcoptes scabiei*, which attacks infants and children as well as adults. Although clinical descriptions of scabies date back to civilization's earliest records, it was not until 1687 that Bonomo first teased the mite out of a scabietic lesion and, with the aid of a light microscope, described the responsible organism and its etiologic role in scabies.[1] Unfortunately, either through ignorance or prejudice, two centuries passed before the parasite was officially acknowledged as the true cause of this disorder.

Over 50 years ago John Stokes commented that scabies was both the easiest and yet the most difficult diagnosis in dermatology. This is just as true today as it was in 1936.[2] Epidemics of scabies seem to occur in 30-year cycles, each one lasting about 15 years, with a 15-year gap between the end of each cycle and the beginning of the next. It appears that we are presently in the midst of a worldwide pandemic, one that began in 1964; although the current epidemic is widespread, it does not appear to be of sufficient intensity to limit the cycle to the usual 15 years and therefore has persisted longer than originally anticipated.[3, 4]

Infestation begins with a newly fertilized female

mite. Pinpoint in size and barely visible to the unaided eye, the oviporous parasite is oval, eight legged, translucent, and pearly gray, measuring less than 0.5 mm in length (Fig. 14–1). It tunnels into the stratum corneum and lives in cutaneous burrows, which may measure several millimeters to a few centimeters in length.[2] What determines the area of the burrow is unknown; apparently the parasite favors areas with a low concentration of pilosebaceous follicles and a thin stratum corneum.[5] This seems to account for a difference in the distribution of lesions in infants and young children as compared with that seen in older children and adults.

During the years from 1970 to 1976 I had the opportunity to see over 400 infants and children with scabies, ranging in age from 2 months to 18 years of age.[6] The first of these was a 3-month-old white female infant who started with a pruritic, scaly, erythematous papular eruption on the trunk, the postauricular areas, and extremities at 2 months of age (Fig. 14–2). Microscopic examination of skin scrapings and fungal cultures were done, and the eruption was treated as a seborrheic dermatitis with frequent shampoos and topical fluocinolone acetonide cream.

Two weeks later the rash had spread to the back of the head and neck, the entire trunk, and all extremities, including the palms and soles. A 3-mm cutaneous punch biopsy revealed a nonspecific dermatitis with focal parakeratosis and a mild dermal mononuclear infiltrate. A second skin biopsy several days later revealed a more severe der-

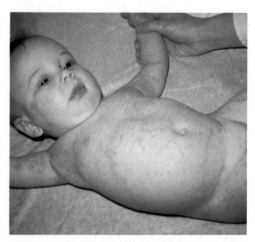

Figure 14–2. A 3-month-old infant with a scaly erythematous papular eczematoid eruption due to scabies. (Hurwitz S: Scabies in babies. Am. J. Dis. Child. *126*:226, 1973.)

mal mononuclear infiltrate, hyperkeratosis and parakeratosis of the stratum corneum, and a burrow within the hyperkeratotic stratum corneum, which suggested the presence of *Sarcoptes scabiei* (Fig. 14–3). Microscopic examination of skin scrapings subsequently confirmed the diagnosis of scabies.

The infant's parents and two babysitters were examined and found to have excoriated papules and nodules of the trunk, axillae, wrists, and interdigital spaces of the fingers, with involvement of the areolae of the mother, both babysitters, and the genital area of the father. Subsequently a total of 32 cases were detected through direct or indirect exposure to this infant, including my wife and myself. The initial source of exposure to the scabies mite was never determined, but the disease must have been contracted either in the hospital during the newborn period or shortly thereafter by other personal contacts, possibly babysitters.

Clinical Manifestations. The eruption in scabies presents as a distinctive clinical syndrome of pruritic papules, vesicles, and linear burrows. Unfortunately most patients do not present this pure a picture, but rather a mixture of primary lesions, intermingled with or obliterated by excoriation, eczematization, crusting, or secondary infection (Table 14–1). Primary lesions of scabies consist of burrows, papules, and vesicular lesions (Fig. 14–4). Burrows represent the home of the invading female parasite (Fig. 14–5), the papules appear to represent temporary invasion by the larval stages of the parasite, and the vesiculation is believed to be the result of sensitization of the host. The severe itching that accompanies this disorder takes 4 to 6 weeks to develop and also is believed to be related to sensitization. Until this sensitization occurs, the disorder is usually unrecognized and almost never diagnosed.

In adults and older children lesions tend to involve the webs of the fingers (Table 14–2; Fig.

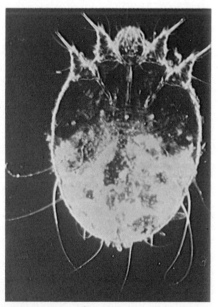

Figure 14–1. Microscopic appearance of an adult female mite of *Sarcoptes scabiei*. Pinpoint in size (less than 0.5 mm in length) and barely visible to the unaided eye, the parasite is oval, eight-legged, translucent, and pearly gray. (Courtesy of Reed & Carnrick.)

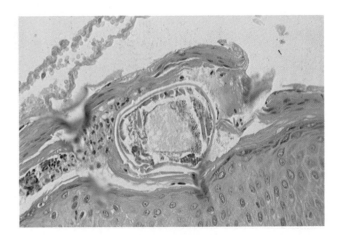

Figure 14–3. Scabies. Microscopic examination of a cutaneous biopsy reveals a burrow containg an adult female mite (*S. scabiei*) within the stratum corneum.

14–6), the axillae, the flexures of the arms and wrists, the beltline, and the areas around the nipples, genitals, and lower buttocks. In infants and young children the distribution is altered and includes the palms (Fig. 14–7), soles, head, neck, and face (Figs. 14–8 and 14–9).[6] Although bullous lesions are uncommon, vesicles are often found in infants and young children, owing to the predisposition for blister formation seen in this age group. The recurrent crops of vesicles and pustules seen on the hands and feet and occasionally elsewhere appear to represent hypersensitivity reaction and may sometimes persist for weeks to months despite repeated scabicidal therapy. Bullous lesions, however, are unusual and generally suggest secondary infection (Fig. 14–10).

The burrow, long considered a pathognomonic sign of scabies, unfortunately is demonstrable in a mere 7 to 13 per cent of adult patients.[6–8] In infants and children this is even less convenient a clue, owing to frequent obliteration by vigorous hygiene, excoriation, and secondary eczematization, crusting, or infection.[6]

Nodular Scabies. A high percentage of children who develop scabies have been found to develop persistent reddish brown infiltrated nodules, particularly on the covered parts of the body (the axillae, shoulders, groin, buttocks, and genital area (Figs. 14–11 and 14–12). These lesions represent a hypersensitivity reaction to the scabies mite, often persist for months despite therapy, and when present may be misdiagnosed, both clinically and on histopathologic examination, as forms of histiocytosis or lymphoma.[9]

An increased frequency of scabies, varying between 5 and 10 per cent, possibly even higher, has been noted in foreign-born children, principally from Korea and South Vietnam, who have been brought to this country for adoption. It has been noted that high numbers of these children seem to develop the granulomatous nodular lesions.[10]

Crusted (Norwegian) Scabies. This distinctive form of scabies is characterized by extensive heavily crusted skin lesions, with thick hyperkeratotoic areas on the scalp, ears, elbows, knees, palms, soles, and buttocks. Crusted scabies is highly contagious, even on casual contact, because of the vast numbers of mites in the exfoliating scales and the lengthy period of time until the diagnosis is established. The predilection of this disease for the physically debilitated, mentally retarded, and immunologically deficient remains unknown.[11, 12]

Animal-Transmitted Scabies. Children can be infested by *Sarcoptes* from domestic animals. This infestation is not permanent and dies out in a few

Table 14–1. CLINICAL APPEARANCE OF SCABIES

A. Primary Lesions
  1. Pruritic papules
  2. Vesicles
  3. Burrows
B. Secondary Lesions
  1. Excoriations
  2. Eczematization
  3. Crusts
  4. Secondary infection

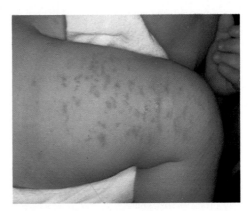

Figure 14–4. Papulovesicular lesions of scabies in a 2½-year-old child.

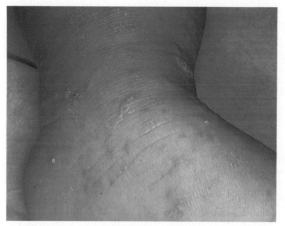

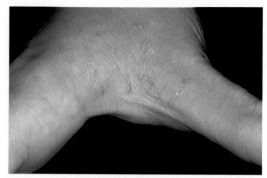

Figure 14–6. Scabietic lesions in the web between the thumb and index finger of an 11-year-old child.

Figure 14–5. Scabies on the foot and ankle of a 10-month-old infant.

weeks. Although persons may be susceptible to mites from a variety of domestic animals, the human's close relationship to the dog makes the canine form of animal scabies the most common type transmitted to humans.[13–17] Canine scabies, or sarcoptic mange, causes patchy loss of hair with scaling in the dog. It is seen most commonly in undernourished, heavily parasitized puppies. A presumptive diagnosis of canine scabies can be made on the basis of exposure to a pet with a pruritic papular eruption, alopecia involving mainly the head, ears, and intertriginous folds, and the characteristic mouse-like odor of animals with extensive sarcoptic infestation.

In children with canine scabies the eruption is most common on the forearms, lower region of the chest, abdomen, and thighs. The distribution usually differs from that of human scabies in that it spares the interdigital webs and the genitalia. Absence of burrows and rare reports of finding the mite on microscopic examination of skin scrapings appear to be related to the fact the the mite of canine scabies does not reproduce on human skin. The infestation, therefore, is usually self-limiting and generally clears spontaneously within 4 to 6 weeks if the patient is not reexposed to the animal source.

Secondary Complications. Eczematous changes due to scratching and rubbing of involved areas or to topical therapeutic agents are common complications of scabies in infants and children. They are frequently aggravated by excessive bathing, overzealous attempts at hygiene, and associated dryness and pruritus. In infants, young children, and atopic individuals, such complications may be particularly severe and widespread.[6] Urticaria, although infrequently reported, has also been recognized as a complication of scabietic infestation and may at times be diagnosed only after careful examination of affected persons.[18]

Corticosteroid administration (topical or systemic) may further mask the diagnosis of scabies by amelioration of signs and symptoms while the infestation and its transmissibility persist. This frequently results in unusual clinical presentations, atypical distributions, and unusual extents of involvement, in some instances closely simulating a variety of other entities (Fig. 14–13). It has been suggested that unusual features of scabies associated with the use of topical corticosteroids may be related to a suppression of hypersensitivity cell-

Table 14–2. DISTRIBUTION OF LESIONS IN SCABIES

A. Older Children and Adults
 1. Interdigital webs
 2. Flexures of wrists and arms
 3. Axillae
 4. Belt line
 5. Areolae
 6. Genitalia
 7. Buttocks
B. Infants and Small Children
 1. Trunk and extremities
 2. Head, neck, palms, and soles

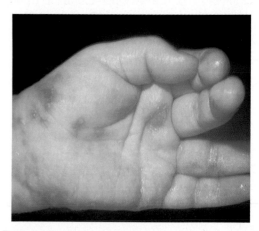

Figure 14–7. Infected scabies on the hand of an 18-month-old child (Hurwitz S: Scabies in babies. Am. J. Dis. Child. *126*:226, 1973.)

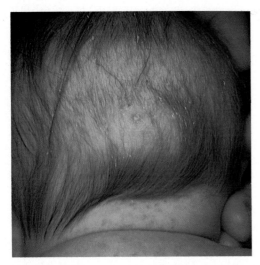

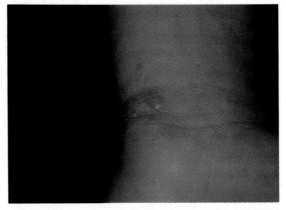

Figure 14–10. A bullous lesion on the wrist of a 9-year-old child with scabietic infestation.

Figure 14–8. Papulovesicular and crusted lesions on the scalp and nape of the neck of an infant with scabies.

mediated immunity.[19, 20] The term *scabies incognito* has been suggested for this phenomenon.[10]

Secondary infection, seen as pustulation, bullous impetigo, severe crusting, or ecthyma, is frequently seen as a complication of scabies in young children (Fig. 14–7). Recent epidemics of nephritis suggest that scabietic lesions are particularly favorable for the growth of virulent M-strains of nephritogenic streptococci. These are distinctive from the *Streptococcus* found in the throat and are associated with a high incidence of nephritis, reportedly in the neighborhood of 12 per cent.[21] This nephritogenic strain of *Streptococcus* is not as common in the northern part of the United States

as it is in the south, the Island of Trinidad in the West Indies, and parts of Africa.[22]

Diagnosis. The diagnosis of scabies is best made by the history of itching, a characteristic distribution of lesions, the recognition of primary lesions, particularly the pathognomonic burrow when present, and the presence of disease among the patient's family or associates (Table 14–3). In infants and children, however, the diagnosis of scabies is often overlooked because of a lower index of suspicion, an atypical distribution that includes the head, neck, palms, and soles, and obliteration of demonstrable primary lesions as a result of vigorous hygienic measures, excoriation, crusting, eczematization, and secondary infection.

Rapid and definitive confirmation can be made by microscopic examination of scrapings of suspicious lesions, with demonstration of the adult mite, ova, larva, or fecal matter (Fig. 14–14). The best

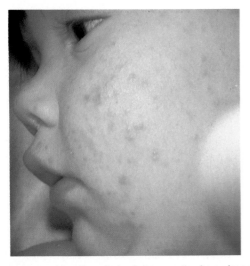

Figure 14–9. Papulovesicular lesions on the face of an 18-month-old child with scabies. (Hurwitz S: Scabies in babies. Am. J. Dis. Child. *126*:226, 1973.)

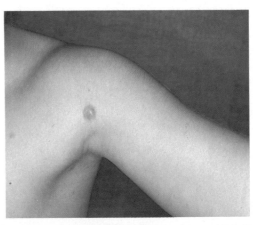

Figure 14–11. Postscabietic nodules (nodular scabies). The result of a hypersensitivity to the mite, these pruritic, reddish brown, infiltrated nodules generally appear on covered parts of the body (the axillae, shoulders, groin, buttocks, and genital area) and often persist for months.

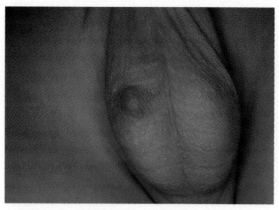

Figure 14–12. Postscabietic nodule, a hypersensitivity reaction to the scabies mite on the scrotum of a 6-year-old boy.

Table 14–3. DIAGNOSIS OF SCABIES

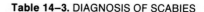

1. History of intractable itching
2. History of exposure to other cases
3. Character and distribution of lesions
4. Burrows (when present)
5. Microscopic examination of skin scrapings
6. Cutaneous biopsy

lesions for microscopic examination are fresh papules or identifiable burrows, ideally those where potential organisms and ova have not been scratched or excoriated. Potassium hydroxide, time-honored for microscopic examination of skin scrapings, dissolves the organisms, their ova, and excreta, thus making the diagnosis even more difficult and less reliable. In practical application, a drop of mineral oil on the suspected lesion will allow easier scraping of the lesion and more definitive identification of the pathogenic organism.[23]

Although positive microscopic identification of the parasite is dramatic, convincing, and helpful to the physician, I find the yield of such examinations in infants and small children to be particularly low, frustrating, and frequently unrewarding. When lesions are atypical or obliterated, therefore, diagnosis must be made by the history of intractable, particularly nocturnal pruritus, the character and distribution of the eruption, and the presence of associated contact cases. Despite the low yield and the time required for careful microscopic examination, I firmly believe that all suspected lesions should be scraped and minutely examined.

In patients in whom the true nature of the dermatosis remains undiagnosed, a cutaneous punch biopsy, although not always diagnostic, may rule out other diagnoses and assist in establishing the final correct diagnosis (see Fig. 14–3). Most skin biopsies of scabies demonstrate intracellular and intercellular edema, with or without vesicle formation, and a nonspecific lymphocytic infiltrate in the dermis. The histopathologic demonstration of a sarcoptic burrow within the stratum corneum is uncommon and frequently fortuitous. Except in overwhelming infestations such as crusted scabies, it is often found only after multiple sectionings and repeated biopsies.

In the differential diagnosis of scabies in infants and young children, atopic, contact, and irritant dermatitides are the most frequently confused and misdiagnosed. Other common misdiagnoses include Letterer-Siwe disease (histiocytosis X), seborrheic dermatitis, dermatitis herpetiformis, and papular urticaria. An awareness of scabies, the morphology and distribution of lesions, a history of itching or lesions in other members of the family, microscopic examination of skin scrapings, and histopathologic examination of lesions usually will

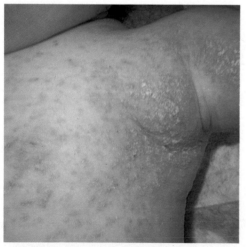

Figure 14–13. Eczematoid scabies (scabies incognito) following long-term topical corticosteroid therapy.

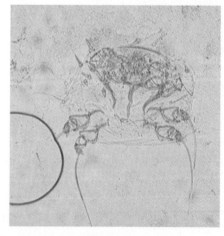

Figure 14–14. A gravid female of *S. scabiei* as seen on microscopic examination of a skin scraping of a patient with scabies. (Hurwitz S: Scabies in babies. Am. J. Dis. Child. *126*:226, 1973.)

help differentiate scabies from these cutaneous disorders.

Treatment. Present-day therapy for scabies consists of topical application of 1.0 per cent gamma benzene hexachloride (lindane, available as Kwell), 10 per cent crotamiton (Eurax), 6 to 10 per cent precipitate of sulfur in petrolatum, a suspension of benzyl benzoate in a 12.5 to 25 per cent concentration, and 5 per cent permethrin cream (Elimite) (Table 14–4).

Gamma Benzene Hexachloride (Lindane). Lindane, for years the most extensively used scabicide in the United States, because of reports of possible drug resistance and potential toxicity (particularly in infants and young children) has been supplanted by 5 per cent permethrin cream (Elimite) as the treatment of choice for scabietic therapy.[24] Although the majority of untoward effects attributed to the use of lindane have been associated with inappropriate, prolonged, or repetitive use, the problem of possible toxic effects becomes more acute in infants and small children, owing to a relatively greater skin surface and possibly higher blood level accumulations in this age group. Reactions attributed to the use of lindane include eczema, urticaria, aplastic anemia, possible alopecia, muscular spasms, and central nervous system toxicity, manifested by irritability, nausea, vomiting, amblyopia, headache, dizziness, and convulsions.[25–33]

Although studies by Taplin have shown that a 6-hour application is sufficient, current recommendations for the use of lindane suggest an 8- to 12-hour period of application for this preparation in a 1 per cent cream or lotion. Following the prescribed time of application the preparation should be washed off thoroughly, and a second application may be required 1 week later to destroy recently hatched larvae not eliminated by the initial treatment. There is no justification, however, for repeated treatment at more frequent intervals. This practice, which is unfortunately all too common, may result in toxicity due to abnormally high blood levels of this potentially toxic agent.[27, 28] Crusted lesions, if present, can be removed more easily following a tepid bath. If a bath is deemed necessary, the skin should be allowed to dry and cool in an effort to limit transcutaneous permeability and possible excessive levels of absorption. Although older children and adults should be treated from the neck down, in infants and young children, since the head and neck may also be affected, these areas should also be treated, with appropriate pre-

caution to avoid the eyes, nose, and mouth. Signs and symptoms of scabies may not clear for weeks, since the hypersensitivity state does not cease immediately after eradication of the infection. The patient and family should be alerted to this possibility so that they will know what to expect and will not be tempted to continue excessive, unnecessary, and potentially hazardous therapy.

Studies have shown that the scabies mite is unable to live for more than 5 minutes in temperatures above 120°F (50°C), or when away from its human host for periods of 2 days or more. Thus, if personal clothing and bedclothing of treated individuals are changed, laundered in a washing machine and dryer, or stored for a period of several days, reinfestation can usually be prevented.[34] Since symptoms and signs of infestation may not develop for 1 or 2 months after initial exposure, and asymptomatic or undiagnosed individuals may harbor mites and thus continue to transmit the disease, simultaneous treatment is generally recommended for all household members and close contacts in an effort to prevent reinfestation. When epidemics or localized outbreaks occur in institutions, hospitals, or nursing homes, patients, staff members, and visitors who have prolonged personal (skin-to-skin) contact with infested patients should also be considered for treatment.[35]

Permethrin Topical Cream. Permethrin 5 per cent cream (Elimite; AllerganHerbert), approved as a treatment for scabies by the U.S. Food and Drug Administration in September 1989, is recommended as the treatment of choice for infants, as young as 2 months of age, and children as well as adults.[36–38] Although scabies rarely infests the scalp of adults, but may infest the hairline, neck, temples, and forehead in infants and geriatric patients and the scalp, face and neck of infants and young children, this product should be applied and massaged into the skin from the neck down in older children and adults, and from the head to toes in infants and young children (including the palms and soles) and left on for 8 to 14 hours. When treating patients with permethrin, as with other agents, particular attention should be applied to the intertriginous areas, including the intergluteal cleft, and subungual areas.[39] As recommended with other forms of therapy, it is generally advisable to treat close family or personal contacts whether or not they show evidence of infestation. Rapidly metabolized, this agent can be safely repeated, if necessary, 2 weeks after initial treatment.

Crotamiton. Crotamiton (Eurax) has no reported systemic effects and may be used as a safe alternative for the treatment of pregnant women, infants, and small children. It should be noted, however, that crotamiton, currently recommended in a 2-day dose application of 24 hours each, even when used in a longer 5-day application regimen, only has a 69 per cent success rate. Crotamiton, however, can be irritating on raw or denuded skin and reportedly has caused sensitization after prolonged use in pa-

Table 14–4. TREATMENT OF SCABIES

1. 1.0% lindane (gamma benzene hexachloride, Kwell)
2. 10% crotamiton (Eurax)
3. 6% to 10% sulfur in petrolatum
4. 12.5% to 25% benzyl benzoate
5. 5% permethrin cream (Elimite)
6. Antipruritics (systemic and topical)
7. Appropriate antibiotics when necessary

tients with eczema. This agent, therefore, should be used with caution in patients with acutely inflamed, weeping cutaneous surfaces or atopic dermatitis, and is not recommended as a treatment of choice for scabietic infestation. [38, 40 41]

Benzyl Benzoate. Used extensively in the past for the management of scabies in the United Kingdom and Canada, although not readily available in the United States, benyzl benzoate can be compounded and used in concentrations of 12.5 to 25 per cent. Applied nightly or every other night for three applications, this preparation is effective and cosmetically acceptable but can result in an increase in pruritus or irritation. In such cases, topical or systemic antipruritic agents can be beneficial. Particular care should be exerted in the use of benzyl benzoate so as to avoid conjunctivitis or irritation to the eyes.

Sulfur. Although somewhat messy, odoriferous, and staining to clothing, 6 per cent sulfur precipitate in petrolatum or Aquaphor appears to be safe, effective, and well tolerated, even in infants and young children. This preparation can be applied nightly for 3 nights and, if evidence of infestation persists, may be repeated in 1 week. With the availability of 5 per cent permethrin cream, precipitate of sulfur is no longer recommended as a treatment of choice.

Treatment of Scabietic Nodules. A high percentage of children with scabies may at times develop persistent reddish brown infiltrated nodules, particularly on the covered parts of the body (the axillae, groin, buttocks, and genital areas). These lesions, termed *nodular scabies* (see Figs. 14–11 and 14–12), are associated with a hypersensitivity and may persist for months despite adequate antiscabietic therapy. If treatment is desired, scabietic nodules respond to topical coal tar preparations, intralesional corticosteroids, and/or corticosteroids under occlusion.

Precautions. Once a diagnosis of scabies has been made, many patients or their parents will embark on a regimen of frequent bathing and overzealous attempts at hygiene. This frequently leads to excessive dryness of the skin, secondary eczematization, and persistent pruritus. Often the generalized itch will persist long after the parasite has been eliminated by antiscabietic therapy. This itching, perhaps due to an acquired sensitivity to the mite or its products, should not be confused with resistance of the mite to therapy. Repeated examinations and skin scrapings, therefore, should also be performed in these cases to ensure that infestation is no longer present.

Reports of infants with extensive scabietic infestation and unusual clinical presentation (scabies incognito), apparently promoted by extended topical use of potent corticosteroids, suggest avoidance of such preparations in the routine treatment of scabies. Systemic antipruritic agents, topical antipruritic formulations (such as Prax, PrameGel, or Sarna Lotion), and low-potency hydrocortisone preparations may be used for the management of persistent pruritus and secondary eczematization associated with scabietic infestation.

Although evidence suggests that adequate treatment may fail to reduce the incidence of nephritis following streptococcal disease, it seems reasonable to treat all scabies infestations complicated by cutaneous streptococcal infection with appropriate systemic antibiotics.[42] Simple and effective in promptly eradicating the infecting organism, antibiotics clear the clinical infection and limit the spread of this organism to others. Because of the risk of nephritis, it is further recommended that urinalyses be done for 2 or 3 weeks in all patients suspected of harboring nephritogenic strains of this organism.

OTHER MITES

Harvest Mites (Chiggers). The chigger, *Trombicula alfreddugesi*, or red bug, a member of the American harvest mite family, is commonly seen in the southern United States. The chigger is distinct from other mites in that only the larva is parasitic to humans and animals. The eight-legged adult and nymphal stages are spent in a nonparasitic existence. They live in grain stems, in grasses, or in areas overgrown with briars or blackberry bushes, where they exist and feed on vegetable matter, minute arthropods, and insect eggs. The six-legged larvae are responsible for the characteristic eruption seen in this disorder. They attach themselves to the skin of a passing human or animal host, inject an irritating secretion that causes itching, and then drop to the ground or are scratched off within 1 or 2 days after the itching begins.[43]

Areas affected by chiggers depend to a certain extent on the type of clothing worn, for they tend to attach themselves to areas where they meet an obstacle in the clothing, such as a belt, brassiere, garter, or boot or shoe top. A few hours after exposure itching, which may be intense, occurs. The itching reaches its peak of intensity on the second day and gradually decreases over the next 5 or 6 days. The eruption, chiefly seen on the legs and at the beltline, is characterized by pruritic discrete bright-red papules, 1 to 2 mm in diameter, often with hemorrhagic puncta. At times there may be scratch marks, urticarial lesions, and diffuse erythema. In children the eruption is often widespread, the pruritus may persist for months, purpuric lesions or bullae may develop, and secondary excoriation and impetiginization are common. In sensitized persons wheals, followed by papules, papulovesicles, or nodules, may be noted. In severe cases, fever may be present, and an eczematous reaction may complicate the picture.

Treatment of chigger bites consists of antihistamines, cool baths or compresses, and topical corticosteroids. Clear nail polish applied to the individual chigger bites appears to be a simple yet highly effective measure for immediate relief.[43] Bullous lesions readily become infected, particularly in children, and may be treated with appropriate antibiotics as well as antihistamines. Materials used for protection against chiggers function more as toxicants than true repellents.[44] The good mosquito repellents—diethyltoluamide (DEET), ethylhexanediol dimethyl phthallate, and dimethyl carbate—are good chigger toxicants. They provide the best protection when applied to the clothing, but if inadequate clothing is worn, it may be necessary to apply the protective material to the skin as well. Benzyl benzoate is an excellent chigger toxicant and is the only one that remains effective after rinsing, washing, or submersion in water.[44]

Grain Mites. Of medical interest is the grain itch mite (*Pyemotes ventricosus*), which feeds on the larvae of insects, infesting seeds, grains, and plant stems. Persons coming into contact with infested straw and grain are particularly susceptible to this form of dermatitis.[45] The eruption is seen as seasonal, severely pruritic, pale pink to bright red, macular, papulovesicular, or pustular lesions followed by urticarial wheals, and, at times, a purpuric eruption. In severe cases involving the entire body, constitutional reactions with fever can be confused with the eruption of varicella (chickenpox). The eruption is self-limiting and generally managed by antihistamines and topical antipruritic preparations (calamine lotion or topical corticosteroids).

Fowl Mites ("Pigeon-Mite" Dermatitis). *Dermonyssus gallinae*, a common ectoparasite of chickens and wild or domesticated birds (swallows, canaries, pigeons), may temporarily infest humans and produce troublesome skin lesions at the site of skin puncture. The eruption is characterized by urticarial wheals, papules, or vesicles that develop at areas of bites (Fig. 14–15).

Cheyletiella and other Mites. Other mites often present a therapeutic challenge in the diagnosis and management of patients with pruritus of undetermined origin. As transient visitors barely visible to the naked eye, these mites are rarely found on the patient's skin, either by close inspection or with meticulous scrapings, thus frequently leaving the physician with a puzzling pruritus of undetermined origin. In such patients, the search for a cause should extend to the ubiquitous reservoirs of mites found on animals, birds, plants, foods, furniture, and bedding. Nonburrowing mite bites produced by *Cheyletiella* species include *C. yasguri* (the dog mite), *C. parasitovirax* (the rabbit mite), *C. blakei* (the cat mite), *Notoedres cati* (an itch mite that causes persistent and at times fatal mange in cats and also infests domestic rabbits), house dust mites (*Dermatophagoides* species), *Ophinyssus natricis* (the snake mite), *Liponyssoides sanguinous* (the house mouse mite), and *Ornithonyssus bacoti* (the tropical rat mite) can produce pruritic, papular, and eczematous eruptions. In such instances, the clinician must maintain a high degree of suspicion and the possibility of mite infestation must be sought by careful history-taking and microscopic examination of specimens from possible reservoirs, including underclothing, household vacuumings, and family pets.[15–17, 46–49]

TICKS

Ticks are large, globular arachnids with short legs and hard leathery skin and mouth parts adaptable for sucking blood from mammals, birds, and reptiles. They are important vectors of diseases such as relapsing fever, rickettsial infection (typhus fever, rickettsialpox, Rocky Mountain spotted fever, Q fever, and ehrlichiosis), erythema chronicum migrans (erythema migrans) and Lyme disease (Fig. 14–16), babesiosis, tularemia, acrodermatitis chronica atrophicans, and perhaps morphea, lichen sclerosus et atrophicus, and lymphocytoma cutis.

Classified into two family groups, hard ticks (Ixodidae) and soft ticks (Argasidae), they are found in grass, shrubs, vines, and bushes, from which they attach themselves to dogs, cattle, and humans. The female tick attaches to the intended victim by sticking its proboscis into the skin to suck blood from the superficial vessels (Figs. 14–16 and 14–17). The local bite is painless and innocuous, and thus the tick is frequently undetected or noted only after several days of attachment. The local bite often results in an infiltrated lesion with a distinct surrounding erythematous halo, which may persist for 1 or 2 weeks or more (Fig. 14–18). The bites are often followed by small, often pruritic nodules (a local foreign body reaction if the mouth parts are carelessly left in the skin or improperly removed). The resulting pruritic granulomatous nodule may persist for months or even years.

Tick bite pyrexia, manifested by fever, chills,

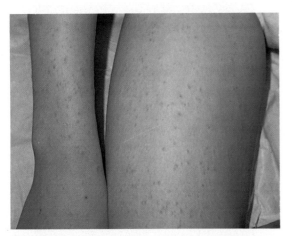

Figure 14–15. "Pigeon-mite" dermatitis. Urticarial wheals, papules, and vesicles occur in the areas of bites by *Dermonyssus gallinae* (a common parasite of chickens, swallows, canaries, and pigeons).

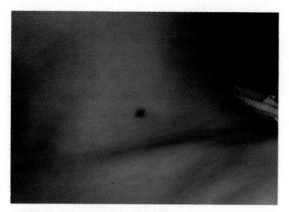

Figure 14–16. *Ixodes dammini,* the deer tick vector of Lyme disease, on the neck of a 5-year-old boy.

headache, vomiting, and abdominal pain, is presumably caused by a toxin secreted by the female tick. Removal of the engorged tick results in improvement of symptoms, usually within a period of 12 to 36 hours.

Tick paralysis, a reversible disease of the nervous system, manifested by incoordination, weakness, and flaccid paralysis, is due to a neurotoxin that is injected into the victim while the tick is engorging. In this disorder it appears that the tick must feed for several days before paralysis occurs. Although there is wide variation in individual susceptibility, paralysis generally occurs about 6 days after attachment of the tick. The paralysis usually starts in the legs and gradually ascends upward over the body. Bulbar paralysis, dysarthria, dysphagia, and death from respiratory failure may occur unless the tick is found and removed. Most cases of tick paralysis occur in children, especially girls. The tick is usually attached to the scalp, where it is hidden by the hair, but it may attach to any part of the skin, especially the ear, axilla, back, groin, or vulva (Fig. 14–17). Prompt recovery from tick paralysis generally occurs, often within 24 hours, after the tick is removed.[50]

Various methods of tick removal have been advocated. Recommended methods include heat from a previously lighted match; covering the area with nail polish, mineral oil, or petrolatum; a few drops of chloroform or ether; ethyl chloride spray; cryotherapy with liquid nitrogen; and, perhaps the easiest and most efficient method, mechanical removal by firmly grasping the tick with forceps, tweezers, or fingers, preferably protected with gloves, and gentle pulling straight upward with steady even pressure.[51] It is important that ticks not merely be plucked off but that care be exercised to ensure that no fragments of mouth parts or proboscis be left within the skin. Should a portion be retained, a cutaneous punch biopsy generally will effectively remove it. In infested areas protection from tick bites is best accomplished by the use of repellents in clothing—diethyltolua-

mide (DEET), butopyronoxyl (Indalone), dimethyl carbate, dimethyl phthalate, benzyl benzoate, and permethrin. It should be noted, however, that DEET-containing repellents may cause allergic and toxic effects, especially when used in high concentrations (see Chapter 10).[52–54] In addition, the wearing of protective clothing with long sleeves and pants tucked into socks, careful inspection for ticks after exposure, and early removal appear to provide the greatest degree of protection against tick bites and their sequelae.

SPIDERS

Spiders, because of their menacing appearance, are frequently unjustifiably blamed for more damage than they actually create. Virtually all the serious spider bites on the North American continent are caused by *Lactrodectus mactans* (the black widow spider) and *Loxosceles reclusa* (the brown recluse spider).

Black Widow Spider. The female black widow spider, the dangerous spider of southern Canada, the United States, Cuba, and Mexico, is recognized by its coal-black color and globular body (1 cm across) with a red or orange hourglass marking on the underside of its abdomen. A webspinner (in contrast to burrowing spiders), it lives in cool dark places in outbuildings and little used structures and often spins its web across outdoor privy seats. Therefore, a large number of bites in the southern United States are received around the genitalia and buttocks.

The black widow spider bites humans only in self-defense. Two red punctate marks and local swelling may be seen, and burning or stinging develops at the site of the bite. This is followed, within 10 minutes to an hour, by severe cramping pain, which increases to a maximum in about 3

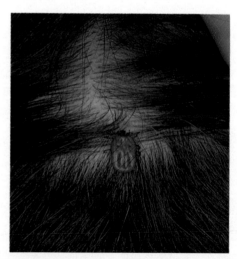

Figure 14–17. A tick embedded in the scalp of an 11-year-old child. In the removal of ticks, care must be exercised to ensure that fragments of mouth parts are not left within the skin.

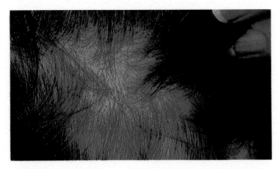

Figure 14–18. Infiltration with surrounding erythema (cutaneous reaction to a tick bite on the scalp of a 4-year-old child).

hours. Although the bite may be fatal in approximately 5 per cent of children, most patients recover spontaneously in 2 or 3 days.

Treatment consists of specific antivenin, intravenous calcium gluconate, muscle relaxants such as methocarbamol (Robaxin) or intravenous diazepam (Valium), morphine or meperidine (Demerol) for analgesia, tetanus prophylaxis, and appropriate antibiotics to cover skin flora if evidence of infection develops. Although the safety and effectiveness of methocarbamol in children younger than the age of 12 years have been established only in the treatment of tetanus, the injectable form can be administered intravenously (10 ml over a 5-minute period, with a second 10-ml ampule in 250 ml of a glucose or saline drip solution intravenously at 20 drops per minute). Neostigmine methylsulfate may help relieve muscle spasm, and in severe cases adrenocorticotropic hormone or systemic corticosteroids may be helpful.

Brown Recluse Spider. The brown recluse spider has an oval light-fawn to dark chocolate-brown body (about 1 cm in length and 4 to 6 mm in width) and a leg span greater than 25 mm. A dark brown violin-shaped band (extending from the eyes back to the end of the cephalothorax) and three pairs of eyes, rather than the four seen in other spiders, differentiate the brown recluse from other brown spiders. The spider has been found and bite reactions have been reported from Colorado to the eastern coast of the United States, from southern Illinois to the Gulf coast, and in the western states of California and Arizona. When in the house, the brown recluse spider is found in storage closets (among clothing); when outdoors, it generally resides in grasses, rocky bluffs, and barns. Because of its normal shyness and predilection for dark recesses, it bites only in self-defense when molested.

The venom of the *Loxosceles* spider is hemolytic and necrotizing and contains a spreading factor. Two types of reaction, a localizing cutaneous response and a severe, potentially grave systemic reaction, may occur. These reactions are not mutually exclusive and individual patients may exhibit either or both reactions. In localized reactions the initial symptom may be a mild itching or stinging at

the time of the bite. Mild to severe pain begins after 2 to 8 hours, followed by swelling and tenderness, a hemorrhagic vesicle or blister, and finally a gangrenous eschar with surrounding zones of edema, erythema, and ischemia (Figs. 14–19 and 14–20). Lymphangitis, manifested by a linear erythema along the course of the lymphatics, is not uncommon when the bite occurs on an extremity. In about a week the central portion becomes dark, demarcated, and gangrenous and may produce a large necrotic ulceration that can extend many centimeters in width and may last for months before healing occurs. In 25 per cent of patients, the bite evokes a systemic reaction in addition to the cutaneous reaction. This reaction may include nausea, vomiting, chills, fever, malaise, muscle aches and pains, a generalized erythematous, often purpuric macular eruption, thrombocytopenia, hemolytic anemia, hemoglobinuria, shock, coma, and eventual renal failure. Severe systemic reactions are noted more often in children and adults. Fatal cases, although rare, are usually preceded by intravascular hemolysis, hemolytic anemia, thrombocytopenia, hemoglobinuria, and renal failure.

Most brown recluse spider bites are fortunately not serious and tend to heal without incident. Mild or moderate bites (those with necrotic centers less than 2 cm in diameter), therefore, generally require no treatment other than tetanus prophylaxis, medication for the relief of pain, application of ice or cold packs to the bite site, and elevation of the injured area.[55] Large or massive bites, those with necrotic centers greater than 2 cm in diameter, however, are more likely to result in systemic loxoscelism, severe necrosis, and, at times, invasion of adjacent muscle tissue. These should be treated with systemic corticosteroids, at least during the first 5 days (the damaging active phase is usually completed after approximately 1 week), particularly if systemic loxoscelism with renal or coagulation problems seems to be emerging.[56] In addition, the administration of aspirin and antibiotics such as erythromycin or cephalosporin appears to be associated with a more favorable clinical course, and dapsone (presumably for its anti-inflammatory effect and inhibition of polymorphonuclear cell accumulation in the dermis) is often recommended as a treatment of choice. The use of intralesional corticosteroids is controversial, and since early

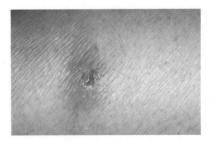

Figure 14–19. Cutaneous reaction 8 days after a spider bite on the arm of a young woman.

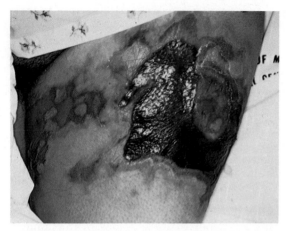

Figure 14–20. Eschar due to the bite of a brown recluse spider. (Courtesy of Larry M. Millikan, M.D., and Richard Berger, M.D.)

surgical excision may inhibit wound healing and produce an inferior clinical result, surgical repair and skin grafts, when required, should be delayed for at least 2 months or more.[55, 56]

SCORPIONS

Scorpions are tropical photophobic arachnids that hide by day and hunt by night. They differ from other arachnids in that they have an elongated abdomen ending in a stinger. Found all over the world, particularly in the tropics, in North America they are generally seen in the southern United States and Mexico. Other than the *Centruroides* species (found in the desert regions of Arizona and its neighboring states), scorpion stings in the United States are usually not dangerous and generally do not warrant definitive medical care. Stings in children, however, should be watched carefully, particularly during the first 4 hours since an occasional child will react adversely. The venom apparatus of the scorpion is carried in its curved stinger at the tip of the tail, which is swung over the scorpion's head to penetrate the victim's skin. During the day scorpions hide in shoes, closets, clothing, and crevices. Some species of ground scorpions, however, may burrow and hide in gravel or children's sandboxes. They rarely attack humans but will sting humans when accidentally disturbed, brushed against, or stepped upon.

The sting of the scorpion releases two noxious agents: a localized hemolytic toxin and a dangerous neurotoxic venom. The hemolytic toxin may cause a painful burning sensation, with pronounced redness, swelling, discoloration, lymphangitis, severe necrosis, and, in some patients, disseminated intravascular coagulation or renal failure. The degree of damage at the site of the sting varies; the variations are most likely due to polypeptide variations in the different venoms and the amount of venom injected.[57, 58] The neurotoxic

venom may produce local numbness and a severe generalized reaction consisting of sweating, salivation, tightness in the throat, abdominal cramps, cyanosis, convulsions, and, particularly in small children, respiratory paralysis and death. In a tabulation of deaths according to age, 75 per cent are in infants and children younger than 3 years of age.

Treatment of scorpion stings consists of immediate application of a tourniquet above the area whenever possible, applications of ice or cold water, and, in severe reactions, the administration of epinephrine, specific antivenin (available from the Antivenom Production Laboratoy, Arizona State University), and/or systemic corticosteroids. The site of the sting should not be incised, and neither opiates nor paraldehyde should be given. Shock, when present, is treated with parenteral fluids, and barbiturates should be administered to patients with extreme irritability or convulsions, or both.

Insects

Insects are the class of arthropods characterized by division into three parts (a head, thorax, and abdomen). Noxious insects are ubiquitous, affecting all humans in some manner at one time or another. The insects of medical significance include lice, bugs, bees, wasps, ants, fleas, moths and their larvae, flies, and mosquitoes.

LICE (PEDICULOSIS)

Lice have plagued humans since ancient times. Although infection is most common during times of stress, such as war, crowded situations in schools, camps, or institutions, following widespread use of DDT after the end of World War II there were relatively few reports of pediculosis in the United States. Subsequent to restrictions in the use of DDT in this country since January 1973, however, the number of cases has increased, particularly pediculosis capitis and, with our present climate of sexual permissiveness, pediculosis pubis. Lice occur wherever there are humans. They spend their entire life as ectoparasites, living on humans, depending on the blood they extract from their victims for sustenance. Their existence, therefore, independent of humans is impossible. They are small, six-legged, wingless insects with translucent, almost gray or grayish white bodies, which become red when engorged with blood. Barely visible to the naked eye, they measure 1 to 4 mm. The head contains a pair of eyes and a pair of short segmented antennae. The mouth parts consist of stylets modified for piercing and sucking (retractable when not in use) and six pairs of hooks by which they attach to the skin while feeding (Fig. 14–21). In general, body lice are 10 to 20 per cent longer than head lice and are often lighter in color.

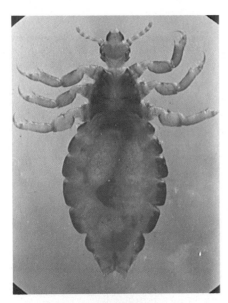

Figure 14–21. The head louse (*Pediculus humanus capitis*). This six-legged wingless insect (1 to 4 mm in size) has a translucent grayish white body that becomes red when engorged with blood. Body lice are lighter in color and 10 to 20 percent larger than head lice. (Courtesy of Reed & Carnrick.)

Three varieties of pediculi attack humans. These include *Pthirus pubis* (the crab louse), *Pediculus humanus capitis* (the head louse), and *Pediculus humanus corporis* (the body louse). Although the official designation of the crab louse is *Pthirus pubis*, *Phthirus pubis* is the spelling one frequently sees in medical dictionaries and articles on the subject.[59]

Although the crab louse is a distinct genus and species, some doubt exists as to the status of the two forms of *Pediculus humanus*. Most authorities believe that the head louse represents the ancestral type and that the body louse evolved when humans began wearing clothes. Each variety has a predilection for certain parts of the body and rarely migrates to other regions. In piercing the skin they exude a poisonous salivary secretion, which, together with the mechanical puncture, produces a pruritic dermatitis. In addition, the body louse is the carrier of certain rickettsial diseases (louse-born typhus and trench fever) and a spirochetal disorder (relapsing fever).

Head and body lice may be acquired by personal contact or by putting on infested clothing. Head lice may also be acquired by contact with upholstered chairs and the use of infested combs or brushes.

Crab lice are spread chiefly by sexual contact and perhaps occasionally by close personal contact or the proverbial toilet seat. The crab louse has a shorter abdomen, bearing hairy lateral tufts, and large second and third legs, which give it its crab-like appearance (Fig. 14–22). Small children may become infected with crab lice on their eyebrows or eyelashes from their mothers or by close contact with infested adults. For some unknown reason, perhaps the characteristic shape and configuration of the hairs, blacks are relatively resistant to head and crab louse infestation.

The ova or nits are oval, are grayish or yellowish white, and are seen as tiny pinhead specks measuring 0.3 to 0.8 mm. They may be found in the scalp in pediculosis capitis, the pubic and anal regions in pediculosis pubis, and on the seams of clothing in pediculosis corporis (Figs. 14–23 and 14–24). They are laid within 24 to 48 hours after mating and, incubated by the heat of the body, hatch in about 8 days. It takes another 8 days for the emerging larvae to reach maturity. The ova can be identified by fluorescence under Wood's light and by examination under the microscope. They have a chitinous ring at the base by which they are fastened securely to the hair. The egg may have an embryo visible inside and a cap at the free end (operculum) for breathing purposes (Fig. 14–25).

Pediculosis Corporis. The body louse is slightly larger (10 to 20 per cent) than the head louse, generally lives in clothing or bedding, lays eggs along the seams of clothing, and only visits the human host long enough to feed. Its nits attach firmly to

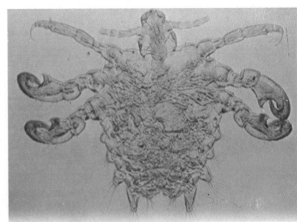

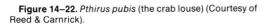

Figure 14–22. *Pthirus pubis* (the crab louse) (Courtesy of Reed & Carnrick).

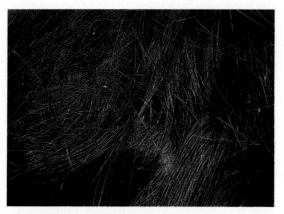

Figure 14–23. Pediculosis capitis. Oval grayish to yellowish white nits are present in the hair of the scalp.

the fibers of clothing (where they may remain viable for several weeks) and hatch out, owing to body warmth when the clothing is worn by the human host. The parasite is rarely observed on the skin; it obtains its nourishment by clinging to the patient's clothing and piercing the skin by its proboscis. The primary lesion is a small pinpoint red macule, papule, or urticarial wheal, with a characteristic hemorrhagic central punctum. Due to the intense generalized pruritus associated with this disorder, primary lesions are frequently obliterated by scratching and, therefore, are seldom seen. Diagnosis is established by a generalized pruritus, parallel scratch marks (particularly in the interscapular region), fleeting wheals, secondary eczematization, bacterial infection, bloody crusts, and, in cases of prolonged duration, postinflammatory hyperpigmentation. The diagnosis can be confirmed by the finding of lice or nits in the seams of clothing (Fig. 14–24).

Pediculosis Capitis. Pediculosis capitis, except during situations that cause crowding and insanitary conditions, is the most common form of louse infestation. Children, particularly girls, are more

susceptible to infestation than adults. Presumably the higher incidence in females is due to their usually longer hair styles. In addition, since it appears that North American head lice are poorly adapted to the thick curly hair of blacks, pediculosis capitis is less common in blacks in the United States. This phenomenon, however, does not appear to be the case in Africa where the lice have apparently adapted to this situation and are therefore able to grasp the hair shafts of affected individuals. Itching is the principal symptom of pediculosis capitis and infestation should not be overlooked when overshadowed by impetigo of the scalp, furunculosis, postoccipital lymphadenopathy, dermatitis of the neck, shoulders (Fig. 14–26), and postauricular areas, or urticaria.

Head lice can survive for as long as 55 hours off the scalp of an infested individual. Pediculosis capitis, therefore, may be transmitted by shared hats, headsets such as those used with cassette players, clothing, towels, combs, hair brushes, and, at times, bedding, clothing, or upholstery. Although traditionally confined to the scalp, the head louse may sometimes be responsible for pediculosis of the eyelids, particularly in children, and *Pthirus pubis* may also be responsible for scalp or eyelid infestation in adults and children.[60–62]

Nits are chiefly found in the hairs above the ears and in the occipital region, initially one-fourth inch or so from the scalp (Fig. 14–23). The nits are small, oval, and whitish and measure about 0.5 mm in length. They are laid close to the scalp near the bottom of the hair shaft and, as hairs grow out, are carried outward. Nits present away from the scalp and along the shafts or tips of long hairs signify long-standing infection or residual nits from previously treated infestation. It is important not to mistake epidermal scales or hair casts as pediculosis capitis or nits. Such errors may have severe psychological consequences for the patients, their families, and, at times, even school authorities.[63] Of diagnostic importance is the fact that nits fluoresce under Wood's light examination and are not easily flicked off or moved along the shaft with the

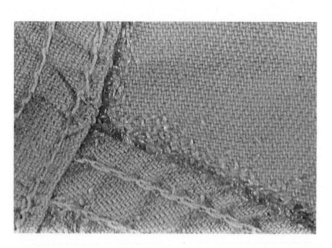

Figure 14–24. Nits in the seams of clothing are diagnostic of *Pediculus humanus corporis*. (Courtesy of Reed & Carnrick.)

fingers. If the differentiation is doubtful, snipping of the hair and low power microscopic examination of suspected nits will usually clarify the diagnosis (Fig. 14–25).

Pediculosis Pubis. Pediculosis pubis is caused by the crab louse (*Pthirus pubis*) (see Figs. 14–22 and 14–27). As stated previously, the scientific name of the insect is often misspelled as *Phthirus pubis*.[59] This parasite normally inhabits the hairs of the pubic region but may also involve the eyelashes, beard, mustache, axillary, and other body hairs. Infestation of the pubic region is most frequently seen in adolescents and young adults as the result of transmission by sexual intercourse, although it may also be transmitted by clothing, bedding, or towels. The crab louse is shorter and broader than the head and body louse. Itching may be the initial symptom, but in persistent cases eczematization or secondary infection may occur (Fig. 14–27). A heavy infestation is occasionally accompanied by asymptomatic bluish or slate-colored macules, 0.5 to 1.0 cm in diameter (maculae cerulae), that do not blanch on pressure with a glass slide. They may be seen on the trunk, thighs, or upper arms and often last for months. Although frequently described in clinical descriptions of pediculosis pubis, they are not commonly seen in mild infestations and therefore should not be relied on as a clinical feature in the differential diagnosis of this disorder.

Pediculosis Palpebrarum. In children *Pthirus pubis* (occasionally *Pediculus humanus capitis* or *corporis*) may locate in the eyelashes or eyebrows

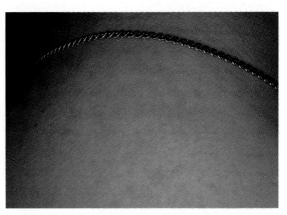

Figure 14–26. Dermatitis, as seen on the neck of this 6-year-old girl, should not be overlooked as a clinical sign of pediculosis capitis.

(pediculosis palpebrarum). When the eyelids are involved it usually is related to infestation in an adult, often the mother; but when seen in children and caused by *Pthirus pubis*, the condition must be considered as a sign of possible molestation or sexual abuse.[64] In pediculosis palpebrarum the nits must also be differentiated from the scaling seen in blepharitis associated with seborrheic dermatitis.

Treatment. Since the body louse ordinarily does not inhabit the body, the treatment of pediculosis corporis mainly consists of proper hygiene and frequent showering or bathing, with change of underclothes and bedding. Underclothing and bedding should be laundered with hot water or boiled. Dry cleaning destroys lice in articles that cannot be laundered. Pressing woolens with a hot iron is also satisfactory, but special attention should be given to the seams of the clothing. All likely contacts (members of the household and close contacts in institutions) should be examined and treated if there is evidence of infestation.

Although the incidence of pediculosis capitis is unknown, it is estimated that 6 to 10 million schoolchildren are infested annually in the United States, thus often producing a problem for physicians, teachers, school and health officials, affected children, and their families. Agents for the treatment of pediculosis capitis include lindane, pyrethrins combined with piperonyl butoxide, malathion, and permethrin, synthetic pyrethroid. Although lindane (Kwell) has been used for years, in view of potential toxicity associated with overuse or accidental ingestion and reports of lindane resistance in Europe, but not believed to be widespread in North America, other forms of therapy are frequently recommended.[62]

Pyrethrins, over-the-counter remedies derived from chrysanthemum plants available as RID, A-200 Pediculocide Shampoo or Gel Concentrate, and permethrin (Nix), appear to be equally if not more effective than lindane.[65–68] Since the incubation of louse eggs is 6 to 10 days and lindane and pyrethrin products are not totally ovicidal and lack

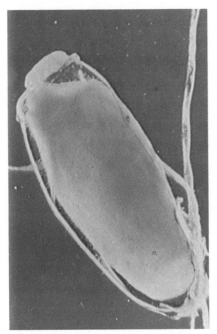

Figure 14–25. *Pediculus humanus capitis.* Note chitinous attachment to the hair shaft, an embryo in situ, and the intact operculum. Microscopic examination of nits readily establishes the proper diagnosis. (Courtesy of Reed & Carnrick.)

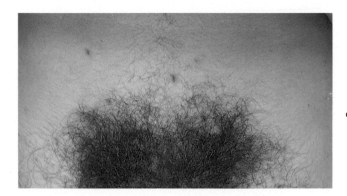

Figure 14–27. *Pediculosis pubis.* Excoriated cutaneous lesions and nits can be seen.

residual activity, a second treatment 7 to 14 days later and removal of nits with a fine-toothed comb is often recommended.[62] Although pyrethrin pediculocides carry a warning of possible allergic reaction in patients sensitive to ragweed, modern refining techniques make this complication extremely unlikely; and there is no evidence that multiple treatments are hazardous. Thus, a permethrin 1 per cent creme rinse (Nix), with its high pediculocidal and ovicidal activities and low mammalian toxicity and residual effect, currently appears to be the treatment of choice for pediculosis capitis.[65–68] Since its pediculocidal activity continues for 10 to 14 days, although currently recommended as a single treatment, a second application may be used after 2 weeks, thus extending the period of protection and ensuring that newly hatched nymphs are killed.

Used successfully for many years in the United Kingdom and continental Europe, 0.5 per cent malathion (Ovide lotion [GenDerm Corporation]) currently appears to be the most effective ovicidal pediculocide. When used, it should be sprinkled onto dry hair, rubbed in gently until the scalp is thoroughly moistened, allowed to dry naturally (avoiding open flames or hair dryers since the product is flammable) and removed after 8 to 12 hours with a nonmedicated shampoo. Although malathion binds to the hair shaft for periods of up to 4 weeks, a second application, although generally not required, may be applied 7 to 9 days later. Adverse systemic effects have not been reported following the use of 0.5 per cent malathion, but its alcoholic vehicle may cause stinging, especially of the eyes, and its main drawbacks are the odor associated with the release of sulfhydryl compounds through hydrolysis and the fact that this product is flammable until the alcoholic base has dried.

Whatever the method of therapy, other family members and close contacts should be examined and those with evidence of infestation should be treated. Live (viable) nits can be differentiated from dead ones by use of a Wood's lamp in a completely darkened room (live nits glow with a pearly fluorescence while dead nits do not) or by microscopic examination of nits (the absence of an em-

bryo or operculum in ova that have hatched). Since nits are firmly attached to the hair shaft, removal (although not necessary) may be made easier by the use of a fine-toothed comb, or tweezers, or by soaking the hair with white vinegar or a 3 to 5 per cent acetic acid solution, followed by wrapping with a damp towel soaked in the same solution. The towel may be removed after about an hour, and removal of the nits can be facilitated by a shampooing and the use of a fine-toothed comb (the acetic acid dissolves the chitin, which binds the nits to the hair shafts). Also effective is a commercial rinse (Step 2 [GenDerm]), a formulation containing 8 per cent formic acid.[69] Information regarding management and control of this disorder is available from the National Pediculosis Association, Box 149, Newton, MA 02161 (617-969-5623).

In an effort to minimize and prevent spread of pediculosis capitis, floors, play areas, and furniture can be vacuumed and bedding, clothing, and head gear may be machine washed on a hot cycle and dried in a domestic dryer. Items that cannot be washed may be dry cleaned or placed in plastic bags in a warm place for 2 weeks. Hats, combs, brushes, grooming aids, towels, school lockers and hooks, and other items that come into contact with the head or head coverings should not be shared. Combs and brushes may be coated with the pediculicide for 15 minutes or soaked in rubbing alcohol or 2 per cent Lysol for 1 hour, followed by washing in hot soapy water.

For pediculosis pubis, lindane (Kwell) shampoo, which requires only a 5-minute application time to the infested and adjacent hairy areas, with particular attention to the mons pubis and perianal region, is currently recommended as the treatment of choice. Sexual contacts should be treated simultaneously, but other household members need not be treated. At the conclusion of therapy, treated individuals should change their underclothing, pajamas, sheets, and pillow cases. These articles should be washed by machine, automatically dried or laundered, ironed, or boiled to destroy remaining ova or parasites.

Pediculosis of the eyelashes (pediculosis palpebrarum) may be treated by petrolatum applied thickly to the eyelashes twice daily for 8 days, followed by mechanical removal of remaining nits. Although petrolatum applied to the eyelashes is the treatment of choice, physostigmine ophthalmic preparations (Eserine) are also effective if applied topically to the eyelid margin (twice daily for 24 to 48 hours). Because of the parasympathetic effects of physostigmine, miosis should be watched for as a possible side effect. In addition, freshly prepared 20 per cent fluorescein eye drops (one or two drops) applied to the lid margins and eyelashes has been recommended as a treatment for this disorder.[70]

MOSQUITOES AND FLIES

Flies and mosquitoes belong to the order Diptera. One of the largest orders of insects, it includes the two-winged biting flies, gnats, and mosquitoes. Of these, mosquitoes, worldwide in distribution, are the most important from the standpoint of human health. They are vectors of many important diseases (encephalitis, malaria, yellow fever, and filariasis). In the United States the most common insect bites of infants and children are those of mosquitoes.

Mosquitoes are attracted to bright clothing, heat, humidity, and human odors, particularly those of young children. In unsensitized individuals, the ordinary mosquito bite only produes a local irritation. Following the initial bite there may be a slight stinging sensation and a small pruritic erythematous papule with some transient discomfort. In sensitized individuals, however, bites may produce itching; urticarial wheals, which may last for several hours to several days; or firm papules or nodules, which may persist for longer periods of time. Occasionally, particularly in the young, mosquito bites may produce blisters or hemorrhagic lesions, and, owing to pruritus and excoriation, may result in secondary eczematization and impetiginization. Although the diagnosis of insect bites is often obvious, differentiation from other papular, vesicular, and pruritic eruptions can be assisted by a characteristic grouping of lesions, a central punctum when present, and the seasonal incidence of the disorder.

Treatment of mosquito bites consists of oral antihistamines, cool compresses, topical antipruritic agents (see Chapter 3), calamine lotion, and topical corticosteroids. Insect repellents are recommended for individuals who are sensitive to mosquito bites. When out of doors, children prone to insect bite reactions should wear a head covering, shoes, trousers, clothing with long sleeves, and garments of smooth-finished fabrics of neutral colors (white, green, tan, and khaki do not, as a rule, attract insects). Scented hair sprays, tonics or pomades, soaps, lotions, powders, colognes, and perfumes may attract all forms of stinging insects. Although results are not definite, in some individuals thiamine hydrochloride taken orally in dosages of 25 to 50 mg three times a day appears to help repel insects. This innocuous vitamin apparently produces an odor that is imperceptible to the human host but theoretically disagreeable and repelling to insects.[71, 72]

Various species of biting flies (sandflies, gnats, black flies, deerflies, horseflies) are known to attack the exposed areas of the face, neck, arms, and legs, with the production of painful, irritating, or pruritic papules or nodules, often with vesiculation. Although lesions often disappear in a few hours, they may persist for several days and can be very annoying, particularly in small children. Treatment consists of the prophylactic use of insect repellent (6-12, DEET, or Off), with appropriate precautions (see Chapter 10), and symptomatic relief by acetaminophen, antihistamines, calamine lotion, or topical corticosteroids.

Nonbiting flies, including common houseflies, tend to feed at open wounds, exudates, and cutaneous ulcers and may produce *myiasis*, a far less common, but severe cutaneous disorder. Uncommon in areas where high standards of hygiene prevail, fly larvae may burrow into normal or injured skin (wounds or ulcers), invade the epidermis, and wander in the cutaneous tissues with a resulting migratory inflammatory pattern (migratory myiasis). Treatment of myiasis consists of injection of a local anesthetic, simple incision and covering of the area with petrolatum (which interferes with larval respiration, thus prompting the larvae to crawl out, generally within 48 hours), surgical removal of the larvae, and antibiotics, when necessary, to control secondary infection. In addition, topical application of a 20 per cent aluminum salt solution (available in most household antiperspirants) or Burow's solution, which appears to inactivate the venom, can be used to help relieve the pain and discomfort associated with this disorder.[73]

FLEAS

Fleas (Siphonaptera) exist universally among animals and humans. Those that most commonly attack humans in the United States are the human flea (*Pulex irritans*), the cat flea (*Ctenacephalides felis*), and the dog flea (*Ctenacephalides canis*). The eruption produced by a flea bite in a sensitized individual is an urticarial wheal or papule, often, but not invariably, centered by a hemorrhagic punctum (Fig. 14–28). In highly susceptible individuals, particularly young children, wheals may progress and develop into bullae. Bites are usually multiple and grouped together in linear or irregular clusters on the arms, forearms, or legs or on areas where clothing fits snugly (the thighs, buttocks, waist, and lower abdomen). Treatment consists of antihistamines, calamine lotion, or topical corticosteroids and elimination of fleas by treatment of suspected animal carriers and spraying of carpets, floors, crevices, and other potentially infested areas (such as stuffing of furniture and bedding), with 5 per cent malathion powder, 1 per cent

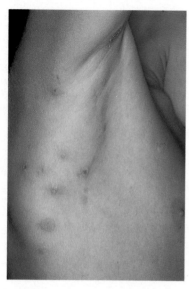

Figure 14–28. Flea bites on the upper trunk, axilla, and shoulder of a young child. Note the characteristic clustering, central hemorrhagic puncta, and urticarial wheals.

lindane dust, or, if available, 5 per cent DDT powder. It should be noted that for every flea seen on the pet there are 10 to 100 more in the environment, that flea collars, although extremely popular, are not completely effective, and that animal flea sprays and powders, if used, must be repeated every 2 weeks during the summer months to be effective.[74]

BEDBUGS

Bedbugs, *Cimex lectularius* (Hemiptera), are reddish brown blood-sucking insects, 3 to 5 mm in size, wingless, with flattened oval bodies and three pairs of legs. They secrete themselves in crevices of floors and walls and in bedding or furniture and normally emerge to feed only in darkness. Under normal conditions feeding takes place about once a week; in cold weather it is less frequent. The time required for feeding varies from 5 to 12 minutes, after which the insect leaves its victim as quickly as possible. The bedbug is capable of traveling long distances in search of food, often from one house to another, and has been known to survive without food for up to 6 months to a year.

The bites are commonly seen on exposed areas of the face, neck, arms, or hands, often two or three in a line. Usually the host does not feel the bite. In individuals not sensitized by previous exposure the only manifestation is a symptomless purpuric macule at the site of the bite. In previously sensitized individuals, intensely pruritic papules, or wheals, often with central hemorrhagic puncta, are characteristic. A vesicle may surmount the papule or wheal. Frequently the initial lesion may evolve into a nodule that may last up to 14 days or more. Bullae are frequently seen in children, and exco-

riated lesions, associated eczematization, or secondary infection may alter the clinical picture.

Treatment is directed at elimination of the bug from the environment by DDT, chlordane, or lindane. Although individual lesions require no direct therapy, oral antihistamines and topical corticosteroids or calamine lotion may give subjective relief.

PAPULAR URTICARIA

Papular urticaria (lichen urticatus) is a common disease of childhood manifested by a chronic or recurrent papular eruption caused by a sensitivity reaction to the bites of mosquitoes, fleas, bedbugs, and other insects. Although cases have been described in infants as young as 2 weeks of age, it is seen primarily in children between 2 and 7 years of age, particularly in those with an atopic background. The disorder appears in summer and late spring; lesions may occur on any part of the body but tend to be grouped in clusters on exposed areas, particularly the extensor surfaces of the extremities. Although they may occur to a lesser extent on the face and neck, trunk, thighs, and buttocks, they generally spare the genital, perianal, and axillary regions.

Individual lesions are seen as 3- to 10-mm firm urticated papules with wheals, or wheals surmounted by papules, often with a central punctum (Fig. 14–29). Lesions may be rubbed or irritated, excoriated, lichenified, or secondarily infected with impetiginized crusts or inflammatory ulcerations.[75] The lesions recur in crops, and all stages of development and regression may be noted. Most lesions persist for 2 to 10 days and, after resolution, may result in temporary postinflammatory erythema or pigmentation. If exposure to the parasite is allowed to continue, the attacks may persist for an average of 3 to 4 years, perennially or recurring seasonally; occasionally they may persist into adolescence or later.

On histopathologic examination the lesions of papular urticaria are identical to those of insect bites. Affected persons give a delayed papular reaction when injected intradermally with flea, bedbug, or mosquito antigens and run a course that parallels that of papular urticaria. There is no feature of the disease, clinical, histopathologic, immunologic, or epidemiologic, that is not consistent with the theory that parasite bites in specifically sensitized subjects are the cause of this disorder.

The differentiation of papular urticaria from true urticaria and arthropod infestations is seldom difficult, but when indeterminate, microscopic examination of skin scrapings, examination of other household members, and skin biopsy may be indicated. In some cases the early lesions of granuloma annulare resemble nodular lesions of papular urticaria; this, too, can be differentiated by histopathologic examination of a cutaneous biopsy. The histopathologic changes in papular urticaria consist of

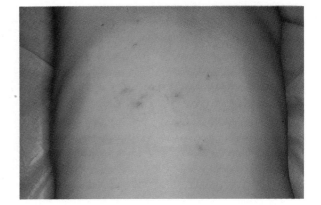

Figure 14–29. Papular urticaria. Recurrent crops of grouped papules are shown with central puncta and urticarial wheals.

intercellular and intracellular edema, spongiotic vesicles in the epidermis, and moderate to heavy infiltration of lymphocytes, with many eosinophils around vesicles and epidermal appendages in the middle and lower dermis.[76]

Therapy for papular urticaria consists of insect control in the household, with particular attention to baseboards, basements, bed frames, and upholstered furniture and treatment of affected dogs and cats. Antihistamines appear to be of limited value; in most cases disinfestation, simple sedation, and topical calamine lotion or corticosteroids are adequate for relief of symptoms. In patients with bullous lesions or secondary impetiginization, bacterial culture and appropriate antibiotics are indicated.

BEES, WASPS, AND ANTS

Bees, wasps, and ants belong to the order Hymenoptera, a large order of insects that contains about 100,000 species, of which about half are parasitic on insects or other invertebrates. Like most other insects they have three pairs of legs and four wings and are recognized by the narrow isthmus separating the abdomen from the thorax.

Bees, the only insects that produce food eaten by humans, live in almost every part of the world except the North and South Poles. Honey bees live and work together in large groups and do not sting unless frightened or hurt. Wasps, among the most interesting and intelligent of insects, may live together and cooperate with one another, as the so-called social wasps (hornets and yellow jackets), or may live as solitary wasps (those that build separate nests and do not live in communities). Most wasps are helpful to humans. Although they sometimes damage fruit, they also destroy large numbers of flies, caterpillars, and other insects harmful to humans. Wasps, just as bees, ordinarily do not sting humans unless they are bothered or frightened.

Symptoms of bee or wasp stings vary from mild local pruritus, pain, and edema to general anaphylactic reactions with associated difficulty in breathing and swallowing, hoarseness, thickened speech, gastrointestinal disturbances, abdominal pain, dizziness, weakness, confusion, generalized edema, collapse, unconsciousness, and, at times, even sudden death.

Ants, like bees and wasps, have large glands at the tip of the abdomen from which they introduce venom into wounds produced by their bites. The fire ant (*Solenopsis saevissima, richteri,* and *invicta*), imported from South America, has spread rapidly in the southern part of the United States and produces a venom more potent than that of other hymenoptera. Fire ants are particularly ferocious and, when molested, produce many burning and painful stings within seconds. Pivoting about the grasping jaws, which produce two hemorrhagic sites of puncture, the fire ant inserts its sting into multiple areas producing intense pain, followed by an almost immediate flare, which generally measures from 2.5 to 5.0 cm in diameter. This is rapidly followed by a wheal, which may measure from 2.0 mm to 1 cm in diameter. Eight to 10 hours later cloudy and then purulent fluid develops at the puncture site. The bites generally occur in clusters, and frequently result in systemic reactions (fever, gastrointestinal distress, urticaria, angioedema, and asthma) and, although rare, life-threatening injury (particularly in infants) can be expected from a small percentage of these encounters.[77–79]

The treatment of ordinary bee, wasp, or ant stings consists of local application of antipruritic shake lotions (calamine lotion), cool compresses or cool baths, and oral antihistamines. A papain solution made up of 1 part meat tenderizer to four parts of water will frequently help relieve local symptoms of pain or discomfort. Epinephrine, oxygen, antihistamines, and systemic corticosteroids should be administered to patients with severe allergic reactions. Patients known to suffer systemic reactions to the sting of a bee, wasp, hornet, or yellow jacket should be desensitized and should have an insect sting kit readily available as a prophylactic measure. An effective insect sting kit should contain a tourniquet (to be applied above the sting when possible), a 15-mg sublingual tablet of isoproterenol for immediate use, an oral antihistamine, and a hypodermic syringe (preferably preloaded with epinephrine) for intramuscular or subcutaneous injection.

Although immunotherapy is not necessary for most children with insect sensitivity, if a child has a generalized reaction to a hymenoptera sting, whether mild or severe, desensitization is recommended. A history of repeated stings with progressively larger local reactions also invites a program of hypersensitization. Severe local reactions and delayed reactions, particularly with angioedema and generalized urticaria, place the patient in the same category.[80]

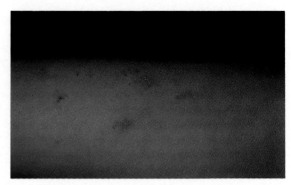

Figure 14–30. Gypsy moth caterpillar dermatitis.

BLISTER BEETLES

Blister beetles (Coleoptera) contain cantharidin, a volatile substance most concentrated in the beetles' genitalia. The lesions produced accidentally by crushing blister beetles, by discharge of their body fluid on the skin, or by external therapeutic use of cantharidin (as in the treatment of verrucae) consist of slowly forming blisters that involve the outer layers of the skin. Treatment depends on the extent and location of lesions. Simple aseptic drainage of large bullae and cool compresses generally give adequate relief of symptoms. If vesicles are not traumatized, they usually resolve in 3 or 4 days, and the overlying epidermis usually flakes off within a period of 6 or 7 days, requiring no further therapy.

CATERPILLARS AND MOTHS

Caterpillars represent the larval stage of butterflies and moths of the order Lepidoptera. The hairs of certain moths and caterpillars are known to produce a dermatitis, often severe and incapacitating to both children and adults. In the United States, the most frequently seen and most irritating of these are those due to the hairs of the brown-tail moth (usually seen in the northeastern part of this country) and the hairs of the puss caterpillar (the larva of the "flannel" moth, *Megalopyge opercularis*), seen from Virginia southward to the states bordering the Gulf of Mexico.[81–84]

Reactions produced by contact with the hairs and spines of these moths and caterpillars appear to be associated with the release of histamine and other vasoactive substances and mechanical irritation by caterpiller hairs (setae) that become imbedded in the pores of affected individuals.[85] These reactions range in severity from a local dermatitis characterized by discrete pruritic, burning, or stinging maculopapular lesions, to localized pruritic, vesicular, or excoriated papular lesions, or urticarial wheals with vesicular or shallow necrotic centers (Figs. 14–30 and 14–31). Systemic reactions may consist of severe local pain, nausea, fever, swelling of the affected area, numbness, severe muscle cramps, intense headache, shock, and convulsions. Not only do the hairs themselves penetrate the skin, but slender delicate hairs are also often detached and transported through air or clothing, thus resulting in widespread dermatitis or painful nodular conjunctivitis.

The diagnosis of moth or caterpillar dermatitis can be confirmed by microscopic examination of Scotch tape strippings or scrapings of involved areas with demonstration of offending hairs. Although the disorder is self-limiting and in almost all instances resolves within a period of several days to 2 weeks, relief can be obtained by the use of oral antihistamines, topical corticosteroids, and topical antipruritic agents such as Prax, PrameGel, or Sarna Lotion. Immediate application of Scotch tape or adhesive over the sting may be helpful in the removal of broken-off spines. Ice packs to

Figure 14–31. Gypsy moth caterpillar dermatitis. Urticarial wheals are evident on the arm of a 15-year-old boy.

the involved areas may help to relieve discomfort in some patients; in others narcotics may be required to control severe pain, and intravenous calcium gluconate and systemic corticosteroids may be of distinct benefit in patients with severe generalized reactions.[81]

OTHER CUTANEOUS PARASITES

Cutaneous Larva Migrans (Creeping Eruption)

Creeping eruption is a distinctive skin disorder that results from invasion of the epidermis and subsequent migration within the superficial layers of skin by larval parasites (cutaneous larva migrans). This produces a tortuous linear eruption characterized by bizarre serpentine pink or skin-colored tracts, 2 to 3 mm in diameter (Fig. 14–32). Although the majority of cases are caused by larvae of the dog or cat hookworm (*Ancylostoma braziliense*), other species of parasitic nematodes have been described in this disorder. Infections are most common in warm, humid, and sandy coastal areas of tropical and subtropical regions and in travelers to and from these areas.[86] In the United States it occurs in states bordering the Gulf of Mexico and the Atlantic Ocean from Texas to Rhode Island. Infections are most common in children and adolescents, although infestations have been noted in adults strolling barefoot or walking in these areas. Infections are also frequently acquired by workmen such as plumbers ("plumbers' itch"), electricians, carpenters, pest exterminators exposed to the larvae in warm, moist sandy areas such as the crawl spaces of houses, and gardeners and fishermen working in infested areas.

Adult nematodes live in the intestines of their unnatural host (dogs or cats). Ova are deposited in the animal feces and, under favorable conditions of humidity and temperature, hatch into infective larvae. The larvae, perhaps with the aid of a collagenase or other enzyme, may then penetrate human skin that has been in contact with contaminated sandy areas. Unable to proceed

through the bloodstream to the lungs and ultimately the intestines of the unnatural host, the larvae remain in the skin, wander aimlessly along the dermal-epidermal junction, and produce the characteristic serpentine tracts seen in this disorder.

The onset of creeping eruption is characterized by pruritus at the site of larval penetration (usually the feet, lower legs, buttocks, or hands). The larvae may lie quietly for weeks or months or may begin a tortuous serpentine migration along the dermal-epidermal junction. Their migration may vary from 1 mm to 1 or 2 cm a day, with resultant slightly elevated pink or flesh-colored tortuous or serpentine tracts (see Fig. 14–32). The number of tracts is variable (in one study the number ranged from 1 to 50, with an average of 10.9 tracts per patient). The disease is self-limiting. In most patients the parasites may wander aimlessly for periods of a few days to several weeks. In some patients they may persist for 6 months or longer. In one study it was noted that 81 per cent of lesions disappeared spontaneously within 4 weeks.[87]

For years the management of creeping eruption was inadequate and ineffective. It consisted of an attempt at larval destruction by caustic agents (trichloroacetic acid), by cryotherapy (ethyl chloride spray, carbon dioxide, or liquid nitrogen), or by electrodesiccation. These methods are effective only if the skin is damaged sufficiently to cause sloughing of the ensheathed parasite. This requires therapy aimed at a site just ahead of the advancing burrow. Unfortunately, advance of the parasite beyond the site of inflammation frequently complicates attempts at localization and destruction.

Since 1963 the broad-spectrum antihelminthic thiabendazole has been used successfully in the managment of creeping eruption. The treatment of choice consisted of oral thiabendazole (Mintezol) in a dosage of 25 mg/kg, given twice a day for 2 to 4 days, with a maximum dosage of 2 to 4 g/day.[87] Unfortunately, 30 to 40 per cent of patients treated in this manner develop side effects consisting of dizziness, nausea, cramps, and vomiting. These side effects, therefore, dictated the desirability of an

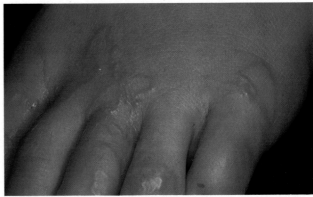

Figure 14–32. Creeping eruption (cutaneous larva migrans) with characteristic serpiginous tracts.

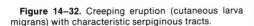

effective topical preparation. A 2 per cent solution of thiabendazole in dimethyl sulfoxide (DMSO) was effective, but difficulties with this combination limited its use to research purposes. The topical use of thiabendazole suspension (Mintezol) under an occlusive plastic film has been shown to be effective but produced pruritus and stinging in a substantial number of patients. Addition of a topical corticosteroid cream to topical thiabendazole (under occlusion with Saran Wrap for 24 to 48 hours) has been shown to be a most effective method of therapy,[86, 88] and albendazole (Zentel), a broad-spectrum antihelminthic not yet available in the United States or United Kingdom that appears to be as effective as thiabendazole and virtually free of side effects, can be given as a single 400-mg oral dose daily, regardless of age, for 3 consecutive days.[89]

Jellyfish

Jellyfish (the common name of a type of invertebrate sea animal) are classified as Coelenterata, a phylum that includes corals, sea anemones, and hydras. The Portuguese man-of-war is a jellyfish that floats on the surface of tropical seas and the Gulf Stream. All coelenterates possess tentacles that bear numerous stinging structures (nematocysts). On contact each nematocyst discharges a small barb and a neurotoxin that seems to paralyze fish on contact. In humans this toxin produces a toxic linear papulovesicular eruption within a few minutes after contact, erythematous or urticarial ulcerations, burning pain, vesiculation, necrotic cutaneous ulcerations, and systemic reactions characterized by fever, vomiting, collapse, shock, and, at times, death.[90]

Treatment consists of immediate bathing of affected areas to wash away the barbs, analgesics, applications of topical corticosteroids, soaking the area with vinegar for 30 minutes, followed by application of a mixture of baking soda for 10 minutes, and topical application of meat tenderizer (one in four parts of water) to affected areas to relieve local discomfort. In patients with systemic reactions, antihistamines, application of tourniquets on the affected limb or limbs in an effort to reduce venous return, intravenous calcium gluconate, and systemic corticosteroids are often beneficial.

Cercariae (Cercarial Dermatitis)

Cercarial dermatitis (also known as swimmer's itch, clam diggers' itch, or sea bather's eruption) is an acute pruritic papular cutaneous response that follows penetration of the skin by parasitic cercariae of the *Schistosoma* genus. Although global in its distribution, in North America this disorder has been noted most frequently in bathers in fresh water lakes in the north central part of the United States, with humans as the accidental host of schistosomes of birds, ducks, or cattle that use snails as their intermediate host. When it occurs after bathing in salt water, particularly in the Caribbean area and along the beaches of Florida, the disorder has been termed *sea bathers' eruption*, and when seen along the coastal areas of New England, Long Island Sound, and the Eastern shore of the United States it is often referred to as clam diggers' itch (Fig. 14–33). Although swimmers' itch, sea bather's eruption, and clam diggers' itch are often separated as distinct entities, this distinction is artificial and sometimes confusing and these probably represent variants of the same disorder.[91]

Affected individuals have no difficulty after initial exposure. Subsequent exposures, however, stimulate an allergic response to a protein residue deposited by the invading cercariae. A pricking or itching sensation may be noted at the time of cercarial penetration. This itching, which may last for periods of 5 minutes to 1 hour, is generally associated with 1- or 2-mm macules at each penetration site. The initial macules often persist or may disappear after a few hours, only to be followed, 10 to 15 hours later, by a more severe, intensely pruritic eruption characterized by 3- to 5-mm papules surrounded by variable zones of erythema. These papular lesions may or may not progress, with a resulting erythematous reaction consisting of edema, vesicles, and/or urticarial wheals. In most

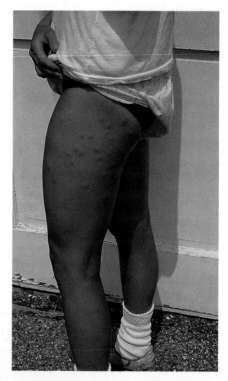

Figure 14–33. Cercarial dermatitis. A pruritic eruption on the legs of a teenager developed after wading in Long Island Sound at low tide. (Courtesy of George Kraus, M.D.)

individuals this stage of the eruption reaches its peak in 2 or 3 days, resolves within a week, and leaves a residual brown hyperpigmentation, which may persist for several months or more. Children are likely to have a more extensive eruption than that seen in adults and may at times have systemic reactions such as nausea, vomiting, and fever.

Prophylaxis of cercarial dermatitis consists of avoidance of prolonged immersion in polluted water and treatment of polluted fresh lakes or streams with a mixture of copper sulfate and carbonate, or sodium pentochlorphenate. Brisk towel drying can help remove or destroy the cercariae before penetration can occur, and the use of waterproof boots will help prevent infestation. In addition, some degree of protection can be gained by allowing a 20 per cent solution of copper sulfate to evaporate on the skin prior to bathing or wading in infested waters. Since cercarial dermatitis is self-limiting, treatment is generally palliative and consists of prevention of secondary infection, topical corticosteroids, topical antipruritic agents, oral antihistamines, and systemic corticosteroids, which although seldom necessary, are at times helpful for individuals with systemic reactions or severe involvement.

References

1. Mellanby K: Scabies, 2nd ed. E. W. Classey, Ltd., Hampton, England, 1972.

   Reissue of a classic review of scabies originally published in 1943 as one of a series of "Oxford War Manuals."

2. Stokes JH: Scabies among the well-to-do. J.A.M.A. 106:674–678, 1936.

   Scabies affects individuals from all walks of life.

3. Mellanby K: The development of symptoms, parasitic infection and immunity in human scabies. Parasitology 35:197–206, 1944.

   Studies on human volunteers suggest hypersensitivity as an explanation of some features of the clinical picture and cyclic epidemic nature of scabies.

4. Orkin M: Resurgence of scabies. J.A.M.A. 217:593–597, 1971.

   A forecast of global resurgence of scabies in epidemic proportions.

5. Madsen A: Why Acarus scabiei avoid the face. Acta. Derm. Venereol. 45:167–168, 1965.

   The author suggests that female mites avoid the head and face because of a greater density of hair follicles in this region (16 times that of the extremities and trunk).

6. Hurwitz S: Scabies in babies. Am. J. Dis. Child. 126:226–228, 1973.

   Scabies in infants and young children may be misdiagnosed because of a low index of suspicion, the frequent lack of burrows, secondary eczematization suggesting other conditions, and an atypical distribution in this age group.

7. Sehgal VN, Rao TL, Rege VL, Vadiraj SN: Scabies: A study of incidence and treatment method. Int. J. Dermatol. 11:106–111, 1972.

   Analysis of 1,015 cases of scabies revealed the most common lesions (in order of frequency) to be papules, vesicles, crusted lesions, pustules, burrows and wheals; burrows were seen in a mere 7 per cent of patients.

8. Friedman R: Atypical scabies: Diagnosis by the scrape and smear method. Penn. Med. J. 47:39–41, 1943.

   The burrow, the so-called pathognomonic clinical sign of scabies, is demonstrated in only 13 per cent of patients.

9. Berge T, Krook G: Persistent nodules in scabies. Acta Derm. Venereol. 47:20–24, 1967.

   Histologic study of five cases of nodules that persisted after apparent successful treatment of scabies suggest a possible allergic origin to these lesions.

10. Orkin M: Today's scabies. J.A.M.A. 233:882–885, 1975.

    A review of scabies, with emphasis on diagnosis and management.

11. Hubler WR Jr, Clabaugh W: Epidemic Norwegian scabies. Arch. Dermatol. 112:179–181, 1976.

    An epidemic of Norwegian scabies in a 25-patient ward of physically handicapped (mostly mongoloid) individuals.

12. Jucowics P, Raman ME, Stone RK, et al.: Norwegian scabies in an infant with acquired immunodeficiency syndrome. Arch. Dermatol. 125:1670–1671, 1989.

    A report of a 6-month-old infant with acquired immunodeficiency syndrome (AIDS) and hyperkeratotic scabies.

13. Smith EB, Claypoole TF: Canine scabies in dogs and humans. J.A.M.A. 199:95–100, 1967.

    A review of 22 patients with canine scabies.

14. Norins AL: Canine scabies in children. "Puppy dog" dermatitis. Am. J. Dis. Child. 117:239–242, 1969.

    Canine scabies in humans is characterized by small red papular and papulovesicular lesions with predilection for the chest, abdomen, and forearms.

15. Shelley ED, Shelley WB, Pula JF, et al.: The diagnostic challenge of nonburrowing mite bites. Cheyletiella yasguri. J.A.M.A. 251:2690–2691, 1984.

    The cause of an undiagnosed pruritic eruption was established only after the 6-year-old girl experienced an explosive attack of pruritus after taking a nap in the dog's sleeping box.

16. Cohen SR: Cheyletiella dermatitis: A mite infestation of rabbit, cat, dog, and man. Arch. Dermatol. 116:435–437, 1980.

    A report of two patients with recurring episodes of intensely pruritic, grouped, red papular lesions on the chest, abdomen, and thigh in which the diagnosis was established by careful examination of fur brushings of household pets.

17. Chakrabarti A: Human notoendric scabies from contact with cats infested with Notoedres cati. Int. J. Dermatol. 25:646–648, 1986.

    Hyperemia, pruritus, papulovesicular eruptions, and eczematous lesions in 30 patients following exposure to cats infested with Notoedres cati.

18. Chapel TA, Krugel L, Chapel J, et al.: Scabies presenting as urticaria. J.A.M.A. 246:1440–1441, 1981.

    The cause of generalized urticaria was only established after careful examination and recognition of an underlying scabietic infestation in three patients.

19. MacMillan AL: Unusual features of scabies associated with topical fluorinated steroids. Br. J. Dermatol. 87:496–497, 1972.

    An infant with scabies treated topically with potent fluorinated corticosteroids for 4 months manifested extensive scabietic infestation attributable to an adverse effect of topical corticosteroids.

20. Burgess I: Unusual features of scabies associated with topical fluorinated steroids. Br. J. Dermatol. 88:519–520, 1973.

    The prolonged application of potent topical corticosteroids appears to suppress cell-mediated immunity, thus upsetting the normal pattern of response to scabietic infestation.

21. Wannamaker LW: Differences between streptococcal infections of the throat and skin. N. Engl. J. Med. 282:23–31, 78–85, 1970.

Streptococcal infection of the skin does not lead to rheumatic fever.

22. Svartman M, Potter EV, Finklea JF, et al.: Epidemic scabies and acute glomerulonephritis in Trinidad. Lancet 1:249–251, 1972.

Cutaneous infection due to nephritogenic strains of streptococci is responsible for epidemics of acute glomerulonephritis following scabies.

23. Muller GH, Jacobs PH, Moore NE: Scraping for human scabies. Arch. Dermatol. 107:70, 1973.

A drop of mineral oil on suspected lesions allows easier scraping and more definitive identification of scabies.

24. Purvis RS, Tyring SK: An outbreak of lindane-resistant scabies treated successfully with permethrin 5% cream. J. Am. Acad. Dermatol. 25:1015–1016, 1991.

Of 12 persons exposed to a hospitalized patient with lindane-resistant Norwegian (hyperkeratotic) scabies, in whom resistance was documented in 7 of 10 patients treated with lindane, 1 responded to 10 per cent crotamiton cream and the remaining were cured by a single treatment of permethrin 5 per cent cream.

25. Feldman RJ, Maibach HI: Percutaneous penetration of some pesticides and herbicides in man. Toxicol. Appl. Pharmacol. 28:126–132, 1974.

Studies reveal that 9.3 per cent of gamma benzene hexachloride applied to adult skin can be recovered in the urine.

26. Lee B, Groth P, Turner W: Suspected reactions to gamma benzene hexachloride. J.A.M.A. 236:2846, 1976.

Reports of adverse reactions following *imprudent* use of gamma benzene hexachloride.

27. Lee B, Groth P: Letters to the editor: Scabies: Transcutaneous poisoning during treatment. Pediatrics 59:643, 1977.

Case reports of suspected central nervous system toxicity due to excessive or inappropriate use of gamma benzene hexachloride (lindane).

28. Ginsburg CM, Lowry W, Reisch JS: Absorption of lindane (gamma benzene hexachloride) in infants and young children. J. Pediatr. 91:998–1000, 1977.

Concentrations of lindane in the blood of 20 children who received treatment with 1 per cent lindane lotion were inversely related to the body weight and surface area of the treated patients.

29. Pramanik A, Hansen RC: Transcutaneous gamma benzene hexachloride absorption and toxicity in infants and children. Arch. Dermatol. 115:1224–1225, 1979.

Central nervous system toxicity in an infant following one topical application of gamma benzene hexachloride (lindane) to a premature malnourished infant; the level of gamma benzene hexachloride was 17 times greater than mean levels reported in children 48 hours after topical application of this agent.

30. Matsuoka LY: Convulsions following application of gamma benzene hexachloride. J. Am. Acad. Dermatol. 5:98–99, 1981.

A 7-year-old boy with tuberous sclerosis developed two petite mal seizures within 12 hours following one topical application of lindane for the treatment of scabies.

31. Berry DH, Brewster MA, Watson R, et al.: Untoward effects associated with lindane abuse. Am. J. Dis. Child. 141:125, 1987.

A report of a 14-year-old boy who developed a transient episode of blindness, dysarthria, syncope, and pancytopenia following repeated use of lindane (on at least eight occasions) for the treatment of scabies.

32. Davies JE, Dadhia HW, Morgade C, et al.: Lindane poisoning. Arch. Dermatol. 119:142–144, 1983.

A report of two lindane-related deaths: a 16-year-old retarded boy who accidentally ingested lindane and a 2-month-old infant treated with spot applications of lindane for 2 days and one total body application in which the medication was left on for 18 hours.

33. Friedman SJ: Lindane neurotoxic reaction in nonbullous congenital ichthyosiform erythroderma. Arch. Dermatol. 123:1056–1058, 1987.

A 3-year-old boy with nonbullous congenital ichthyosiform erythroderma developed nausea, vomiting, muscular spasms, and convulsions following a single treatment with lindane; the fact that the child was found to have elevated blood levels (54 mg/ml) reaffirms the need for caution in the use of this modality for patients with compromised epidermal barrier function.

34. Arlian LG, Runyan RA, Aschar S, et al.: Survival and infectivity of Sarcoptes scabei var. canis and var. hominis. J. Am. Acad. Dermatol. 11:210–215, 1984.

High temperatures and low relative humidity lead to early death of Sarcoptes mites (scabies mites require water from a host to avoid dehydration and death).

35. Yonkosky D, Ladia L, Gackenheimer L, et al.: Scabies in nursing homes: An eradication program with permethrin 5% cream. J. Am. Acad. Dermatol 23:1133–1136, 1990.

In a study in which scabies had plagued three large nursing homes, mass treatment of all residents, staff, frequent visitors, and family members who were symptomatic or known to be exposed to scabies resulted in an overall cure rate of 98 per cent after three or more treatments with 5 per cent permethrin cream.

36. Taplin D, Meinking TL, Porcelain SL, et al.: Permethrin 5% dermal cream: A new treatment for scabies. J. Am. Acad. Dermatol. 15:995–1001, 1986.

Five per cent permethrin cream gave a 91 per cent 1-month cure rate (vs. 65 per cent for lindane) in a heavily populated community in which scabies had been endemic for years and lindane had an unacceptable level of treatment failures.

37. Schultz MW, Gomez M, Hansen RC, et al.: Comparative study of 5% permethrin cream and 1% lindane lotion for the treatment of scabies. Arch. Dermatol. 126:167–170, 1990.

Following a multicenter controlled study comparing 5 per cent permethrin cream and 1 per cent lindane lotion, permethrin cream was recommended as the treatment of choice for scabies in children, and possibly in adults as well.

38. Taplin D, Meinking TL, Chen JA, et al.: Comparison of crotamiton 10% cream (Eurax) and permethrin 5% cream (Elimite) for the treatment of scabies in children. Pediatr. Dermatol. 7:67–73, 1990.

In a study comparing the treatment of scabies in children 2 months to 5 years of age in which Elimite was found to be more effective than Eurax, the authors recommended the permethrin formulation as a safe, efficacious, and cosmetically acceptable form of therapy for the treatment of this disorder in infants and children.

39. Witkowski JA, Parish JC: Scabies: Subungual areas harbor mites. J.A.M.A. 252:1318–1319, 1984.

Until the nails were trimmed and lindane was applied to the subungual areas, a patient with subungual involvement was thought to be resistant to lindane.

40. Cubela V, Yawalker SJ: Clinical experience with crotamiton cream and lotion in treatment of infants with scabies. Br. J. Clin. Pract. 32:229–231, 1978.

In a study of 50 infants and small children with scabies treated with 10 per cent crotamiton cream or lotion, a 5-day regimen resulted in a cure rate of 69 per cent (and a benefit rate of 85 per cent), and the cream formulation was found to be more effective than the lotion.

41. Konstantinov D, Stanoeva L, Yawalker SJ: Crotamiton cream and lotion in the treatment of infants and young children with scabies. J. Inter. Med. Res. 7:443–448, 1979.

A comparison of crotamiton cream or lotion given over a 5-day period in 50 hospitalized infants and small children from 3 months to 2 years of age found the cream formulation to be more effective and a 5-day treatment in a hospital more effective than treatment at home.

42. Lasch EE, Frankel V, Pardy PA, et al.: Epidemic glomerulonephritis in Israel. J. Infect. Dis. 124:141–147, 1971.

Early treatment of streptococcal infection did not appear to prevent the development of acute glomerulonephritis.

43. Selfon PM: The red mite among our field personnel. Milit. Med. 127:479–484, 1962.

Clear nail polish appears to be effective for relief of chigger bites.

44. Gouck, HK: Protection from ticks, fleas, chiggers, and leeches. Arch. Dermatol. 93:112–113, 1966.

Mosquito repellents are good chigger toxicants; benzyl benzoate is also effective and withstands washing and submersion in water.

45. Betz TG, Davis BL, Fournier PV, et al.: Occupational dermatitis associated with straw itch mites (*Pyemotes ventricosus*). J.A.M.A. 247:2821–2823, 1982.

An outbreak of itch mite dermatitis was traced to occupational exposure to infested wheat.

46. Westrom DR, Milligan MP: Rodent mite dermatitis. J. Assoc. Milit. Dermatol. 10:19–20, 1984.

A 23-year-old woman presented with a pruritic rash traced to exposure to rodent mites from a bed and an adjacent wall acquired during a stay at a hotel.

47. Shelley WB, Shelley ED, Welbourn WC: Polypodium fern wreaths (Hagnaya): A new source of occupational mite dermatitis. J.A.M.A. 253:3137–3138, 1985.

Successful treatment of mite dermatitis depends on careful evaluation and detection of all potential sources of infestation.

48. Fishman HC: Rat mite dermatitis. Cutis 42:414–416, 1988.

A report of an elderly woman with a severe excoriated pruritic eruption found to be the result of an infestation by the rat mite (*Ornithonyssus bacoti*).

49. Lee BW: *Cheyletiella* dermatitis: A report of fourteen cases. Cutis 47:111–114, 1991.

A report of 14 cases of *Cheyletiella* dermatitis over an 8-year period in a small community.

50. Jellison WL, Gregson JD: Tick paralysis in northwestern United States and British Columbia. Rocky Mountain Med. J. 47:28–53, 1950.

An undertaker who picked ticks off a cadaver subsequently died of tick paralysis.

51. Needham GR: Evaluation of five popular methods for tick removal. Pediatrics 75:997–1002, 1985.

Straight upward pulling with forceps, tweezers, or protected fingers (as close to the skin as possible, in an effort to remove the mouth parts) is suggested as the method of choice for tick removal.

52. Revveni H, Yaguspy P: Diethyltoluamide-containing insect repellent: Adverse effects in worldwide use. Arch. Dermatol. 118:582–583, 1982.

A report of 10 soldiers with eruptions in the antecubital fossae, burning, erythema, blistering, and, in some instances, ulcerations and scarring, following the use of an insect repellent containing 50 per cent DEET.

53. Heick HMC, Peterson RG, Dalpe-Scott M, et al.: Insect repellent, *N*, *N*-diethyl-m-toluamide, effect on ammonia metabolism. Pediatrics 82:373–376, 1988.

A review of three possible mechanisms for systemic reaction to diethyltoluamide.

54. Insect repellents. Med. Lett. 31:45–47, 1989.

A comparison of various insect repellents with emphasis on their efficiency and possible side effects.

55. King LE Jr, Rees RS: Treatment of brown recluse spider bites. J. Am. Acad. Dermatol. 14:691–692, 1986.

Therapeutic recommendations based on observations in 31 patients with severe brown recluse spider bites.

56. Wong RC, Hughes SE, Voorhees JJ: Review in depth: Spider bites. Arch. Dermatol. 123:98–104, 1987.

A comprehensive review of spiders and spider bites, their diagnosis and management.

57. Chadha JS, Leviav A: Hemolysis, renal failure, and local necrosis following scorpion sting. J.A.M.A. 241:1038, 1979.

Renal failure associated with severe hemolysis following a scorpion sting.

58. Rimsza ME, Zimmerman DR, Bergeson PS: Scorpion envenomation. Pediatrics 66:298–302, 1980.

A review of signs, symptoms and management of scorpion stings.

59. Arnold HL Jr: Correspondence: Reply to a letter: P(h)thirus pubis. J. Am. Acad. Dermatol. 14:282, 1986.

Although *Phthirus pubis* should have been the designation for the pubic louse, an error by the International Committee on Zoological Nomenclature inadvertently accepted a misspelling (*Pthirus pubis*) as the official designation of the crab louse.

60. Silburt BS, Parsons WL: Scalp infestation by *Pthirus pubis* in a 6-week-old infant. Pediatr. Dermatol. 7:205–207, 1990.

A report of a 6-week-old infant with *P. pubis* infestation of the scalp in which the mother and her partner both had pubic lice.

61. Signore RJ, Love J, Boucree MC: Scalp infection with *Phthirus pubis*. Arch. Dermatol. 125:133, 1989.

A report of *Pthirus pubis* scalp infestation in a 25-year-old woman and her three children.

62. Rasmussen JE: Pediculosis and the pediatrician. Pediatr. Dermatol. 2:74–79, 1984.

The epidemiology, clinical appearance, and treatment of pediculosis in childhood.

63. Kohn SR: Hair casts or pseudonits. J.A.M.A. 238:2058–2059, 1977.

Hair casts, or pseudonits, are 2 to 7 mm long, discrete, firm, shiny, white, freely movable accretions that encircle the hair shafts of the scalp and may be responsible for pseudoepidemics of pediculosis capitis.

64. Scott MJ, Esterly NB: Eyelash infestation by *Phthirus pubis* as a manifestation of child abuse. Pediatr. Dermatol. 1:179, 1983.

A 4-year-old girl with *Pthirus pubis* infestation of the eyelids, which appeared to be the result of sexual molestation by her mother's boyfriend.

65. Meinking TL, Taplin D, Kalter DC, et al.: Comparative efficacy of treatments for pediculosis capitis infestations. Arch. Dermatol. 122:267–271, 1986.

A comparison of six pesticides commonly used for the treatment of pediculosis capitis.

66. Taplin D, Meinking TL, Castillero PM, et al.: Permethrin 1% creme rinse for the treatment of *Pediculus humanus* var. *capitis* infestation. Pediatr. Dermatol. 3:344–348, 1986.

Permethrin 1 per cent demonstrates high pediculicidal and ovicidal activities that, in combination with its low toxicity, residual activity, and cosmetic properties, makes it an excellent treatment for pediculosis capitis.

67. Brandenberg K, Deinerd AS, DiNapoli J, et al.: 1% permethrin creme rinse vs. 1% lindane shampoo in treating pediculosis capitis. Am. J. Dis. Child. *140*:894–896, 1986.

Of 257 patients treated with 1 per cent permethrin creme rinse, 99 per cent were free of pediculosis 14 days after treatment.

68. Carson DS, Tribble PW, Weart CW: Pyrethrins combined with piperonyl butoxide (RID) vs. 1 per cent permethrin (Nix) in the treatment of head lice. Am. J. Dis. Child. *142*:768–769, 1988.

In a randomized controlled trial, permethrin creme rinse was found to be more effective than RID for the eradication of head lice.

69. DeFelice J, Rumsfield JQ, Bernstein JE, et al.: Clinical evaluation of an after-pediculocide nit removal system. Int. J. Dermatol. *218*:468–470, 1989.

A creme rinse containing formic acid that loosens the bond between the nit and hair greatly facilitated nit removal.

70. Mathew M, D'Souza P, Mehta DK: A new treatment of pthiriasis palpebrarum. Ann. Ophthalmol. *14*:439–441, 1982.

One or two drops of freshly prepared 20 per cent fluorescein eye drops, when applied to the lid margins, was shown to be lethal to pubic louse infestation of the eyelids and its nits; reapplication 10 days later, however, was recommended to eliminate possible newly hatched lice.

71. Shannon WR: Thiamine chloride—an aid in the solution of the mosquito problem. Minn. Med. *26*:799, 1943.

Although studies on oral thiamine give conflicting results, this vitamin may offer value as a mosquito repellent.

72. Marks MB: Stinging insects: Allergy implications. Pediatr. Clin. North Am. *16*:191, 1969.

Fifty to 70 per cent of children with histories of severe local response to insect bites appear to improve with thiamine hydrochloride (25 mg three times a day).

73. Kenney RL, Baker FJ: Botfly (*Dermatobia hominis*) myiasis. Int. J. Dermatol. *23*:676–677, 1984.

A 43-year-old man who had been working in Panama had three 1.5- to 3.0-cm erythematous nodules, each with a central orifice, as a manifestation of myiasis.

74. Medleau L, Miller WH Jr: Flea infestation and its control. Int. J. Dermatol. *22*:378–379, 1983.

A comprehensive review of flea infestation and valuable tips on control measures for the management of this disorder.

75. Blank, H, Shaffer B, Spencer MC, et al.: Papular urticaria: A study of the role of insects in its etiology and the use of DDT in its treatment. Pediatrics *5*:408–412, 1950.

Seventy-seven per cent of 30 patients with papular urticaria, in contrast to 2 of 124 in a control series, proved to be sensitive to flea and bedbug antigens, thus supporting the theory of hypersensitivity as the cause of papular urticaria.

76. Shaffer B, Jacobson C, Beerman H: Histopathologic correlation of lesions of papular urticaria and positive skin test reactions to insect antigens. Arch. Dermatol. Syph. *70*:437–442, 1954.

Histologic examination of lesions of papular urticaria display similarity to ordinary insect bites and urticarial and delayed skin reactions to insect antigens.

77. Caro MR, Derbes VJ: Skin responses to the study of the imported fire ant (*Solenopsis saevissima*). Arch. Dermatol. *75*:475–488, 1957.

The fire ant imported from South America, a particularly destructive insect, has spread rapidly in the southern part of the United States.

78. Ginsburg CM: Fire ant envenomation in children. Pediatrics *73*:689–692, 1984.

A review of fire ant infestation, its diagnosis and management.

79. deShazo RD, Butcher BT, Banks WA: Reactions to the stings of the fire ant. N. Engl. J. Med. *323*:462–466, 1990.

A comprehensive review of fire ant reactions and their management.

80. Valentine MD, Schuberth KC, Kagey-Sobotka A, et al.: The value of immunotherapy with venom in children with allergy to insect stings. N. Engl. J. Med. *323*:1601–1603, 1990.

Although venom immunotherapy prevents recurrences of systemic reactions, only 9.2 per cent of insect stings lead to systemic reactions.

81. McMillan CS, Purcell W: Hazards to health: the puss caterpillar, alias wooly slug. N. Engl. J. Med. *271*:147–149, 1964.

More than 50 species of caterpillars possess irritative hairs. Depending on the species, their effects range from a local dermatitis to a dangerous disorder with systemic signs and symptoms.

82. Daly JJ, Derrick BL: Puss caterpillar sting in Arkansas. South Med. J. *68*:893–894, 1975.

Toxin from the hairs of the puss caterpillar can produce numbness and swelling of the affected areas, severe radiating pain, regional lymphadenopathy, nausea, and fever.

83. Zaias N, Ioannides G, Taplin D: Dermatitis from contact with moths (genus *Hylesia*). J.A.M.A. *207*:525–527, 1969.

Histopathologic examination of dermatitis from exposure to *Hylesia* moths suggests toxic injury as the principal cause of caterpillar dermatitis.

84. McGovern JP, Barkin GD, McElhenney TR, et al.: *Megalopyge opercularis*: Observations of its life history, natural history of its sting in man, and report of an epidemic. J.A.M.A. *175*:1155–1158, 1961.

The symptoms of exposure to the puss caterpillar include marked local pain and swelling, lymphadenopathy, headache, shock-like symptoms and convulsions.

85. Beaucher WB, Farnham JE: Gypsy moth caterpillar dermatitis. N. Engl. J. Med. *306*:1301–1302, 1982.

A review of gypsy moth caterpillar dermatitis, a disorder believed to be a form of delayed contact dermatitis caused by irritation and release of histamine by the setae (hairs) of the gypsy moth caterpillar.

86. Edelglass JW, Douglass MC, Stiefler R, et al.: Cutaneous larva migrans in northern climates: A souvenir of your dream vacation. J. Am. Acad. Deramtol. *7*:353–358, 1982.

A report of three women who developed creeping eruption during their Caribbean vacations successfully treated with topical thiabendazole.

87. Kata R, Ziegler J, Blank H: The natural course of creeping eruption and treatment with thiabendazole. Arch. Dermatol. *91*:420–424, 1965.

Systemic thiabendazole effective in the treatment of creeping eruption.

88. Davis CM, Israel RM: Treatment of creeping eruption with thiabendazole. Arch. Dermatol. *97*:325–326, 1968.

In 15 patients with creeping eruption, 160 of 164 tracts cleared in 1 week with topical treatment with 10 per cent thiabendazole suspension; symptomatic relief of pruritus was noted within 3 days.

89. Orihuela AR, Torres JR: Single dose of albendazole in the treatment of cutaneous larva migrans. Arch. Dermatol. *126*:398–399, 1900.

Eight patients with cutaneous larva migrans successfully treated with oral albendazole without side effects.

90. Bengston K, Nicholas MM, Schnadig V, et al.: Sudden death

in a child following envenomation by *Chiropsalmus quadru-manus.* J.A.M.A. *266:*1404–1406, 1991.

A report of a 4-year-old child in Texas who died within 40 minutes after an encounter with a jellyfish.

91. Fisher AA: Atlas of Aquatic Dermatology. Grune & Stratton, New York, 1978.

A comprehensive pictorial and descriptive review of water-related dermatoses, their diagnosis and management.

BULLOUS DISORDERS OF CHILDHOOD

Blisters or bullae are rounded or irregularly shaped lesions of the skin or mucous membranes that result from the accumulation of fluid between the cells of the epidermis or between the epidermis and underlying corium. The term *bullae* refers to blistering lesions 0.5 to 1 cm or more in diameter; those less than 0.5 cm in diameter are termed *vesicles*. Owing to our limited knowledge, the classification of bullous or vesiculobullous disorders was initially based on clinical morphology and light microscopic examination, differed according to the national background and training of individual authors, and implied neither an etiologic nor a pathogenic basis to the disease process.

Although our knowledge as to pathogenetic mechanisms remains limited, current classification is based on clinical features, electron microscopic examination, and, whenever possible, immunopathologic mechanisms. It is well recognized that the skin of infants and children is more susceptible to blister formation than that of adults. With the exception of epidermolysis bullosa, however, the blistering group of diseases in general are a relatively uncommon group of disorders in childhood.

EPIDERMOLYSIS BULLOSA

The term *epidermolysis bullosa* refers to a group of inherited disorders characterized by bullous lesions that develop spontaneously or as a result of varying degrees of friction or trauma. Although categorization of types of epidermolysis bullosa in the past has been controversial and often confusing, approximately 20 phenotypes of inherited epidermolysis bullosa have now been delineated. They may be divided into three major inherited forms (simplex, junctional, and dystrophic), based on the presence or absence of scarring, the mode of inheritance, and the level of skin cleavage following minor trauma, and an acquired form (epidermolysis bullosa acquisita).[1] In epidermolysis bullosa simplex (epidermolytic EB, EB simplex) the blister cleavage occurs within the epidermis and healing occurs without scarring. In junctional epidermolysis bullosa the skin separates in the lamina lucida of the dermal-epidermal junction and blistering leads to mild atrophic changes. In dermolytic (dystrophic, scarring) epidermolysis bullosa the blister forms in the papillary dermis, below the basement membrane. (Table 15–1). Although the exact prevalence of epidermolysis bullosa is not known, mild variants have been estimated to occur as frequently as 1 in every 50,000 births and the more severe varieties are believed to occur in 1 per 500,000 population per year.[2–4]

Nonscarring Forms of Epidermolysis Bullosa

EPIDERMOLYSIS BULLOSA SIMPLEX

Epidermolysis bullosa simplex, an autosomal dominant disorder associated with defective kera-

Table 15–1. CLASSIFICATION OF EPIDERMOLYSIS BULLOSA

Type	Inheritance	Blister Location	Structural Defect
1. *Simplex (Epidermolytic, Nondystrophic)*			
Localized (Weber-Cockayne)	AD	Basal and suprabasal cells	Keratinocyte lysis
Generalized (Koebner)	AD	Basal cells	Keratinocyte lysis
Herpetiformis (Dowling-Meara variant)	AD	Basal cells	Basal cell cytolysis with clumping of tonofilaments
Ogna	AD	Intraepidermal	Keratinocyte lysis
Epidermolysis bullosa simplex with mottled pigmentation, with or without keratoderma	AD	Intraepidermal	Basal cell cytolysis
2. *Junctional*			
Lethal (gravis, Herlitz)	AR	Lamina lucida	Reduced number and abnormal structure of hemidesmosomes
Nonlethal (mitis, non-Herlitz)	AR	Lamina lucida	Hemidesmosome abnormality not consistent
Junctional epidermolysis bullosa inversa	AR	Lamina lucida	Hypoplasia of hemidesmosomes
3. *Dystrophic (Dermolytic)*			
Dominant dystrophic	AD	Below basal lamina	Reduced number of anchoring fibrils
Recessive dystrophic, generalized	AR	Below basal lamina	Absence of anchoring fibrils, collagenolysis
Recessive dystrophic, localized	AR	Below basal lamina	Reduced number of anchoring fibrils

AD, autosomal dominant; AR, autosomal recessive. Modified from Hurwitz S, Eady RAJ: Epidermolysis bullosa. *In* Rook A, Parish LC, Beare JM (Eds.): Practical Management of the Dermatologic Patient. J. B. Lippincott Co., Philadelphia, 1986.

tin filaments, is characterized by blisters that develop in areas of trauma. Since the blister cleavage is intraepidermal, lesions tend to heal without scarring. Forms of epidermolysis bullosa simplex include localized epidermolysis bullosa (Weber-Cockayne disease), epidermolysis bullosa simplex of the generalized (Koebner) type, epidermolysis bullosa simplex herpetiformis (the Dowling-Meara type), an Ogna variant described in Norwegian kindreds, and epidermolysis bullosa with mottled pigmentation with or without keratoderma (Table 15–2).

Localized epidermolysis bullosa simplex (epidermolysis bullosa simplex of the hands and feet, the Weber-Cockayne variant) is a clinical variant that requires a relatively high threshold of frictional trauma to induce blister formation and bullae. It is usually confined to the hands and feet (primarily the palms and soles) and is associated with hyperhidrosis and hyperkeratosis (Fig. 15–1). Probably the most common form of epidermolysis bullosa simplex, blisters can occur in the first 2 years of life but frequently do not appear until adolescence or early adulthood. The bullae, usually associated with trauma, particularly in hot weather, in general are not seriously debilitating. Hyperhidrosis is common, and hyperkeratosis of the palms and soles, although often present, is usually mild. Although the pathophysiology is not fully understood, it appears to represent an exaggeration of the normal mechanism for production of friction blisters, possibly related to activation of a cytolytic enzyme (or enzymes) and an associated dyskeratosis of squamous cells in the epidermis. Lesions heal rapidly without scarring, nail involvement rarely occurs, and the teeth and mucous membranes (except for occasional scattered oral erosions) are not involved. In young children, blisters develop on the knees from the frictional trauma of crawling. In adolescents and young adults, blisters may occur on the feet after long hikes or on the hands following a game of tennis or golf. Although an autosomal dominant mode of inheritance is generally described for this subset, an autosomal recessive form may also exist.[5]

Cytolysis of epidermal cells is the essential histologic feature of epidermolysis bullosa simplex. Epidermal cleavage usually occurs in the mid-squamous area but it may be noted anywhere from the suprabasal to the lower granular cell layers of the epidermis.

Generalized epidermolysis bullosa simplex (Koebner variant) is an autosomal dominant disorder in which the bullae generally heal without scarring. Although erosions of the mucous membranes (as a result of vigorous sucking) may be seen in the newborn, mucosal involvement is generally mild and the nails are rarely affected. If nails are shed, they regrow without dystrophy, but on rare occasions longitudinal striations or brittleness may occur. Involvement of the conjunctiva and cornea may also be present but is uncommon. The disorder generally tends to improve at puberty, and patients usually have a normal life span. In some

Table 15–2. EPIDERMOLYSIS BULLOSA SIMPLEX

Type	Clinical Manifestations
Localized epidermolysis bullosa simplex (Weber-Cockayne disease, recurrent bullous eruption of hands and feet)	May be present in first 2 years of life, but usually before adolescence or early adulthood; bullae usually confined to hands and feet
Generalized epidermolysis bullosa simplex (Koebner variant)	Bullae usually present at birth or early infancy; generally improves in adolescence; little to no mucosal involvement; nail involvement in 20%
Epidermolysis bullosa herpetiformis (Dowling-Meara disease)	Onset at birth or early infancy; may be severe and, when extensive, life threatening; herpetiform pattern on trunk and extremities; nails may be shed but regrow; warm temperatures do not exacerbate blistering
Epidermolysis bullosa simplex (Ogna variant)	Described in Norwegian kindreds; onset in infancy; hemorrhagic and serous blisters on hands and feet and occasionally elsewhere; heal without scarring; onychogryphosis; a bruising tendency of the skin; linkage with erythrocyte glutamic pyruvic transaminase locus
Epidermolysis bullosa simplex with mottled pigmentation, with or without keratoderma	Onset at birth or early infancy; association with mottled hyperpigmentation and hypopigmentation; usually evident at birth or early childhood; may fade with increasing age

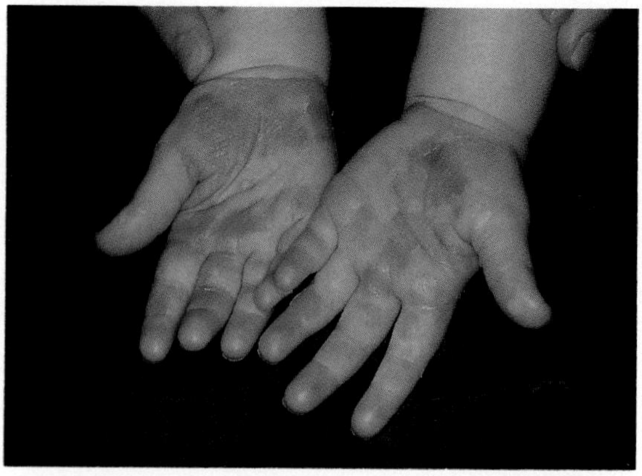

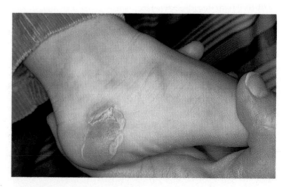

Figure 15–1. Localized epidermolysis bullosa simplex (Weber-Cockayne disease, recurrent bullous eruption of the hands and feet) on the hands of a 2½-year-old girl.

cases, however, the disease may be severe and life threatening in early infancy.[4]

Epidermolysis bullosa simplex usually begins at birth or shortly thereafter. In the neonatal period blisters or large erosions tend to involve areas of friction, namely, the hands, feet, neck, and lower aspect of the legs. As the infant begins to crawl and walk, the knees, ankles, feet, buttocks, elbows, and hands are the principal areas of involvement, and blisters, owing to rubbing from clothing, may also occur in other locations (Fig. 15–2). After age 3 years usually only the hands and feet are affected. Heat and trauma, as in other forms of epidermolysis bullosa, aggravate the disorder. Hyperhidrosis is common, and mild to moderate hyperkeratosis of the soles is often present. Palmar hyperkeratosis, however, if present, is usually mild.

Electron microscopic examination shows cleavage through the basal layer (above the periodic acid–Schiff-positive basement membrane of the epidermis), formation of vacuoles in the basal cells adjacent to areas of separation, and displacement of nuclei to the epidermal end of involved cells. Although the pathogenesis of this disorder has not been fully delineated, the disorder appears to be related to defects in a gene resulting in abnor-

mal keratin, mechanical trauma, and an associated temperature-sensitive activation of cytolytic enzymes. Deficiencies of galactosylhydroxylysyl glucosyltransferase and gelatinase (an enzyme involved in collagen degradation) in skin fibroblast cultures have been reported to exist, but the significance of these enzyme defects is as yet unknown.[3]

Epidermolysis bullosa simplex herpetiformis (Dowling-Meara variant) is a rare autosomal dominant disorder characterized by herpetiform clustering of blisters (often extensive) at birth or in early infancy and palmoplantar keratoderma.[6] A pronounced inflammatory reaction followed by transient formation of milia may occur early in life, large serosanguineous blisters appear on the hands and feet, and spontaneous blisters develop in a herpetiform pattern on the proximal extremities and trunk. After the age of 6 or 7 years hyperkeratosis of the palms and soles may develop; and although involvement of the mucosae and nail may occur during the neonatal period, the nails regrow without dystrophy. The Dowling-Meara variant, which is associated with an intrinsic abnormality in keratinocytes,[6] has a relatively good overall

Figure 15–2. Epidermolysis bullosa simplex. Blisters develop in areas of trauma and heal without subsequent scar formation.

prognosis but can mimic severe dystrophic or junctional forms of the disorder early in its course. With extensive blistering, the disease may prove life threatening and there is significant morbidity and mortality during the neonatal period. After this period the blistering is rarely a threat to life, and blistering tends to decrease during later childhood and adulthood.[7, 8] In contrast to other types of epidermolysis bullosa simplex, it has been suggested that warm temperatures do not appear to exacerbate blistering and that dramatic clearing may follow high fevers. Warm salt water bathing, therefore, is often suggested as a form of therapy.[2, 9] Blister cleavage in this variant occurs within the epidermis and begins with clumping of tonofilaments and basal cell cytolysis.

Epidermolysis bullosa simplex (Ogna variant) is an autosomal dominant disorder originally recognized in a large pedigree from Ogna, Norway. It has its onset in infancy and is characterized by small hemorrhagic and serous blisters that occur, particularly during the summer months, on the hands and feet, and occasionally elsewhere, and heal without scarring. The distinguishing features of this disorder are onychogryphosis of the great toenails (which occurs later in life), an associated bruising tendency, and genetic linkage to the erythrocyte glutamic pyruvic transaminase (GPT) locus.[2, 4]

JUNCTIONAL EPIDERMOLYSIS BULLOSA

Junctional epidermolysis bullosa is a mechanobullous disorder in which the cleavage plane occurs in the lamina lucida at the junction of the epidermis and dermis (Table 15–3). Encompassing a spectrum from severe life-threatening disease to relatively mild involvement, various subtypes of this disorder have been described, each transmitted in an autosomal recessive manner. In the most severe form, usually referred to as Herlitz disease, blistering begins at birth and death frequently occurs during the first 2 years of life. Not all types of junctional epidermolysis bullosa, however, have the dismal prognosis of the Herlitz variety.[1, 9–11]

Junctional epidermolysis bullosa (Herlitz variant), the most severe form of junctional epidermolysis bullosa, is characterized by blistering and large erosions (Fig. 15–3) mainly on the buttocks, trunk, and scalp without scarring and milia formation unless complicated by secondary infection. Although approximately 50 per cent of patients with this disorder die within the first 2 years of life, some patients survive into adulthood. It is therefore suggested that the term *epidermolysis bullosa letalis* no longer be used to describe this disorder. Healing results in mild atrophic changes, generally without milia formation; and although the hands and feet are usually spared, the oral mucous membranes are affected and pyloric atresia may be seen. There is involvement of the nail folds with

Table 15–3. JUNCTIONAL EPIDERMOLYSIS BULLOSA

Type	Clinical Manifestations
Epidermolysis bullosa letalis (Herlitz variant)	Onset at birth; 50% of patients die within first 2 years of life; perioral involvement with sparing of lips; blisters, unless complicated by infection, heal without scarring or milia; nails may show paronychia; teeth may be dysplastic; patients who survive tend to have severe growth retardation and anemia; laryngeal involvement is often an unrecognized cause of death
Generalized atrophic benign epidermolysis bullosa (nonlethal, mitis variant)	Serosanguineous blistering at birth; atrophic scarring; dystrophic or absent nails; palmoplantarhyperkeratosis and scarring alopecia may be present; blisters predominate on extemities, but may occur on scalp, trunk, or face; normal growth; patients improve with age
Junctional epidermolysis bullosa inversa	At birth or early infancy; pyoderma-like generalized blistering early; later affects inverse sites (axillae, groin, neck, and perineal areas); nail dystrophy, dysplastic teeth; hoarseness from laryngeal involvement

blistering of the fingertips (an important, if not diagnostic, feature) and, at times, loss of nails. The teeth may be dysplastic, and a cobblestone appearance to the dental enamel is characteristic. Perioral involvement with sparing of the lips is reported to be pathognomonic, and severe growth retardation and recalcitrant anemia are common. Hoarseness and laryngeal involvement are common, and the latter, often unrecognized, is a frequent complication and cause of death in infants and young children with this disorder.[12]

Light microscopy reveals subepidermal cleavage above the basement membrane and, as in all forms of junctional epidermolysis bullosa, electron microscopy shows blister formation in the lamina lucida. Reduced numbers and abnormal structures of hemidesmosomes have been noted in the Herlitz variant, but aside from the ultrastructural abnormalities, the pathogenesis is unknown.[3]

Nonlethal (mitis, non-Herlitz) junctional epidermolysis bullosa begins with serosanguineous blistering at birth and results in cutaneous atrophy and fragility without scarring or milia formation.[13] Alopecia, dystrophic or absent nails, hyperkeratotic palms and soles, and scalp atrophy are all features of this disorder. Mucous membrane (oral, conjunctival, esophageal, laryngeal, or tracheal) involvement is mild to moderate, but esophageal

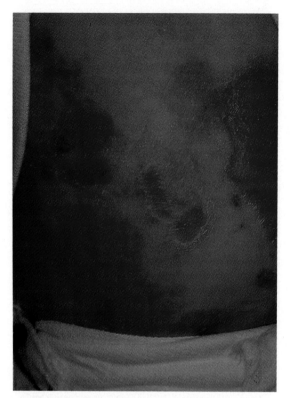

Figure 15–3. Junctional epidermolysis bullosa encompasses a spectrum from severe life-threatening disease (the Herlitz variant) to a benign nonlethal disorder.

strictures, excessive granulation tissue, and growth retardation are not present, and anemia is rarely seen. Affected individuals generally tend to have normal growth and life span, and the histologic features of this disorder are identical to those of the Herlitz variant.

Other reported forms of junctional epidermolysis bullosa include (1) a localized form, in which nails are dystrophic at birth, blisters occur primarily on the soles and lower extremities, the mucosae of the mouth and esophagus are spared, and all teeth show enamel dysplasia; (2) an inverse form in which blisters and erosions occur primarily in body folds, notably axillary areas and groins[14]; (3) a rare progressive form (epidermolysis bullosa progressiva, epidermolysis bullosa neurotropica), in which the skin and nails are normal until the age of 5 to 8 years when blistering and traumatic nail loss and nail dystrophy occur; and (4) cicatricial junctional epidermolysis bullosa, a disorder that has its onset at birth and in which the blisters, which appear predominantly on the hands, feet, knees, elbows, and trunk, heal with scarring and eventually result in acral mitten deformities; in this cicatricial form at times the patient may have dysplastic teeth, absent nails, contractures of the anterior nares, and/or subglottic stenosis.[9, 11]

Scarring Forms of Epidermolysis Bullosa

The scarring (dysplastic or dystrophic) types of epidermolysis bullosa are divided into dominant and recessive forms (Table 15–4). Although the term *epidermolysis bullosa* is retained, since bullae are subepidermal rather than epidermal, *dermolytic bullous dermatosis* is often used as a more accurate term for these disorders. The dominant disease is less severe. Affected individuals are generally healthy, are of normal stature, and have little or no involvement of hair and teeth. The recessive form, conversely, is severe and incapacitating. Growth and development are retarded, the teeth are abnormal, and hypotrichosis or alopecia is common (Figs. 15–4 through 15–9).

Histopathologic examination of involved skin in dystrophic forms of epidermolysis bullosa reveals separation at the dermal-epidermal junction, fragmentation of collagen bundles in the floor of blisters, and a lymphohistiocytic infiltrate with extravasation of erythocytes. Electron microscopy shows separation beneath the basal lamina (on the dermal side of the dermal-epidermal junction) and decrease or absence of anchoring fibrils in normal as well as blistered skin. The abnormality resides in the dermis.

The absence of anchoring fibrils (the apparent primary structural defect in recessive forms of dystrophic epidermolysis bullosa) allows disruption of the structural integrity of the dermal-epidermal junction and subsequent blister formation. Although anchoring fibrils are decreased or lacking in damaged skin of patients with dominant forms of dystrophic epidermolysis bullosa, studies of a large kindred revealed normal fibrils in the nonin-

Table 15–4. DYSTROPHIC (DERMOLYTIC) EPIDERMOLYSIS BULLOSA

Type	Clinical Manifestations
Dominant dystrophic epidermolysis bullosa	Early in infancy and later; of intermittent severity (between that of the simplex and recessive forms); little or no involvement of hair and teeth; 20% have mucous membrane lesions; 80% have nail dystrophy; albopapuloid form occurs later
Recessive dystrophic epidermolysis bullosa	Present at birth; widespread dystrophy, scarring, and deformity; digital fusion, contractures, and mitten deformities common; severe involvement of mucous membranes and nails; retardation of growth and development, poor nutrition, anemia, and mottled carious teeth common; predisposition to squamous cell carcinoma in heavily scarred areas

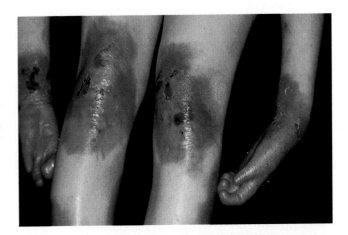

Figure 15–4. Epidermolysis bullosa, recessive dystrophic form (recessive dermolytic bullous dermatosis). Note hemorrhagic bullae, dystrophic scars, pseudosyndactyly and claw-like deformities of the hands. (Courtesy of Department of Dermatology, Yale University School of Medicine.)

volved skin of three individuals with this disorder. This suggests a possible means of differentiating dominant from recessive forms of this disorder, but it requires confirmation.

The most likely defect that would account for the pathologic alterations seen in dystrophic forms of epidermolysis bullosa therefore appears to be a structural abnormality of intradermal type VII collagen, with an associated impaired function of anchoring fibrils.[15–21]

Dominant Dystrophic Epidermolysis Bullosa.
Dominant dystrophic epidermolysis bullosa (dominant dermolytic bullous dermatosis), a disorder of intermediate severity, is characterized by atrophic scarring, nail dystrophy, and milia formation (Fig. 15–10). It is more severe than epidermolysis bullosa simplex and considerably milder than the recessive dystrophic disease. Although the onset of bullae in mild cases may occur later in life, blisters generally appear at birth or shortly thereafter. About 20 per cent of patients show changes before the age of 1 year. Improvement seems to occur with

age, and only rarely is there deformed scarring of the hands and feet approaching that seen in recessive disease. Dependent on the subset of dominant dystrophic epidermolysis bullosa present, scarring may be hypertrophic (the Cockayne-Touraine variant) or atrophic (the Pacini variant). Although mucous membrane lesions appear in 20 per cent of cases, they do not present the severe problems seen in patients with recessive dystrophic disease. Bullae generally appear on the dorsal aspect of extremities, milia are present, and atrophic scars occur. The teeth are generally not affected, the hair is not affected, physical development is normal, and the conjuctiva and cornea are less likely to be involved. In 80 per cent of cases, the nails may be thickened, dystrophic, or completely destroyed.

Albopapuloid Form of Epidermolysis Bullosa.
A unique variant of epidermolysis bullosa, the albopapuloid form is occasionally seen as a variant of

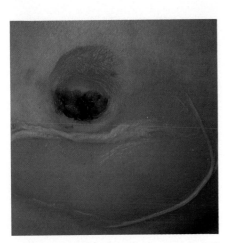

Figure 15–5. Recessive dystrophic epidermolysis bullosa (recessive dermolytic bullous dermatosis). A large blister is present on the lower aspect of the abdomen of a newborn.

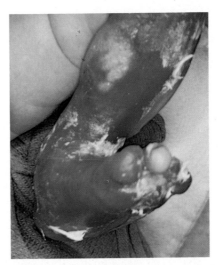

Figure 15–6. Recessive dystrophic epidermolysis bullosa (recessive dermolytic bullous dermatosis). Erosive lesions are seen on the foot and lower aspect of the leg of a newborn.

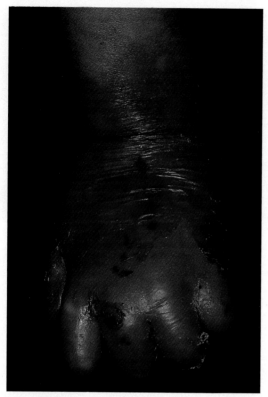

Figure 15-7. Recessive dystrophic epidermolysis bullosa (recessive dermolytic bullous dermatosis). Note hemorrhagic blisters, crusts, erosions, superficial, crinkled tissue paper–like appearance and mitten-like deformities of the hands and feet.

area of the skin may be involved in infants, the most commonly affected areas are the hands, feet, buttocks, scapulae, face, occiput, elbows, and knees. In older children the hands, feet, knees, and elbows are most commonly involved. Bullae may be hemorrhagic, and large areas, especially on the lower extremities, may be completely devoid of skin (similar to that seen in epidermolysis bullosa letalis) (see Fig. 15–6). When a blister ruptures or its roof peels off, a raw painful surface is evident. The Nikolsky sign (production or enlargement of a blister by slight pressure or the production of a moist abrasion by slight pressure on the skin) is often positive. Fluid contained in bullae, although at first sterile, may become secondarily infected, which can lead to sepsis; and in older children, nephritis has been seen as a sequela to streptococcal infection.

Bullae are often followed by atrophic scars or varying degrees of hyperpigmentation or hypopigmentation, or both. Milia are frequently seen (see Fig. 15–9), and in severely affected individuals large areas of the skin surface may show a fine superficial crinkled tissue-paper appearance (see Fig. 15–7). Repeated cycles of blistering, secondary infection, and healing leave wide areas of superficial scars and, at times, deep or hypertrophic cicatrices. The hands and lower aspects of the legs are particularly susceptible to severe involvement. With repeated scarring the fingers and toes may become fused, with resultant pseudosyndactyly. As the fingers become immobile (usually over prolonged periods of time), the hands and arms may become fixed in a flexed position, with resulting contractures (see Figs. 15–4 and 15–7). During fusion and with recurrent scarring, the digits may be bound together by a glove-like epidermal sac,

dominant dystrophic disease (Fig. 15–11). Although it may be present in infancy, this disorder usually begins in later childhood, early adolescence, or adult life. It is characterized by small, firm, raised, ivory-white perifollicular papules that vary from several millimeters to 1 cm or more in diameter. They appear independent of bullae and are generally seen on the trunk, particularly the lower back. Although generally associated with dominant dystrophic epidermolysis bullosa, similar lesions occasionally may be found in the recessive form of this disorder.

Recessive Dystrophic Epidermolysis Bullosa.
Recessive dystrophic epidermolysis bullosa (recessive dermolytic bullous dermatosis) can be divided into a mild localized form (mitis), a severe generalized disorder (gravis, Hallopeau-Siemens variant), or an inverse variant (recessive epidermolysis inversa).[14] Generalized recessive dystrophic epidermolysis bullosa is a severe distressing bullous disease characterized by widespread dystrophic scarring and deformity and by severe involvement of mucous membranes. In this disorder, erosions and blisters are usually manifested at or shortly after birth (see Fig. 15–5). Some blisters may appear to occur spontaneously, but most seem to arise at sites of pressure or trauma. Although any

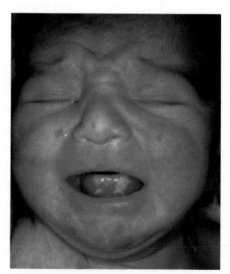

Figure 15-8. Involvement of the oral mucosa in an infant with recessive dystrophic epidermolysis bullosa (recessive dermolytic bullous dermatosis).

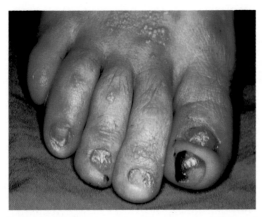

Figure 15–9. Recessive dystrophic epidermolysis bullosa (recessive dermolytic bullous dermatosis). Hemorrhagic bullae, milia, and nail dystrophy are seen.

with resulting claw-like clubbing or mitten-like deformities.

In recessive forms of dystrophic epidermolysis bullosa the nails may show extreme involvement, with severe dystrophy or complete absence of nails due to degeneration of the nail bed (see Fig. 15–9). The eyes may develop a number of characteristic changes, including blepharitis, symblepharon, and conjunctivitis or keratitis or both, with associated vesicle formation and corneal opacity. Hoarseness, aphonia, dysphagia, or all three may occur as a result of blistering of the larynx or pharynx. Laryngeal stenosis, although rare, may occur in varying degrees as the result of blistering and subsequent scarring of the larynx. Oral mucosal involvement occurs soon after birth, and erosions of the esophagus may at times result in segmental stenosis (most often in the upper half) with consequent difficulty in swallowing (see Fig. 15–8). Scarring in such cases is common and may resemble that seen after corrosive poisoning. Such children are reluctant to eat and, as a result, often fail to thrive. As the child grows older there is a tendency for the disease to become less severe, but the affected person soon learns to avoid hot drinks, rough foods, large particles, and anything that might produce blistering of the mouth, pharynx, or esophagus.

The teeth in the recessive dysplastic disorder are frequently delayed in eruption, are malformed, and are particularly susceptible to early and frequently severe caries. Even routine dental care may cause the eruption of bullae on the lips, gums, and oral mucosa, and the children soon come to recognize the sequelae associated with even slight abrasions from normal toothbrushing procedures. The face often has a "puckered" appearance about the mouth due to intraoral scarring. The ears may be mildly scarred or bound down to the scalp. Scalp and body hair may be sparse, and there may be patches of cicatricial alopecia.

In some cases the dystrophy may be minimal, and differentiation from milder forms of epider-

molysis may be difficult. In more severely affected individuals, death may occur during infancy or childhood as a result of septicemia, pneumonia, fluid loss from extensive areas of denuded skin, amyloidosis due to chronic and recurrent infection, renal failure (possibly due to chronic pyelonephritis), or malnutrition secondary to esophageal strictures. Other complications associated with this disorder include poor nutrition, secondary bacterial or candidal infection, erosions and scarring of the anal area (often resulting in severe discomfort, chronic constipation, or soiling), urethral stenosis, and, at times, urinary retention, hypertrophy of the bladder, and occasionally hydronephrosis, refractory anemia, hyperglobulinemic purpura, and clotting abnormalities. Those patients who have had epidermolysis for years may show a predisposition to carcinomas (both basal and squamous cell types) of the skin. The cause of this complication appears to be related to abnormal collagen in heavily scarred areas with continuing blister activity. The pathogenesis is probably similar to that seen in neoplastic disorders that arise in thermal burns and other chronic scars.

Treatment. As in any inherited disorder, it is the responsibility of the physician to inform parents of the risks associated with transmitting genetic abnormalities. When the condition is determined by a dominant gene (as in dominant dystrophic epidermolysis bullosa), if one parent is affected, there is a 50 per cent risk that each child will be so afflicted. In a family in which a child manifests abnormalities due to a recessive gene (as in recessive dystrophic epidermolysis bullosa), parents must be prepared to risk a 25 per cent possibility of this severe disorder occurring in future offspring. Appropriate genetic counseling, however, depends on accurate diagnosis. Since there is vari-

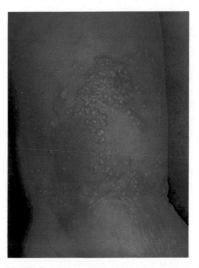

Figure 15–10. Dominant dystrophic epidermolysis bullosa. Erosions and milia formation are evident on the lower leg and foot of a 1½-year-old infant.

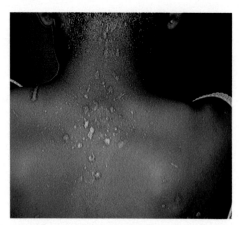

Figure 15–11. Albopapuloid form of epidermolysis bullosa. Small firm ivory-white perifollicular papules occur on the trunk of a patient with dominant dystrophic epidermolysis bullosa (dominant dermolytic bullous dermatosis). (Courtesy of Robert A. Briggaman, M.D.)

ability in the clinical course of many forms of epidermolysis bullosa, it is recommended that patients be carefully evaluated, appropriate family histories be obtained, and cutaneous biopsy, electron microscopy, and, in selected cases, immunofluorescent mapping and monoclonal studies be performed in an effort to establish an appropriate diagnosis.

The treatment of epidermolysis bullosa is palliative, with avoidance of trauma and control of secondary infection. Since blisters result from mechanical injury, measures should be taken to relieve pressure and prevent unnecessary trauma. A cool environment, avoidance of overheating, and lubrication of the skin to decrease the surface coefficient of friction are helpful in the reduction of blister formation. When blisters occur, extension may be prevented by aseptic aspiration of blister fluid. The roofs of blisters should be trimmed with a sterile scissors whenever feasible, and no ragged edges should be left under which organisms may flourish and lead to secondary infection.

A water mattress and a soft fleece covering will help to limit friction and trauma. Daily baths, topical protective antibiotic dressings, or sterile petrolatum-impregnated gauze applied with sterile precautions may help reduce topical bacterial infection and assist spontaneous healing of involved areas. Large denuded areas should be treated, whenever possible, by the open method (as in treatment of burns) with intravenous fluids, appropriate systemic antibiotics when indicated, and protection of injured areas by nonadherent dressings, petrolatum-impregnated gauze or commercially available synthetic dressings, with tape applied only to the occlusive covering (never to the skin).

Although it has been stated that high concentration topical corticosteroid preparations may facilitate healing of chronically blistered areas, this has not been verified. If sepsis is to be prevented or controlled, especially in the newborn and young infant, careful monitoring of the skin and mucosal florae is essential. In severe dystrophic forms of epidermolysis bullosa, topical antibiotic ointments and prophylactic antibiotics such as penicillin and erythromycin are valuable. They lessen the tendency to local infection, sepsis, and severe scarring and help prevent the risk of glomerulonephritis secondary to cutanous streptococcal infection.

Oral vitamin E (DL-α-tocopherol) has been suggested for the treatment of patients with epidermolysis.[22] Vitamin E is an antioxidant that enhances the activity of some enzymes and perhaps induces the synthesis of others. Although there are reports of favorable responses to oral vitamin E in dosages of up to 2,000 units/day, most studies do not seem to confirm its value in the prevention of blistering and scarring. Vitamins, iron, and protein supplements, however, are advisable if nutritional compromise exists.

Dysphagia is the major symptom of esophageal involvement in recessive dystrophic epidermolysis bullosa. It may result from a reversible inflammatory reaction or from a permanent stricture. Barium studies demonstrate esophageal lesions; endoscopy, however, is not recommended. Softening of the diet for several weeks may result in modest to marked improvement of symptoms. If conservative management fails to result in proper nourishment, bougienage, surgery, or both should be considered.[23, 24] Once bougienage has been initiated, however, some patients may require the procedure at frequent intervals. In those instances when surgery must be considered, colon transplant procedures have been successful. With repeated blistering, ulceration, and scar formation, carcinomas may sometimes develop on the involved skin or mucous membrane. Although the cause of carcinoma is unknown, abnormal collagen formation in heavily scarred areas with continuous blistering activity appears to predispose to this complication.

Systemic corticosteroids have been tried in all forms of epidermolysis bullosa. Although they appear to have value in the management of junctional bullous dermatosis (epidermolysis bullosa, Herlitz variant), present studies do not substantiate reports that high doses of systemic corticosteroids prevent the scarring and mutilation in severe dystrophic forms of this disorder. Moynahan, however, has stated that systemic corticosteroids in high doses (140 to 160 mg of prednisone or its equivalent per day) may be lifesaving in some cases of severe dystrophic forms during the neonatal period.[25] Since high doses may be required for several weeks or months, if this form of therapy is initiated, it should be used only with recognition of the potential risks of associated complications, particularly sepsis, poor wound healing, and growth suppression and that patients treated with corticosteroids tend to relapse once this form of therapy is discontinued.

In 1978, oral phenytoin (Dilantin) was suggested for the treatment of dystrophic forms of epidermolysis bullosa.[26] This form of therapy is based on the fact that phenytoin in pharmacologic doses has been shown to cause significant inhibition of collagenolytic activity both in vivo and in vitro. Although phenytoin in dosages of 2.5 to 5.0 mg/kg/day, to a maximum dose of 300 mg/day (a dosage high enough to obtain serum levels of 5 to 12 μg/ml), resulted in a reduction of tissue collagenase activity correlating with a reduction in the number of blisters and enhancement of the healing time in such patients, a double-blind placebo-controlled study has failed to demonstrate a statistically significant benefit in the majority of patients with this disorder.[27]

The nursing care of patients with severe epidermolysis bullosa is time consuming and difficult, and appropriate oral and dental care and aggressive nutritional supplementation are recommended.[28] In addition, restoration of function in severe fusion and flexion deformities of the hands and feet can often be helped by physiotherapy and appropriate plastic surgery. Mild cases of the dystrophic and nondystrophic types may be compatible with a nearly normal life. The severe dystrophic forms remain a challenge and require cooperation by patient, parents, and physician.

Prenatal ultrastructural diagnostic study of fetoscopic skin samples can be used in an effort to assist the prenatal diagnosis of junctional epidermolysis bullosa; and although more experience must be gained before this approach becomes widely used, chemical markers from fetal cells, immunohistochemical markers, and fetoscopy will probably become valuable tools for the prenatal diagnosis of severe forms of epidermolysis bullosa.[29]

A national epidermolysis bullosa registry has been established, and information and support groups are beneficial to many families who have children with epidermolysis bullosa. The Academy of Dentistry for the Handicapped (1240 East Main Street, Springfield, OH 45503) maintains a national referral system of specialists who deal specifically with dental care for patients with severe forms of the disorder,[30] and the Dystrophic Epidermolysis Bullosa Research Association (DEBRA), a national and international group dedicated to research and support for patients with all forms of epidermolysis bullosa and their families, is available. For information on this organization contact DEBRA of America, Inc., 141 Fifth Avenue, Suite 7-S, New York, NY 10010 (212-995-2220) or Mrs. Mary Freeland, MBE, 7 Sandhurst Lodge, Wokingham, Crowthorne, Berkshire, RG11 7QD, England.

BART'S SYNDROME

In 1966, Bart and associates recognized a mechanobullous syndrome consisting of skin defects (congenital localized absence of skin) that affected the lower extremities, blistering of the skin and mucous membranes, and congenital absence or dystrophy of the nails (Table 15–5). Although the etiology of Bart's syndrome is unknown, the disorder appears to be a variant of epidermolysis bullosa with features consistent with the dystrophic dominant form with variable penetrance and, in some instances, perhaps spontaneous mutation.[31, 32]

Some patients have only mouth erosions; others have deformed nails, recurrent blistering, or the complete syndrome, with characteristic localized, sharply marginated skin defects on the hands and feet (Fig. 15–12). Other skin defects, apparently due to mechanobullous phenomena induced by local shearing trauma, may appear as extensive erosions on the extensor aspects of the extremities, intertriginous areas, neck, and buttocks. Although skin and mucous membrane erosions heal with minimal or no scarring, milia and occasional residual hypopigmentation may be noted.

Histologically, skin lesions show loss of the epidermis, an intact dermis with the basement membrane on the dermal side of the split, and normal adnexa and subcutaneous tissue. A tendency toward progressive spontaneous improvement without residual defects emphasizes the importance of early recognition and conservative management of individuals with this disorder.

Table 15–5. OTHER SYNDROMES ASSOCIATED WITH EPIDERMOLYSIS BULLOSA

Type	Clinical Manifestations
Congenital localized absence of skin with blistering and nail dystrophy (Bart's syndrome)	Autosomal dominant with variable penetrance and expressivity; blister cleavage on dermal side of basement membrane; extensive erosions on extensor aspects of extremities, intertriginous areas, neck, and buttocks; spontaneous improvement with at times residual hypopigmentation
Acquired epidermolysis bullosa	Nonhereditary; blisters subepidermal (below basement membrane); affects ears, elbows, knees, hands, and feet; mucous membrane erosion and nail dystrophy common
Kindler's syndrome	Progressive poikiloderma-like changes on face and neck; photosensitivity; congenital blistering of acral skin; progressive diffuse macular atrophy; nail dystrophy, syndactyly, and hyperkeratosis of palms and soles
Transient bullous dermatosis	A fetal response to a variety of autoimmune disorders of the mother during pregnancy temporarily manifested during the neonatal period

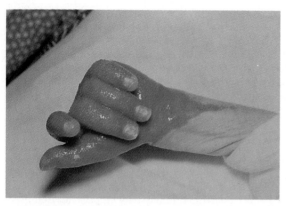

Figure 15–12. Bart's syndrome (congenital localized absence of skin), a disorder that, although usually seen on the feet, can also be seen on the hands of affected persons. (Courtesy of William J. Nyhan, M.D.)

ACQUIRED EPIDERMOLYSIS BULLOSA

Acquired epidermolysis bullosa (epidermolysis bullosa acquisita) is an acquired bullous disorder manifested in children and adults characterized by IgG autoantibodies that bind to the subepidermal anchoring fibril zone.[33–35] Ultrastructural findings are similar to those seen in the hereditary forms of dystrophic epidermolysis and most closely resemble those of the dominantly inherited disease. Patients with acquired epidermolysis bullosa generally appear with a peculiar susceptibility to blister formation following trauma or pressure. The disorder is manifested by vesicles, bullae, and erosions over the pressure areas of the ears, elbows, knees, and particularly hands and feet. Scarring, milia, and nail dystrophy occur. Although the teeth are normal and mucous membrane erosions are frequently seen, the conjunctival, esophageal, and genitoanal mucous membranes are not involved.

Epidermolysis bullosa acquisita has been associated with poison oak dermatitis, dermatitis herpetiformis, inflammatory bowel disorders (Crohn's disease), impetigo, scarlet fever, tuberculosis, porphyria, cutaneous amyloidosis, Ehlers-Danlos syndrome, and ingestion of sulfonamides, arsenic, and penicillamine. Although patients may have localized and relatively asymptomatic disease activity and reports of spontaneous or drug-induced remissions have been noted, these situations are relatively uncommon and many individuals experience extensive and at times disabling involvement. Therapy with topical corticosteroids, prednisone, azathioprine, cyclosporine, colchicine, methotrexate, plasma exchange, cyclophosphamide, and dapsone, given singly or in combination, has been used with varying success.

KINDLER'S SYNDROME

In 1954 Theresa Kindler described a clinical syndrome characterized by generalized progres-

sive poikiloderma, diffuse cutaneous atrophy, congenital acral skin blistering, webbing of the fingers and toes, nail dystrophy, oral mucosal lesions, and photosensitivity.[36] Since this original report there have been additional accounts of this syndrome with principal features including trauma-induced blisters involving mainly the hands and feet, photosensitivity, progressive poikiloderma-like changes on the face and neck, diffuse macular atrophy, involving at times large areas of the skin, nail dystrophy, syndactyly, hyperkeratosis of the palms and soles, leukokeratosis, red friable gums, and esophageal, laryngeal, anal, and urethral meatal stenosis. Although the photosensitivity and the blister formation seem to decrease with age, treatment of this disorder requires the avoidance of trauma and the proper use of emollients, appropriate sun protection, and the judicious use of antibiotics to prevent secondary infection.[37]

TRANSIENT BULLOUS DERMOLYSIS OF THE NEWBORN

In 1985 Hashimoto and others reported a case of an infant with a neonatal blistering disease that healed spontaneously within several months. Although the nosology of this disorder remains unclear, it appears that transient bullous dermolysis of the newborn may represent a rare variant of dominant dystrophic epidermolysis bullosa or a fetal response to an autoimmune disorder similar to that seen in infants born to pregnant women with pemphigus vulgaris.[38]

CHRONIC NONHEREDITARY BLISTERING DISEASES OF CHILDHOOD

The chronic nonhereditary bullous diseases of childhood have given rise to nosologic confusion owing to their varying responses to sulfapyridines and sulfone preparations, usually negative results from immunofluorescent studies, and histologic patterns no more characteristic than subepidermal bulla formation. In 1971 Bean and colleagues emphasized the usefulness of immunofluorescent techniques as a diagnostic aid and suggested a classification based on the clinical, histologic, and immunologic features of each disorder.[39] In 1974, on the basis of information regarding the clinical course, immunologic characteristics, and appropriate therapy for these diseases in children, dermatitis herpetiformis, bullous pemphigoid, benign chronic bullous dermatitis of childhood, pemphigus vulgaris, and pemphigus foliaceus were grouped under the inclusive term *chronic nonhereditary blistering diseases of children*.[40] Although previously regarded as a form of bullous pemphigoid or dermatitis herpetiformis, or a combination of the two, chronic bullous dermatosis of childhood and adult linear IgA dermatosis currently appear to represent variants of the same disorder.[41, 42]

Childhood Dermatitis Herpetiformis

Dermatitis herpetiformis (Duhring's disease) is a chronic recurrent cutaneous disease of unknown cause characterized by an intensely pruritic papulovesicular and, at times, bullous eruption that responds dramatically to orally administered doses of sulfones or sulfapyridine. Although the disorder may affect individuals of all ages, dermatitis herpetiformis generally occurs during the second to fifth decades of life. It is relatively uncommon in infancy and early childhood, affects males more frequently than females, and is relatively uncommon in blacks.

Dermatitis herpetiformis in childhood usually occurs in children older than five years of age, persists into adulthood, and is fundamentally the same disease as that seen in adults. Diagnosis of this disorder, just as in adults, should not be based solely on the morphologic aspects and distribution of lesions, but on the constellation of clinical appearance, histopathologic characteristics, immunofluorescent findings, and response to therapy.[43, 44]

Dermatitis herpetiformis is characterized by an extremely pruritic, symmetrically grouped papulovesicular eruption that affects the extensor surfaces: the elbows, knees, sacrum, buttocks, and shoulders, and occasionally the face, eyelids, facial hairline, posterior nuchal area, and scalp. In association with the onset of intense pruritus or burning, erythematous and, at times, urticarial lesions may develop. Characteristic of this disorder are minute, clear, relatively tense vesicles that measure from 0.3 to 4.0 mm in diameter. These vesicles rupture easily, either spontaneously or when scratched, and frequently erythematous lesions, small grouped papules and vesicles, superficial hyperpigmented macules, and hypopigmented scars exist at the same time. In addition, tender purpuric lesions and unusual palmar blisters and brown macules have been reported on the palms of some children and adults.[45, 46] The general course of this disorder is chronic (often lasting 5 to 10 years or more) with frequent exacerbations and remissions.

The most useful diagnostic histologic changes in dermatitis herpetiformis are seen in the vicinity of new blisters. Whenever possible, cutaneous biopsy should include the newest vesicle and a piece of the surrounding erythematous portion of the lesion. The initial changes are first noted in the tips of the dermal papillae and consist of subepidermal microabscesses with accumulations of neutrophils and eosinophils. Immunofluorescent studies suggest the best criteria for diagnosis of dermatitis herpetiformis to be the finding of IgA and complement deposits at the tips of the dermal papillae in a granular or specked distribution (or, less frequently, in a linear pattern) along the basement membrane at the dermal-epidermal junction of normal-appearing skin, without detectable circulating antibody to the basement membrane.

Dermatitis herpetiformis is generally manifested as a purely cutaneous disorder. Studies, however, have demonstrated that 60 to 90 per cent of patients with this disorder also have small bowel abnormalities indistinguishable from those seen in celiac-type gluten-sensitivity enteropathy.[47, 48] Although the cutaneous abnormality may not be caused by the same agent as that of gluten-sensitive enteropathy, it appears that there are strong genetic links with an unusually high frequency of leukocyte antigen HLA-B8, HLA-Dr3, and HLA-Dr7 in patients with both disorders.[49-51] In addition, an association with renal disease has appeared sporadically in the literature, antithyroid antibodies have been detected, case reports suggest an association with thyroid disease in some patients, and hoarseness and laryngeal involvement have at times been reported.[52, 53]

Although the cause of dermatitis herpetiformis remains unknown, there is increasing evidence that, in some individuals at least, immunologic processes may be involved in the pathogenesis of dermatitis herpetiformis and adult celiac disease. Since the immunoglobulin in the skin of patients with adult-type dermatitis herpetiformis has been shown to be IgA, it has been suggested that immunoglobulins formed in the gut lodge in the skin and produce the characteristic cutaneous lesions seen in this disorder.

Treatment. Clinical experience has shown that sulfapyridine and the sulfones are effective in relieving the symptoms and suppressing the eruption of dermatitis herpetiformis in children as well as adults. Dramatic relief from the use of these agents, therefore, frequently as early as 24 to 48 hours, is often helpful in the diagnosis of this disorder.

Sulfapyridine is frequently considered to be the drug of choice. The initial dose of sulfapyridine is usually 100 to 200 mg/kg/day for children, in four divided doses (with a maximum total of 2 to 4/day). Once existing lesions have been suppressed, the dosage may be tapered at weekly intervals, with a maintenance level of 0.5 g or less as the daily required dose for most patients. Nausea and vomiting are usually the first signs of sulfapyridine toxicity. Other side effects include anorexia, headache, fever, leukopenia, agranulocytosis, hemolytic anemia, serum sickness–type reactions, hepatitis, exfoliative dermatitis, and renal crystalluria. A screening test for glucose-6-phosphate dehydrogenase deficiency should be performed prior to the initiation of therapy, and close observation of the patient with pretreatment and follow-up blood cell counts at monthly intervals is recommended. Patients should be encouraged to drink large quantities of fluid to avoid renal complications, and since the disease may remit spontaneously, gradual attempts at reduction of treatment should be attempted at intervals of 3 to 6 months.

Various sulfone derivatives of dapsone are better tolerated and more economical than sulfapyridine. Their side effects, however, are more severe, and because of an increased tendency to hemolytic anemia in patients with glucose-6-phosphate dehydrogenase deficiency, as with sulfapyridine therapy, a screening test should be done prior to initiation of therapy. Available in 25- and 100-mg tablets, dapsone treatment may be initiated with 2 mg/kg/day, with an increase or decrease in dosage depending on the clinical response and the side effects associated with therapy. If side effects do not occur, a maximum of 400 mg/day may be reached, (the required dosage, however, is usually in the range of 50 mg three times daily).

Once a favorable response is achieved (usually within a week) the dose is decreased gradually to a minimum level (generally 25 to 50 mg/day). In addition to hemolysis, side effects include methemoglobinemia (manifested by bluish discoloration of the face, mucous membranes, and nails), nausea, vomiting, headache, giddiness, tachycardia, psychoses, anemia, fever, exfoliative dermatitis, liver necrosis, lymphadenitis, and peripheral neuropathy. Although leukopenia rarely occurs, complete blood cell counts and urinalyses should be performed at monthly intervals during the first year of therapy (after that about 3-month intervals appear to be adequate). Since the disease has a tendency to remission after a period of years, periodic gradual decrease in dosage levels should be attempted, as with sulfapyridine therapy.

A high percentage of patients with dermatitis herpetiformis have an associated gluten-sensitive enteropathy. Accordingly, it has been recommended that patients should have studies of the small intestine for the possibility of this association. Although conflicting data exist, adherence to a strict gluten-free diet (avoiding foods containing wheat, rye, and barley flour) after variable periods of time (from 5 months to 1 year) may reduce or eliminate the need for systemic drug therapy. It should be noted, however, that only highly motivated individuals will adhere to this diet. If a gluten-free diet is chosen, patients and their families should be advised that consultation with a dietitian is recommended and strict adherence to the diet is necessary.[54, 55]

Local applications of corticosteroid creams or shake lotions such as calamine lotion with menthol or phenol may diminish pruritus and permit control of the disorder with lower doses of systemic preparations. For patients who can tolerate neither sulfapyridine nor sulfone therapy, systemic corticosteroids (although not very effective) may be the only available form of treatment.

Bullous Pemphigoid

Bullous pemphigoid, a blistering disorder characterized by large, tense, subepidermal bullae that appear on normal-appearing or erythematous skin, although most commonly seen in elderly persons, may also occur occasionally in young adults and young children. In children, however, fewer than 40 cases have been reported and the youngest patient reported to date is a 2½-month-old infant.[56–62] Although in aged and debilitated individuals the disorder may result in death, the condition generally subsides after several months to 2 or 3 years.

Juvenile bullous pemphigoid resembles the adult type of bullous pemphigoid except that the incidence of oral lesions is higher in children. The clinical features of bullous pemphigoid are dominated by large bullae that are more tense and inflamed but otherwise similar to those of pemphigus vulgaris (Fig. 15–13). The course of bullous pemphigoid, however, is more indolent than that of pemphigus vulgaris, and the Nikolsky sign is usually absent. Denuded areas tend toward spontaneous healing and do not extend or increase in size as they do in patients with pemphigus vulgaris. The disorder is characterized by mild pruritus and by large, tense, sometimes hemorrhagic, bullae that measure 0.25 to 2.0 cm in diameter and generally involve the lower abdomen, anogenital region, posterior aspect of the thighs, and sometimes the face. Lesions may appear on normal skin or on an erythematous base, and they frequently occur at the periphery of annular or polycyclic erythematous plaques.

Variants include cicatricial pemphigoid, which affects mucosal surfaces, and a localized form (chronic pemphigoid of Brunsting-Perry), which is generally limited to the head and neck. Although other variants (vesicular pemphigoid and hyperkeratotic pemphigoid) have been described, their nosology is unclear at this time. In cicatricial pemphigoid, recurrent bullae are seen in the oral mucosa and conjunctiva and other mucous membranes such as those of the nasopharynx, esophagus, larynx, genitalia, and anal canal. Oral involvement often takes the form of a desquamative gingivitis, and the ocular form may not occur until many years after the onset of the condition. Conjunctival involvement can lead to entropion, trichiasis (ingrowing eyelashes), sym-

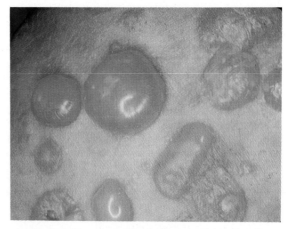

Figure 15–13. Large tense bullous lesions on the lower aspect of the abdomen of a 3½-year-old boy with juvenile bullous pemphigoid.

blepharon, dryness of the cornea, corneal ulceration, and, at times, eventual blindness. Esophageal lesions may result in stricture formation, and laryngeal lesions, when present, can sometimes be life threatening.[57]

The clinical and immunologic features of bullous pemphigoid of childhood are indistinguishable from those in adults. Biopsy specimens of cutaneous lesions show subepidermal blister formation, generally without papillary microabscesses (an important diagnostic feature of dermatitis herpetiformis); direct immunofluorescence reveals deposition of C_3 and IgG at the lamina lucida of the basement membrane zone; and although indirect testing of serum for circulating IgG anti-basement membrane zone antibodies is positive in approximately 70 per cent of patients, antibody titers do not correlate with clinical disease activity. Although the etiology of bullous pemphigoid is unknown, at times it appears that this cutaneous reaction may represent an antigen–antibody complex precipitated by administration of certain drugs or antibiotics.

The response to treatment of bullous pemphigoid of childhood is variable. Systemic corticosteroids may suppress the eruption; and in severe and resistant cases a combination of sulfones, sulfapyridine, or chlorambucil in conjunction with corticosteroids may be helpful, and cyclosporine and cyclophosphamide (alone or with low doses of corticosteroids), at least in some patients, appear to have been effective.[56–58] Topical corticosteroids, cool baths with colloidal oatmeal, erythromycin, tetracycline, and systemic antipruritics can also be beneficial in the management of this disorder.

Linear IgA Bullous Disease of Childhood

Linear IgA bullous disease of childhood (chronic bullous disease of childhood, benign chronic bullous dermatosis of childhood, bullous disease of childhood) is a subepidermal blistering disease that frequently is indistinguishable both clinically and histologically from bullous pemphigoid and dermatitis herpetiformis. Although this disorder has long been confused with other chronic nonhereditary bullous skin disorders of childhood, immunofluorescent and immunoelectron microscopic techniques have established this childhood bullous disorder as a distinct clinical entity. Most authors currently consider chronic bullous dermatosis of childhood and linear IgA bullous dermatosis of adults and childhood to be expressions of the same process.[41]

Linear IgA bullous disease of childhood is usually a disorder of the first decade of life, with onset occurring most frequently during the preschool years and spontaneous remission occurring after several months to 3 years of activity. The eruption is characterized by large, tense, clear or hemorrhagic bullae measuring 1.0 to 2.0 cm in diameter on a normal or erythematous base. The eruption is widespread, and areas of predilection include the face, scalp, lower part of the trunk (including the genitalia and pubis), buttocks, inner thighs, legs, and dorsal aspect of the feet. The bullae may form annular or rosette-like lesions composed of sausage-shaped blisters resembling a cluster of jewels surrounding a central crust, the "string of pearls" sign (Fig. 15–14). Pruritus is a variable feature and may be mild to moderate, intense and distressing, or completely absent.

Histologically, linear IgA bullous disease of childhood is characterized by subepidermal bullae with edema of adjacent dermal papillae and a dermal infiltrate of neutrophilic polymorphonuclear leukocytes, eosinophils, and mononuclear cells. The histology, however, is not diagnostic and will not differentiate this disorder from dermatitis herpetiformis or bullous pemphigoid. The immunofluorescent findings of linear IgA deposits in the lamina lucida zone of the dermal-epidermal junction obtained from tissue adjacent to a vesicle or bulla, and of circulating IgA basement membrane zone antibody (found in 70 to 80 per cent of patients with this disorder), correlated with clinical and histologic data, however, will frequently help establish the appropriate diagnosis.[63, 64]

Although most children with linear IgA dermatosis of childhood have a self-limiting disorder and disease-free remissions (which spontaneously resolve after several months to several years, generally within 2 to 4 years, and almost always before puberty), the course of the disorder may at times be prolonged and it may occasionally last for decades. Response to therapy is generally favorable. Sulfapyridine, as in dermatitis herpetiformis, is the drug of choice. If response to sulfapyridine is inadequate, it is discontinued and dapsone is begun. Although the disorder may respond to potent topical and systemic administration of corticosteroids, use of these agents can generally be avoided in childhood.[65, 66]

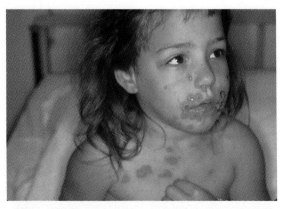

Figure 15–14. Linear IgA bullous dermatosis of childhood (chronic bullous dermatosis of childhood). Bullae with annular or rosette-like sausage-shaped blisters resemble a cluster of jewels. (Courtesy of Department of Dermatology, Yale University School of Medicine.)

Pemphigus in Childhood

Pemphigus is a term applied to a group of severe, chronic, sometimes fatal blistering disorders characterized by flaccid bullae that develop on normal-appearing skin and mucous membranes. Although four types of pemphigus have been described (vulgaris, vegetans, foliaceus, and erythematous), on the basis of histologic criteria it now appears that this disease can be simplified into two basic disorders, pemphigus vulgaris and pemphigus foliaceus and their variants, a drug-induced pemphigus, and paraneoplastic pemphigus, an autoimmune mucocutaneous disease of adults associated with neoplasia, particularly lymphoreticular malignancies.

PEMPHIGUS VULGARIS

Pemphigus vulgaris is a chronic vesiculobullous disease characterized by flaccid bullae and persistent erosions, with a predilection for middle-aged individuals (Fig. 15–15). Although the etiology is unknown, a genetic predisposition is suspected and the finding of intercellular antibodies in the serum of patients suggests an autoimmune basis to pemphigus and its variants (Fig. 15–16).

An extremely uncommon disorder of childhood, the apparent rarity of pemphigus in childhood may be related to difficulty in diagnosis and a low index of suspicion in this age group.[67] In addition, a transient form of pemphigus vulgaris (neonatal pemphigus vulgaris) has been seen in infants of pregnant women afflicted with pemphigus vulgaris,[38, 68, 69] and a rare type of pemphigus characterized by the presence of IgA rather than IgG antibodies in the intracellular areas of the epidermis has been reported in a child.[70]

Clinical Manifestations. The cutaneous lesions of pemphigus vulgaris favor the seborrheic areas (the face, scalp, neck, sternum, axillae, groin, and periumbilical regions) and pressure areas of the feet and back, and mucous membranes are affected in 95 per cent of patients. In more than half the patients the disorder starts with erosions of the oral mucosa, which are frequently present for several months before the appearance of skin lesions. Intact blisters are rarely seen on the oral mucosa, since they rupture soon after formation, leaving raw denuded painful erosions that heal slowly. Other mucosal surfaces, the anogenital areas, conjunctivae, vermilion borders of the lips, pharynx, and larynx may also be similarly involved. Since a majority of patients with proven pemphigus vulgaris present with painful oral erosions for weeks to months before they develop the characteristic bullous eruption, children with severe recurrent mucocutaneous lesions or chronic erosive mucous membrane disease should be examined carefully, and mucosal biopsy should be performed to rule out the possibility of this severe debilitating disorder.

The primary cutaneous lesions of pemphigus vulgaris appear as vesicles or bullae that arise on erythematous plaques or normal-appearing skin (see Fig. 15–15). The initial lesions may remain localized to one area of the skin or mucous membrane for weeks or months before other areas of the skin are involved. With the onset of new lesions, the patient may experience some pruritus, burning, or local discomfort. Blisters generally measure 1 cm or less at onset but may increase by peripheral extension to several centimeters in diameter. Vertical pressure may produce peripheral extension of lesions. The blisters rupture easily, and the resultant erosions are painful, bleed easily, and heal slowly. Scaling and crusting are common, and patients frequently are misdiagnosed as having impetigo or infected seborrheic dermatitis.

The diagnosis of pemphigus vulgaris depends on awareness that the disorder can occur in children and on the clinical picture, histologic examination of lesions, and immunofluorescent studies. Dislodgement of the outermost layer from the basal layer of the epidermis by gentle sliding pressure of involved as well as uninvolved skin (the Nikolsky sign) is invariably demonstrable in patients with pemphigus vulgaris. This phenomenon, a manifestation of defective epidermal cohesion, however, is not pathognomonic of this disorder, since it may also be seen in patients with epidermolysis bullosa, bullous pemphigoid, severe erythema multiforme (Stevens-Johnson disease), and toxic epidermal necrolysis. An ancillary sign of pemphigus vulgaris, however, is the peripheral enlargement of blisters by peripheral extravasation of fluid into the layers of the epidermis.

The Tzanck test is useful for the rapid demonstration of acantholytic epidermal cells in vesicles or bullae of pemphigus. After careful removal of the roof of a blister, smears from the base of the lesions stained with Giemsa's or hematoxylin and eosin stain show typical detached acantholytic cells. Since acantholytic epidermal cells may also be seen in other disorders, this examination is a

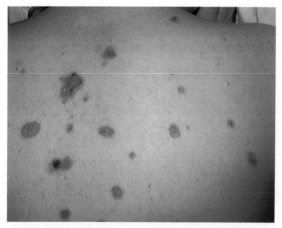

Figure 15–15. Pemphigus vulgaris. Seldom seen in childhood, this dermatosis is characterized by flaccid bullae that develop on normal-appearing skin and mucous membranes.

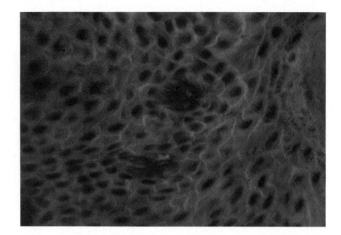

Figure 15–16. Pemphigus vulgaris. Immunofluorescent stains with IgG and complement are bound to intercellular areas of the epidermis. (Courtesy of Irwin M. Braverman, M.D.)

preliminary test and requires histopathologic confirmation.

For diagnostic purposes it is essential that a new bulla be examined histologically, preferably a small one that can be totally excised together with some surrounding skin. Light freezing of the bulla with an aerosol refrigerant prior to biopsy permits removal without damage to its architecture. The earliest histologic change is intercellular edema, with loss of cohesion between epidermal cells. In pemphigus vulgaris this results in the formation of clefts and bullae in a suprabasal location. The basal cells, although separated from one another, remain attached to the dermis, with a resultant "row of tombstones" appearance, and frequently the base of the bulla may be irregular when layers of epidermal cells (villi) project into the bullous cavity.

Although the etiology of pemphigus is unknown, the demonstration of intercellular antibodies in the serum of patients with all forms of pemphigus suggests an autoimmune phenomenon as the basis of pemphigus vulgaris and its variants. Direct immunofluorescent tests show IgG and complement bound to intercellular areas of the epidermis (Fig. 15–16). Indirect immunofluorescent studies of the serum of patients with pemphigus vulgaris containing antibodies against an intercellular substance of the stratified squamous epithelial cells help confirm the diagnosis. The level of serum antibodies against the intercellular substance reflects the severity or extent of the disease; it is particularly helpful in diagnosis of very early cases and appears to be a good index of response to therapy.

Pemphigus Vegetans. Pemphigus vegetans is a variant of pemphigus vulgaris in patients who have an increased resistance to their disease. Some authorities recognize two types of pemphigus vegetans: one is the *Neumann* and the other is the *Hallopeau* type (pyodermite végétante). Pemphigus vegetans differs from pemphigus vulgaris in that it starts at an earlier age and is characterized by flaccid bullae, particularly on the face and genitals and in intertriginous areas, that become eroded and heal with papillomatous proliferation (the so-called vegetations). The Hallopeau type has a prolonged course, and pustules rather than bullae represent the usual primary lesions. The pustules are followed rapidly by verrucous vegetations, which have a tendency to peripheral extension; and older vegetations no longer show the pustules seen in earlier stages, but appear more papillomatous and hyperkeratotic.

Prior to the use of corticosteroids, the course of pemphigus vegetans was more protracted than that of pemphigus vulgaris. It tends to pursue a chronic course, and although spontaneous remission and even permanent healing may occur in some patients, it nearly always ends in death if not treated with corticosteroids.

PEMPHIGUS FOLIACEUS

Pemphigus foliaceus is a more superficial and less severe form of pemphigus. The disease most commonly affects middle-aged persons and, although rare in children, is more common than pemphigus vulgaris of childhood and follows a more benign and less aggressive course than the adult form of the disorder.[71–73] The youngest child with this disorder was an 18-month-old reported in 1971.[74]

Histologic findings in pemphigus foliaceus are similar to those of pemphigus vulgaris and demonstrate epidermal bullae and intercellular acantholysis of the epidermis. The acantholysis seen in pemphigus foliaceus, however, is more superficial and occurs in the upper epidermis, usually in the granular layer or just beneath it, with resultant formation of clefts in a superficial, often subcorneal, location.

Oral lesions are rarely seen in pemphigus foliaceus and, when present, usually consist of small, superficial, often inconspicuous erosions. Bullae, when seen, are usually small and flaccid. They break easily, and because of their superficial location, leave shallow erosions. Common areas of involvement include the scalp, face, upper chest, abdomen, and back; and, in addition to small bullae, patients often describe a slowly spreading eczematoid patch as the initial cutaneous manifestation (Figs. 15–17 and 15–18). Patients generally are not severely ill but complain of pruritus, pain, and burning. At times, however, the clinical picture may progress to resemble that of a severe generalized exfoliative dermatitis.

Pemphigus Erythematosus. The first lesions of pemphigus foliaceus often localize to the center of the face. When the butterfly area of the face, the scalp, upper chest, and back are involved, the disorder has been termed *pemphigus erythematosus*. In 1926, Senear and Usher described this as an unusual form of lupus erythematosus (the Senear-Usher syndrome). Clinical course and histopathologic patterns, however, confirm pemphigus erythematosus and the Senear-Usher syndrome as variants of pemphigus foliaceus.[75]

Fogo Selvagem. Fogo selvagem (Brazilian pemphigus) is a variant of pemphigus foliaceus found in tropical regions. Endemic in Brazil, and to a lesser extent in other South American countries, it occurs in children and young adults, particularly women. It affects native Brazilians and immigrants and commonly affects more than one member of a

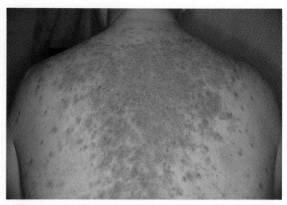

Figure 15–18. Spreading eczematoid eruption with shallow erosions, scaling, and crusting on the back of a patient with pemphigus foliaceus. (Courtesy of Department of Dermatology, Yale University School of Medicine.)

family. Approximately 15 per cent of patients are children, and women younger than age 30 comprise 65 per cent of all patients with this variant of pemphigus. Although it is indistinguishable from nonendemic pemphigus, its localization to small foci point to an infectious agent borne by an arthropod (a black fly, *Simulium prurinosum*) as the etiologic vector responsible for this disorder.[76] The striking distribution of lesions on sun-exposed skin, its burned appearance, and the painful burning sensation in lesions are responsible for the name *fogo selvagum* (Portuguese, meaning "wildfire") used to describe the disease.

The cutaneous eruption in individuals with fogo selvagum is characteristically seen in the seborrheic areas of the face and trunk and is similar to that of the more familiar form of pemphigus foliaceous. Both disorders are characterized by superficial blistering and erosive lesions that affect the skin and rarely involve mucosal surfaces. Although lesions may at times suggest a diagnosis of cutaneous lupus erythematosus, they lack the follicular prominence (the "carpet tack" sign), atrophy, and hypopigmentation seen in patients with lupus erythematosus. In all clinical forms, when the disease is active, Nikolsky's sign can be elicited. In contrast to pemphigus vulgaris, neonatal pemphigus has not been observed in infants born to mothers with active fogo selvagum. The disorder, however, is often associated with systemic features (a dystrophic form of the disease characterized by lack of muscular development and demineralization of bones). Patients often assume a sitting position, and maintain it day and night, in response to the severe burning in the skin; and the skin may become malodorous and so offensive to others that affected children are often ostracized.

The onset of Brazilian pemphigus is similar to that of pemphigus foliaceus. In chronic cases hyperpigmentation, hyperkeratosis, and loss of hair over the scalp and body are prominent features of

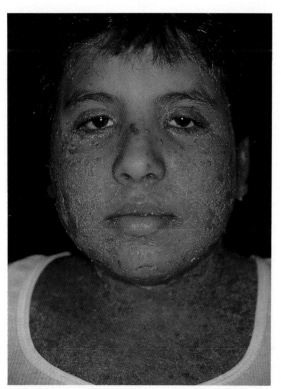

Figure 15–17. Crusted eczematoid eruption on the face and neck of a child with pemphigus foliaceus. (Courtesy of Department of Dermatology, Yale University School of Medicine.)

this disorder. In younger patients the natural course of pemphigus foliaceus is to recede gradually and subside completely. The prognosis prior to the availability of corticosteroids was dependent on the age of the patient and whether the disease took an acute or chronic course. Once the disease has cleared, pemphigus foliaceus has less tendency to recurrence than pemphigus vulgaris.

TREATMENT OF PEMPHIGUS VULGARIS AND PEMPHIGUS FOLIACEUS AND THEIR VARIANTS

Systemic corticosteroids at present are the treatment of choice for patients with pemphigus vulgaris and pemphigus foliaceus and their variants. Childhood pemphigus, although rare, can be just as virulent as its adult counterpart. Without appropriate treatment the disease almost invariably terminates fatally in several months to years. Prompt diagnosis, therefore, is particularly important so that therapy can be instituted early in the course of the disease.

In recent years successful treatment of pemphigus vulgaris in adults has consisted of high-dose prednisone (100 to 200 mg/day or more) or its equivalent. In children the recommended dose is 3 to 6 mg/kg/day (up to 60 to 120 mg of prednisone or its equivalent), depending on the severity of the disorder. This dose is continued until healing occurs (often 2 to 5 months after the onset of therapy in severe cases). Treatment of pemphigus foliaceus is similar to that of pemphigus vulgaris except that patients with pemphigus foliaceus and its variants generally respond to lower corticosteroid dosages. Although patients with Brazilian pemphigus (fogo selvagem) may respond to antimalarial therapy (quinine or quinacrine), systemic corticosteroids continue to be the treatment of choice.

Adverse reactions associated with prolonged high-dose corticosteroid therapy are a major hazard in long-term management of patients with pemphigus vulgaris. Once a maintenance dosage is attained, therefore, treatment should be reduced (by about 20 per cent every 2 weeks), and alternate-day therapy is preferred once the disease is controlled. Dapsone, gold, and intravenous corticosteroid pulse therapy followed by plasmapheresis and immunosuppressive agents such as methotrexate, azathioprine, or cyclophosphamide have also been used, alone or as ancillary therapeutic agents, for patients with severe disease whose disease cannot be controlled by corticosteroids alone or when prolonged use of high doses of corticosteroids is undesirable.[77-79] Because of potential adverse effects, cytotoxic drugs and gold should be used with caution in children. Patients with pemphigus foliaceus or its variants may also respond to topical corticosteroids.[80] Topical corticosteroids are advisable, therefore, in an attempt to limit long-term use of systemic corticosteroid therapy in mild cases of pemphigus foliaceus and its variants.

SUBCORNEAL PUSTULAR DERMATOSIS

Subcorneal pustular dermatosis (Sneddon-Wilkinson disease) is a chronic vesiculopustular disorder of undetermined etiology first described in 1956.[81] It is characterized by pustules in an annular and serpiginous arrangement and generally involves the abdomen, axillae, and groin. This relatively rare disease occurs most frequently in middle-aged women but can also appear in childhood. The youngest reported case is that of a child who had the onset of the disease at 7 weeks of age.[82] Although some authorities have considered this disorder to be an atypical form of dermatitis herpetiformis, lack of changes in the jejunal mucosa and absence of IgA in the tips of dermal papillae suggest that it is distinct from and unrelated to dermatitis herpetiformis.

Comparison of the disease in children and adults indicates no difference in clinical appearance, course, and histologic findings except that children frequently have a more severe toxic reaction with high fever and leukocytosis during the acute stage of the disorder.[82] The disease generally begins with small pustules or vesicles on an erythematous base. Occasionally only vesicles may be present, but these soon change into sterile pustules. The pustules tend to appear in crops and spread to large parts of the body, forming large circinate or gyrate patterns that coalesce to form serpiginous patterns (Fig. 15–19). The eruption favors the groin, abdomen, axillae, and flexural aspects of the proximal extremities. The hands, feet, face, and mucous membranes are rarely affected. Although most patients experience a mild degree of pruritus, severe itching with excoriation is uncommon. Individual lesions tend to last for periods of 5 days, with new lesions appearing as others disappear. As the pustules resolve they are replaced by a superficial leafy scale or crust. After the eruption resolves, a faint blotchy brown hyperpigmentation, without atrophy or scarring, remains. The condition is benign and is characterized by remissions and exacerbations that may last for 5 to 8 years.

Histopathologic examination of an intact lesion reveals a subcorneal blister filled almost entirely with neutrophilic polymorphonuclear leukocytes. The more intense itching and the subepidermal location of blisters in dermatitis herpetiformis help differentiate these two conditions. Subcorneal pustular dermatosis may be differentiated from impetigo, which has a similar histologic picture, by history, absence of pathogenic bacteria on culture, and failure to respond to antibiotics. Differentiation from pemphigus foliaceus can be made by immunofluorescent studies.

Dapsone and sulfapyridine are the drugs of choice. Although the response is slower than that seen in dermatitis herpetiformis, the majority of patients obtain partial, if not complete, relief. Dosage in children and precautions with dapsone or sulfapyridine therapy are similar to those used in the management of dermatitis herpetiformis.

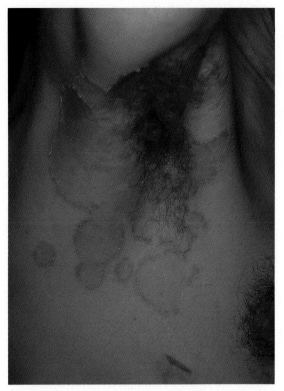

Figure 15–19. Subcorneal pustular dermatosis. Pustules occur in an annular and serpiginous arrangement in the axillary area, a common location for this disorder. (Courtesy of Department of Dermatology, Yale University School of Medicine.)

FAMILIAL BENIGN PEMPHIGUS

Familial benign pemphigus (benign familial chronic pemphigus, Hailey-Hailey disease) is an autosomal dominant genodermatosis characterized by recurrent vesicles and bullae, which most commonly appear on the sides and back of the neck, in the axillae, in the groin, and in the perianal regions. It appears equally in males and females, occurs most frequently in whites, and is relatively uncommon in blacks and Asians. First described by two brothers, Howard and Hugh Hailey in 1939, the disorder is not seen before puberty and usually has its onset in the late teens or early 20s.[83]

Most cases of familial benign pemphigus have a fairly constant course. The primary lesions are small vesicles that occur in groups on normal or erythematous skin. The vesicles may enlarge to form bullae and rupture easily, leaving an eroded base; they exude serum and develop crusts resembling impetigo or pyoderma. Nikolsky's sign may or may not be present. Lesions tend to spread peripherally, with an active, often serpiginous border, and central resolution with peripheral extension often results in circinate lesions. In the intertriginous areas lesions tend to form erythematous plaques with dry crusting and soft, flat, and moist granular vegetations. Burning or pruritus is

common, and, particularly in the intertriginous areas, lesions tend to become irritating, painful, and exceedingly uncomfortable.

Although lesions of the mucous membranes rarely occur, keratoconjunctivitis and papular lesions of the vulva and oral mucosa have been described and esophageal involvement has been demonstrated by esophagoscopy and histopathologic changes.[84] Some patients may have spontaneous improvement, but the disease generally does not clear completely. It may run a chronic course characterized by exacerbations and remissions and by age 50 tends to become less severe.[85]

The basic disturbance in familial benign pemphigus is a defect in the desmosome–filament complex similar to that seen in patients with Darier's disease.[86] The cutaneous lesions of familial benign pemphigus are induced by numerous external stimuli, namely, heat, humidity, friction, exposure to ultraviolet light, and bacterial or candidal infection.[87, 88] Although at times the clinical picture may resemble that of impetigo or pemphigus vegetans, the disorder can be differentiated on the basis of family history (present in 70 per cent of patients with familial benign pemphigus) and the recurring nature of the disorder.

Biopsy of the advancing border of a lesion is particularly helpful in establishing the proper diagnosis. The histologic picture is characterized by vesicle formation in a suprabasal location, separation of the epidermal cells with neighboring cells still adhering loosely one to another, producing a "dilapidated brick wall" appearance, and upward protrusion of villi (papillae lined by a single layer of basal cells) into the vesicular spaces. In some instances corps ronds (large round dyskeratotic masses surrounded by a clear halo as the result of shrinkage) similar to those in Darier's disease may be seen in the granular layer or vesicular spaces. Although some dermatologists have suggested that familial benign pemphigus may represent a vesicular form of Darier's disease, differences in histologic findings, lack of response of Darier's disease to antibiotic therapy, and independent inheritance patterns appear to differentiate the two disorders.

As yet there is no effective treatment that will arrest the basic defect of familial benign pemphigus. An effort should be made to avoid the precipitating factors of heat, humidity, and the friction associated with tight or ill-fitting clothing. Although topical antibiotics may be helpful in some cases, systemic antibiotics chosen on the basis of bacterial culture and sensitivity studies appear to be most effective in the treatment of this disorder.[89] Topical cyclosporine and topical and systemic corticosteroids may also be effective in some cases. Systemic corticosteroids, however, are not recommended since the disorder frequently recurs when the dosage levels are reduced. In persistent cases when patients have been disabled by painful eroded plaques unresponsiveness to other therapeutic measures, carbon dioxide laser therapy[90, 91] and excision of involved regions followed by split-thickness skin grafts have been helpful.[92]

HERPES GESTATIONIS

Herpes gestationis is an uncommon blistering disorder that occurs during pregnancy and the postpartum period and tends to recur in subsequent pregnancies. Its cause is unknown, and its pruritic eruption consists of grouped erythematous edematous papules and plaques, target lesions, annular wheals, grouped vesicles on erythematous bases, and tense bullae. The onset of the eruption most commonly occurs during the fourth or fifth month of gestation but has occurred as early as 2 weeks after conception and as late as the day before delivery, and even during the first few weeks of the postpartum period. The course of herpes gestationis is cyclic but generally tends to abate spontaneously during the last few weeks of gestation. Although the eruption tends to clear in the majority of patients within a few days of delivery, the eruption can persist for many months after delivery, and mild recurrences occasionally have been noted to appear at the time of menstruation, in women who take oral contraceptives, and in women with choriocarcinomas and hydatidiform moles (Fig. 15–20).[93–95] Cutaneous involvement of the newborn has been noted in about 10 per cent of infants born to mothers with this disorder (Fig. 15–21); and, on the basis of immunofluorescent findings, a high percentage of newborns have been noted to have subclinical forms of herpes gestationis.

Speculations regarding the cause of herpes gestationis vary. In view of its clinical and histologic resemblance to erythema multiforme, the possibility that it may represent a hypersensitivity or toxic reaction to fetal or placental products or to hormones or their metabolites must be considered. The immunopathologic hallmark of herpes gestationis is the presence of the third component of complement (C_3), with or without IgG, in a linear band-like distribution along the basement membrane zone.[96] A circulating factor in the serum of patients with this disorder, termed the *herpes gestationis factor*, can cause the deposition of C_3 in

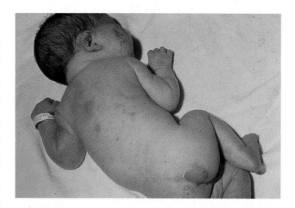

Figure 15–21. Herpes gestationis. Bullous lesions are evident on the face, trunk, and extremities of an infant of the mother with herpes gestationis shown in Figure 15–20. (Courtesy of Wilson Grubb, M.D.)

the same region (this factor has been shown to be IgG).[97]

The histopathologic features of this disorder, although resembling those of dermatitis herpetiformis and erythema multiforme, are said to be distinctive and are characterized by a subepidermal vesicle, spongiosis, focal necrosis of basal cells overlying the tips of dermal papillae, and a dense perivascular infiltrate containing lymphocytes, histiocytes, and numerous eosinophils.

Owing to the relative rarity of herpes gestationis (currently estimated at approximately 1 in 50,000 cases of pregnancy), the question of whether there is an increased fetal morbidity and mortality in women with this disorder varies from estimates of little to no fetal risk to studies suggesting an incidence of morbidity as high as 30 per cent.[97, 98] Current studies, however, suggest that there is no increase in the incidence of premature deliveries and that there is no evidence of increased risk to either mother or child in patients with this disorder.[93] The course of herpes gestationis is characterized by alternating exacerbations and remissions. The pruritus is not relieved by sedatives, antihistamines, or sulfones. When therapy for this disorder is prescribed, the possibility of drug-induced fetal damage, particularly during the first trimester of pregnancy, must be carefully considered. Systemic corticosteroids are the most reliable mode of therapy and, with certain precautions, are generally considered safe for both mother and fetus. To avoid potential risk of fetal developmental abnormality, however, they should be withheld, if possible, during the first trimester of pregnancy. Prednisone (in dosages of 20 to 40 mg/day) or its equivalent, is generally effective and well tolerated. The patient, however, should be monitored, particularly in regard to weight gain, hypertension, and possible fluid retention. Alternate-day dosage, if possible, is preferable to daily treatment; and to avoid adrenal suppression to the fetus, dosages should be re-

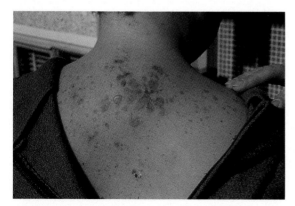

Figure 15–20. Bullous lesions on the upper back of a woman with herpes gestationis. (Courtesy of Wilson Grubb, M.D.)

duced to a minimum during the final weeks of pregnancy. The cutaneous lesions in infants with this disorder generally remit within several weeks and do not require therapy. Infants born to mothers treated with high doses of systemic corticosteroids, however, require careful monitoring for evidence of adrenal insufficiency.

Pyridoxine and plasmapheresis have also been reported to be effective in the management of women with this disorder. One advantage of pyridoxine therapy is that it can be administered safely without risk of fetal damage within the first trimester of pregnancy. Initially it may be administered intravenously or intramuscularly in dosages of 50 mg once or twice a day. Oral pyridoxine, in dosages of 100 to 400 mg, may be administered simultaneously. After good control has been achieved, the parenteral administration may be discontinued and oral pyridoxine continued in dosages varying from 25 to 400 mg/day. If there is no reponse to pyridoxine within 10 days, it is wise to abandon this form of therapy in favor of another modality. It must be remembered that no form of therapy has been curative. Therefore, whatever mode of treatment is prescribed it must be continued throughout the time of pregnancy and during the first few postpartum weeks.

References

1. Fine J-D, Bauer EA, Briggaman RA, et al.: Revised clinical and laboratory criteria for subtypes of inherited epidermolysis bullosa. J. Am. Acad. Dermatol. 24:119–135, 1991.

   A consensus report of the subcommittee on diagnosis and classification of the National Epidermolysis Bullosa Registry.

2. Pearson RW: Clinicopathologic types of epidermolysis bullosa and their nondermatological complications. Arch. Dermatol. 124:718–725, 1988.

   A comprehensive review of epidermolysis bullosa, its cutaneous manifestations, and extracutaneous complications.

3. Cooper TW, Bauer EA: Epidermolysis bullosa: A review. Pediatr. Dermatol. 1:181–188, 1983–1984.

   An overview of epidermolysis bullosa, its pathogenesis, classification, and therapy.

4. Hurwitz S, Eady RAJ: Epidermolysis bullosa. In Rook A, Parish LC, Beare JM (Eds.): Practical Management of the Dermatologic Patient. J. B. Lippincott Co., Philadelphia, 1986, 62–66.

   An overview of epidermolysis bullosa, its classification, diagnosis, and management.

5. Fine J-D, Johnson L, Wright T, et al.: Epidermolysis bullosa simplex: Identification of a kindred with autosomal recessive transmission of the Weber-Cockayne variety. Pediatr. Dermatol. 6:1–5, 1989.

   A report of a family in which four members were afflicted with an autosomal recessive form of epidermolysis bullosa simplex of the Weber-Cockayne variety.

6. Ishida-Yamamoto A, McGrath JA, Chapman SJ, et al.: Epidermolysis bullosa simplex (Dowling-Meara type) is a genetic disease characterized by an abnormal keratin-filament network involving keratins K5 and K14. J. Invest. Dermatol. 97:959–968, 1991.

   Careful analyses of skin biopsy specimens from a large number of patients with the Dowling-Meara type of epidermolysis bullosa simplex provide evidence that the disorder is associated with an intrinsic abnormality of the keratin-filament network resulting in impaired resistance of basal epidermal cells to external shearing forces.

7. Buchbinder LH, Lucky AW, Ballard E, et al.: Severe infantile epidermolysis bullosa simplex: Dowling-Meara type. Arch. Dermatol. 122:190–193, 1986.

   A review of eight infants with epidermolysis bullosa simplex (Dowling-Meara) who were originally thought to have recessive dystrophic epidermolysis bullosa.

8. Hacham-Zadeh S, Rappersberger K, Livshin R, et al.: Epidermolysis bullosa herpetiformis Dowling-Meara in a large family. J. Am. Acad. Dermatol. 18:702–706, 1988.

   A review of four generations of patients with epidermolysis bullosa of the Dowling-Meara type.

9. Briggaman RA: Hereditary epidermolysis bullosa with special emphasis on newly recognized syndromes and complications. Dermatol. Clin. 1:263–280, 1983.

   An authoritative review of the hereditary forms of epidermolysis bullosa.

10. Egan N, Ward R, Olmstead PM, et al.: Junctional epidermolysis bullosa and pyloric atresia in two siblings. Arch. Dermatol. 121:1186–1188, 1985.

    A report of two brothers with junctional epidermolysis bullosa and pyloric atresia.

11. Haber RM, Ramsay CA, Boxall LBH: Cicatricial junctional epidermolysis bullosa. J. Am. Acad. Dermatol. 12:836–844, 1985.

    A report in which electron microscopic examination of the skin of three patients led the authors to describe a seventh type of junctional epidermolysis bullosa emphasizes the need for electron microscopic examination of the skin in all patients with dystrophic features of epidermolysis bullosa.

12. Davies H, Atherton DJ: Acute laryngeal obstruction in junctional epidermolysis bullosa. Pediatr. Dermatol. 4:98–101, 1987.

    A report of a child with junctional epidermolysis bullosa with hoarseness since early infancy who died as a result of acute laryngeal obstruction at the age of 29 months.

13. Paller AS, Fine J-D, Kaplan S, et al.: The generalized atrophic benign form of junctional epidermolysis bullosa: Experience with four patients in the United States. Arch. Dermatol. 122:704–710, 1986.

    Two of four patients with the generalized atrophic benign form of junctional epidermolysis bullosa experienced laryngeal involvement during childhood.

14. Bruckner-Tuderman L, Pfaltz M, Schnyder UW: Epidermolysis bullosa dystrophica inversa in a child. Pediatr. Dermatol. 7:116–121, 1990.

    A report of a 4-year-old child with dystrophic epidermolysis bullosa inversa in which ultrastructural analysis suggested that a mutation preventing appropriate aggregation of collagen VII into anchoring fibrils may underlie this subtype of dystrophic epidermolysis bullosa in some patients.

15. Briggaman RA, Wheeler CA Jr: Epidermolysis bullosa dystrophica-recessive: A possible role of anchoring fibrils in the pathogenesis. J. Invest. Dermatol. 65:203–211, 1975.

    A review of ultrastructural defects and the role of anchoring fibrils in the pathogenesis of recessive epidermolysis bullosa dystrophica.

16. Eisen AZ: Human skin collagenase: Relationship to the pathogenesis of epidermolysis bullosa dystrophica. J. Invest. Dermatol. 52:449–453, 1969.

    Additional studies on collagenase activity in patients with dystrophic epidermolysis bullosa suggest overproduction of collagenase in the role of blister formation.

17. Bauer EA: Recessive dystrophic epidermolysis bullosa: Evidence for an altered collagenase in fibroblast cultures. Proc. Natl. Acad. Sci. USA 74:4646–4650, 1977.

Studies in two patients with recessive dystrophic epidermolysis bullosa suggest that the altered collagenase present in patients with this disorder may be the result of a structural gene mutation, a defect in post-translational modification of the enzyme, or mutation in a gene that regulates the normal degradation of collagenase.

18. Lazarus G: Collagenase and connective tissue metabolism in epidermolysis bullosa. J. Invest. Dermatol. 58:242–249, 1972.

Studies of 19 patients with various types of epidermolysis bullosa suggest that increased local levels of collagenase may merely represent a secondary tissue reaction to chronic injury.

19. Rusenko KW, Gammon WR, Fine J-D, et al.: The carboxyl-terminal domain of type VII collagen is present at the basement membrane in recessive dystrophic epidermolysis bullosa. J. Invest. Dermatol. 92:623–627, 1989.

Studies suggest that the absence of anchoring fibrils in patients with recessive dystrophic epidermolysis bullosa may be due to an abnormality of type VII collagen.

20. Bruckner-Tuderman L, Mitsuhashi Y, Schnyder UW, et al.: Anchoring fibrils and type VII collagen are absent from skin in severe recessive dystrophic epidermolysis bullosa. J. Invest. Dermatol. 93:3–9, 1989.

Studies of the skin of patients with severe generalized recessive dystrophic epidermolysis bullosa suggest a genetic defect in synthesis, secretion, or molecular assembly of type VII collagen in patients with this disorder.

21. Fine J-D, Horiguchi Y, Stein DH, et al.: Intradermal type VII collagen. J. Am. Acad. Dermatol. 22:188–195, 1990.

A defect in the intracytoplasmic packaging or transport of type VII collagen within basilar and suprabasilar keratinocytes appears to have an important role in the pathogenesis of dystrophic epidermolysis bullosa.

22. Smith EG, Michener WM: Vitamin E treatment of dermolytic bullous dermatosis. Arch. Dermatol. 108:254–256, 1973.

Controlled double-blind crossover studies in two sisters with mild recessive dystrophic epidermolysis bullosa demonstrate reduced blister formation while on 1,600 IU daily of vitamin E (DL-α-tocopherol).

23. Absolon KB, Finney LA, Waddill GM Jr, et al.: Esophageal constriction—colon transplant—in two brothers with epidermolysis bullosa. Surgery 65:832–836, 1969.

Colon transplants in the esophagus were successful in two patients unresponsive to conservative management and bougienage.

24. Gryboski JD, Touloukian R, Campanella RA: Gastrointestinal manifestations of epidermolysis bullosa in children. Arch. Dermatol. 124:746–752, 1988.

Case histories of four patients and review of the management of esophageal and anal lesions in patients with recessive dystrophic epidermolysis bullosa.

25. Moynahan EJ: Epidermolysis bullosa affecting the buccal and pharyngeal mucosae. Proc. R. Soc. Med. 56:885–887, 1963.

A review of seven cases of dystrophic epidermolysis bullosa treated with corticosteroids.

26. Eisenberg M, Stevens LH, Schofield PJ: Epidermolysis bullosa: New therapeutic approaches. Aust. J. Dermatol. 19:1–8, 1978.

Parenteral phenytoin, an apparently effective form of therapy for two children with dystrophic epidermolysis bullosa.

27. Caldwell-Brown D, Lin AN, Stern RS, et al.: Lack of efficacy of phenytoin in recessive dystrophic epidermolysis bullosa. N. Engl. J. Med. 327:163–167, 1992.

Although occasional patients with recessive dystrophic epidermolysis bullosa may demonstrate a reduced number of erosions as a clinical response to the use of phenytoin, a study of 36 patients with the disorder failed to show a significant therapeutic benefit for most patients with this disorder.

28. Gruskay DM: Nutritional management in the child with the epidermolysis bullosa. Arch. Dermatol. 124:760–761, 1988.

A review of the nutritional management of children with epidermolysis bullosa.

29. Heagerty AHM, Kennedy AR, Gunner DB, et al.: Rapid prenatal diagnosis and exclusion of epidermolysis bullosa using novel antibody probes. J. Invest. Dermatol. 86:603–605, 1986.

Prenatal diagnosis of recessive dystrophic epidermolysis bullosa was successfully achieved at 19 weeks' gestation by indirect immunofluorescent examination of fetal skin biopsy specimens.

30. Pessar A, Verdicchio JF, Caldwell D: Epidermolysis bullosa; The pediatric dermatologic management and therapeutic update. Adv. Dermatol. 3:99–120, 1988.

An authoritative review and update on the management of patients with epidermolysis bullosa.

31. Bart BJ, Gorlin RJ, Anderson VE, et al.: Congenital localized absence of the skin, blistering and abnormality of nails. Arch. Dermatol. 93:296–304, 1966.

Congenital localized defects of the skin, mechanoblisters, and nail deformities described in a large kinship suggest a distinct mechanobullous disorder of autosomal dominant inheritance with variable penetrance.

32. Sirota L, Dulitzky F, Metzker A: Bart's syndrome: A mechanobullous disease of the newborn: Report of five cases and review. Clin. Pediatr. 25:252–254, 1986.

A review of five children, three of them siblings, with Bart's syndrome.

33. Rubinstein R, Esterly NB, Fine J-D: Childhood epidermolysis bullosa acquisita: Detection in a five-year-old girl. Arch. Dermatol. 123:772–776, 1987.

Description of a 5½-year-old girl with a blistering disease involving the oral, ocular, and anogenital mucosae and comments on previous reports of children, one of whom was taking penicillamine and another who had chronic ulcerative colitis, with childhood forms of epidermolysis bullosa acquista.

34. Arpey CJ, Elewski BE, Moritz DK, et al.: Childhood epidermolysis bullosa acquisita. J. Am. Acad. Dermatol. 24:706–714, 1991.

A report of three children with epidermolysis bullosa acquisita, a review of three previously reported cases, and a description of the disease in children as contrasted to that in adults.

35. Mooney E, Gammon WR: Heavy and light chain isotopes of immunoglobulin in epidermolysis bullosa acquista. J. Invest. Dermatol. 95:317–319, 1990.

Studies demonstrate epidermolysis bullosa acquista antibodies belonging to all IgG subclasses in the sera of most patients with this disorder.

36. Kindler T: Congenital poikiloderma with traumatic bulla formation and progressive cutaneous atrophy. Br. J. Dermatol. 66:104–11, 1954.

A report of a 14-year-old girl with a clinical syndrome characterized by acral bullae, generalized progressvie poikiloderma, and cutaneous atrophy.

37. Forman AB, Prendiville JS, Esterly NB, et al.: Kindler's syndrome: Report of two cases and review of the literature. Pediatr. Dermatol. 6:91–101, 1989.

In a report of two patients with Kindler's syndrome the authors suggest that this disorder and Weary's hereditary acrokeratotic poikiloderma may be variants of the same condition.

38. Hashimoto K, Burk JD, Bale GF, et al.: Transient bullous dermolysis of the newborn: Two additional cases. J. Am. Acad. Dermatol. 21:708–713, 1989.

A report of two infants with a neonatal blistering disease that healed spontaneously and a review of their clinical, histologic, and ultrastructural features.

39. Bean SF, Jordon RE, Winkelman RK, et al.: Chronic non-hereditary blistering disease in children. Am. J. Dis. Child. 122:137–141, 1971.

Immunofluorescent staining techniques suggest benign chronic bullous dermatosis of childhood to be a distinct disorder rather than a variant of bullous pemphigoid or a bullous form of childhood dermatitis herpetiformis.

40. Bean SF, Jordon RE: Chronic non-hereditary blistering disease in children. Arch. Dermatol. 110:941–944, 1974.

Immunofluorescent studies help clarify the classification of dermatitis herpetiformis and bullous pemphigoid in childhood.

41. Chorzelski T, Jablonska S: Evolving concept of IgA linear dermatosis. Semin. Dermatol. 7:225–232, 1988.

Chronic bullous dermatosis of childhood and linear IgA bullous dermatosis of adults appear to be variants of the same disease.

42. Wojnarowska F, Marsden RA, Bhogal B, et al.: Chronic bullous disease of childhood, childhood cicatricial pemphigoid, and linear IgA disease of adults: A comparative study demonstrating clinical and immunopathologic overlap. J. Am. Acad. Dermatol. 19:792–805, 1988.

A comparative study of 25 patients with adult linear IgA disease, 25 patients with chronic bullous disease of childhood, and four cases of childhood cicatricial pemphigoid.

43. Ackerman AB, Tolman MM: Papular dermatitis herpetiformis in childhood. Arch. Dermatol. 100:286–290, 1969.

Clinical, histologic, and therapeutic evaluation of a 6-year-old girl with a vesiculobullous disorder lends support to the hypothesis that dermatitis herpetiformis is fundamentally the same disease in children as it is in adults.

44. Hertz DC, Katz SI, Aaronson C: Juvenile dermatitis herpetiformis: An immunologically proven case. Pediatrics 59:945–948, 1977.

A 2½-year-old boy both clinically and histologically fits the classification of juvenile bullous pemphigoid; therapeutic response to dapsone and the presence of IgA at the basement membrane of normal and perilesional skin, however, are characteristic of the adult-type small blister variety of dermatitis herpetiformis.

45. Pierce DK, Parcell SM, Spielvogel RL: Purpuric papules and vesicles of the palms in dermatitis herpetiformis. J. Am. Acad. Dermatol. 16:1274–1276, 1987.

Purpuric papules and vesicles—a sign of dermatitis herpetiformis in children as well as adults.

46. Karpati S, Torok E, Kosnai I: Discrete palmar and plantar symptoms in children with dermatitis herpetiformis Duhring. Cutis 37:184–186, 1986.

Thirty of 47 children with dermatitis herpetiformis had discrete reddish brown spots or small blisters on the palms and volar aspect of the fingers, and 3 patients had similar lesions on the soles and plantar surfaces of the toes.

47. Marks J, Shuster S, Watson AJ: Small bowel changes in dermatitis herpetiformis. Lancet 2:1280–1282, 1966.

Patients with dermatitis herpetiformis are frequently noted to have villous flattening in the small intestine similar to the histologic findings seen in patients with gluten-sensitivity enteropathy.

48. Marks J, Shuster S: Dermatitis herpetiformis: The role of gluten. Arch. Dermatol. 101:452–457, 1970.

Although some patients with dermatitis herpetiformis have an enteropathy that responds to a gluten-free diet, in this study the cutaneous eruption does not appear to be altered.

49. Katz SI, Hertz KC, Rogentine GN, et al.: The association between HLA-B8 and dermatitis herpetiformis in patients with IgA deposits in skin. Arch. Dermatol. 113:155–156, 1977.

A discussion of the relationship of leukocyte HLA-B8 antigen, dermatitis herpetiformis, and gluten-sensitive enteropathy.

50. Seah PP, Fry L, Kearney JW, et al.: Comparison of histocompatibility antigens in dermatitis herpetiformis and adult celiac disease. Br. J. Dermatol. 94:131–138, 1976.

Significantly elevated incidences of HL-A8 and HL-A1 suggest a common etiology in the pathogenesis of dermatitis herpetiformis and adult celiac disease.

51. Hall RP: The pathogenesis of dermatitis herpetiformis: Recent advances. J. Am. Acad. Dermatol. 16:1129–1144, 1987.

A review of the pathogenesis of dermatitis herpetiformis emphasizes its association with HLA antigens, IgA deposition in normal and perilesional skin, and gluten-sensitive enteropathy.

52. Greenberg RD: Laryngeal involvement in dermatitis herpetiformis: Case report. J. Am. Acad. Dermatol. 20:690–691, 1989.

A report of a patient with laryngeal involvement suggests that hoarseness in a patient with dermatitis herpetiformis, as in other blistering diseases, should be carefully investigated so that therapy can be begun promptly.

53. McFadden JP, Powles AV: Laryngeal involvement in dermatitis herpetiformis. J. Am. Acad. Dermatol. 22:325–326, 1990.

A report of laryngeal involvement in a patient with dermatitis herpetiformis.

54. Reunala T, Kosnai I, Karpati S, et al.: Dermatitis herpetiformis: Jejunal findings and skin response to gluten-free diet. Arch. Dis. Child. 59:517–522, 1984.

In a study in which most children with dermatitis herpetiformis had jejunal villous atrophy, the cutaneous eruption as well as the small bowel disorder responded to dietary withdrawal of gluten.

55. Ermacora E, Prampolini L, Tribbia G, et al.: Long-term follow-up of dermatitis herpetiformis in children. J. Am. Acad. Dermatol. 15:24–30, 1986.

In a review of 76 children with dermatitis herpetiformis (in whom enteric changes were present in over 90 per cent of the patients) a gluten-free diet led to reversal of the intestinal abnormality in 100 per cent and the disappearance of cutaneous lesions in 82 per cent of treated patients.

56. Gould WM, Zlotnick DA: Bullous pemphigoid in infancy: A case report. Pediatrics 59:942–945, 1977.

Improvement on systemic prednisone in a 3½-month-old infant with bullous pemphigoid.

57. Korman N: Bullous pemphigoid. J. Am. Acad. Dermatol. 16:907–924, 1987.

A comprehensive review of bullous pemphigoid, its clinical manifestations, diagnosis, and management.

58. Oranje AP, Vuzevski VD, Van Joost T, et al.: Bullous pemphigoid in children. Int. J. Dermatol. 30:339–342, 1991.

The juvenile form of this disorder, although rare, does not differ in many respects from its adult counterpart.

59. Tani M, Tani M, Komura A, et al.: Bullous pemphigoid of childhood: Report of a case and immunoelectron microscopic studies. J. Am. Acad. Dermatol. 19:366–367, 1988.

A report of a 4-month-old baby girl with bullous pemphigoid of childhood.

60. Nemeth AJ, Klein AD, Gould W, et al.: Childhood bullous pemphigoid. Arch. Dermatol. 127:378–386, 1991.

A report of a 2½-month-old infant with bullous pemphigoid and a review of the literature of this disorder as manifested in childhood.

61. Rosenbaum MM, Esterly NB, Greenwald MJ, et al.: Cicatricial pemphigoid in a six-year-old child: Report of a case and review of the literature. Pediatr. Dermatol. 2:13–22, 1984.

    A review of the literature and a report of a 6-year-old boy with cicatricial pemphigoid and upper airway obstruction.

62. DeCastro P, Jorizzo JL, Rajaraman S, et al.: Localized vulvar pemphigoid in a child. Pediatr. Dermatol. 2:302–307, 1985.

    A case of bullous pemphigoid in a 9-year-old girl in whom the cutaneous lesions were limited to the vulvar area.

63. Horiguchi Y, Toda K, Okamoto H, et al.: Immunoelectron microscopic observations in a case of linear IgA bullous dermatosis of childhood. J. Am. Acad. Dermatol. 14:593–599, 1986.

    A 16-month-old boy diagnosed as having linear IgA bullous dermatosis of childhood by immunofluorescence microscopy.

64. Peters MS, Rogers RS III: Clinical correlations of linear IgA deposition at the cutaneous membrane zone. J. Am. Acad. Dermatol. 20:761–770, 1989.

    Studies illustrate that although features of bullous dermatoses tend to overlap, detailed clinical, histologic, and immunologic evaluations can help establish an appropriate diagnosis, classification, and prognosis of patients with this group of disorders.

65. Westerhof W: Treatment of bullous pemphigoid with topical clobetasol propionate. J. Am. Acad. Dermatol. 20:458–461, 1989.

    In a review of 10 patients with bullous pemphigoid, in which all 10 achieved complete epithelialization within 4 to 17 days after the initiation of topical clobetasol treatment, most patients remained in remission for periods of 5 weeks to 13 months by the use of less potent topical corticosteroid maintenance therapy.

66. Surbrugg SK, Weston WL: The course of chronic bullous disease of childhood. Pediatr. Dermatol. 2:213–315, 1985.

    A report of three children with chronic bullous disease of childhood (linear IgA dermatosis) in which all three were able to discontinue treatment within 2 months to 2 years.

67. Smitt JHS: Pemphigus vulgaris in childhood: Clinical features, treatment and prognosis. Pediatr. Dermatol. 2:185–190, 1985.

    A review of pemphigus vulgaris in children with case reports of 31 patients younger than 18 years of age.

68. Merlob P, Metzker A, Hazaz B, et al.: Neonatal pemphigus vulgaris. Pediatrics 78:1102–1105, 1986.

    The 13th case report of an infant with neonatal pemphigus vulgaris.

69. Moncada B, Sondoval-Cruz JM, Baranda L, et al.: Neonatal pemphigus. Int. J. Dermatol. 28:123–124, 1989.

    A 28-year-old woman with oral and vulvar erosions of 4 months' duration was delivered of an infant with neonatal pemphigus.

70. Caputo R, Pistritto G, Gianni E, et al.: IgA pemphigus in a child. J. Am. Acad. Dermatol. 25:383–386, 1991.

    Although 11 cases of IgA pemphigus had been reported previously, this review of an 11-year-old child appears to be the first report of a child with this variant.

71. Schroeter A, Sams M Jr, Jordan RE: Immunofluorescent studies of pemphigus foliaceus in a child. Arch. Dermatol. 100:736–740, 1969.

    Experience in management of a 3-year-old boy with pemphigus foliaceus suggests that immunofluorescent studies, in addition to aiding in diagnosis, help predict relapse before the appearance of clinical lesions.

72. Yorav S, Trau H, Shewach-Millett M: Pemphigus foliaceus in an eight-year-old girl. Int. J. Dermatol. 28:125–126, 1989.

    A report of an 8-year-old girl with pemphigus foliaceus who was treated successfully with prednisone (40 mg daily for 3 weeks followed by 20 mg every other day for 2 months).

73. Jones SK, Schwabb HP, Norris DA: Childhood pemphigus foliaceus: Case report and review of the literature. Pediatr. Dermatol. 3:459–463, 1986.

    Report of a 4-year-old white boy with pemphigus foliaceus and a review of the literature of reported childhood forms of this disorder.

74. Kahn G, Lewis HM: True childhood pemphigus: Pemphigus foliaceus in an 18-month-old child: Immunofluorescence as a diagnostic aid. Am. J. Dis. Child 121:253–256, 1971.

    Report of an 18-month-old child with pemphigus foliaceus treated with topical high-potency corticosteroids.

75. Usher B: Pemphigus erythematosus—forty years later. Cutis 3:230, 1967.

    Forty years after its original description, the disease called pemphigus erythematosus (Senear-Usher syndrome) appears to be a localized form of pemphigus foliaceus.

76. Diaz LA, Sampaio SA, Rivitti EA, et al.: Endemic pemphigus foliaceus (fogo selvagem): I. Clinical features and immunopathology. J. Am. Acad. Dermatol. 20:657–669, 1989.

    The etiology, clinical, histopathologic, and ultrastructural features of fogo selvagem, and a review of its treatment and prognosis.

77. Basset N, Guillot B, Michel B, et al.: Dapsone as initial treatment in superficial pemphigus: Report of nine cases. Arch. Dermatol. 123:783–785, 1987.

    Dapsone therapy was successful in five of nine patients with superficial pemphigus vulgaris.

78. Fine J-D, Appell ML, Green LK, et al.: Pemphigus vulgaris: Combined treatment with intravenous corticosteroid pulse therapy, plasmapheresis and azathioprine. Arch. Dermatol. 124:236–239, 1988.

    A 13-year-old girl with generalized pemphigus vulgaris unresponsive to high doses of oral corticosteroids improved following treatment with intravenous corticosteroid pulse therapy followed by plasmapheresis and combination prednisone and azathioprine therapy.

79. Poulin YO, Perry HO, Muller SA: Pemphigus vulgaris: Results of treatment with gold as a steroid-sparing agent in a series of thirteen patients. J. Am. Acad. Dermatol. 11:851–857, 1984.

    Seven of 13 patients with pemphigus vulgaris treated with gold salts in addition to prednisone demonstrate that this combination can be useful as initial therapy, can maintain patients in complete remission, and can be used when other adjuvants to prednisone have failed, even in children.

80. Hempstead RW, Marks JG Jr.: Pediatric pemphigus vulgaris: Treatment with topical adrenal steroids. Arch. Dermatol. 120:962–963, 1984.

    Pemphigus vulgaris confined to the mouth of a 13-year-old girl was successfully treated by Kenalog in Orabase.

81. Sneddon IB, Wilkinson DS: Subcorneal pustular dermatosis. Br. J. Dermatol. 63:385–394, 1956.

    Six patients with subcorneal pustular dermatosis are reported, with a description of the clinical features and a review of the literature.

82. Johnson SAM, Cripps DC: Subcorneal pustular dermatosis in children. Arch. Dermatol. 109:73–77, 1974.

    Of two 3-year-old children with subcorneal pustular dermatosis, one appeared to have the onset of disease at 7 weeks of age.

83. Hailey H, Hailey H: Familial benign chronic pemphigus. Arch. Dermatol. Syph. 39:679–685, 1939.

    The first description of a previously unrecognized disorder characterized by chronic and recurring eruptions in the neck and axillae.

84. Schneider W, Fischer H, Wiehl R: Zur Frage der Schleimhautbeteiligung beim pemphigus benignus familiaris chronicus. Arch. Klin. Exp. Dermatol. 225:74–81, 1966.

Oral lesions in a mother and daughter with familial benign pemphigus.

85. Palmer DD, Perry HO: Benign familial chronic pemphigus. Arch. Dermatol. 86:493–502, 1962.

A review of 23 patients with benign familial chronic pemphigus.

86. Gottlieb SK, Lutzner MA: Hailey-Hailey disease: An electron microscopic study. J. Invest. Dermatol. 54:368–376, 1970.

Electron microscopic examination of 18 lesions from four patients reveals a genetic defect in adhesion of epidermal cells one to another.

87. Montes LF, Narkates AJ, Hunt D, et al.: Microbial flora in familial benign chronic pemphigus. Arch. Dermatol. 101:140–144, 1970.

Studies confirm the fact that bacterial infection due to *Staphylococcus aureus* can act as a precipitating factor in the etiology of familial benign chronic pemphigus.

88. Cram DL, Muller SA, Winkelmann RK: Ultraviolet-induced acantholysis in familial benign chronic pemphigus: Detection of the forme fruste. Arch. Dermatol. 96:636–641, 1967.

Ultraviolet light induces histologic acantholysis in patients with familial benign pemphigus.

89. Shelley WB, Pillsbury DM: Specific systemic antibiotic therapy in familial benign pemphigus. Arch. Dermatol. 80:554–556, 1959.

Bacterial cultures and sensitivities are essential to appropriate antibiotic therapy in this disorder.

90. Don PC, Carney PS, Lynch S, et al.: Carbon dioxide laserabrasion: A new approach to management of familial benign chronic pemphigus (Hailey-Hailey disease). J. Dermatol. Surg. Oncol. 13:1187–1194, 1987.

Successful carbon dioxide laserabrasion of familial benign chronic pemphigus spared the underlying adnexae, thus contributing to the reepithelialization of the epidermis.

91. McElroy JA, Mehregan DA, Roenigk RK: Carbon dioxide laser vaporization of recalcitrant symptomatic plaques of Hailey-Hailey disease and Darier's disease. J. Am. Acad. Dermatol. 23:893–897, 1990.

Patients with recalcitrant intertriginous plaques of Hailey-Hailey disease and Darier's disease showed significant clinical improvement following treatment by carbon dioxide laser vaporization.

92. Thorne FL, Hall JH, Mladick RA: Surgical treatment of familial chronic pemphigus (Hailey-Hailey disease). Arch. Dermatol. 98:522–524, 1968.

Excision and grafting proved to be helpful in the management of a 29-year-old man with severe persistent familial benign pemphigus.

93. Shornick JK: Herpes gestationis. J. Am. Acad. Dermatol. 17:539–556, 1987.

A comprehensive review of herpes gestationis, its pathophysiology, clinical manifestations, and therapy.

94. Fine J-D, Omura EF: Herpes gestationis: Persistent disease activity 11 years post partum. Arch. Dermatol. 121:924–926, 1985.

A report of herpes gestationis that developed during the sixth month of a young woman's first pregnancy and recurred 18 months later with a subsequent pregnancy and periodically despite therapy for a period of 13 years.

95. Holmes RC, Williamson DM, Black MM: Herpes gestationis persisting for 12 years post partum. Arch. Dermatol. 122:375–376, 1986.

A report of a 25-year-old patient who developed herpes gestationis in whom the disease continued to be active, despite therapy, until she died of metastatic carcinoma of the rectum 12 years later.

96. Hertz KC, Katz SI, Maize J, et al.: Herpes gestationis: Clinicopathologic study. Arch. Dermatol. 112:1543–1548, 1976.

Herpes gestationis in three patients verified by immunofluorescence of IgG and C_3 deposits along the basement membrane zone.

97. Lawley TJ, Stingl G, Katz SI: Fetal and maternal risk factors in herpes gestationis. Arch. Dermatol. 114:552–555, 1978.

Review of 41 cases of immunologically proven herpes gestationis suggests a definite increased risk of fetal morbidity and mortality.

98. Keaty C, Jones PE, Lamb JH: Progesterone therapy in dermatoses of pregnancy (herpes gestationis). Arch. Dermatol. Syph. 63:675–686, 1951.

A review of 10 patients with herpes gestationis suggests a tendency to recurrence with increased severity in successive pregnancies and possible grave prognosis to the fetus.

16

DISORDERS OF PIGMENTATION

Although chiefly of cosmetic significance, disorders of pigmentation are among the most conspicuous and, at times, among the most cosmetically and psychologically annoying and persistent of cutaneous disorders.

Melanin is the black or brown pigment that is responsible for the color in hair and for the natural and, at times, abnormal pigmentation of the skin. Its presence in the epidermis helps protect against ultraviolet radiation and associated cutaneous damage, of which the most serious type is skin cancer. The synthesis of melanin occurs in melanocytes, which are specialized dendritic secretory cells derived from the neural crest that migrate to the basal layer of the epidermis during embryogenesis.

The amino acid tyrosine is the substrate inside the melanocytes from which melanin is formed. In the presence of tyrosinase and a small amount of oxygen, tyrosine is converted into another amino acid, dihydroxyphenylalanine (dopa). This is then oxidized to dopaquinone and, through a complex series of steps, is eventually converted to melanin. Although the mechanism by which melanin is transferred from epidermal melanocytes to keratinocytes is uncertain, it appears to be brought about through active phagocytosis of the distal processes of melanocytes by keratinocytes. The cell walls of the phagocytized dendritic processes then disappear, and the melanin particles are dispersed throughout the cytoplasm of keratinocytes.

Normal skin color depends on the deposition of

melanin in epidermal cells, the thickness of the stratum corneum, the presence of carotene in the epidermis, and variations in blood flow. Pigmentation of the skin involves the formation and packaging of melanin within the melanosomes of the epidermal cells. The intensity of skin coloration is determined by the size and total number of melanosomes present within the keratinocytes and melanocytes of the epidermis, by the rate of melanogenesis within the melanocytes, and by the rate of transport within the keratinocytes.

There are two major classes of hormones that affect pigmentation: (1) sex steroids, especially estrogen and progestational agents, and (2) peptide hormones, including α- and β-melanocyte stimulating hormone (MSH) and adrenocorticotropic hormone (ACTH). Genetic factors play a primary role in the degree of normal pigmentation for each individual and the capacity of the melanocytes to respond to local stimuli that influence melanogenesis.

In all races the dorsal and extensor surfaces are relatively hyperpigmented, and the ventral surfaces are less pigmented. This is most evident in dark races (blacks and Asians). The separation of the dorsal and ventral pigmentation is most conspicuous on the extremities and more or less follows Voight's lines. Termed *Futcher's* or *Ito's line*, this differentiation of dorsal and ventral pigmentation is present from infancy and persists throughout adulthood. Although early studies suggested a high female-to-male ratio, subsequent reports reveal that 79 per cent of black women, 75 per cent of black men, and 10 per cent of whites have at least one line of pigmentary demarcation (Fig. 16–1).[1–3]

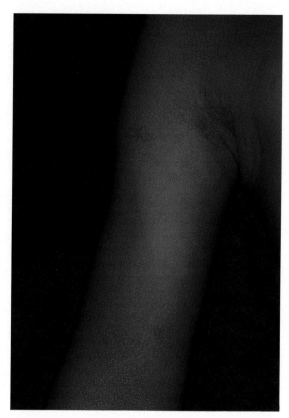

Figure 16–1. Futcher's line. A line of demarcation separates the relatively more deeply pigmented dorsal and lighter ventral surfaces.

DISORDERS OF HYPOPIGMENTATION

Disorders of hypopigmentation may be grouped into two major classifications as follows: (1) genetic or developmentally controlled disorders in which normal amounts of melanin were never present in affected areas and (2) disorders associated with depigmentation or loss of previously existing melanin. Congenital diseases of hypopigmentation include tuberous sclerosis, nevus achromicus, hypomelanosis of Ito, and partial or total albinism. Acquired disorders of hypopigmentation include vitiligo, postinflammatory hypopigmentation, pityriasis alba, and tinea versicolor. Hypopigmentary disorders may be further divided into patterned and unpatterned groups. Patterned forms of leukoderma include pityriasis alba, tinea versicolor, postinflammatory hypopigmentation, leprosy, pinta, tuberous sclerosis, hypomelanosis of Ito, vitiligo, partial albinism, and the Waardenburg and Vogt-Koyanagi syndromes. Unpatterned disorders include albinism and the leukoderma seen in association with nevus achromicus, phenylketonuria, kwashiorkor, hypopituitarism, the Chédiak-Higashi and Alezzandrini syndromes, incontinentia pigmenti, chemically induced hypopigmentation, and sarcoidosis.

Vitiligo

Vitiligo is a common genetically determined patterned loss of pigmentation that follows the destruction of melanocytes and is characterized by oval or irregular ivory-white patches of skin surrounded by a well-demarcated or hyperpigmented, often convex, border (Figs. 16–2 and 16–3). Seen in about 1 per cent of the population, or approximately 2 million people in the United States and 40 million in the world, the disorder appears to be inherited as an autosomal dominant trait of variable penetrance. One fourth of affected individuals have a history of leukoderma, and at least 30 per cent of affected persons have a positive family history of vitiligo, halo nevi, traumatic depigmentation of the skin, or markedly premature graying of the hair.[4, 5]

Although the etiology of vitiligo is unknown, three different hypotheses have been advanced to explain the cause of this disorder. In one theory, the *self-destruction* or *autocytotoxic theory*, an intermediate or metabolite in melanin synthesis such as dopa, dopachrome, or 5,6-dihydroxydrox-

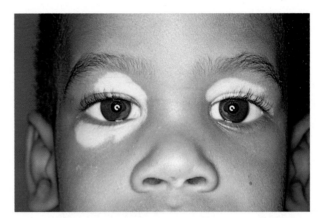

Figure 16–2. Vitiligo. Completely depigmented oval ivory-white areas with convex hyperpigmented borders are evident.

yindole causes melanin destruction, or the normal mechanism for melanin destruction proceeds unchecked to cause melanocyte dysfunction or death.[4, 5]

The *immune hypothesis* implies an autoimmune process as the cause of vitiligo, and circulating antibodies appear to be responsible for the melanocyte destruction.[6] The incidence of vitiligo in patients with some form of autoimmune disease may be as high as 10 to 14 per cent, compared with 1 per cent in the general population. Patients with various abnormalities of the immune system such as lymphomas, thymomas, myasthenia gravis, and mucocutaneous candidiasis tend to develop vitiligo.[4]

Most patients with vitiligo are in good general health. The incidence of this disorder, however, is higher (8 to 20 per cent) in individuals with disorders such as hyperthyroidism, hypothyroidism, Hashimoto's thyroiditis, adrenocortical insufficiency, pernicious anemia, polyendocrine deficiencies, parathyroid abnormalities, myasthenia gravis, dysgammaglobulinemia, and certain types of uveitis, including Vogt-Koyanagi and Harada's syndromes; and the incidence of vitiligo in patients with sympathetic ophthalmia and adult-onset and juvenile-type diabetes appears to be higher than that in the general population. Vitiligo and alopecia areata also appear to be linked, and, since ear as well as eye melanocytes can be damaged, a significant number of patients with vitiligo have ophthalmic abnormalities (discrete depigmentation and pigment hyperplasia involving the choroid and retinal pigment epithelium, discrete atrophic areas of the fundus, posterior chorioretinitis, uveitis, iritis, and vitreous inflammation, with at times loss of vision) or a neurosensory hearing loss associated with destruction of pigment cells of the hearing apparatus.[7–10] Patients with scleroderma or morphea have an increased incidence of vitiligo; approximately 50 per cent of patients with vitiligo have halo nevi; and, perhaps most significant of all, there appears to be a link between vitiligo and melanoma (20 per cent of patients with melanoma have vitiligo).[4, 7] Since vitiligo often appears in patients with melanoma who have been ill and have an advanced stage of their disorder, the onset of vitiligo in such patients may suggest a poor prognostic sign. Actually, most patients with melanoma who develop vitiligo have had their melanoma for a long period of time. The onset of vitiligo in such patients, therefore, may actually imply an immunologic response, with an attempt at the destruction of all melanocytes within the individual system.

In the third or *neural hypothesis*, neurochemical factors such as acetylcholine, epinephrine, or norepinephrine from nerve endings are implicated. This theory can help provide an explanation for the distribution of vitiligo in patients with segmental forms of the disorder. The actual mechanism of inhibition or destruction of melanocytes that results in vitiligo, however, may be much more complex than any of these mechanisms suggest. Thus, a combination or interreaction of the above factors may be found to be incriminated in the causation of this disorder.

Vitiligo may begin at any age. Its onset is most common in young adults; in about half of the patients it begins prior to the age of 20 years, and in one fourth of patients it develops before the age of 8 years. Although vitiligo is relatively uncommon during infancy, patients with congenital vitiligo have been observed.[7] In 75 per cent of affected individuals the first lesions occur as depigmented spots on exposed areas such as the dorsal surfaces

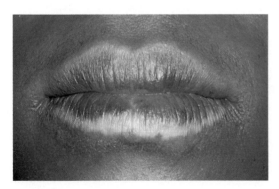

Figure 16–3. Vitiligo with depigmentation of the lips.

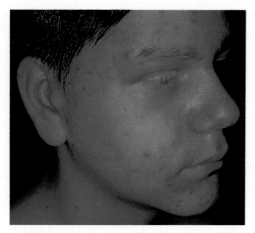

Figure 16–4. Segmental vitiligo of the eyebrow and eyelashes.

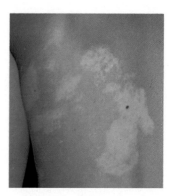

Figure 16–6. Segmental vitiligo on the left upper back with partial spontaneous repigmentation.

of the hands, face, and neck. Other sites of predilection include the body folds (the axillae and groin), body orifices (the eyes, nostrils, mouth, navel, areolae, genitalia, and perianal regions), and areas over bony prominences such as the elbows, knees, knuckles, and shins.

The location, size, and shape of individual lesions vary considerably, yet the overall picture is characteristic. Lesions appear as partially or completely depigmented ivory-white macules or patches, usually with well-defined, frequently hyperpigmented, convex borders. They frequently have an oval or linear contour and vary from several millimeters or less to large, occasionally segmental areas or almost total depigmentation of the body. The latter form is termed *universal* or *total vitiligo*. Although usually considered to be a bilateral disorder, vitiligo is often asymmetrical and frequently may be confined to an area supplied by a nerve segment (this variant, seen more commonly in children than adults, is termed *segmental vitiligo*) (Figs. 16–4 through 16–6).

Many patients date the onset of their disorder to an exposure to the sun, and 15 per cent of patients relate sunburn as a factor in the initiation or as a cause of the disorder. Other individuals associate the onset of vitiligo with periods of severe physical or emotional trauma. In instances in which the onset of vitiligo appears to follow a sunburn or intense tan, the possibility exists that vitiligo may have been present and became apparent only after the patient developed a tan in the surrounding area, thus accentuating the contrast with the depigmented area. It appears, however, that sunburn with vesiculation frequently will precipitate vitiligo. Therefore, although ultraviolet exposure is used in the treatment of this disorder, patients must be forewarned to initiate sunlight or ultraviolet exposure judiciously in an effort to avoid excessive sunburn reactions, particularly in depigmented areas where protective melanin pigment is absent.

Ordinarily the diagnosis of vitiligo is not difficult, especially when there is symmetrical hypopigmentation about the eyes, nostrils, mouth, nipples, umbilicus, or genitalia. In fair-skinned individuals it may be difficult to differentiate areas of vitiligo from the adjacent normal skin. In such cases examination under Wood's light in a darkened room may help to delineate a contrast between normal and hypopigmented skin. When the diagnosis is in doubt, the distribution of lesions, the age at onset, the presence of a convex hyperpigmented border, and the characteristic sites of

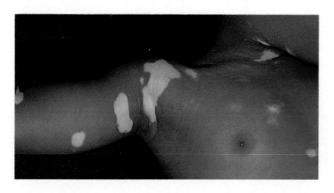

Figure 16–5. Segmental vitiligo on the arm, neck, and chest. Note areas of spontaneous follicular repigmentation.

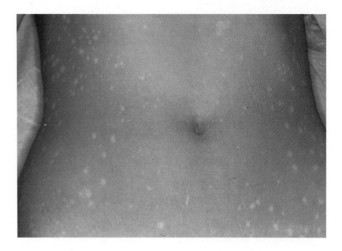

Figure 16–7. Postinflammatory hypopigmentation following resolution of guttate psoriasis.

predilection may help establish the correct diagnosis.

Lesions of postinflammatory hypopigmentation reveal irregular mottling of hyperpigmentation and hypopigmentation (Figs. 16–7 and 16–8). Pityriasis alba may be differentiated by its distribution on the face, upper arms, neck, and shoulders; its characteristic light-pink color; and its fine adherent scale (see Figs. 3–21 and 16–9). Lesions of tinea versicolor may be differentiated by their fine scales and their typical distribution on the trunk, neck, and at times the face (see Fig. 13–31) and upper arms and by the demonstration of hyphae on microscopic examination of epidermal scrapings.

Albinism, either generalized or partial, may be difficult to distinguish from total vitiligo. The diagnosis of albinism, however, may be established by its presence at birth and by the facts that normal eye color is retained in vitiligo (whereas the pigment may be diluted in albinism) and that hair on glabrous skin in the vitiliginous patient, in contrast to that in the patient with albinism, often tends to retain pigment (Figs. 16–10 and 16–11). In partial albinism the diagnosis can be more difficult (Fig. 16–12). The presence of a white forelock and the pattern of hypopigmentation suggests a diagnosis of partial albinism.

The hypopigmented macules of tuberous sclerosis lack the characteristic milk-white appearance of lesions of vitiligo, are present at birth or during the early neonatal period, do not change with age, and have a normal number of melanocytes (with reduc-

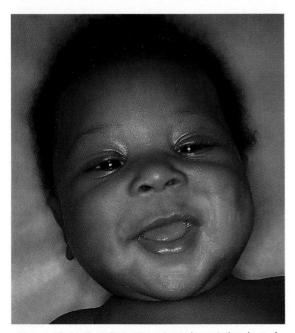

Figure 16–8. Postinflammatory hypopigmentation in a 4-month-old black child with atopic dermatitis.

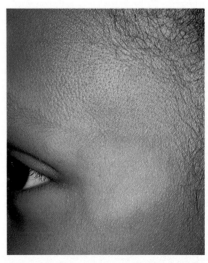

Figure 16–9. Pityriasis alba. Ill-defined hypopigmented oval patches are generally seen on the face, upper arms, neck, and shoulders of affected persons. This disorder can be differentiated from vitiligo by its fine adherent scale, partial hypopigmentation, and distribution.

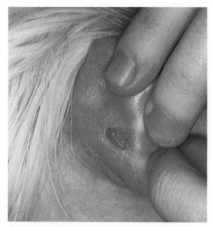

Figure 16–10. Albinism. This patient has light skin, yellowish white hair, and a lack of pigmentation in nevi. (Courtesy of Department of Dermatology, Yale University Shool of Medicine.)

tion in size of melanosomes and melanin granules within them) in contrast to the absence or decrease in number of melanocytes in patients with vitiligo (Fig. 16–13).

Biopsy specimens taken from the depigmented skin of vitiligo reveal a partial to total loss of epidermal pigment cells, and at the borders of lesions the melanocytes are often large and have long dendritic processes.[7] On electron microscopic examination the number of Langerhans' cells seems to be increased, and many are found in the basal portion of the epidermis rather than in the mid epidermis.

The course of vitiligo is variable. Long periods of quiescence may be interrupted by periods of extension or partial improvement. Extension of vitiliginous areas, however, frequently tends to occur when the patient experiences severe emotional or physical stress. Complete spontaneous repigmentation is unusual. Some temporary and partial repigmentation, however, may be detectable in vitiliginous lesions less than 2 years old (particularly in children) during the summer months. In such cases small, freckle-like spots of repigmentation may appear in the white patches during periods of prolonged sun exposure (Figs. 16–14 and 16–15) but occasionally may fade again in temperate climates during the winter months. Complete repigmentation of all involved areas, however, is the exception rather than the rule, and recurrences are common.

The repigmentation process proceeds slowly, and children usually tend to respond with more permanent and complete repigmentation than adults. Since repigmentation, when it occurs, is primarily due to migration of melanocytes from the hair bulbs, sites lacking or poor in hair follicles such as the dorsal surfaces of the fingers, hands, and feet and the volar aspect of the wrists do not respond as well as other areas.[10] The face and, to a lesser extent, the trunk, however, often tend to

have a better response (Fig. 16–16). Vitiligo, therefore, should never be dismissed as only a cosmetic disorder and, although there is no completely satisfactory treatment, all patients deserve an explanation of the disorder, emotional support, and a full discussion of options for therapy.[9–11] Repigmentation can frequently be accomplished by the use of topical corticosteroids or the administration of psoralen compounds followed by gradually increasing exposure to sunlight or long-wave ultraviolet light (UVA) (see Fig. 16–15). Since treatment of vitiligo is long and difficult, only those patients who are highly motivated and completely informed about their chances for improvement should begin such therapy.[12–14] This therapy is most effective in young patients, particularly those who have a relatively short history of the disorder. Trimethylpsoralen tablets, 5 mg (Trisoralen), or 8-methoxypsoralen capsules, 10 mg (Oxsoralen), may be administered 2 hours prior to sunlight or long-wave ultraviolet light exposure. Normal sunlight (particularly between the hours of 11 AM and 4 PM) is an excellent source of natural ultraviolet light for this form of therapy. If sunlight is impractical or unavailable, black-light bulbs or fluorescent tubes rich in wavelengths from 320 to 400 nm (the action spectrum of the psoralens) two or three times a week may be used. Photochemotherapy with oral psoralens and UVA (PUVA),

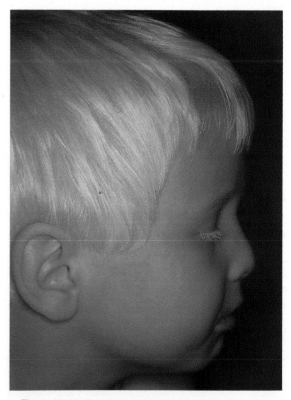

Figure 16–11. Oculocutaneous albinism. Milk-white skin and white hair are seen in a child with photophobia and photosensitivity.

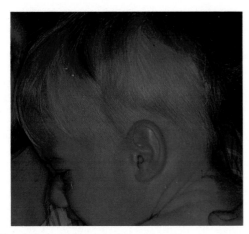

Figure 16–12. Partial albinism and piebaldism were present in a child with tuberous sclerosis.

however, is generally not recommended for children younger than 10 years of age in whom compliance may present a problem. Since aspirin helps block the action of prostaglandins and other mediators that may interfere with repigmentation, some authorities suggest the oral administration of aspirin (up to 5 grains three times a day on the day of therapy) for patients undergoing photochemotherapy for vitiligo. Studies to date, however, are incomplete, and further evaluation is required before concomitant aspirin therapy is universally recommended for the treatment of this disorder.

When trimethylpsoralen was first introduced during the 1950s, some laboratory animals showed abnormalities of liver function tests. The manufacturers of this preparation accordingly include a warning of possible hepatic damage and recommend that these preparations be avoided in the treatment of children younger then age 12. Extensive use of psoralens in children as well as adults, however, has failed to reveal evidence of liver toxicity, and there have been no reported adverse effects, even in young children.[15]

The usual recommended dose of trimethylpsoralen is one to four tablets (5 to 20 mg) and that for 8-methoxypsoralen is one or two capsules (10 to 20 mg) 2 hours before ultraviolet light exposure. With such therapy reasonably good repigmentation may occur in up to one third of cases, some repigmentation may occur in one third of cases, and poor results occur in the other third. In general, significant repigmentation (greater than 75 per cent) can be expected in the head and neck region and on the trunk of 40 to 60 per cent of patients, especially those with more darkly pigmented skin.[14] If patients show no response after 3 months of PUVA therapy or are not significantly better after 60 or more PUVA treatments, their chances of getting better are fairly limited and treatments should be discontinued. Patients should be forewarned that sunburn may develop, particularly in areas of depigmentation, during the

early phases of therapy. The duration of exposure, accordingly, should be initiated gradually and increased as tolerated. When sunlight is used as the source of ultraviolet light, I recommend that a sunscreen with a sunscreen protective factor (SPF) of 8 be used in all areas of vitiligo and a sun-blocking agent with an SPF of 15 or more be used in all other ultraviolet light–exposed areas. Blacks, however, may use sunscreens with an SPF of 6 or 8 on nonvitiliginous ultraviolet light–exposed areas. Although repigmentation may begin after a few weeks, significant results frequently take as long as 6 months or more, and treatment during the summer months may have to be continued for several years or more.

Before beginning treatment of vitiligo with oral psoralens, patients should have a careful eye examination to detect any existing abnormalities of the retina or lens. Although the potential for cataracts and visual loss after PUVA therapy is very low, patients undergoing psoralen and ultraviolet therapy should wear UVA-opaque protective goggles or wraparound glasses during daylight hours for up to 18 hours after ingesting psoralen. Patients requiring therapy for vitiligo of eyelids should keep their eyes closed during their treatment periods, and those using Tripsoralen therapy should wear protective glasses throughout the remainder of the day. Patients undergoing PUVA therapy with Oxsoralen should wear their protective glasses during daylight hours for 48 hours after Oxsoralen is ingested. The goal in using psoralen and ultraviolet light for repigmentation therapy is to achieve a slightly pink color in the depigmented skin, an indication of mild phototoxicity. Marked erythema, however, should be avoided.[16] Although some physicians prefer not to treat children

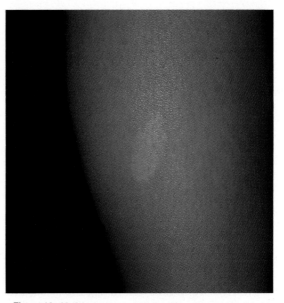

Figure 16–13. A lance-ovate (ash-leaf) white macule on the leg of a child with tuberous sclerosis.

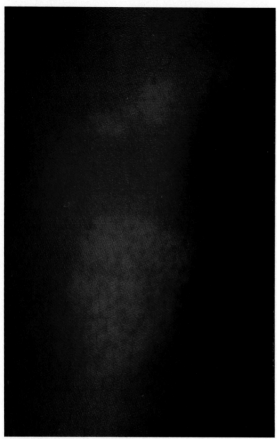

Figure 16–14. Partial repigmentation of lesions of vitiligo on the leg of a 14-year-old child at the end of a summer of sun exposure.

sunburn may follow such therapy, this approach should be initiated with extreme caution, and it is advisable that patients be treated only under the careful supervision of the physician. Topical psoralens are highly phototoxic and should only be used for patients who can comply with the precautions required to minimize severe blistering reactions. It is recommended, therefore, that topical psoralen therapy be used with UVA phototherapy rather than natural sunlight. Although methoxsalen comes as a 1 per cent solution, when used it should be diluted to a 0.05 to 0.1 per cent concentration. Trained personnel should apply the solution precisely to depigmentend patches about 15 minutes before UVA exposure, and after treatment the area should be washed with soap and water followed by application of a sunscreen or other opaque coverup in an effort to avoid sunburn or local reaction in the treated areas. Patients who use this form of therapy must also avoid additional direct ultraviolet or UVA exposure (from direct sunlight, through window glass or car windshields) for the remainder of that day.[10]

Autologous skin grafts and topically applied 5 per cent fluorouracil followed by epidermal abrasion have also been used in patients with relatively localized areas of vitiligo unresponsive to other modes of therapy.[19–22] Such therapy, however, requires further evaluation and is not currently recommended for general use at this time.

younger than 10 years of age, with appropriate eye protection, sunburn precautions, and motivation, treatment can be accomplished safely, even in this age group.

Topical corticosteroids are also useful in the treatment of children or adults who have only a few patches of vitiligo, and during the fall and winter months for individuals who live in temperate climates. Although high-potency topical corticosteroids have been used for this purpose,[17] corticosteroid formulations such as 0.1 per cent triamcinolone acetonide (Kenalog) or mometasone furoate (Elocon) applied once daily for 4 to 6 months can produce repigmentation in one third to one half of patients. Less potent preparations are recommended for topical corticosteroid therapy for the face, eyelids, and intertriginous areas.[10] Patients treated in this manner should be examined at regular intervals to detect side effects associated with topical corticosteroid use.

If vitiligo is localized to a small area, topical application of methoxsalen lotion (Oxsoralen lotion, 1 per cent) followed by short exposure to ultraviolet light (after waiting 45 minutes to 1 hour) or black light (UVA) may be considered.[18] Since

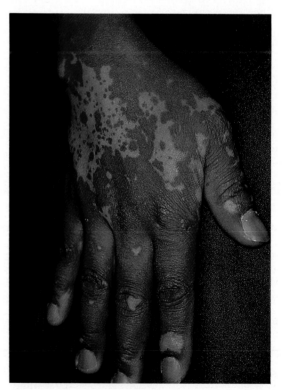

Figure 16–15. Partial repigmentation of vitiligo following psoralen–ultraviolet light (PUVA) therapy. (Courtesy of Department of Dermatology, Yale University School of Medicine.)

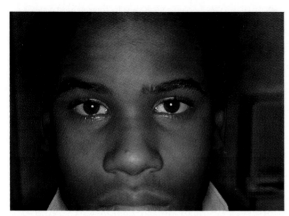

Figure 16–16. Permanent repigmentation after 2 years of photochemotherapy (tripsoralen followed by sunlight exposure) in the patient with vitiligo shown in Figure 16–2.

When treatment of vitiligo is unsatisfactory, lesions can be hidden by the use of cosmetic make-ups or aniline dye stains such as Dy-O-Derm (Owen) or Vitadye (Elder), quick-tan preparations, or cosmetic camouflages (Dermablend or Covermark). In those few cases in which vitiligo has progressed to such an extent that more than 50 per cent of the body is involved (particularly in those persons in whom only a few islands of normal skin remain), an attempt at depigmentation with 20 per cent monobenzyl ether of hydroquinone (Benoquin) may be used.[10] Such patients should be reminded to use appropriate sunscreens and protective clothing and to avoid excessive sun exposure, since, once treated, they lack their usual melanin protection and are more susceptible to sunburn.

Albinism

Albinism is an uncommon inherited disorder of melanin synthesis manifested by a congenital lack of pigmentation of the skin, hair, and eyes. It occurs in two forms: oculocutaneous and ocular. Oculocutaneous albinism comprises a group of 10 heritable disorders with decreased or absent melanin biosynthesis in the melanocytes of the skin, hair follicles, and eyes. All forms except one (autosomal dominant oculocutaneous albinism) are inherited as autosomal recessive traits. In addition there are five types of ocular albinism in which only the eye pigmentation is consistently abnormal.

OCULOCUTANEOUS ALBINISM

Oculocutaneous albinism is an autosomal recessive congenital disorder in which there is a generalized decrease or absence of pigment in the eyes, skin, and hair (see Fig. 16–11). Seen in 1 in 17,000 persons in the United States, the highest incidence (1 to 7:100) occurs in the Cuna tribe of Indians on the San Blas Islands off the coast of Panama. The disorder is characterized by varying degrees of unpatterned reduction of pigment in the skin and hair, translucent irides, hypopigmented ocular fundi, and an associated nystagmus. Melanocytes and melanosomes are present in the affected skin and hair in normal numbers, but although they are tyrosine positive, they fail to produce normal amounts of melanin in the areas of leukoderma or poliosis.

Although at least 10 variants of oculocutaneous albinism have been described, tyrosinase-negative and tyrosinase-positive oculocutaneous albinism, so designated on the basis of pigment production in plucked hair incubated in tyrosine, are the most common. Forms of oculocutaneous albinism having distinct clinical characteristics are the Hermansky-Pudlak syndrome (oculocutaneous albinism with a hemorrhagic diathesis secondary to a platelet storage pool defect and ceroid or wax-like depositions within the reticuloendothelial system, oral and intestinal mucosae, lung, and urine), a yellow mutant form (first recognized in Amish communities and subsequently in most populations throughout the world, in which the hair color turns to yellow within the first few years and a golden blond to light brown by the end of the second decade, and nystagmus, photophobia, and reduced visual acuity are variable), and the Chédiak-Higashi syndrome. Most commonly seen in Hispanics from Puerto Rico, in persons of Dutch origin, and in East Indians from Madras, the platelet defect in patients with the Hermansky-Pudlak syndrome does not produce a severe problem in children. Its expression, however, can be aggravated by aspirin ingestion, and special precautions must be taken to avoid excessive bleeding after minor trauma or dental surgery.[23, 24]

The Chédiak-Higashi syndrome is a rare autosomal recessive lethal form of oculocutaneous albinism characterized by diffuse oculocutaneous hypopigmentation, photophobia, hepatosplenomegaly, abnormal granulation of leukocytes, and recurrent pyogenic infections. Patients with this condition have fair skin; pale retinae; translucent irides; light-blond, frosted, or silvery hair; recurrent respiratory and cutaneous infections; and hematologic, neurologic, and renal abnormalities.

There are giant lysosomal inclusion bodies in all circulating granulocytes, as well as in many other cells of the body, and the large size of the inclusion bodies reflects a functional abnormality that leads to improper handling or distribution of normal lysosomal enzymes.[25] Characteristic cytoplasmic inclusions resembling lysosomes within nerve cells, muscle weakness, and progressive cranial and peripheral neuropathy have been seen in individuals with this disorder, and a lymphoma-like phase with hepatosplenomegaly, lymphadenopathy, and widespread organ infiltrates has been noted.[26]

Most patients die in early childhood of overwhelming infection, hemorrhage, or a lymphoma-like process, with over 50 per cent succumbing before the end of the first decade of life.[26] The management of this disorder accordingly consists of supportive measures to prevent recurrent infection. Combined prednisone and vincristine therapy has been suggested in the management of the accelerated lymphoma-like phase, and ascorbic acid (possibly combined with a cholinergic agent) appears to be beneficial. Ascorbic acid appears to help, not because of a possible nutritional deficiency but because of a lowering effect on cyclic adenosine monophosphate and an associated improvement in leukocyte function.[27]

In whites with oculocutaneous albinism the skin may be milk-white, the hair is white to yellow or light brown, the pupils are pink, the irides are gray or blue, and photophobia and photosensitivity are common (see Figs. 16–10 and 16–11). In blacks the skin color may be tan or may resemble that of whites; freckles can appear on exposure to light; the hair is blond to red; and the eyes are blue or hazel. Patients have a typical appearance not only because of the decrease in skin color but also because of a typical facial expression that results from photophobia, central scotomas, and the associated tendency to habitual squinting and nystagmus. Although the degree of pigment dilution in affected individuals is variable, the diagnosis is easily established in those who have striking pigment loss or relative pigment dilution when compared with unaffected siblings or parents.

The incidence of oculocutaneous albinism is much higher among the Cuna Indians of the San Blas Islands off the east coast of Panama than it is among the general population. This form of oculocutaneous albinism appears to be transmitted by a non-sex-linked autosomal recessive gene; and although the true incidence in this group is not established, it has been estimated to approach 1:100 to 7:100. Affected children have been called "moon children" because they have marked photosensitivity and photophobia and prefer to go outdoors only at night.

The skin of Cuna "moon children" becomes freckled and wrinkled and is easily blistered by the tropical sunshine. Malignant skin tumors are common, and life expectancy is short. Actinic keratoses, atrophy, telangiectasia, and actinic cheilitis appear early, and actinic keratoses occur in most affected Cuna Indian children, unless carefully protected from the sun, by 7 years of age. Malignant changes generally occur by age 30 and often prove fatal, and few Cuna albinos live beyond 40 years of age.[28]

Other abnormalities reported in association with albinism include congenital deafness, small stature, retardation, spasticity, and coagulation disorders. The Tietz syndrome is a rare autosomal dominant disorder characterized by albinism, complete deaf-mutism, hypoplasia or absence of the eyebrows, and normal eye color. Since the irides of the eyes have normal pigmentation, photophobia and nystagmus are not seen as features of this disorder.[29] An oculocerebral syndrome with hypopigmentation (the Cross-McKusick-Breen syndrome), characterized by oculocutaneous albinism, microphthalmus, spasticity, and mental retardation, has also been reported.[30]

OCULAR ALBINISM

In addition to the various types of oculocutaneous albinism, there are five types of ocular albinism in which only the eye pigment is consistently abnormal. Affected males have translucency of the iris, photophobia, nystagmus, and head-nodding similar to that seen in patients with oculocutaneous albinism. Affected females and female carriers have a milder clinical picture, with decreased pigmentation of the iris and posterior fundus and typical retinal changes (stippling, alternating dark and light patches, giving a salt and pepper, grouped, mottled, or striped appearance to the retina, and easily visible choroid vasculature).[31] Except for the frequent presence of myopia, visual acuity in affected individuals is generally normal.

Other than contact lenses and tinted glasses to ameliorate photophobia there is no effective treatment for patients with ocular forms of albinism. Since early actinic changes, keratoses, basal cell tumors, and squamous cell carcinomas are common, even in children and adolescents, those with cutaneous albinism must learn to avoid sunlight exposure and to use protective clothing and sunscreen preparations on exposed surfaces.

Partial Albinism (Piebaldism)

Partial albinism, also termed *piebaldism,* is an uncommon but widely distributed dominantly inherited disorder. Associated with a white lock of hair above the forehead (the white forelock) in 85 to 90 per cent of affected individuals, this disorder is characterized by congenital patterned areas of depigmentation and varying shades of normal skin color that are usually present at birth. Partial albinism occasionally may occur without a white forelock; a white forelock without some degree of leukoderma of the underlying scalp or other parts of the body may also occur, but this seems to represent a forme fruste of the disorder (see Fig. 16–12).[32]

The clinical manifestation of partial albinism may be explained either by incomplete migration of melanoblasts from the neural crest to the ventral midline or by a defect in the differentiation of ventral melanoblasts to melanocytes. The most striking features of partial albinism include distinctive patterns of hypopigmentation or depigmentation, which generally persist unchanged throughout life. These include the white forelock, a hypopigmented triangular patch of the scalp and forehead (widest at the forehead, with the apex pointing backward) that occurs in 80 to 90 per cent of piebald individuals, and hypopigmented or depigmented areas on the chin, anterior neck, and anterior portion of the thorax and abdomen and, at times, on both the anterior and posterior aspects of the midarm to the wrist and the midthigh to midcalf. There may be islands of normal pigment within the hypomelanotic areas, and the borders and islands of pigmentation within the unpigmented areas may be hyperpigmented.

In many individuals the areas of unpigmented skin on the forehead include the whole or inner portions of the eyebrows and eyelashes and extend to the root of the nose. The leukoderma may begin again on the chin or front of the chest and abdomen, and it often spreads to the flanks and back in the form of scattered white patches. The occiput, back of the neck, dorsal aspect of the trunk, and the hands and feet are less commonly involved, and there is little tendency to symmetry of the hypopigmented areas.

The patterns of hypopigmentation of partial albinism can be differentiated from those of vitiligo by their usual presence at birth, lack of convex borders, and predilection for ventral surfaces as opposed to exposed areas, body orifices, areas of trauma, and intertriginous regions. The clinical features that distinguish partial albinism from oculocutaneous albinism are its dominant mode of inheritance, lack of ocular manifestations, and characteristic distribution of lesions, with a predilection for the ventral areas.

Although most individuals with piebaldism are healthy and can anticipate a normal life span, heterochromia irides, mental retardation, ataxia, motor incoordination, Hirschsprung's disease, and Griscelli's syndrome (partial albinism with silvery hair, recurrent cutaneous and systemic pyogenic infections, hepatosplenomegaly, neutropenia, thrombocytopenia, and defective cell-mediated immunity) have been associated with this disorder.

Electron microscopic examination of lesions reveals an absence or lower than normal density of melanocytes, markedly deformed melanosomes, Langerhans cells in the amelanotic areas, and an increase of melanin granules in the hyperpigmented borders.

Treatment consists of cosmetic masking of areas of leukoderma with aniline dyes (as in the treatment of vitiligo), the protection of hypopigmented and depigmented areas from sun damage by proper clothing, and the use of appropriate sunscreen preparations on exposed surfaces.

Waardenburg's Syndrome

Waardenburg's syndrome (also termed *Klein-Waardenburg syndrome*) is a rare autosomal dominant disorder characterized by congenital deafness, lateral displacement of the medial canthi and lacrimal puncta of the lower eyelids (dystopia cantharum), broad nasal root, white forelock, heterochromia irides, and cutaneous depigmentation similar to that seen in patients with piebaldism.[33]

Other features include excessive and occasionally confluent eyebrows, hypoplasia of the ala nasi, mild mandibular prognathism, impaired speech with or without cleft lip or cleft palate, and a variety of skeletal deformities.

Measurements of the interocular distance can help determine the presence or absence of dystopia cantharum, a highly diagnostic feature of this disorder, which is seen in 69 per cent of patients. If the inner canthal distance divided by the interpupillary distance is greater than 0.6, this lateral displacement of the inner canthi may help confirm the diagnosis.

Tuberous Sclerosis

Partially depigmented white macules (the earliest cutaneous feature) are present in 78 to 90 per cent of individuals affected with tuberous sclerosis (see Fig. 16–13 and, in Chapter 23, Figs. 23–8 through 23–10). Since these hypopigmented spots are present at birth or first noted in the neonatal period, they may permit an early diagnosis of tuberous sclerosis in a child with seizures or mental retardation, long before the development of the usual recognized cutaneous and radiologic signs.[34–37]

The hypopigmented macules of tuberous sclerosis are seen on the trunk, arms, and legs and generally spare the face, palms, and soles. Most lesions average 1 to 3 cm in diameter; they may number one to several hundreds and are usually oval with irregular margins. Occasionally there may be numerous small, freckle-sized hypopigmented lesions ("white freckles") on the anterior aspects of the legs.[35] Although the white spots of tuberous sclerosis have been termed *vitiliginous* by many authors, they are unrelated to vitiligo and can be differentiated from it by many characteristics (see discussion under Vitiligo). Of further interest is the fact that in addition to the characteristic hypopigmented macules there also appears to be an increased incidence of tuberous sclerosis in patients with partial albinism (see Fig. 16–12). In fair-skinned individuals the detection of characteristic hypopigmented macules is aided by a powerful Wood's light in a completely darkened room. This procedure may be of value in the differentiation of lesions of tuberous sclerosis from the less discrete hypopigmentation of postinflammatory hypomelanosis and pityriasis alba (see Chapter 23 for a more detailed discussion of tuberous sclerosis).

Incontinentia Pigmenti

Incontinentia pigmenti (Bloch-Sulzberger syndrome) is a hereditary disorder affecting the skin, central nervous system, eyes, and skeletal system. Although the genetics of this disorder have not been delineated, it appears to be an autosomal dominant or X-linked dominant disorder, prenatally lethal to males (see Chapter 23 for a more detailed discussion of incontinentia pigmenti).

In addition to the well-recognized vesiculobullous, verrucous, and highly characteristic pigmentary stages of this disorder (see Figs. 23–12 through 23–16), a fourth manifestation consisting of depigmented lesions has also been recognized (see Fig. 23–17).[38] Observed as isolated lesions or seen in conjunction with other dermatologic manifestations, they have been reported on the arms, thighs, and trunk. More characteristically, however, they appear on the calves of children as well as adults with this disorder. Although the histologic features of these hypopigmented lesions are poorly defined and their incidence and pathogenesis are unknown, the presence of streaked hypopigmented macules in family members related to children with incontinentia pigmenti may provide clues to the hereditary pattern and may play a role in the genetic counseling of families of individuals with this disorder.

Incontinentia Pigmenti Achromians (Hypomelanosis of Ito)

Among nevoid causes of hypopigmentation, incontinentia pigmenti achromians (more appropriately termed hypomelanosis of Ito) is a neurocutaneous syndrome characterized by distinctive macular, linear, or irregular whorls and swirls of hypopigmentation (see Fig. 23–20).

This disorder is unrelated to incontinentia pigmenti. The loss of pigment is present at birth or may begin in early childhood, may spontaneously remit at a later age, and is of particular significance because of the fact that approximately 50 per cent of patients have associated internal manifestations (seizure disorders, delayed development, musculoskeletal anomalies, or ocular disturbances).[39–43] Microscopic examination of affected areas reveals normal numbers of melanocytes. The melanocytes contain less melanin, are less dopa-positive, and have smaller melanosomes than those in the adjacent normal skin. Since the hypopigmented lesions appear early, the appearance of hypopigmentation in a whorled or swirled pattern should alert physicians to the possible association with systemic disease.

Nevus Achromicus

Nevus achromicus (nevus depigmentosus) is a congenital disorder characterized by single macular lesions, bands, or bizarre streaks of hypopigmentation (Fig. 16–17).[44] Affected areas may be quite small or may cover large segments of the body, and present at birth, they grow only with the growth of the individual. This disorder may be seen in association with hemihypertrophy and severe mental retardation.[45]

Nevus achromicus is probably seen more fre-

Figure 16–17. Nevus achromicus, achromic nevus (a congenital area of partial hypopigmentation that remains unchanged throughout life). This disorder is probably more common than the literature indicates.

quently than the literature indicates. The hypopigmented areas are usually confined to one side of the body and are most often located on the trunk. They are generally irregular, frequently tend to occur in long bands or streaks, and show varying degrees of melanin deficiency and a reduced number of functional melanocytes.

Nevus Anemicus

Nevus anemicus is a developmental anomaly characterized by a circumscribed round or oval patch of pale or mottled skin. Appearing at birth or in early childhood, the area of involvement appears to be pale owing to a decreased sensitivity of the vessels to endogenous vasodilatory mediators such as acetylcholine, histamine, and serotonin[46] or to a localized hypersensitivity of the α-adrenergic receptor sites of cutaneous blood vessels within the lesion to constricting catecholamines.[47] When the diagnosis is in doubt, rubbing makes the pale area stand out in contrast to the adjacent unaffected skin, and its border can be obscured by gentle pressure with a translucent plastic or glass slide (diascopy). In addition, Wood's lamp examination does not accentuate lesions of nevus anemicus (in fact, the lesion may become inapparent) and friction and cold or heat applications fail to induce the erythema normally seen on uninvolved skin. Although there is no effective therapy other than cosmetic camouflage, the lesion, usually in a covered area, is generally so slight that treatment is rarely required.

Vogt-Koyanagi Syndrome

The Vogt-Koyanagi syndrome (Vogt-Koyanagi-Harada syndrome) is a rare, possibly autoimmune disorder characterized by bilateral uveitis, alopecia, vitiligo, poliosis (which may be limited to the eyebrows and eyelashes or may also involve the scalp and body hair), dysacousia (a condition in which certain sounds produce discomfort), and deafness. Usually seen in adults in the third and fourth decades of life, the disorder also occurs in children and adolescents. Although the etiology is unknown, it has been hypothesized that this syndrome is associated with an abnormal host response to an infective agent, possibly a virus, with an allergic sensitization to uveal melanocyte antigens and destruction of melanin in the hair and skin.[48] The Vogt-Koyanagi and the Vogt-Koyanagi-Harada syndromes appear to be the same, except that meningeal irritation or encephalitic symptoms are described in association with the latter condition. In this variant a prodromal febrile episode, with encephalitic or meningeal symptoms, lymphocytosis, and increased pressure of the cerebrospinal fluid, is followed by bilateral uveitis (often with choroiditis and optic neuritis).

In all patients there is a bilateral uveitis, which is self-limiting. As the uveitis begins to subside, poliosis (in 80 to 90 per cent), temporary auditory impairment, vitiligo, usually symmetrical (in 50 to 60 per cent), and alopecia (in 50 per cent) develop. The hearing usually returns to normal, but the pigmentary changes, which generally appear 3 weeks to 3 months after the onset of the uveitis, tend to be permanent. The uveitis generally takes a year or more to clear, and although most patients show some recovery of visual acuity, only partial recovery may occur at times, and some individuals may be left with a residual visual defect.

Alezzandrini's Syndrome

Alezzandrini's syndrome is a rare disorder of unknown origin primarily seen in adolescents and young adults. Possibly related to the Vogt-Koyanagi syndrome, it is characterized by unilateral degenerative retinitis with visual impairment, which is followed, at times, after an interval of months or years, by bilateral deafness and unilateral vitiligo and poliosis, which appear on the same side of the face.

Chemically Induced Hypopigmentation

A number of chemical agents are known to cause depigmentation. Among these compounds, the rubber antioxidant monobenzyl ether of hydroquinone, hydroquinone photographic developer, sulfhydryl compounds, phenolic germicidal agents (paratertiary butylphenol and amylphenol), hydroxyanisole, and 4-tertiary butyl catechol (an additive to polyethylene film) have been recognized as causes of leukoderma (Fig. 16–18).[49] The biochemical mechanism by which phenolic chemicals induce such hypopigmentation appears to be the competitive inhibition of tyrosinase[50] or the release of toxic metabolites that produce injury to the melanocytes.

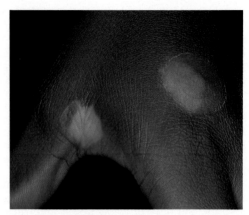

Figure 16–18. Chemical depigmentation due to a germicidal detergent. Patients with this disorder usually improve after discontinuation of the offending agent. (Courtesy of Department of Dermatology, Yale University School of Medicine.)

Postinflammatory Hypopigmentation

Postinflammatory leukoderma may be associated with a wide variety of inflammatory dermatoses or infections. This relative pigmentary deficiency may be noted following involution of certain inflammatory skin disorders, particularly burns, bullous disorders, infections, eczematous or psoriatic lesions, and pityriasis rosea (see Figs. 16–7 and 16–8). The inflammatory reactions in some secondary syphilitic lesions and pityriasis lichenoides (Mucha-Habermann syndrome) in particular may result in postinflammatory hypopigmentation. In the inflammatory dermatoses the intensity of the inflammatory reaction may bear little relationship to the development of postinflammatory leukoderma, and such hypopigmentation is generally self-limiting.

Although the pathophysiology of postinflammatory hypopigmentation is unclear, it is postulated that the hypopigmentation is caused when keratinocytes injured by the inflammatory process are temporarily unable to accept melanosomes from the melanocyte dendrites. Since the defect is primarily epidermal, postinflammatory hypopigmentation generally improves with time, without need for active therapy.

Other Types of Hypopigmentation

Pityriasis alba is a common cutaneous disorder characterized by asymptomatic scaly hypopigmented patches on the face, neck, upper trunk, arms, shoulders, and at times the lower aspect of the trunk and extremities of children and young adults (see Figs. 3–21 and 16–9). Seen predominantly in children 3 to 16 years of age, individual lesions vary from 1 to several centimeters in diameter and have sharply delineated margins and a fine branny scale. Although the cause is unknown, this disorder appears to represent a nonspecific dermatitis (possibly a form of atopic dermatitis).

Phenylketonuria (phenylpyruvic oligophrenia) represents a group of inborn errors of phenylalanine metabolism characterized by pigmentary dilution of the skin, hair, and eyes and, if not treated early, by mental retardation. Patients with this disorder typically have an oculocutaneous pigmentary dilution characterized by blonde hair, fair skin, and blue eyes, mental retardation, seizures, hyperreflexia, dermatitis, and, in rare instances, scleroderma-like skin lesions (see Chapter 22).

Tinea versicolor (pityriasis versicolor), a common condition frequently found on the upper part of the trunk and neck of young adults and caused by *Pityrosporum orbiculare* (*Malassezia furfur*), is characterized by either hypopigmented or hyperpigmented macules on the upper part of the trunk and neck of young adults (occasionally infants and young children) and at times the face, scalp, extremities, and lower part of the trunk (see Chapter 13).

Sarcoidosis is a disorder of unknown origin with widespread manifestations involving the skin and many of the internal organs. In addition to the characteristic yellowish brown, flesh-colored, pink, red, and reddish brown to black or blue lesions, subcutaneous nodules, and infiltrated plaques (see Chapter 24), the spectrum of sarcoidal skin lesions has been extended to include hypomelanotic macules and papules. Measuring up to 1.0 to 1.5 cm in diameter, these depigmented lesions reveal sarcoid-type granulomas on cutaneous biopsy and accordingly have been suggested as another cutaneous manifestation of this disorder.[51]

Leprosy (Hansen's disease), a chronic infection in which the acid-fast bacillus *Mycobacterium leprae* has a special predilection for the skin and nervous system, can be divided into several types depending on the patient's cellular immune response to *M. leprae* (see Chapter 10). Lepromatous leprosy is generally manifested by symmetrically arranged lesions, which, at first macular, develop nodules or diffuse infiltrates (especially on the eyebrows and ears), resulting in a leonine facies. Tuberculoid leprosy, conversely, shows characteristic well-defined anesthetic hypopigmented lesions and thickened and palpable peripheral nerves. Intermediate leprosy, an early stage of the latter, is manifested by one or a few macules or edematous papules that are erythematous and may show loss of pigment.

When the diagnosis is indeterminate, the presence of thickened tender superficial nerves, anesthetic hypopigmented macules, a granulomatous infiltrate on microscopic examination of cutaneous lesions, and demonstration of *M. leprae* on cutaneous smear or biopsy specimen generally help confirm the diagnosis.

Pinta, a treponemal infection caused by *Treponema carateum*, seen almost exclusively among the dark-skinned population of Cuba and Central and South America, is frequently seen in children of parents afflicted with this disorder.

The cutaneous manifestations may be divided into primary, secondary, and tertiary stages (these are described in Chapter 10). The late dyschromic stage takes several more years to develop. These lesions have an insidious onset and usually appear during adolescence or young adulthood. They consist of slate-blue hyperpigmented lesions, which, after a period of years, become widespread and are replaced by depigmented macules resembling those seen in patients with vitiligo. Located chiefly on the face, waist, and areas close to bony prominences (elbows, knees, ankles, wrists, and the dorsal aspect of the hands), these depigmented lesions of pinta can be differentiated from those of vitiligo by the presence of the other pigmented lesions, microscopic examination of cutaneous lesions, isolation of *T. carateum* by serologic testing, darkfield examination, and their histopathologic features.

DISORDERS OF HYPERPIGMENTATION

Disorders of hyperpigmentation may be external or internal in origin. The diagnosis and therapy for some of these disorders are described below.

Postinflammatory Melanosis

Postinflammatory melanosis (postinflammatory hyperpigmentation), one of the most common causes of hyperpigmentation, is characterized by an increase in melanin formation following cutaneous inflammation. Ordinary postinflammatory hyperpigmentation is of relatively short duration and tends to persist for several weeks or months after the original cause has subsided. Examples include the pigmentation following physical trauma, friction, primary irritants, eczematoid eruptions, lichen simplex chronicus, and dermatoses such as pityriasis rosea, psoriasis, dermatitis herpetiformis, fixed drug eruptions, photodermatitis, and pyoderma (Fig. 16–19). Individuals with dark complexions and those who tan easily following ultraviolet light exposure show the greatest degree of this form of melanosis. In cases in which the dermal-epidermal junction and basal layer become disrupted (lupus erythematosus, lichen planus, lichenoid drug eruptions) melanin incontinence occurs. The melanin tends to drop from its normal epidermal position and passes into the melanophages of the epidermis, and the discoloration is frequently longer lasting and more pronounced.

If areas of postinflammatory hyperpigmentation can be protected from further ultraviolet light exposure, fading gradually occurs over a period of months. In blacks and other heavily melanized individuals, however, the disorder may persist for longer periods of time. In cases in which hyperpigmentation is prolonged and therapy is desired,

Melanosis of the Face and Neck

MELASMA

Melasma (formerly referred to as *chloasma*) is a term applied to a patchy dark-brown to black hyperpigmentation located primarily on the cheeks, the forehead, and occasionally the temples, upper lip, and neck. Seen in up to 20 per cent of women who take anovulatory drugs or who are pregnant, this disorder has been termed the *mask of pregnancy*. Since sun exposure tends to trigger and intensify this hyperpigmentation, the disorder characteristically becomes more prominent in the summer months.

Typical melasma also can occur in males and in females who are neither pregnant nor taking oral contraceptives. Occasionally it may also appear in patients of both sexes taking phenytoin (Dilantin) or its derivatives.[55] Dermatoses considered in the differential diagnosis of melasma include berloque dermatitis, postinflammatory hyperpigmentation, Riehl's melanosis, poikiloderma of Civatte, and cases of vitiligo in which the depigmented skin may appear to be normal while the surrounding normal skin may appear to be abnormal or "hyperpigmented."

The histopathologic features of melasma include increased melanization of the epidermis without melanocytic proliferation. When the melasma is induced by oral anovulatory preparations, a mild perivascular and perifollicular lymphocytic infiltrate may be present.

Once melasma has developed it generally tends to persist for long periods of time, and treatment is generally not very satisfactory. Melasma of pregnancy usually clears within a few months after delivery, only to recur with subsequent pregnancies. Oral contraceptive pill–induced melasma may not clear or may clear slowly after cessation of oral intake of the anovulatory preparation, and pigmentation may persist for up to 5 years after discontinuation of the medication. The treatment of melasma consists of discontinuation of potentially responsible medications, protection from sun or ultraviolet light exposure by the use of appropriate clothing and sunscreen preparations, and the topical application of hydroquinones (as described for the treatment of postinflammatory hyperpigmentation).

RIEHL'S MELANOSIS

Riehl's melanosis represents a spotty hyperpigmentation of the face and occasionally of the neck and arms. Primarily seen in adult women with a history of exposure to cosmetics, it may also appear in men and children of all ages. Approximately half the reported cases result from the use of cosmetics containing coal tar derivatives. Other possible etiologic factors include avitaminosis, malnutrition, and contact with hydrocarbons (especially impure mineral oil).

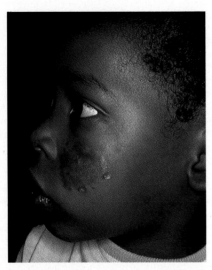

Figure 16–19. Postinflammatory hyperpigmentation following resolution of lymphocytoma cutis on the cheek of a black child.

a low-potency corticosteroid (hydrocortisone in a 1.0 per cent concentration) may be helpful. In patients who desire more active therapy, quicker improvement may be seen with hydroquinone formulations, available as Artra, Porcelana, or Esoterica (a 2 per cent over-the-counter preparation); Melanex (Neutrogena); or Eldoquin, Eldopaque, or Solaquin (Elder Pharmaceuticals). Since continuous use of hydroquinone bleaching creams or lotions can result in excessive pigmentary loss or ochronosis-like hyperpigmentation,[52, 53] once the desired degree of depigmentation is achieved, hydroquinone therapy should be discontinued.

If these preparations do not achieve the desired result, higher concentrations of hydroquinone, available as Benoquin ointment (20 per cent monobenzyl ether of hydroquinone) or a formulation consisting of tretinoin (retinoic acid) 0.1 per cent, hydroquinone 5 per cent, and dexamethasone (or triamcinolone) 0.1 per cent in a hydrophilic ointment (which can be compounded by a pharmacist), applied once daily for 5 to 7 weeks may be beneficial.[54] Since irreversible depigmentation can occur with the use of 20 per cent monobenzyl ether of hydroquinone, this preparation should be used with extreme caution and probably should be reserved for the depigmentation of residual areas of normal pigment in patients with extensive vitiligo (that involving 50 per cent or more of the cutaneous surface).

Hydroquinones act by the inhibition of tyrosinase. These preparations, therefore, act slowly and frequently require 3 to 4 months before a therapeutic effect is achieved. Since the ability of the sun to darken areas of postinflammatory hyperpigmentation is greater than the lightening effect of hydroquinones, ultraviolet light exposure should be avoided and appropriate sun-blocking agents should be used.

The disorder is characterized by a distinctive brownish gray, spotty pigmentation on the forehead and malar areas, behind the ears, on the sides of the neck, and, at times, other sun-exposed areas such as the scalp, arms, chest, forearms, and hands. Although most cases appear to be associated with a photocontact-type reaction, pigmentation on covered parts of the body (e.g., the anterior axillary folds and umbilicus) exposed to friction has also been associated with this disorder.

Histopathologic examination of affected areas reveals liquefactive degeneration of the basal layer of the epidermis in the early stages, large amounts of melanin within melanophages located in the dermis, and a perivascular band-like dermal infiltrate. Treatment is dependent on identification of the cause of the dermatosis, the use of suitable sunscreen preparations, and, if desired, the topical application of hydroquinone preparations.

POIKILODERMA

The term *poikiloderma* (poikiloderma atrophicans vasculare) is used to describe a triad of telangiectasia, atrophy, and dyschromia (hyperpigmentation and hypopigmentation). The disorder may be seen in patients with poikiloderma congenitale (Rothmund-Thomson syndrome), xeroderma pigmentosum, congenital telangiectatic erythema and stunted growth (Bloom's syndrome), dyskeratosis congenita, connective tissue disorders, lymphomatous diseases, and myocosis fungoides. It may also be seen as cutaneous changes associated with actinic, thermal, or radiation damage.

Poikiloderma of Civatte (thought by many to be a variant of Riehl's melanosis) appears over light-exposed areas in women of middle age or older. Characterized by uneven, frequently reticulated, reddish brown pigmentation, superficial telangiectasia, and atrophy in irregular, more or less symmetrical patches on the cheeks, sides of the neck, and upper chest, the disorder persists indefinitely. Photosensitivity is believed to be involved in the pathogenesis of this disorder.

Histopathologic examination of areas of poikiloderma reveals varying degrees of epidermal hyperkeratosis and atrophy, hydropic degeneration of the basal layer, varying numbers of pigment-laden melanophages, and a lymphocytic band-like or perivascular infiltration in the dermis. Management consists of early recognition, avoidance of sun exposure, and the use of protective clothing and topical sunscreen preparations in an attempt to arrest progression of the dermatosis.

Erythema Dyschromicum Perstans

Erythema dyschromicum perstans (dermatosis cinecienta, ashy dermatosis) is an acquired chronic, progressive bluish to ash-gray hyperpigmentation first described in patients in San Salvador in 1957, but also recently described in Central and South America and the United States.[56, 57] This disorder affects individuals of both sexes from childhood through adulthood. Although nearly all reported patients have been dark-complexioned Hispanics or Indians from Central America, reports in Native Americans, East Indians, blacks, and Scandinavians and other fair-skinned individuals suggest that erythema dyschromicum perstans may be more widespread than previously recognized and that mild variants of the disorder probably occur.

Because of its distinctive ashen color, the name occasionally ascribed to patients with this disorder is *los cenicientos* (the ash-colored ones). Although many etiologies have been suggested, the cause of erythema dyschromicum perstans remains unknown.[58] Lesions usually begin as erythematous macules and gradually assume a slate-gray hue and a thin, slightly raised erythematous border. Generally seen on the face, trunk, and upper limbs, lesions may also occur on other areas, with the exception of the scalp, mucous membranes, palms, and soles. Lesions vary from a few millimeters to many centimeters in diameter, and larger lesions, formed by the merging of small macules, may cover extensive areas.

This disorder must be differentiated from lesions of tinea versicolor, erythema annulare centrifugum, melasma, poikiloderma, fixed drug eruption, leprosy, and pinta by its characteristic slate-gray macular lesions with a peripherally spreading erythematous border and characteristic but not diagnostic histologic features of spongiosis, microvesicle formation, hydropic degeneration of epidermal cells, and pigmentary incontinence. The dermatosis is asymptomatic but chronic. There are frequent exacerbations, with extension into previously uninvolved areas, and there is no known effective therapy.

Familial Progressive Hyperpigmentation

Progressive hyperpigmentation, seen in the "carbon baby" described in 1978,[59] or as a familial disorder (familial progressive hyperpigmentation), is an uncommon but distinctive dominantly inherited genodermatosis that presents at birth as irregular patches and streaks of hyperpigmentation, which increase in size, number, and confluence with age. Hyperpigmentation later appears in the conjunctivae and buccal mucosa and, with time, extensive areas of the skin and mucous membrane become involved.[60] The most distinctive histopathologic manifestation consists of heavy melanization of the basal cell layers, particularly the tips of the rete ridges, and a diffuse scattering of pigmented granules throughout the epidermal layers, including the stratum corneum.

Linear and Whorled Nevoid Hypermelanosis

In 1988 a congenital, asymmetrical, patterned epidermal hypermelanosis in streaky configurations along Blaschko's lines was described. This disorder, which appears without associated anomalies or preceding inflammation (termed *linear and whorled nevoid hypermelanosis*), generally develops at birth or shortly thereafter, gradually spreads during the first 2 years of life, and then stabilizes, and occasionally becomes less prominent with time (Figs. 16–20 and 16–21).[61] It should be differentiated from the third stage of incontinentia pigmenti; epidermal nevi; hypomelanosis of Ito; nevoid hypermelanosis seen in human chimeras; reticulated acropigmentation of Kitamura (an autosomal dominant pigmentary disorder characterized by slightly depressed round macules, palmar pits, and breaks in the epidermal rete ridge patterns); Dowling-Degos disease, a rare benign genodermatosis characterized by an acquired reticular pigmentation of the flexural areas; and reticular erythematous mucinosis, a sharply

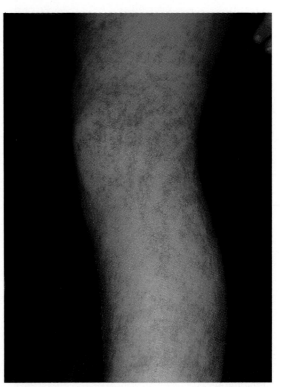

Figure 16–21. Linear and whorled nevoid hypermelanosis on the leg.

marginated bluish red eruption usually seen in the center of the chest and upper back composed of reticulated erythema, confluent papules, and plaque-like dermal mucinosis. The histologic pattern of linear and whorled hypermelanosis consists of increased pigmentation of the basal layer and prominence or vacuolation of melanocytes without increase in dermal melanophages or pigment incontinence.

Metabolic Causes of Hyperpigmentation

Cutaneous changes frequently are helpful in the diagnosis of underlying metabolic or endocrine disorders. Hepatobiliary disorders, hemochromatosis, Addison's disease, hyperthyroidism, hypothyroidism, acromegaly, and Cushing's syndrome are prime examples of metabolic disorders in which hyperpigmentation may be seen as a cutaneous manifestation.

HEPATOBILIARY HYPERPIGMENTATION

More than two thirds of patients with chronic hepatic disease (cirrhosis or prolonged bile duct obstruction) have some degree of cutaneous hyper-

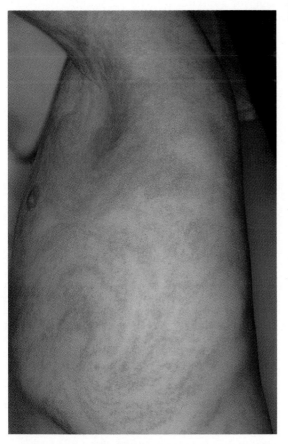

Figure 16–20. Linear and whorled nevoid hypermelanosis on the trunk of a 3-year-old child, a benign pigmentary disorder without associated anomalies.

pigmentation. Of these, diffuse darkening of the skin is perhaps the most common. Blotchy areas of brown hyperpigmentation occasionally may be seen, and accentuation of normal freckling and areolar hyperpigmentation may appear. Although the actual cause of hyperpigmentation associated with chronic liver disease is uncertain, it appears to be associated with humoral mechanisms that result in stimulation of melanogenesis, such as is seen with ACTH, MSH, or endocrine abnormalities,[62] or perhaps hepatic dysfunction may lead to biochemical abnormalities of the epidermal melanin unit with a resultant increase in pigment.

ADRENAL INSUFFICIENCY (ADDISON'S DISEASE)

Addison's disease (chronic adrenocortical insufficiency) is characterized by weakness, anorexia, hypotension, loss of body hair, low values of serum sodium and chloride, high levels of serum potassium, and melanin hyperpigmentation of the skin and mucous membranes. Hyperpigmentation, apparently the result of increased production of MSH by the pituitary gland (a compensatory phenomenon associated with decreased cortisol production by the adrenals), is most intense in the flexures, at sites of pressure and friction, in creases of the palms and soles, in sun-exposed areas, and in normally pigmented areas such as the genitalia and areolae.[63] Pigmentation of the conjunctivae and vaginal mucous membranes is common, and pigmentary changes of the oral mucosae include spotty or streaked blue-black to brown hyperpigmentation of the gingivae, tongue, hard palate, and buccal mucosa.

The diagnosis of chronic adrenocortical insufficiency is suggested by the clinical features and may be confirmed by serum electrolyte studies and cortisol level detemations following stimulation by ACTH (the ACTH-stimulating test).

HYPERTHYROIDISM

The cutaneous changes in hyperthyroidism consist of warm, moist, smooth, and elastic skin, and, in some patients, increased pigmentation (believed to be caused by increased MSH secretion from the pituitary). Vitiligo develops in about 7 per cent of thyrotoxic individuals, and pretibial myxedema, due to the presence of long-acting thyroid stimulating substance (LATS), may also be seen in patients with this disorder.

Pretibial myxedema is manifested by plaques on the shins, exophthalmos, and clubbing, with or without associated osteoarthropathy. Hyperpigmentation, seen in about 10 per cent of patients with primary thyrotoxicosis, is usually diffuse and generally appears in a pattern similar to that seen in patients with Addison's disease, except that the eyelids may occasionally be conspicuously hyperpigmented and involvement of the mucous membranes, areolae, and genitalia is less prominent.

HYPERPITUITARISM

The excessive secretion of growth hormone by pituitary tumors produces gigantism in children whose epiphyses have not yet closed and acromegaly in adults whose normal bone growth has ceased.

Acromegaly is rare in children, but transitional acromegalic features at times may be seen in adolescents. In addition to cutis verticis gyrata (coarse furrowing of the skin on the posterior aspect of the neck and the vertex of the scalp) (see Fig. 21–9), a large and sometimes deeply furrowed tongue, thick lips, large nose, lantern jaw, broad spade-like hands with squatty fingers, hirsutism, and hyperpigmentation in a pattern similar to that observed in patients with Addison's disease may be seen in approximately 40 per cent of patients with acromegaly. Although the cause of hirsutism is not well understood, the hyperpigmentation appears to be related to increased secretion of MSH.[63]

CUSHING'S SYNDROME

Addison-like pigmentation (particularly on the face and neck) has also been noted in 6 to 10 per cent of individuals with Cushing's syndrome. Other associated features include a characteristic plethoric "moon" facies, with telangiectasia over the cheeks; patchy cyanosis over the upper arms, breast, abdomen, buttocks, thighs, and legs; increased presence of fine lanugo hair on the face and extremities; fatty deposits over the back of the neck ("buffalo hump"); increased fat deposits on the torso with a contrasting thinning of the arms and legs; purplish atrophic striae at points of tension such as the lower abdomen, thighs, buttocks, upper arms, and breasts; fragility of dermal blood vessels with increased tendency to bruisability and ecchymoses at sites of slight trauma; poor wound healing; frequent and recurrent pyoderma; and steroid acne.

HEMOCHROMATOSIS

Hemochromatosis, occasionally termed *bronze diabetes,* is a familial iron storage disorder characterized by cutaneous hyperpigmentation, hepatic cirrhosis, diabetes mellitus, and, at times, cardiac failure. This is an uncommon disorder generally seen in males between 40 and 60 years of age, but also occasionally seen in childhood (particularly during adolescence). The pathogenesis is uncertain but appears to be associated with an increase in iron absorption attributable perhaps to an as yet undemonstrated enzymatic defect.

Hemochromatosis is thought to be inherited as a mendelian dominant trait with incomplete penetrance. Hyperpigmentation is seen in almost every patient and is the presenting sign in 25 to 40 per cent of affected individuals. The increased pigmentation is produced by melanin and not by the deposition of iron in the skin.[64, 65] It appears initially in the exposed areas before it becomes diffuse and is most intense in the skin of the face, arms, body folds, and genitalia. Mucous membranes (the gums, palate, and buccal mucosa), and sometimes the conjunctivae, are involved in 15 to 20 per cent of affected persons. The skin is soft, dry, thin, shiny, and of fine texture. Spider angiomas are present in 60 to 80 per cent of affected individuals; icterus is unusual; palmar erythema is common; hypogonadism may be present; and facial, axillary, thoracic, and pubic hairs are scant or absent.[63, 66]

Secondary hemochromatosis (hemosiderosis) may be seen in patients with anemia who receive numerous blood transfusions. This disorder occurs in individuals of both sexes and all ages. In such instances, visceral fibrosis is unusual, diabetes mellitus is uncommon, and hypogonadism is not present.

The diagnosis of metabolic hemochromatosis is suggested by the presence of cutaneous hyperpigmentation in patients with hepatic cirrhosis and a history of diabetes mellitus. Elevated serum iron and saturation of serum iron-binding globulin help confirm the diagnosis. The demonstration of parenchymal iron distribution by skin, liver, and gastric biopsies, and the presence of hemosiderin in urinary sediment are particularly helpful. Histopathologic examination of involved skin is characterized by a normal epidermis, increased melanin in the basal layer, and deposition of iron in the upper cutis (especially in macrophages, endothelial cells of capillaries, and the propria of eccrine glands).

The clinical course of untreated hemochromatosis is characterized by tissue destruction, malfunction of involved organs, and eventual death. Symptomatic treatment of the diabetes, liver dysfunction, and cardiac symptoms and repeated phlebotomies, when initiated early, frequently result in clinical and pathologic improvement. Dietary restriction of iron is impractical, and chelating agents to date have been of little value. Since individuals with hemochromatosis accumulate about 3 mg of iron daily in excess of body losses, to maintain normal iron balance, quarterly phlebotomies of about 500 ml are generally necessary throughout life.

OCHRONOSIS

Ochronosis (alkaptonuria) is an inborn error of tyrosine metabolism in which homogentisic acid, an intermediate product in the metabolism of phenylalanine and tyrosine, accumulates in the tissues and is excreted in the urine because of a lack of homogentisic acid oxidase. A rare or autosomal recessive disorder, the condition is characterized by homogentisic aciduria, dark urine, blue to bluish brown or black-brown cartilaginous pigmentary changes and dermal deposition of pigment (ochronosis), degenerative joint disease, and vascular abnormalities (see Chapter 22).

HYPERMELANOSIS IN OTHER SYSTEMIC DISORDERS

Increased pigmentation may also appear as an inconstant feature of a wide variety of other systemic disorders. In most instances the mechanism is obscure, and a number of factors may be involved.

Hyperpigmentation may occur in chronic infections. Whether the hyperpigmentation is due to the infection, associated malnutrition, or other factors, however, is uncertain. Hyperpigmentation also may be seen as a manifestation of lymphomas and may be noted in 10 per cent of cases of Hodgkin's disease and in 1 or 2 per cent of cases of lymphosarcoma or lymphatic leukemia. It has been noted that attacks of asthma may be preceded by 3 or 4 days of diffuse darkening of the skin and an increase in the size and number of melanocytic nevi. Rheumatoid arthritis, particularly the juvenile variety (Still's disease), also may be associated with a generalized cutaneous hyperpigmentation.

Generalized hyperpigmentation may also be noted in patients with progressive systemic sclerosis or dermatomyositis (accompanying or following the cutaneous lesions) and on light-exposed skin in about 10 per cent of patients with systemic lupus erythematosus.

Polycystic kidney disease and other forms of chronic renal disease with nitrogen retention may also be accompanied by pruritus and, at times, a diffuse yellowish brown discoloration of the skin that is most pronounced on the face and hands. Although urinary chromogens and carotenemia may be present, melanin pigmentation also has been implicated as a cause of this discoloration.

Exogenous Causes of Pigmentation

HYPERPIGMENTATION DUE TO HEAVY METALS

The systemic absorption of chemicals can also cause discoloration of the skin. Although the incidence of hyperpigmentation due to exogenous heavy metals has decreased in recent years, limited exposure to such preparations still occurs, and metallic hyperpigmentation may still be seen in children as well as adults.

Argyria is a localized or widespread bluish gray or slate-colored discoloration of the skin produced by the deposition of silver within the dermis. The condition is more pronounced on exposed parts of the body, namely the face, forearms, and hands, but may also occur in the sclerae, oral mucous membranes, and lunulae of the nails. Most cases develop as a result of long-continued use of eye drops (Argyrol S.S.) or ophthalmic preparations containing silver, the degree of discoloration being proportional to the duration of exposure to the preparation and the duration and intensity of light exposure to the areas of involvement.

The diagnosis of argyria is based on clinical examination and history of exposure and may be confirmed by cutaneous biopsy of affected areas. Histopathologic examination is characterized by fine, small round refractive silver granules, which may be seen throughout the dermis, particularly the hyaline basement zone and membrana propria surrounding eccrine glands. In addition to silver, increased amounts of melanin may be seen in the basal layer of the epidermis and also within macrophages in the upper dermis. Treatment of argyria depends on recognition of the disorder, discontinuation of the use of the silver-containing preparation, and avoidance of sunlight exposure.

Chrysiasis (gold-induced hyperpigmentation) is a rare cutaneous disorder induced by the administration of gold salts followed by exposure to ultraviolet light. The pigmentation is bluish gray or purplish and is similar to that seen in argyria except that the hyperpigmentation is more prominent around the eyes, is limited to areas of sunlight exposure, and does not affect the sclerae and oral mucous membranes. Other cutaneous manifestations are seen in up to 20 per cent of individuals on gold therapy. These include morbilliform, eczematous, urticarial, bullous, purpuric, lichen planus–like, and pityriasis rosea–like eruptions. The histopathologic features of gold-induced hyperpigmentation consist of small, black, round or oval, irregularly shaped gold particles that are located in a perivascular distribution and in dermal histiocytes.

Mercury-induced hyperpigmentation also may result in the deposition of the metal in the dermis, with a slate-gray pigmentation in areas of topical application. The discoloration is exaggerated in the areas of skinfolds, and the resulting pigmentation is permanent.[67]

DRUG-INDUCED HYPERPIGMENTATION

Hyperpigmentation may be induced by chronic long-term chlorpromazine (Thorazine) administration (dosages of 300 to 500 mg/day for 3 to 5 years or more).[68] The bluish gray discoloration is most prominent about the face (particularly the tip of the nose, malar prominence, forehead, and cheeks), the "V" of the neck, the dorsal aspect of the hands, and exposed areas of the legs (Fig. 16–22). A brownish pigmentation of the conjunctivae occurs in only a small percentage of patients and has been described primarily in those on long-term therapy, such as might be seen in psychiatric care hospitals. Although the mechanism is uncertain, it has been suggested that chlorpromazine may have a specific affinity for melanin-containing tissues.

About 25 per cent of patients receiving antimalarial preparations (quinacrine, chloroquine, or hydroxychloroquine) for long periods of time develop a bluish gray pigmentation of the face, neck, oral mucous membranes (particularly the soft palate), forearms, legs, and nail beds.[69] Of interest and occasional diagnostic significance is the fact that antimalarials (chloroquine) may at times produce a sil-

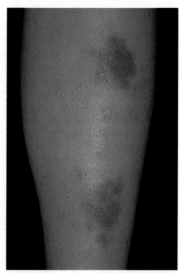

Figure 16–22. Fixed drug eruption. This disorder tends to recur in the same areas on readministration of the offending drug.

very or white bleaching at the eyebrows, eyelids, or temples of red-headed, blond, or fair-haired individuals.

Circumscribed plaques of purplish to purplish red pigmentation, usually round or oval, sometimes bullous, are commonly associated with fixed drug eruptions. Drug-induced hyperpigmentation tends to recur in the same location following the readministration of certain drugs, particularly phenolphthalein, barbiturate derivatives, and antineoplastic agents such as busulfan and cyclophosphamide. Other occasionally incriminated drugs include aspirin, phenacetin, phenytoin, gold, arsenic, sulfonamides, tetracycline, and minocycline.

The diagnosis of a drug eruption is based almost entirely on history and physical examination. Histopathologic examination of lesions reveals subepidermal bullae with degeneration of the detached portion of the epidermis in early lesions. The late hyperpigmented stage is characterized by an increase in the amount of melanin in the basal layer of the epidermis and within macrophages of the upper dermis.

CAROTENEMIA

Carotenemia is a yellowish orange discoloration of skin due to the ingestion of excessive quantities of carotene-containing foods, particularly carrots, squash, pumpkins, yellow turnips, sweet potatoes, peaches, apricots, papayas, mangos, or egg yolk. The condition is seen primarily in infants and occasionally in older children and adults. The color is most prominent on the palms and soles, in the nasolabial grooves, on the forehead, chin, upper eyelids, postauricular areas, and anterior axillary folds, and over areas of pressure such as the elbows, knees, knuckles, and ankles. Lack of involvement of the sclerae and mucous membranes, coupled with the absence of pruritus and lack of color change in the urine or stool, helps rule out the presence of hepatic or biliary jaundice. Lycopene, a red-colored carotenoid pigment found in fruits and vegetables, especially ripened tomatoes, beets, chili beans, and various fruits and berries, may cause a reddish yellow discoloration of the skin (lycopenemia). In addition, ingestion of red palm oil, a cooking product with high carotenoid content, can result in a diffuse guttate papulosquamous dermatitis and orange discoloration of the palms and soles.[70, 71] This disorder, termed *xanthoderma* or *carotenoderma*, should not be confused with "the red man syndrome" (a transient orange-red discoloration of the skin, mucous membranes, urine, feces, sweat, and tears associated with overdosage with rifampin or vancomycin therapy) or acrodynia (pink disease), a disorder of infants and young children characterized by leg cramps, headaches, hypertension, excessive perspiration, itching, swelling, redness and peeling of the hands, feet, and nose, weakness of the pectoral and pelvic girdles, and nerve dysfunction in the lower extremities, occurring as a result of chronic exposure to mercury or mercury-containing compounds.[72–75]

The diagnosis of carotenemia is confirmed by the presence of high carotene levels in the presence of normal serum bilirubin. Reduction of dietary intake of carotene-containing foods to normal levels results in gradual improvement (usually within a period of 4 to 6 weeks). A few persons have been found in whom carotenemia develops despite a normal diet; these patients appear to have a genetic inability to convert carotenoids into vitamin A to the same degree as normal persons. For patients who cannot convert carotenoids to vitamin A, the vitamin should be given if its serum levels are found to be below the normal range. In such individuals control of the carotenoderma may be difficult. Such patients, under the supervision of a dietitian, should try to decrease red and yellow vegetable and fruit intake, making sure that the diet is otherwise well balanced.[76]

References

1. Futcher PH: A peculiarity of pigmentation of the upper arms of Negroes. Science 88:570–571, 1938.

   A distinctly darker dorsolateral and lighter anteromedial pigmentation noted on the upper arms bilaterally in 17.5 per cent and unilaterally in 2.0 per cent of 200 blacks.

2. Ito K: The peculiar demarcation of pigmentation along the so-called Voigt's line among the Japanese. Dermatol. Int. 4:45–47, 1965.

   A pigmentary peculiarity (similar to that described by Futcher in 1938 and Matsuomoto in 1913) is seen in 130 of 3,000 Japanese; this peculiarity appeared 10 times more frequently in females than in males.

3. James WD, Carter JM, Rodman OG: Pigmentary demarcation lines: A population survey. J. Am. Acad. Dermatol. 16:584–590, 1987.

   In a study of 380 patients, 79 per cent of black females, 75 per cent of black males, and about 10 per cent of whites had at least one type of pigmentary demarcation line.

4. Lerner AB: Vitiligo. J. Invest. Dermatol. 32:285–310, 1959.

   A classic reference for vitiligo, a chronic disorder of depigmentation affecting 2 million people in the United States.

5. Bolognia JL, Pawelek JM: Biology of hypopigmentation. J. Am. Acad. Dermatol. 19:217–255, 1988.

   A comprehensive review of pigment cell biology, pathophysiology, and clinical characteristics of various disorders of hypopigmentation.

6. Naughton GK, Reggiardo D, Bystryn J-C: Correlation between vitiligo antibodies and extent of depigmentation in vitiligo. J. Am. Acad. Dermatol. 15:978–981, 1986.

   Studies of antibody levels in 32 patients with vitiligo support the role of antimelanocytic antibodies in the pathogenesis of vitiligo.

7. Nordlund JJ, Lerner AB: Vitiligo: Its relationship to systemic disease. In: Moschella SL (Ed.): Dermatology Update: Review for Physicians. Elsevier North Holland, Inc., New York, 1979, 411–432.

   A review of the pathogenesis of vitiligo and its relationship to other disorders.

8. Tosti A, Bardazzi F, Tosti G, et al.: Audiologic abnormalities in cases of vitiligo. J. Am. Acad. Dermatol. 17:230–233, 1987.

   The eye and inner ear contain a substantial number of melanocytes that can be damaged in patients with vitiligo.

9. Lerner AB, Nordlund JJ: Vitiligo: What is it? Is it important? J.A.M.A. 239:1183–1187, 1978.

   An update of the clinical features, classification, and physiology of vitiligo.

10. Cline DJ, Nordlund JJ: Vitiligo. In Greer KE (Ed.): Common Problems in Dermatology. Year Book Medical Publishers, Inc., Chicago, 1988, 421–430.

    An authoritative review of vitiligo and its management.

11. Porter J, Beuf AH, Lerner A, et al.: Response to disfigurement in patients with vitiligo. Cutis 39:493–494, 1987.

    In response to a questionnaire, 326 patients with vitiligo describe the anxieties, embarrassment, and frustration experienced with this disorder.

12. El-Mofty AM: The treatment of vitiligo with a combination of psoralens and quinolines. Br. J. Dermatol. 76:56–62, 1964.

    Psoralens and quinolone derivatives produced good to excellent repigmentation (over 50 per cent) in 84 per cent of 55 patients with vitiligo.

13. Parrish JA, Fitzpatrick TB, Shea C, et al.: Photochemotherapy of vitiligo: Use of orally administered psoralen and a high-intensity long-wave ultraviolet system. Arch. Dermatol. 112:1531–1534, 1976.

    An artificial light source that provides high-intensity ultraviolet light (UVA, 300 to 400 nm) to the entire body, with orally administered psoralen as an adjunct to the treatment of patients with vitiligo.

14. Pinto FJ, Bolognia JL: Disorders of hypopigmentation in children. Pediatr. Clin. North Am. 38:991–1017, 1991.

    An authoritative update of the disorders of hypopigmentation in childhood with emphasis on their diagnosis and management.

15. Kenny JA Jr: Pigmentary disturbances. In Conn HF (Ed.): Current Therapy, 1978. W. B. Saunders Co., Philadelphia, 1978, 641–643.

    A practical approach to the therapy of pigmentary disorders.

16. Gupta AK, Anderson TF: Psoralen and photochemotherapy. J. Am. Acad. Dermatol. 17:703–734, 1987.

    A review of psoralen photochemotherapy (PUVA) and its use in a variety of dermatologic disorders.

17. Kumari J: Vitiligo treated with clobetasol propionate. Arch. Dermatol. *120*:631–635, 1984.

Clobetasol propionate, applied twice a day for 2 months, with a maximum of four courses over a 3-year period, achieved 92 to 100 per cent repigmentation in 80 per cent of patients with facial vitiligo.

18. Fulton JE, Leyden JE, Papa C: Treatment of vitiligo with topical methoxsalen and blacklight. Arch. Dermatol. *100*:224–229, 1969.

Fourteen of 15 patients with vitiligo respond to topical application of 10 per cent methoxsalen in hydrophilic ointment followed by exposure to long-wave ultraviolet light.

19. Orentreich N, Selmanowitz VJ: Autograft repigmentation of leukoderma. Arch. Dermatol. *105*:734–736, 1972.

Autotransplantation of melanocytes from pigmented skin lead to repigmentation in the skin of a black woman with long-standing leukoderma following a chemical burn.

20. Falabella R: Repigmentation of segmental vitiligo by autologous minigrafting. J. Am. Acad. Dermatol. 9:514–521, 1983.

Successful repigmentation of segmental vitiligo by autologous minigrafting.

21. Hatchome N, Kato T, Takami H: Therapeutic success of epidermal grafting in generalized vitiligo is limited by the Koebner phenomenon. J. Am. Acad. Dermatol. *22*:87–91, 1990.

Except for generalized lesions in which a Koebner phenomenon may prove to be a problem, epidermal grafting can be used as a therapeutic approach for the treatment of selected individuals with vitiligo.

22. Tsuji T, Hamada T: Topically administered fluorouracil in vitiligo. Arch. Dermatol. *119*:722–727, 1983.

Following abrasion of vitiliginous areas, topical 5 per cent fluorouracil, applied daily and covered with a polyethylene occlusive dressing for 7 to 10 days, produced complete or almost complete repigmentation in 18 of 28 patients within 2 months after reepithelization occurred.

23. Hermansky F, Pudlak P: Albinism associated with hemorrhagic diathesis and unusual pigmented reticular cells in the bone marrow: Report of two cases with histochemical studies. Blood *14*:162–169, 1959.

Two unrelated patients with oculocutaneous albinism with prolonged bleeding time and unusual pigment-containing macrophages in the bone marrow suggest a syndrome of pseudohemophilia and albinism.

24. Depinho DA, Kaplan KL: The Hermansky-Pudlak syndrome: Report of three cases and review of the pathophysiology and management considerations. Medicine *64*:192–202, 1985.

A comprehensive report of three patients with the Hermansky-Pudlak syndrome and a comprehensive review of the pathophysiology and management of individuals with this disorder.

25. Windhorst DB, Zelickson AS, Good RA: Human pigmentary dilution based on heritable subcellular structural defect: Chédiak-Higashi syndrome. J. Invest. Dermatol. *50*:9–18, 1968.

A failure in the control of the size of melanin granules relates to the color defect in the giant granules seen in leukocytes, leukocyte precursors, and other cells of children with the Chédiak-Higashi syndrome.

26. Blume RS, Wolff SM: The Chédiak-Higashi syndrome: Studies in four patients and review of the literature. Medicine *51*:247–280, 1972.

A thorough analysis of the Chédiak-Higashi syndrome with a description of four patients and review of 59 cases from the literature.

27. Boxer LA, Wanatabe AM, Rister M, et al.: Correction of leukocyte function in Chédiak-Higashi syndrome by ascorbate. N. Engl. J. Med. *295*:1041–1045, 1976.

The effect of ascorbic acid on cyclic adenosine monophosphate in leukocytes of patients with the Chédiak-Higashi syndrome may be associated with differences in leukocyte membrane structure.

28. Jeliffe DB, Jeliffe EFP: The children of the San Blas Islands of Panama. J. Pediatr. *59*:271–285, 1961.

A comprehensive analysis of the children of the San Blas Islands from birth to 4 years of age.

29. Tietz W: A syndrome of deaf-mutism associated with albinism showing dominant autosomal inheritance. Am. J. Hum. Genet. *15*:259–264, 1963.

A family pedigree of 14 individuals combining the features of albinism with deaf-mutism as an autosomal dominant disorder.

30. Cross H, McKusick J, Breen W: A new oculocerebral syndrome with hypopigmentation. J. Pediatr. *70*:398–406, 1967.

Three siblings affected with mental retardation, spastic diplegia, hypopigmentation with many characteristics of true albinism, and multiple ocular anomalies appear to comprise a unique autosomal recessive syndrome.

31. Falls HF: Sex-linked ocular albinism displaying typical fundus changes in the female heterozygote. Am. J. Ophthalmol. *34*:41–50, 1951.

Ophthalmic examination in two families with sex-linked ocular albinism reveals typical retinal changes in the heterozygote female carrier.

32. Mosher DB, Fitzpatrick TB: Editorial: Piebaldism. Arch. Dermatol. *124*:364–365, 1988.

An authoritative update on piebaldism and its pathogenesis.

33. Waardenburg PJ: A new syndrome combining developmental anomalies of the eyelids, eyebrows and nose root with pigmentary defects of the iris and head hair with congenital deafness. Am. J. Hum. Genet. *3*:195–253, 1951.

A clinical description of 161 individuals with Waardenburg's syndrome.

34. Fitzpatrick TB, Szabo G, Hori Y, et al.: White leaf-shaped macules, earliest visible sign of tuberous sclerosis. Arch. Dermatol. *98*:1–6, 1968.

Of 31 individuals with tuberous sclerosis, 10 had white leaf-shaped macules as the only cutaneous manifestation of their disorder.

35. Hurwitz S, Braverman IM: White spots in tuberous sclerosis. J. Pediatr. *77*:587–594, 1970.

Hypopigmented macules, the earliest signs of tuberous sclerosis: Their clinical variations and differentiation from lesions of vitiligo.

36. Nickel WR, Reed WB: Tuberous sclerosis. Arch. Dermatol. *85*:209–226, 1962.

In 40 of 61 patients with tuberous sclerosis who had associated areas of leukoderma or poliosis, 29 had leukoderma alone, 2 had poliosis alone, and 9 had a combination of both.

37. Hurwitz S: Discussion on Tuberous Sclerosis, Society Transactions. Arch. Dermatol. *104*:336–337, 1971.

Report of a patient with partial albinism and hypopigmented macules and a discussion of leukoderma in tuberous sclerosis.

38. Wiley HE III, Frias JL: Depigmented lesions in incontinentia pigmenti: A useful diagnostic sign. Am. J. Dis. Child. *128*:546–547, 1974.

Streaked hypopigmented macules on the calves or other areas in relatives of individuals in families with incontinentia pigmenti serve as a clue to the familial genetic pattern of patients with this disorder.

39. Ito M: Studies on melanin: I. Incontinentia pigmenti achromians: A singular case of nevus depigmentosus systematicus bilateralis. Tohoku J. Exp. Med. *55*(suppl I):57–59, 1952.

Description of a woman with a distinctive, depigmented, systematized, bilateral "nevus" that took the form of bizarre irregular hypopigmented patches on the trunk and extremities.

40. Hamada T, Saito T, et al.: Incontinentia pigmenti achromians (Ito). Arch. Dermatol. 96:673–676, 1967.

A 3-month-old Japanese girl with incontinentia pigmenti achromians.

41. Rubin MB: Incontinentia pigmenti achromians. Arch. Dermatol. 105:424–425, 1972.

Multiple cases of incontinentia pigmenti achromians in a family suggests an autosomal dominant mode of inheritance.

42. Jelinek JE, Bart RS, Schiff GM: Hypomelanosis of Ito ("incontinentia pigmenti achromians"): Report of three cases and review of the literature. Arch. Dermatol. 107:596–601, 1973.

Three children with hypopigmented asymmetric whorls and streaks in a marble-cake pattern representing a negative picture of incontinentia pigmenti.

43. Schwartz MF, Esterly NB, Fretzin DF, et al.: Hypomelanosis of Ito (incontinentia pigmenti achromians): A neurocutaneous syndrome. J. Pediatr. 90:236–240, 1977.

The identification of 10 patients with hypomelanosis of Ito within a relatively brief period suggests that this entity probably is more common than the literature would indicate.

44. Coupe RL: Unilateral systematized achromic nevus. Dermatologica 134:19–35, 1967.

Congenital systematized hypopigmentation—an embryonic error of melanocytic migration from the neural crest.

45. Solomon LM, Esterly NB: Pigmentary abnormalities, nevus achromicus. In: Neonatal Dermatology. W. B. Saunders Co., Philadelphia, 1973, 106.

The authors note the case of an infant with an achromic nevus, hemihypertrophy, and retardation.

46. Fleisher TL, Zeligman I: Nevus anemicus. Arch. Dermatol. 100:750–755, 1969.

Nevus anemicus may be due to a defect at the motor end plate or smooth muscle effector cell of blood vessels associated with increased stimulation of vasoconstrictor or inhibition of vasodilator fibers of arterioles.

47. Mountcastle EA, Distelmeier MR, Lupton GP: Nevus anemicus. J. Am. Acad. Dermatol. 14:628–632, 1986.

A report of three patients with nevus anemicus, its differential diagnosis, and a review of proposed theories of pathogenesis.

48. Hammer H: Lymphocyte transformation test in sympathetic ophthalmitis and the Vogt-Koyanagi-Harada syndrome. Br. J. Ophthalmol. 55:850–852, 1971.

Lymphocyte transfer tests in two patients with Vogt-Koyanagi syndrome and three with sympathetic ophthalmitis stimulated with bovine uveal pigment suggests that delayed autoaggressive allergic response to uveal pigment plays a role in the pathogenesis of these disorders.

49. Kahn G: Depigmentation caused by phenolic detergent germicides. Arch. Dermatol. 102:177–187, 1970.

Eighteen patients with patchy depigmentation from contact with paratertiary butyl phenol or paratertiary amyl phenol in commercial disinfectants.

50. McGuire J, Hendee J: Biochemical basis for depigmentation of skin by phenolic germicides. J. Invest. Dermatol. 57:256–261, 1971.

The depigmentation caused by phenol-containing germicides appears to be due to competitive inhibition of tyrosinase by phenolic compounds.

51. Cornelius CE III, Stein KM, Hanshaw WL, et al.: Hypopigmentation and sarcoidosis. Arch. Dermatol. 108:249–251, 1973.

Microscopic examination of cutaneous biopsies of hypopigmented lesions in patients with sarcoidosis suggest hypopigmentation as another cutaneous clue to the diagnosis of this disorder.

52. Hoshaw RA, Zimmerman KG, Menter A: Ochronosis-like pigmentation from hydroquinone bleaching creams in American blacks. Arch. Dermatol. 121:105–108, 1985.

Hydroquinone bleaching cream–induced hyperpigmentation in dark-skinned individuals in the United States.

53. Hardwick N, Van Gelder LW, Van Der Merwe CA, et al.: Exogenous ochronosis: An epidemiological study. Br. J. Dermatol. 120:229–238, 1989.

A study of 195 black outpatients in Pretoria, South Africa, revealed a 69 per cent incidence of ochronosis-like pigmentation following prolonged use of hydroquinone skin-lightening agents.

54. Kligman AM, Willis I: New formulation for depigmenting human skin. Arch. Dermatol. 111:40–48, 1975.

A new formulation containing 0.1 per cent tretinoin (vitamin A acid), 5 per cent hydroquinone, 0.1 per cent dexamethasone, and hydrophilic ointment effective in the management of cosmetically objectionable freckles, postinflammatory hypopigmentation, and melasma.

55. Kuske H, Krebs A: Hyperpigmentation of chloasma-type after treatment with hydantoin preparations. Dermatologica 129:121–139, 1964 (in German).

Chloasma-type hyperpigmentation developed in 13 patients on hydantoin and its derivatives (particularly mesantoin).

56. Knox JM, Dodge BG, Freeman RG: Erythema dyschromicum perstans. Arch. Dermatol. 97:262–272, 1968.

Report of six patients from Houston, Texas, with erythema dyschromicum perstans.

57. Byrne DA, Berger RS: Erythema dyschromicum perstans: Report of two cases in fair-skinned patients. Acta Derm. Venereol. 54:65–68, 1974.

Erythema dyschromicum perstans on the trunk, arms, neck, and thighs of two fair-skinned 12-year-old girls suggests that this condition may be more widespread than generally recognized and that relatively mild variants of this disorder apparently occur.

58. Miyagawa S, Komatsu M, Okuchi T, et al.: Erythema dyschromicum perstans: Immunopathologic studies. J. Am. Acad. Dermatol. 20:882–886, 1989.

Immunopathologic studies in a 14-year-old girl appear to support the concept that erythema dyschromicum perstans and lichen planus involve a common disease process.

59. Ruiz-Maldonado R, Tamayo L, Fernàndez-Dies J: Universal acquired melanosis: The carbon baby. Arch. Dermatol. 114:775–778, 1978.

A unique case of dark black pigmentation that began at the age of 15 days and progressed to include the entire cutaneous surface and ocular and mucous membranes of a Mexican child.

60. Chernosky ME, Anderson DE, Chang JP, et al.: Familial progressive hyperpigmentation. Arch. Dermatol. 103:581–598, 1971.

Four patients in a black family with irregular patchy areas of hyperpigmentation that progressed in number, size, and confluence with the patients' increasing age.

61. Kalter DC, Griffiths WA, Atherton DJ: Linear and whorled nevoid hypermelanosis. J. Am. Acad. Dermatol. 19:1037–1044, 1988.

A report of two patients with congenital, asymmetrical, patterned epidermal hypermelanosis.

62. Lerner AB, McGuire JS: Melanocyte stimulating hormone and adrenocorticotrophic hormone. N. Engl. J. Med. 270:539–564, 1964.

Homogeneous pig ACTH and α-MSH given separately in large quantities to a bilaterally adrenalectomized patient resulted in true pigment darkening of the skin.

63. Braverman IM: Skin Signs of Systemic Disease, 2nd ed. W. B. Saunders Co., Philadelphia, 1981.

A comprehensive review of the systemic disorders and their effect on the skin.

64. Cawley EP, Hsu T, Wood BT, et al.: Hemochromatosis and the skin. Arch. Dermatol. *100*:1–6, 1969.

The cutaneous pigmentation in patients with hemochromatosis is related to epidermal thickening and the amount of epidermal melanin, not iron.

65. Perdrup A, Poulsen H: Hemochromatosis and vitiligo. Arch. Dermatol. *90*:34–37, 1964.

A patient who had both vitiligo and hemochromatosis vividly demonstrates that melanin rather than iron is the cause of hyperpigmentation in hemochromatosis.

66. Cherant-Breton J, Simon M, Bourel M, et al.: Cutaneous manifestations of idiopathic hemochromatosis: Study of 100 cases. Arch. Dermatol. *113*:161–165, 1977.

Skin pigmentation, one of the earliest signs of hemochromatosis.

67. Lamar LM, Bliss BO: Localized pigmentation of the skin due to topical mercury. Arch. Dermatol. *93*:450–451, 1966.

Lichen planus–like and pityriasis rosea–like eruptions in patients on topical mercuric preparations.

68. Hays GB, Lyle CB Jr, Wheeler CE: Slate-gray color in patients receiving chlorpromazine. Arch. Dermatol. *90*:471–476, 1964.

Five white women in a mental hospital who had taken large amounts of chlorpromazine (500 to 3,000 mg/day for 1 to 5 years) developed a bluish discoloration on exposed areas resembling the slate-gray discoloration seen in patients with argyria.

69. Tuffanelli D, Abraham RK, Dubois EJ: Pigmentation from antimalarial therapy. Arch. Dermatol. *88*:419–426, 1963.

Localized cutaneous blue-black pigmentation on the pretibial, facial, and subungual areas in 8 per cent (25) of 300 patients receiving antimalarial therapy.

70. Person JR: Red palms and orange palms. Arch. Dermatol. *117*:757, 1981.

A 28-year-old man with a diffuse guttate papulosquamous dermatitis and orange discoloration of the palms and soles following the use of red palm oil for cooking purposes.

71. Stack KM, Churchwell MA, Skinner RB, Jr: Xanthoderma: Case report and differential diagnosis. Cutis *41*:100–102, 1988.

A 29-year-old man with a 3-year history of "yellow jaundice" was found to have carotenoderma resulting from long-term red palm oil ingestion used in cooking. The patient's siblings and mother also had similar discoloration on the palms and soles.

72. Bolan G, Laurie RE, Broome CV: Red man syndrome: Inadvertent administration of an excessive dose of rifampin to children in a day-care center. Pediatrics 77:633–635, 1986.

A common complication of excessive dosage of rifampin.

73. Gross DJ: Red/orange person syndrome. Cutis *42*:175–177, 1988.

An 18-year-old Hispanic woman's skin turned red overnight following an attempt to commit suicide by a massive overdose of rifampin.

74. Levy M, Koren G, Dupys L, et al.: Vancomycin-induced red man syndrome. Pediatrics 86:572–580, 1990.

A review of 11 cases of vancomycin-induced "red man syndrome": a flushed erythematous rash on the face, neck, and around the ears; hypotension; watery puffy eyes; tachycardia; respiratory distress; dizziness; agitation; and mild temperature increase.

75. Agocs MM, Etzel RA, Parrish RG, et al.: Mercury exposure from interior latex paint. N. Engl. J. Med. *323*:1096–1101, 1990.

Symptoms of acrodynia developed in a 4-year-old boy 10 days after the inside of his home was painted with an interior latex paint containing mercury.

76. Mathews-Roth MM: Answer to a question on carotenemia. J.A.M.A. *241*:1835, 1979.

Although overindulgence in carotenoid-containing vegetables, fruit, and fruit juices is the most common cause of carotenemia, hypothyroidism, diabetes, renal failure, and a genetic inability to convert carotenoids into vitamin A also should be considered as possible causes of this disorder.

17

DISORDERS OF HAIR AND NAILS

HAIR

Hair is a protein byproduct of follicles that are distributed everywhere on the body surface except the palms, soles, vermilion portion of the lips, glans penis, penile shaft, nail beds, and sides of the fingers and toes. Although hair is of minimal functional benefit to humans, the psychological effects of disturbances of hair growth are frequently a source of great concern to children, adolescents, and their parents.

In the human fetus, groups of cells appear in the epidermis at about the 8th week of gestation. These differentiate to form the hair follicles, and hair begins to develop between the 8th and 12th weeks of fetal life. This growth continues throughout fetal development, and although there are indications that some hair is lost during gestation and at the time of birth, the majority of hairs on the newborn are 5 to 6 months old.[1]

Although the terms *lanugo* and *vellus* are frequently used synonymously, lanugo hairs, except in the rare hereditary syndrome hypertrichosis lanuginosa, are seen only in fetal and neonatal life. They are fine, soft, unmedullated, and poorly pigmented, and they appear as a fine dense growth over the entire cutaneous surface of the fetal infant. Lanugo hair is normally shed in utero in the 7th or 8th month of gestation but may cover the entire cutaneous surface of the newborn premature infant. Postnatal hair may be divided into vellus and terminal types. Vellus hairs are the fine, lightly pigmented hairs seen on the arms and faces of children and faces of women. Terminal hairs are the mature thick dark hairs on the scalp, eyebrows, eyelashes, and areas of secondary sexual hair distribution.

The number and distribution of individual hair follicles are genetically determined, and under most circumstances new follicles are not formed after birth. As the infant grows, however, the density of hair follicles becomes reduced as the skin grows to accommodate the enlarging body. In the newborn the average density of scalp hairs is $1,135/cm^2$, in infants 3 to 12 months of age the density is reduced to $795/cm^2$, and by the age of 20 to 30 years, it is decreased to $615/cm^2$.[2]

The hair root is characterized by three definable cyclic stages of growth—anagen, catagen, and telogen (Table 17–1). The anagen or active growth phase lasts for 2 to 6 years, with an average of about 3 years. The follicle then undergoes a short period of partial degeneration (the catagen phase). This generally lasts for 10 to 14 days and is immediately followed by a resting or telogen phase, which lasts for 3 to 4 months.[3] What triggers the resumption of the active growing stage is yet to be determined.

Neonatal Hair

The first crop of terminal scalp hairs is in the actively growing anagen phase at birth, but within the first few days of life there is a physiologic conversion to the telogen phase. Consequently, a high proportion of neonatal scalp hairs are shed during the first 4 months of life. This telogen shedding (telogen effluvium of the newborn) may occur as a sudden hair loss, leading to almost complete alopecia or, in a more common gradual form, may be scarcely perceptible. Whether sudden or gradual, replacement of the first terminal hairs is generally completed before the first 6 months of life.[3] Some infants do not become significantly bald. Presumably these individuals retain the telogen club hairs until anagen replacement takes over. The neonatal hairline frequently extends along the forehead and temples to the lateral margin of the eyebrows. These terminal hairs gradually convert to vellus hairs during the first year of life (the influence at birth on vellus hair, however, is not fully explained).

Premature infants are frequently covered by lanugo hairs, which are more densely distributed on the face, limbs, and trunk. This probably is related to the cyclic activity in utero and the normal shedding of telogen vellus hairs in the fetus during the last few weeks of gestation. The thickness of infant scalp pelage varies among individuals and, depending on habits such as hair rubbing or head banging, is determined by how rapidly trauma results in destruction of terminal hairs and the rate at which telogen hairs are rubbed away.

Congenital Disorders

A variety of congenital and hereditary disorders are associated with abnormalities of hair growth. These include a congenital, triangularly patterned alopecia seen at the frontotemporal aspect of the hairline, aplasia cutis, acrodermatitis enteropathica, Leiner's disease, Rothmund-Thomson syndrome, the hereditary ectodermal dysplasias, progeria, the Hallermann-Streiff syndrome, hereditary trichodysplasia (Marie-Unna hypotrichosis), the oral-facial-digital syndromes (OFD I and II), Coffin-Siris syndrome, the trichodental and trichodento-osseous syndromes, and Sensenbrenner's syndrome.

Congenital triangular alopecia is characterized by an area of alopecia that, although present at birth, may not be noticed until the child is 2 or 3 years of age or older (Fig. 17–1).[4] The area is triangular and overlies the frontotemporal suture, with the base of the triangle directed forward and frequently impinging on the anterior hairline. Gener-

Table 17–1. CYCLIC STAGES OF HAIR GROWTH

1. Anagen phase (active growth phase) lasts 2 to 6 years (average 3 years)
2. Catagen phase (stage of partial degeneration) lasts 10 to 14 days
3. Telogen phase (resting stage) lasts 3 to 4 months

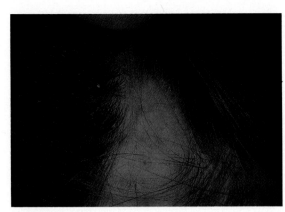

Figure 17–1. Congenital triangular alopecia on the frontotemporal area of the scalp of a 12-year-old boy.

ally measuring 3 to 5 cm from base to apex, the area may be completely bald or partially covered by vellus hairs and remains unchanged throughout life. Although generally unilateral, it may be bilaterally symmetrical, and, on rare occasions, similar triangular patches may be noted on the nape of the neck.

Extreme *unruliness of the hair,* a disorder seen in 2 per cent of normal infants, may also be seen at times in individuals with microcephaly. It is characterized by hair that tends to stand up from the area of the posterior parietal whorl toward the frontal hairline. Although the finding of scalp hair unruliness in an otherwise normal infant (except perhaps for patients with the uncombable hair syndrome) should evoke little concern, this finding should be added to those of upsweep of anterior scalp hair and aberrant parietal whorl position, which are potential indicators of abnormal brain growth and morphogenesis that may occur in infants during the 10th to 16th weeks of fetal life.[5]

The *Hallermann-Streiff syndrome* (oculomandibulocephaly) is characterized by dwarfism, beaked nose, and brachycephaly, often accompanied by frontal and parietal bossing, mandibular hypoplasia, microphthalmia, low-set ears, thin and small lips, high-arched palate, atrophy of the skin of the face, congenital cataracts, blue sclerae, motor and occasionally mental retardation, dental abnormalities, irregularly implanted or supernumerary teeth, and hypotrichosis of the scalp, eyebrows, and eyelids. Alopecia is most prominent about the frontal and occipital areas and is especially marked along suture lines. Axillary and pubic hair may also be scant, and cutaneous atrophy, largely limited to the scalp and nose, may be seen as thin taut skin and prominence of underlying blood vessels.

Hereditary trichodysplasia (Marie Unna hypotrichosis) is a rare autosomal dominant disorder manifested by almost complete congenital absence of scalp hair, eyebrows, and eyelashes; decreased body hair; and widespread facial milia. In early childhood, hair growth may occur but the hair soon becomes coarse, flattened, or twisted. During puberty the hair becomes very sparse, particularly on the vertex and scalp margins, resulting in a high frontal and nuchal hairline. Scattered follicular horny plugs may be associated with this disorder, and histologic examination of cutaneous biopsy specimens of involved areas reveals an abnormal proliferation of the internal root sheath in many of the follicles. When examined under the dissecting microscope, abnormal hairs are seen as flat, twisted, and ribbon-like. Electron microscopic examination of hair may reveal peeling of the cuticle, increased interfibrillar cortical matrix, and intracellular fractures of the cuticular cells, cortical cell fibrils, and medullary cells.[6]

The *oral-facial-digital syndrome* consists of two distinct disorders (*OFD I* and *OFD II*). OFD I was originally described as a condition of hypoplasia of nasal cartilages, lobulated cleft tongue, cleft lip and palate, maldeveloped frenula, hypertelorism, trembling, mental retardation, and various malformations of the hands. It is a rare dominant X-linked disorder limited to females and lethal to males. It occurs in approximately 1 in 50,000 live births and is characterized by a distinctive facies with frontal bossing, a hooked pug-nose with hypoplasia of the nasal cartilages, lateral displacement of the inner canthi (dystopia canthorum), micrognathia, cleft lip, a high-arched or cleft palate, lobulated clefts of the tongue, hyperplasia of the frenulum with thick bands in the lower buccal fold, dental abnormalities, mental retardation, hydrocephalus, kyphoscoliosis, equinovarus, conductive hearing loss, and various malformations of the hands (brachydactyly, syndactyly, clinodactyly, polydactyly). Cutaneous abnormalities seen in association with this disorder include numerous milia at birth, alopecia (secondary to a decrease in the number of hair follicles), and sparse fine or coarse, dry and lusterless hair.

Oral-facial-digital syndrome II, an autosomal recessive trait that affects both sexes, may be differentiated from OFD I by a broad bifid nasal tip, occasional flaring of the alveolar ridge, a tendency toward hexadactyly, bilateral polysyndactyly of the halluces, and a lack of cutaneous or appendageal changes.[7]

The *cartilage-hair hypoplasia syndrome* is an autosomal recessive disorder with reduced penetrance seen primarily in inbred Amish and at times non-Amish individuals, characterized by short limbs, hyperextensible digits, and sparse, fine scalp and body hair. In addition to hair and skeletal abnormalities, defective cell-mediated immunity, seen in most patients, results in relative anergy, altered T-cell responses, increased susceptibility to viral infections, infantile neutropenia, Diamond-Blackfan anemia, severe combined immunodeficiency, and, at times, celiac syndrome and toxic megacolon.[8]

In 1970, Coffin and Siris described three patients with the *Coffin-Siris* syndrome, a distinct pattern of severe mental retardation, a characteristic coarse-appearing facies, scalp hypotrichosis with eyebrow and eyelash hypertrichosis, hypotonia, absent fifth fingernails, smallness or hypoplasia of other nails, postnatal growth deficiency, microcephaly, lax joints, smallness for gestational age, feeding problems, recurrent lower respiratory tract infections during early life, and congenital heart defects. Although the sparsity of reported cases makes its inheritance pattern uncertain, occurrence in siblings of unaffected parents suggests the possibility of an autosomal recessive mode of inheritance.[9]

Trichorhinophalangeal syndrome I is an uncommon inherited disorder characterized by fine, brittle, sparse, slow-growing hair; a distinctive facies with pear-shaped nose, high philtrum, supernumerary incisors, and receding chin; and skeletal abnormalities (brachyphalangeal dysostosis that results in fusiform swelling of the proximal interphalangeal joints). Although the inheritance of this disorder is usually determined by an autosomal dominant gene of variable expressivity, there also appears to be a recessive form of the disorder. A second sporadic form of this disorder, *trichorhinophalangeal syndrome II*, is characterized by a bulbous nose, an elongated prominent philtrum, a thin upper lip, large protruding ears, sparse scalp hair, microcephaly, mild to moderate mental retardation, and multiple cartilaginous exostoses.[9]

The *trichodento-osseous syndrome* is an autosomal dominant disorder characterized by tight, curly hair that tends to become straighter during childhood; small, widely spaced, pitted, eroded, and discolored teeth with early caries as a result of defective enamel; thickness and splitting of the nails; dolichocephaly, frontal bossing, and square jaw, giving affected persons a distinctive facies; normal physical development; and slight to moderately increased bone density. The *trichodental syndrome*, also known as the tooth and nail syndrome, is an autosomal dominant disorder characterized by fine, dry, slow-growing lusterless hair; sparseness or absence of the lateral halves of the eyebrows; hypotonia; and slow-growing, small, spoon-shaped nails (especially toenails).

Sensenbrenner's syndrome is a rare, probably autosomal recessive disorder manifested by small stature; dolichocephaly; an unusual facies characterized by frontal bossing, hypertelorism, prominent epicanthal folds, antimongoloid palpebral fissures, eversion of the lip, and full rounded cheeks; small, gray, widely spaced teeth; and short, fine, hair.[9]

Nonscarring Alopecia

Hair loss disorders can be divided into nonscarring (noncicatricial) or scarring (cicatricial) groups (Table 17–2). Causes of nonscarring alopecia include alteration of the hair growth cycle, structural abnormalities of the hair, and inflammatory cutaneous disease.

Table 17–2. CLASSIFICATION OF HAIR LOSS

1. Scarring (cicatricial)
   a. Developmental defects
   b. Infectious disorders
   c. Chemical or thermal injury
   d. Dermatologic disorders
2. Nonscarring (noncicatricial)
   a. Androgenetic alopecia
   b. Telogen effluvium (physiologic)
   c. Anagen effluvium
   d. Alopecia areata
   e. Traumatic alopecia
   f. Hair shaft abnormalities
   g. Inflammatory disease

TELOGEN EFFLUVIUM

It is calculated that the average human scalp contains 100,000 hairs. The average growth rate of terminal hair is approximately 2.5 mm/week (1 cm/month). The hair shaft is a nonliving structure and is not susceptible to biologic activity once it has formed. Although the hair shafts are the clinical focus of interest, it is the follicle itself that is responsible for the changes seen in most abnormalities of hair growth. The human hair follicle has a fairly long phase of regular growth (the anagen phase), which lasts 2 to 6 years, with an average of 3 years. The hairs then undergo a period of involution (the catagen phase), lasting about 3 weeks, followed by a resting (telogen) club phase. The telogen phase of the follicle lasts for about 3 months. At the end of this time new growth is initiated; and as new hairs grow, they push out the old club hairs that have remained in the resting follicles. In healthy individuals, 80 to 90 per cent of the scalp is in the actively growing (anagen) stage, 5 per cent is in the brief transitional (catagen) stage, 10 to 15 per cent is in the resting or telogen stage, and 50 to 100 hairs are shed and simultaneously replaced each day.[3]

During the period of hair growth, the normal cyclic pattern may be interrupted by a variety of different stimuli and may result in a highly characteristic form of alopecia termed *telogen effluvium*. Second in incidence only to male-pattern baldness, this disorder represents the most common type of alopecia. The stimuli capable of producing an interruption in the normal growing (anagen) phase of the hair follicles include febrile illness (Fig. 17–2), parturition, surgical shock, crash diets, injury, emotional stress, anticoagulant drugs, excessive ingestion of vitamin A (hypervitaminosis A) (Fig. 17–3), and discontinuation of an estrogen-dominated oral contraceptive. The proportion of follicles affected and the severity of the subsequent alopecia depend on the duration and severity of the stress and individual variations in susceptibility.

It must remembered that 50 to 100 hairs are lost from the average scalp per day (in individuals who groom infrequently, shampooing may yield up to

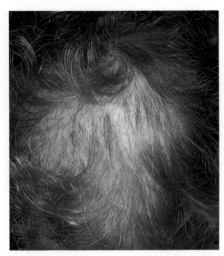

Figure 17–2. Telogen effluvium. Temporary diffuse alopecia was initiated by a stressful situation (a severe viral infection) in a 4-year-old girl.

200 lost hairs per day), and that 25 per cent (25,000 hairs) must be shed before unmistakable thinning becomes apparent; club hairs do not fall out but are pushed out as new hairs drive their way through the anchoring fibrils. Accordingly, the shedding seen in telogen effluvium actually marks the end, not the beginning, of the disorder.[3]

The diagnosis of telogen effluvium may be suggested by a history of a stressful event preceding the onset of alopecia by 6 to 16 weeks (generally 2 to 4 months) and can be confirmed by counting the number of hairs shed each day and by determining the percentage of telogen hairs in the scalp. Daily hair counts can be accomplished by counting the number of hairs lost each day (broken hairs without roots should not be included). Loss of over 100 hairs a day can be considered excessive. The ratio of resting to growing hairs (the "telogen-anagen" ratio) can be determined by gently plucking approximately 50 hairs from the patient's temporo-parietal scalp and examining them under a hand lens or low-power microscope. This can be accomplished by clamping approximately 50 hairs about 1 cm from the skin surface with a hemostat (the jaws of which have been covered by rubber tubing to prevent trauma to the hair shafts), followed by a gentle but short tug.

Hairs thus obtained can be placed on a microscope slide and examined under low magnification. Anagen hair roots can be recognized by the fact that the outer and inner hair sheaths are intact, with or without a portion of the dermal papilla adherent to the tip of the root. Telogen hair roots have uniform shaft diameters, contain no pigment, and are club shaped, much like the tip of a cotton-tipped applicator. The ratio of telogen to anagen hairs varies from one person to another, with an average telogen count of 15 per cent and an aver-

age anagen count of 85 per cent. A telogen count of 25 per cent or more is considered to be diagnostic of telogen effluvium.

There is no effective treatment for telogen effluvium, and since spontaneous regrowth is characteristic of this disorder, unless the stressful event is repeated, complete regrowth takes place almost invariably within about 6 months. Exceptionally prolonged illness with high fevers, however, may destroy some follicles completely, so that in some cases only partial recovery may be possible. Careful explanation of the cause of this disorder and its favorable prognosis, with careful instructions to the patient to avoid manipulation such as vigorous shampooing, combing, and brushing until new growth has occurred, is generally all that is required.

ANAGEN EFFLUVIUM

Anagen effluvium is a far less common disorder of hair loss that follows the use of antimitotic agents such as those used in the therapy for cancer or leukemia. These agents include folic acid antagonists (aminopterin and amethopterin), purine antagonists such as 6-mercaptopurine, alkylating agents (cyclophosphamide and nitrogen mustard), and natural alkaloids such as vincristine. In addition, anagen effluvium may be associated with excessive x-irradiation to the scalp and the ingestion of various chemicals such as lead, thallium, arsenic, bismuth, and coumadin. During the period of drug administration, the follicle remains in a modified growth phase, and in contrast to telogen effluvium, the disorder occurs with follicles in the anagen growing stage.

The clinical features of anagen alopecia depend on the degree of toxicity created by the causative agent. Since an average of 85 per cent of scalp hairs in a healthy individual are in anagen stage at a given time, severe toxicity may result in profound hair loss. The usual change in the hair root is quite

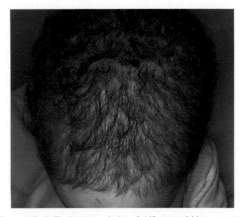

Figure 17–3. Toxic alopecia in a 2 1/2-year-old boy caused by the ingestion of excessive amounts of vitamin A.

characteristic in this disorder and consists of tapered hair root tips and sharp thinning or constriction of the hair shaft (at which point the hairs simply separate). With lower doses there may be only segmental thinning or narrowing, without actual fracture of the hair shaft.[3] A careful history, documented evidence of hair loss, microscopic examination of spontaneously shed and manually epilated hairs, and appropriate physical and toxicologic examinations help establish the correct diagnosis. Cessation of the responsible drug generally results in regrowth of hair.

There is no effective treatment for anagen effluvium except removal of the precipitating cause. The use of a simple occlusive scalp tourniquet, however, is frequently effective in protecting against this disorder during the intravenous use of vincristine (as in the treatment of children with acute leukemia, Wilms' tumor, neuroblastoma, lymphoma, and rhabdomyosarcoma). With this technique, a specially constructed scalp tourniquet placed around the head just above the ears and inflated to 10 mm Hg above systolic pressure immediately before injection of the drug frequently helps minimize the toxic effects of vincristine on the hair follicles of the scalp.[10]

ALOPECIA AREATA

Alopecia areata, a common disorder with an incidence of 17.2 per 100,000 population (affecting 1:1,000 individuals at any one time), is characterized by the sudden appearance of sharply defined round or oval patches of hair loss. Although the condition occurs at all ages, the first attack usually appears in patients younger than 25 years of age; there is a history of familial occurrence in 10 to 20 per cent of affected individuals. Although occasional reports of simultaneous occurrence in identical twins have been published, the genetic status of this disorder is unclear at this time.

The cause of alopecia areata remains unknown, but various causes have been proposed. Recent evidence suggests an immune mechanism (an autoimmunologic process) as a possible cause of this disorder. In support of this hypothesis several studies indicate an interrelationship with chronic lymphocytic thyroiditis (Hashimoto's disease), pernicious anemia, adrenal disease, vitiligo, myasthenia gravis, autoimmune polyendrocrinopathy, idiopathic hypoparathyroidism, chronic mucocutaneous candidiasis, diabetes, and atopy.[11, 12] An increased incidence has also been noted in patients with Down's syndrome, and there also seems to be more than a coincidental association with cataracts.

Clinical Manifestations. The typical clinical picture of alopecia areata generally consists of a sudden (frequently overnight or over a period of several days) appearance of one or more round or oval well-circumscribed and clearly defined patches of hair loss (Figs. 17–4 and 17–5). Occasionally, particularly in children, the initial patches may be

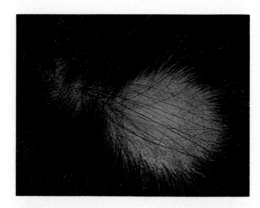

Figure 17–4. Alopecia areata with sharply defined oval patches of hair loss.

atypical, may lack a regular outline, and, at times, may demonstrate scattered long hairs within the bald areas. In other instances the initial loss may be diffuse, with patches of alopecia being apparent only after 1 or 2 weeks, if at all. The primary patch may appear on any hairy cutaneous surface but usually occurs on the scalp. The skin is smooth, soft, occasionally slightly pink or violaceous and, in white individuals, ivory white, and almost totally devoid of hair. Rarely, slight erythema or edema may be found at an early stage, and older patches frequently contain depigmented hair shafts, simulating poliosis (Fig. 17–6). Discrete islands of hair loss sometimes are separated by completely uninvolved or partially involved scalp, and around the margins of patches of alopecia, pathognomonic "exclamation-mark" hairs may be detected. These loose hairs, with attenuated bulbs and short stumps, are easily plucked out of the scalp. Examination of such hairs under a low-power microscope reveals an irregularity in diameter and a poorly pigmented hair shaft that tapers to

Figure 17–5. Multiple lesions of alopecia areata. Short stubby "exclamation mark" hairs may be plucked out and identified under low-power microscopic examination.

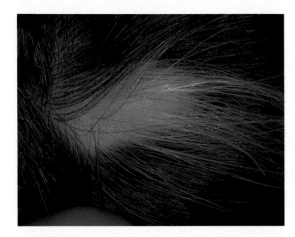

Figure 17–6. Alopecia areata with depigmented hairs simulating poliosis.

an attenuated bulb. The telogen bulb represents the dot of the exclamation point.

A clinical form of alopecia termed *ophiasis* occasionally occurs, particularly in children. This unusual form of alopecia, which begins as a bald spot on the posterior occiput and extends anteriorly and bilaterally in a 1- to 2-inch wide band above the ear, at times extending to meet on the anterior aspect of the scalp, is generally associated with a poor prognosis.

It is stated that alopecia totalis (loss of all scalp hair) may ultimately develop in 5 to 10 per cent of cases of partial alopecia. This figure may be high in view of the fact that a high percentage of cases of mild alopecia resolve spontaneously, thus never being seen by a physician. Progression to the totalis form occurs more slowly, but more frequently in children than in adults. If, in addition, there is complete or virtually complete loss of body hair, the disorder is termed *alopecia universalis* (Fig. 17–7).

Nail defects are seen in 10 to 20 per cent of cases. While it is true that the more extensive the disease, the more likely the possibility and severity of nail involvement, some patients may have gross nail dystrophy with little hair change. The most characteristic nail abnormality is a fine grid-like stippling, regularly arranged in horizontal or vertical rows or both, with pits smaller and more shallow than those seen in patients with psoriasis (Fig. 17–8). Proximal shedding (onychomadesis), longitudinal ridging, opacification, serration of the free edges and severe dystrophy, although less common, appear to be more likely in patients with alopecia totalis and universalis. Ridging and dystrophy may, at times, be quite marked but, when present, are generally confined to only a few nails.

Diagnosis. The diagnosis of alopecia areata is based on its clinical picture. The sudden appearance and circumscribed nonscarring, patterned nature of hair loss will frequently distinguish it from other disorders of alopecia. Trichotillomania is typically associated with bizarre, irregular patches of hair loss, with areas of broken hairs of different lengths. The absence of signs of inflammation and scaling will generally help distinguish this disorder from that of tinea capitis. Alopecia due to secondary syphilis may be recognized by its moth-eaten appearance, irregular borders, incomplete loss of hair within individual patches, and a predilection for the posterior scalp. When the diagnosis is in doubt, microscopic examination of hairs with potassium hydroxide, fungal cultures, serologic testing, and cutaneous punch biopsy will frequently help establish the proper diagnosis.

In newly formed patches of alopecia areata the vast majority of hair follicles are in telogen phase. When a patch of alopecia has been present for a period of many months, however, most hairs are in the anagen phase. Histopathologic examination of affected areas is characterized by small hair structures and hair bulbs located higher in the scalp than normally seen. The most characteristic microscopic feature consists of a nonspecific inflammatory infiltrate of the hair follicles and a round cell "swarm of bees" infiltration surrounding the hair bulbs.

Course. The course of alopecia areata is variable and difficult to predict. Extension may continue for a few weeks. Frequently new patches of hair loss appear within 4 to 6 weeks; and, occasionally, after 4 to 10 months, spontaneous regrowth may occur (Fig. 17–9). In general, when the process is limited to a few patches, the prognosis is good, with complete regrowth occurring within 1 year in 95 per cent of children; the earlier the onset, however, the

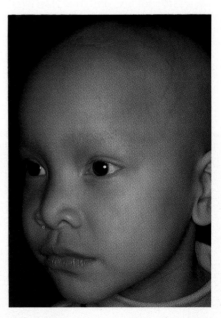

Figure 17–7. Alopecia universalis. Note loss of scalp hair, eyebrows, and eyelashes.

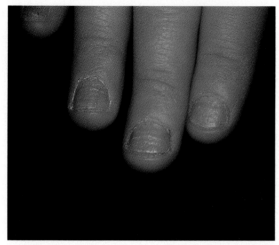

Figure 17–8. Grid-like stippling of the nails in a patient with alopecia areata.

poorer the prognosis. When the disorder is extensive or total (Fig. 17–7), the possibility of complete and permanent recovery is poor, and about 30 per cent of patients will have future episodes of alopecia areata.

Management. The therapy for alopecia areata consists of topical corticosteroids alone or under occlusion (such as may be achieved under a wig, bathing cap, or Saran Wrap)[13, 14] or multiple intradermal corticosteroid injections, which frequently result in regrowth in tufts at injection sites within 4 to 6 weeks. When an intralesional corticosteroid is used, a syringe with a 30-gauge needle or jet-injection may be used. All anti-inflammatory insoluble corticosteroids are effective. However, triamcinolone acetonide in concentrations of 2.5 to 10 mg/ml is the most practical for acute cases, with a maximum of 1 or 2 ml total at 4- to 6-week intervals (no more than one injection per site per month) (Figs. 17–10 and 17–11).[15] Efficacy appears to be greatest in those who have less than 75 per cent hair loss, in children, and in those with a relatively short duration of hair loss. It should be noted, however, that up to 5 to 10 per cent of individuals with extensive (including 100 per cent) scalp hair loss, even after long duration (up to 26 years), have had good cosmetic regrowth following treatment.[16]

Although not recommended for general use, systemic corticosteroids may be considered for carefully selected patients with severe involvement and an associated psychological handicap who do not respond to topical and intralesional corticosteroid therapy. In such instances, prednisone, in dosages of 20 to 30 mg/day for 4 to 6 weeks, followed by alternate-day therapy, may be beneficial and causes relatively few significant side effects. It must be emphasized that close follow-up evaluation is indicated in such cases and that the potential side effects associated with systemic corticosteroid therapy must be explained to the patient and his or her parents.[17, 18]

Experimental studies have suggested a possible therapeutic approach using contact sensitization with weekly applications of dinitrochlorobenzene (DNCB) sufficient to produce a mild contact dermatitis. Although the mechanism of the therapeutic effect is unknown, it has been suggested that the induced contact dermatitis may produce an accumulation of suppressor cells that neutralize the effects of lymphocytes surrounding the hair bulbs (an "antigenic-competitive phenomenon"). Studies suggest a possible mutagenic response to DNCB. This form of therapy, therefore, is not recommended.[19]

Other therapeutic approaches include the induction of irritant dermatitis with compounds such as anthralin,[20] allergic contact dermatitis with squaric acid dibutyl ester or diphencyprone (agents that appear to be as effective as DNCB but do not demonstrate mutagenicity),[21, 22] topical minoxidil (Rogaine), which appears to have some degree of success (in up to one third of patients),[23] the administration of inosiplex (a synthetic immunomodulator),[24] photochemotherapy with sys-

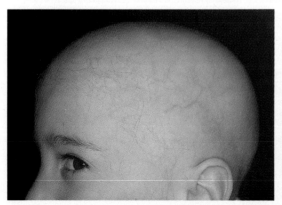
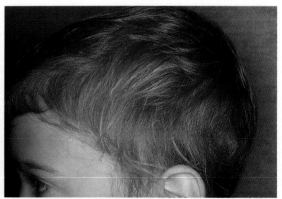

Figure 17–9. A. Alopecia totalis in a 3 1/2-year-old boy. B. Spontaneous regrowth of hair in the same boy 5 months later.

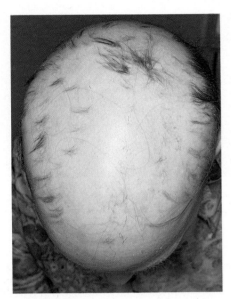

Figure 17-10. Alopecia totalis. Early regrowth of hair follows intradermal corticosteroid injections.

temic psoralen followed by ultraviolet A (PUVA) therapy,[25] and topical or oral cyclosporine. Although PUVA and cyclosporine therapy have been successful in some adults with this disorder, their efficacy and safety have not been established in children. Since the social and psychological implications suffered by patients with alopecia areata are many, wigs can frequently help those with severe forms of the disorder. The National Alopecia Areata Foundation (714 C Street, Suite 202, San Rafael, California) is available as a support group for affected children and their families.[26]

TRAUMATIC ALOPECIA

Traumatic alopecia results from the forceful extraction of hair or the breaking of hair shafts by friction, traction, or other physical trauma. The usual causes are trichotillomania (a self-induced alopecia caused by plucking, pulling, or cutting the hair in a bizarre manner) and cosmetic practices, such as tight braiding or pony-tails; the use of tight rollers, barrettes, head bands, or rubber bands; hair-straightening practices such as teasing or pulling, or frequent brushing with nylon bristles; and the use of hot combs and petrolatum (Figs. 17-12 through 17-16). Other common causes of traumatic alopecia include pressure, such as is seen on the occiput of infants who lie on their backs or are in the habit of "head-banging" (Fig. 17-17); prolonged bed rest in one position such as may be seen in chronically ill patients; postoperative alopecia (as a result of pressure-induced ischemia during long surgical procedures); thermal or electric burns; repeated vigorous massage; a severe blow to the scalp (Fig. 17-18); occipito-parietal alopecia such as may be induced by

spinning on the crown of the head during "breakdancing"; or prolonged use of wide-strapped heavy headphones, such as those frequently used by individuals while jogging.[27, 28]

Traction Alopecia. Traction alopecia is characterized by oval or linear areas of hair loss at the margins of the hair line, along the part, or scattered through the scalp, depending on the type of traction or trauma. Peripheral scalp hair loss may occur in individuals who wear their hair in pony-tail style, and the hair loss from hair rollers is usually most conspicuous in the frontocentral area or around the margins of the scalp. Hot comb alopecia, seen primarily in black individuals who straighten their hair for cosmetic purposes, generally occurs on the vertex or marginal areas of the scalp. In severe chronic forms, however, the entire scalp may be involved.

Trichotillomania. Trichotillomania is a self-limiting form of traction alopecia produced either consciously or subconsciously as the result of habit. Seen in children and young adults of both sexes, it is most common in children between 4 and 10 years of age and young adolescents. The scalp is the most common site of involvement, but the eyebrows and eyelashes may also be affected as the patient plucks, twirls, or rubs hair-bearing areas, resulting in the epilation or breakage of hair shafts.

The habit is usually practiced in bed before the child falls asleep (when the parent does not notice the habit) or when the child is reading, writing, or watching television. In young individuals the con-

Figure 17-11. Regrowth of hair following intradermal corticosteroid injections in a patient with alopecia areata.

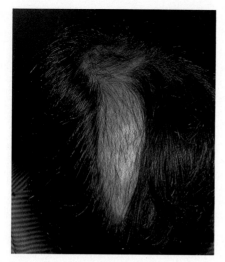

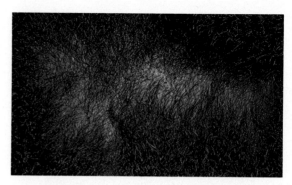

Figure 17–14. Traumatic alopecia produced by tight braiding of hair.

Figure 17–12. Trichotillomania of the scalp—a self-induced traumatic alopecia.

dition is frequently associated with a habit of finger or thumb sucking. Although many authors emphasize severe psychological problems in patients with this disorder, most affected individuals are merely under varying degrees of emotional stress or have developed a habit that generally can be managed by a sympathetic physician and understanding parent.

Trichotillomania usually begins insidiously as an irregular linear or rectangular area of partial hair loss. Affected areas are generally single, often frontal, frontotemporal, or frontoparietal, and frequently appear on the contralateral side of right- or left-handed individuals. The affected patches have irregularly shaped angular outlines and are never completely bald. Within the involved regions the hair is short or stubbly and broken off at varying lengths (see Figs. 17–12, 17–13, and 17–19).[29]

If one maintains a high index of suspicion, trac-

tion alopecia can generally be distinguished from other forms of hair loss by its characteristic configuration and distribution. Occasionally the diagnosis can be confirmed by the finding of wads of hair under the pillow or bed or by observation of the habit by a parent, teacher, or physician. When the diagnosis is suspected, regrowth of hair in a carefully shaved or occluded patch of scalp in the involved area (to prevent manipulation) frequently will confirm the correct diagnosis (Fig. 17–20). Clinical differentiation from alopecia areata is usually based on the bizarre configuration, irregular outline, and presence of short stub-like broken hairs. Differentiation from tinea capitis may require Wood's light examination, microscopic examination of plucked hairs with potassium hydroxide (occasionally revealing node-like swellings of the hair shaft and broken hairs), and fungal culture (see Chapter 13). Of particular significance is the fact that the broken hairs of trichotillomania, unlike those of certain forms of tinea capitis, remain firmly rooted in the scalp, and the cutaneous surface is normal and stubbled rather than erythematous or scaly.

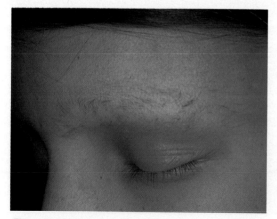

Figure 17–13. Trichotillomania of the eyebrow with characteristic short broken hairs.

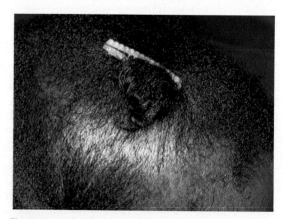

Figure 17–15. Traction alopecia caused by frequent use of hair curlers.

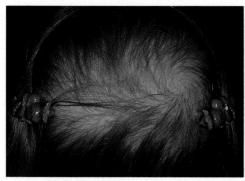

Figure 17–16. Traction alopecia caused by barrettes.

If the diagnosis remains in doubt, biopsy of the involved area is frequently helpful. The histopathologic features of trichotillomania consist primarily of catagen hairs, evidence of traumatic damage (often with evidence of hemorrhage), the presence of keratin plugs and dilated follicular infundibula, the replacement of some hair follicles by fibrosis, and absence of significant inflammation or scarring.[30] In taking biopsy specimens from suspected patients with trichotillomania it is best to carefully select the precise site of most recent hair loss.

The management of trichotillomania is often difficult and requires a strong doctor, patient, and parent relationship. Although patients occasionally will admit to touching the affected areas, they frequently will deny plucking, rubbing, or excessive manipulation. Direct confrontation and accusation is frequently detrimental and rarely helpful. Psychopathologic changes are reported to be present in some 50 to 75 per cent of affected individuals. These changes are usually mild and require no special management. Deep emotional and psychological disorders occur in fewer than 5 per cent of patients with trichotillomania.

If patients are reassured, given an opportunity to express their emotional needs, and offered a reasonable therapeutic regimen such as a mild shampoo and scalp lotion (perhaps hydrocortisone in a 1.0 per cent concentration as a placebo or to "relieve pruritus or possible irritation"), the tic will frequently disappear. For those individuals with persistent or severe obsessive-compulsive or emotional problems, however, antidepressants such as clomipramine (Anafranil [Ciba]) or fluoxetine (Prozac]) and professional psychological assistance should be considered,[31] and in those with a persistent habit, particularly nervous young females with long hair, the possibility of trichophagia and trichobezoar should be considered.[32]

ANDROGENETIC ALOPECIA

Androgenetic alopecia occurs in both men and women and appears to be inherited as an autosomal dominant trait with variable expression. The onset of this androgenically induced disorder has been noted as early as 14 years of age; the earlier the onset, the more profound the subsequent alopecia.

Male Pattern Alopecia. The mildest and often earliest form of androgenetic male pattern alopecia is seen as a symmetrical triangular recession of the hairline in the frontoparietal and occasionally frontal scalp margins. Uniform recession of the frontal hairline is seen during adolescence in 96 per cent of males and in about 80 per cent of females; it does not represent the first stage of male pattern alopecia and does not signify the onset of profound or premature baldness (Fig. 17-21). In 5 per cent of white males, alopecia is first observed before the age of 20, usually as symmetrical frontotemporal recession. It is generally not until the third or fourth decade that the incidence of this pattern increases and is associated with some loss of hair in the crown of the scalp (Fig. 17–22). In women the loss in rare instances progresses to the total crown involvement of males but otherwise appears to be a diminutive form of the disease as seen in males.

In a young man the onset of male pattern alopecia frequently causes severe distress and anxiety. Careful examination and repeated reassurance are required to discourage recourse to expensive and ineffective proprietary therapeutic regimens. Un-

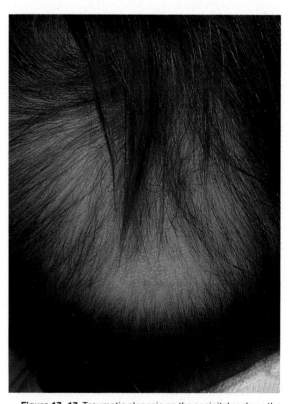

Figure 17–17. Traumatic alopecia on the occipital scalp as the result of a head-rubbing habit in a 7-month-old infant.

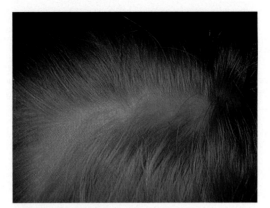

Figure 17–18. Traumatic alopecia. Alopecia was induced by a severe blow to the scalp.

fortunately modern medicine has found no universally effective form of therapy for male pattern alopecia. Massage and topical stimulating agents have no value, and the use of estrogenic creams and other hormonal approaches are ineffective or potentially hazardous. Until recently treatment has been limited to reassurance or to the recommendation of artificial hair pieces. Currently, topical minoxidil, [33, 34] plastic surgery techniques, implantation of nylon filaments, and multiple-punch autografting hair transplant techniques may be considered.[35] Punch-graft hair transplants can be performed in the physician's office, and, although not a panacea, when properly performed by an experienced dermatologist or plastic surgeon, a cosmetically satisfactory redistribution of hair can generally be achieved (Fig. 17–23). The response rates for cosmetically acceptable hair growth for patients with male pattern alopecia with topical minoxidil currently appears to be 15 to 25 per cent, and if successful, the therapy must be continued throughout the patient's lifetime. Good prognostic factors for hair regrowth with minoxidil include a balding history of less than 5 years, such as seen in young individuals with frontal recession, and an area of baldness on the vertex measuring less than 10 cm (4 inches) in diameter. Males in the 40-year age group appear to do better than older men with this disorder.[33, 34]

Female Androgenetic Alopecia. Androgenetic alopecia in women is generally less severe than that seen in men. The frontal hair line is relatively unaffected, with only slight recession. The process may become apparent at any time after puberty (during the second to fourth decades of life); progress is slow, and male-type baldness is rare. Although genetic susceptibility and androgenic stimulation are essential factors in the pathogenesis of female androgenetic alopecia, women may be endocrinologically normal or may exhibit mild, moderate, or severe abnormalities of androgen metabolism. In women with severe

forms of androgenetic alopecia, especially if there is evidence of hirsutism, acne, menstrual disturbance, or other evidence of virilization, evaluation for possible elevation of dehydroepiandrosterone sulfate, free plasma testosterone, and testosterone-binding globulin levels is recommended. When endocrinologic abnormality is present and hormonal therapy with dexamethasone or spironolactone appears to be indicated, therapy is best carried out in cooperation with an endocrinologist.[36, 37]

LOOSE ANAGEN HAIR OF CHILDHOOD

Loose anagen hair of childhood (loose or short anagen syndrome) is a recently described occasionally autosomal dominant disorder characterized by actively growing anagen hairs that, loosely anchored, can be easily and painlessly pulled from the scalp. Although the majority of patients with this disorder have been described as blond girls 2 to 5 years of age, patients of both sexes and individuals with dark hair may also be affected. Affected children generally have sparse short scalp hairs that seldom require cutting (Fig. 17–24) and a predominance (98 to 100 per cent) of actively growing anagen hairs with ruffled hair shafts and heavily pigmented misshapen bulbs. Diffuse or patchy alopecia may at times be

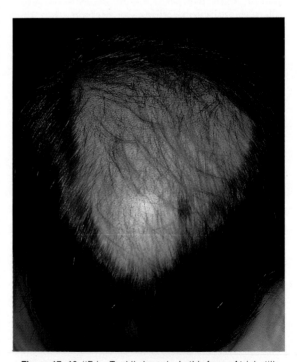

Figure 17–19. "Friar Tuck" alopecia. In this form of trichotillomania the hair is pulled from an initial starting point, resulting in an area of alopecia surrounded by a rim of unaffected hair. Its resemblance to the shaven crown of the head of a monk has suggested the term *Friar Tuck* to designate this form of trichotillomania.

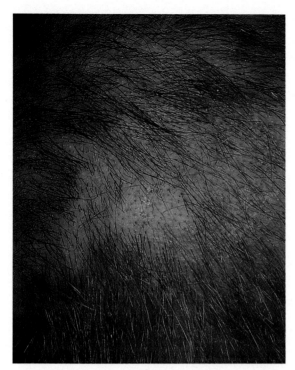

Figure 17–20. If the diagnosis remains in doubt, regrowth of normal hair density (because the hair is too short to manipulate) in a small shaved area of the scalp in the middle of a region of the alopecia after a period of 3 to 4 weeks can help confirm the diagnosis of trichotillomania.

present; and although no treatment is available for this disorder, it is reassuring for patients and their families to know that other abnormalities are not associated with this disorder and that individuals with this condition generally tend to improve with time.[38, 39]

Scarring Alopecia

Scarring or cicatricial alopecia is the end result of a wide number of inflammatory processes in and about the pilosebaceous units, resulting in irreversible destruction of tissue and consequent permanent scarring alopecia of the affected areas. The scarring may be the result of a developmental defect (aplasia cutis) (see Figs. 2–17 and 2–18); inflammatory changes of infective origin, such as severe bacterial, viral, or fungal infection; physical trauma (irradiation, trichotillomania practiced over a long period of time, thermal or caustic burns); neoplastic disorders; various dermatoses (lichen planus, lupus erythematosus, localized or systemic scleroderma); or various dermatologic syndromes, such as keratosis pilaris atrophicans, folliculitis decalvans, dissecting cellulitis of the scalp, acne keloidalis, pseudopelade, and alopecia mucinosa. This latter group of dermatologic disorders is described below.

KERATOSIS PILARIS ATROPHICANS

Numerous terms have been used to describe a group of interrelated syndromes characterized by inflammatory keratotic follicular papules and later by atrophy. Frequently described as atrophic variants of keratosis pilaris, these include keratosis pilaris atrophicans faciei (ulerythema ophryogenes), atrophoderma vermicularis, and keratosis follicularis spinulosa decalvans (keratosis pilaris decalvans). These disorders occur sporadically and are presumed to be the result of inborn defects. The major histologic features include plugging and distention of hair follicles, dilatation of dermal vessels, perifollicular and perivascular lymphocytic infiltration, dermal atrophy, and horn cysts.

Ulerythema Ophryogenes. Ulerythema ophryogenes (keratosis pilaris atrophicans faciei) is a disorder primarily affecting infants, boys, and young men and is characterized by persistent reticular erythema, small horny papules, atrophy, and permanent loss of the involved hairs in the outer halves of the eyebrows. Occasionally the disorder extends to include the adjacent skin, adjacent scalp, and cheeks. To date there is no effective therapy for this disorder.

Atrophoderma Vermicularis. Atrophoderma vermicularis (folliculitis ulerythema reticulata, atrophodermia vermiculata) is a variant of keratosis pilaris atrophicans that usually has its onset between 5 and 12 years of age and occasionally later. This disorder is characterized by the formation of numerous tiny symmetric atrophic and, at times, erythematous pits on the cheeks, and occasionally the forehead and eyebrows. Generally measuring 1 to 2 mm across and 1 mm deep, these cribriform lesions are separated from each other by narrow ridges of normal-appearing skin. Although there is no effective treatment for this disorder, dermabra-

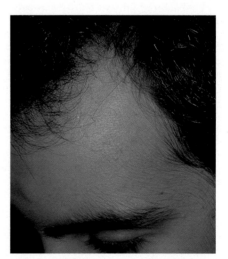

Figure 17–21. Triangular recession of the hairline in the frontotemporal scalp margin, the earliest and mildest form of male pattern alopecia (seen in 5 per cent of males before age 20).

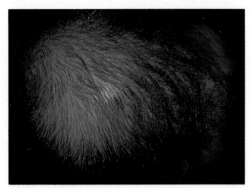

Figure 17–22. Androgenic male pattern baldness on the crown of the scalp of an adult man.

sion can frequently improve the cosmetic appearance of affected individuals.

The variant termed *keratosis pilaris decalvans* occurs in infancy or early childhood. It is characterized by numerous milia and prominent follicular plugs on the nose and cheeks and, later, on the limbs and neck. Various exfoliants and keratolytics have been used for this disorder, but with limited success.

FOLLICULITIS DECALVANS

Folliculitis decalvans is a rare form of cicitricial alopecia characterized by erythematous scaling and small rounded or oval patches of scarring surrounded by perifollicular pustules. The etiology is unknown, but it appears to be associated with a long history of seborrheic dermatitis and a low grade pustular reaction in hair follicles of the scalp, occasionally of the bearded, axillary, pubic, or other cutaneous areas, resulting in a peripherally spreading inflammatory disease and alopecia. Although a bacterial folliculitis, such as caused by *Staphylococcus aureus*, at times is associated with this disorder, virulent pyococcal organisms are often not demonstrated. In many forms of this disorder the condition tends to persist indefinitely, and although the inflammation and cosmetic disability are frequently limited, severe forms, especially in males, may be particularly disfiguring.

In the pustular phase the histologic picture is characterized by polymorphonuclear microabscesses in the upper half of the pilosebaceous follicle and a perifollicular infiltrate that contains numerous plasma cells. In the atrophic phase the histology of the disorder is frequently indistinguishable from that seen in the atrophic phase of lichen planus or lupus erythematosus.

The treatment of folliculitis decalvans consists of topical antibiotics, systemic antibiotics, and, in severe or protracted cases, a combination of topical, intralesional, and systemic corticosteroids and long-term antibiotics. Unfortunately, in many

individuals the disorder persists and may result in severe alopecia and scarring despite long-term and intensive therapy.

DISSECTING CELLULITIS OF THE SCALP

Dissecting cellulitis of the scalp, also termed *perifolliculitis capitis abscedens et suffodiens,* is a rare dissecting cellulitis of the scalp that leads to the formation of burrowing abscesses and fluctuant nodules connected by tortuous ridges or elevations. Seropurulent drainage may persist indefinitely, and cicatricial alopecia and keloid formation frequently develop. Seen primarily in individuals between 18 and 40 years of age, the disease occurs in whites and blacks, with a greater incidence in the latter, and men are affected more frequently than women.

The disease appears to have a slightly increased incidence in patients with chronic hidradenitis or acne conglobata. There is no specific therapy for this disorder. Local and sytemic antibiotics, intralesional corticosteroids, incision and drainage of abscesses, and radiation therapy have been used with varying results, but the course is generally chronic, with remissions and relapses over many years.

ACNE KELOIDALIS

Acne keloidalis (folliculitis keloidalis) is a chronic scarring folliculitis and perifolliculitis of the nape of the neck (occasionally the bearded area) that leads to the formation of keloidal papules, nodules, and plaques.

Seen most frequently in postpubertal males, especially blacks between the ages of 14 and 25, it has also been noted in white males and black women (Fig. 17–25). Although the precise cause of this disorder is not clear, it appears to be related to a persistent infection (frequently but not

Figure 17–23. Hair transplants in an area of cicatricial alopecia.

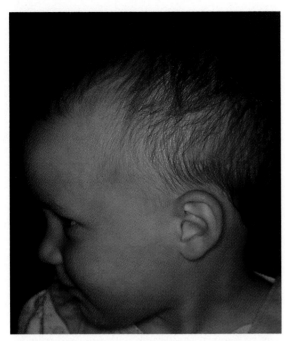

Figure 17–24. Loose anagen hair syndrome. The hair is short, loosely anchored, and easily pluckable in this 6-year-old girl.

necessarily streptococcal or staphylococcal), with a tendency toward granulomatous change followed by eventual destruction of normal structures and their replacement by hypertrophic connective tissue and plasma cell infiltrate.

Treatment of this disorder is difficult and consists of long-term systemic antibiotics, intralesional corticosteroids, and, in some cases, perhaps radiation therapy. In long-term cases with severe scarring, excision and plastic repair are occasionally beneficial.

PSEUDOPELADE

Pseudopelade is a nonspecific scarring form of alopecia of the scalp generally seen in adults. It is characterized by multiple small, round, oval, or irregularly shaped hairless cicatricial patches of varying sizes. Affected areas are shiny, ivory white or slightly pink, and atrophic. Interspersed between the patches may be a few hair-containing dilated hair follicles. The etiology is unknown, and the onset of the disorder is insidious and asymptomatic. Lesions generally appear at the vertex of the scalp. They frequently coalesce to form finger-like projections and have been compared to "footprints in the snow" (Fig. 17–26).

The histopathologic examination of involved areas reveals perifollicular and perivascular infiltrates composed almost entirely of lymphocytes and a few histiocytes. Slight follicular hyperkeratosis may be present; and, in late stages, extensive fibrosis of the dermis predominates.

There is no specific or effective therapy for this disorder. Infiltration of triamcinolone acetonide in a 2.5-mg/ml concentration into active areas at 6- to 8-week intervals may be temporarily beneficial; and, in persistently unresponsive cases, a reasonable cosmetic improvement frequently can be achieved by the multiple-punch autograft technique of hair transplantation.

ALOPECIA MUCINOSA

Alopecia mucinosa (follicular mucinosis) is an inflammatory disorder characterized by sharply defined follicular papules or infiltrated plaques, with scaling, loss of hair, and accumulation of mucin (acid mucopolysaccharide) in sebaceous glands and the outer root sheaths of affected hair follicles. A relatively uncommon condition affecting children as well as adults, the disorder presents three morphologic forms: (1) flat rough patches consisting of grouped follicular papules, (2) scaly plaques formed through the coalescence of follicular papules, and (3) nodular boggy infiltrated plaques with overlying erythema and scaling. Distributed primarily on the face, scalp, neck, and shoulders (occasionally the trunk and extremities), lesions are usually devoid of hair. Except in the scalp or eyebrows, this is generally not a conspicuous feature.

The cause of follicular mucinosis is unknown. In the majority of cases (in those younger than age 40) it is a benign idiopathic condition. In persons older than age 40, however, the presence of boggy infiltrated plaques of alopecia mucinosa may be the first sign of an accompanying reticulosis, usually mycosis fungoides (an uncommon neoplastic disorder of the lymphoreticular system generally affecting adults and but rarely seen in childhood).

In the benign form, lesions of alopecia mucinosa generally appear as grouped skin-colored papules or firm and coarsely rough plaques of erythema measuring 2 to 5 cm in diameter (sometimes larger with prominent follicles and fine

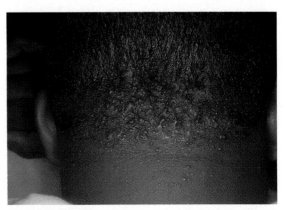

Figure 17–25. Acne keloidalis on the nape of the neck of an 18-year-old black young man.

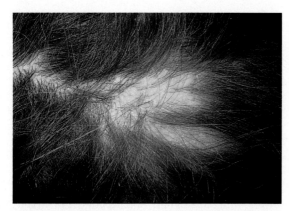

Figure 17–26. Pseudopelade. Cicatrical patches of alopecia ("footprints in the snow") are seen on the scalp of a 9-year-old boy.

scaling, and, in some instances, anesthesia in the affected areas.[40] In patients with solitary or few lesions, clearing usually occurs spontaneously within 2 years. In the chronic form, lesions are more numerous and more widely distributed and the plaques may be flat, domed, or elevated. Destruction of follicles may give rise to permanent alopecia, and the disorder may persist, with new lesions continuing to appear over a period of many years.

Alopecia mucinosa must be differentiated from lichen spinulosus, pityriasis rubra pilaris, tinea infection, pityriasis alba, granulomatous diseases, and the papulosquamous group of disorders. When the diagnosis remains in doubt, cutaneous biopsy of an affected area is generally confirmatory. The histopathologic picture is characterized by intracellular edema, loss of cohesion between cells, formation of cystic spaces, and accumulation of mucin within the external root sheaths and sebaceous glands. This substance shows metachromatic staining with Giemsa's stain, is periodic acid–Schiff negative, stains with alcian blue, and is digested by hyaluronidase.

Generally, especially in children and young adults, lesions of alopecia mucinosa involute spontaneously. Although some cases appear to benefit from topical or intralesional corticosteroids or radiation therapy, such claims are difficult to evaluate since spontaneous healing is the rule.[41]

Hair Shaft Abnormalities With Increased Fragility

Variations in the structure of the hair shaft are a common occurrence and, at times, may provide clues to other pathologic abnormalities. Because each hair shaft anomaly has a distinctive morphology, the diagnosis frequently can be established in the office by microscopic examination of preferably snipped rather than pulled hairs.

MONILETHRIX

Monilethrix (beaded hair) is a rare autosomal dominant disorder affecting both sexes equally (Fig. 17–27). It is characterized by variation in hair shaft thickness, with small node-like deformities that produce a beaded appearance, internodal fragility, breakage, and partial alopecia.

In this disorder, normal neonatal lanugo hairs are shed during the first few weeks of life and subsequent hair growth, generally at about the second month of life, becomes dry, lusterless, and brittle, failing to grow to any appreciable length. In severe cases the infant may remain bald or the scalp hair may be sparse, easily fractured, and stubble-like. Although generally a disorder of scalp hair, body hairs may also be affected. Occasionally this disorder is not apparent during infancy, only to become apparent later in childhood or during adult life.

The cause of monilethrix is unknown, but autosomal dominant transmission with high penetrance and variable expressivity has been demonstrated in large pedigrees. It is not characteristic of any systemic disease or metabolic defect but may be seen in association with physical retardation, syndactyly, keratosis pilaris, trichorrhexis nodosa, brittle nails, cataracts, or dental abnormalities.[9] Although argininosuccinic aciduria has been reported in patients with this disorder, this association requires confirmation. A tendency to spontaneous improvement or remission may occur at puberty or during pregnancy and, in some cases, may continue during adult life. In some individuals, however, the disease may persist unchanged throughout adulthood. Prognosis, accordingly, is guarded, and there is no effective therapy for this disorder.

PSEUDOMONILETHRIX

Pseudomonilethrix is an autosomal dominant disorder with variable penetrance that differs from monilethrix in that it begins at a later age (the age of 8 years or older). There is no follicular hyperkeratosis, and the hair shaft shows irregular flattened and thickened areas with an indented appearance, at times twisting of the longitudinal axis, and distal fractures similar to those seen in trichorrhexis nodosa. In addition, as in monilethrix, mechanical procedures such as combing, brushing, or massaging cause fragility and breakage of hairs. Treatment of this disorder consists of reassurance and gentle hair grooming with minimal manipulation.[42]

TRICHORRHEXIS NODOSA

Trichorrhexis nodosa, the most common hair shaft anomaly, is a distinctive disorder manifested by increased fragility owing to the presence of grayish white nodules, which, under a light microscope, give the appearance of two interlocking

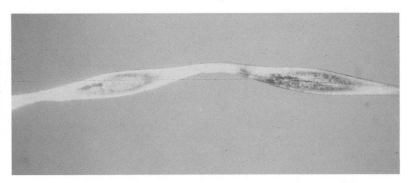

Figure 17–27. Monilethrix (beaded hair, nodose hair). Variable hair shaft thickness and node-like deformities occur. (Courtesy of Joseph McGuire, M.D.; reprinted from Hurwitz S: Hair disorders. *In* Schachner LA, Hansen RC (Eds.): Pediatric Dermatology. Churchill-Livingstone, New York, 1988.)

brushes or brooms, an appearance based on segmental longitudinal splitting of fibers without complete fracture (Fig. 17–28).

The disorder features dry lusterless short hair that is easily fractured and may be seen in a congenital or familial form. In affected individuals scalp hair breaks easily and leaves short stubbly broken ends and areas of partial alopecia. This disorder may be associated with tooth or nail abnormalities, and the occasional associaton of congenital or familial forms of trichorrhexis nodosa in mentally retarded children with argininosuccinic aciduria is of particular import. In such cases the amino acid arginine can be measured in the erythrocytes as well as skin fibroblasts, and marked elevations of argininosuccinic acid may be detected in the urine, blood, and cerebrospinal fluid. It must be remembered that this is a relatively uncommon disorder, and most patients with trichorrhexis nodosa have no underlying disease.

The most common type of hair loss secondary to structural hair shaft abnormality is that seen in patients with *acquired* forms of trichorrhexis nodosa. This disorder is seen in two clinical varieties, proximal trichorrhexis nodosa (a common condition seen in the black population) and distal trichorrhexis nodosa (a disorder observed mostly in whites and Asians).

Proximal trichorrhexis nodosa appears to be associated with a genetic predisposition and trauma from hair straightening, tight caps, or harsh brushing and combing techniques. Distal trichorrhexis nodosa is a disorder that occurs in otherwise normal hair as a result of cumulative cuticular damage (vigorous combing and brushing, repeated salt-water bathing, prolonged sun exposure, and frequent shampooing). Cream rinses and protein conditioners are helpful, and if hair-straightening procedures, vigorous grooming habits, and thermal and chemical trauma to the hair are discontinued, the acquired forms of trichorrhexis nodosa generally improve within 2 to 4 years.

TRICHORRHEXIS INVAGINATA

Trichorrhexis invaginata (bamboo hair) is a peculiar nodular defect caused by abnormal intussusception or telescope-like invagination along the hair shaft, which microscopically resembles the ball-and-cup joints of bamboo (Fig. 17–29). A relatively rare disorder, it is more common in females than in males, may involve all body hairs, and clinically is characterized by dry, lusterless, easily fractured, sparse and short hair. This disorder has been found in a rare, apparently autosomal recessive genodermatosis known as Netherton's disease, which is a combination of trichorrhexis invaginata, various forms of ichthyosis, and, at

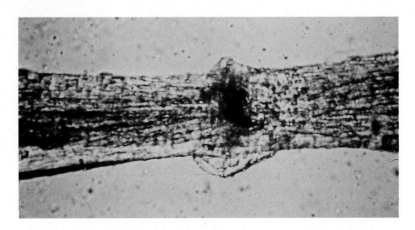

Figure 17–28. Trichorrhexis nodosa. Increased fragility occurs owing to the presence of grayish white nodules that, under a light microscope, give the appearance of two interlocked brushes or brooms pushed end to end. (Courtesy of Joseph McGuire, M.D.; reprinted from Hurwitz S: Hair disorders. *In* Schachner LA, Hansen RC (Eds.): Pediatric Dermatology. Churchill-Livingstone, New York, 1988.)

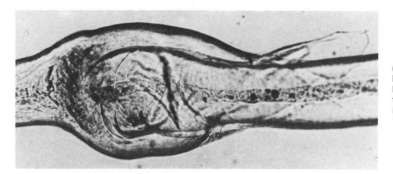

Figure 17–29. Trichorrhexis invaginata (bamboo hair). A nodular defect is caused by intussusception of the hair shaft. (From Hurwitz S, Kirsch N, McGuire J: Reevaluation of ichthyosis and hair shaft abnormalities. Arch. Dermatol. *103:*266, Copyright © 1971, American Medical Association.)

times, atopy, manifested by flexural eczema, allergic vasomotor rhinitis, asthma, angioneurotic edema, urticaria, or anaphylactic reaction. Although ichthyosis linearis circumflexa (see Chapter 7) is the form of ichthyosis most frequently seen in patients with this disorder, studies suggest that the original patient reported by Netherton probably had a form of lamellar ichthyosis and that some patients had ichthyosis vulgaris, ichthyosis linearis circumflexa, or both.

The hair defect in trichorrhexis invaginata is believed to be related to an incomplete conversion of sulfhydril groups into disulfide bonds in cortical fibers. This results in softening of the hair cortex and allows the distal portion of the hair shaft to intussuscept into the softer proximal portion. Beginning in infancy, all hair is affected to some degree, and there is no specific therapy for this hair abnormality. Although spontaneous remission of the hair defect can occur (generally between 6 and 15 years of age), many cases will persist into adulthood.

PILI TORTI

Pili torti (twisted hairs) is an autosomal dominant congenital hair defect of variable expression characterized by dry, fragile, twisted hairs (Fig. 17–30A). It affects females (chiefly blondes) more often than males and generally is observed in infancy as a patchy or diffuse hair loss. Although twisted hairs may be found in some individuals, the hair of children with classic pili torti, in contrast to those with pili torti associated with copper deficiency (Menkes' kinky hair syndrome), is clinically normal at birth, but by 2 or 3 years of age or later is replaced by brittle hair. The hairs shimmer in reflected light, and the twisted feature of this disorder often creates a "spangled" appearance. The disorder has also been seen in normal individuals; in association with ectodermal defects such as keratosis pilaris; and in individuals with dental abnormalities; dystrophic nails; corneal opacities; congenital sensorineural hearing loss; citrullinemia; arginine deficiency; Björnstad's syndrome (a disorder of probably autosomal dominant inheritance characterized by sensorineural deafness and pili torti); Basex syndrome (twisted hairs, basal cell carcinoma of the face, abnormal nails, follicular atrophoderma, eczematous and psoriasiform lesions on the ears, nose, cheeks, hands, feet, and knees, hyperkeratosis of the palms and soles, and carcinomas of the upper respiratory and digestive tracts in adults); Crandall's syndrome, consisting of twisted hairs with alopecia, deafness, and hypogonadism (probably a sex-

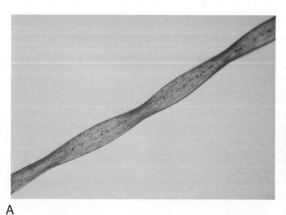
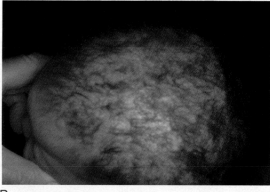

A   B

Figure 17–30. A. Pili torti (twisted hairs). B. Trichothiodystrophy. Sparse, short, brittle hair with variable degrees of alopecia. (A, Courtesy of Joseph McGuire, M.D.; reprinted from Hurwitz S: Hair disorders. *In* Schachner LA, Hansen RC (Eds.): Pediatric Dermatology. Churchill-Livingstone, New York, 1988.)

linked recessive disorder); hypohidrotic ectodermal dysplasia; and pseudomonilethrix.

The scalp hair in patients with pili torti becomes more normal with time, and although twisted hairs can still be found in the adult scalp, the cosmetic appearance may be normal by puberty. Those who still manifest the disorder at puberty, however, are unlikely to show significant improvement with age.

The diagnosis of pili torti is confirmed by microscopic examination of snipped hairs. Although a dry mount is frequently satisfactory, immersion of the hairs in water or a weak solution of potassium hydroxide (10 per cent) often allows swelling of the hairs, which may assist in the microscopic differentiation of abnormal from normal hairs. Other than reduction of trauma to reduce breakage, there is no effective treatment for this disorder.

PILI BIFURCATI

Pili bifurcati is an uncommon anomaly of hair growth characterized by intermittent bifurcation of the hair shaft in which affected hairs divide into two separate shafts that subsequently become rejoined along the hair shaft. This bifurcation is repeated at intervals, and the anomaly appears to be transitory, with only a small percentage of hairs exhibiting the bifurcation. This disorder should not be confused with *pili multigemini*, a disorder in which multiple hairs project from a single hair follicle.

MENKES' KINKY HAIR SYNDROME

Menkes' kinky hair syndrome (trichopoliodystrophy) is a rare, sex-linked recessive neurodegenerative disorder that affects male infants and is characterized by coarse facies, pili torti, temperature instability, seizures, psychomotor retardation, arterial intimal changes, low or absent plasma copper and ceruloplasmin levels, growth failure, increased susceptibility to infection, and death, generally by age 3 or 4 years.[43-45] Clinical features often include premature birth, hypothermia, and relatively normal development until 2 to 6 months of age, when drowsiness and lethargy are noted, intractable seizures begin, and growth and development cease. Usually the hair is fine, dull, sparse, and poorly pigmented in infancy; it stands on end, and looks and feels like steel wool. Additional features include a seborrheic rash, which may be coincidental; tortuous cerebral and other medium-sized arteries; osteoporosis; frequent subdural hematomas; widening of the metaphyses, with spurring; and frequent fractures, at times simulating the radiologic findings characteristic of patients with the battered child syndrome. Although pili torti is generally a prominent feature of this disorder, other less frequently reported hair abnormalities include monilethrix and trichorrhexis nodosa.

The combination of clinical features, bone abnormalities, and low plasma copper and ceruloplasmin levels establishes the correct diagnosis in patients with this disorder. Since the demonstration of a defect in intestinal absorption and utilization of copper, parenteral copper and ceruloplasmin therapy have been attempted, with results varying from a temporary arrest to clinical worsening of the disorder. Although treatment has raised plasma copper and ceruloplasmin levels to normal, possible irreversible damage prior to diagnosis (presumably in utero) cautions against undue optimism in using intravenous copper therapy for this disorder.[45]

TRICHOTHIODYSTROPHY

Trichothiodystrophy is a rare disorder of autosomal recessive inheritance in which patients have sulfur-deficient, sparse, short, dry, brittle, transversely broken hairs (trichoschisis), variable degrees of alopecia, physical and intellectual impairment, and a wide spectrum of other developmental defects (Fig. 17–30B). Polarizing microscopy shows a typical appearance of alternating light and dark bands. Syndromes seen in patients with trichothiodystrophy include (1) *BIDS syndrome*, a disorder characterized by *b*rittle hair, *i*mpaired intelligence, *d*ecreased fertility, and *s*hort stature; (2) a similar disorder to which ichthyosis has been added (the *IBIDS* or *Tay syndrome*); (3) the *PIBIDS syndrome*, a term used to describe patients who have trichothiodystrophy and photosensitivity; (4) the *Marinesco-Sjögren syndrome*, a rare condition in which affected individuals have cerebellar ataxia, dysarthria, cataracts, physical and mental retardation, abnormal teeth, flat, thin, and fragile nails, and fine, light, brittle, and unruly hair; and (5) the *PIBI(D)S syndrome*, a disorder in which features of trichothiodystrophy are combined with a defect of the DNA excision repair system (xeroderma pigmentosum group D mutation).[46-51] There is no known therapy for trichothiodystrophy. Although avoidance of cosmetic trauma and the use of hair conditioners are sometimes helpful, its course and prognosis depend on the specific physical features manifested in individuals with this disorder and its specific variants.

Hair Shaft Abnormalities Without Increased Hair Fragility

FRAGILITAS CRINIUM

Splitting of the hair shaft along its long axis (fragilitas crinium, trichoptilosis) is a common condition occurring particularly in the hair of girls and women who subject their hairs to various chemical and physical agents in the course of cosmetic treatment. Although the disorder may occur anywhere along the length of the shaft, splitting and fraying at the ends of dry and heavily bleached hair is a particularly common manifestation of this disorder.

The condition is readily distinguished by examination with a hand lens or low-power microscope, and therapy consists of gentle grooming techniques and the application of oils or cream rinses.

PILI ANNULATI

Pili annulati (ringed hair) is a rare familial defect of keratin synthesis involving the cortex of the hair shaft of scalp hair and is characterized by alternating bands of dark and light hair. The banding is due to an irregular distribution of air-filled cavities within the cortex of the hair shaft, which appear lighter by reflected light and darker by transmitted light.[52] The disorder is noted shortly after birth and is of equal sex distribution. The hair shaft is structurally strong, and the bright rings tend to produce an attractive highlight. There are no associated defects, and therapy is unnecessary.

Pseudopili annulati is an unusual variant of normal hair in which bright bands are seen at intervals along the hair shaft. Secondary to periodic twisting or curling of the hair shaft, this banding is conspicuous only in blond hairs and represents an optical effect due to reflection and refraction of light by flattened and twisted hair surfaces. This too is generally an attractive phenomenon and does not require therapy.[53]

WOOLLY HAIR

The subject of woolly hair is confused by the use of such terms as *woolly, kinky, spun glass, crimped, frizzy,* and *steely* to define the clinical appearance of peculiar hair that will not group in locks or lie down flat and is difficult to comb or brush.[54] The term woolly hair should be reserved to describe unruly scalp hair that curls readily in spirals but does not form locks and shows a slow twist on its long axis. It is an autosomal dominant inherited disorder in which the entire scalp hair is distinctly different from that of nonaffected family members in an individual who is not black. Hair shafts are usually ovoid in cross section, and the shaft diameter may at times be reduced. The individual scalp hairs are fine and dry, light in color, and corrugated at intervals, and resemble the crimp found in the wool of sheep. There is no known means of altering the manner of hair growth in this disorder, but it usually improves during adult life.

WOOLLY HAIR NEVUS

The woolly hair nevus is a rare condition and, in contradistinction to woolly hair of the entire scalp, is without familial correlation. It arises on the scalp as one or more patches of unruly hair that are quite different in color, shape, and consistency from the normal surrounding scalp hair. The hairs on the affected area are usually smaller in diameter and lighter in color and appear more sparse than those on the rest of the scalp. They are normally not fragile; and when examined under a dissecting microscope, the individual hairs are noted to twist about their long axis. The majority of reported cases of woolly hair nevus have been recognized during the first few months of life, but some have appeared in young adulthood. The cause of this disorder is unknown. In about 50 per cent of cases, woolly hair nevus coexists with a linear nevus in the same area or elsewhere.[55] Ocular involvement has been described as an associated feature, and a persistent pupillary membrane has been described; however, no other cutaneous or systemic disorders have been associated with this condition. There is no known treatment.

UNCOMBABLE HAIR SYNDROME

The uncombable hair syndrome (pili trianguli canaliculi, spun glass hair syndrome) is a unique hair disorder characterized by very pale, silvery, blond, or straw colored hair that is dry, frizzy, and unruly, and does not lie flat on the scalp, thus making combing impossible (Fig. 17-31). It is caused by a characteristic structural defect (the presence of canalicular depressions along the hair shaft). Although a familial incidence suggesting an autosomal dominant mode of inheritance has been reported, the genetics of this abnormality have yet to be defined. Diagnosis is made by demonstration of triangular hairs with characteristic longitudinal grooves along the hair shafts under light or electron microscopy. Although there is no definitive treatment, the unruly character of the hair generally resolves with time, and biotin (0.3 mg three times a day) has been reported to reverse the scaling, hair loss, hair fragility, and uncombability seen in individuals with this disorder.[56-58]

ACQUIRED PROGRESSIVE KINKING OF THE HAIR

Acquired progressive kinking of the hair is a rare disorder of scalp hair, with onset in adolescence or in young adulthood, characterized by a rapid onset of extreme curliness of the hair (mainly on the frontoparietal region of the scalp and vertex) often in association with an increased coarse texture, diminished luster, and striking unruliness. More common in males than in females, the hair may become darker or remain unaltered in color, and the rate of growth may be decreased or unchanged.[59]

Although the etiology of this disorder is unknown, it may develop at times following retinoid (isotretinoin or etretinate) therapy, and it has been

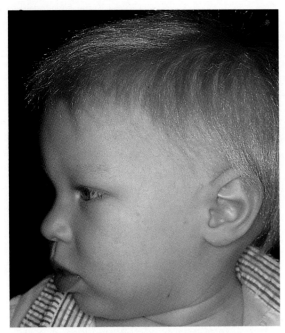

Figure 17–31. The uncombable hair syndrome in an 11-month-old boy. The spangled, upright, unruly spun glass appearance is characteristic of this disorder.

suggested that androgenic hormonal changes at puberty are somehow related to its pathogenesis.[60] Examination of abnormal hairs by light microscopy reveals alterations in hair shaft diameter, partial twisting of the hair on its longitudinal axis, and a beaded appearance attributed to twisting and consequent changes in diameter. Cross sections of affected hairs reveal an elliptical or irregular configuration with partial twists and spindle-shaped broadening of the shafts, occasional fractures, and sporadic canalicular grooves that extend for variable lengths along the hair shafts. There is no known effective therapy for this disorder, and, although the condition may persist for a period of many years, spontaneous reversion to normal hair has been reported in some individuals.

FELTED HAIR SYNDROME

Felted hair ("bird's nest hair") is a rare condition involving sudden and severe tangling of the scalp hair. Although its cause is unknown, the disorder appears to be associated with shampooing, chemical treatments, and damaged hair. Characterized by sudden massive tangling of the scalp hair, mild felting of the hair is probably common and can be remedied by cutting out the affected areas. Separation of the tangled hairs, although long and arduous, can also be used as an alternative option for patients unwilling to cut out the affected area and allow the hair to regrow normally.[61]

Hypertrichosis and Hirsutism

Excessive hairiness may be localized or diffuse, congenital or acquired, and normal or pathologic. The terms *hypertrichosis* and *hirsutism* are frequently used inappropriately and synonymously to describe a presence of excessive hair on the body. *Hirsutism* implies an excessive growth of body hair in women or children (mostly girls) in an androgen-induced hair pattern (upper lip, chin, sideburn areas, neck, anterior chest, breasts, linea alba, abdomen, upper inner thighs, and legs) (Fig. 17–32). The most common form of hirsutism is not a disease but merely represents a physiologic variant of hair growth in persons in a civilization that considers hairiness in women to be cosmetically undesirable. *Hypertrichosis*, conversely, refers to a generalized or localized pattern of *non-androgen-dependent* excessive hair growth in a male or female without evidence of masculinism or menstrual abnormality (Fig. 17–33).

CONGENITAL HYPERTRICHOSIS

Generalized hypertrichosis in the newborn generally represents a temporary normal condition. Except in the rare inherited disorder hypertrichosis lanuginosa, the first fine soft unmedullated and usually unpigmented lanugo hairs are generally shed in utero during the seventh or eighth month of gestation. Premature infants, however, frequently display this fine coat of lanugo hair, particularly on the face, limbs, and trunk. In such infants the fine lanugo hairs are shed during the first months of life and replaced by normal terminal hair growth, generally before the first 6 months.

Hypertrichosis Lanuginosa. Hypertrichosis lanuginosa is an exceedingly rare inherited disorder

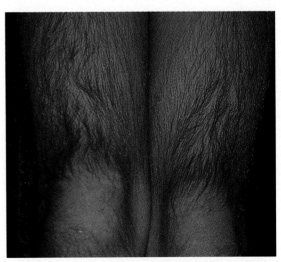

Figure 17–32. Hirsutism. Excessive hair is seen on the legs of a 12-year-old girl with excessive body hair in an adult male-pattern distribution.

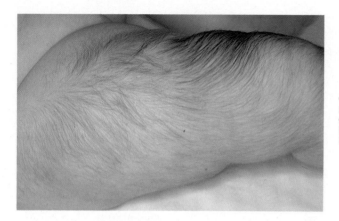

Figure 17–33. Hypertrichosis (a localized pattern of excessive hair growth) in an infant with hemihypertrophy of the right leg. (From Hurwitz S, Klaus SN: Congenital hemihypertrophy with hypertrichosis. Arch. Dermatol. *103*:98, 1971. Copyright © 1971, American Medical Association.) (See Chapter 2.)

in which there is persistence, or an acquired excessive production, of lanugo hairs. Affected infants, accordingly, may be unusually hairy at birth or may develop hirsutism in early childhood. This type of hairiness has attracted considerable attention over the years, and those afflicted by this disorder have been labeled by derogatory terms such as "dog-face men and women," "human Skye terriers," or "monkey-men."

There are two clinical forms of congenital hypertrichosis lanuginosa. The dog-face type is transmitted as an autosomal dominant trait. In this form, affected persons develop typical lanugo growth, reaching several inches in length over the first years of life. This persists and is associated with other congenital anomalies. The second, or monkey-face, variety is of uncertain heredity and is associated with a high incidence of infant mortality. Lanugo hair is present at birth, and surviving patients develop a simian-like facies.

In adults, acquired forms of hypertrichosis lanuginosa appear to have a strong association with internal malignancy (adenocarcinoma). Prominent red papillae on the tip and distal third of the tongue have been described and appear to be a prominent feature of the adult form of this disorder associated with underlying malignancy.[62]

The Cornelia de Lange Syndrome. The Cornelia de Lange syndrome is a congenital disorder consisting of marked hirsutism; cutis marmorata; hypoplastic genitalia, nipples, and umbilicus; growth and skeletal abnormalities; mental retardation; and a characteristic low-pitched and growling cry. Instances of affected siblings have been reported, but most cases have been sporadic and the disorder appears to be the result of an autosomal dominant inheritance (with a low recurrence risk as a result of inability of severely affected individuals to reproduce), or perhaps a homozygous recessive mutation. The face of afflicted individuals is characterized by overgrowth of the eyebrows, long eyelashes, high upper lip, saddle-nose, and a cyanotic hue about the eyes, nose, and mouth. Children with this disorder often have recurrent respiratory tract infections and gastrointestinal upsets;

seizures have been observed in about 20 per cent of reported cases, and most patients die before the age of 6 years.

Nevoid Hypertrichosis. Growth of hair abnormal in length, shaft diameter, or color for the site, size, and age of the patient may occur in association with other nevoid abnormalities or as isolated circumscribed developmental defects. Abnormal tufts of hair in the lumbosacral and, at times, the cervical or thoracic areas (the faun-tail nevus) may be associated with an underlying kyphoscoliosis or duplication of a portion of the spinal cord (diastematomyelia).[63] Although neurologic signs of this disorder generally apear to appear during early childhood, they may be delayed until the affected person's teenage or adult years.

Hypertrichosis may also be a characteristic of melanocytic nevi, Becker's nevus, linear epidermal nevus, nevoid circumscribed hypertrichosis (Fig. 17–34), a hair follicle nevus (which clinically may be misdiagnosed as a congenital pigmented nevus) (Fig. 17–35),[64] chronic low-grade physical trauma or wearing a cast over an affected area, thrombophlebitis, stasis dermatitis, x-ray or ultraviolet light irradiation, chemical irritation, or hormonal stimulation. Although for years individuals have been advised not to pluck, cut, or shave areas of hypertrichosis, it now is apparent that cutting, shaving, or epilation of such areas does not produce faster or thicker growth or increased predisposition to neoplastic change.

GENERALIZED HYPERTRICHOSIS

Generalized hypertrichosis may be associated with nervous system disorders (postencephalitic hypertrichosis, multiple sclerosis), anorexia nervosa, Hurler's syndrome, the Cornelia de Lange syndrome, and hypertrichosis lanuginosa. Other disorders that may be associated with hypertrichosis include acrodynia, hypothyroidism, porphyria, POEMS (or PEP) syndrome,[65] dermatomyositis in some children, gross malnutrition, and various forms of drug-induced hypertrichosis.

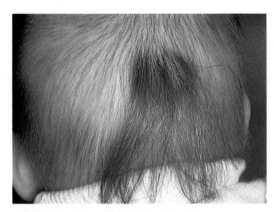

Figure 17–34. Nevoid circumscribed hypertrichosis. A congenital growth of thicker, darker, and longer hairs is seen on the occipital scalp of a 4-month-old infant.

Drug-induced hypertrichosis may be seen following the administration of phenytoin (usually after 2 or 3 months of treatment); hexachlorobenzene, as in the classic epidemic of drug-induced porphyria cutanea tarda in Turkey (see Chapter 4); occasionally following the systemic use of testosterone propionate, streptomycin, cortisone, diazoxide, minoxidil, cyclosporine, or penicillamine; or in association with hyperpigmentation in some individuals treated with systemic psoralens and ultraviolet light exposure.

IDIOPATHIC HIRSUTISM

The terms *heterosexual* and *idiopathic hirsutism* are used to describe the presence in females of excessive body hair in a male sexual pattern (the face, particularly the upper lip, chest, abdomen, arms, and legs) in the absence of clinical evidence of disturbed endocrine or metabolic function. Unaccompanied by other physical signs or symptoms, idiopathic hirsutism is assumed to be related to increased stimulation of the hair follicles of genetically predisposed females by normal levels of androgenic hormones.

The incidence of hirsutism in any population is difficult to assess, since the range of normal is quite wide, subject to individual acceptance, and includes that which is not always socially acceptable in a particular culture. Latin, Jewish, and Welsh women in general have more hair than their counterparts of Northern European, Japanese, and Indian heritage. In such cases the physician should be cognizant as to what is normal and acceptable to some individuals, yet unacceptable and a source of anguish to others.

A detailed history and thorough physical examination will help the physician decide whether a full endocrinologic investigation is indicated. When hirsutism is observed in a postpubertal female without other signs of masculinity (receding hairline, deepening of the voice, or evidence of menstrual disturbance) there is little likelihood of endocrine disease. When the disorder does not appear to be physiologic, abnormalities of the pituitary, adrenals, and ovaries must be ruled out. Of these, ovarian tumors and the adrenogenital, Cushing, Stein-Leventhal (polycystic ovary), and Achard-Thiers (diabetes, hypertension, and hirsutism in women) syndromes are the most frequently implicated. If endocrine abnormality is suspected, minimal laboratory testing for excessive androgen production should include urinary 17-ketosteroids, free plasma testosterone, dehydro-epiandrosterone sulfate levels, and morning and evening cortisol levels; at times, luteinizing hormone and follicle-stimulating hormone ratios and pelvic ultrasound (to rule out small ovarian cysts) may be useful.

Once endocrine or local factors have been ruled out, there are several ways in which the appearance of excessive hair may be modified. Cutting with a scissors or shaving with a razor or electric shaver, although occasionally not psychologically acceptable to the patient, are the simplest methods and least likely to irritate the skin, and bleaching by a 6 per cent hydrogen peroxide solution (20 volume peroxide) or a commercial bleach may be used to render the objectionable hair less conspicuous. Contrary to a popular misconception, there is no evidence that cutting, plucking, or shaving leads to neoplastic potential or increases the growth or coarseness of hair.

Gentle rubbing with a pumice stone will help remove fine hairs. Plucking or wax epilation (essentially a form of widespread plucking) by application of a warm wax preparation to the affected areas, although slightly uncomfortable, is effective but may at times distort the follicles, thereby making electrolysis more difficult. Depilatories consist of sulfides of alkali metals or alkaline earths or of thioglycolate-containing agents that destroy the projecting hair shafts by degradation of disulfide bonds. Of these, the sulfide-containing prepara-

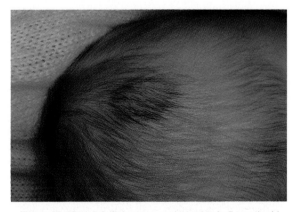

Figure 17–35. Hair follicle nevus on the scalp of a 7-month-old child. Histologic examination of a cutaneous punch biopsy specimen can differentiate this benign hair follicle hamartoma from a congenital pigmented hairy nevus.

tions are more effective, but more irritating, and produce a disagreeable hydrogen sulfide odor. The thioglycolate-containing agents are less irritating but slower in action and less effective on coarse hairs.

Electrolysis is a tedious procedure and, even in the best of hands, one can expect up to 25 per cent regrowth. Although not all patients with excessive facial hair are suitable candidates and overaggressive electrolysis may produce perceptible scarring, when done carefully by knowledgeable individuals this procedure generally offers a satisfactory approach.

Drugs used to control hirsutism are best administered under the guidance of a gynecologist or endocrinologist. These include oral contraceptives, preferably ones containing 35 to 50 mg of estrogen (ethinyl estradiol), even if androgen levels are not elevated (but they must be administered early to increase the chances of success); low-dose prednisone (5 mg/day) or dexamethasone (0.5 mg/day); cyproterone acetate, 50 to 100 mg/day (available in Europe) with ethinyl estradiol (0.5 mg/day); spironolactone in doses of 50 to 200 mg/day; or cimetidine (300 mg, five times a day).[66]

Eruptive Vellus Hair Cysts

Eruptive vellus hair cysts are characterized by 1- to 2-mm skin-colored to variably pigmented follicular papules, most commonly on the anterior chest, but in some instances on the upper and lower extremities, face, neck, abdomen, axillae, posterior trunk and/or buttocks. Although usually seen in children between 4 and 18 years of age, these cysts can occur at any age. The lesions are soft and sharply demarcated and may be skin colored, yellow, blue, red, or hyperpigmented; although a follicular orientation is common, there is usually no tendency to grouping. Most of the lesions are smooth surfaced with a round or domed shape, but central puncta, umbilication, and hyperkeratotic crusts have been noted. Although the etiology has not been proved, an autosomal dominant developmental abnormality of the vellus hair follicles, predisposing them to occlusion at their infundibular level, has been hypothesized as the cause of this disorder.[67] The histologic picture of eruptive vellus hair cysts is characterized by small, mid to upper dermal keratinizing cysts filled with lamellar keratin and small-diameter nonpigmented or lightly pigmented hair shafts. Although spontaneous resolution is the rule, this generally takes place within a few months to years but may at times take much longer. Patients desiring therapy can be treated by incision of individual cysts and expression of their contents followed by gentle curettage, light electrodesiccation, therapy with topical vitamin A acid (tretinoin, Retin-A) or lactic acid (Lac-Hydrin 12 per cent lotion), and carbon dioxide laser vaporization.[68–70]

Pigmentary Changes of Hair

PREMATURE GRAYING

Graying of human hair is caused by a reduction in the activity of melanocytes within hair follicles. Premature graying of hair, termed *canities*, refers to a loss of color, especially of scalp hair, at an age earlier than that generally accepted as physiologic (before the age of 20 in whites and 30 in blacks). It may be seen as an early sign of pernicious anemia and in hyperthyroidism and other thyroid disorders, progeria, Werner's disease, Rothmund-Thomson disease, vitiligo, alopecia areata, poliosis, tuberous sclerosis, neurofibromatosis, and the Waardenburg and Vogt-Koyanagi syndromes.

Premature graying may be readily masked, if desired, by chemical rinses and dyes. Since the possibility of carcinogenesis or chromosomal damage due to chemical hair dyes has been suggested, the possibility of this risk may be avoided by the use of vegetable dyes.

GREEN DISCOLORATION

The spontaneous appearance of green discoloration in the hair of light haired individuals may occur as a result of exposure to copper used as an algae-retardant in swimming pools, copper exposure in industry, or household tap water containing excesssive amounts of copper.[71, 72] In patients with copper tinting of hair from household plumbing, the introduction of fluoride into a town water supply (thus acidifying the water and causing copper to be leached from the plumbing system) or a ground wire connecting a faulty electrical apparatus to the copper water pipes (thus diverting sufficient flow of electric current through the water system to dissolve copper) has been implicated as a possible cause of this condition.

Knowledgeable swimming pool owners and swimming enthusiasts are often aware of this problem. In such cases, the use of a copper-based algicide should be discontinued. In cases related to household tap water, electrical grounding of household plumbing and adjustment of the pH of the tap water will help prevent recurrences. Copper-induced discoloration of the hair can be treated by topical application of a chelating agent containing EDTA (edetic acid, Melatex), a product sold as a reconditioner for hairs that have been discolored by overexposure to the sun, application of an aqueous solution of 1.5 per cent 1-hydroxyethyl diphosphonic acid, or a penicillamine-containing shampoo followed by a non-copper-containing water rinse.[73–75]

NAILS

The nails are convex horny structures originating from a matrix that develops from a groove formed by epidermal invagination on the dorsum of the distal phalanges at 9 weeks' gestation. At 10 weeks' gestation a smooth shiny quadrangular area can be recognized on the distal dorsal surface of each digit, and formation is completed by 20 weeks' gestation. While the nail plate is translucent and essentially colorless, most of the exposed nail appears pink as the result of transmission of color from the adherent richly vascular underlying nail bed. Usually in the thumbs, and in a variable number of digits, a white crescent-shaped lunula may be seen projecting from under the proximal nail folds. The white color of the lunula is believed to be the result of incomplete keratinzation of this portion of the nail plate and the looseness of the underlyng connective tissue in this region of the nail bed.

Unlike hairs, the nails grow continuously throughout life and normally are not shed. Although the nails of individual fingers grow at different rates, the normal rate of growth of fingernails varies between 0.5 and 1.2 mm (approximately 1.0 mm) per week; the rate of toenail growth is one-third to one-half that of the fingernails. Many dermatoses that characteristically involve the skin and hair may also affect the nails. These include disorders such as eczema, psoriasis, lichen planus, Darier's disease, alopecia areata, onychomycosis, ectodermal dysplasia, dyskeratosis congenita, and epidermolysis bullosa.

Congenital and Hereditary Diseases

Atrophic nails range from complete absence of the nail to nails that are poorly or partially developed. They frequently result from generalized congenital disorders but also may develop as the result of trauma, infection, or acquired cutaneous conditions.

MEDIAN NAIL DYSTROPHY

Median nail dystrophy (dystrophia unguium mediana canaliformis) (Fig. 17–36) is an uncommon temporary nail disorder in which a split or canal-like dystrophy develops in one or more nails, usually those of the thumb. Often described as having an inverted fir tree or Christmas tree appearance, with feathery cracks extending laterally from the split outward but not reaching the nail edge, the cause is unknown but appears to be related to a temporary defect in the matrix that interferes with nail formation. The split occurs at the cuticle, generally slightly off the midline, and proceeds outward as the nail grows. The disorder may at times improve spontaneously after a period of several years, and other than avoidance of trauma there is no effective treatment for this disorder.

FRAGILE NAILS

Fragile, britttle, or split nails (fragilitas unguium) are a common complaint of children (par-

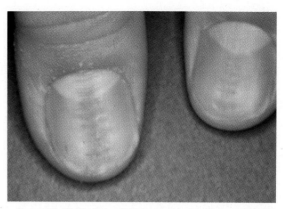

Figure 17–36. Median nail dystrophy (dystrophia unguium mediana canaliformis). In this uncommon disorder a canal-like dystrophy develops in one or more nails.

ticularly adolescent girls) and women (frequently housewives who often have their hands in soap and water). There is evidence that the underlying defect is an architectural abnormality that frequently is aggravated by excessive manicuring and the frequent use of solvents to remove nail polish. Although gelatin administration (Knox gelatin, one envelop daily, mixed with water, juice, or some other beverage) or other forms of gelatin (such as those available in capsule forms) have been recommended, there is no evidence that this form of therapy helps the disorder. Since nail brittleness results from dehydration, nail polish removers are particularly damaging. The regular use of a moisturizer or emollient hand cream to the nail and its cuticles, the avoidance of excessive manipulation, and the use of several layers of nail polish in an effort to splint the nail, with avoidance of all but oily polish removers, although not curative, appear to be somewhat beneficial.

CONGENITAL MALALIGNMENT OF THE GREAT TOENAILS

Congenital malalignment of the great toenails, a cause of onychogryphosis and ingrown toenail, is characterized by lateral rotation of the nail matrix, a lateral deviation of the great toenail from the longitudinal axis of the distal phalanx, and, at times, thickening, discoloration, and shortening of the nail plate. Believed to be an autosomal dominantly inherited disorder or perhaps an acquired or intrauterine malformation, although spontaneous improvement has been reported, the disorder can be treated by surgical realignment of the nail into its proper position, often with the use of local anesthesia, preferably before age 2 years.[76, 77]

TWENTY-NAIL DYSTROPHY

Twenty-nail dystrophy is an idiopathic disorder characterized by dystrophy of all 20 nails that begins most commonly but not exclusively in early

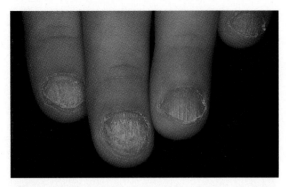

Figure 17–37. Twenty-nail dystrophy. Opalescent discoloration, excessive ridging, and longitudinal striations of all 20 nails occurred in childhood.

childhood and becomes less obvious with increasing age (Fig. 17–37). The disorder is characterized by excessive ridging, longitudinal grooves and striations, opalescent discoloration, a rough sandpaper-like quality of the nails (trachyonychia), a tendency toward breakage and fragmentation (onychorrhexis), and splitting at the free margins. Congenital, familial, and hereditary cases have been described in both children and adults, and the disorder has been regarded by various authors as a distinct clinical entity or a manifestation of a number of other clinical entities, such as lichen planus, psoriasis, or alopecia areata.[78–80] Since twenty-nail dystrophy is generally self-limiting, treatment, other than regular manicuring and perhaps application of a nail lacquer to improve the appearance, is often unnecessary and unrewarding.

NAIL-PATELLA SYNDROME

The nail-patella syndrome, also termed the *nail-patella-elbow syndrome* or *osteo-onychodysplasia*, is characterized by the absence or hypoplasia of the patella and nails, subluxation of the radial heads, and, in some pedigrees, renal dysplasia, which presents as a chronic glomerulonephritis (Fig. 17–38). Other bone features include thickened scapulae, hyperextendable joints, and iliac horns. It is inherited as an autosomal dominant disorder of variable expressivity, with high penetrance and linkage between the loci controlling the syndrome and ABO blood groups.[81]

The nail dystrophy may vary from nothing more than a triangular lunula, especially of the thumbs and index fingers, to moderate to severe dysplasia of the medial and distal aspects of the index and thumb nails; occasionally nails of other fingers and sometimes the toes may also be affected. The nail changes, seen in 98 per cent of affected patients, consist of triangle-shaped lunulae, softening, spooning, discoloration, central grooving, splitting and cracking, narrowing, and less commonly, thickening.[82] The thumbnails and great toenails, and occasionally the nails of the index fingers, are

the most severely affected, often with severe hypoplasia or partial or total absence of the nails of the thumbs and index fingers. The remaining nails, if involved, are progressively damaged, from index to little finger, and the hands show symmetrical nail involvement.

The renal involvement has been reported in up to 42 per cent of patients with this disorder.[83] Patients with renal lesions are asymptomatic and show proteinuria, reduced renal clearance, and hematuria. Although many affected individuals with this complication do well, the prognosis remains guarded.

PACHYONYCHIA CONGENITA

Pachyonychia congenita (the Jadassohn-Lewandowsky syndrome) is an unusual congenital and sometimes familial disorder, usually inherited in an autosomal dominant fashion with high penetrance and variable expressivity, characterized by dyskeratosis of the fingernails and toenails, hyperkeratosis of the palms and soles, follicular keratosis (especially about the knees and elbows), hyperhidrosis of the palms and soles, and oral leukokeratosis. Frequently not all features of the disorder are present in affected individuals and an autosomal recessive form and a variant with cutaneous amyloidosis and hyperpigmentation have also been described.[84–86]

Finger and toenail changes, usually present at birth or during the first year of life, consist of thickened, tubular, and hard nails, the undersurface being filled with a horny, yellowish brown material that causes the nail to project upward from the nail bed at the free margin (Fig. 17–39). Paronychial inflammation and recurrent loss or shedding of nails are common.

Hyperhidrosis of the palms and soles nearly always occurs, and the rest of the skin is frequently quite dry and often described as ichthyotic. Hyper-

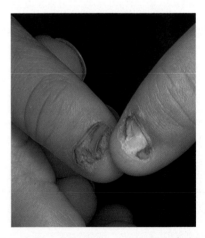

Figure 17–38. Nail-patella syndrome (osteo-onychodysplasia). Triangular-shaped lunulae are seen along with severe dystrophy of the thumb nail.

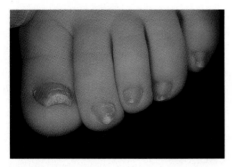

Figure 17–39. Pachyonychia congenita. Note thickened, tubular hard nails with subungual keratin and upward projection of the distal portion of the nail plate.

keratosis of the palms and soles, seen in up to 65 per cent of cases, generally appears during the first few years of life. Bullae frequently appear, particularly during warm weather, on the toes, heels, sides of the feet, and occasionally palms.

Pinhead-sized grayish black follicular papules appear in over 50 per cent of cases in areas of trauma, on the extensor surfaces of the extremities, and on the popliteal fossae, lumbar region, and buttocks, and less commonly on the face and scalp. The hair is frequently noted to be dry; and when the follicular papules are numerous, alopecia has been seen in association with this disorder. In some cases there may be malformation of the teeth manifested by natal teeth with poor dentition.

Early oral lesions are frequently present in the form of opaque white or grayish white plaques (leukokeratosis) on the dorsum of the tongue or the buccal mucosa at the interdental line or as neonatal teeth. Less frequently associated findings include cheilitis, scrotal tongue, corneal dystrophy, hoarseness, and steatocystoma multiplex, which is manifested as large epidermal cysts of the head, neck, and upper chest (a complication not readily evident until puberty).

The differential diagnosis includes the hereditary mucosal syndromes that produce leukokeratotic lesions of the oral mucosa. Of these, dyskeratosis congenita and Darier's disease, in particular, should be ruled out. The characteristic nail changes and associated findings generally allow proper identification of this disorder. Histopathologic examination of the leukokeratotic oral lesions shows thickening of the oral epithelium and extensive intracellular vacuolization, similar to that seen in the white sponge nevus.

Subungual hyperkeratosis persists for life, and treatment is directed toward relief of the hyperkeratosis by the use of oral vitamin A in large doses (potentially toxic and not universally successful); 20 per cent urea in an emollient cream, available as Ureacin Creme (Pedinol Pharmacal); 60 per cent propylene glycol in water under occlusion; 6 per cent salicylic acid in a gel containing propylene glycol (Keralyt gel); or 10 per cent salicylic acid or urea in petrolatum followed by occlusion (which

aids in the débridement of the excessive keratin); and trimming of the nails with professional nail clippers. As a last resort, surgical avulsion and matrix destruction followed by scarification of the nail bed to prevent regrowth can be done.

Other Nail Dystrophies

HABIT-TIC DYSTROPHY

Injuries to the base of the nail and nail matrix may result in longitudinal ridging or splitting of the nail. A common form of nail injury is that caused by a habit or tic. Habit-tic dystrophy is caused by continuous picking of the nail cuticle of the affected digit with a finger (usually the index finger) of the same hand and is generally characterized by a depression down the center of a nail with numerous horizontal ridges extending across it (Fig. 17–40).

BEAU'S LINES

Beau's lines are transverse grooves or furrows that originate under the proximal nail fold (Fig. 17–41). They develop as a nonspecific reaction to any stress that temporarily interrupts nail formation and become visible on the surface of the nail plate several weeks or more after onset of the disease that caused the condition. They first appear at the cuticle and move forward with the growth of the nail; and since normal nails grow at a rate of approximately 1 mm per week, the duration and time of the illness frequently can be estimated by the width of the furrow and its distance from the cuticle. In addition, Beau's lines may also appear in infants, probably as a result of birth trauma. These grow out at about 4 weeks of age, leaving a

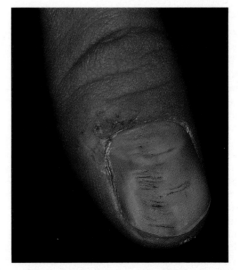

Figure 17–40. Habit-tic dystrophy. Depression and horizontal ridging of the thumbnail are caused by a continuous picking habit of the nail cuticle.

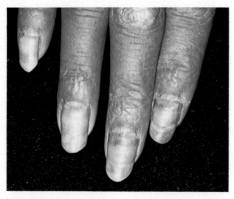

Figure 17–41. Beau's lines. Transverse grooves originate under the nail plate and move forward with the growth of the nail (this was caused by drug-induced toxic epidermal necrolysis). (Courtesy of Department of Dermatology, Yale University School of Medicine.)

normal nail by the time the infant reaches the age of 4 months.

ONYCHOGRYPHOSIS

Onychogryphosis is a hypertrophic nail deformity most commonly seen in the toenails. Some cases of nail hypertrophy are developmental, the nails becoming thick and circular in cross section instead of flat (thus resembling a claw). In more severe forms of onychogryphosis one or more nails become grossly thickened, and with failure to cut the nails frequently and at regular intervals, increase in length results in a curved ram's horn type of deformity (Fig. 17–42). Management requires regular paring or trimming and, when severe, treatment by a podiatrist using files, nail clippers, or mechanical burrs.

SPOON NAIL

Spoon nail (koilonychia) is a common deformity in which the normal contour of the nail is lost. The nail is thin, depressed, and concave from side to side, with turned-up distal and lateral edges. Often a congenital or hereditary disorder, this condition is occasionally associated with the Plummer-Vinson syndrome (a disorder of middle-aged women characterized by dysphagia, glossitis, hypochromic anemia, and spoon nails). Although hypochromic anemia occasionally does predispose to this disorder, this relationship is probably exaggerated, and in some cases spoon nails may persist into adult life without any evidence of associated disease. Other causes include psoriasis, lichen planus, trichothiodystrophy, pachyonychia congenita, focal dermal hypoplasia, hypohidrotic ectodermal dysplasia, local trauma (seen in rickshaw boys), and, at times, habitual trauma associated with frequent water immersion and walking barefoot.[87]

RACKET NAIL

The term *racket nail* refers to an abnormality of the thumbs in which the phalanx is shorter and wider than normal. The nail is correspondingly short, wide, and fatter than normal, and there is loss of curvature (Fig. 17–43). This disorder is dominantly inherited, may be bilateral or unilateral, and is more common in females than in males.

ONYCHOLYSIS

Onycholysis refers to separation of the nail plate from the underlying hyponychium. The disorder may be seen in patients with psoriasis, atopic dermatitis, lichen planus, congenital abnormalities, trauma, infection, hyperthyroidism or hypothyroidism, pregnancy, porphyria, pellagra, syphilis, and tetracycline-induced photo-onycholysis (see Fig. 6–17).

ONYCHOMADESIS

As result of temporary arrest of the function of the nail matrix, onychomadesis (proximal separation of the nail) has been described in patients with penicillin anaphylaxis, keratosis punctata palmaris et plantaris, pemphigus vulgaris, and epidermolysis bullosa and as a possible complication of carbamazepine therapy.[88]

Ingrown Nails

Ingrown toenails are a common disorder in which the lateral edge of the nail is curved inward and penetrates the underlying tissue, with resulting erythema, edema, pain, and in chronic forms,

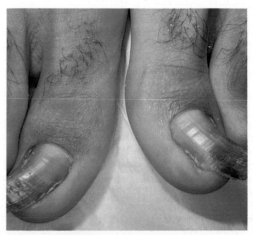

Figure 17–42. Onychogryphosis. In this hypertrophic nail deformity the nails become thick and circular in cross section. Failure to cut the nails at regular intervals frequently results in a curved ram's horn deformity.

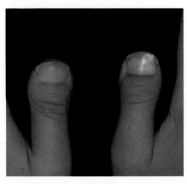

Figure 17–43. Racket nails. The distal phalanx is shorter and wider than that of a normal thumb. The nail is correspondingly short and wide, with a loss of normal curvature.

the formation of granulation tissue. Generally seen on the great toes of affected individuals, the main cause of the deformity is compression of the toe from side to side by ill-fitting footwear and improper cutting of the nail (in a half-circle rather than straight across). Ingrown toenails, also seen as a transient deformity in newborns, are a common phenomenon and are generally self-corrected by the time the child reaches the age of 12 months.[89] The treatment of ingrown toenails, other than the transient congenital form of the disorder that requires no therapy, consists of the wearing of properly fitting footwear, allowing the nail to grow out beyond the free edge, control of acute infection by compresses, topical and, at times, systemic antibiotics, and in many instances (once the infection has subsided) surgical treatment. In recurring cases, excision of the lateral aspect of the nail with the use of local anesthesia followed by curettage or chemical destruction of the nail matrix with liquid phenol will prevent regrowth of the offending portion of the nail.

Disorders of Pigmentation

Abnormal nail pigmentation may be seen in systemic diseases or in association with the ingestion of various chemicals or medications.

Brown pigmentation of nails may be associated with the ingestion of phenolphthalein, as a reaction to antimalarials, minocycline, or gold therapy, or as a manifestation of Addison's disease. In argyria the lunulae show a distinctive slate blue discoloration, and in hepatolenticular degeneration (Wilson's disease) the lunulae may present an azure blue discoloration. Lithium carbonate can cause brownish black transverse bands at the margins of the lunulae,[90] and pigmentation in the form of transverse bands has been reported in patients receiving idovidine, bleomycin, and doxorubicin (Adriamycin).[91] Gray or blue-gray nails can occur in individuals with ochronosis or argyria or as a

reaction to quinacrine (Atabrine) or phenolphthalein. Brown-black pigmentation of the nail fold and nail matrix can be seen as a sign of melanoma of the nail bed (Hutchinson's sign), Addison's disease, and Peutz-Jeghers syndrome. When a green discoloration is seen in association with onycholysis, *Pseudomonas aeruginosa* infection must be considered.

Red lunulae can be seen in patients with alopecia areata, lupus erythematosus, dermatomyositis, congestive heart failure, reticulosarcoma, psoriasis, carbon monoxide poisoning, twenty-nail dystrophy, and lymphogranuloma venereum.[92] When the distal 1- 2 mm portion of the nail has a normal pink color and the rest of the nail has a white appearance, the disorder has been termed *Terry's nails.* Seen in patients with cirrhosis, chronic congestive heart failure, adult-onset diabetes, and POEMS syndrome,[65] Terry's nails may also be seen in normal children younger than 4 years of age, in the very elderly, and at times in normal individuals without evidence of cirrhosis or other systemic disease.

The term *leukonychia* (white nails) is used to describe a disorder in which a portion or all of the nail becomes white (Fig. 17–44). The white color may be seen as punctate, leukonychia striata (believed to be due to local trauma such as might be seen from frequent or excessive manipulation or grooming techniques) (Fig. 17–45) or superficial onchomycosis; as paired narrow white bands (seen in patients with cirrhosis and hypoalbuminemia); as transverse 1- to 2-mm white bands (Mees' bands), suggestive of arsenic or heavy metal poisoning, septicemia, dissecting aortic aneurysm, and renal failure; as white transverse bands in the nail bed occurring in pairs (Muehrcke's nails) as a sign of hypoalbuminemia; or as the half-and-half nail, a disorder characteristic of renal disease and azotemia in which the proximal nail bed is white and the distal half is red, pink, or brown (Lindsay's nails).

The yellow nail syndrome is a disorder associated with severe long-term lymphedema and, at times, chronic bronchitis, bronchiectasis, intersti-

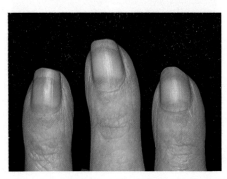

Figure 17–44. Leukonychia (white nails) in a patient with hepatic cirrhosis.

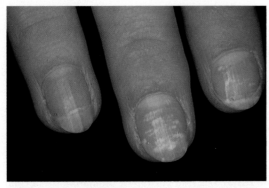

Figure 17–45. Leukonychia striata. Punctate white discoloration of the nails caused by local trauma (excessive manipulation and grooming techniques).

tial pneumonitis, pleural effusion, persistent hypoalbuminemia, thyroid disease, immunologic deficiencies, lymphoreticular malignancy, rheumatoid arthritis, lupus erythematosus, Hodgkin's or Raynaud's disease, mental retardation, and the nephrotic syndrome. Most often a phenomenon of middle-aged individuals, but also described in young children, it is characterized by a pale yellow or greenish yellow to brown discoloration of the nails associated with slow growth, thickening and excessive curvature from side to side (on its long axis), increased hardness, onycholysis, or spontaneous shedding of the nails; absence of lunulae and cuticles; and swelling of the periungual tissues, as might be seen in patients with chronic paronychia (Fig. 17–46). Although the nail changes, once established, are usually permanent, oral and topical vitamin E have been reported to be effective in some individuals and complete spontaneous reversion to normal may occur at times.[93,94]

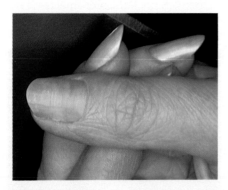

Figure 17–46. Yellow nail syndrome. A yellowish discoloration of the nails associated with slow growth, thickening, excessive curvature, and an absence of lunulae and cuticles, as seen in patients with lymphedema, bronchitis, pleural effusion, hypoalbuminemia, and at times other disorders.

References

1. Saadat M, Khan M, Gutberlet RL, et al.: Measure of hair in normal newborns. Pediatrics 57:960–962, 1976.

   Studies of morphology and physiology of hair roots and hair shafts in 63 newborns.

2. Rook A, Dawber R: Diseases of the Hair and Scalp. Blackwell Scientific Publishers, Oxford, England, 1982.

   A comprehensive overview of hair and scalp disorders in infants, children, and adults.

3. Kligman AM: Pathologic dynamics of human hair loss: I. Telogen effluvium. Arch. Dermatol. 83:175–198, 1961.

   A review of the dynamics of hair growth and the general problems encountered in analysis of hair loss.

4. Tosti A: Congenital triangular alopecia: Report of fourteen cases. J. Am. Acad. Dermatol. 16:991–993, 1987.

   The clinical and histologic features of congenital triangular alopecia in 14 patients.

5. Jones KL: Smith's Recognizable Patterns of Human Malformation, 4th ed. W.B. Saunders Co., Philadelphia, 1988.

   A comprehensive update of David W. Smith's textbook on dysmorphogenesis.

6. Solomon LM, Esterly NB, Medenica M: Hereditary trichodysplasia: Marie-Unna's hypertrichosis. J. Invest. Dermatol. 57:389–400, 1971.

   Light and electron microscopic findings in patients with Marie-Unna hypotrichosis (hereditary trichodysplasia).

7. Solomon LM, Fretzin D, Pruzansky S: Pilosebaceous dysplasia in the oral-facial-digital syndrome. Arch. Dermatol. 102:598–602, 1970.

   Eight female patients with oral-facial-digital syndrome type I and delineation of the cutaneous features of this disorder.

8. Brennan TE, Pearson RW: Abnormal elastic tissue in cartilage-hair hypoplasia. Arch. Dermatol. 124:1411–1414, 1988.

   A 29-year-old white Amish woman with cartilage-hair hypoplasia was found to have abnormal dermal elastic fibers, hypermobile digits of the hands, and hyperextensible skin.

9. Hurwitz S: Hair disorders. In Schachner LA, Hansen RC (Eds.): Pediatric Dermatology. Churchill Livingstone, New York, 1988, 575–613.

   A review of hair disorders in infants and children.

10. O'Brien R, Zelson JH, Schwartz AO, et al.: Scalp tourniquet to lessen alopecia after vincristine. N. Engl. J. Med. 238:1496, 1970.

    A simple tourniquet technique to prevent alopecia in children treated with intravenous vincristine therapy.

11. Galbraith GMP, Thiers BH, Vasily DB, et al.: Immunological profiles in alopecia areata. Br. J. Dermatol. 110:163–170, 1984.

    Cell-mediated and autoimmune phenomena in 60 patients with alopecia areata offer support, at least in part, for an immunologic basis for some patients with this disorder.

12. Perret CM, Stijlen PM, Happle R: Alopecia areata: Pathogenesis and topical immunotherapy. Int. J. Dermatol. 29:83–88, 1990.

    An authoritative review of alopecia areata supporting an autoimmune pathogenesis and a discussion of topical immunotherapy with diphenylcyclopropenone (diphencyprone) and squaric acid dibutylester.

13. Pascher F, Kurtin S, Andrade R: Assay of 0.2 per cent fluocinolone acetonide cream for alopecia areata and totalis. Dermatologica 141:193–202, 1970.

    Paired comparisons of fluorinated corticosteroid and a blank vehicle applied topically on opposite areas of the scalp in patients with alopecia areata and alopecia totalis revealed a satisfactory response to therapy in 17 of 28 patients.

14. Montes LF: Topical halcinonide in alopecia areata and alopecia totalis. J. Cutan. Pathol. *4*:47–50, 1977.

Dramatic results in 10 patients with alopecia areata treated twice daily with topical applications of halcinonide cream in a 0.1 per cent concentration with and without occlusion.

15. Abell E, Munro DD: Intralesional treatment of alopecia areata with triamcinolone acetonide by jet injector. Br. J. Dermatol. *88*:55–59, 1973.

Of 84 patients treated by intradermal corticosteroid injection, 71 per cent of patients with limited alopecia and 28 per cent of those with extensive alopecia achieved hair regrowth in 12 weeks.

16. Fiedler VC: Alopecia areata: Current therapy. J. Invest. Dermatol. *96*:69s–70s, 1991.

An overview of currently available therapeutic agents for the management of alopecia areata.

17. Kern F, Hoffman WH, Hambrick GW Jr, et al.: Alopecia areata, immunologic studies and treatment with prednisone. Arch. Dermatol. *107*:407–412, 1973.

Twenty-seven patients with alopecia areata who received alternate-day corticosteroid therapy demonstrated a significant hair growth and relatively few adverse effects.

18. Unger WP, Schemmer RJ: Corticosteroids in the treatment of alopecia totalis: Systemic effects. Arch. Dermatol. *114*:1486–1490, 1978.

Seven of 15 patients with alopecia totalis or alopecia universalis treated with a combination of topical, intralesional, and oral corticosteroids with relatively insignificant side effects regrew all or virtually all of their scalp hair and were able to discontinue oral corticosteroids without recurrence of the alopecia for 3 months to 7 1/2 years.

19. Happle R: The potential hazards of dinitrochlorobenzene. Arch. Dermatol. *121*:330–331, 1985.

An editorial on dinitrochlorobenzene (DNCB), a potent contact allergen, recommends that DNCB be abandoned for the treatment of recalcitrant warts and extensive alopecia areata until a lack of mutagenicity has been demonstrated.

20. Fiedler-Weis VC, Buys CM: Evaluation of anthralin in the treatment of alopecia areata. Arch. Dermatol. *123*:1491–1493, 1987.

A cosmetic response in 25 per cent of 68 patients with alopecia areata treated with 0.5 to 1.0 per cent anthralin cream suggests that this modality may be effective for many individuals with persistent forms of this disorder.

21. Case PC, Mitchell AJ, Swanson NA, et al.: Topical therapy of alopecia areata with squaric acid dibutylester. J. Am. Acad. Dermatol. *10*:447–451, 1984.

In a study of 21 patients with alopecia areata treated with squaric acid dibutylester, 52 per cent had good results. Complete hair regrowth occurred in 6, and 5 had cosmetically acceptable regrowth.

22. Kietzmann H, Hardung H, Christophers E: Treatment of alopecia areata with diphenylcyclopropenone. Hautartz *36*:331–335, 1985.

Diphenycyclopropenone was successful in the regrowth of hair in 17 of 20 patients with alopecia areata.

23. Weiss VC, West DP, Fu TS, et al.: Alopecia areata treated with topical minoxidil. Arch. Dermatol. *120*:457–476, 1984.

Although 25 of 48 patients (24 with patchy alopecia areata and 24 with alopecia totalis or universalis) developed terminal hair growth within 2 to 15 months following twice-a-day applicatons of 1 per cent minoxidil solution, only 11 of the 25 experienced cosmetically acceptable regrowth.

24. Galbraith GMP, Thiers BH, Jensen J, et al.: A randomized double-blind study of inosiplex (Isoprinosine) therapy in pa-

tients with alopecia totalis. J. Am. Acad. Dermatol. *16*:977–983, 1987.

In a trial of inosiplex therapy for alopecia totalis of at least 1 year's duration, 11 of 25 patients showed a clinical response to this modality.

25. Claudy AL, Gagnaire D: PUVA treatment of alopecia areata. Arch. Dermatol. *119*:975–978, 1983.

Eleven of 17 patients with multiple patches of alopecia areata, alopecia totalis, or alopecia universalis treated with oral methoxsalen and UVA therapy had complete or more than 90 per cent hair regrowth.

26. Beard HO: Social and psychological implications of alopecia areata. J. Am. Acad. Dermatol. *14*:697–700, 1986.

The social and psychological effects of alopecia areata on the lives of children, teenagers, and adults.

27. Wiles JC, Hansen RC: Postoperative (pressure) alopecia. J. Am. Acad. Dermatol. *12*:195–198, 1985.

A report of three patients with postoperative pressure alopecia that apparently resulted from pressure-induced ischemia during surgery.

28. Cooperman SM: Two new causes of alopecia. J.A.M.A. *252*:336, 1984.

A report of two young men with occipitoparietal hair loss associated with break dancing and the wearing of wide-strapped heavy head phones while jogging.

29. Dimino-Emme L, Camisa C: Trichotillomania associated with the "Friar Tuck" sign and nail-biting. Cutis *47*:107–110, 1991.

A report of three patients with trichotillomania demonstrating the "tonsure pattern" ("Friar Tuck" sign) and onychophagia (nail-biting), which the authors describe as clinical identifying features of this syndrome.

30. Mehregan AH: Trichotillomania: Clinicopathologic study. Arch. Dermatol. *102*:129–133, 1970.

Clinical and histopathologic features of trichotillomania.

31. Oranje AP, Peereboom-Wynia JDR, De Raeymacker DMJ: Trichotillomania in childhood. J. Am. Acad. Dermatol. *15*:614–619, 1986.

In a review of 21 patients with trichotillomania in children 2 to 15 years of age, 4 patients required psychological assistance.

32. Hurwitz S, McAlleney PF: Trichobezoar in children: Review of the literature and report of two cases. Am. J. Dis. Child. *81*:753–761, 1951.

Two patients with trichobezoars (hairballs), a disorder generally seen in nervous young girls who have an uncontrollable habit of biting or chewing the hair.

33. Savin RC: Use of topical minoxidil in the treatment of male pattern baldness. J. Am. Acad. Dermatol. *16*:696–704, 1987.

In a 12-month double-blind placebo-controlled study of 96 patients with male pattern baldness, 50 per cent of the patients achieved a modest or moderate degree of hair growth.

34. Stern RS: Topical minoxidil: A survey of use and complications. Arch. Dermatol. *123*:62–65, 1987.

In a survey of 900 members of the American Academy of Dermatology, the response rate for cosmetically acceptable hair regrowth for patients with androgenic alopecia treated with topical minoxidil appeared to be less than 25 per cent, probably 15 per cent or less when only those who continued therapy for 1 year or less were considered.

35. Orentreich N: Autografts in alopecias and other selected dermatologic conditions. Ann. N. Y. Acad. Sci. *83*:463–479, 1960.

Multiple punch autografts afford a new approach to the therapy of male pattern and other forms of alopecia.

36. Futterweit W, Dunaif A, Yeh H-C, et al.: The prevalence of

hyperandrogenism in 109 consecutive female patients with diffuse alopecia. J. Am. Acad. Dermatol. *19*:831–836, 1988.

In a study of endocrine function in 109 female patients with moderate to severe alopecia in which 42 per cent demonstrated endocrine dysfunction, the most common endocrine disorder was polycystic ovarian disease.

37. Weigand DA: Androgenic alopecia. In Greer KE: Common Problems in Dermatology. Year Book Medical Publishers, Chicago, 1988, 30–34.

A practical approach to the diagnosis and management of androgenic alopecia in the female.

38. Hamm H, Traupe H: Loose anagen hair of childhood: The phenomenon of easily pluckable hair. J. Am. Acad. Dermatol. *20*:242–248, 1989.

A report of 2 boys with easily pluckable hair, a disorder termed the *loose anagen* or *loose anagen hair syndrome.*

39. Price VH, Gummer CL: Loose anagen syndrome. J. Am. Acad. Dermatol. *20*:249–256, 1989.

A report of 22 children and five adults with a distinctive hair condition in which the hair pulled out easily, did not appear to grow (or grew very slowly), and rarely required cutting.

40. Matuska MA, Weigand DA: Anesthesia in alopecia mucinosa. Cutis *40*:46–47, 1987.

A report of a patient with a solitary hypoanesthetic lesion of alopecia mucinosa.

41. Fahrner LJ, Solomon AR: Persistent papular plaques on the face. Pediatr. Dermatol. *6*:254–255, 1989.

Lesions of alopecia mucinosa on the face of a 2-year-old girl who responded within 4 weeks to a preparation containing equal parts of desonide cream and 0.05 per cent tretinoin cream applied to the affected areas daily at bedtime.

42. Whiting DA: Structural abnormalities of the hair shaft. J. Am. Acad. Dermatol. *16*:1–25, 1988.

A comprehensive review of hair shaft abnormalities and the value of careful hair shaft examination in the evaluation of patients with hair disorders.

43. Menkes JH, Alter M, Steigleder GK, et al.: A sex-linked recessive disorder with retardation of growth, peculiar hair, and focal cerebral and cerebellar degeneration. Pediatrics *29*:764–779, 1962.

The first description of a syndrome characterized by slow growth, progressive cerebral degeneration, pili torti, X-linked inheritance, and death, usually before age 3 years.

44. Danks DM, Campbell PE, Stevens BJ, et al.: Menkes's kinky hair syndrome. An inherited defect in copper absorption with widespread effects. Pediatrics *50*:188–201, 1972.

The recognition of seven patients with Menkes' syndrome born in five families during a 3-year period suggests that this disease is not as rare as believed and that infants with this disorder may die undiagnosed.

45. Bucknall WE, Haslan RHA, Holtzman NA: Kinky hair syndrome: Response to copper therapy. Pediatrics *52*:653–657, 1973.

Failure of clinical response to purified human ceruloplasmin and oral and intravenous copper administration suggests irreversible damage, possibly in utero.

46. Tay CH: Ichthyosiform erythroderma, hair shaft abnormalities and mental and growth retardation: A new recessive disorder. Arch. Dermatol. *104*:4–13, 1971.

Three members of a Chinese famiy with growth retardation, a progeria-like appearance, mental deficiency, nonbullous congenital ichthyosiform erythroderma, and hair shaft abnormalities.

47. Happle R, Traupe H, Grobe H, et al.: The Tay syndrome (congenital ichthyosis with trichothiodystrophy). Eur. J. Pediatr. *141*:147–152, 1984.

A 5-year-old boy with the Tay syndrome and a review of 12 cases previously reported under a different designation.

48. Jorizzo JL, Atherton DJ, Crounse RG, et al.: Ichthyosis, brittle hair, impaired intelligence, decreased fertility, and short stature (IBIDS syndrome). Br. J. Dermatol. *106*:705–710, 1982.

A patient with ichthyosis, brittle hair, intellectual impairment, decreased fertility, and short stature (the IBIDS syndrome).

49. Itin PH, Pittelkow MR: Trichothiodystrophy: Review of sulfur-deficient brittle hair syndromes and association with the ectodermal dysplasias. J. Am. Acad. Dermatol. *22*:707–717, 1990.

A comprehensive review of trichothiodystrophy, its clinical features and frequent association with disorders in organs of ectodermal or neuroectodermal origin.

50. Lucky PA, Kirsch N, Lucky AW, et al.: Low-sulfur hair syndrome associated with UVB photosensitivity and testicular failure. J. Am. Acad. Dermatol. *11*:340–346, 1984.

A report of a patient with low-sulfur brittle hair, mental retardation, deafness, contracture of the fifth finger, UVB-photosensitive dermatitis, and testicular failure suggests that photosensitivity and testicular dysfunction may be seen as important features of the low-sulfur hair syndrome.

51. Rebora A, Crovato F: PIBI(D) syndrome —trichothiodystrophy with xeroderma pigmentosum (group D) mutation. J. Am. Acad. Dermatol. *16*:940–947, 1987.

An autosomal recessive syndrome is described that associates extreme photosensitivity with a defect of the DNA excision repair system, mild congenital ichthyosis, brittle cystine-deficient hair, impaired intelligence, neurologic disorders, and short stature.

52. Price VH, Thomas RS, Jones FT: Pili annulati: Optical and electron microscopic studies. Arch. Dermatol. *96*:640–644, 1968.

Light and electron microscopic studies demonstrate air-filled cavities in affected hair shafts as the cause of the disorder.

53. Price VH, Thomas RS, Jones FT: Pseudopili annulati: An unusual variant of normal hair. Arch. Dermatol.*102*:354–358, 1970.

Pseudopili annulati: Flattened external surfaces of twisted hair shafts act as mirrors and variable cylindrical lenses, which reflect, refract, and focus incidental light on the posterior wall of the hair shaft.

54. Lantis SDH, Pepper MC: Woolly hair nevus: Two case reports and a discussion of unruly hair forms. Arch. Dermatol. *114*:233–238, 1978.

Two case reports of woolly hair nevus with discussion of the features distinguishing this disorder from other types of unruly hair.

55. Peteiro C, Oliva NP, Zulaica A, et al.: Woolly-hair nevus: Report of a case associated with a verrucous epidermal nevus in the same area. Pediatr. Dermatol. *6*:188–190, 1990.

While the association of woolly-hair nevus with a localized or systematized epidermal nevus is not infrequent, this report of their localization in the same site appears to be unique.

56. Matis WL, Baden H, Green R, et al.: Uncombable-hair syndrome. Pediatr. Dermatol. *4*:215–219, 1987.

In a study of four children with short unmanageable pale blond hair, electron microscopic examination of hairs from all children revealed longitudinal grooves in the hair shaft, a finding believed to be diagnostic of the uncombable-hair syndrome.

57. McCullum N, Sperling LC, Vidmar D: The uncombable hair syndrome. Cutis *46*:479–483, 1990.

A report of three children with the uncombable hair syndrome and a comprehensive review of the disorder and its clinical features.

58. Shelley WB, Shelley ED: Uncombable hair syndrome: Observations on response to biotin and occurrence in siblings with ectodermal dysplasia. J. Am. Acad. Dermatol. *13*:97–102, 1985.

Biotin (0.3 mg three times a day) reversed scaling, hair loss, hair fragility, and uncombability of the hair within 4 months in a 2-year-old boy.

59. Esterly NB, Lavin MP, Garancis JC: Acquired progressive kinking of the hair. Arch. Dermatol. *125*:813–815, 1989.

A report of a 14-year-old girl with acquired progressive kinking of the hair.

60. Cullen SI, Fulghum DD: Acquired progressive kinking of the hair. Arch. Dermatol. *125*:252–255, 1989.

A report of three female patients with acquired progressive kinking of the hair (a disorder in which the hair changes are similar to those of woolly hair nevus) and a review of all previously reported cases.

61. Marshall J, Parker C: Felted hair untangled. J. Am. Acad. Dermatol. *20*:688–689, 1989.

A report of a 40-year-old white woman whose hair became extensively tangled immediately after shampooing (the condition improved after 2 1/2 months of daily lubricating of the mass with olive oil and tedious separation of the tangled hairs with a knitting needle).

62. Hegedus SI, Schorr WF: Acquired hypertrichosis lanuginosa and malignancy. Arch. Dermatol. *106*:84–88, 1972.

A review of hypertrichosis lanuginosa and description of two adults displaying the acquired form of this disorder as a cutaneous sign of internal malignancy.

63. Reed OM, Malette JR, Fitzpatrick JR: Familial cervical hypertrichosis with underlying kyphoscoliosis. J. Am. Acad. Dermatol. *20*:1069–1072, 1989.

Report of a 63-year-old woman and four other family members with cervical hypertrichosis and kyphoscoliosis. This, to the authors' knowledge, is the first report of a familial incidence of the faun tail nevus.

64. Pippione M, Aloi F, Depaoli MA: Hair follicle nevus. Am. J. Dermatopathol. *6*:245–247, 1984.

A report of a child with a hair follicle nevus, a benign disorder that at times may be clinically misdiagnosed as a congenital pigmented nevus.

65. Shelley WB, Shelley ED: The skin changes in the Crow-Fukase (POEMS) syndrome; Arch. Dermatol. *123*:85–87, 1987.

Generalized hypertrichosis, hypothyroidism, thickening of the skin, and Terry's nails in a patient with POEMS (or PEP) syndrome; acronyms used to describe individuals with *p*olyneuropathy, *o*rganomegaly, *e*ndocrinopathy, *M*-proteins, and *s*kin changes; or *p*eculiar progressive polyneuritis with pigmentation, *e*dema, and *p*lasma cell dyscrasia.

66. Lucky AW: Hirsutism. In Greer KE (Ed.): Common Problems in Dermatology. Year Book Medical Publishers, Chicago, 1988, 174–184.

A practical approach to the diagnosis and management of hirsutism.

67. Esterly NB, Fretzin DF, Pinkus H: Eruptive vellus hair cysts. Arch. Dermatol. *113*:500–503, 1977.

The term *eruptive vellus hair cysts* was suggested to describe a disorder characterized by papular cystic eruptions in the mid-dermis containing multiple vellus hair shafts.

68. Fisher DA: Retinoic acid in the treatment of eruptive vellus hair cysts. J Am. Acad. Dermatol. *5*:221, 1981.

Topical application of tretinoin solution resulted in resolution of vellus hair cysts that had been present since birth and remained until the time of consultation when the patient was 11 years of age.

69. Hurerter CJ, Wheeland RG: Multiple eruptive vellus hair cysts with carbon dioxide laser vaporization. J. Dermatol. Surg. Oncol. *13*:260–263, 1987.

Eruptive vellus hair cysts on the face of a 46-year-old woman successfully treated with carbon dioxide laser therapy.

70. Mayron R, Grimwood RE: Familial occurrrence of eruptive vellus hair cysts. Pediatr. Dermatol. *5*:94–96, 1988.

A report of a 15-year-old boy with extensive eruptive vellus hair cysts whose father and brother also had similar lesions. The patient's lesions achieved 50 per cent improvement by twice daily topical applications of 12 per cent lactic acid (Lac-Hydrin) within 4 weeks.

71. Lampe RM, Henderson AL, Hansen GH: Green hair. J.A.M.A. *237*:2092, 1977.

A report of two children with green discoloration of the hair acquired from swimming in pools, due to copper, not chlorine.

72. Nordlund JJ, Hartley C, Fister J: On the cause of green hair. Arch. Dermatol. *113*:1700, 1977.

Two postgraduate nursing students with green hair from tap water containing excessive amounts of copper.

73. Goldschmidt H: Green hair. Arch. Dermatol. *115*:1288, 1979.

Green hair was successfully treated with a commercial product containing a chelating agent (EDTA, Melatex), a product sold as a reconditioner for overbleached hairs caused by overexposure to the sun.

74. Melnik BC, Plewig G, Daldrup T, et al.: Green hair: Guidelines for diagnosis and therapy. J. Am. Acad. Dermatol. *15*:1065–1068, 1986.

A 26-year-old woman with green discoloration of her scalp hair was successfully treated by the application of an aqueous solution of 1.5 per cent 1-hydroxyethyl diphosphonic acid.

75. Person JR: Green hair: Treatment with a penicillamine shampoo. Arch. Dermatol. *121*:717–718, 1985.

Since the commercial shampoo containing EDTA was difficult to obtain, a shampoo made by dissolving a 250-mg capsule of penicillamine in 5 ml of water and 5 ml of shampoo was successfully used to remove the green discoloration of the hair of a 20-year old light brunette.

76. Barth JH, Dawber RPR, Ashton RE, et al.: Congenital malalignment of great toe nails in two sets of monozygotic twins. Arch. Dermatol. *122*:379–380, 1986.

A report of two sets of monozygotic twins with congenital malalignment of the great toes appears to confirm the congenital nature of this disorder.

77. Cohen JL, Scher RK, Rappaport AS: Congenital malalignment of the great toenails. Pediatr. Dermatol. *8*:40–42, 1991.

A report of 6-year-old boy and his father with congenital malalignment of the great toenails.

78. Scher RK, Fischbein R, Ackerman AB: Twenty-nail dystrophy: A variant of lichen planus. Arch. Dermatol. *114*:612–613, 1978.

A biopsy of the nail of a 7-year-old boy with twenty-nail dystrophy revealed a microscopic picture of lichen planus.

79. Silverman RA, Rhodes AR: Twenty-nail dystrophy of childhood: A sign of localized lichen planus. Pediatr. Dermatol. *1*:207–210, 1984.

A bipsy of the oral mucosa confirmed a diagnosis of lichen planus in a 9 1/2-year-old-girl with twenty-nail dystrophy.

80. Commens CA: Twenty nail dystrophy in identical twins. Pediatr. Dermatol. *5*:117–119, 1988.

Lifelong twenty-nail dystrophy in 12-year-old identical female twins suggests a localized congenital malformation as one of the causes of this disorder.

81. Lucas GL, Opitz JM: The nail-patella syndrome: Clinical and genetic aspects of five kindreds with 38 affected family members. J. Pediatr. *68*:273–288, 1966.

A review of the nail-patella syndrome, with discussion of the genetic and clinical aspects of this disorder.

82. Daniel CR, III, Osment LS, Noojin RO: Triangular lunulae: A clue to the nail-patella syndrome. Arch. Dermatol. *116*: 448–449, 1980.

A review of nail abnormalities associated with the nail-patella syndrome (NPS) and a reminder that although trauma and various other causes of matrix damage may cause triangular lunulae, the presence of triangular lunulae, especially with a sharp apex pointing distally, should suggest a diagnosis of NPS and prompt the physician to look for other associated abnormalities.

83. Carbonara P, Alpert M: Hereditary osteo-onycho-dysplasia (HOOD). Am. J. Med. Sci. *248*:139–151, 1964.

Review of 60 well-documented and two personal cases of the nail-patella-syndrome (hereditary osteo-onycho-dysplasia).

84. Haber RM, Rose TH: Autosomal recessive pachyonychia congenita. Arch. Dermatol. *122*:919–923, 1986.

Two brothers with pachyonychia congenita from a family of consanguineous parents suggest the presence of an autosomal recessive form of this disorder.

85. Tidman MJ, Wells RS, MacDonald DM: Pachyonychia congenita with cutaneous amyloidosis and hyperpigmentation: A distinct variant. J. Am. Acad. Dermatol. *16*:935–940, 1987.

A report of five cases of pachyonychia congenita from two kindreds manifesting an unusual variant of cutaneous hyperpigmentation resembling macular amyloidosis.

86. Feinstein A, Friedman J, Schewach-Millet M: Pachyonychia congenita. J. Am. Acad. Dermatol. *19*:705–711, 1988.

A comprehensive review of 168 patients with pachyonychia congenita.

87. Yinnon AM, Matalon A: Koilonychia of the toenails in children. Int. J. Dermatol. *27*:685–687, 1988.

A report of koilonychia in 55 of 171 children living on the shore of the Dead Sea suggests that habitual trauma associated with walking barefoot and frequent water immersion can also be a cause of the koilonychia.

88. Mishra D, Singh G, Pandey SS: Possible carbamazepine-induced reversible onychomadesis. Int. J. Dermatol. *28*:460, 1989.

A report of a patient who developed shedding of the finger nails on all fingers and onycholysis of all toenails while on carbamazepine.

89. Honig PJ, Spitzer A, Bernsten R, et al.: Congenital ingrown toenails: Clinical significance. Clin. Pediatr. *21*:424, 1982.

Congenital ingrown toenails are a common disorder that can affect up to 13 per cent of infants and usually self-corrects by the time the child reaches the age of 12 months.

90. Don PC, Silverman RA: Nail dystrophy induced by lithium carbonate. Cutis *41*:19–20, 1988.

A 62-year-old black man treated with lithium carbonate for manic depression developed wide, brownish-black transverse bands on several nails at the margins of the lunulae, followed, 2 weeks later, by transverse ridges proximal to the pigmentation.

91. Giacobetti R, Esterly NB, Morgan ER: Nail hyperpigmentation secondary to therapy with doxorubicin. Am. J. Dis. Child. *135*:317–318, 1981.

Two black children with dense brown pigmentation of the nail plate and transverse dark brown bands on the nail beds associated with chemotherapy with doxorubicin (Adriamycin) given for treatment of osteogenic sarcoma.

92. Wilkerson MG, Wilkin JK: Red lunulae revisited: A clinical and histopathologic examination. J. Am. Acad. Dermatol. *20*:453–457, 1989.

Four patients with red lunulae and a review of potential mechanisms by which this phenomenon can develop.

93. Norton L: Further observations on the yellow nail syndrome with therapeutic effects of oral alpha-tocopherol. Cutis *36*:457–462, 1985.

Oral vitamin E in dosages of 800 to 1200 IU daily for 6 months was associated with clearing of the yellow nail syndrome in four of six patients.

94. Williams HC, Buffham R, du Vivier A: Successful use of topical vitamin E solution in the treatment of nail changes in yellow nail syndrome. Arch. Dermatol. *127*:1023–1028, 1991.

In a double-blind controlled study of a patient with long-standing yellow nail syndrome, marked clinical improvement was noted in nails treated with topical vitamin E in a dimethyl sulfoxide solution.

18

THE HYPERSENSITIVITY SYNDROMES

The hypersensitivity syndromes are a group of disorders mediated by immunologic or hypersensitivity reactions to foreign proteins such as food or drugs; to infectious agents, immunizations, and malignancies; and, in some instances, to other dermatologic conditions. Although diagnosis of these disorders is often relatively easy, difficulties frequently arise in determining the etiology because each entity may be associated with innumerable underlying factors.

ALLERGIC REACTIONS

Allergy may be defined as a specific acquired alteration in the capacity of an individual to react to an antigen. Mediated by circulating or cellular antibodies, allergic reactions may be classified as IgE-mediated hypersensitivity (type I), cytotoxic (type II), Arthus-type toxic immune complex reactions (type III), and delayed-type hypersensitivity (type IV).

Type I. Anaphylactic reactions include local and systemic manifestations of the interaction between antigen and tissue cells previously sensitized with skin-sensitizing reaginic antibody, usually IgE. This interaction of antigen and antibody results in the release of pharmacologically active substances that produce urticaria, angioedema, anaphylaxis, hay fever, and asthma.

Type II. Cytotoxic reactions include those reactions initiated by antibody interacting with an antigenic component of tissue–cell surface. The antigen may be a natural component of the cell or an unrelated antigen that has become associated with the cell. Examples include hemolytic disease of the newborn, transfusion reactions, hemolytic anemia, leukopenia, or thrombopenia due to the reaction of antibody with drugs attached to blood-cell surfaces.

Type III. Toxic immune complex reactions (Arthus-type reactions) are associated with the deposition of immune microprecipitates in or around blood vessels, which results in tissue damage through activation of complement or toxic products from leukocytes attracted to the areas. Examples include serum sickness, glomerulonephritis, and local Arthus reactions following injection of antigens into the skin, subcutaneous tissue, or muscle.

Type IV. Delayed-type hypersensitivity is due to the interaction between antigen and specifically sensitized lymphocytic cells, which results in a mononuclear cell infiltration and the elaboration of toxic lymphoid cell products. Examples include tuberculin and other skin test reactions, contact dermatitis, and graft-versus-host–type reactions.

515

URTICARIA

Urticaria, a systemic disease with cutaneous manifestations, occurs at some time in the life of about 15 per cent of the population.[1] It is characterized by the appearance of transient well-circumscribed wheals that are seen as erythematous, intensely pruritic elevated swellings of the skin (Fig. 18–1) or mucous membranes.

The etiology of urticaria is often not well understood and may be related to a multitude of factors. Therefore it can be thought of as a symptom-complex in which multiple factors can cause and perpetuate the condition. Individual lesions are due to extravasation of fluid from small blood vessels, a reflection of increased permeability of capillaries and small venules. Various pharmacologically active agents appear to be capable of mediating these changes (i.e., kinins, prostaglandins, serotonin, and histamine). [1, 2]

Clinical Manifestations. Typical lesions have a white palpable center of edema with a variable halo of erythema. They vary from pinpoint-sized papules to large lesions several centimeters in diameter. Central clearing, peripheral extension, and coalescence of individual lesions result in a clinical picture of oval, annular, or bizarre serpiginous configurations. They may be localized to one small area or may become so extensive and generalized as to cover almost the entire skin surface. Subcutaneous extension may result in large giant wheals. In infants and young children, swelling of the distal extremities with acrocyanosis may be a prominent feature of the urticarial reaction. Occasionally, particularly in infants and young children, bullae may form in the center of the wheal, usually on the legs and buttocks. Individual wheals rarely persist longer than 12 to 24 hours. Those lasting more than 24 hours are probably not true urticaria and may represent another vascular pattern, such as vasculitis or erythema multiforme.

The terms *angioedema, giant urticaria,* and *Quincke's edema* occasionally are used to describe large giant wheals and diffuse swellings of the eyelids, hands, genitalia, and mucous membranes (the lips and tongue). Although angioedema may occur on its own, it often accompanies and shares a common etiology with ordinary urticaria.

For convenience, urticaria of less than 6 weeks' duration is considered *acute.* Acute urticaria due to food or drugs is generally of brief duration (a few days to weeks). Urticaria that recurs frequently and lasts longer than 6 weeks is termed *chronic.* The exact etiology in a particular patient is often unknown and may be associated with hypersensitivity to a multitude of possible agents such as foods, drugs, infections, immunizing agents, serum injections, insect bites, inhalant or contact allergens, and psychogenic factors. Many physicians still regard urticaria as characteristically and almost invariably allergic in origin. Although an allergic cause can be determined in many cases, in 70 to 80 per cent of patients, particularly those with chronic urticaria, no definite etiology can be established.

Although seldom life-threatening, chronic urticaria has been noted to be an important sign of underlying systemic disease. It may occur in association with malignancy or may be an important sign of connective tissue disease. It may be seen as the first sign of Still's disease (juvenile rheumatoid arthritis), in 7 to 23 per cent of cases of lupus erythematosus,[3] and in 10 per cent of patients with acute rheumatic fever. When urticaria is observed in a patient with arthralgia and fever of unknown origin, it should alert the physician to the possibility of serum hepatitis.[4] Diagnosis and treatment of a patient with chronic urticaria, therefore, demand a complete history and physical examination, appropriate laboratory evaluation, and an awareness of possible underlying disease.

Diagnosis. It is seldom difficult to make a diagnosis of urticaria, even in the absence of a visible eruption at the time of examination. However, patients may confuse wheals with blisters or insect bites with hives. Although rapid onset and the self-limiting nature of urticarial and angioedematous eruptions are distinguishing features, other reaction patterns may be confused with urticaria. The differential diagnosis of urticaria, therefore, should include dermographism, arthropod bites, papular urticaria, atopic dermatitis, contact dermatitis, cutaneous mastocytosis, erythema multiforme, and allergic vasculitis.

Histopathologic examination of urticarial lesions reveals dilatation and engorgement of venules and capillaries, edema, and perivascular infiltration of

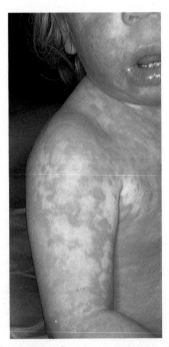

Figure 18–1. Urticaria. Transient well-circumscribed erythematous wheals are present.

the dermis composed of round cells, polymorphonuclear leukocytes, and a variable number of eosinophils. Urticarial wheals are characterized by edema of the dermis; in lesions of angioneurotic edema the edema extends into the subcutaneous and submucosal tissues without infiltrating inflammatory cells.

Treatment. Effective treatment of urticaria depends on identification of the etiologic factor and its elimination whenever possible. Symptomatic treatment consists of antihistamines, of which hydroxyzine (Atarax or Vistaril) appears to be the most effective and is the drug of choice. When antihistamines are used, they provide symptomatic relief in about 80 per cent of patients, but their use should not be stopped prematurely. In an effort to prevent recurrences and the development of chronic urticaria, continuing therapy with antihistamines for 1 or 2 weeks after all signs of urticaria have cleared followed by gradual tapering of the dosage is recommended.

Antihistamines may be divided into seven pharmacologic groups, all having somewhat similar properties. Histamine produces its various effects through receptors on the cell membranes and blood vessels containing H_1 and H_2 receptors. H_1 receptors are blocked by classic antihistamines; H_2 receptors are blocked by cimetidine (Tagamet) or ranitidine (Zantac), and doxepin (Adapin, Sinequan), a tricyclic antidepressant with H_1 and H_2 antagonistic effects, although not approved for use in children under the age of 12 years, has been utilized for the treatment of chronic urticaria. When one antihistamine proves ineffective, the dosage may be gradually increased or an agent from another pharmacologic group may be administered. In cases in which H_1 antihistamines are unable to control the disorder, a combination of an H_1 and an H_2 antagonist may be considered. However, an H_2 antagonist such as cimetidine should not be used alone since it may aggravate the urticarial problem[5] and long-term cimetidine therapy (longer than 6 weeks) has been associated with antiandrogen effects, neutropenia, and, especially in the elderly, confusion. When sedation associated with the administration of antihistamines proves to be a problem, terfenadine (Seldane), 60 mg twice a day, and astemizole (Hismanal), 10 mg/day, which have less penetration through the blood-brain barrier and a lower affinity for brain H_1 receptors, with appropriate precautions, can be used (see Chapter 3).[6] The dosages of terfenadine and astemizole for children younger than the age of 12 years have not yet been established, and since the administration of astemizole with food significantly decreases its absorption and bioavailability, it is recommended that astemizole be taken on an empty stomach (at least 1 hour before or 2 hours after eating).

The subcutaneous administration of 0.1 to 0.5 ml of epinephrine 1 : 1,000) or 0.1 to 0.3 ml of SusPhrine (1 : 200) is often effective and particularly beneficial in patients with angioedema and acute or severe urticaria. Although frequently effective in patients with severe or persistent urticaria, because of the side effects associated with prolonged corticosteroid therapy, administration of systemic corticosteroids should be reserved for those patients who are unresponsive to other modes of therapy.

PHYSICAL URTICARIAS

The physical urticarias are a group of disorders in which wheals occur in response to various physical stimuli. These include dermographism (factitious urticaria) and pressure, cholinergic, aquagenic, solar, and cold urticaria. Dermographism and cholinergic urticaria are quite common, cold urticaria is less common, and other patterns of physical urticaria are relatively rare.

Dermographism (dermatographism) is manifested by a sharply localized edematous or wheal reaction with a surrounding zone of erythema that occurs locally within seconds after firm stroking of the skin. Seen in approximately 5 per cent of the normal population, more vigorous or repeated stroking will produce the response in 25 to 50 per cent of normal subjects.

Pressure urticaria is a related disorder characterized by the development of hives or a deeper swelling simulating angioedema that is often painful and occurs immediately or after a 4- to 6- hour delay following local pressure produced by clothing, jewelry, or weight bearing. Because of this delay in appearance, patients frequently fail to appreciate the cause of the disorder.[4]

Cholinergic urticaria (micropapular urticaria) is a very distinctive type of urticaria. It usually starts in adolescence and is associated with heat, exertion, or emotional stress. Reported in 5 to 7 per cent of the cases of urticaria, it is considered to be a physical allergy and not a sign of systemic disease.[7, 8] Cholinergic urticaria is characterized by a generalized eruption, usually on the trunk and arms, which consists of discrete, papular wheals, 1 to 3 mm in diameter with or without a surrounding area of erythema (Fig. 18–2). The duration of the eruption varies from 30 minutes to several hours.

Acetylcholine, released through some unknown mechanism (perhaps liberated when sweat glands are stimulated by heat, exertion, emotional, or taste stimuli), may stimulate histamine release, thus causing the lesions.[4] The diagnosis is made on the basis of history and the appearance of the eruption several minutes after exercise. Once cholinergic urticaria occurs, the condition may recur for periods of months to years, and then tends toward spontaneous improvement and resolution. Treatment consists of systemic antihistamines, particularly cyproheptadine (Periactin), hydroxyzine (Atarax or Vistaril), or ketotifen (an H_1 histamine receptor antagonist and stabilizer of mast cell mediator release not yet available in the United States)[9]; awareness of potential precipitating fac-

Figure 18–2. Cholinergic urticaria (induced by heat, exertion, or emotional stress). Discrete micropapular wheals are surrounded by a wide area of erythema.

tors; and avoidance of heat, excessive exertion, and excitement whenever possible. After a severe attack of cholinergic urticaria, further exertion frequently fails to cause urticaria for periods of 24 hours or more. Some patients thus find that they can induce attacks by exercise or hot showers and in this way achieve freedom from symptoms for varying periods of time.

Aquagenic urticaria, a disorder that resembles but is not identical to cholinergic urticaria, occurs most frequently in adolescence and is characterized by small, intensely pruritic, perifollicular papular wheals with surrounding axon reflex erythema (with sparing of the palms and soles). The disorder is precipitated by contact with water or perspiration (irrespective of temperature). Exercise and other cholinergic factors do not precipitate this disorder, and patients can drink water without adverse reaction.[10] Although the etiology remains unknown, aquagenic urticaria may be related to a toxic substance created by a combination of water and sebum, resulting in local histamine release from the perifollicular mast cells.[11] The administration of H_1 blockers, H_1 blockers combined with H_2 blockers, or anticholinergics seems to reduce the whealing tendency and lessen the severity of the disorder.

Solar urticaria is a rare disorder in which minimal exposure to sunlight at different wavelengths in the visible or ultraviolet light range provokes an almost immediate localized urticarial reaction, with "burning" followed by erythema, wheal, and flare sharply confined to light-exposed sites (see Chapter 4, Fig. 4–1). Although the reaction generally fades within 15 or 30 minutes to 1 or 2 hours, scratching and rubbing may lead to secondary eczematization with persisting cutaneous changes.

Solar urticaria is a chronic disease and has been described in individuals from 3 to 52 years of age. It appears to be a disorder dependent on a variety of mechanisms, and although the wavelength of light causing the urticarial response varies considerably from person to person, the majority of patients react within wavelengths in the 290- to 480-nm range. Although therapy is generally unsatisfactory, oral antihistamines occasionally may be helpful for individuals with this disorder. Repeated gradual exposure to sunlight, oral administration of a psoralen followed by UVA (PUVA) radiation (alone or in combination with terfenadine), antimalarials, adrenocorticosteroids, and plasmapharesis have been beneficial for some patients, and measures should be directed toward diminishing exposure to sunlight. Sunscreen preparations, which are occasionally beneficial when the precipitating wavelengths are in the sunburn and UVA range, appear to be the most consistently helpful form of therapy available at this time.

Cold urticaria is a disorder characterized by localized or generalized urticaria that develops within a few minutes or hours of exposure to cold air or water. In highly sensitive persons, in whom whealing may be widespread or severe, cold showers or swimming in cold water may produce hypotension and, on occasion, syncope, loss of consciousness, and drowning.[12] If the cold extends to the mucous membranes, respiratory symptoms such as nasal stuffiness, cough, and dyspnea, and gastrointestinal symptoms such as swelling of the lips, swelling of the oral mucous membranes, dysphagia, and abdominal cramps may occur.

Cold urticaria can be divided into two forms: (1) a rare congenital or familial type inherited on an autosomal dominant basis and (2) a more common acquired form. Although not sex-linked, familial cold urticaria is more common in females. The disorder may be present at birth or may occur during infancy and usually develops in early childhood. It is characterized by an urticarial or papular eruption, fever, chills, arthralgia, headache, malaise, muscle tenderness, and, at times, a significant leukocytosis.[13] Although the tendency to familial cold urticaria generally persists for life, the severity of symptoms may decrease with advancing age. The urticarial reaction is usually induced by a generalized body cooling, more often in cold air than cold water. It generally develops after a latent period of several hours and, once it develops, may persist for up to 48 hours.

The acquired form of cold urticaria often appears suddenly, usually in children, but may occur at any age and has an equal incidence in both sexes. Once symptoms develop they are generally short-lived and, although they may persist indefinitely, usually disappear after a few months or years.

Secondary forms of cold urticaria may also be associated with cold hemolysin and cold agglutinin syndromes. These forms, generally seen in adults, cause Raynaud's phenomenon, acrocyanosis, and cutaneous ulcers. Some cases of cold urticaria manifested by itching, erythema, purpura, atypical Raynaud's phenomenon, and ulceration due to cryoglobulins may also be associated with multiple myeloma, leukemia, kala-azar, systemic lupus erythematosus and melanoma.

The diagnosis of cold urticaria requires a careful

history and investigation for other possible etiologic factors. When the diagnosis remains in doubt, patients should be evaluated for other systemic diseases, particularly lupus erythematosus, cryoglobulinemia, and hereditary angioneurotic edema. Diagnosis of cold urticaria may frequently be assisted by reproduction of symptoms by local applications of an ice cube for periods of 2 to 10 minutes. The best areas for this testing are the face, neck, and particularly the arms (Fig. 18–3). Some patients fail to respond to ice but do respond to cold water or generalized cooling of the body.[14]

Patients with a severe or widespread urticarial reaction should be forewarned of the risk of drowning following loss of consciousness when swimming or bathing in cold water. The treatment of cold urticaria is aided by oral administration of antihistamines, particularly cyproheptadine (Periactin).[15] For those patients who are unresponsive to systemic antihistamines, desensitization to cold may be attempted by gradually cooling an extremity in cold water for 5 to 10 minutes a day with a gradual increase in the time of exposure and decrease of the temperature over a period of weeks or months. This treatment is not regularly effective and must be done cautiously in an effort to minimize the risk of systemic reaction.

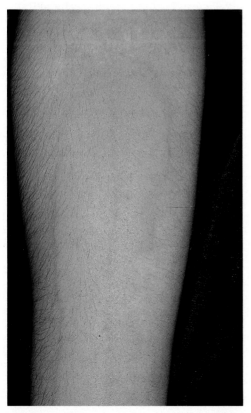

Figure 18–3. The diagnosis of cold urticaria can be assisted by the local reproduction of symptoms following an application of an ice pack to an extremity for a period of 2 to 10 minutes.

HEREDITARY ANGIONEUROTIC EDEMA

Hereditary angioneurotic edema (hereditary angioedema) is a serious but rare form of urticaria characterized by recurrent episodes of edema of the subcutaneous tissue, particularly the hands, feet, and face, and of the gastrointestinal or upper respiratory tracts. An autosomal dominant disorder occurring in approximately 1 in 150,000 persons, the defect appears to be due to a deficiency of the α_2-globulin inhibitor of the first component of complement (C_1-esterase inhibitor [C_1-INH], which results in transient episodes of increased vascular permeability. Although the pathogenesis of this disorder is not fully understood, it appears that a kinin-like permeability factor generated by the action of C_1-esterase on C_4 and C_2, the episodic activation of Hageman factor working through a kinin-forming system of plasma or plasmin, and an elevated capillary filtration rate in affected areas may be physiologic mediators of attacks.[16–18]

Two genetic variants of hereditary angioneurotic edema have been described. In the more common type, seen in an estimated 85 per cent of affected kindreds, serum levels of C_1-esterase inhibitor are extremely low because of decreased synthesis in the liver. In the variant form, normal or elevated levels of C_1-esterase inhibitor are present, but the inhibitor is apparently nonfunctional. Trauma, a major known precipitating factor in many attacks, induces activation of factor XII (the Hageman factor). Attacks of hereditary angioedema, therefore, may be the result of malfunction of both the contact phase of coagulation and complement system dysfunction. In addition, acquired C_1-INH deficiency caused by paraproteinemia, cutaneous or systemic lupus erythematosus, scleroderma, focal lipodystrophy, and certain neoplastic diseases (lymphomas, carcinoma of the lungs and colon, and multiple myeloma) may have a syndrome similar to that seen in hereditary angioedema. Unlike patients with hereditary angioedema, patients with these conditions have decreased levels of C_1 and C_{1q} in addition to decreased C_4, C_2, and C_1-INH. Acquired angioedema can be distinguished from hereditary angioedema by the absence of complement abnormalities in other family members and the finding of reduced levels of the first component of complement (which is present in normal concentrations in patients with hereditary angioedema).[19, 20]

Clinical Manifestations. The earliest symptoms of hereditary angioneurotic edema (Table 18–1) often begin in infancy or early childhood, usually before the age of 10 years, and rarely as late as the third decade of life.[19] The frequency and severity of attacks are typically exacerbated during adolescence and subside in the fifth decade. Mottling of the skin often occurs early in life and may be the first evidence of the disorder. Affected individuals are prone to sudden attacks of circumscribed subcutaneous edema. The swelling evolves very quickly. It usually affects the face or an extremity,

Table 18–1. HEREDITARY ANGIONEUROTIC EDEMA

1. Earliest symptoms often in infancy or early childhood.
   a. Usually before age 10.
   b. Rarely as late as the third decade of life.
2. Mottling of skin may be first sign.
3. Sudden attacks of circumscribed subcutaneous edema.
   a. Precipitated by minor trauma, especially extraction of teeth, infection, strenuous exercise, menses, the use of oral contraceptives, extremes of temperature, psychic disturbances or emotional excitement.
   b. Usually on the face or an extremity.
4. Reduced levels of C_4 or C_1-esterase inhibitor (C_1-INH), or both; reduced serum levels of C_4 and/or C_2; and demonstration of a functional lack of C_1-esterase inhibitor.
5. Asphyxiation in up to 25 per cent of patients.

may be severe enough to cause remarkable disfiguration of the affected parts, and generally subsides within 1 to 5 days. The skin and mucosal lesions may appear spontaneously or may be precipitated by minor trauma, especially extraction of teeth, strenuous exercise, infection, menses, the use of oral contraceptives, extremes of temperature, psychic disturbances, or emotional excitement. There is no pitting, discoloration, redness, pain, or itching associated with the edema, and a rash similar to erythema marginatum is noted in some patients, particularly children.

Gastrointestinal involvement, second in order of frequency, is marked by nausea, vomiting, or diarrhea, sometimes with recurrent colic and severe abdominal pain simulating a surgical emergency. Involvement of the mucous membranes of the hypopharynx and larynx, although seen less often, may be particularly severe and result in asphyxiation, the leading cause of death in patients with this disorder. This complication, usually seen in the third decade of life, may occur in 25 per cent of patients.

Treatment. Diagnosis of hereditary angioneurotic edema can be confirmed by the finding of reduced levels of C_4 or C_1-esterase inhibitor, or both. The finding of reduced serum levels of C_4 and/or C_2 is a reliable indirect way to screen patients for the possibility of hereditary angioneurotic edema. However, if these levels are reduced in the presence of normal levels of C_1 inhibitor protein, confirmation must rely on demonstration of a functional lack of C_1-esterase inhibitor (C_1-INH) by hemolytic or biochemical assay.

Although up to 25 per cent of patients with hereditary angioneurotic edema may die of suffocation during attacks of laryngeal edema, the development of better diagnostic techniques and therapy now offers a more favorable prognosis. Antihistamines and corticosteroids have not been effective in the management of patients. Epinephrine is beneficial in the control of swelling in only a very few patients. Intravenous administration of diuretics such as metalluride (Mercuhydrine) or ethacrynic acid is helpful in halting the progression of severe angioedema. Tracheostomy frequently is lifesaving in patients with laryngeal ob-

struction. Although methyltestosterone linguets (in dosages of 10 to 25 mg once daily) may prevent attacks in one third to one half of patients, they can produce masculinization in women patients and their use is not recommended for children. The semisynthetic androgens danazol (Danocrine) and stanozolol (Winstrol) have fewer androgenic side effects than methyltestosterone, but their safety and efficiency in children have not been established.[21, 22]

ε-Aminocaproic acid (EACA) inhibits the conversion of plasminogen to plasmin (a known C_1 activator). Its safety in long-term therapy has not been established; in short-term use its major side effect has been muscle weakness with associated elevation of creatine phosphokinase and aldolase and an increased predisposition to thrombosis and phlebitis. Its analogue tranexamic acid (Cyclokapron) has also been effective in aborting attacks of angioedema, but since this drug can cause severe toxicity, its use is not recommended.[20]

SERUM SICKNESS

Serum sickness is an allergic reaction characterized by urticaria, malaise, fever, lymphadenopathy, splenomegaly, and swollen and tender joints. The syndrome, originally noted and most commonly seen following the administration of antiserum of horse or rabbit origin, is now most frequently encountered following treatment with drugs. Although penicillin accounts for most cases of serum sickness reactions, other antibiotics, thiouracils, p-aminosalicylic acid, hydralazine, sulfonamides, salicylates, and a wide variety of other drugs may be responsible for this disorder. Serum sickness develops gradually, generally within 8 to 14 days following antigenic exposure of nonsensitive individuals, with shorter latent periods when presensitization exists. It is believed to be mediated largely by circulating antigen–antibody complexes (a type III Arthus reaction), in which IgG is the predominant immunoglobulin.

The clinical manifestations of serum sickness are urticaria, malaise, fever, lymphadenopathy, splenomegaly, and swollen and tender joints (Fig. 18–4). Localized or generalized edema is common. Although temperatures up to 105°F (40.6°C) may occur, the fever is usually slight or moderate. Skin eruptions, the most common and characteristic feature, are present in over 80 per cent of cases. In 90 per cent the rash is urticarial. Morbilliform and scarlatiniform eruptions are less common, and erythema multiforme, erythema nodosum, and vasculitic purpura are rarely seen. Lymphadenopathy, the second most common manifestation, often appears initially in the epitrochlear region, but it may be generalized or regional. The latter is particularly common when the allergic reaction is secondary to an injection.

Joint symptoms occur in about 50 per cent of patients and vary in severity from a mild arthralgia

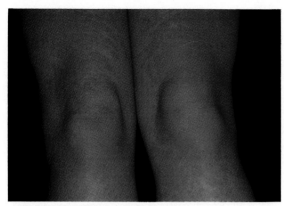

Figure 18–4. Serum sickness. Urticaria and swollen, tender knees were present in a 16-year-old girl. (From Hurwitz S: The hypersensitivity syndromes. *In:* The Skin and Systemic Disease in Children. Year Book Medical Publishers, Chicago, 1985.)

to severe polyarthritis. Neurologic manifestations, when present, include peripheral neuritis, radiculitis, optic neuritis, and cerebral edema. A more severe form of serum sickness–like reaction is associated with glomerulonephritis caused by the deposition of antigen–antibody complexes in the kidney. In other instances, serum sickness can result in hypersensitivity angiitis involving multiple organ systems.

Serum sickness generally is a self-limiting disease that subsides within 2 to 3 weeks. Although rarely fatal, death may occur as a consequence of coronary artery vasculitis or severe neuropathy. Treatment consists of ephedrine, antihistamines, and analgesics. Hydroxyzine appears to be the most effective antihistaminic and antipruritic agent. It may be administered to children in dosages of 2 mg/kg/24 hr in three or four divided doses (this amount may be increased twofold for severe cases) and 50 to 100 mg four times a day for adults. If this fails to make the patient more comfortable, systemic corticosteroids are effective; and in severe cases and for individuals with facial or epiglottic edema, epinephrine or ephedrine is indicated. In cases in which glottal edema is severe, tracheostomy may be lifesaving.

ANAPHYLAXIS

Anaphylaxis is an immediate hypersensitivity reaction to the administration of an antigen that has previously produced a specific sensitization. It is characterized within a few seconds to 1 hour after injection of the antigen by weakness, dyspnea, pruritus of the palms, soles, and scalp, urticaria, hypotension, and circulatory collapse.

The treatment of anaphylaxis consists of the administration of 0.1 to 1.0 ml of 1 : 1,000 aqueous epinephrine (0.01 ml/kg) followed by the intravenous administration of antihistamines such as di-

phenhydramine (Benadryl), 1.25 mg/kg; chlorpheniramine (Chlor-Trimeton), 0.25 mg/kg; or promethazine (Phenergan), 1 mg/kg. Aminophylline (7 mg/kg) given slowly intravenously over a 10-minute period is often helpful in cases in which anaphylaxis cannot be managed effectively with epinephrine and antihistamine alone. However, since there is a 6- to 12-hour delay before the onset of its effectiveness, an oral corticosteroid is not the drug of choice for initial therapy. If hypotension is present, intravenous fluids (5 per cent glucose in water) should be initiated to permit the ready use of plasma volume expanders, fluids, and electrolytes. Corticosteroids should be given intravenously for severe cases, and once shock is overcome and oral fluids are well tolerated, oral corticosteroids may be initiated.

ANNULAR ERYTHEMAS

The annular erythemas (erythema marginatum, erythema annulare centrifugum, erythema migrans, and erythema annulare of infancy) represent a group of reactive vascular dermatoses that are distinguished primarily by their oval, annular, arcuate, circinate, polycyclic, reticular, or serpiginous configurations with individual characteristics that allow differentiation into distinctive clinical categories. Although it is not yet proved, it appears that these disorders may be related to cell-mediated urticarial reactions. Their individual appearances and behaviors are characteristic and, therefore, frequently helpful in the clinical diagnosis of various systemic disorders.

Erythema Marginatum and Rheumatic Fever

Erythema marginatum is a distinctive form of annular erythema that occurs on the trunk (especially on the abdomen) and the proximal extremities in about 10 per cent of patients with active rheumatic fever and occasionally in patients with juvenile rheumatoid arthritis. Lesions appear as evanescent pink macules or papules that fade centrally (leaving a pale or sometimes pigmented center) and rapidly expand to form nonpruritic rings or segments of rings with elevated reticular, polycyclic, or serpiginous borders.

Often easily overlooked, erythema marginatum is associated with active carditis. It is seen more frequently in children than in adults with rheumatic fever, frequently follows the onset of migratory arthritis by a few days, but at times may also occur many months after the carditis. Lesions are evanescent (fading in a few hours to several days), spread rapidly, and may recur in crops in different areas. Unlike the characteristic rash of juvenile rheumatoid arthritis, lesions of erythema marginatum are larger, spread centrifugally with central clearing, and are limited to the trunk and sometimes the proximal limbs. Although the eruption seldom lasts more than several weeks, occasionally it may recur at sporadic intervals for several months to years.

Erythema marginatum presents a clinical picture that characteristically resembles a variety of dermatoses, including urticaria, erythema multiforme, and other transient figurate erythemas. Frequently seen more easily in the afternoon, coalescence of polycyclic lesions often results in a characteristic chickenwire-like appearance. Believed to represent a vascular reaction to a preceding streptococcal infection, gentle warming of the skin often enhances visualization of pale or barely perceptible lesions. Histologic features consist of a perivascular infiltrate of neutrophils in the papillary dermis. These findings are helpful and frequently will enable the physician to rule out or to suspect a diagnosis of rheumatic fever, often before other clinical and/or laboratory features of the disease become evident (Table 18–2).

Another type of erythema seen in rheumatic fever consists of small, 2- to 5-mm, dull red macules and urticarial papules that occur on the arms, elbows, buttocks, or knees. Seen in 2 to 3 per cent of patients with rheumatic fever, these lesions do not form rings or develop in crops, are less transient than lesions of erythema marginatum, and last from hours to days.

Occurring in 20 per cent to less than 2 per cent (in more recent series) of patients, subcutaneous nodules present another characteristic cutaneous manifestation of rheumatic fever (Table 18-3). Most prevalent in children with extensive cardiac involvement, subcutaneous nodules can coexist with erythema marginatum and are a late manifestation of rheumatic fever. They usually portend serious disease and are observed in no other diseases except granuloma annulare and rheumatoid arthritis. The nodules of rheumatic fever are smaller than those seen in rheumatoid arthritis and last for shorter periods of time, usually less than 1 month. They tend to occur in crops and often appear in a symmetric distribution on the extensor tendons of the hands, feet, knees, and scapulae, on the occiput, and on the spinous processes of the vertebrae. They are never painful and vary from

Table 18-2. ERYTHEMA MARGINATUM

1. Pink macules or papules fade centrally and expand to form rings or segments of rings, often with a chickenwire-like appearance.
2. The lesions are limited to proximal limbs and trunk.
3. The lesions are evanescent (fading in a few hours to several days), spread rapidly, and may recur in crops in different areas.
4. Associated with fever and active carditis in 10% to 15% of children with acute rheumatic fever, it also occurs occasionally in patients with juvenile rheumatoid arthritis.
5. Histopathology: Perivascular infiltrate of neutrophils in the papillary dermis.

Table 18–3. SUBCUTANEOUS NODULES IN RHEUMATIC FEVER

1. Seen in up to 20% of patients with rheumatic fever
2. Occur in crops (often in a symmetric distribution) on extensor tendons of hands, feet, knees, and scapulae and on the occiput and spinous processes of the vertebrae
3. Lesions are small (2 mm to 2 cm in diameter) and last for shorter periods of time than those of juvenile rheumatoid arthritis, usually less than 1 month
4. Most prevalent in children with extensive cardiac involvement

2 mm to 2 cm in diameter. Lying deep in the connective tissue, over bony prominences with freely movable skin over them, they are more readily felt than seen, and, unless a careful search is made, are frequently overlooked. The differentiation of subcutaneous nodules of rheumatic fever from rheumatoid nodules and granuloma annulare is not possible on clinical or histologic grounds alone. The diagnosis of rheumatoid nodules, however, can usually be established if the patient has other cutaneous and systemic features of rheumatic fever.

Currently accepted criteria for the diagnosis of rheumatic fever include two major or one minor manifestation and evidence of recent group A streptococcal disease. The major manifestations include erythema marginatum, carditis, polyarthritis, chorea, and subcutaneous nodules. The minor manifestations include fever, arthralgias, previous rheumatic fever or rheumatic heart disease, leukocytosis, elevated erythrocyte sedimentation rate or positive C-reactive protein, and prolonged PR interval.

Erythema Annulare Centrifugum

Erythema annulare centrifugum is an eruption characterized by persistent, occasionally pruritic, erythematous annular lesions, each with a clear center and a raised, thin, wall-like border that slowly enlarges centrifugally (Fig. 18–5; Table 18–4). At times the palpable border of the expanding ring may be topped by microvesicles or may show a fine collarette scale on its trailing edge, suggesting a diagnosis of tinea corporis. Synonyms for erythema annulare centrifugum include *gyrate erythema* and *erythema perstans*. The latter term is used when the figurate erythema arising as an erythematous plaque persists for weeks to months without centrifugal spread.[4]

The etiology of erythema annulare centrifugum is unknown. Although it often occurs without apparent cause, most cases appear to be related to hypersensitivity to an underlying inflammatory or neoplastic disease. In infants it may be associated with autoimmune disorders in their mothers (see Erythema Annulare of Infancy). In such instances, the possibility of neonatal lupus erythematosus must be considered. Thus, erythema annulare centrifugum may occur as a cutaneous sign of hyper-

Figure 18–5. Erythema annulare centrifugum. Slowly expanding annular lesions have dusky centers and palpable scaly erythematous borders.

sensitivity to drugs, molds, foods, fungus infection, blood dyscrasia, immunologic disorders, or neoplastic disease.

Primary lesions of erythema annulare centrifugum tend to be single or multiple erythematous, edematous papules with a predilection for the trunk, buttocks, thighs, and legs. They are asymptomatic except for occasional mild pruritus. The rings extend peripherally, usually slowly, 1 to 3 mm per day, sometimes up to 4 cm in a week. New lesions may form within the original circle. The resulting overall shape may be irregular, oval, circinate, semiannular, target-like, or polycyclic. The borders may eventually reach a size of 10 cm or more in diameter. The duration of the disease is extremely variable and may go on for weeks or months and, with new lesions appearing in successive crops, frequently for years.

Erythema annulare centrifugum must be differentiated from lesions of pityriasis rosea, erythema multiforme, tinea corporis, early lesions of lupus erythematosus, granuloma annulare, and erythema chronicum migrans (erythema migrans). Fungal infections can be distinguished by their more pronounced epidermal changes, with vesiculation or scaling or both at the edge of the lesions, by microscopic examination of skin scrapings, and by fungal culture. When the diagnosis is indeterminate, histopathologic examination of cutaneous lesions showing focal infiltration of lymphocytes around the blood vessels and dermal appendages in a "coat sleeve" arrangement may help establish the true nature of the disorder.

Since erythema annulare centrifugum represents a hypersensitivity reaction, treatment depends on the determination and removal of the underlying cause. Antihistamines produce variable and usually incomplete relief. Although systemic corticosteroids may aid the temporary resolution of lesions, unless the underlying cause is removed, the disorder frequently recurs as soon as medication is discontinued.

Erythema Annulare of Infancy

Erythema annulare of infancy may at times be seen as a distinct or undiagnosed entity with a benign, self-limiting symptom-free course; as a manifestation of urticaria; as a neonatal or infantile manifestation of an immunologic disorder of the infant or its mother (e.g., neonatal lupus); as a familial disorder (erythema gyratum atrophicans) originally described by Colcott Fox in 1881 that occurs as annular erythematous patches that become atrophic over a period of several weeks and persists for many years; and as erythema annulare centrifugum, erythema multiforme, or erythema migrans. Although the etiology of annular erythema of infancy is not yet completely resolved, it has been suggested that this disorder may represent a unique clinical entity with a benign self-limiting symptom-free course or a neonatal or infantile manifestation of an autoimmune maternal disorder.[23–25]

Erythema Migrans

Erythema migrans (erythema chronicum migrans), the earliest symptom of Lyme disease, is a cutaneous eruption that follows a tick bite and is

Table 18–4. ERYTHEMA ANNULARE CENTRIFUGUM

1. Erythematous annular lesions with a clear center and a raised, thin wall-like border that slowly enlarges centrifugally
2. A sign of hypersensitivity to drugs, molds, foods, fungus, infection, blood dyscrasia, immunologic disorders, or neoplastic disease
3. Varying duration of weeks to months (new crops may appear for years)
4. Histopathology: focal infiltration of lymphocytes around blood vessels and dermal appendages in a "coat-sleeve" arrangement

characterized by single or multiple erythematous expanding lesions with advancing indurated borders and central clearing (see Chapter 10). Erythema migrans is caused by the tick-borne spirochete *Borrelia burgdorferi* (see Figs. 10–30 through 10–34).

ERYTHEMA NODOSUM

Erythema nodosum represents a delayed cell-mediated hypersensitivity syndrome characterized by red, tender, nodular lesions that are usually on the pretibial surface of the legs (Fig. 18–6) and occasionally on other areas of the skin where subcutaneous fat is present (Table 18–5). Although etiologic causes are numerous, the most common are β-streptococcal infection, sarcoidosis, and tuberculosis. In children, streptococcal and other respiratory tract infections and primary tuberculosis are the most common cases of erythema nodosum. Thus, any child younger than the age of 5 years with erythema nodosum, a positive tuberculin test, and no evidence of streptococcal infection or other respiratory illness should be considered to have tuberculosis until proven otherwise.[4] Other disorders that may cause erythema nodosum include leprosy, coccidioidomycosis, histoplasmosis, leishmaniasis, cat-scratch disease, *Mycobacterium marinum* infection, and fungal infection. Noninfectious disorders that cause erythema nodosum are sarcoidosis, Behçet's disease, internal malignant disease, ulcerative colitis, regional ileitis, and reactions to various drugs, particularly sulfonamides, phenytoin (Dilantin), and contraceptive

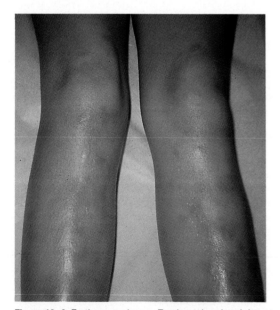

Figure 18–6. Erythema nodosum. Tender red oval nodules on the extensor aspect of the legs.

Table 18–5. ERYTHEMA NODOSUM

1. Red, tender, nodular lesions, usually on the pretibial surface of the legs
   a. A delayed cell-mediated hypersensitivity
   b. Although respiratory tract infection is the most common cause in children, noninfectious causes such as sarcoidosis, ulcerative colitis, and drugs may be incriminated
2. Ten per cent of cases are recurrent
3. Histopathologic features:
   a. Lymphocytic perivascular infiltrate in the dermis
   b. Lymphocytes and neutrophils (with histiocytes, giant cells, and, at times, plasma cells) in the fibrous septa in the subcutaneous fat

pills containing ethinyl estradiol and norethynodrel.[26–29]

The disease has its greatest incidence in the spring and fall and is less common in summer. Although most cases occur in the third decade of life, the disorder may be seen in children, particularly those older than 10 years of age.[27] During childhood girls are affected slightly more than boys, but in adult life women are affected three to four times as often as men. Lesions, which are 1 to 5 cm in diameter, occur symmetrically, usually on the pretibial areas, occasionally on the knees, ankles, thighs, extensor aspects of the arms, the face, and neck, and rarely on the palms. Initially they appear as bright to deep red, warm and tender, oval, slightly elevated nodules. After a few days they develop a brownish red or purplish bruise-like appearance (this has been termed *erythema contusiformis*). The eruption usually lasts 3 to 6 weeks but may recede earlier if the patient remains in bed. Recrudescences may occur over a period of weeks to months, but attacks are seldom recurrent[28] and arthralgias may precede, coincide with, or follow the eruption in as many as 90 per cent of cases. In the 10 per cent of patients in whom the condition may present as a recurring disorder, recurrences are frequently associated with repeated streptococcal infection.[4]

Erythema nodosum has a characteristic clinical picture, and diagnosis generally can be made on the basis of physical examination alone. Although diagnosis is usually not difficult, common bruises, cellulitis or erysipelas, deep fungal infections (such as Majocchi's granuloma or sporotrichosis), insect bites, deep thrombophlebitis, angiitis, erythema induratum, and fat-destructive panniculitides can be confused with this disorder. When the diagnosis is in doubt, bacterial and fungal cultures and histologic examination of skin biopsy specimens generally will help clarify the diagnosis.

The principal histologic changes of erythema nodosum are located in the deep dermis and subcutaneous tissue. They consist primarily of lymphocytes and neutrophils (with histiocytes, giant cells, and at times plasma cells) in the fibrous septa between fat lobules as well as in individual fat cells. The dermis shows a moderate degree of perivascular infiltrate composed primarily of lymphocytes.

The management of erythema nodosum is directed at identification and treatment of the underlying cause. Bed rest, with elevation of the patient's legs, helps reduce pain and edema. When pain, inflammation, or arthralgia is prominent, salicylates and other nonsteroidal anti-inflammatory drugs (such as indomethacin or naproxen), potassium iodide, or colchicine may be helpful.[30–33] In chronic or recurrent cases, detailed investigations must be performed to uncover the underlying cause. Intralesional corticosteroids frequently cause rapid involution of individual lesions, and in persistent or recurrent eruptions oral corticosteroids may be beneficial.

ERYTHEMA MULTIFORME

Erythema multiforme is a distinctive acute hypersensitivity syndrome characterized by skin and mucous membrane lesions and, in its more severe form, mucosal lesions, constitutional symptoms, and, at times, visceral involvement (Table 18–6). Although its pathogenesis remains unknown, it appears to represent the end result of a hypersensitivity reaction to any number of etiologies: hypersensitivity to viral, bacterial, protozoal, fungal, or *Mycoplasma pneumoniae* (Eaton agent) infection; sensitivity to food or drugs; immunizations; connective tissue disorders; and a wide variety of other systemic diseases and physical agents. Whereas drug reactions and malignancies are important causes of erythema multiforme in older persons, infectious diseases are the most prominent precipitants in children and young adults. The most common cause of erythema multiforme appears to be the virus of herpes simplex, with a history of cold sores preceding the development of other lesions by 3 to 14 days. Recurrences are particularly common in this form of erythema multiforme.[34, 35]

The clinical spectrum of erythema multiforme ranges from a localized eruption of the skin and mucous membranes (erythema multiforme minor)

Table 18–6. ERYTHEMA MULTIFORME

1. A distinctive acute hypersensitivity syndrome
   a. Viral, bacterial, protozoal, fungal, or *Mycoplasma pneumoniae* infection
   b. Food or drugs, immunizations, systemic disease
2. A symmetric eruption with predilection for the palms, soles, extensor surfaces of arms and legs, and backs of hands and feet
3. Macular, urticarial, and vesiculobullous (the predominant lesions are dull red to dusky flat macules or sharply marginated wheals)
4. Target lesions (the hallmark of the disorder)
5. May be divided into two variants (erythema multiforme minor and erythema multiforme major)

Table 18–7. ERYTHEMA MULTIFORME MINOR

1. Erythema multiforme minor is a relatively benign, acute, self-limiting, or recurrent disorder with few complications.
2. Cutaneous lesions consist of symmetrically distributed erythematous macules, papules, and urticarial and target lesions.
3. Mucous membrane involvement may be absent or limited to one surface (usually the mouth).
4. In this relatively benign illness, involvement of organ systems besides the skin and mucosa rarely, if ever, occurs.
5. The mortality is low.

to a severe multisystemic disorder (erythema multiforme major) with widespread blisters and severe erosions of the mucous membranes (Stevens-Johnson syndrome). Some authors also place Lyell's disease (toxic epidermal necrolysis) under the classification of erythema multiforme major (Tables 18–6 through 18–9).[34, 35]

Erythema Multiforme Minor

Erythema multiforme minor occurs at any age, with the most severe forms occurring most frequently in children and young adults. The disorder may occur at any time of year but appears to have its highest incidence in the spring and fall. The eruption is symmetric and may be noted on any part of the body, with a predilection for the palms and soles, backs of the hands and feet, and extensor surfaces of the arms and legs. As the disorder progresses, lesions often extend to the trunk, face, and neck. Oral lesions may occur alone or in conjunction with cutaneous lesions (Fig. 18–7).

The term *erythema multiforme* is often confusing to nondermatologists and should not be applied indiscriminately to any polymorphic eruption. Erythema multiforme is a specific hypersensitivity syndrome with a distinctive clinical pattern, the hallmark of which is the erythematous ring (the so-called iris or target lesion) (Figs. 18–8 and 18–9). Although a single type of lesion might predominate during a particular attack, the basic lesions of erythema multiforme are macular, urticarial, and vesiculobullous. The clinical diagnosis can be made readily if these characteristics are kept in mind.[4] The evolution and resolution of individual lesions lasts about a week, but the erup-

Table 18–8. ERYTHEMA MULTIFORME MAJOR (STEVENS-JOHNSON DISEASE)

1. Starts abruptly with high fever, prostration, extensive eruption, and widespread bullae
2. Severe involvement of mucous membranes (at least two surfaces)
3. Much more prolonged and severe course than that of erythema multiforme minor
4. Mortality of 5% to 15%

Table 18–9. TOXIC EPIDERMAL NECROLYSIS
(LYELL'S DISEASE)

1. A hypersensitivity reaction (usually to drugs or a manifestation of graft-versus-host disease)
2. Universal erythema with subepidermal separation of the skin (between the dermis and epidermis)
   a. Nikolsky's sign is positive
   b. With extensive involvement patients should be watched for evidence of shock, electrolyte imbalance, and secondary infection
3. High mortality (25–70%)
4. Uncommon in young children
5. Can be differentiated from staphylococcal scalded skin syndrome by a Tzanck test or cutaneous punch biopsy
   a. In staphylococcal scalded skin syndrome the blister cleavage plane is intraepidermal
   b. In toxic epidermal necrolysis the separation is in the upper dermis, below the basement membrane

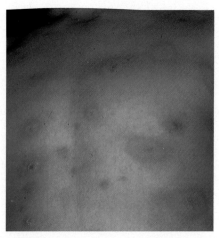

Figure 18–8. Erythema multiforme. Target lesions and marginated wheals with central vesicles are characteristic.

tion may continue to appear in crops for as long as 2 or 3 weeks, thus contributing to the variable multiform appearance of the eruption.

The primary lesion of erythema multiforme is a dull red to dusky flat macule, or a sharply margined wheal, in the center of which a papule or vesicle develops, thus creating the multiformity of lesions. The central area then flattens and develops clearing. As a result it is not unusual to see iris or target lesions consisting of concentric circles whose bright red rings alternate with cyanotic or violaceous ones. Although occasionally seen in erythema annulare centrifugum and Kawasaki disease, target lesions are highly characteristic of erythema multiforme. Careful inspection of the eruption in erythema multiforme may disclose fine petechiae, the clinical feature that distinguishes lesions of erythema multiforme from those of urticaria and erythema annulare centrifugum.

Erythema multiforme minor is characterized by a symmetric eruption on any part of the body with a predilection for the palms, soles, backs of the hands, tops of the feet, and the extensor surfaces of the arms and legs. As the disorder progresses, lesions often extend to the trunk, face, and neck. Oral lesions, seen alone or in conjunction with cutaneous lesions in 25 per cent of patients with erythema multiforme minor, first appear as bullae that break

soon after formation, accompanied by swelling and crusting of the lips and erosions of the buccal mucosa and tongue (Figs. 18–10 and 18–11). Gingival involvement, however, is quite rare; this is an important criterion for distinguishing erythema mul-

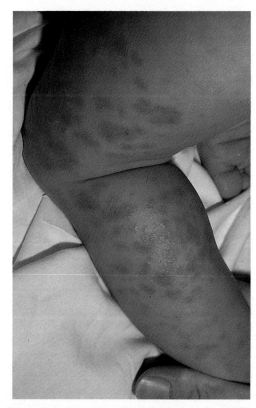

Figure 18–9. Target lesions and marginated wheals with central vesicles are noted in an infant with erythema multiforme. (From Hurwitz S: The hypersensitivity syndromes. *In:* The Skin and Systemic Disease in Children. Year Book Medical Publishers, Chicago, 1985).

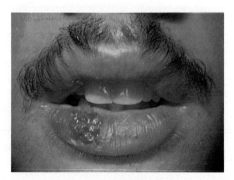

Figure 18–7. Blisters, crusting, and swelling of the lower lip in a patient with erythema multiforme.

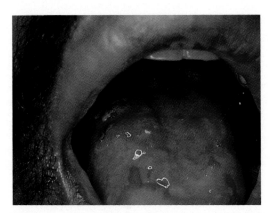

Figure 18–10. Erythema multiforme. Blisters, crusting, swelling of the lips, and erosions of the tongue are evident. (From Hurwitz S: The hypersensitivity syndromes. *In:* The Skin and Systemic Disease in Children. Year Book Medical Publishers, Chicago, 1985.)

tiforme from herpes simplex infection of the mouth, a disorder in which gingival involvement is characteristic.

In contrast to erythema multiforme major, erythema multiforme minor is a relatively benign disorder, involvement of organ systems besides the skin and mucosa rarely if ever occurs, and systemic manifestations, when present, are mild and consist of low-grade fever, malaise, and, in rare cases, myalgia or arthralgia (see Table 18–7). In most cases, skin lesions erupt over a period of less than a week and resolve over another 1 or 2 weeks. The course from the onset of lesions to healing, therefore, is generally less than 4 weeks. When mucosal involvement is present it is limited to one surface (usually the mouth) and, in instances of recurrent disease, one episode may closely follow a preceding one.

The reasons for the typical distribution of skin lesions in erythema multiforme are not entirely understood. Two factors that may play a part in determining the distribution are ultraviolet light and trauma to the skin. This phenomenon appears to be the result of an isomorphic response (koebnerization) and the development of lesions at sites of injury. Since photoaccentuation of erythema multiforme is relatively common, appreciation of this fact may require careful examination of lesion distribution and inquiry into recent light exposure.

The cutaneous lesions of erythema multiforme appear in various forms, but all have an identical histologic picture; the severity of the histologic reaction determines the clinical appearance of lesions. Microscopic examination of skin lesions reveals edema just below the epidermis, which when mild or moderate produces urticarial lesions; when the edema is severe, bullae are formed. Other histologic features consist of dilatation of blood vessels, accompanied by a perivascular infiltration composed mainly of lymphocytes, nuclear dust resulting from disintegration of neutro-

phils and eosinophils (leukocytoclasis), edema, and extravasation of erythrocytes (Fig. 18–12).

The diagnosis of erythema multiforme can generally be made by the clinical features and distribution of lesions. The following criteria can be used to diagnose erythema multiforme minor: (1) an acute self-limiting or recurrent course with a duration, from onset to healing, of 1 to 4 weeks; (2) symmetrically distributed, fixed (lasting more than 7 days), discrete, round, erythematous skin lesions; (3) concentric color changes in at least some of the lesions (iris or target lesions); (4) absent mucous membrane involvement or involvement that is limited to one surface (usually the mouth); and (5) a histopathologic appearance compatible with the diagnosis.[34, 35]

Erythema Multiforme Major

Erythema multiforme major (Stevens-Johnson syndrome), named after the two physicians who first described this variant of the disorder,[36] is a severe bullous form of erythema multiforme with high fever, pronounced constitutional symptoms, widespread bullae, and involvement of two or more mucous membrane surfaces (Figs. 18–13 through 18–15). The disorder lasts as long as 6 weeks and is characterized by a sudden onset; a prodromal period of 1 to 14 days, which can include fever, malaise, headache, cough, coryza, sore throat, vomiting, diarrhea, chest pain, myalgia, and arthralgias; and a mortality rate of 5 to 15 per cent (see Table 18–8). Although recurrent herpes simplex infection appears to be an important etiologic factor in erythema multiforme minor (and is seen

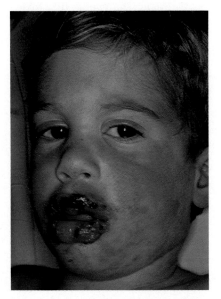

Figure 18–11. Stevens-Johnson syndrome. Mucous membrane involvement with severe swelling and hemorrhagic crusting of the lips.

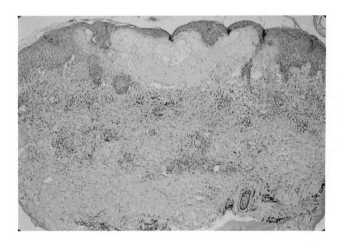

Figure 18–12. Bullous erythema multiforme. Dilatation of blood vessels, perivascular round cell infiltration, extravasation of erythrocytes, and edema of the upper dermis with subepidermal blister formation are shown.

in more than 50 per cent of individuals with this variant of the disorder), in the more severe form (Stevens-Johnson syndrome), *Mycoplasma* infections and drugs appear to be more common.

In Stevens-Johnson syndrome the mucous membranes of the lips, eyes, nose, genitalia, and rectum may show extensive bullae with grayish white membranes, characteristic hemorrhagic crusts, and superficial erosions and ulcerations. The eye changes may be particularly serious, including severe conjunctivitis, corneal ulcerations, keratitis, uveitis, and panophthalmitis; and sequelae may be grave, with a possibility of corneal ulceration and partial or even complete blindness. Pulmonary involvement may occur as an extension from the oropharynx and tracheobronchial tree or may be due to pneumonitis associated with an initiating viral infection or secondary infection. There are patients with what appears to be classic Stevens-Johnson syndrome who evolve into toxic epidermal necrolysis and, in extreme cases, renal involvement with hematuria, nephritis, and, in some

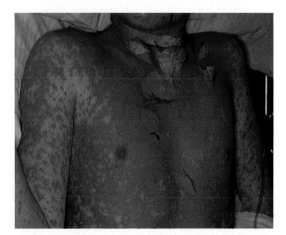

Figure 18–13. Bullous erythema multiforme (Stevens-Johnson syndrome). Confluent erythema, target lesions, blisters, and exfoliation of the epidermis are present.

cases, progressive renal failure may result. In other instances, esophageal or tracheal ulceration, pyoderma, and/or septicemia may complicate the disorder.

Toxic Epidermal Necrolysis

Toxic epidermal necrolysis (Lyell's disease) is a severe exfoliative disorder believed by many to be a variant of erythema multiforme major characterized by the rapid onset of widespread erythema and epidermal necrolysis. Originally described by Lyell in 1956, and by Lang and Walker in 1956 and 1957,[7] in the original descriptions the term *Lyell's disease* was mistakenly used to describe two distinct entities: a subcorneal staphylococcal-induced exfoliative disorder (staphylococcal scalded skin syndrome) and a subepidermal drug-induced exfoliative dermatosis (toxic epidermal necrolysis).[7, 37, 38] Thus, the pathogenesis of toxic epidermal necrolysis involves a drug (or graft-versus-host)-induced necrosis of the basal cell layer of the epidermis, with the production of a subepidermal separation rather than the more superficial (epidermal) split seen in patients with staphylococcal scalded skin syndrome. This distinguishing feature is important in the clinical differentiation of the two disorders.[34, 35]

Usually seen in older children and adults 40 years of age or older, and only rarely in young children, toxic epidermal necrolysis is frequently, but not necessarily, related to a hypersensitivity to drugs, such as phenylbutazone and other nonsteroidal anti-inflammatory drugs, phenolphthalein, procaine, sulfonamides, penicillin or other antibiotics, barbiturates, tranquilizers, vaccines, salicylates, aminopyrine, allopurinol, phenytoin, and griseofulvin, and at times is a manifestation of human immunodeficiency virus infection or graft-versus-host reaction.[39–42] The reason for the decreased incidence of drug-induced toxic epidermal necrolysis in infants and young children appears to be related to the fact that infants and young chil-

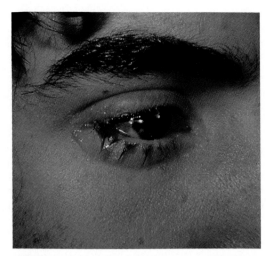

Figure 18–14. Stevens-Johnson syndrome with ophthalmic involvement.

dren have less exposure to potentially sensitizing drugs and therefore less opportunity to develop sensitization.

In toxic epidermal necrolysis a widespread macular erythema and stomatitis may be common features, with exfoliation of the skin occurring in limited areas or, in severe cases, along the entire body surface. As the erythema becomes more universal, the skin begins to develop areas of separation between epidermis and dermis (these superficial blisters are usually first noticed on the face and upper trunk) (Fig. 18–16). During this stage of the disease the upper layer of the epidermis may become wrinkled or may be removed, often peeling off like wet tissue paper, by light stroking—the characteristic Nikolsky sign. The Nikolsky sign, however, is not specific for drug-induced toxic epidermal necrolysis; it may be seen in other bullous disorders (pemphigus, Stevens-Johnson disease, epidermolysis bullosa, and the staphylococcal scalded skin syndrome). Shortly thereafter, the patient develops flaccid bullae and eventual exfoliation; and death, when it occurs, is usually the result of sepsis and fluid and electrolyte imbalance. Secondary infection of denuded areas is common and may lead to scarring. When there is extensive involvement, severe dehydration, electrolyte imbalance, and impaired ability to regulate body temperature effectively, toxic epidermal necrolysis can result in a mortality rate as high as 25 to 70 per cent (see Table 18–9).

The diagnosis of toxic epidermal necrolysis should be considered when there is generalized or focal erythema with exquisite tenderness, bullae, a positive Nikolsky sign, and large areas of exfoliation (more than 30 per cent of the cutaneous surface). History of ingestion of a drug known to provoke toxic epidermal necrolysis in an older child or adult is additional evidence. When the diagnosis is indeterminate, toxic epidermal necrolysis can be differentiated from staphylococcal scalded skin syndrome by a Tzanck test or by histopathologic examination of a cutaneous punch biopsy specimen. In the staphylococcal disorder, the disruption shows cleavage in the epidermis; in toxic epidermal necrolysis, separation is seen in the upper dermis below the basement membrane (similar to the cleavage plane seen in patients with bullous erythema multiforme). Histopathologic examination of a cutaneous punch biopsy specimen also demonstrates eosinophilic necrosis of epidermal cells with a paucity of cellular infiltrates; the latter features, however, are not diagnostic of this disorder.

TREATMENT OF ERYTHEMA MULTIFORME

The management of all forms of erythema multiforme depends on the clinical status of the patient. A thorough search for the identification and elimination of the cause of the disorder is imperative. If a drug is suspected it should be discontinued, and infection, if present, should be treated. Mild forms of erythema multiforme resolve spontaneously, generally within 5 to 15 days, or may respond to antihistamines, and the mortality is low. Local therapy depends on the type and extent of lesions. Simple erythema usually requires no treatment.

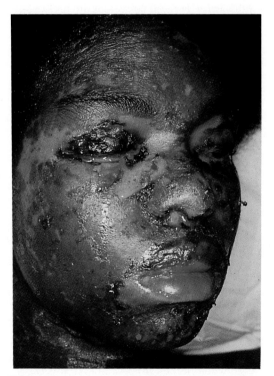

Figure 18–15. Stevens-Johnson form of erythema multiforme (Stevens-Johnson syndrome). Note hemorrhagic crusts of the mucous membranes, extensive bullae, and severe ophthalmic involvement. (From Hurwitz S: The hypersensitivity syndromes. *In:* The Skin and Systemic Disease in Children. Year Book Medical Publishers, Chicago, 1985).

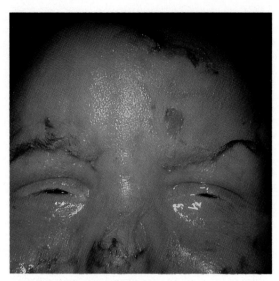

Figure 18–16. Toxic epidermal necrolysis in an 18-month-old child. (Courtesy of Patricia Treadwell, M.D.)

Patients with vesicular, bullous, or erosive lesions can frequently be made more comfortable by colloidal oatmeal baths or the use of open wet compresses, and oral histamines such as hydroxyzine or diphenhydramine (Benadryl) can be beneficial. Mouthwashes for oral lesions with half-strength hydrogen peroxide are helpful; severe oropharyngeal involvement, however, often requires soothing formulations such as a half-and-half mixture of Kaopectate or Maalox and elixir of diphenhydramine, topical application of dyclonine 0.5 per cent or 1 per cent (Dyclone), or topical use of lidocaine (Xylocaine 2% viscous solution) as an anesthetic. Although typical erythema multiforme minor is usually a benign illness with no significant complications, severe oral involvement may be accompanied by difficulty in taking food and fluids and can result in dehydration.

Considerable controversy exists regarding the use of systemic glucocorticosteroids and their role, if any, in the treatment of patients with erythema multiforme, Stevens-Johnson disease, and toxic epidermal necrolysis.[35, 43–47] Many authorities feel that a short vigorous course of systemic corticosteroids, however, may at times be justified in the early treatment of severe progressive or recurrent herpes simplex–induced or progressive drug-induced forms of these disorders.[35, 46, 47] In addition, many clinicians believe that early institution of oral acyclovir and high-dose corticosteroids is effective in the management of patients with recurrent erythema multiforme and Stevens-Johnson disease when herpes simplex infection is the precipitating cause of the disorder.[48] Others, however, strongly champion the approach that corticosteroids have no place in the management of these disorders and, in view of their possible disadvantages, should be discontinued in patients already receiving therapy unless unequivocally indicated for a coexisting condition.[43, 45, 47] Those who believe that systemic corticosteroids have a role in the management of some patients recommend that, if there is no response to this form of therapy within 3 to 5 days, the corticosteroid should be abruptly discontinued in an effort to avoid the risk of associated morbidity and complications associated with their use.

Patients with severe forms of Stevens-Johnson disease are difficult to manage. They frequently require hospitalization and bear a mortality rate of 5 to 15 per cent. As in patients with erythema multiforme minor, all drugs administered before the eruption should be discontinued, appropriate cultures and serologic studies should be performed, and antibiotics should be initiated when indicated. Severe oropharyngeal involvement often necessitates frequent mouthwashes and local application of a topical anesthetic (as in the treatment of patients with erythema multiforme minor), and when ocular involvement is present, ophthalmologic consultation should be obtained. The eyes should be cleansed frequently, with separation of the eyelids, and topical antibacterial agents should be used to prevent secondary infection. Topical use of corticosteroids, however, is contraindicated in this area, since they may produce thinning of the cornea and eventual ulceration or perforation.

A liquid diet and replacement intravenous fluid therapy may be required in extreme cases of erythema multiforme major (Stevens-Johnson syndrome), and patients with severe Stevens-Johnson syndrome with more than 30 per cent skin denudation and patients with toxic epidermal necrolysis should be treated with aggressive supportive care and reverse isolation technique, either in a burn unit or equivalent intensive care unit.[43] Although some clinicians admit patients with severe Stevens-Johnson and toxic epidermal necrolysis into hospital burn units for surgical debridement of the skin under general anesthesia, many feel that this may lead to further infection and that only skin that becomes folded back on itself and serves as a focus for infection should be debrided. Fluid lost through the skin must be considered and, when extensive, should be treated in a manner similar to that used for patients with extensive burns. In patients who are severely ill, and in whom the cutaneous and mucosal damage is extreme and progressive (particularly early in the course of the illness), some clinicians believe that a trial of systemic corticosteroids may sometimes be justified, although many authorities decry the use of corticosteroids in patients with erythema multiforme and toxic epidermal necrolysis. The risks and potential benefit of such therapy, therefore, must be carefully analyzed and evaluated on a case-by-case and day-by-day basis.[43, 47, 49] When a trial of systemic corticosteroids is deemed necessary, a dosage of 1 to 2 mg/kg/day of prednisone or its equivalent is recommended, with tapering of the dosage over a period of 1 to 3 weeks during the healing phase of the illness. If there is no response to corticosteroid therapy within 3 to 5 days, systemic corticosteroids should be abruptly discontinued in an effort to minimize the risk of complications such as delayed wound healing, increased susceptibility to infection, masking of early signs of sepsis, or possible gastrointestinal hemorrhage.

In patients with toxic epidermal necrolysis and possible drug-induced erythema multiforme, all drugs administered before onset of the eruption should be discontinued. Ophthalmologic consultation and appropriate ocular care, as in patients with Stevens-Johnson disease, is recommended, and if damage to the epidermis is extensive, treatment should be similar to that advocated for burn victims (with special attention to fluid requirements, electrolyte balance, and avoidance of secondary infection). Although topical applications of silver sulfadiazine cream (Silvadene) are frequently beneficial, the risk of absorption and possible bone marrow suppression must be considered as a potential side effect.[7] Systemic corticosteroids should not be used as standard therapy. If they are started early (particularly in the first 24 to 48 hours in drug-induced forms of the disorder), however, many authorities believe that they can help prevent extension of the disease process. After large areas of the dermis (more than 20 per cent of the body surface) are uncovered, unless indicated for a coexisting medical disorder, the advantages of systemic glucocorticosteroids are far outweighed by their drawbacks.

HYPEREOSINOPHILIC SYNDROME

The hypereosinophilic syndrome is a multisystemic disorder characterized by persistent peripheral blood and bone marrow eosinophilia associated with diffuse infiltration of various organs by eosinophils. Although virtually any organ system can be involved, affected patients generally demonstrate hepatosplenomegaly and cardiac, pulmonary, renal, nervous system, or dermatologic involvement.[50, 51] The pathogenesis of the hypereosinophilic syndrome remains unknown. It has been suggested that a hypersensitivity reaction to an unidentified antigen or antigens with abnormal immune reactivity may be involved in the production of eosinophilia and the mediation of organ damage seen in patients with this disorder.

Seen primarily in midde-aged men, the hypereosinophilic syndrome most often occurs in the 20- to 50-year age group, and, at times, it is reported in infants, children, and adolescents (Table 18–10).[52] Clinical features include lethargy, anorexia, weight loss, dyspnea, cough, fever, night sweats, chest pain, diarrhea, arthralgia, hepatosplenomegaly, lymphadenopathy, cardiac disease, and eosinophilia greater than 1500 eosinophils/mm³ lasting for 6 months or longer. Except for the blood and bone marrow involvement, cardiovascular disease,

which occurs in 50 per cent of patients, is the major cause of morbidity and mortality.

Cutaneous lesions are found in up to 50 per cent of patients and may present as pruritic erythematous or hyperpigmented macules, papules, and serpiginous lesions with vesicles or as nodules, some of which may have an associated ulceration. These lesions may appear anywhere on the body but are generally present over the trunk and extremities. Urticaria or angioedema may appear on the face and extremities, and, in its most benign form, erythematous papules may be seen in a patchy and at times perifollicular distribution over the trunk.[50]

Pulmonary complications (seen in 40 per cent of patients) include interstitial infiltrates, a persistent nonproductive cough, and pleural effusion. Neurologic findings include hemiparesis, dysesthesias or paresthesias, slurred speech, confusion, and, at times, coma. Hepatic dysfunction and diarrhea, with or without malabsorption, and renal involvement with persistent hematuria and hypouricemia have also been reported.[51]

Historically, the hypereosinophilic syndrome has been associated with a poor prognosis and a mortality rate of 81 to 95 per cent within 3 years of diagnosis. Some patients, however, have no progression of the disease and seem to do well without treatment, and currently up to 80 per cent of patients have a 5-year survival. Factors associated with a poor prognosis include congestive heart failure, infections, bleeding, renal or liver disease, peripheral leukocytosis (90,000/mm³ or more), and the finding of myeloblasts in the peripheral blood with cases described as "eosinophilic leukemia" appearing at the severe end of the clinical spectrum.

The diagnosis of the hypereosinophilic syndrome is dependent on its clinical features, an increased leukocyte count, eosinophilia of greater than 1500 eosinophils/mm³ for longer than 6 months (with lack of parasitic, allergic, or other

---

Table 18–10. THE HYPEREOSINOPHILIC SYNDROME

1. A group of disorders characterized by persistent idiopathic eosinophilia of the blood and bone marrow with diffuse infiltration of various organs by eosinophils
   a. A hypersensitivity reaction?
   b. Male-to-female ration of 9:1
   c. Uncommon in children
2. Anorexia, weight loss, dyspnea, cough, fever, night sweats, chest pain, diarrhea and arthralgia associated with hepatosplenomegaly, lymphadenopathy, renal, cardiac, or neurologic features
3. Cutaneous lesions:
   a. Pruritic erythematous or hyperpigmented macules, papules, nodules, or serpiginous lesions (often with secondary ulceration)
   b. Urticaria or angioedema (particularly on face and extremities)
   c. Erythematous papules over the trunk in a patchy sometimes perifollicular distribution
4. Except for the blood and bone marrow involvement, cardiovascular disease (seen in 50% of affected patients) is the major cause of morbidity and mortality

disease associated with eosinophilia), and signs and symptoms consistent with organ involvement. The histopathologic features of cutaneous lesions include a predominantly perivascular infiltrate of mature eosinophils, mononuclear cells, and, at times, polymorphonuclear cells. Although patients with hypereosinophilic syndrome with mild disease and little or no evidence of organ involvement may require no therapy, systemic corticosteroids are the treatment of choice for patients with progressive organ-system involvement. For patients unresponsive to corticosteroids, the addition of chemotherapeutic agents such as hydroxyurea, vincristine, and cytarabine has been beneficial.

SCOMBROID AND CIGUATERA FISH POISONING

Scombroid fish poisoning (scombrotoxism) is a clinical syndrome that results from the ingestion of spoiled (improperly refrigerated) fish of the Scombroidea family (tuna, mackerel, and bonito) and certain other fish such as bluefish, mahi-mahi, amberjack, herring, sardines, and anchovies.[53–56] The disorder, believed to be related to high levels of histamine and saurine produced when these fish are improperly refrigerated, is characterized by a diffuse erythema of the face and upper body, somewhat resembling a sunburn, and, at times, giant hive-like lesions that develop within minutes to hours after ingestion of the toxic fish. Symptoms resemble a histamine reaction and frequently include a hot burning sensation rather than pruritus such as might be seen in urticaria. The conjunctivae are often markedly injected, and many patients have a severe throbbing headache, tachycardia, palpitations, nausea, vomiting, abdominal cramps, diarrhea, dryness and a burning sensation or peppery taste in the mouth, urticaria, angioneurotic edema, oral blistering, hypotension, blurred vision, and asthma-like symptoms. Although superficially resembling an allergic reaction, patients with scombroid fish poisoning can be reassured that they do not have fish allergy and that scombroidosis will not occur when fish are handled properly. Symptoms are generally self-limiting and even if untreated tend to resolve within 8 to 10 hours. Most patients treated with oral antihistamines or cimetidine become asymptomatic within 2 or 3 hours.

In contrast to scombroid fish poisoning, *ciguatera fish poisoning*, a common disorder endemic throughout the Caribbean and Indo-Pacific islands and the most frequently reported seafood-related disease in the United States, is caused by the ingestion of ciguatoxin, a toxin originating from a dinoflagellate (*Gambierdiseus toxicus*) in affected fish that acts on sodium channels and causes changes in electrical potential and permeability of the cells. Present in certain fish such as the red snapper, amberjack, and surgeon fish, ingestion of affected fish (whether cooked, raw, or frozen) may result in this disorder. Clinical symptoms, which usually appear within 12 hours but sometimes within minutes after ingestion of ciguatoxin, include abdominal pain, cramping, diarrhea, nausea, vomiting, paresthesias, pain or burning when cold water is touched, arthralgia, myalgia, and, in severe cases, hypotension, shock, respiratory depression, paralysis, coma, and death. The duration of illness averages 8½ days but may be prolonged. Treatment consists of supportive measures, and intravenous mannitol has been found, at least in one report, to be extremely effective, lessening the neurologic and muscular dysfunction of affected patients within minutes of administration.[57]

AUTOIMMUNE PROGESTERONE DERMATITIS AND PREGNANCY-RELATED DERMATOSES

Autoimmune progesterone dermatitis is an autosensitive form of dermatitis characterized by urticarial vesiculobullous papules, pustules, erythema multiforme, and dyshidrotic eczema–like eruptions in a follicular and perifollicular distribution on the extensor surfaces of the thighs, forearms, hands, and buttocks. This disorder, which may begin at menarche and thereafter occurs during the mid-menstrual and premenstrual period, is believed to represent an autosensitivity reaction to progesterone; it may also be seen in individuals on anovulatory hormone therapy and in pregnant women during the first trimester of pregnancy. Although urticaria is the predominant cutaneous lesion, the disorder may be severe enough to produce laryngeal spasms requiring epinephrine administration.

The diagnosis of autoimmune progesterone dermatitis can be confirmed by a positive intradermal skin test to aqueous progesterone suspension (100 mg/ml, diluted with normal saline to concentrations of 0.1, 0.01, and 0.001 mg/ml) with the production of a positive urticarial response within a few minutes or a delayed hypersensitivity reaction at the site of the skin test after 48 hours. Treatment consists of estrogens such as ethinyl estradiol, 0.025 to 0.05 mg three times a day, from the 4th to the 24th day of the menstrual cycle, the administration of 1.25 mg of conjugated estrogen (Premarin) for 21 days of each cycle, or 30 mg of the nonsteroidal antiestrogen tamoxifen (Nolvadex). Oophorectomy proved to be the ultimate cure for a patient who was unresponsive to other modes of therapy.[58–60]

Although a number of dermatoses have been associated with pregnancy and the natural histories of many of these disorders are fairly well understood, controversies over nomenclature and clinical reports of overlapping disorders often present a problem in nomenclature and classification.

Herpes gestationis, also referred to as pemphigoid gestationis, is an intensely pruritic blistering eruption that occurs in pregnancy and the postpartum period and tends to recur in subsequent pregnancies. Although its precise pathogenesis is unknown, the disorder is characterized by a pruritic eruption consisting of grouped erythematous edematous papules and plaques, grouped vesicles on erythematous bases, and tense bullae affecting pregnant women (with at times recurrences at the time of menstruation), women taking oral contraceptives, infants born to mothers with this disorder, and women with hydatidiform moles or choriocarcinomas (Figs. 15–20 and 15–21) (see Chapter 15).

Pruritic urticarial papules and plaques of pregnancy (PUPPP) is a common intensely pruritic dermatitis that occurs late in the third trimester in approximately 1 in 200 pregnancies. Seen at least in one instance in a mother-and-infant pair, and generally in primigravidas (75% of the time), the disorder begins as 1- to 2-mm lesions on the abdomen, often within the abdominal striae, which soon coalesce to form large erythematous plaques centered around the umbilicus and then spread to involve the abdomen, buttocks, thighs, and, in some cases, the arms and legs (Fig. 18–17), with sparing

of the upper chest, face, and mucous membranes. Although pruritus is frequently extreme and patients are often unable to sleep, excoriations are rare. Other pruritic papular eruptions of pregnancy have been described. Although they tend to differ somewhat from one another, they also show distinct similarities and therefore are frequently united under the nonspecific term *pruritus of pregnancy*. These include toxemic rash of pregnancy (Bourne's disease), toxic erythema of pregnancy, prurigo of pregnancy of Nurse, prurigo annularis of Davies, polymorphic eruption of pregnancy, papular dermatitis of pregnancy of Spangler, and pruritus gravidarum (prurigo gestationis) of Besnier.[61-64] Although the etiology of pruritic urticarial papules and plaques of pregnancy and its variants is unknown, current studies suggest an allergic response to hormonal factors.

The histopathologic features of PUPPP, although not specific, include a moderately pronounced mononuclear infiltrate with a variable number of perivascular collections of lymphohistiocytes and eosinophils. Epidermal changes, although not always present, consist of focal spongiosis and parakeratosis in association with mild acanthosis. Topical application of corticosteroids usually provides symptomatic relief and frequently prevents the formation of new lesions, and in instances where the condition is severe or unresponsive brief courses of systemic corticosteroids (20 to 40 mg of prednisone daily with rapid tapering) are frequently beneficial.

Pruritic folliculitis of pregnancy is a term used to describe patients with a pruritic follicular papular and pustular eruption that appears between the fourth and ninth months of pregnancy and generally resolves within a few weeks after delivery. Clinical and histologic features of acute folliculitis with focal spongiosis and exocytosis of polymorphonuclear cells suggest that this disorder represents a form of hormonal acne similar to that seen in patients with corticosteroid acne rather than a hypersensitivity reaction. Topical applications of benzoyl peroxide and hydrocortisone are helpful in the management of patients with this disorder.[61, 65]

BOWEL BYPASS SYNDROME

Intestinal bypass disease (bowel bypass syndrome, bowel-associated arthritis-dermatosis syndrome) is a disorder characterized by a flu-like illness (chills, malaise, and myalgia), asymmetric polyarthritis, tenosynovitis, thrombophlebitis, retinal vasculitis, and crops of skin lesions most often seen on the arms and hands and less often on the shoulders and flanks. The lesions are generally asymptomatic or mildly pruritic and begin as 3- to 10-mm macules, which develop into vesiculopustules and undergo central necrosis resembling insect bites. Lesions over acral areas may be painful and often mimic pustulovesicular le-

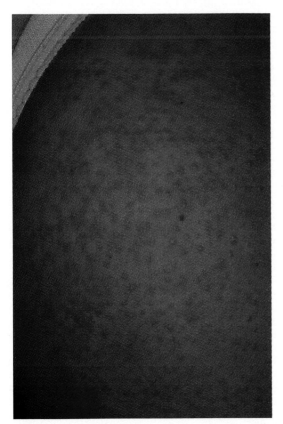

Figure 18–17. Pruritic urticarial papules and plaques of pregnancy.

sions of gonococcemia; and lesions on the legs, which are generally red and tender and usually present on the shins or ankles, often appear as a panniculitis resembling erythema nodosum. The eruption usually lasts for 2 to 6 days and recurs at varying intervals for weeks to months. It is apparently an immune complex disorder, in which bacterial overgrowth in blind intestinal loops and bacterial peptidoglycans produce circulating immune complexes. The diagnosis is suggested by the presence of vesiculopustules, polyarthralgia, polymyalgia, tenosynovitis, and malaise of an intermittent nature in a patient who has undergone bypass surgery producing an intestinal blind loop and, at times, in patients with bowel disease without bowel bypass.[66]

The histologic picture in early lesions reveals a massive dermal infiltrate of neutrophils showing leukocytoclasia without vascular destruction, and sometimes a necrotizing vasculitis with fibrin deposition within and around the vessel walls. Low-dose systemic corticosteroids (10 to 20 mg/day of prednisone or its equivalent) markedly ameliorate symptoms of this disorder and tetracycline, minocycline, metronidazole, clindamycin, sulfisoxazole, and dapsone have been suggested for both acute exacerbations and chronic prophylaxis. Reconstruction of the normal bowel anatomy is curative.

SWEET'S SYNDROME (ACUTE FEBRILE NEUTROPHILIC DERMATOSIS)

Acute febrile neutrophilic dermatosis (Sweet's syndrome), originally described by Sweet in 1961, is a rare disorder characterized by raised painful papules, nodules, or plaques on the limbs, face and neck, accompanied by fever and leukocytosis (Table 18–11). Although the etiology of this disorder is unknown, it appears to represent a hypersensitivity reaction to a bacterial or viral infection or an immunologic response to a leukemic or preleukemic state or other malignancy. The disorder has been described in an infant as young as 7

Table 18–11. ACUTE FEBRILE NEUTROPHILIC DERMATITIS (SWEET'S SYNDROME)

1. High persistent fever
2. Irregular, somewhat nodular, red, tender nodules or plaques on face, neck, and limbs
3. An immunologic response to infection, leukemia, or a preleukemic state?
4. Histologic features
   a. Edema, polymorphonuclear leukocytes, and nuclear dust with an exploding hand grenade appearance in the dermis
   b. Older lesions less characteristic (less infiltrate, and lymphocytes replace polymorphonuclear leukocytes)
5. Rapid response to systemic corticosteroids (potassium iodide, clofazimine, colchicine, indomethacin, and dapsone have also been recommended)

weeks of age but is rare in children; it is most frequent in women between 35 and 66 years of age.[67–69]

The presence of upper respiratory tract infection, high antistreptolysin titers, positive intracutaneous tests with bacterial antigens, and occasional kidney and joint involvement in affected patients suggests an Arthus-like response to an infectious agent as the cause in many individuals. In adults the disorder may also be associated with malignancy, presumably as a hypersensitivity reaction to tumor antigen. The eruption, therefore, in adults can frequently serve as a cutaneous sign of malignancy. Although Sweet's syndrome appears to represent a hypersensitivity reaction with deposition of antigen–antibody complexes in dermal vessel walls and nuclear dust, histopathologic examinations of cutaneous lesions lack the characteristic vascular damage seen in lesions of leukocytoclastic angiitis.

Patients with acute febrile neutrophilic dermatosis usually have a spiking fever associated with raised, brightly erythematous, painful papules, plaques, or nodules on the face, neck, and limbs (particularly the upper arms), with sparing of the areas between the upper chest and thighs. Although the lesions develop almost exclusively in sun-exposed regions, there is no evidence to implicate a role for photosensitivity. Elevated plaques measure 1 cm or more in diameter, are distributed in an asymmetric pattern, and tend to develop partial clearing, resulting in an arcuate configuration as the border of the lesion advances. They are indurated, red to plum-colored, and heal without scarring, often leaving a residual reddish brown color as a result of hemosiderin deposition. Larger plaques frequently have a mammillated surface simulating vesicles, and the borders of the plaques may develop vesicles or sterile pustules (Fig. 18–18).

Leukocytosis ranging from 15,000 to 20,000 (with 80 to 90 per cent polymorphonuclear leukocytes) is common and myalgia, polyarthalgia, and polyarthritis of large joints have been reported in 15 to 25 per cent of patients afflicted with this disorder. In at least 50 per cent of patients there is a history of a preceding febrile illness. Conjunctivitis and episcleritis may be present, and leukemia and carcinoma have been reported in adult patients.

Acute febrile neutrophilic dermatosis generally presents a fairly characteristic clinical picture that can be confirmed by cutaneous biopsy. Two major and four minor criteria have been proposed for the diagnosis of Sweet's syndrome. To establish the diagnosis, it has been suggested that patients must fulfill both major criteria and at least two of the minor criteria. The suggested major criteria include abrupt onset of tender or painful erythematous or violaceous plaques or nodules and predominantly neutrophilic infiltration in the dermis without leukocytoclastic vasculitis. Minor criteria include an illness preceded by fever or infection; fever accompanied by arthralgia, conjunctivitis, or

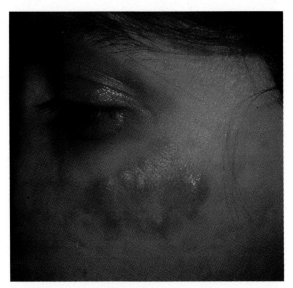

Figure 18–18. Sweet's syndrome. A raised erythematous plaque has a mammillated vesiculopustular surface. (Courtesy of Louis Fragola, M.D.; reprinted from Hurwitz S: The hypersensitivity syndromes. *In:* The Skin and Systemic Disease in Children. Year Book Medical Publishers, Chicago, 1985.)

underlying malignancy; leukocytosis greater than 10,000/mm^3; and a good response to systemic corticosteroids and lack of response to antibiotics.[70] The histologic features of cutaneous lesions consist of edema and a dense perivascular infiltration of polymorphonuclear leukocytes with occasional eosinophils and some lymphoid cells in the upper and mid dermis without vasculitis. As the disorder becomes more pronounced, the infiltrate frequently extends throughout the dermis and nuclear dust and, at times, polymorphonuclear involvement (described as an "exploding hand grenade") becomes apparent. Older lesions present a less characteristic appearance, with lessening of the infiltrate and lymphocytes replacing the polymorphonuclear leukocytes.

If untreated, lesions of Sweet's syndrome may increase and can persist for 1 to 12 months, eventually resolving spontaneously without residual scarring.[4] Patients generally respond to systemic corticosteroids (2 mg/kg/day, up to a dosage of 30 to 60 mg/day of prednisone or its equivalent for 10 days). Once the patient responds, the systemic corticosteroids should be tapered gradually over 1 to 2 months in an effort to prevent recurrences. Potassium iodide, clofazimine (Lamprene), colchicine, indomethacin, and dapsone have also been recommended for the treatment of Sweet's syndrome. Although the reason for the response to iodides is not clear, it appears to be related to an inhibitory effect on hypersensitivity in patients with this disorder. In chronic and relapsing cases unresponsive to other modalities, pulsed methylprednisolone and chlorambucil have also been shown to be effective.[70]

References

1. Champion RH, Roberts SOB, Carpenter RG, et al.: Urticaria and angioedema. Br. J. Dermatol. *81*:588–597, 1969.

    Clinical features, pathogenesis, and management of urticaria and angioedema.

2. Serafin WE, Austin KF: Mediators of immediate hypersensitivity reactions. N. Engl. J. Med. *317*:30–34, 1987.

    A review of histamine, proteases, proteoglycans, arachidonic acid metabolites, prostaglandins, and leukotrienes and their roles in the pathophysiology of immediate hypersensitivity.

3. O'Laughlin S, Schroeter AL, Jordon RE: Chronic urticaria-like lesions in systemic lupus erythematosus: A review of 12 cases. Arch. Dermatol. *114*:879–883, 1978.

    Twelve of 54 patients (23 per cent) with systemic lupus erythematosus had chronic urticaria-like lesions; biopsies in 9 of 11 of these patients revealed necrotizing vasculitis with leukocytoclasis as the major histologic finding.

4. Braverman IM: Skin Signs of Systemic Disease, 2nd ed. W.B. Saunders Co., Philadelphia, 1981.

    A valuable, well-written text emphasizing cutaneous features and their role in the diagnosis of systemic disease.

5. Monroe EW, Cohen SH, Kalbfleisch J, et al.: Combined H$_1$ and H$_2$ antihistamine therapy in chronic urticaria. Arch. Dermatol. *117*:404–407, 1981.

    In a study of 18 patients with refractory chronic idiopathic urticaria, combined H$_1$ and H$_2$ antihistamines were shown to be statistically more effective than H$_1$ antihistamine alone in controlling the symptoms of this disorder.

6. Monroe EW: Chronic urticaria: Review of nonsedating H$_1$ antihistamines in treatment. J. Am. Acad. Dermatol. *19*:842–849, 1989.

    A review of the nonsedating antihistamines, their safety, convenience, and clinical efficacy in the treatment of chronic urticaria.

7. Hurwitz S: The hypersensitivity syndromes. In: The Skin and Systemic Disease in Children. Year Book Medical Publishers, Chicago, 1985, 1–34.

    A review of hypersensitive reactions and their relationship to cutaneous disease in children with emphasis on their pathogenesis, clinical manifestations, and treatment.

8. Hirschmann JV, Lawlor F, English JSC, et al.: Cholinergic urticaria: A clinical and histologic study. Arch. Dermatol. *123*:462–467, 1987.

    A comprehensive review of cholinergic urticaria, its clinical features, natural history, and histologic findings.

9. McLean SP, et al.: Refractory cholinergic urticaria successfully treated with ketotifen. J. Allergy Clin. Immunol. *83*:738–741, 1989.

    Four patients with cholinergic urticaria refractory to conventional antihistamine therapy demonstrated symptomatic improvement after the administration of 3 to 8 mg of ketotifen per day.

10. Chalamidas SL, Charles R: Aquagenic urticaria. Arch. Dermatol. *104*:541–546, 1971.

    Studies in a 49-year-old man with a 3-year history of hives on contact with water support the hypothesis that aquagenic urticaria probably is due to a histamine-induced phenomenon.

11. Shelley WB, Rawnsley HM: Aquagenic urticaria. J.A.M.A. *189*:895–898, 1964.

    An unusual form of perifollicular urticaria caused by a toxic substance formed by a combination of water and sebum that induces degranulation of perifollicular mast cells and subsequent histamine release.

12. Juhlin L, Shelley WB: Role of mast cell and basophil in cold urticaria with associated systemic reactions. J.A.M.A. *177*:371–377, 1961.

With the use of an in vitro technique, circulating basophils and cutaneous mast cells in cold urticaria patients were shown to discharge their granules upon cooling.

13. Tindall JP: Cold urticaria. Postgrad. Med. 50:133–137, 1971.

A review of acquired and familial forms of cold urticaria.

14. Sarkany I, Gaylarde PM: Negative reactions to ice in cold urticaria. Br. J. Dermatol. 85:46–48, 1971.

Some patients with cold urticaria who do not respond to application of ice to the skin may be diagnosed by generalized cooling of the body, or by a positive response to cold water.

15. Wanderer AF, St. Pierre J, Ellis E: Primary acquired cold urticaria. Arch. Dermatol. 113:1375–1377, 1977.

Patients unresponsive to chlorpheniramine responded to treatment with cyproheptadine (Periactin).

16. Klemperer MR, Rosen FS, Donaldson VH: A polypeptide derived from the second component of human complement (C2) which increases vascular permeability. J. Clin. Invest. 48:44a–44b, 1969.

An esterase derived from the first component of human complement (C_{1s}) demonstrated increased vascular permeability when incubated with human C_4 and C_2.

17. Donaldson VH: Mechanisms of activation of C1 esterase in hereditary angioneurotic edema plasma in vitro: The role of Hageman factor, a clot promoting agent. J. Exp. Med. 127:411–429, 1968.

Studies of C_1 esterase activity in plasma obtained from individuals with hereditary angioneurotic edema suggest a role of Hageman factor in the activation of C_1 in this disorder.

18. Hyman C, Wong WH, Janklow HM, et al.: Physiologic studies of the peripheral circulation in a patient with Quincke's disease. J. Invest. Dermatol. 49:533–536, 1967.

Blood flow studies in a 23-year-old man suggest an elevated capillary filtration coefficient in the pathogenesis of the edema in hereditary angioneurotic edema.

19. Massa MC, Connolly SM: An association between C_1 esterase inhibitor deficiency and lupus erythematosus: Report of two cases and review of the literature. J. Am. Acad. Dermatol. 7:255–264, 1982.

A report of two patients and review of data from 11 previously reported patients with hereditary angioneurotic edema and lupus erythematosus suggest a possible relationship between these two disorders.

20. Farnam J, Grant JA: Angioedema. Dermatol. Clin. 3:85–95, 1985.

A comprehensive review of angioedema, its pathogenesis and management.

21. Gelfand JA, Sherrin RJ, Alling DW, et al.: Treatment of hereditary angioedema with danazol. N. Engl. J. Med. 295:1444–1448, 1976.

A double-blind study in nine patients demonstrates a significant decrease in attacks of angioedema in patients treated with danazol.

22. Sheffer AL, Fearon DT, Austen KE: Hereditary angioedema: A decade of management with stanozolol. J. Allergy Clin. Immunol. 80:855–860, 1987.

A review of 37 patients with hereditary angioedema carefully monitored to define the minimal effective dose and duration of therapy for patients treated with stanozolol.

23. Peterson AO Jr, Jarrat M: Annular erythema of infancy. Arch. Dermatol. 117:145–148, 1981.

A report of a 6-month-old boy with a history of an intermittent urticarial eruption whose clinical course and histologic features did not fit well into previously described annular lesions of infancy.

24. Hebert AA, Esterly NB: Annular erythema of infancy. J. Am. Acad. Dermatol. 14:339–343, 1986.

A report of a 7-month-old girl with urticarial annular erythema that began when she was 6 weeks of age and completely resolved by the age of 14 months and a review of the annular erythemas of infancy and childhood.

25. Toonstra J, De Wit FE: "Persistent" annular erythema of infancy. Arch. Dermatol. 120:1069–1072, 1984.

A report of a child with persistent annular cutaneous lesions that were present between the ages of 6 and 11 months, with each of the lesions lasting for periods of months.

26. Baden HP, Holcomb FD: Erythema nodosum from oral contraceptives. Arch. Dermatol. 98:634–635, 1968.

Noninfectious disorders that cause erythema nodosum are ulcerative colitis and regional ileitis, and reactions to various drugs, particularly sulfonamides, phenytoin, and contraceptive pills containing ethinyl estradiol and norethynodrel.

27. Aetiology of erythema nodosum in children: A study by a group of pediatricians. Lancet 2:14–16, 1961.

In a study of 105 children in England, β-hemolytic streptococcal infection proved to be the most common cause of erythema nodosum.

28. Kibel MA: Erythema nodosum in children. S. Afr. Med. J. Sci. 44:873–876, 1970.

A review of 21 cases of erythema nodosum in children from 1958 to 1969.

29. Simon S, Azvedo SJ, Byrnes JJ: Erythema nodosum heralding recurrent Hodgkin's disease. Cancer 56:1470–1472, 1985.

A report of two young men with recurrent Hodgkin's disease heralded by erythema nodosum.

30. Lehman CW: Control of chronic erythema nodosum with naproxen. Cutis 26:66–67, 1980.

The administration of naproxen (Naprosyn), 250 mg twice daily for 1 month, gave prompt resolution and complete clearing of chronic erythema nodosum of 7 years' duration in a 28-year-old woman; although several relapses occurred 6 months after the naproxen was discontinued, the disorder promptly responded to repeated courses of therapy.

31. Horio T, Imamura S, Danno K, et al.: Potassium iodide in the treatment of erythema nodosum and nodular vasculitis. Arch. Dermatol. 117:29–31, 1981.

Eleven of 15 patients with erythema nodosum received symptomatic relief in 24 hours, and complete resolution within 10 to 14 days, after starting oral potassium iodide (300 mg three times a day).

32. Barr WG, Robinson JA: Chronic erythema nodosum treated with indomethacin. Ann. Intern. Med. 95:659, 1981.

Indomethacin (25 mg three times a day for 1 month) completely cleared chronic erythema nodosum of 3 years' duration in a 32-year-old-woman.

33. Wallace SL: Erythema nodosum treatment with colchicine (letter to the editor). J.A.M.A. 202:1056, 1967.

Colchicine was found to be helpful in the management of erythema nodosum.

34. Huff JC, Weston WL, Tonnesen MG: Erythema multiforme: A critical review of characteristics, diagnostic criteria, and causes. J. Am. Acad. Dermatol. 8:763–775, 1983.

A comprehensive review of erythema multiforme, its causes, diagnosis, and clinical spectrum.

35. Hurwitz S: Erythema multiforme: A review of its characteristics, diagnostic criteria and management. Pediatr. Rev. 11:217–222, 1990.

A comprehensive review of the diagnosis, classification, and management of erythema multiforme, Stevens-Johnson disease, and toxic epidermal necrolysis.

36. Stevens AM, Johnson FC: A new eruptive fever associated with stomatitis and ophthalmia: Report of two cases in children. Am. J. Dis. Child. 24:526–533, 1922.

Review of the clinical manifestations of two children suggested that this disorder deserved consideration as a specific clinical entity, Stevens-Johnson disease.

37. Lyell A: Toxic epidermal necrolysis: An eruption resembling scalded skin. Br. J. Dermatol. 68:355–361, 1956.

    The original description of a disorder somewhat similar to what is now termed *staphylococcal scalded skin syndrome*.

38. Goldstein SM, Wintroub BW, Elias PM, et al.: Toxic epidermal necrolysis: Unmuddying the waters. Arch. Dermatol. 123:1153–1156, 1987.

    A review of the pathogenesis of toxic epidermal necrolysis and the debate over its nosology and relationship to erythema multiforme major.

39. Guillaume J-C, Roujeau J-C, Revuz J, et al.: The culprit drugs in 87 cases of toxic epidermal necrolysis (Lyell's syndrome). Arch. Dermatol. 123:1166–1170, 1987.

    In a review of 87 patients with toxic epidermal necrolysis in which the culpable drug was determined in 67 patients, nonsteroidal anti-inflammatory drug therapy was implicated as the principal cause of drug-induced Lyell's syndrome.

40. Taylor B, Duffil M: Toxic epidermal necrolysis from griseofulvin. J. Am. Acad. Dermatol. 19:565–568, 1988.

    A report of a 40-year-old woman with toxic epidermal necrolysis presumed to be associated with the taking of griseofulvin.

41. Peck GL, Herzig JP, Elias PM: Toxic epidermal necrolysis in a patient with graft-vs-host reaction. Arch. Dermatol. 105:561–569, 1972.

    A 22-year-old man with acute lymphatic leukemia developed graft-vs.-host disease and toxic epidermal necrolysis following allogeneic bone marrow transplantation.

42. Stern RS, Chan H-L: Usefulness of case report literature in determining drugs responsible for toxic epidermal necrolysis. J. Am. Acad. Dermatol. 21:317–322, 1989.

    A literature review of toxic epidermal necrolysis from January 1966 to April 1987 and the drugs apparently responsible for 73 cases of this disorder.

43. Prendiville JS, Hebert AA, Greenwald MJ, et al.: Management of Stevens-Johnson syndrome and toxic epidermal necrolysis in children. J. Pediatr. 115:881–887, 1989.

    A retrospective analysis of 21 consecutive patients hospitalized with Stevens-Johnson syndrome or toxic epidermal necrolysis in which the authors concluded that systemic steroids have no place in the management of these disorders.

44. Roujeau J-C, Chosidow O, Saiag P, et al.: Toxic epidermal necrolysis (Lyell syndrome). J. Am. Acad. Dermatol. 23:1039–1058, 1990.

    A comprehensive overview of toxic epidermal necrolysis, its pathogenesis and management.

45. Rasmussen JE: Erythema multiforme in children—response to treatment with systemic corticosteroids. Br. J. Dermatol. 95:181–185, 1976.

    Review of 32 patients with Stevens-Johnson disease suggest that treatment with systemic corticosteroids may be associated with delayed recovery and significant side effects.

46. Renfro L, Grant-Kels JM, Feder HMJ, et al.: Controversy: Are systemic steroids indicated in the treatment of erythema multiforme? Pediatr. Dermatol. 6:43–50, 1989.

    A review of the controversy of steroids and the value of their use, if at all, in erythema multiforme and a report of two children and one adolescent successfully treated with systemic corticosteroids.

47. Esterly NB (Ed.): Corticosteroids for erythema multiforme? Pediatr. Dermatol. 6:229–250, 1989.

    In a review of the controversy over the role of corticosteroid therapy, 15 recognized authorities were asked to describe their preferred management for patients with erythema multiforme and toxic epidermal necrolysis.

48. Lemak MA, Duvic M, Bean SF: Oral acyclovir for the prevention of herpes-associated erythema multiforme. J. Am. Acad. Dermatol. 15:50–54, 1986.

    A report of four patients in whom oral acyclovir was successfully used to prevent herpes simplex–associated erythema multiforme.

49. Avakian R, Flowers FP, Araujo DE, et al.: Toxic epidermal necrolysis: A review. J. Am. Acad. Dermatol. 25:69–79, 1991.

    A comprehensive review of toxic epidermal necrolysis, its pathophysiology and management.

50. Kazmierowski JA, Chusid MJ, Parillo JE, et al.: Dermatologic manifestations of the hypereosinophilic syndrome. Arch. Dermatol. 114:531–535, 1978.

    A review of the histopathologic and dermatologic manifestations in eight of 15 patients with hypereosinophilic syndrome.

51. Lugassy G, Michaeli J: Hypouricemia in the hypereosinophilic syndrome: Response to treatment. J.A.M.A. 250:937–938, 1983.

    A report of a patient with severe hypouricemia associated with the hypereosinophilic syndrome.

52. Wynn SR, Sachs MI, Keating MU, et al.: Idiopathic hypereosinophilic syndrome in a 5 1/2 -month-old infant. J. Pediatr. 111:94–97, 1987.

    A report of an infant with hypereosinophilic syndrome successfully treated with prednisone, vincristine, and hydroxyurea.

53. Morrow JD, Margolies GR, Rowland J, et al.: Evidence that histamine is the causative toxin of scombroid-fish poisoning. N. Engl. J. Med. 324:716–720, 1991.

    Studies of histamine content of fish and urinary histamine levels in patients with scombroid-fish poisoning incriminate histamine as the toxin responsible for this disorder.

54. Blakesley ML: Scombroid poisoning: Prompt resolution of symptoms with cimetidine. Ann. Emerg. Med. 12:104–106, 1983.

    A report of four patients with scombroid poisoning and a discussion of the pathophysiology, clinical features, and management of this disorder.

55. Kasha EE Jr, Norins AL: Scombroid fish poisoning with facial flushing. J. Am. Acad. Dermatol. 18:1363–1364, 1988.

    A report of two patients with scombroid fish poisoning and a review of the pathophysiology, clinical features, and treatment of this disorder.

56. Etkind P, Wilson ME, Gallagher K, et al.: Bluefish-associated scombroid poisoning: An example of the expanding spectrum of food poisoning from seafood. J.A.M.A. 258:3409–3410, 1987.

    Five persons who attended a medical conference developed symptoms of scombroid poisoning following the ingestion of improperly handled frozen bluefish; elevated levels of histamine, putrescine, and cadaverine were detected in samples of the uncooked fish.

57. Palafox NA, Jain LG, Pinano AZ, et al.: Successful treatment of ciguatera fish poisoning with intravenous mannitol. J.A.M.A. 259:2740–2742, 1988.

    In a report of 24 patients with acute ciguatera poisoning, each patient improved dramatically within minutes following the administration of intravenous mannitol.

58. Shelley WB, Preucel RW, Spoont SS: Autoimmune progesterone dermatitis: Cure by oophorectomy. J.A.M.A. 190:35–38, 1964.

    An extensive pruritic vesiculobullous eruption of 5 years' duration that did not respond to various forms of therapy was ultimately cured by oophorectomy.

59. Bierman SM: Autoimmune progesterone dermatitis of pregnancy. Arch. Dermatol. 107:896–901, 1973.

The administration of conjugated aqueous estrogen dramatically reduced the symptoms of autoimmune progesterone dermatitis in a 25-year-old patient with this disorder.

60. Hart R: Autoimmune progesterone dermatitis. Arch. Dermatol. *113*:426–430, 1977.

Five of seven woman with autoimmune progesterone dermatitis responded to cyclic administration of Premarin in a dosage of 1.25 mg/day for a period of 21 days.

61. Holmes RC, Black MM: The specific dermatoses of pregnancy. J. Am. Acad. Dermatol. 8:405–412, 1983.

A review of the dermatoses of pregnancy and an attempt to rationalize the nomenclature by a critical review of the literature and personal study of 64 patients.

62. Yancey KB, Hall RP, Lawley TJ: Pruritic urticarial papules and plaques of pregnancy. J. Am. Acad. Dermatol. *10*:473–480, 1984.

In a review of 25 patients with features of pruritic urticarial papules and plaques of pregnancy, high potency topical corticosteroids were found to be effective in relieving pruritus and controlling the eruption associated with this disorder.

63. Michaud RM, Jacobson D, Dahl MV: Papular dermatitis of pregnancy. Arch. Dermatol. *118*:1003–1005, 1982.

A report of a widespread pruritic urticaria-like papular eruption in a woman during the third trimester of her pregnancy in whom urinary chorionic gonadotropin levels were found to be elevated.

64. Uhlin SR: Pruritic urticarial papules and plaques of pregnancy: Involvement of mother and infant. Arch. Dermatol. *117*:238–239, 1981.

A report of a 19-year-old mother with pruritic urticarial papules and plaques of pregnancy in which similar lesions also occurred on her newborn.

65. Zoberman E, Farmer ER: Pruritic folliculitis of pregnancy. Arch. Dermatol. *117*:20–22, 1981.

Since histopathologic examinations of pruritic erythematous papular lesions in 5 of 6 pregnant women revealed features of acute folliculitis, the authors suggested that the term *pruritic folliculitis of pregnancy* be used to identify patients with this cutaneous disorder.

66. Dicken C: Bowel-associated dermatosis-arthritis syndrome: Bowel bypass syndrome without bowel bypass. J. Am. Acad. Dermatol. *14*:792–796, 1986.

In a report of a 24-year-old woman and a review of 7 previously reported patients with bowel-associated dermatosis-arthritis syndrome, none of the patients had undergone ileojejunal bypass surgery.

67. Hazen PG, Kask EC, Davis BR, et al.: Acute neutrophilic dermatosis in children. Arch. Dermatol. *119*:998–1002, 1983.

A report of two children, both younger than 1 year of age, who developed Sweet's syndrome; both infants acquired their disease during or after an upper respiratory tract illness.

68. Kibbi AG, Zaynoun ST, Kurban AK, et al.: Acute febrile neutrophilic dermatosis (Sweet's syndrome): Case report and review of the literature. Pediatr. Dermatol. 3:40–44, 1985.

A report of an 8-month-old infant with Sweet's syndrome and a review of the literature.

69. Dunn TR, Saperstein HW, Biederman A, et al.: Sweet's syndrome in a neonate with aseptic meningitis. Pediatr. Dermatol. 9:288–292, 1992.

A 7-week-old infant with antecedent otitis media, upper respiratory infection, and aseptic meningitis and Sweet's syndrome, the youngest of 17 children with this syndrome reported to date, and the first in whom the syndrome was associated with aseptic meningitis.

70. Su WPD, Liu H-N: Diagnostic criteria for Sweet's syndrome. Cutis 38:167–172, 1986.

A report of five patients with Sweet's syndrome and a review of proposed diagnostic criteria for this disorder.

71. Case JD, Smith SZ, Callen JP: The use of pulse methylprednisolone and chlorambucil in the treatment of Sweet's syndrome. Cutis *44*:125–129, 1989.

A report of a patient with an unusual variant of Sweet's syndrome in whom the course of the disease was chronic and relapses of the disorder were successfully treated with methylprednisolone pulse therapy.

VASCULITIC DISORDERS

The vasculitic disorders are a heterogeneous group of conditions characterized by inflammation and necrosis of blood vessels, deposition of fibrinoid material in blood vessel walls, and the presence of scattered nuclear fragments, referred to as nuclear dust, resulting from disintegration of neutrophilic nuclei (leukocytosis) within the necrotic areas of the vessel wall and surrounding tissues. The classification of cutaneous vasculitis is based on gross and morphologic features and encompasses a wide spectrum of vascular reactions to a variety of noxious stimuli and associated systemic disease. The vasculitic disorders discussed in this chapter include leukocytoclastic vasculitis (Henoch-Schönlein purpura), hemorrhagic edema of infancy (a possible variant of Henoch-Schönlein purpura), pediatric and adult types of periarteritis nodosa, Kawasaki disease, vasculitides with granulomatosis, erythema elevatum diutinum, urticarial vasculitis, and Behçet's syndrome.

HENOCH-SCHÖNLEIN (ANAPHYLACTOID) PURPURA

Henoch-Schönlein purpura, also known by its synonym *anaphylactoid purpura*, is a well-defined systemic disorder of children and young adults. An inflammatory disorder of multiple causes, it appears to represent a diffuse vasculitis caused by hypersensitivity to a variety of etiologic factors. Although the nature of the immunologic reaction is not completely clear, a history of frequent antecedent upper respiratory tract infections preceding the onset of symptoms suggests a hypersensitivity phenomenon resulting in localized or widespread vascular damage. Bacterial or viral infections appear to be the most frequently implicated precipitating causes; drugs, food, insect bites, immunizations, cold exposure, foods, and chemical toxins have also been suggested as possible etiologic factors.

Clinical Manifestations. The clinical picture of Henoch-Schönlein vasculitis is distinctive. Mainly a disease of children and young adults (particularly those between 3 and 10 years of age), the disorder is characterized by a distinctive rash (erythematous papules followed by purpura), abdominal pain, and joint symptoms. Renal disease occurs frequently, but other organ involvement is relatively less common. Generally the disease subsides within a few weeks, with frequent recurrences often related to an upper respiratory tract infection or reexposure to the offending agent. The disorder appears to represent a variety of leukocytoclastic angiitis initiated by deposition of immune complexes, mainly of the IgA class, which produces a vasculitis of the capillaries and precapillary and postcapillary vessels in the upper dermis, gastrointestinal tract, synovial membranes, renal glomeruli, and lungs.[1-4] IgA complexes, however, are not a necessary requirement for the development of Henoch-Schönlein purpura and their absence should not exclude the diagnosis. In addition, the presence of IgA in skin biopsy specimens in patients with hematuria following an upper respiratory tract infection without cutaneous lesions (Berger's disease) suggests an association between these two disorders.

Cutaneous Lesions. The skin lesions of Henoch-Schönlein purpura consist of small, 2- to 10-mm hemorrhagic macules, papules, and/or urticarial

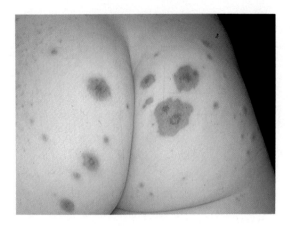

Figure 19–1. Henoch-Schönlein purpura (anaphylactoid purpura). Hemorrhagic macules, papules, and urticarial lesions appear in a symmetric distribution over the buttocks of a young child.

lesions, which appear in a symmetric distribution over the buttocks (Fig. 19–1) and extensor surfaces of the extremities (particularly the elbows and knees) (Fig. 19–2).[5] In some instances, skin lesions may develop in patterns at pressure sites; and in more severe cases, hemorrhagic, purpuric, or necrotic lesions may be prominent. The disease usually consists of a single episode, which may last for several days to several weeks. In some cases, however, recurrent attacks may occur at intervals for weeks or months.

Individual lesions occur in crops, tend to fade after about 5 days, and eventually are replaced by areas of brownish pigmentation, purpura, or ecchymoses. New crops of lesions frequently occur over the fading lesions of a previous episode, thus giving a polymorphous appearance to the disorder. Although the lesions may be misinterpreted as drug reactions, erythema multiforme, or urticaria, the presence of *palpable purpura* (the hallmark of leukocytoclastic angiitis) will usually clarify the true nature of the disorder. This characteristic finding, created by edema and extravasation of erythrocytes, gives individual lesions their diagnostic palpable and purpuric appearance.

Rarely, the face, mucous membranes of the mouth and nose, and the anogenital regions may show petechial involvement. Children younger than 3 years of age often have an associated edema of the scalp, hands, feet, scrotum, and periorbital tissues. This edema occurs in the absence of renal or cardiac disease and appears to reflect an increased capillary permeability due to the underlying vasculitis.

The diagnosis of Henoch-Schönlein purpura is seldom difficult when all the components of the syndrome are present or when the typical eruption with palpable purpura is present. When the diagnosis remains in doubt, histopathologic examination of a cutaneous biopsy specimen generally helps clarify the nature of the eruption. Histopathologic changes of Henoch-Schönlein purpura are characterized by leukocytoclastic vasculitis, with fibrinoid degeneration of vessel walls and a peri-

vascular infiltrate consisting of neutrophils, some eosinophils, and only a few lymphocytes. Extravasation of erythrocytes is present in purpuric lesions, with deposits of hemosiderin in lesions of long duration. A highly characteristic feature is the presence of scattered nuclear fragments (nuclear dust), which result from the disintegration of the neutrophils.

Systemic Manifestations. Systemic involvement is seen in up to 80 per cent of children with severe forms of Henoch-Schönlein purpura. Since proper diagnosis depends on the characteristic cutaneous eruption, a significant diagnostic challenge occurs when systemic manifestations appear alone or precede the appearance of skin lesions.[6] The degree of systemic involvement may vary, with arthritic or gastrointestinal symptoms reportedly seen in as many as two thirds of affected children. Gastrointestinal symptoms resulting from edema of the bowel wall and hemorrhage as a result of vasculitis occur in approximately 75 per cent of

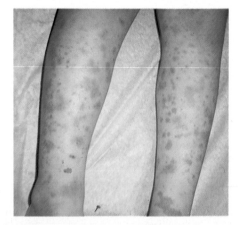

Figure 19–2. Henoch-Schönlein purpura. Small hemorrhagic symmetric papules are seen on the lower extremities. Edema and extravasation of erythrocytes give individual lesions their diagnostic palpable and purpuric appearance.

patients. They usually include colicky abdominal pain and in severe cases may consist of vomiting, visceral infarction or perforation, pancreatitis, cholecystitis, esophageal involvement, colitis, protein-losing enteropathy, chronic intestinal obstruction with ileal stricture, intussusception, hemorrhage, or shock.[7, 8] Intussusception, seen in up to 2 per cent of patients, is more frequently seen in boys, particularly those about 6 years of age. Since intussusception (when not associated with Henoch-Schönlein purpura) generally occurs in children younger than 2 years of age, when seen in older children, Henoch-Schönlein purpura must be strongly considered as a diagnostic possibility.[9] Intramural hematomas also may occur in the small or large bowel, and on rare occasions ischemic necrosis and spontaneous intestinal perforation have been noted. Hepatosplenomegaly may be present, and although bowel involvement is the major cause of abdominal signs and symptoms, other abdominal complications such as pancreatitis and cholecystitis may contribute to the abdominal pain and vomiting seen in individuals with this disorder.

Joint involvement, affecting 60 to 84 per cent of patients, is characterized by warm, tender, painful swelling of joints, with or without overlying purpura. It is generally believed that joint symptoms are due to periarticular edema rather than a true arthritis. Although the ankles and knees are most frequently affected, arthropathy of the elbows, hands, and feet may also be seen in association with this disorder. Arthritic symptoms, when present, generally persist for several days and are frequently recurrent.

Renal involvement is probably the most frequent and serious complication of anaphylactoid purpura. It occurs in 25 per cent of children younger than age 2 and in 50 per cent of those older than 2 years of age.[10] Nephritis may be demonstrated by gross or microscopic hematuria, with or without casts and proteinuria. Although often self-limited, if hematuria persists, it may progress to advanced glomerular disease and a poor prognosis, with death resulting from acute or chronic renal failure.

Central nervous system involvement may result in headache and diplopia, and rarely subarachnoid hemorrhage may occur, with coma, seizures, and/or paresis.[11, 12] Respiratory involvement, also uncommon, may range from an asymptomatic pulmonary infiltrate to recurrent episodes of pulmonary hemorrhage. Testicular and scrotal hemorrhage may occur in up to 20 per cent of boys with this disorder. This may cause intense pain, scrotal swelling, and, at least in one instance, torsion of the testis requiring surgical intervention.

The prognosis for most patients with Henoch-Schönlein vasculitis is excellent, with full recovery without residue in most instances. In younger children the disease is generally milder and of shorter duration, with fewer renal and gastrointestinal manifestations and few recurrences. In approximately 5 per cent of patients with nephritis, the disorder progresses to end-stage renal disease. Serious gastrointestinal lesions and extensive kidney disease account for a mortality rate of up to 1 to 3 per cent.

There is no specific therapy for Henoch-Schönlein purpura. Bed rest and general supportive care are helpful. Throat cultures and appropriate antibiotics are indicated if a specific respiratory illness is identified. Since many cases of chronic glomerulonephritis in adults may be related to anaphylactoid purpura during childhood, serial urinalyses are indicated. The efficacy of corticosteroids is debatable. Although there is little evidence that corticosteroids influence the prognosis of Henoch-Schönlein purpura, they suppress the acute manifestations and may be justified for short periods in severe cases, particularly those with significant gastrointestinal complications or chronic glomerulonephritis.[13] Corticosteroids, alone or in combination with cytotoxic agents, and anticoagulants have also been used in the treatment of Henoch-Schönlein nephritis; and since it has been reported that the level of factor XIII activity declines during the acute phase of childhood Henoch-Schönlein purpura, factor XIII concentrate therapy has been found to be effective for severe abdominal pain, at least in some patients with adult Henoch-Schönlein purpura with low factor XIII activity during the acute phase of the disorder.[14]

ACUTE HEMORRHAGIC EDEMA OF INFANCY

Acute hemorrhagic edema of infancy (acute hemorrhagic vasculitis, Finkelstein's disease) is an acute form of cutaneous leukocytoclastic vasculitis in children between 5 and 24 months of age characterized by fever, large purpuric lesions, and edema. The cutaneous lesions often have a cockade (medallion-like) pattern on the face, auricles, and extremities with a rapid onset and a short benign course followed by complete recovery. The disorder resembles Henoch-Schönlein purpura, and some believe it to be a variant of Henoch-Schönlein purpura without intestinal, renal, or arthritic manifestations. Its frequent association with a preceding infection suggests a cell-mediated response to an infectious agent or a hypersensitivity to medication as a cause of the disorder. Although no specific therapy is available, antibiotics are recommended when there is evidence of concurrent infection.[15, 16]

PERIARTERITIS (POLYARTERITIS) NODOSA

Periarteritis nodosa, also known as polyarteritis nodosa, is a relatively uncommon systemic disorder characterized by a severe necrotizing inflammation of small and medium-sized arteries. Classified as adult or infantile types, periarteritis nodosa has two disease spectra. The adult form affects older children and adults; the infantile disorder characteristically affects children in the first 2 years of life (Table 19–1). Although the cause of periarteritis nodosa is unknown, it is presumed to represent a hypersensitivity-type immune-complex vasculitis with deposits of IgM, C_3, or both, in affected vessel walls.[17]

Pediatric Periarteritis (Polyarteritis) Nodosa

Pediatric periarteritis nodosa (infantile or pediatric polyarteritis), a disorder characteristically affecting children in the first 2 years of life, usually manifests as an overwhelming acute illness diagnosed at autopsy by coronary artery occlusion and vasculitis. It frequently begins as a febrile illness (suggesting a viral infection) and, in contrast to the strong male predominance characteristic of adult periarteritis nodosa, affects both sexes equally. As the disorder progresses, cardiac arteritis leads to aneurysms, infarction, cardiomegaly, congestive heart failure, and renal peripheral artery and nervous system involvement, resulting in hypertension, abnormal urinary findings, peripheral ischemia, neuritis, paralysis, and seizures. Prognosis is poor, and death is usually related to cardiac decompensation. Although the small number of reported cases and high rate of mortality of infants with infantile periarteritis nodosa appear to distinguish this disorder from Kawasaki disease, many authorities suggest that Kawasaki disease may represent an infantile form of periarteritis nodosa.[18, 19]

Adult-Type Periarteritis (Polyarteritis) Nodosa

Adult-type periarteritis (polyarteritis) nodosa, a disorder of older children and adults with strong male predominance, is characterized by crops of subcutaneous nodules along the course of the superficial arteries of the trunk and extremities with fever, calf pain, arthritis, abdominal pain,

Raynaud's phenomenon, hypertension, peripheral neuropathy, and myocardial infarction.

Cutaneous lesions, seen in about half the cases, are usually limited to the lower extremities and range from livedo reticularis, purpura, urticaria, and bullae to maculopapular eruptions, necrotic vesicles, pustules, and, at times, tender subcutaneous nodules or ulcerations that follow the course of medium-sized arteries of the trunk and extremities (Fig. 19–3). The nodules vary from 0.5 to 1.0 cm, are tender to palpation, and are usually red to purple. They may persist for days or months, often disappear spontaneously, or, as a result of acute infarction (depending on the degree of necrosis), may go on to develop ulceration and scar formation. Other cutaneous manifestations include ecchymoses and peripheral gangrene of fingers and toes.

Benign cutaneous periarteritis nodosa is a clinical variant in which cutaneous lesions predominate and there is no visceral involvement. In some instances, however, fever, peripheral neuropathy, myalgia, or arthralgia may be present. After many years' duration, the disorder gradually subsides. The term *nodosa* refers to the fact that the arteritis is focal, thus causing nodose swellings in the affected blood vessels. Since subcutaneous nodules are present in the benign cutaneous form and are rarely encountered in the systemic disorder, they generally suggest a good prognosis.

In the systemic disease, coronary arteritis may lead to aneurysms and infarction, thus producing cardiomegaly, congestive heart failure, and (in 70 to 80 per cent of patients) kidney disease. Peripheral artery and nervous system involvement may result in hypertension, abnormal urinary sediment, peripheral ischemia, paralysis, and convulsions. Death, when it occurs, is usually associated with renal failure, intracranial or intra-abdominal hemorrhage, hypertensive heart failure, and myocardial involvement.

The diagnosis of adult-type periarteritis nodosa is suggested by the presence of renal and visceral arterial involvement with dilatation of medium-sized arteritis demonstrable by angiography. Histopathologic examination of cutaneous lesions reveals a necrotizing vasculitis (a panarteritis) in medium-sized and small muscular arteries with

---

Table 19–1. PERIARTERITIS NODOSA

1. Infantile form (usually in first 2 years of life)
   a. An overwhelming acute illness (usually begins with fever)
   b. Bears pathologic similarity to Kawasaki disease
   c. Prognosis is poor and death usually is related to cardiac decompensation
   d. Possibly the severe fatal end of the Kawasaki disease spectrum?
2. Adult form (older children and adults)
   a. A necrotizing arteritis of small and medium-sized muscular-type arteries (gastroinestinal tract, pancreas, kidney, heart, muscles, and skin)
   b. Death, when it occurs, usually associated with renal failure, cardiac involvement or intracranial or intra-abdominal hemorrhage
   c. Cutaneous features in 25% to 50% of patients (livedo reticularis, purpura, bullae, necrotic vesicles or pustules, urticaria, and tender subcutaneous nodules or ulcerations along course of medium-sized arteries)

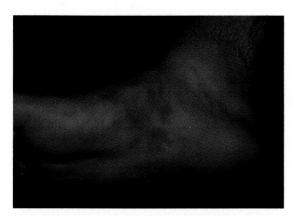

Figure 19–3. Periarteritis nodosa of the adult type. Livedo reticularis, purpura, and subcutaneous nodules are seen on the foot of a 20-year-old young man. (From Hurwitz S: Vasculitic syndromes. *In:* The Skin and Systemic Disease in Children. Year Book Medical Publishers, Chicago, 1985.)

fibrinoid necrosis of the media, endothelial proliferation, and predominantly polymorphonuclear leukocytic infiltration of affected vessel walls.

Untreated, the adult-type periarteritis nodosa follows an intermittent course and used to be uniformly fatal within a few months to a few years. With present-day therapy, however, the prognosis is not as grim and half of the patients currently survive. Management consists of general supportive therapy and corticosteroids (1-2 mg/kg/day of prednisone or its equivalent). In patients in whom the disease persists or worsens despite the use of systemic corticosteroids, immunosuppressive agents (azathioprine or cyclophosphamide) may be used, with cyclophosphamide appearing to be the more effective drug. Since systemic corticosteroids appear to be contraindicated for patients with Kawasaki disease, nonsteroidal anti-inflammatory agents such as aspirin in combination with intravenous γ-globulin currently are a more logical choice for the treatment of the infantile form of periarteritis nodosa.

KAWASAKI DISEASE

Kawasaki disease (Kawasaki syndrome, mucocutaneous lymph node syndrome) is an acute febrile disorder of unknown etiology affecting infants and young children in Japan since around 1950. First reported by Dr. Tomisaku Kawasaki in 1967, the disorder is referred to as Kawasaki disease in honor of the Tokyo physician who contributed so much to our recognition of the syndrome.[20] The first cases in the United States were reported from Hawaii in 1974,[21, 22] and patients with this multisystemic disease have now been described worldwide. Despite the vast numbers of well-documented case histories, the etiology of Kawasaki disease remains unknown. It currently appears to represent an immunologic disorder triggered by an infectious or perhaps toxic agent, with a possible relationship to a collagen vascular disorder.[22, 23] The presence of generalized vasculitis, circulating immune complexes, and occasional hypocomplementemia suggests an immunologic reaction and an association with collagen vascular disease; the acute onset, fever, and occasional association with aseptic meningitis suggest an infectious agent; and epidemics following exposure to shampooed or spot-cleaned rugs or carpets[24, 25] suggest a possible relationship to a toxic agent.

Because this disease is most prevalent in Japan and its incidence is much higher in Japanese than in whites or blacks, and because Chinese, Polynesian, and Filipino children have an intermediate incidence, a unique genetic susceptibility has been hypothesized for this disorder. This genetic susceptibility appears to be further supported by an increased frequency of antigens that have a higher incidence in Japanese than in other races (i.e., HLA-B22 and HLA-B22 subtype J2 antigens) in patients with Kawasaki disease.[23] From a pathologic viewpoint, Kawasaki disease is an arteritis involving the small and medium-sized arteries with a predilection for involvement of the main coronary vessels.

Kawasaki disease resembles the infantile form of periarteritis nodosa in many respects. Although it has been suggested that the small number of reported cases and the high rate of mortality in infantile periarteritis nodosa distinguish this disorder from mucocutaneous lymph node syndrome, children with infantile periarteritis nodosa may represent the more severe fatal end of the Kawasaki disease spectrum. However, infantile periarteritis nodosa should not be confused with the adult form of periarteritis nodosa.

Clinical Manifestations. Although occasional cases of Kawasaki disease have been reported in adults and children older than 10 years of age, most patients (85 per cent) are younger than 5, and 50 per cent are younger than 2 1/2 years of age.[20] Few cases of Kawasaki disease are actually seen in individuals older than the age of 10 years, and most reports of Kawasaki syndrome in adults probably represent cases of toxic shock syndrome.[26]

The clinical course of Kawasaki disease may be described as triphasic (Table 19–2) with phase I, *the acute febrile period*, lasting for approximately 12 days. It begins abruptly with the onset of fever and is followed (usually within 1 to 3 days) by most of the other principal diagnostic criteria: bilateral conjunctival vascular dilatation (conjunctival injection), changes on the lips and in the mouth, an erythematous rash, and lymphadenopathy. Associated features seen during this period include diarrhea, hepatic dysfunction, and aseptic meningitis.

Phase II, *the subacute phase*, lasts until approximately day 30 of the illness. It encompasses the period characterized by resolution of fever, desquamation, and thrombocytosis. Arthritis, arthralgia, and carditis, when present, usually appear in

Table 19–2. CLINICAL PHASES OF KAWASAKI DISEASE

Phase I The acute febrile period
  a. Begins abruptly with the onset of fever
  b. Lasts approximately 12 days
  b. Is followed (usually within 1 to 3 days) by most of the other principal
     features
Phase II The subacute phase
  a. Lasts approximately until day 30 of illness
  b. Resolution of fever, thrombocytosis, desquamation, and (when present)
     arthritis, arthralgia, and carditis
  c. Highest risk for sudden death during this period
Phase III The convalescent period
  a. Usually begins within 8 to 10 weeks after onset of illness
  b. Begins when all signs of illness have disappeared and ends when
     erythrocyte sedimentation rate returns to normal
  c. A small number of deaths occur during this period

this period. This stage has the highest risk for sudden death due to coronary thrombosis.

Phase III, *the convalescent period,* begins when all signs of illness have disappeared, and lasts until the sedimentation rate returns to normal, usually 8 to 10 weeks after the onset of illness. A small proportion of reported patients died suddenly during the convalescent phase (at a time when they were thought to be recovering from their illness).

Principal Criteria. The diagnosis of Kawasaki disease is based on clinical criteria, together with the exclusion of other clinically similar diseases. To make a diagnosis, the patient should meet five of six criteria (Table 19–3). These include fever persisting at least 5 days, with no other reasonable explanation for the illness, and four of the following five features: (1) changes in peripheral extremities, including acute erythema and edema of the hands and feet followed by convalescent desquamation of the fingertips; (2) a polymorphous exanthem; (3) bilateral, painless bulbar conjunctival injection without exudate; (4) changes in lips and oral cavity, such as erythema and cracking of lips, strawberry tongue, and diffuse injection of oral and pharyngeal mucosae; and (5) acute, usually unilateral nonpurulent cervical lymphadenopathy (equal to or greater than 1.5 cm in diameter).[27] In practice, most patients have all of the first five criteria while the sixth, lymphadenopathy, is seen in approximately 70 per cent of patients in Japan and 50 to 86 per cent of patients in the United States.[23]

It should be noted, however, that some patients, particularly those younger than 6 months of age, do not meet the full spectrum of criteria for the diagnosis of Kawasaki syndrome. It has been recommended, therefore, that echocardiography be performed 3 to 4 weeks after the onset of unexplained febrile illnesses fulfilling partial but not complete criteria for this disorder.[28] Although at least five of the previously cited clinical features generally satisfy a diagnosis of Kawasaki disease, patients with four of the features can be diagnosed as having the disorder when coronary aneurysm is recognized by two-dimensional echocardiography or coronary angiography.[29] In addition, it has been noted that siblings of children with Kawasaki disease have a significantly greater chance of acquiring this disorder than children of the same age in the general population.[30] The fact that more than half of second case reports develop 10 days or less after the first, coupled with a high incidence and short interval between onset in twins, suggests a likelihood of common exposure and the possibility of genetic susceptibility.[31]

Fever. For a diagnosis of Kawasaki disease, the patient should have a fever lasting more than 5 days (with no other reasonable explanation of the illness). Fever, the first sign and principal symptom of this disorder, begins abruptly without prodromal signs. Seen in most patients (95 per cent), it has a remittent pattern with several spikes in temperature up to 104°F (40.0°C) each day, does

Table 19–3. DIAGNOSTIC CRITERIA OF KAWASAKI DISEASE

1. Fever lasting at least 5 days
2. At least four of the five following features:*
   a. Changes in peripheral extremities, including acute erythema and edema of the
      hands and feet, followed by convalescent desquamation of the fingertips
   b. Polymorphous exanthem
   c. Bilateral painless bulbar conjunctival injection without exudate
   d. Changes in lips and oral cavity (erythema and cracking of lips, strawberry tongue
      and diffuse injection of oral and pharyngeal mucosae)
   e. Acute nonpurulent cervical lymphadenopathy, usually unilateral, equal to or greater
      than 1.5 cm in diameter

* Although at least five of the above clinical features generally satisfy a diagnosis of Kawasaki disease;
patients with four of the above features can be diagnosed as having Kawasaki disease when coronary
aneurysm is recognized by two-dimensional echocardiography or coronary angiography.

not respond to antibiotics or intermittent doses of antipyretics, and lasts 1 to 3 weeks (5 to 23 days, with an average duration of 11 days).

Conjunctival Injection. Painless discrete bilateral injection of the bulbar conjunctivae with relative sparing of the area around the limbus (seen in 88 per cent of patients) generally appears within 2 days of the onset of fever and persists for 1 to 3 weeks (throughout the febrile course of the illness) (Fig. 19–4). This is not a true conjunctivitis and consists chiefly of discrete dilatation of the bulbar conjunctival vessels without evidence of exudative discharge or corneal ulceration.

Oral Cavity Changes. Changes in the mouth consist of erythema, fissuring, and, at times, bleeding and severe crusting of the lips. The lip changes (seen in 90 per cent of patients) may last for 1 to 3 weeks. Erythema and protruberance of the papillae of the tongue (seen in 77 per cent of patients) produces a "strawberry tongue" appearance. When present, strawberry tongue and erythema of the oropharynx appear within 1 to 3 days after the onset of fever (Figs. 19–5 and 19–6).

Exanthem. On the third to fifth day of illness a macular erythematous skin eruption appears (in 92 per cent of patients) (Fig. 19–7). Usually occurring simultaneously with or soon after the onset of fever, it generally begins with pronounced reddening of the palms and soles and gradually spreads to involve the entire trunk and extremities within 2 days. The rash is polymorphous and usually begins on the extremities as erythematous macules measuring 5 mm or more in diameter. Individual lesions become increasingly larger and often coalescent. Although frequently pruritic, the eruption is never accompanied by vesicles, bullae, or crusts. Deeply erythematous and widespread, the rash may be maculopapular or morbilliform, urticarial (Fig. 19–8), scarlatiniform (Fig. 19–9), or erythema multiforme–like (Fig. 19–10) and generally persists for the duration of the fever. Of these, symmetric pruritic urticaria-like plaques are the most common, maculopapular morbilliform le-

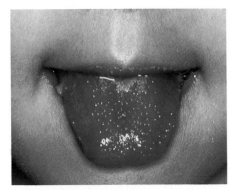

Figure 19–5. Strawberry tongue in mucocutaneous lymph node syndrome (Kawasaki disease). (Courtesy of Tomisaku Kawasaki, M.D.)

sions are the second most common, and less than 5 per cent are scarlatinal or erythema multiforme–like eruptions. In some patients, scattered areas of desquamation may appear some time between the 10th and 15th days of the illness. The eruption is not purpuric (it blanches with pressure), and the presence of an erythematous desquamating perineal rash early in the disorder, most severe and coalescent in the perineal area, appears to be a valuble clinical finding that when recognized may lead to more rapid diagnosis and treatment of this disorder (see Fig. 19–9).[32, 33]

The histopathologic features of the cutaneous eruption are nonspecific. Microscopic findings reveal an arteritis involving small and medium-sized vessels, marked edema of the dermal connective tissue, swelling of the endothelial cells in postcapillary venules, dilatation of small blood vessels, and lymphocytic and monocytic perivascular infiltration in arteries and arterioles of the dermis.

Changes in the Extremities. Reddening of the palms and soles (seen in 90 per cent of patients) and a firm indurative edema of the hands and feet develop (in 75 per cent of patients). The edema is characterized by deeply erythematous to violaceous brawny swelling of the palms and soles, fusiform swelling of the digits, and tightly stretched skin on the dorsal aspect of the hands and feet (Fig. 19–11).

Generally 14 to 20 days after the onset of fever a highly characteristic pattern of desquamation begins. Seen in 94 per cent of patients, it lasts approximately 1 week. The desquamation generally begins at the tips of the fingers and toes at the junction of the nails and skin (just beneath the tips of the nails) and, over a period of 10 days, gradually progresses to include the fingers, toes, and areas of the palms and soles (Fig. 19–12).

As with many other severe illnesses, Beau's lines (transverse furrows on the nail surface) may develop 1 or 2 months after the onset of the illness. This horizontal groove, although seen in almost all patients with Kawasaki disease, is not diagnostic of this disorder; these horizontal grooves develop as a

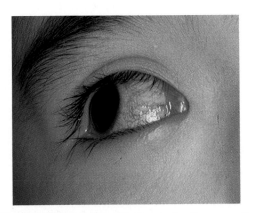

Figure 19–4. Congestion of bulbar conjunctiva in a patient with mucocutaneous lymph node syndrome (Kawasaki disease). (Courtesy of Tomisaku Kawasaki, M.D.)

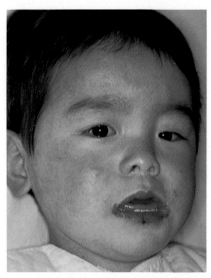

Figure 19–6. Kawasaki disease (mucocutaneous lymph node syndrome). Note characteristic facies with congestion of the bulbar conjunctivae and hemorrhagic crusts and erosions of the lips. (Courtesy of Tomisaku Kawasaki, M.D.)

nonspecific reaction to any stress that temporarily interrupts nail growth and become visible on the surface of the nail several weeks later (Fig. 19–13).

Lymphadenopathy. Cervical lymphadenopathy (the least reliable clinical feature of this disorder) is said to occur in 70 per cent of patients with Kawasaki disease in Japan and in 50 to 86 per cent of patients seen in the United States.[23]

When present it is unilateral and is generally seen as a single enlarged lymph node in the cervical region. Measuring more than 1.5 cm in diameter, the enlarged node is usually not warm, red, tender, or fluctuant; and in most cases, the lymphadenopathy disappears as the fever subsides. Histopathologic examinations of lymph nodes from patients with Kawasaki disease are nonspecific and reveal hypertrophy of germinal centers, medullary

edema, and an inflammatory infiltrate consisting of lymphocytes and large atypical mononuclear cells.

Other Clinical Features. Other clinical features include cardiac manifestations, central nervous system involvement, extreme irritability, lethargy, aseptic meningitis, pyuria, uveitis, rheumatic complications (arthritis and arthralgia), peripheral gangrene, and gastrointestinal manifestations. The prognosis of mucocutaneous lymph node syndrome is good in most cases, with improvement usually beginning about the 14th day of illness. Electrocardiographic abnormalities (prolongation of the PR and QT intervals, and ST segments and T-wave changes), however, have been found in 70 to 90 per cent of children with this disorder, and 27 per cent of patients demonstrate abnormalities in coronary angiography 1 to 6 months after the onset of disease.

Cardiac Effects. Clinical cardiac disease occurs in at least 20 per cent of patients with Kawasaki syndrome. During the acute febrile phase of the disease, severe tachycardia and gallop rhythm are the most common manifestations. Toward the end of the febrile phase (at a mean time of 11 days) more serious cardiac abnormalities appear, including congestive heart failure, pericardial effusion, mitral insufficiency, and cardiac arrhythmias manifesting as first- and second-degree atrioventricular block, premature ventricular contractions, or paroxysmal atrial tachycardia.

Sudden death due to coronary occlusion was originally reported in 1 to 2 per cent of patients, generally young infants with Kawasaki disease. More recent studies, however, indicate that such deaths in Japan have decreased to 0.2 per cent. Male infants are at special risk (80 per cent of fatalities have been in boys). Although death due to coronary occlusion has been noted a short time after apparent recovery from the illness, most deaths (90 per cent) occur suddenly, between 3 and 7 weeks after the onset of the disease. Deaths have been reported 2 to 4 and occasionally many years after apparent recovery, and 16 per cent of survivors have experienced a second infarction (27

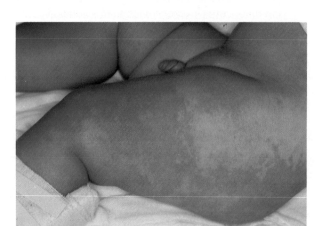

Figure 19–7. Urticaria-like rash in mucocutaneous lymph node syndrome (Kawasaki disease). (Courtesy of Tomisaku Kawasaki, M.D.)

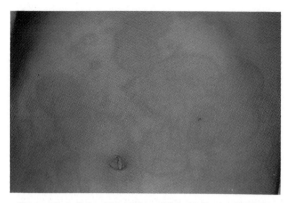

Figure 19–8. Urticarial rash in a child with Kawasaki disease. (Courtesy of Tomisaku Kawasaki, M.D.)

per cent of these occurred more than 1 year later.[34–36] Children with the greatest risk of sudden death or carditis are boys younger than 1 year of age, particularly those who have prolonged or recurrent fever and rash, extreme elevation of the erythrocyte sedimentation rate, and cardiac signs such as gallop rhythm, arrhythmia, cardiomegaly, and electrocardiographic abnormality. These factors, however, are only a guide and are not always reliable in predicting the prognosis for patients with Kawasaki syndrome.

Pathologic examination of the hearts of patients who died of Kawasaki syndrome reveals acute perivasculitis of the arterioles, capillaries, and venules of the small arteries, acute perivasculitis and endarteritis of the major coronary arteries, myocarditis, coagulation necrosis, lesions of the conduction system, pericarditis, and endocarditis with vasculitis. The causes of sudden death in such individuals are myocarditis, inflammation of the atrioventricular conduction systems, ischemic heart disease, and rupture of aneurysms.[37]

Arthritis and Arthralgia. Arthritis and arthralgia (seen in 20 and 40 per cent of patients, respectively) occur later in the febrile stage of the illness or shortly thereafter. Large joints such as the knees, hips, and elbows are the most commonly affected. Although ultimately self-limiting, arthritis and effusion may last for 2 to 4 weeks.

Central Nervous System Effects. Central nervous system effects are seen in nearly all patients with Kawasaki disease. They consist of negativistic behavior, sleep disturbances, severe irritability, frequent episodes of crying and whining, and, at times, sensorineural hearing loss. Approximately one third of patients have severe lethargy, semicoma, or coma during the acute febrile stage. One fourth of patients are found to have an associated aseptic meningitis with mononuclear pleocytosis (25 to 100 leukocytes/mm³) with normal glucose and normal to slightly elevated protein values.[23]

Gastrointestinal Manifestations. Gastrointestinal manifestations (diarrhea and abdominal pain) are seen in approximately one fourth of affected patients, and hepatitis, with modest to moderate bilirubin elevation and moderate elevations of serum aspartate aminotransferase (SGOT) and alanine aminotransferase (SGPT), occurs in about 10 per cent of patients during the acute febrile stage of the illness. Diarrhea (consisting of frequent watery stools, generally without blood, pus, or mucus), pancreatitis, and acute hydrops of the gallbladder have also been reported. Appearing late in the acute febrile phase of the illness or early in convalescence, the hydrops is frequently self-limiting, may disappear spontaneously in 2 or 3 weeks and can be monitored by repeated ultrasound evaluations.

Pyuria. Pyuria, seen in 70 per cent of patients, occurs in the acute stage of the disease. It appears to be urethral in origin, and although a small portion of patients may have a transient hematuria, proteinuria is not a feature of the disease. A number of boys have also been found to have small meatal ulcers during the acute stage of the illness.

Laboratory Studies. Laboratory tests show leukocytosis, polycythemia, a mild anemia, normal flora in the throat and stools, and sterile cultures of the blood and cerebrospinal fluid. Thrombocytosis is a universal laboratory finding in Kawasaki disease, and it appears to coincide with the period of highest risk of coronary thrombosis. In most instances the leukocyte count is over 18,000/mm³, and most patients have an elevated number of polymorphonuclear leukocytes and an elevated sedimentation rate. Unlike the sedimentation rate and leukocyte count, platelet counts are usually normal during the acute febrile phase of the illness. Thrombocytosis generally rises after the 10th day of illness, reaches a peak of 600,000 to 1.8 million/mm³ between the 15th and 25th days, and then falls to normal values by the 30th day of the disorder.[23] Other laboratory findings may include a positive C-reactive protein value, increased serum α₂-protein levels, elevated IgM and IgE levels, and reduced serum protein levels with reversal of the albumin–globulin ratio.

Diagnosis. The diagnosis of Kawasaki disease depends on the previously described clinical cri-

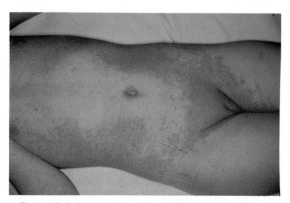

Figure 19–9. A scarlet fever–like rash in a child with Kawasaki disease. (Courtesy of Tomisaku Kawasaki, M.D.)

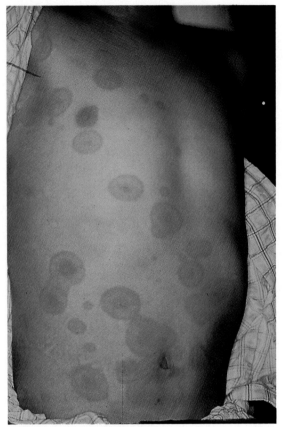

Figure 19–10. Erythema multiforme in a child with Kawasaki disease. (Courtesy of Tomisaku Kawasaki, M.D.)

teria (see Table 19–3) and the exclusion of other disorders considered in its differential diagnosis. These include scarlet fever, viral exanthems, leptospirosis, erythema multiforme and Stevens-Johnson syndrome, rickettsial disease, atypical measles, juvenile rheumatoid arthritis, systemic lupus erythematosus, toxic epidermal necrolysis, staphylococcal scalded skin syndrome, herpetic stomatitis, drug reactions, acrodynia (mercury poisoning, pink disease), Lyme disease, and toxic shock syndrome.

Management. Currently the most important problem in the management of patients with Kawasaki disease appears to be the ability to diagnose the disorder and prevent coronary aneurysm and myocardial infarction. Present treatment requires a careful program of repeated clinical and laboratory evaluation to detect and manage potentially serious cardiac and vascular complications. All patients should be hospitalized during the acute febrile stage to facilitate diagnostic testing; and as soon as the disease is diagnosed, patients should have a baseline echocardiogram and receive intravenous γ-globulin, 2 g/kg given in a 10- to 12-hour infusion. This dosage schedule has been demonstrated to be equally if not more efficacious in reducing the risk of coronary disease than 400 mg/

kg/day given in 2-hour infusions for 4 consecutive days.[38–41]

On the same day that γ-globulin is given, the patient should start on aspirin therapy. Although the appropriate dose of aspirin has been controversial, the dosage generally used in Canada and the United States is 100 mg/kg/day, until the fever is controlled or until day 14 of the illness, followed by a dosage of 5 to 10 mg/kg/day until the sedimentation rate and platelet count are normal. This usually occurs within 6 to 12 weeks after the onset of the illness. Salicylate levels should be obtained if vomiting, hyperpnea, lethargy, or liver function abnormalities develop.[38, 42] In Japan a dose of 50 mg/kg/day is recommended in the febrile phase rather than high-dose aspirin. Salicylate levels should be monitored 48 hours after the initiation of aspirin therapy, aiming for a level of between 18 and 28 mg/dl, with adjustment upward or downward as indicated by the clinical picture. Although the question of the possibility of Reye's syndrome as a complication of aspirin therapy in Kawasaki disease has been raised, the benefits of aspirin in this disorder greatly outweigh the risks.[43] To decrease the risk, however, aspirin can be interrupted if patients develop varicella or influenza during the follow-up phase. In addition, dipyridamole (Persantine), although not recommended for this purpose, can be used to inhibit platelet aggregation when given in dosages of 4 mg/kg/day in addition to low doses of aspirin for patients known to have coronary aneurysms, or it can be used for those patients who have persistent coronary abnormalities or cannot take aspirin for other reasons.

Once the child's fever has decreased, it is unlikely that significant congestive failure or myocardial dysfunction will occur. The patient should be evaluated within a week after discharge and have an echocardiogram between 21 and 28 days after onset of fever. If baseline and 3- to 4-week echocardiograms are normal with no evidence of coro-

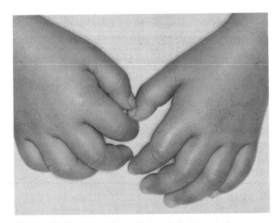

Figure 19–11. Indurative edema of the hands in mucocutaneous lymph node syndrome (Kawasaki disease). (Courtesy of Tomisaku Kawasaki, M.D.)

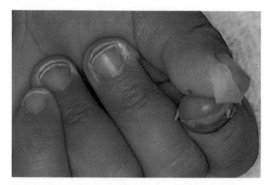

Figure 19–12. Desquamation of the fingers in a patient with mucocutaneous lymph node syndrome (Kawasaki disease). (Courtesy of Tomisaku Kawasaki, M.D.)

nary abnormality, further echocardiograms are unnecessary. Patients, however, should have periodic follow-up examinations, even if coronary aneurysms are not present, and if symptomatic, a maximal exercise stress test is recommended during adolescence to look for signs of ischemia.

Although systemic corticosteroids have been shown to be effective for the treatment of infantile periarteritis nodosa, corticocosteroids in patients with Kawasaki disease are contraindicated since there appears to be a higher incidence of coronary aneurysms and/or thrombosis in patients so treated. Careful, long-term follow-up of all patients with Kawasaki disease, however, is necessary. At present, the disease appears to be self-limiting and the short-term outlook for most children is hopeful. Delayed deaths, however, have been reported up to 14 years after onset of the illness, and the ultimate outcome of this multisystemic vasculitis remains unknown.[35, 36]

NECROTIZING VASCULITIS WITH GRANULOMATOSIS

There are three systemic diseases in which necrotizing vasculitis is seen in association with necrotizing granulomas: Wegener's granulomatosis, allergic granulomatosis (Churg-Strauss syndrome), and lymphomatoid granulomatosis (Table 19–4). Primarily seen as adult disorders, Wegener's disease may also be seen in pediatric patients, lymphomatoid granulomatosis has been seen in children as young as 7 and 8 1/2 years of age, and Churg-Strauss syndrome has been described in an adolescent boy and pediatric cases have been reported in retrospective studies of individuals with this disorder.

Wegener's Granulomatosis

Wegener's granulomatosis (giant cell granulomatosis) is a rare systemic disease characterized by necrotizing granulomatous vasculitis of the small vessels of the upper and lower respiratory tract (the nose, nasal sinuses, nasopharynx, glottis, trachea, bronchi, and lungs) and focal necrotizing glomerulitis of the kidneys. Although the etiology is unknown, the presence of granulomatous inflammation with vasculitis and circulating immune complexes suggests a hypersensitive or immunologic basis to this disorder.

Presenting features are usually related to the upper respiratory tract and include rhinorrhea, paranasal sinus drainage and pain, nasal mucosal ulcerations, blocked tear ducts, slight changes in the contour of the face, and, at times, otitis media, cough, hemoptysis, and pleurisy.[44–46] Cutaneous lesions are present in the early stage of the disease in about one fourth, and at the height of the disease in about one half, of patients with this disorder.[47] Mucocutaneous involvement appears as crusting, bleeding, and nonhealing sores on the nostrils or nasal septum. Ophthalmologic findings (occurring in more than 50 per cent of patients) include conjunctivitis, dacryocystitis, episcleritis, corneoscleral ulceration, retinal artery thrombosis, uveitis, proptosis, cavernous sinus thrombosis, and pseudotumor of the orbits. Cutaneous lesions consist of petechiae, palpable purpura or ecchymoses (sometimes in association with ulcerations or blisters on the face, upper limbs, and trunk), and erythematous papulonodular lesions measuring 1 to 5 cm in diameter, subcutaneous nodules, vesicles, pustules, and ulcerations on the extremities, neck, upper chest, and trunk caused by necrotizing vasculitis with thrombosis and necrosis. Large, deep, punched-out ulcers, with undermined violaceous borders, similar in appearance to lesions of pyoderma gangrenosum, and gingival granulomas (strawberry gums) are particularly characteristic (Fig. 19–14). Gingivitis, although rarely reported in the literature, in some cases can be the presenting sign. Although not pathognomonic, the gingival changes have distinctive features; the tissue is magenta in color, spongy, friable, and exuberant with, at times, petechiae with preferential involvement of the interdental papillae. These features

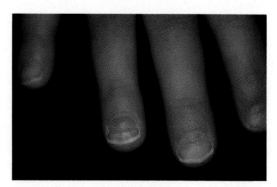

Figure 19–13. Beau's lines, a horizontal groove on the nails of a patient with Kawasaki disease.

Table 19–4. NECROTIZING VASCULITIC GRANULOMATOSES

1. Wegener's granulomatosis
   a. A necrotizing granulomatous vasculitis of small vessels of upper and lower respiratory tracts with necrotizing glomerulitis of kidneys
   b. Cutaneous lesions in 25% to 50%
      (1) Crusting, bleeding, nonhealing sores on nostrils or nasal septum; distinctive gingival changes
      (2) Petechiae, purpura, or ecchymoses (at times with ulcerations or blisters) on face, upper limbs, and trunk
      (3) Papulonodular lesions, subcutaneous nodules, vesicles, pustules, and ulcerations on neck, upper chest, trunk, and extremities
2. Churg-Strauss syndrome (allergic granulomatosis)
   a. Asthma, pneumonitis, peripheral eosinophilia, and vasculitis of skin, gastrointestinal tract, and nervous system (generally sparing renal glomeruli)
   b. Cutaneous lesions in two thirds of patients
      (1) Erythema multiforme–like and hemorrhagic lesions (occasionally with necrotic ulcers); cutaneous and subcutaneous nodules
      (2) Nodular lesions reveal histologic picture of allergic granulomatosis
3. Lymphomatoid granulomatosis
   a. A serious systemic disease primarily affecting the lungs, but also affects the skin, kidney, liver, and nervous system
   b. Skin lesions in 40% to 45%
      (1) Often the first clinical sign of disease
      (2) Symmetric erythematous macules, papules, annular plaques with central clearing, and dermal or subcutaneous nodules that tend to ulcerate
   c. Lymphomas develop in 15%

should suggest the possibility of Wegener's granulomatosis when other manifestations of the disease are present and no other explanation for the severe gingivitis is found. Pericarditis, endocarditis, and pancarditis with coronary vasculitis have been reported, and peripheral neuropathy and cerebral vasculitis, with or without subarachnoid or intracerebral hemorrhage, have also been noted in approximately 25 per cent of patients.

The diagnosis of Wegener's granulomatosis is suggested by cutaneous lesions; involvement of the respiratory tract (particularly cavitating nodules), kidneys, and other organs, often accompanied by arthritis or arthralgias; and necrotizing granulomas with vasculitis on histopathologic examinaton of biopsy specimens of the skin, lungs, or kidneys. Although Henoch-Schönlein purpura

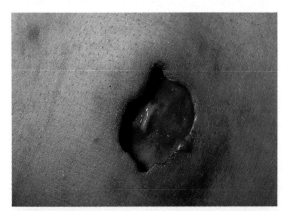

Figure 19–14. Wegener's granulomatosis. An ulcerated lesion caused by necrotizing vasculitis with thrombosis, necrosis, and undermined borders. (Courtesy of Department of Dermatology, Yale University School of Medicine.)

has a clinical picture at times somewhat similar to that of Wegener's granulomatosis (including palpable purpura), it lacks the characteristic necrotizing vasculitis of the upper and lower respiratory tract.

Prior to the advent of cytotoxic agents, Wegener's granulomatosis was considered to be fatal with a mean survival of 5 months. Untreated patients have a 50 per cent survival at 5 months and a 90 per cent mortality rate at 2 years. Systemic corticosteroids are not very helpful, but immunosuppressive drugs, particularly cyclophosphamide, alone or in combination with prednisolone, offer a better prognosis. The usual starting dose of cyclophosphamide is 1 to 2 mg/kg/day, increased by 25 mg every 10 to 14 days (unless serious hematologic toxicity intervenes) until a favorable clinical response occurs. When an appropriate response is evident, the dose should be gradually reduced in an effort to prevent severe leukopenia. If cyclophosphamide is not well tolerated, azathioprine, although not as effective, can be substituted. Since some patients with Wegener's granulomatosis may also respond to trimethoprim-sulfamethoxazole (Bactrim/Septra), it has been suggested that infectious agents may be related to the pathogenesis of individuals with this disorder.[48]

Churg-Strauss Syndrome

Allergic granulomatosis (Churg-Strauss syndrome), originally believed to be a form of polyarteritis nodosa, is a systemic disorder that can be differentiated from periarteritis nodosa by the presence of respiratory symptoms (usually asthma and pneumonitis); pronounced eosinophilia in the circulating blood and individual lesions; widespread vasculitis that may involve the skin, heart, lungs, kidneys, gastrointestinal tract, and peripheral nervous system; and palisading granulomas in the connective tissue with involvement of small arterioles and venules rather than small and medium-sized arteries. Although the etiology of Churg-Strauss syndrome remains unknown, its frequent association with a history of allergy (with the respiratory tract as a primary target) in the patient and patient's family suggests the possibility of an inhaled antigen or pathogen in the pathogenesis of the disorder.

Respiratory symptoms usually precede the onset of allergic granulomatosis, and cutaneous lesions, seen in about two thirds of patients, consist of erythema multiforme—like lesions, hemorrhagic lesions (varying from petechiae and palpable purpura to extensive ecchymoses), and discrete, generally multiple skin-colored to violaceous papulonodules with a predilection for the elbows, knees, scalp, digits, and buttocks, sometimes accompanied by necrotic ulcers. The presence of granulomas in the dermis and in subcutaneous nodules is of diagnostic value, and histologic examination of nodular lesions shows large numbers of degenerated collagen fibers, disintegrated cells, particularly eosinophils, giant cells, plasma cells, and nuclear debris imparting a bluish tinge to the center of the lesion.

Patients with allergic granulomatosis have a high incidence of abdominal pain, bloody diarrhea, hypertension, mild hematuria, and albuminuria. Although spontaneous resolution of the disorder has been reported, untreated cases usually have a poor prognosis, the most frequent cause of death being congestive heart failure secondary to myocardial damage from the arteritis. Systemic corticosteroids appear to be the treatment of choice (with reports of survival rates of 67 per cent after 5 years); for those patients unresponsive to corticosteroid therapy, the addition of cytotoxic agents may prove to be beneficial.

Lymphomatoid Granulomatosis

Lymphomatoid granulomatosis is a serious sytemic disease primarily affecting the lungs, but also involving the skin, kidney, liver, and nervous system. First described in 1972, the disorder has been seen in children as young as 7 and 8 1/2 years of age, but primarily affects adults (up to the age of 70 years) with an average onset at between 30 and 60 years of age.

The skin is involved in 40 to 45 per cent of patients, with the first clinical sign of disease frequently consisting of symmetric erythematous macules, papules, annular plaques with central clearing, and dermal or subcutaneous nodules that often tend to ulcerate. Petechiae are also occasionally seen, and cutaneous lesions, often extensive, may resemble the cutaneous features (but without the purpura) of Wegener's granulomatosis. Dermal nodules and plaques, frequently the key primary

lesions, can often lead to early diagnosis. Other features include pulmonary symptoms (cough, shortness of breath, chest pain, hemoptysis), fever, malaise, weight loss, myalgias, arthralgias, cranial nerve palsies, peripheral neuritis, ataxia, proptosis, diplopia, deafness, vertigo, hemiparesis, and seizures.[49–51]

Although not considered a true malignant lymphoma, pulmonary lymphomas simulating lymphomatoid granulomatosis have been described, 15 to 18 per cent of patients with lymphomatoid granulomatosis go on to develop a lymphoma, and it has been suggested that lymphomatoid granulomatosis may represent a histologic variant of T-cell lymphoma, termed *angiocentric T-cell lymphoma*. Contrasting to previous reports of a mortality as high as 90 per cent, studies have demonstrated good results in patients when prednisone and cyclophosphamide were included in the management of the disorder.[44, 51]

ERYTHEMA ELEVATUM DIUTINUM

Seen primarily in middle-aged adults, and at times also in children as young as 5 years of age, erythema elevatum diutinum is a rare chronic cutaneous disorder characterized by persistent red purple and yellowish papules, plaques, and nodules with a predilection for the extensor surfaces of the extremities, elbows, knees, dorsal aspects of the hands and feet, pretibial surfaces, buttocks, and skin overlying the Achilles tendon. Although the wrists, ankles, face, ears, palms, and soles may also be affected, the trunk and mucous membranes are generally spared. Lesions tend to vary from a few millimeters to several centimeters in diameter and may be round or oval, soft, and freely movable; and early in development or during exacerbations some patients show areas of erythema with vesicles and bullae. Purpura or petechiae are sometimes seen in early lesions; and with time, nodules or plaques may become firm, fibrotic, and indurated, sometimes resembling xanthomas. Although lesions are typically asymptomatic, they may sometimes be tender or painful and are often accompanied by systemic abnormalities such as arthralgia, fever, and malaise. Involution occurs, generally after a period of years, without scarring, but residual hypopigmentation or hyperpigmentation is common.

Although the pathogenesis of erythema elevatum diutinum is unknown, the presence of C_{1q} binding activity in the serum of some patients, exacerbations after streptococcal infection or skin testing with streptokinase or streptodornase, occasional association with IgA or IgG monoclonal gammopathy or mixed IgG-IgM cryoglobulinemia, and the Arthus-like histology of lesions suggests that elicitation of an immune reaction by bacterial antigens may be the initial event in the histogenesis of this disorder.[52] Histopathologic features consist of leukocytoclasis, with deposition of eosinophilic hyaline material around and within blood vessels, and a sleeve-like perivascular, mainly neutrophilic, dermal infiltrate with lymphocytes, histiocytes, eosinophils, and plasma cells. In older lesions, intracellular and extracellular lipid deposition (extracellular cholesterosis) unassociated with disturbances of lipid metabolism may predominate. Although none of the histologic features is pathognomonic, the constellation of histopathologic and clinical features of the disorder helps distinguish this entity from other forms of leukocytoclastic vasculitis.

The disease tends to be chronic and progressive over 5 to 10 years and eventually tends to resolve spontaneously. Although topical or intralesional corticosteroids may sometimes be of benefit, treatment is generally unsatisfactory. Dapsone, however, with an initial dosage of 2 mg/kg/day up to a total of 100 to 150 mg/day, may, at times, be beneficial,[53] and sulfapyridine (200 to 400 mg/kg/day) for children in four divided doses, with a maximum total dose of 1,000 to 1,500 mg/day, is probably an equally effective form of therapy. Niacinamide and tetracycline have also been reported to be effective in some individuals with this disorder.[54]

URTICARIAL VASCULITIS

Since 1973, a number of patients have been reported with cutaneous necrotizing vasculitis in whom the predominant skin lesions have been blanching erythematous papules or plaques closely resembling or indistinguishable from nonvasculitic (true) urticaria. Although primarily a disorder of young adult women, urticarial vasculitis has also been reported in children as young as 4 years of age. A distinctive clinical syndrome associated with arthritis, arthralgia, angioedema, uveitis, myositis, abdominal or chest pain, and, in some cases, pulmonary or renal involvement, urticarial vasculitis is characterized by erythematous papules, plaques, or wheals, which usually last less than 24 to 72 hours and may be asymptomatic or may itch, burn, or sting. Lesions are usually generalized and may involve the palms and soles, and new lesions may develop daily or as infrequently as once a month for a few weeks or many years.[55]

Although the etiology of urticarial vasculitis is unknown, the condition appears to represent a nonspecific immune complex disorder or a nonspecific reaction pattern caused by multiple etiologic agents. Patients present with variable degrees of severity. Various therapeutic modalities such as prednisone, antihistamines, chloroquine, indomethacin, azathioprine, colchicine, and dapsone have been used for patients with this disorder. Response to these agents, however, has been inconsistent.[55–57]

BEHÇET'S SYNDROME

Behçet's syndrome is a chronic multisystemic disease of unknown etiology characterized by a triad of recurrent oral aphthous stomatitis, recurrent aphthous ulcers in or on the external genitalia, and inflammatory disease of the eye (uveitis, iritis, or iridocyclitis). Originally described in 1937, the spectrum of the disease has broadened with the recognition of multiple organ system involvement: dermal vasculitis, synovitis, arthritis, central nervous system involvement (meningoencephalitis), myocarditis, colitis, phlebitis, and focal necrotizing glomerulonephritis (Table 19–5). Although onset in infants as young as 2 months of age has been noted, this rare syndrome usually begins in patients between 10 and 45 years of age and has a marked predilection (between 2:1 and 5:1) for males. Behçet's syndrome has also been described in infants born to mothers with the disease. This form of the disorder, neonatal Behçet's syndrome, is characterized by aphthous stomatitis and skin phenomena and generally disappears spontaneously by the time the infants reach the age of 6 months.[58, 59]

A precise etiology has not been delineated for Behçet's disease, but genetic factors associated

---

Table 19–5. BEHÇET'S SYNDROME

1. Etiology: an aberration of humoral and cellular immunity?
2. Cutaneous lesions
    a. Widely scattered papules, pustules, furuncles, vesicles, ulcerations, or acneiform lesions
    b. Painful nodose lesions resembling erythema nodosum in severe chronic forms
3. Oral ulcerations frequently the first manifestation
4. Ocular lesions (in up to 80%)
    a. Intense periorbital pain and photophobia
    b. Conjunctivitis, iritis, iridocyclitis, glaucoma, cataracts, optic neuritis, uveitis, vitreous opacification, and hypopyon
5. Genital ulcers in 10%
6. Other clinical findings
    a. Fever, thrombophlebitis, arthralgia, and gastrointestinal symptoms (which may at times be due to an ulcerating hemorrhagic colitis)
    b. Pericarditis, myocarditis, and focal glomerulonephritis
    c. Central nervous system involvement in 20% to 50% (the most severe prognostic feature)

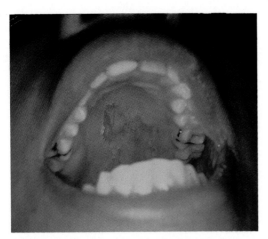

Figure 19–15. Behçet's disease. Aphthous ulcerations appear on the hard palate of the mouth. (Courtesy of Department of Dermatology, Yale University School of Medicine.)

with human lymphocyte antigens HLA-B51, HLA-B27, and HLA-B12, viral infection, exposure to environmental pollutants, cellular and humoral immunologic factors, skin hyperreactivity (pathergy), and the deposition of immunoreactants around blood vessels induced by cutaneous trauma appear to play a pathogenetic role.[60–62]

Clinical Manifestations. Cutaneous and oral lesions are the most common clinical features of Behçet's disease. Oral lesions, an almost constant feature, are the initial manifestations in about 60 per cent of patients. The ulcerations begin as vesicles or pustules, may occur anywhere on the oral mucosa, and present as superficial erosions indistinguishable from aphthous stomatitis or as deeply punched-out necrotic ulcers on the lips, buccol mucosa, tongue, tonsils, and larynx (Fig. 19–15). They tend to appear in crops and are characterized by superficial grayish erosions that vary from a few millimeters to a centimeter in diameter. The ulcer base is covered with a yellowish gray exudate, and the margin is surrounded by a red halo. The aphthous lesions, whether in the mouth or genitalia, generally persist for 7 to 14 days, usually heal without scarring, and recur at intervals varying from weeks to months. Deep crateriform necrotic ulcerations with raised margins, called periadenitis mucosa necrotica recurrens (Sutton's disease), are distinctive, are usually very painful, and frequently heal without scarring. Whether Sutton's disease is a separate entity or a form of Behçet's disease is still uncertain. Features of Behçet's syndrome and relapsing polychondritis have also been described as the MAGIC syndrome (mouth and genital ulcers with inflamed cartilage). Whether the MAGIC syndrome represents a separate and distinct entity or a manifestation of Behçet's disease remains unknown.[63]

Cutaneous lesions of Behçet's syndrome present a varied picture. Seen in approximately 70 per cent of patients, they consist of folliculitis, papules, vesicles, pustules, pyoderma, acneiform lesions, furuncles, abscesses, ulcerations, and angiitic lesions on the legs, suggesting a diagnosis of erythema nodosum. Pathergy, an exaggerated skin response to a needle prick, is typical and often pathognomonic. Genital ulcerations, since they define the disease, are seen in 80 to 100 per cent of patients with Behçet's syndrome. Generally less painful than oral lesions, they are found on the scrotum or penis in males and the vulva and vagina of females, are similar in appearance to the oral ulcerations, and are frequently overlooked.

Ocular lesions, seen in up to 80 per cent of patients, generally begin with intense periorbital pain and photophobia. Conjunctivitis may be an early ocular finding, followed by iritis, iridocyclitis, glaucoma, cataracts, optic neuritis, arteritis of retinal vessels or uveitis, often with loss of vision from vitreous opacification and, eventually, hypopyon. Of these, retinal vasculitis (posterior uveitis) is the most classic lesion of this disorder.

Fever and constitutional symptoms are variable. Other findings include recurrent thrombophlebitis of the superficial veins of the legs (in about 45 per cent of patients), arthralgia and arthritis (in 35 to 60 per cent), gastrointestinal ulceration, pericarditis, orchitis, and epididymitis. Gastrointestinal complaints range from vague abdominal pain and anorexia to diarrhea and may be due to an ulcerating, hemorrhagic colitis. Central nervous system involvement, often the most severe prognostic feature of this disorder, is seen in 20 to 50 per cent of patients (generally an average of 2 to 5 years after the disease has begun). Renal involvement, an uncommon complication, may be seen with a spectrum ranging from asymptomatic abnormalities detected on urinalysis to a rapidly progressive glomerulonephritis and nephrosis.

The diagnosis of Behçet's syndrome in a patient with the full triad of oral and genital ulcers and iritis is not difficult. Two or more major criteria (oral, genital, ocular, or cutaneous involvement) or a combination of major and minor criteria (vascular, neurologic, skeletal, or intestinal), however, may constitute a diagnosis. Although pathergy (the formation of an ulceration at an area of trauma, skin prick, or venipuncture) is common and a helpful criterion to the diagnosis, it may also be seen in patients with pyoderma gangrenosum, paraproteinemia, leukemia, and intestinal bypass syndrome; and a negative pathergy test does not rule out the diagnosis.[61]

Treatment. There is no entirely satisfactory treatment of Behçet's syndrome. Treatment of the aphthous ulcers with tetracycline suspension, topical or intralesional corticosteroids, topical application of silver nitrate, oral rinses with elixir of diphenhydramine (Benadryl), alone or mixed with Maalox or Kaopectate, or viscous lidocaine (Lidocaine Viscous 2%) can give symptomatic relief (see Chapter 11). Although favorable results are inconsistent, antihistamines, indomethacin, dapsone, cyclosporine, antimalarial drugs (e.g., hydroxychloroquine), nonsteroidal anti-inflammatory drugs, and thalidomide may suppress many of the inflammatory features of this disorder. In severe cases, corticosteroids, alone or in combination with immunosuppressive agents such as cyclophosphamide, chlorambucil, or azathioprine, currently appear to be the treatment of choice. Although contraindicated in patients with leukopenia or substantial hepatic or renal disease, colchicine, perhaps due to its inhibition of leukocyte chemotaxis, has also been found to be effective (especially for its cutaneous manifestations) and may have a corticosteroid-sparing effect. Therapy is begun with a dosage of 0.6 mg twice daily for the first week; if the patient has no nausea, vomiting, or diarrhea, the dosage can be increased to three times a day; and, as the patient improves, it is then tapered to once daily and perhaps to an alternate-day regimen.[62, 64]

The overall mortality of Behçet's disease is 3 to 4 per cent. When death occurs, it is usually attributed to intestinal perforation, cardiopulmonary disease, a ruptured aneurysm, central nervous system involvement, or a complication of therapy for central nervous system disease. Although the incidence in childhood is relatively uncommon, except in infants born to mothers with the disease (neonatal Behçet's syndrome), the younger the patient at the onset of illness, the worse the prognosis.

References

1. Saulsbury FT: Henoch-Schönlein purpura. Pediatr. Dermatol. 1:195–201, 1984.

   An excellent review of Henoch-Schönlein purpura in 25 children with particular emphasis on the clinical and laboratory features of the disorder.

2. Vernier RL, Worthen HC, Peterson RD, et al.: Anaphylactoid purpura: I. Pathology of the skin and kidney and frequency of streptococcal infection. Pediatrics 27:181–193, 1961.

   Clinical, experimental, and pathologic features of anaphylactoid purpura support the concept that this disorder is a form of diffuse vascular disease, probably caused by hypersensitivity to a variety of agents.

3. Piette WW, Stone MS: A cutaneous sign of IgA-associated small dermal vessel leukocytoclastic vasculitis in adults (Henoch-Schönlein purpura). Arch. Dermatol. 125:53–56, 1989.

   In a series of seven adults with Henoch-Schönlein purpura, each patient was found to have distinctive cutaneous findings and IgA-associated small dermal vessel vasculitis.

4. Saulsbury FT: IgA rheumatoid factor in Henoch-Schönlein purpura. J. Pediatr. 108:71–76, 1986.

   The finding of elevated concentrations of IgA, increased numbers of IgA-bearing lymphocytes, and IgA-containing circulating immune complexes in patients with Henoch-Schönlein purpura further support the concept of IgA immunoglobulins in the pathogenesis of this disorder.

5. Allen DM, Diamond LK, Howell DA: Anaphylactoid purpura in children (Schönlein-Henoch syndrome). Am. J. Dis. Child. 99:833–854, 1960.

   Characteristic manifestations of anaphylactoid purpura as noted in a comprehensive analysis of 131 patients.

6. Byrn JR, Fitzgerald JF, Northway JD, et al.: Unusual manifestations of Henoch-Schönlein syndrome. Am. J. Dis. Child. 130:1335-1337, 1976.

   Henoch-Schönlein syndrome presents a diagnostic challenge when the abdominal or joint manifestations precede the cutaneous lesions.

7. Lombard KA, Shah PC, Thrasher TV, et al.: Ileal stricture as a late complication of Henoch-Schönlein purpura. Pediatrics 77:396–398, 1986.

   A report of a 3-year old boy with late ileal stricture following Henoch-Schönlein purpura with enteropathy.

8. Hurwitz S: Vasculitic syndromes. In: The Skin and Systemic Disease in Children. Year Book Medical Publishers, Chicago, 1985, 35–64.

   A review of the cutaneous features and systemic manifestations of the vasculitic disorders of childhood.

9. Wolfsohn H: Purpura and intussusception. Arch. Dis. Child. 22:242–247, 1947.

   Intussusception in older children should suggest a diagnosis of Henoch-Schönlein purpura.

10. Wedgewood RJP, Klaus MH: Anaphylactoid purpura (Schönlein-Henoch syndrome)—a long-term follow-up study with special reference to renal involvement. Pediatrics 16:196–206, 1955.

    Ten of 26 children with anaphylactoid purpura were noted to have an apparent latent nephritis after long-term follow-up.

11. Lewis IC, Philpott MG: Neurologic complications in the Schönlein-Henoch syndrome. Arch. Dis. Child. 31:369–371, 1956.

    Two cases of anaphylactoid purpura complicated by subarachnoid hemorrhage.

12. Belman AL, Leicher CR, Moshe SL, et al.: Neurologic manifestations of Schönlein-Henoch purpura: Report of three cases and a review of the literature. Pediatrics 75:687–692, 1985.

    A report of three children with neurologic manifestations of Henoch-Schönlein purpura (status epilepticus, a seizure followed by hemiparesis, left brachial plexopathy, and transient weakness of the left leg).

13. Experience and Reason: Steroid effects in the course of abdominal pain in children with Henoch-Schönlein purpura. Pediatrics 79:1018–1021, 1987.

    A review of 48 children with Henoch-Schönlein purpura suggests that the abdominal pain seen in children with this disorder is self-limiting, and although treatment with corticosteroids may hasten the resolution of pain, their value in altering the course of this complication is questionable.

14. Utani A, Ohta M, Shinya A, et al.: Successful treatment of adult Henoch-Schönlein purpura with factor XIII concentrate. J. Am. Acad. Dermatol. 24:438–442, 1991.

    A report of successful treatment of three adult patients with severe abdominal complications of Henoch-Schönlein purpura who had low activity of factor XIII during the acute phase of the disorder.

15. Legrain V, Jejean S, Taieb A, et al.: Infantile acute hemorrhagic edema of the skin: Study of 10 cases. J. Am. Acad. Dermatol. 24:17–22, 1991.

    A report of 10 children with acute hemorrhagic edema of the skin.

16. Hirschel-Scholz S, Hunziker N: Correspondence: Acute hemorrhagic edema of the infant (Finkelstein's disease). Pediatr. Dermatol. 7:323, 1990.

    A brief report of acute hemorrhagic edema of the infant, a disorder often recognized by Europeans but overlooked in the American literature.

17. Diaz-Perez JL, Schroeter AL, Winkelmann RK: Cutaneous periarteritis nodosa. Arch. Dermatol 116:56–58, 1980.

A study of 10 cases of cutaneous periarteritis nodosa by immunofluorescence microscopy suggests that immune mechanisms may be involved in the pathogenesis of this disorder.

18. Jones SK, Lane AT, Golitz L, et al.: Cutaneous periarteritis nodosa in a child. Am. J.Dis. Child. *139*:920–922, 1985.

A 5-year-old boy with cutaneous periarteritis nodosa in whom prednisone promptly resulted in resolution of signs and symptoms of the disorder.

19. Golitz LE: The vasculitides and their significance in the pediatric age group. Dermatol. Clin. *4*:117–125, 1986.

A review of the vasculitides in the pediatric age group with emphasis on their pathogenesis, classification, and significance in childhood.

20. Kawasaki T, Kosaki F, Okawa S, et al.: A new infantile acute febrile mucocutaneous lymph node syndrome (MLNS) prevailing in Japan. Pediatrics *54*:271–276, 1974.

Clinical and epidemiologic features of what appeared to be a new disorder affecting infants and young children.

21. Melish ME, Hicks RM, Larson E: Mucocutaneous lymph node syndrome (MLNS) in the United States (abstr). Pediatr. Res. *8*:427, 1974.

Nine children in Hawaii with an unusual and highly distinctive multisystemic disease indistinguishable from mucocutaneous lymph node syndrome (Kawasaki disease) as seen in Japan.

22. Melish ME, Hicks RM, Larson EJ: Mucocutaneous lymph node syndrome in the United States. Am. J. Dis. Child. 130:599–607, 1976.

A review of 16 patients with Kawasaki disease seen in Honolulu, Hawaii, during the 4-year period between April 1971 and February 1975.

23. Melish ME: Kawasaki syndrome (mucocutaneous lymph node syndrome). Pediatr. Rev. *2*:107–114, 1980.

A thorough analysis of Kawasaki disease, its clinical characteristics, diagnosis, and treatment.

24. Patriarca PA, Rogers MF, Morens D, et al.: Kawasaki's syndrome: Association with the application of a rug shampoo. Lancet *2*:578–580, 1982.

An epidemic of 26 cases of Kawasaki disease following use of a rug shampoo suggests a toxic etiology for this disorder.

25. Rauch AM, Glode MP, Wiggins JW Jr, et al.: Outbreak of Kawasaki syndrome in Denver, Colorado: Association with rug and carpet cleaning. Pediatrics *87*:663–669, 1991.

A case-controlled study in which 16 (62 per cent) of 26 patients, in contrast to 10 (20 per cent) of 49 matched control subjects, were exposed to rug or carpet clearing prior to the onset of their disease is presented as a third outbreak in which an association between Kawasaki syndrome and rug or carpet cleaning was demonstrated.

26. Raimer S, Tschen EH, Walker MK: Toxic shock syndrome: Possible confusion with Kawasaki's disease. Cutis *28*:33–36, 1981.

A 26-year-old female house officer who experienced an illness initially thought to be Kawasaki disease, on subsequent reassessment, was actually found to have suffered from toxic shock syndrome.

27. American Heart Association Committee on Rheumatic Fever, Endocarditis, and Kawasaki Disease. Diagnostic guidelines for Kawasaki disease. Am. J. Dis. Child. *149*:1218–1219, 1990.

Current recommendations for the diagnosis of Kawasaki disease.

28. Rowley AH, Gonzalez-Crurri F, Gidding SJ, et al.: Incomplete Kawasaki disease with coronary involvement. J. Pediatr. *110*:409–413, 1987.

Characteristic coronary abnormalities found at autopsy in 5 of 27 individuals suggest that Kawasaki syndrome may not always meet the full spectrum of criteria for diagnosis.

29. Levy M, Koren G: Atypical Kawasaki disease: Analysis of clinical presentation and diagnostic clues. Pediatr. Infect. Dis. J. *9*:122–126, 1990.

Studies suggest that children with atypical presentations should have an echocardiogram, erythrocyte sedimentation rate, and platelet count in an effort to identify patients with incomplete clinical features of Kawasaki disease.

30. Yanagawa H, Kawasaki T, Shigematsu I: Nationwide survey on Kawasaki disease in Japan. Pediatrics *80*:58–62, 1987.

In an analysis of patients with Kawasaki disease diagnosed in Japan between July 1982 and December 1984, the proportion of sibling cases was 1.4 per cent and there was a 3.9 per cent incidence of recurrent disease.

31. Fujita Y, Nakamura Y, Sakata K, et al.: Kawasaki disease in families. Pediatrics *84*:666–669, 1989.

An increased rate of second-case Kawasaki disease occurring among 1,788 siblings of children with the disease (often within 10 days) suggests a common exposure and genetic susceptibility in individuals with this disorder.

32. Urbach AH, McGregor RS, Malatack J, et al.: Kawasaki disease and perineal rash. Am. J. Dis. Child. *142*:1174–1176, 1988.

A report of seven children with Kawasaki disease with a distinctive perineal rash 3 to 4 days after the onset of illness suggests that this eruption may provide a valuble clue to the diagnosis and thus allow early initiation of therapy for individuals with Kawasaki disease.

33. Friter BS, Lucky AW: The perineal eruption of Kawasaki syndrome. Arch. Dermatol. *124*:1805–1810, 1988.

The presence of an erythematous desquamating perineal rash, usually within the first week of the onset of symptoms, in 67 per cent of 58 patients with Kawasaki syndrome suggests that this eruption may be far more common than previously recognized and thus may provide an important early clue to the diagnosis of this disorder.

34. Kitamura S, Kawashima Y, Fujita T, et al.: Aortocoronary bypass grafting in a child with coronary artery obstruction due to mucocutaneous lymph node syndrome. Circulation *53*:1035–1040, 1976.

A 4-year-old boy with myocardial infarction and total occlusion of the right coronary and left anterior descending coronary arteries approximately 10 months after mucocutaneous lymph node syndrome underwent a successful double aortocoronary bypass grafting.

35. Kato H, Ichinose E, Kawasaki T: Myocardial infarction in Kawasaki disease. J. Pediatr. *108*:923–927, 1986.

In a review of 195 patients with Kawasaki disease who had myocardial infarctions, usually in the first year of life, 16 per cent of survivors had a second infarction and 27 per cent of these occurred more than 1 year later.

36. Pounder DJ: Coronary artery aneurysms presenting as sudden death 14 years after Kawasaki disease in infancy. Arch. Pathol. Lab. Med. *109*:874–876, 1985.

A 17-year-old young man who collapsed and died was found at autopsy to have coronary aneurysms and evidence of arteritis, presumably a result of an infection at 17 months of age which, in retrospect, was believed to have been Kawasaki disease.

37. Fujiwara H, Hamashima Y: Pathology of the heart in Kawasaki disease. Pediatrics *61*:100–107, 1978.

Pathologic studies of 20 hearts of patients with Kawasaki disease revealed acute perivasculitis and vasculitis of the arterioles, capillaries, venules, and small arteries; acute perivasculitis and endarteritis of the three major coronary arteries; myocarditis; coagulation necrosis; lesions of the conduction system; pericarditis; and endocarditis with vasculitis.

38. Melish ME: Kawasaki syndrome (mucocutaneous lymph node syndrome). In Gellis SS, Kagan BM: Current Pediatric

Therapy 13. W.B. Saunders Co., Philadelphia, 1990, 443–444.

An authoritative approach to the management of patients with Kawasaki syndrome.

39. Furusho K, Nakara H, Shinomiya K, et al.: High-dose intravenous gamma-globulin for Kawasaki disease. Lancet 2:1055–1058, 1984.

In a study of 85 patients with Kawasaki disease, 15 per cent of those who received intravenous gamma globulin and aspirin developed coronary aneurysms as compared with 45 per cent of 45 patients who received aspirin alone for the treatment of this disorder.

40. Newburger JW, Takahashi M, Burns JC, et al.: The treatment of Kawasaki disease with intravenous gamma globulin. N. Engl. J. Med. 315:341–347, 1986.

A multicenter study of 168 patients with Kawasaki disease found that high-dose intravenous gamma globulin was safe as well as effective in reducing the prevalence of coronary artery abnormalities when administered early in the course of the disorder.

41. Newburger JW, Takahaski M, Beiser AS, et al.: A single intravenous infusion of gamma globulin as compared with four infusions in the treatment of acute Kawasaki syndrome. N. Engl. J. Med. 324:1633–1639, 1991.

In children with acute Kawasaki disease, a single dose of intravenous gamma globulin (2 g/kg of body weight over 10 hours) was found to be more effective than the conventional regimen of four smaller daily doses and equally safe.

42. Koren G, Rose V, Lavi S, et al.: Probable efficacy of high-dose salicylates in reducing coronary involvement in Kawasaki disease. J.A.M.A. 254:767–769, 1985.

A study of 36 children with Kawasaki disease treated with high-dose salicylates (80–180 mg/kg/day) compared with a placebo group of 18 children treated with acetaminophen revealed a lower incidence of coronary aneurysms in the salicylate-treated group. The authors found it necessary to give substantially more salicylate during the febrile phase of the disease because of apparent impaired absorption of the drug resulting in serum levels twofold lower than those achieved during the nonfebrile phase of the disorder.

43. Takahashi M, Mason W: Kawasaki syndrome, Reye syndrome, and aspirin. Pediatrics 77:616–617, 1986.

If one assumes the incidence of Kawasaki syndrome to be 1/10,000 children, and that of Reye syndrome to be 1/100,000, the probability of a patient contracting both diseases in the same year can be calculated to be 1 in 1 billion.

44. Yevich I; Necrotizing vasculitis with granulomatosis. Int. J. Dermatol. 27:540–546, 1988.

A review of the clinical features, histopathology, and treatment of Wegener's granulomatosis, Churg-Strauss syndrome, and lymphomatoid granulomatosis.

45. Baliga R, Chang C-H, Bidani AK, et al.: A case of Wegener's granulomatosis in childhood: Successful therapy with cyclophosphamide. Pediatrics 51:286–290, 1978.

A report of an 11-year-old boy who survived Wegener's granulomatosis after immunosuppressive therapy with cyclophosphamide.

46. Orlowski JP, Clough JD, Dyment PG: Wegener's granulomatosis in the pediatric age group. Pediatrics 61:83–90, 1978.

A description of 6 patients and a review of 11 previously reported patients younger than 21 years of age with Wegener's granulomatosis.

47. Chyu JYH, Hagstrom WJ, Soltani K, et al.: Wegener's granulomatosis in childhood: Cutaneous manifestations as the presenting signs. J. Am. Acad. Dermatol. 10:241–246, 1984.

A report of a 16-year-old boy with Wegener's granulomatosis in whom cutaneous lesions were the presenting sign.

48. West BC, Todd JR, King JW: Wegener granulomatosis and trimethoprim-sulfamethoxazole: Complete remission of a twenty-year course. Ann. Intern. Med. 106:840–842, 1987.

A report of a woman with a 20-year history of Wegener's granulomatosis who responded to trimethoprim-sulfamethoxazole reaffirms the possibility that infectious agents may be related to the pathogenesis of this disorder.

49. James WD, Odom RB, Katzenstein AA: Cutaneous manifestations of lymphomatoid granulomatosis: Report of 44 cases and review of the literature. Arch. Dermatol. 117:196–202, 1981.

In a review of the clinical manifestations of 44 patients with lymphomatoid granulomatosis, ulcerations were rare, a maculopapular rash or macular erythema was relatively uncommon, and subcutaneous or dermal nodules were present in 60 per cent of patients with this disorder.

50. Camisa C: Lymphomatoid granulomatosis: Two cases with skin involvement. J. Am. Acad. Dermatol. 20:571–578, 1989.

A report of two cases of lymphomatoid granulomatosis with emphasis on cutaneous manifestations and their importance in the early recognition and diagnosis of this disorder.

51. Gibson LE: Cutaneous vasculitis: Approach to diagnosis and systemic association. Mayo Clin. Proc. 65:221–229, 1990.

A review of the cutaneous vasculitides with emphasis on the clinical manifestations and their clinicopathologic correlation.

52. Katz SI, Gallin JI, Hertz KC, et al.: Erythema elevatum diutinum: Skin and systemic manifestations, immunologic studies, and successful treatment with dapsone. Medicine 56:443–455, 1977.

A detailed study of four patients with erythema elevatum diutinum who responded dramatically within 2 days of starting dapsone (50 to 300 mg/day). Both cutaneous and systemic manifestations, however, recurred rapidly (within 12 to 48 hours) after medication was discontinued.

53. Fort SL, Rodman OG: Erythema elevatum diutinum: Response to dapsone. Arch. Dermatol. 113:819–822, 1977.

A 29-year-old woman who had the onset of chronic erythema elevatum diutinum at the age of 10 years showed a dramatic response to dapsone therapy and also improved spontaneously during each of her three pregnancies.

54. Kohler IK, Lorincz AL: Erythema elevatum diutinum treated with niacinamide and tetracycline. Arch. Dermatol. 116:693–695, 1980.

A 60-year-old woman with recurrent papular and vesiculobullous lesions of erythema elevatum diutinum had a good clinical response to niacinamide (100 mg three times a day) and tetracycline hydrochloride (250 mg four times a day) within 4 weeks.

55. Gammon WR: Urticarial vasculitis. Dermatol. Clin. 3:97–105, 1985.

A comprehensive review of urticarial vasculitis, its etiology, cutaneous and extracutaneous manifestations, and its treatment.

56. Millns JL, Randle HW, Solley GO, et al.: The therapeutic response of urticarial vasculitis to indomethacin. J. Am. Acad. Dermatol. 3:349–355, 1980.

Twenty-five to 50 mg of indomethacin three to four times daily resulted in complete clearing of all disease manifestations in 6 of 10 patients with urticarial vasculitis within 17 days and a partial improvement in three individuals with this disorder.

57. Wiles JC, Hansen RC, Lynch PJ: Urticarial vasculitis treated with colchicine. Arch. Dermatol. 102:802–805, 1985.

Two women with urticarial vasculitis responded dramatically to colchicine after other therapeutic approaches failed.

58. Lewis MA, Priestley BL: Transient neonatal Behçet's disease. Arch. Dis. Child. 61:805–806, 1986.

A report of three neonates with Behçet's syndrome born to mothers with this disorder.

59. Rakover Y, Adar H, Tal I, et al.: Behçet disease: Long-term follow-up of three children and review of literature. Pediatrics *83*:986–992, 1989.

A report of three children with Behçet's syndrome and review of the literature.

60. Arbesfeld SJ, Kurbin AK: Behçet's disease: New prospectives on an enigmatic syndrome. J. Am. Acad. Dermatol. *19*:767–779, 1988.

A comprehensive overview of the epidemiology, clinical manifestations, etiology, pathogenesis, and therapy of Behçet's disease.

61. Gilhar A, Winterstein G, Turani H, et al.: Skin hyperreactivity response (pathergy) in Behçet's disease. J. Am. Acad. Dermatol. *21*:547–552, 1989.

A study of 11 patients with Behçet's disease and the value of minor trauma or pathergy (a nonspecific cutaneous hyperreactivity response to intracutaneous injection of either saline or histamine) as an important diagnostic marker for patients with this disorder.

62. Jorizzo JL, Hudson D, Schmalstieg FC, et al.: Behçet's syndrome: Immune regulation, circulating immune complexes, neutrophil migration, and colchicine therapy. J. Am. Acad. Dermatol. *10*:205–214, 1984.

A study of six patients with Behçet's syndrome supports the hypothesis that circulating immune complexes and a factor in the serum that enhances polymorphonuclear leukocyte migration have a role in the pathogenesis of this disorder.

63. Orme RL, Nordlund JJ, Barich L, et al.: The MAGIC syndrome (mouth and genital ulcers with inflamed cartilage). Arch. Dermatol. *126*:940–944, 1990.

A report of a patient with features of both Behçet's disease and relapsing polychondritis suggests that Behçet's syndrome and the MAGIC syndrome may be manifestations of the same disorder.

64. Jorizzo JL: Behçet's disease: An update based on the 1985 International Conference in London. Arch. Dermatol. *122*:556–558, 1986.

Based on the 1985 International Conference, a combination of systemic prednisone (1 mg/kg/day) and azathioprine appears to be the treatment of choice for severe Behçet's disease (alternative choices include chlorambucil, cyclosporine, and thalidomide).

20

THE COLLAGEN VASCULAR DISORDERS

Juvenile Rheumatoid Arthritis
Lupus Erythematosus
  Neonatal Lupus Erythematosus
Dermatomyositis
Scleroderma
Eosinophilic Fasciitis
Eosinophilia-Myalgia Syndrome
Sjögren's Syndrome
Mixed Connective Tissue Disease

The connective tissue (collagen vascular) disorders represent a group of diseases characterized by inflammatory changes of the connective tissue in various parts of the body. Of these, rheumatoid arthritis, lupus erythematosus, dermatomyositis, scleroderma, eosinophilic fasciitis, eosinophilia-myalgia syndrome, Sjögren's syndrome, and mixed connective tissue disease exhibit a variety of cutaneous findings that act as specific markers for the individual disorders.

JUVENILE RHEUMATOID ARTHRITIS

Juvenile rheumatoid arthritis (Still's disease) is a common generalized systemic disease of unknown etiology that may occur at any age in childhood (Table 20–1). The disorder occurs almost twice as frequently in girls as in boys. The most common age at onset is between 2 and 4 years, with another peak in frequency in girls during adolescence. Although the age at onset is rarely younger than 1 year, it has been reported as early as the first week of life. The term *Still's disease* is used when the onset is abrupt and the child has systemic as well as joint symptoms.

Clinical Manifestations. The onset of juvenile arthritis may be sudden and fulminating, with a high spiking fever (which may last for weeks or months), adenopathy, splenomegaly, and anemia, with or without arthralgia; or it may begin slowly, with insidious involvement of a single joint for weeks or months before the other joints are affected. The type of onset, to a considerable extent, is related to the age of the patient—the younger the patient, generally the more prominent the systemic manifestations.

A highly characteristic rash may be the first clue to the diagnosis of juvenile rheumatoid arthritis.

Seen in 25 to 50 per cent of patients, it may precede other manifestations by up to 3 years. The eruption, generally seen at the height of fever, appears as flat to slightly elevated macules or papules that measure from 2 to 6 mm in diameter. Lesions vary from salmon-pink to red and display a characteristic slightly irregular or serpiginous margin (Fig. 20–1).[1] Some lesions may be slightly raised, edematous, and urticarial, but, unlike true urticaria, they do not itch, migrate, or change in shape. They are often surrounded by a zone of pallor, and larger lesions frequently have a pale center.

The eruption is usually intermittent, is often evanescent, and frequently subsides during periods of remission. The rash may appear at any time during the course of the disease and is associated in particular with spikes in fever, splenomegaly, and lymphadenopathy. Accentuated in areas of local heat or trauma, it may be precipitated by emotional, infectious, or surgical stress. Individual lesions often coalesce to form large plaques 8 to 9 cm in diameter and, in severely affected individuals, the eruption may persist for 1 week to several years.

Histologic examination of the cutaneous eruption reveals edematous collagen fibers and perivascular cell infiltrate in the upper portion of the corium, with polymorphonuclear leukocytes and, to a lesser extent, plasma cells and histiocytes.

Children with juvenile rheumatoid arthritis characteristically have an anxious or worried facial expression and an intense desire to be left alone, perhaps owing to their extreme discomfort and an attempt to guard their joints against movement. Thirty to 50 per cent of affected children initially have involvement of only one joint at a time, usually the knee or ankle, but eventually almost all manifest polyarthritis. When multiple joint involvement occurs, it usually is symmetrical and

Table 20–1. JUVENILE RHEUMATOID ARTHRITIS

1. Cutaneous eruption in 25% to 50% of patients
   a. Usually intermittent and often evanescent with fever, lymphadenopathy, and splenomegaly
   b. Flat to slightly elevated macules, papules, or urticarial lesions
2. Spindling of fingers (in 50%)
3. Subcutaneous nodules (in 6% to 10%)
   a. Barely palpable to several centimeters in size (deep in dermis or subcutaneous tissue)
   b. Near olecranon process, on dorsal aspect of hands, knees, ears, and pressure areas (scapulae, sacrum, buttocks, and heels)
4. Eighty to 85% survive without serious disability (10% have severe crippling arthritis)

Hurwitz S: The Skin and Systemic Disease in Children. Year Book Medical Publishers, Chicago, 1985.

may involve any synovial joint in the body (with the possible exception of joints of the lumbothoracic spine). Joints of the lower extremities are usually affected first, especially the knee joint, which is involved in 90 per cent of patients. Finger joints are involved in approximately 75 per cent and the ankles and wrists are affected in approximately two thirds of all patients. There is limitation of motion, usually due to pain; the joints may be warm but not tender; and redness is not marked. The skin, especially over the affected joint of the extremities, becomes atrophic, smooth, and glossy. The thenar and hypothenar eminences may be red; the palms, however, usually remain cold and damp.

Morning stiffness in adult patients with rheumatoid arthritis is a well-known symptom and frequently is helpful in diagnosis of the disease. This is most common early in the morning, is not the result of pain, and, with activity, completely disappears during the day. Children frequently have the same experience after periods of inactivity or sleep, sometimes to the point that they are unable to rise from bed spontaneously. After a few minutes in a tub with moist heat and activity, however, the stiffness disappears and the child is able to move about more freely. Whether inactivity or pain is responsible for morning stiffness is difficult to determine, but the stiffness proves to be a useful clinical manifestation in the diagnosis of this disorder.[2]

Spindling of the fingers (Fig. 20–2), one of the earliest objective signs of joint involvement, is seen in more than 50 per cent of children with juvenile rheumatoid arthritis. The spindle-shaped deformity of the fingers develops because the proximal interphalangeal joints are affected more severely than the distal joints. This finding, rarely seen in any other childhood disease, is highly characteristic and carries considerable diagnostic significance.

Subcutaneous nodules occur in 6 to 10 per cent of children with rheumatoid arthritis at some time during the course of the disease. Barely palpable to several centimeters in size, they may be the first presenting sign of juvenile rheumatoid arthritis. Their most common location is near the olecranon process on the ulnar border of the forearm. Less commonly they may occur on the dorsal aspect of the hands, on the knees and ears, and over pressure areas such as the scapulae, sacrum, buttocks, and heels. In the areas of fingers and toes, subcutaneous nodules are only a few millimeters in size. Subcutaneous nodules are firm and nontender and may be attached to the periarticular capsules of the fingers. In contrast to lesions of granuloma annulare they may be deep in the dermis or in the subcutaneous tissue. Subcutaneous nodules are associated with severe exacerbation of the disease but are not related to prognosis.

About 5 per cent of patients with rheumatoid arthritis have cuticular telangiectases, a characteristic sign of connective tissue disease also seen in patients with lupus erythematosus, scleroderma, and dermatomyositis. This finding is seen as linear wiry vessels perpendicular to the base of the nail in the overlying cuticular and periungual skin. Cu-

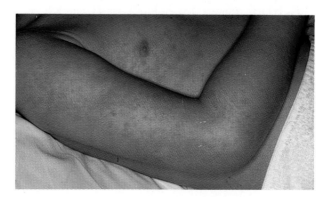

Figure 20–1. A salmon-pink to red maculopapular eruption with irregular or serpiginous margins seen in a child with juvenile rheumatoid arthritis.

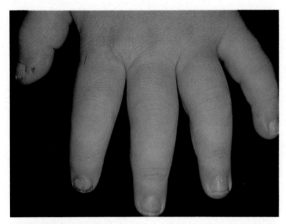

Figure 20–2. Spindling of the fingers—a highly diagnostic feature of juvenile rheumatoid arthritis. The spindle-shaped deformity is related to the fact that the proximal interphalangeal joints are affected more severely than the distal ones.

ticular telangiectases are usually bright red, are not caused by trauma, and, when thrombosed, appear to be black. Cuticular telangiectases are rarely seen in normal individuals and are particularly helpful in the diagnosis of connective tissue disease.

The natural course of juvenile rheumatoid arthritis is variable. The disease may end after a few months and never recur, or it may recur after months or years of remission. The active process often improves by puberty, and because true bony changes are uncommon in children, 80 to 85 per cent of patients achieve remission.[3]

Diagnosis. The diagnosis of juvenile rheumatoid arthritis is based on the clinical features with a history of arthritis (effusion or pain and limitation of motion in at least one joint) lasting for at least 6 weeks, with appropriate studies to exclude other causes of arthritis. Although a number of laboratory tests are helpful in exclusion of other disorders, none is diagnostic of juvenile rheumatoid arthritis. Radiographic changes of joint destruction are helpful in late disease, approximately 80 per cent of patients have a positive rheumatoid factor by latex fixation, and other less specific laboratory tests include an elevated erythrocyte sedimentation rate, leukocytosis, anemia, hyperglobulinemia, and hypoalbuminemia.

Treatment. There is no specific or curative treatment for this disorder. Aspirin (acetylsalicylic acid) is the drug of choice for early treatment, with an attempt to maintain serum salicylate levels between 20 and 30 mg/dl. Such blood levels can be achieved by dosages of 70 to 100 mg/kg/day for children weighing up to 25 kg or less, with total daily doses of 50 to 60 mg/kg/day for heavier children. Once active disease is suppressed, aspirin must be continued for months before it is gradually withdrawn. Although the risk of Reye's syndrome associated with aspirin intake has been empha-

sized, only a handful of case reports have associated high-dose chronic salicylate use with Reye's syndrome. It appears to be prudent, however, to discontinue aspirin temporarily for children with varicella or flu-like syndromes. Other nonsteroidal anti-inflammatory drugs, such as tolmetin sodium (Tolectin) and naproxen (Naprosyn), may also be used for children who either do not respond to salicylates or cannot tolerate a dose required to achieve control.[3] All nonsteroidal anti-inflammatory drugs can cause dyspepsia and gastrointestinal toxicity, including upper gastrointestinal tract bleeding, ulcerations, and perforation, with or without warning symptoms, in patients treated chronically with these agents. Corticosteroids (0.5 to 1.0 mg/kg of prednisone or its equivalent) are indicated only for the seriously ill child or when disease threatens life or sight; and cytotoxic drugs such as methotrexate, cyclophosphamide, azathioprine, and chlorambucil are reserved for those children whose disease is crippling and unresponsive to more conventional therapies. Corticosteroids, however, are vital for protracted iridocyclitis and vasculitis. Intrasynovial corticosteroid injections are helpful in severe joint involvement.

Gold therapy, with weekly doses of 1 mg/kg of the salt for a total of 500 mg, may be useful for patients with nonresponsive polyarthritis. Careful examination, however, for leukopenia, thrombocytopenia, eosinophilia, proteinuria, hematuria, severe pruritus, or cutaneous eruption, particularly exfoliative dermatitis, should be performed at frequent intervals. Corticosteroid drops in association with mydriatics are helpful in the management of iridocyclitis. Appropriate rest, splinting, exercise, and physical therapy are important for the prevention and correction of deformity. Although severe deformities can be corrected by surgery, surgical treatment (synovectomy for removal of granulation tissue) should be considered only after a fair trial of medical therapy has been undertaken. Children 6 years of age or younger are poor surgical risks, however, because of their inability to cooperate effectively with postoperative measures.

LUPUS ERYTHEMATOSUS

Lupus erythematosus (LE) is a chronic inflammatory condition that may affect the skin as well as most other organ systems. Although the etiology is unknown, reports of familial cases and a high concordance for clinical disease in monozygotic, but not dizygotic, twins suggest a strong genetic component and altered cellular immunity in genetically predisposed individuals as factors in its pathogenesis.

Typically a disease of young women, the disorder is seen in all age groups. Up to one fifth (15 to 25 per cent) of all cases of systemic lupus erythematosus (SLE) occur within the first 2 decades of life. The onset in adults usually is during the third and fourth decades of life; in childhood the disorder usually occurs in those older than 8 years of age, the peak incidence occurs between ages 11 and 13, and in 5 per cent of children the disorder appears before the age of 5 years. Although cases have been described in newborns, except for neonatal lupus the disorder is rarely seen before the age of 3 years.[4]

Clinically, two types of LE are often described, but division into only two forms represents an oversimplification of this multifaceted disease complex. The cutaneous form, often referred to as discoid lupus erythematosus (DLE), is without systemic manifestations and occurs at the benign end of the LE spectrum. Systemic LE is a chronic multisystemic disease. In addition, several intermediate types have been described. These have been termed *generalized discoid LE* (a disorder that is evidenced by widespread scarring discoid lesions usually with mild systemic involvement) and *subacute lupus erythematosus,* a subset used to describe individuals who manifest a widespread photosensitive form of cutaneous LE in which systemic involvement tends to be relatively mild, is mainly musculoskeletal (arthritis or arthralgia), and patients have serologic abnormalities without serious renal or central nervous system disease.

Females with SLE outnumber males by ratios varying from 3:1 to 8:1 in all age groups except prepubertal children (in whom the sex incidence appears to be about equal). Cutaneous or DLE is rare in children, and although it has been stated that most childhood cases have been systemic and that SLE appears to have a greater severity in children than in adults (and the younger the patient, the more acute the disorder), reviews suggest that patterns and prognosis in children may indeed be similar to those of adults.[4]

Clinical Manifestations

Cutaneous Manifestations. Although the incidence of cutaneous (discoid) LE is less common in childhood, the cutaneous lesions of discoid LE in children and adults are similar. About 80 per cent of patients with SLE have cutaneous involvement at some time, and in up to 25 per cent of patients cutaneous lesions are the presenting sign of the disorder. A rash often appears over the cheeks and bridge of the nose. This so-called malar or butterfly rash, seen in 30 to 60 per cent of patients with SLE, is neither a specific nor the most frequent sign of the disorder.[5]

The classic discoid lesion of LE is a well-circumscribed, elevated, indurated red to purplish plaque with adherent scale (Fig. 20–3), fine telangiectasia, and areas of atrophy. Discoid lesions can be asymmetrical on the head and face, scalp, arms, legs, hands, fingers, back, chest, or abdomen. At times the openings of hair follicles are dilated and plugged by an overlying scale. If the scale is thick enough, it can be lifted off in one piece. The undersurface then reveals follicular projections that resemble carpet tacks, a characteristic sign of LE.

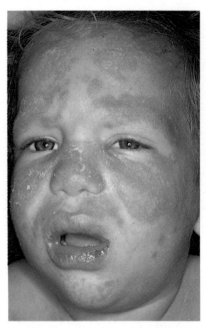

Figure 20–3. Lupus erythematosus. Scaly erythematous urticarial plaques on the face, with scaling and crusting of the lips, are seen in a 2-year-old boy with systemic lupus erythematosus.

Another common lesion of LE is a red to purplish urticarial plaque, which is relatively fixed in shape and does not undergo atrophy or scaling. This lesion, often associated with photosensitivity, usually occurs on the face or other exposed areas of the body (Fig. 20–4). Although cutaneous lesions and photosensitivity are of diagnostic and cosmetic significance, photosensitivity reactions have also been known to precipitate fatal exacerbations of the disease. When untreated, lesions may go on to develop permanent areas of hyperpigmentation or hypopigmentation with atrophy—another commonly seen cutaneous manifestation of LE (Fig. 20–5).

Mucosal membrane lesions (gingivitis, mucosal hemorrhage, erosions, and small ulcerations) are seen in 3 per cent of patients with cutaneous LE and in from 10 to 15 per cent of patients with the systemic form of the disorder. A silvery whitening of the vermilion border of the lips is highly characteristic and pathognomonic of LE. The lips are often involved, with slight thickening, roughness, and redness, with or without superficial ulceration and crusting. One must never neglect, therefore, to examine the nose and mouth of patients for evidence of silvery white scaling and ulcerations (Figs. 20–6 and 20–7). The gingivae may also appear red, edematous, friable, and eroded, or they may exhibit silvery white changes similar to those on the nasal or buccal mucosa.

Scarring alopecia, another important marker of lupus erythematosus, may be seen as single or multiple well-demarcated patches (Fig. 20–8) that ex-

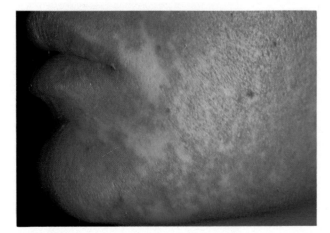

Figure 20–4. Reddish purple plaques on the face following sun exposure in a 17-year-old patient with systemic lupus erythematosus.

hibit erythema, scaling, telangiectasia, atrophy, and plugging (the classic changes of LE). Increased fragility of the hair in LE may produce broken hairs several millimeters from the roots, with a resulting receding hairline with an unruly appearance due to the short broken hairs ("lupus hair").

Livedo reticularis, a peculiar blotchy bluish red discoloration of the skin due to vasospasm of the arterioles, although often normal when seen in young children, may be the earliest sign of lupus erythematosus, rheumatoid arthritis, rheumatic fever, or scleroderma. It can also be seen in patients with leukemia, idiopathic thrombocytopenic purpura, idiopathic thrombocytopenia, atheromatous vascular disease, periarteritis nodosa, cryoglobulinemia, or neurologic abnormalities or in those on immunosuppressive therapy. Aggravated by exposure to cold, the area becomes livid or cyanotic when the arterial supply is reduced. Livedo reticularis, when it affects the entire trunk or limbs in a continuous manner, is often a normal phenomenon. When it develops in a blotchy interrupted configuration, however, it is frequently a sign of systemic disease.

Other vascular phenomena associated with LE include Raynaud's phenomenon and urticaria. Raynaud's phenomenon, seen in 10 to 30 per cent of patients with LE, as in scleroderma may precede the onset of disease by months or years. This phenomenon is described in more detail in the section on scleroderma.

Chronic urticaria-like lesions associated with a leukocytoclastic vasculitis may also be seen as the first sign of LE. The extent of hives, seen at some time in 7 to 22 per cent of patients with LE, frequently reflects the activity of the disease and, at times, may serve as a useful guide to therapy. Generally persisting for a more prolonged period of time than classic urticaria, urticaria seen in association with LE tends to be chronic and is often associated with hypocomplementemia. Probably a manifestation of immune complex deposition, it generally occurs in patients demonstrating clinical or serologic evidence of systemic disease activity.

Telangiectases represent another characteristic

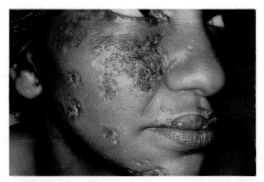

Figure 20–5. Lupus erythematosus. Note atrophic hyperpigmented discoid lesions. (Courtesy of Department of Dermatology, Yale University School of Medicine.)

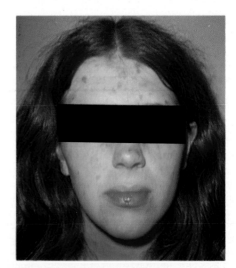

Figure 20–6. A crusted lesion on the lower lip and discoid LE plaques on the face of a 16-year-old girl with systemic lupus erythematosus.

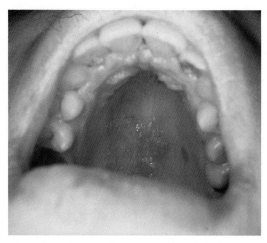

Figure 20–7. Ulcerated mucosal lesions on the palate of a 16-year-old girl with lupus erythematosus. (Hurwitz S: The Skin and Systemic Disease in Children. Year Book Medical Publishers, Chicago, 1985.)

marker of connective tissue disease. Distinctive findings here include erythema and papular telangiectasia of the palms and fingers (Fig. 20–9) and linear telangiectasia of the cuticles and periungual skin (with or without thromboses). Cuticular telangiectasia is not specific for LE; it is also seen in patients with dermatomyositis and scleroderma and in about 5 per cent of patients with rheumatoid arthritis. Diffuse angiitis, with or without ulceration, also occurs in about 10 per cent of patients with LE, and vesiculobullous eruptions may develop as a result of liquefactive degeneration of the basal layer. Although studies of patients with bullous eruptions suggest that individuals with this variant, termed *bullous* (or *vesiculobullous*) LE, seen most frequently in patients who have systemic LE, may display clinical features suggestive of other bullous disorders, a review of reported cases supports the inclusion of this entity in the spectrum of LE.[6–7]

Periorbital edema, probably as a result of loose areolar connective tissue and dermal edema, truncal papulonodular lesions (characterized by diffuse dermal mucin without the usual inflammatory or epidermal charges of LE),[8] and chilblains (chilblain, perniosis) may also be seen in patients with LE (Fig. 20–10). Seen as tender cyanotic to reddish blue nodular swellings on the fingers or toes of some patients with LE, chilblains represents cold-induced chronic vasospasm of digital vessels. Seen in up to 12 per cent of patients with DLE, chilblain lupus may occur some years after lesions of DLE or may precede the onset of DLE or SLE.[9]

Lupus panniculitis (lupus profundus), an uncommon subtype of chronic LE characterized by deep dermal and subcutaneous inflammatory involvement, occurs in approximately 2 per cent of patients with cutaneous LE or SLE. Lesions are seen as firm, asymptomatic or tender, sharply defined, rubbery dermal and subcutaneous plaques or nodules, with a predilection for the scalp, forehead, cheeks, upper arms, breasts, thighs, and buttocks. Although the skin overlying the lesions usually appears normal (Fig. 20–11), it may be drawn inward with cup-shaped depressions, and ulcerations may develop, spontaneously or following nonspecific trauma such as a biopsy or injections of intralesional corticosteroids.[5, 10, 11] The histology of lupus profundus is characterized by a perivascular lymphocytic, plasma cell, and histiocytic infiltration in the deep dermis and subcutaneous fat without accompanying fat necrosis. Direct immunofluorescence is particularly helpful in the diagnosis of this disorder, since immunoglobulins or C_3 deposits are often seen in the basement membrane of affected patients. Approximately 70 per cent of patients with lupus panniculitis also have typical lesions of DLE and 50 per cent eventually develop systemic involvement or symptoms of SLE such as fever, arthralgia, and lymphadenopathy. Lesions of lupus profundus may persist for years; and although they can be confused with those of erythema nodosum, they generally are not tender, are more chronic, and do not have a predilection for the legs.

Patients with *subacute cutaneous lupus erythematosus* (SCLE), which represents 10 to 15 per cent of all cases of LE, manifest a subset characterized by a recurring extensive erythematous, nonscarring, photosensitive form of cutaneous LE. The disorder usually affects young and middle-aged white women in the 15- to 40-year age group and is uncommon in blacks and Hispanics. The cutaneous lesions of SCLE arise quite suddenly, mainly on the upper trunk, extensor part of the arms, and dorsal aspect of the hands and fingers. The lesions may be annular and may enlarge and merge into psoriasiform or polycyclic lesions with thin and easily detached scales (Fig. 20–12). Although arthritis and fatigue are common, patients usually only have mild systemic manifestations and, in most cases, the cutaneous features are completely reversible as the inflammatory process re-

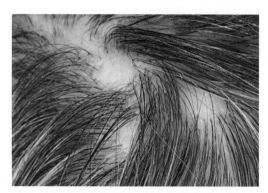

Figure 20–8. Scarring alopecia of the scalp in a patient with systemic lupus erythematosus.

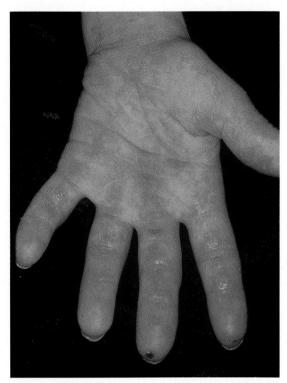

Figure 20–9. Erythema and papular telangiectasia on the palm and fingers of a child with lupus erythematosus. (Hurwitz S: The Skin and Systemic Disease in Children. Year Book Medical Publishers, Chicago, 1985.)

solves.[12–14] The majority of patients with SCLE have antibodies to Ro (SSA), La (SSB), or single-stranded (SS) DNA and carry the HLA-DR3 subtype. The histologic features of SCLE differ only in degree from those seen in patients with DLE, the hydropic degeneration of the basal cell layer and edema of the dermis are more pronounced than those seen in patients with DLE, and the hyperkeratosis and inflammatory infiltrate are less prominent.

Systemic Manifestations. The systemic manifestations of SLE include fever, malaise, weight loss, fatigue, arthralgia (the most common symptom of the disorder), pleurisy, cardiac complications (pericarditis, endocarditis, myocarditis, and extramural and intramural coronary arteritis), gastrointestinal symptomatology, hepatomegaly, ischemic necrosis of bone, renal involvement, and, in 25 per cent of patients, ocular complications (cotton-wool patches, optic neuropathy, perivasculitis, and edema of the optic disk). Lymphadenopathy, although common in adults, is relatively rare in children with SLE. Lupus nephritis (diffuse proliferative glomerulonephritis) is seen at the most severe end of the LE spectrum. Characterized by the abrupt appearance of polyarthritis, leukopenia, alopecia, severe proteinuria, and an evanescent butterfly rash, it may be seen in 50 to 85

per cent of children at the onset of their disease. Anti-DNA antibody is a serologic marker for this complication (the most common cause of mortality for patients with SLE).

Diagnosis. The diagnosis of SLE is chiefly clinical and is based on the presence of cutaneous lesions, systemic manifestations, and confirmatory laboratory tests. A person is said to have SLE if four or more of the following criteria are present: (1) malar rash, (2) discoid rash, (3) photosensitivity, (4) oral ulcers, (5) arthritis, (6) serositis, (7) renal complications, (8) neurologic involvement, (9) hematologic features, (10) immunologic manifestations, and (11) abnormal antinuclear antibody titer (Table 20–2).[15]

In most instances, a histopathologic diagnosis can be established by a combination of histologic findings. These include (1) hyperkeratosis with keratotic plugging; (2) atrophy of the stratum malpighii; (3) liquefactive degeneration of basal cells; (4) a patchy, chiefly lymphoid cell infiltrate with a tendency to arrangement about the cutaneous appendages; and (5) edema, vasodilation, and extravasation of erythrocytes in the upper dermis. However, all five changes are not present in every patient. Of these, focal liquefaction degeneration of the basal layer represents the most significant histologic change. In its absence, a histologic diagnosis is difficult and often impossible. Histopathologic findings of oral lesions consist of parakeratosis, hydropic degeneration of the stratum germinativum, and perivascular lymphocytic infiltration.

Laboratory features include antinuclear antibodies, anti-DNA antibodies, low complement levels, and deposits of immunoglobulin and complement at the dermal-epidermal junction. Leukopenia of less than 5,000/mm³ frequently occurs. Anemia and thrombocytopenia are frequently noted in pa-

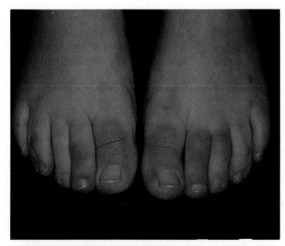

Figure 20–10. Chilblains (perniosis). Tender, reddish blue nodular swellings on the toes of a 21-year-old woman were the initial manifestation of her systemic lupus erythematosus.

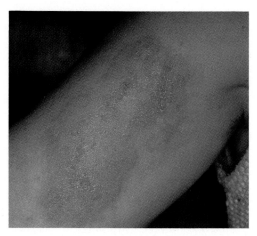

Figure 20–11. Firm, sharply defined, dermal and sub-cutaneous lesions on the arm of a patient with lupus profundus. (Courtesy of Department of Dermatology, Yale University School of Medicine.)

tients with SLE, and serum globulin levels are elevated in about 80 per cent of patients. In patients with active disease a reduced serum complement level may be frequently noted and the erythrocyte sedimentation rate is elevated in all but an occasional patient during periods of clinical activity.

Of all the tests available, antinuclear antibody is the most valuable screening test for SLE, and approximately 90 per cent of patients with systemic disease have an antinuclear antibody titer of 1:32 or greater. Other common serologic abnormalities include elevated levels of immunoglobulin, positive tests for rheumatoid factor, positive Coombs' test, lowered serum complement levels (in patients with active immune-complex disease, particularly nephritis), and other autoantibodies such as anti-single-stranded (SS) DNA, anti-Ro (SSA) or anti-La (SSB), and 20 per cent of patients have positive serologic tests for syphilis. The LE cell test, except for its presence in lupoid hepatitis, rheumatoid arthritis, and, at times, scleroderma and dermatomyositis, is generally specific for the disease. Anti-Ro–positive patients generally demonstrate a prominent widespread photosensitivity dermatitis, a particularly common feature in patients with SCLE and neonatal LE.[16] Detection of antibodies against DNA has been found to be extremely valuable in the evaluation of patients with SLE, and patients with anti-DNA antibodies appear to be at risk for the development of renal disease. Since the test for anti-nDNA is as sensitive and specific as the LE cell test, and has the advantage of being less time consuming and easier to read, it is frequently used to replace the traditional LE test. Double-stranded (dsDNA) tests are highly specific; this occurs in 50 to 60 per cent of patients with SLE, and is responsible for immune-complex SLE renal disease. Sm (Smith) antibodies, found in

approximately 30 per cent of patients with SLE who usually have renal disease, are also specific for SLE, and nuclear ribonuclear protein (nRNP) antibodies, although not specific, are found in approximately 40 per cent of patients with systemic disease and at times in patients with scleroderma and the mixed connective tissue syndrome. Although patients with anti-nRNP antibody have a low incidence of renal disease (hence a good prognosis), the presence of anticardiolipin antibodies appears to place patients with SLE at risk for the development of thromboembolic phenomena such as recurrent deep vein thrombosis, pulmonary emboli, and central nervous system thromboembolic events, and women with SLE who are pregnant and manifest anticardiolipin antibodies appear to have an increased risk for spontaneous abortion.

In patients with SLE, the detection of a band of bright yellow-green fluorescence at the dermal-epidermal junction (the lupus band test) in lesions of cutaneous LE is said to be more specific and sensitive in establishing the diagnosis of LE than routine histologic studies. Thus, when involved skin is tested, immunoglobulins (most commonly IgG and IgM) and complement have reportedly been found in over 90 per cent of specimens of both SLE and DLE (Fig. 20–13). Although direct immunofluorescent testing of involved skin is more sensitive and specific than routine histologic studies of biopsy specimens, the false-positive rate of this test on sun-exposed skin can be as high as 25 per cent, and up to 25 per cent of patients with cutaneous LE lesions may have negative immunofluorescence. Some authors, therefore, believe that positive immunofluorescence from sun-exposed skin is not specific and adds little information to the clinical and histopathologic findings.[18, 19] In addition, a serologic profile composed of antinuclear antibody (ANA), a thready ANA pattern of anti–extractable nuclear antigen (ENA), and anti–single-stranded deoxyribonucleic acid (ssDNA) have also been found to be useful immunologic markers for different clinical presentations of LE.

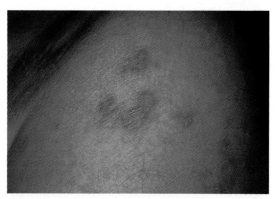

Figure 20–12. Annular lesions of subacute lupus erythematosus. (Courtesy of Department of Dermatology, Yale University School of Medicine.)

Autoantibody profiles consisting of a thready ANA pattern and anti-ENA (Sm) antibodies appear to have a higher incidence of pulmonary, joint, and renal involvement than anti-ENA negative patients with the large speckle-like thready patterns.

Table 20–2. CRITERIA FOR CLASSIFICATION OF SYSTEMIC LUPUS ERYTHEMATOSUS*

Criterion	Definition
1. Malar rash	Fixed erythema, flat or raised, over the malar eminences (tending to spare the nasolabial folds)
2. Discoid rash	Erythematous raised patches with adherent keratotic scaling and follicular plugging; atrophic scarring may occur in old lesions
3. Photosensitivity	A cutaneous rash following exposure to sunlight (by history or observation)
4. Oral ulcers	Oral or nasopharyngeal ulceration
5. Arthritis	Nonerosive arthritis (characterized by tenderness, swelling, or effusion) involving two or more peripheral joints
6. Serositis	Pleuritis (history of pleuritic pain or rub heard by a physician, or evidence of pleural effusion) *or* Pericarditis (by electrocardiogram, pericardial rub, or evidence of pericardial effusion)
7. Renal disorder	Persistent proteinuria greater than 0.5 g/day (greater than 3+ if quantitation not performed) *or* Cellular casts
8. Neurologic disorder	Seizures in the absence of offending drugs or known metabolic derangements *or* Psychosis (in the absence of offending drugs or known metabolic derangements)
9. Hematologic disorder	Hemolytic anemia with reticulocytosis Leukopenia less than 4,000 mm³ on two or more occasions *or* Thrombocytopenia less than 100,000/mm³ (in the absence of offending drugs)
10. Immunologic disorder	Positive LE cell preparation *or* Anti-DNA antibody to native DNA in abnormal titer *or* Anti-Sm (presence of antibody to Sm nuclear antigen) *or* Chronic false-positive serologic test for syphilis, positive for at least 6 months (confirmed by *Treponema pallidum* immobilization or fluorescent treponemal antibody absorption test)
11. Antinuclear antibody	An abnormal titer of antinuclear antibody by immunofluorescence or equivalent assay in the absence of drugs known to be associated with "drug-induced lupus" syndrome

* A person is diagnosed as having systemic lupus erythematosus if any four or more of the above criteria are present, serially or simultaneously, during any interval of observation.

There is a higher incidence of Raynaud's phenomenon in patients with the large speckle-like thready ANA pattern, and photosensitivity appears to be more common in patients with large speckle-like thready patterns.[17–19]

Treatment. Our understanding of LE has improved substantially over the past 35 years. Recent statistics reveal that patients with cutaneous LE have an excellent prognosis, only about 5 per cent of patients go on to develop systemic disease, and the prognosis for children with SLE has changed dramatically from nearly 100 per cent mortality to a survival rate of over 90 per cent. The main causes of death in children are renal failure, central nervous system lupus, myocardial infarction, cardiac failure, or infection. Although previous reports suggested that children had a worse prognosis than adults with SLE, subsequent studies reveal that children with milder disease are now recognized; and although those with renal involvement are indeed seriously ill, SLE in childhood is not always associated with a poor prognosis.[4]

The therapy for LE currently depends on the extent of local and systemic involvement. Avoidance of sun exposure and daylight fluorescent light by hats, clothing, and appropriate broad-spectrum sunscreens with UVA as well as UVB protection is essential. Although only 30 to 40 per cent of patients with lupus erythematosus are photosensitive, ultraviolet light may induce or exacerbate cutaneous lesions or produce a fatal deterioration of systemic disease. Fatigue is also a problem in patients with SLE and is often the last symptom to respond to therapy. Thus, although patients with SLE generally do not need to give up schooling, employment, or recreation, they should adjust their schedules to allow for intervals of rest between periods of activity.

Patients with mild disease without nephritis should be treated with salicylates or other nonsteroidal agents for symptomatic relief of arthritis or other discomforts. Topical corticosteroid preparations are effective for most cutaneous lesions, and antimalarial therapy is beneficial for long-term suppression of the disease. When antimalarials are used, since deposition of the drug in the pigmented portion of the retina can produce irreversible retinopathy following long-term use, the patient should have a pretreatment ophthalmologic examination and periodic follow-up examinations. Although many reviews have mentioned a special sensitivity of children to antimalarial drugs, chloroquine has been shown to be quite safe if used in the recommended dosage range.[20, 21] The average dose of hydroxychloroquine (Plaquenil) for children is 5 to 10 mg/kg/24 hr; for adults it is 400 mg/day with a maintenance dose of 200 to 400 mg/day. It is advisable, however, that chloroquine be dispensed in child-proof containers, and the taking of other medications such as sulfonamides, hydralazine, reserpine, griseofulvin, and oral contraceptives, which may exacerbate the disease, should be discouraged.[22]

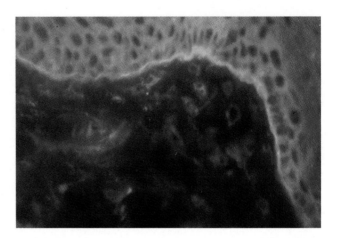

Figure 20–13. Lupus erythematosus. Direct immuno-fluorescence shows globulin deposition at the dermal-epidermal junction. (Courtesy of Irwin M. Braverman, M.D.)

Systemic lupus erythematosus should be considered a lifelong incurable but controllable disease. Although children with mild LE may respond well to mere bed rest, salicylates or other nonsteroidal agents, and the avoidance of excessive sun exposure, they should be carefully evaluated for major organ involvement, particularly for the presence of nephritis (the major cause of death in persons with this disorder). In severe cases, hospitalization may be necessary for diagnostic evaluation as well as for definitive therapy for SLE, and prednisone, the cornerstone of therapy for severe childhood SLE, in dosages of 1 to 3 mg/kg/24 hr, may be lifesaving for patients with renal complication, pericarditis, neurologic involvement, or hemolytic anemia. Once remission is induced, a minimal corticosteroid maintenance dose, preferably alternate-day therapy, is advisable. Although corticosteroid therapy has increased the survival rate, the possibility of complications associated with long-term systemic corticosteroid use must be considered.

Since immunosuppressive agents are beneficial (but carry an increased risk of neoplasia, aplastic anemia, and sepsis), when renal disease is present, the patient is best referred to a center where immunosuppressive therapy is available. The recommended pediatric dose for azathioprine (Imuran) is 2 mg/kg/day; for 6-mercaptopurine, 50 to 100 mg/day; for cyclophosphamide (Cytoxan), 50 mg/day; and for chlorambucil (Leukeran), 0.1 mg/kg/day, with appropriate modification depending on the size and weight of small children.

Several newer therapeutic regimens also deserve mention. Intravenous pulse corticosteroid therapy with methylprednisolone (Solu-Medrol), 30 mg/kg/dose, given as a bolus for 3 days, has been reported to reverse rapid renal deterioration and is frequently beneficial in other acute situations. In addition, isotretinoin, plasmapheresis, clofazimine (Laprene), thalidomide (available in the United States for research purposes only), gold, or oral retinoids may be considered, and renal transplantation may be used for patients with severe (end-stage) renal disease.[2, 23]

Neonatal Lupus Erythematosus

Neonatal LE is a unique variant of LE found in infants born to mothers with or who have a tendency for SLE, rheumatoid arthritis, Sjögren's syndrome, or undifferentiated connective tissue disease (Table 20–3). Affected infants have a lupus-like rash, lupus-associated hematologic and serologic abnormalities, and, in 15 to 30 per cent of patients, congenital atrioventricular heart block.[24–27]

Infants born to mothers with disseminated LE are usually normal but occasionally have some manifestations of neonatal lupus. Although anti-Ro (SSA) antibodies, found in 95 per cent of affected mother–infant pairs, have a major role in the genesis of this disorder, anti-La (SSB) and anti-U$_1$RNP (nRNP) and other autoantibodies have also been reported.[28–30] In addition, an increased frequency of histocompatibility antigens HLA-B8 and HLA-DR3 may be higher in mothers of infants with con-

Table 20–3. NEONATAL LUPUS ERYTHEMATOSUS

1. Seen in infants born to mothers with a tendency for systemic lupus erythematosus, rheumatoid arthritis, or undifferentiated connective tissue disease
2. Lupus-like rash, often in areas of sun exposure; diffuse erythema of face; oval atrophic hypopigmented discoid lesions with telangiectasia
3. Associated with anti-Ro (SSA), anti-La (SSB) and anti-U$_1$RNP (nRNP) antibodies
4. Congenital atrioventricular heart block in 15% to 30%

genital block. Although genetics are important, a report of an infant with neonatal lupus and congenital heart block who shared antibodies to SSA and SSB with her mother, but failed to inherit the chromosome containing HLA-DR3, suggests that the HLA system may not be the sole factor determining susceptibility to neonatal LE.[31]

The majority of infants with neonatal LE are female with a ratio thought to be similar to that of adults with SLE. Cutaneous lesions appear from the time of birth (in two thirds of patients) until about 12 weeks of age, and the majority of infants have spontaneous resolution of their cutaneous lesions by the age of 6 to 12 months. In a few patients, however, the cutaneous lesions disappeared within 1 month and at times the eruption has lasted up to the age of 26 months.[27] The cutaneous lesions of neonatal LE generally appear on the head and neck, the extensor surfaces of the arms, and, less frequently, on the trunk and other areas of the extremities (including the palms and soles). They are manifested as a diffuse erythema of the face (especially the forehead and periorbital regions) (Figs. 20–14 and 20–15), scaly atrophic discoid lesions (Fig. 20–16), and, at times, hypopigmented atrophic plaques with telangiectasia (Fig. 20–17). Although occurring predominantly in areas of sun exposure, particularly following intense sun exposure or sunburn, lesions may also occur in sun-protected areas of the skin.

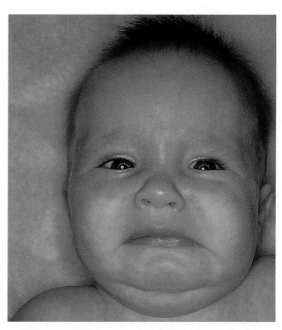

Figure 20–15. Neonatal lupus erythematosus. Diffuse erythema is seen on the forehead and periorbital regions of a 5-month-old infant following sun exposure. (Hurwitz S: The Skin and Systemic Disease in Children. Year Book Medical Publishers, Chicago, 1985.)

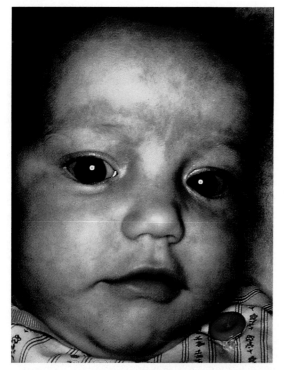

Figure 20–14. Erythematous patches on the scalp, forehead, and periorbital region in a 3 1/2-month-old infant with neonatal lupus erythematosus. (Hurwitz S: The Skin and Systemic Disease in Children. Year Book Medical Publishers, Chicago, 1985.)

Neonatal LE was originally believed to be a transient disease, but it is now apparent that systemic involvement may also occur. Cardiac involvement, the most serious complication, occurs in 75 per cent of cases and congenital heart block occurs in 15 to 30 per cent of affected patients. Unlike other complications of neonatal LE, congenital heart block is usually irreversible, and infants with complete heart block have a high mortality rate, in some instances said to be as high as 20 to 30 per cent, with the greatest risk occurring in the first few months of life. Some infants, however, have only first- or second-degree heart block, and at least one infant had spontaneous resolution of second-degree heart block over the first few months of life.[26] Death may also result from congestive heart failure or other associated complications such as transposition of the great vessels, patent ductus arteriosus, septal defects, and endocardial fibroelastosis.[32] Other systemic complications include liver involvement (generally manifested by hepatomegaly and abnormalities of liver function tests),[33] splenomegaly (in 40 per cent), lymphadenopathy (in 7 per cent), leukopenia, thrombocytopenia (about 20 per cent have significant thrombocytopenia, with or without petechial lesions), Coombs'–test positive hemolytic anemia, and anemia without a positive Coombs' test. In addition, mothers with one child with neonatal LE are at an increased risk for having a second affected child and a few infants with neonatal LE have gone on to develop SLE at later ages.[26]

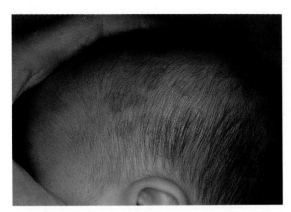

Figure 20–16. Annular discoid lesions on the scalp of a 2-month-old infant with neonatal lupus erythematosus.

The diagnosis of neonatal LE is aided by the presence of typical cutaneous lesions, systemic manifestations, and confirmatory laboratory studies (positive LE preparations, positive anti-Ro, anti-La, or anti-U₁RNP antibody tests of the infants and mothers, lymphocyte tuboreticular inclusions, leukopenia, thrombocytopenia, and Coombs' test–positive hemolytic anemia) in infants born to mothers with or at risk for LE, rheumatoid arthritis, Sjögren's syndrome, or undifferentiated connective tissue disease. Because of the possibility of involvement of internal organs, a thorough physical examination, electrocardiogram, complete blood cell count with platelet count, and liver function tests are often recommended for infants suspected of having neonatal LE.[26]

Cutaneous biopsy of skin lesions of affected infants generally demonstrates the histopathologic features of LE with injury to the basal epidermal cells as a prominent feature. Although immunofluorescent studies have been performed in a relatively low percentage of affected cases, positive immunofluorescence of skin lesions has been demonstrated as immunoreactants of C₃, IgG, or IgM at the dermal-epidermal junction of infants with this disorder, and fluorescent tests for antinuclear antibodies have been shown to be positive with speckled patterns.

Although the natural course of cutaneous lesions suggests spontaneous resolution in most instances, appropriate treatment of neonatal LE suggests avoidance of sun exposure and the topical use of low- to mid-potency glucocorticosteroids on cutaneous lesions. Treatment of heart block, however, is not necessary unless the child has heart failure. In that case, a pacemaker should be used and, inas-much as heart block may at times persist, pacemakers may have to be continued throughout the lifetime of the child. Children who have cutaneous neonatal LE and any infant known to have heart block by in-utero testing, therefore, should be investigated for the possibility of congenital atrial ventricular block and be monitored for signs of active or recurring disease.

DERMATOMYOSITIS

Dermatomyositis is an inflammatory disorder that primarily affects the skin, striated muscles, and occasionally other internal organs in children as well as adults (Table 20–4). In cases in which cutaneous changes are absent or insignificant, the term *polymyositis* is used. Since the clinical and pathologic features of involved skin and muscles are similar, dermatomyositis and polymyositis are believed to be variants of the same disease process.

The etiology of dermatomyositis is unknown. Cell-mediated hypersensitivity appears to play a major role in its pathogenesis, and in children more than one mechanism may be involved. A febrile illness occasionally preceding the onset of childhood dermatomyositis and demonstration of coxsackievirus in muscles suggest an infectious origin, particularly in childhood, and reports of increased frequency of HLA-B8/HLA-DR3 in children and HLA-B14 in adults with dermatomyositis suggest the possibility of a genetic predisposition to the disorder. Thus, genetic, viral, and immunologic mechanisms appear to play a role and dermatomyositis and polymyositis probably have a number of different causes in which cellular immune mechanisms produce tissue injury.[34, 35]

Dermatomyositis occurs twice as frequently in females as in males. Although it may occur at any age, it rarely begins before the second year of life and about 25 per cent of those afflicted are younger than 18 years of age at the time of onset. In adults the disorder occurs most commonly between the ages of 50 and 70; in childhood the highest incidence is between 5 and 12 years, the youngest case reported being that of a 4-month-old infant. Malignancy is associated with adult dermatomyositis in about 20 per cent of cases and is more common in dermatomyositis than polymyositis. Although malignancy has been reported at least three times in children with dermatomyositis, there appears to be no relationship between malignancy and this disorder in the childhood age group.[36, 37] In addition, children rarely have Raynaud's phenomenon; they tend to have more inflammation and necrosis of

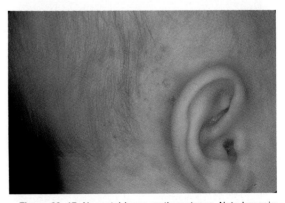

Figure 20–17. Neonatal lupus erythematosus. Note hypopigmented atrophic plaque with telangiectasia.

Table 20–4. DERMATOMYOSITIS

1. An inflammatory disorder of unknown etiology affecting the skin and striated muscles (other organs rarely involved)
2. Erythematous red to purplish heliotrope edematous patches on face (especially eyelids, forehead, cheeks, and temples), extensor surfaces of arms, shoulders, elbows, knees,and dorsal interphalangeal joints
3. Gottron's papules pathognomonic; cuticular telangiectasia and palmar erythema common
4. Association with malignancy in 15% to 20% of adults (but not in children)
5. Cutaneous calcinosis generally a favorable prognostic sign in children

muscle, and in contrast to adults, a respiratory illness often precedes the onset of the dermatomyositis and the mortality is lower.

Clinical Manifestations. The onset of dermatomyositis is usually insidious, with muscle weakness and fatigue. Children often present with fever. Characteristic cutaneous lesions include a violaceous erythema of the upper eyelids and extensor joint surfaces (Figs. 20–18 and 20–19). They may come after polymyositis or may precede muscle disease by an interval of a few weeks to 3 years. When skin markings precede polymyositis, the interval is generally between 3 and 6 months.

A variety of cutaneous findings may be noted in dermatomyositis. The dermatitis may be the most striking feature of the illness, or it may be so minor as to be easily overlooked. The rash in most cases is distinctive and highly suggestive, but not pathognomonic. A purplish red erythema occurs on the face, especially on the eyelids, upper cheeks (Fig. 20–18), forehead, and temples. Frequently associated with photosensitivity, it is often described as a heliotrope erythema, from the flower of the reddish purple plant bearing this name. When present, this color is highly distinctive and often diagnostic. Sometimes the facial lesions are very edematous, leading to a periorbital edema with the reddish or purplish heliotrope color. Within a few weeks a confluent, violaceous, often edematous erythema with fine scaling may also appear over the hairline of the scalp, nape of the neck, extensor surfaces of the arms and shoulders, elbows, knees, and dorsal interphalangeal joints (Fig. 20–20), often suggesting a diagnosis of contact dermatitis or photosensitivity. When the heliotrope erythema on the face is inapparent or not definitive, a simple maneuver of having the child lie on the edge of the examining table, with the head extended beyond the edge at a slightly lower level than the rest of the body, will often bring out the red or purplish hue (personal communication, Dr. Arthur L. Norins, Indianapolis).

In almost every case there is erythema of the cuticles at the base of the nails, with accompanying cuticular linear telangiectasia (see Fig. 20–20). At times, the cuticles may also be thickened, hyperkeratotic, and irregular, giving an appearance of excessive picking or manicuring. Hypertrichosis and hyperpigmentation, independent of corticosteroid therapy, may also complicate previously involved skin, particularly in children, and ulcerations of the fingertips (Fig. 20–21), probably associated with angiitis, may be seen in acute forms of this disorder.

A pathognomonic sign of dermatomyositis is the

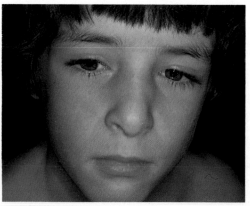

Figure 20–18. Edema of the cheeks and eyelids with a purplish red heliotrope erythema on the eyelids and cheeks of a child with dermatomyositis.

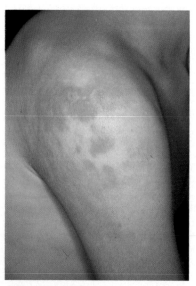

Figure 20–19. Heliotrope eruption on the shoulders and upper arm of an 11-year-old boy with dermatomyositis.

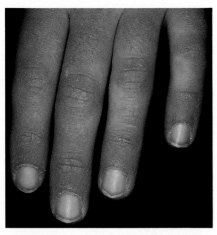

Figure 20–20. Violaceous flat-topped papules (Gottron's papules) on the dorsal interphalangeal joints and erythema and telangiectasia of the cuticles in a patient with dermatomyositis.

Gottron papule, a violaceous flat-topped lesion over the dorsal interphalangeal joints, which usually occurs late in the disease (in about one third of patients) (see Fig. 20–20). When the papule resolves, atrophy, telangiectasia, or hypopigmentation may persist. Other cutaneous features include palmar erythema (Fig. 20–22), cutaneous atrophy, a tight glossy appearance over involved extremities, and poikiloderma (a variegated or multicolored condition of the skin). In longstanding disease there may be cutaneous atrophy and the skin is frequently bound down to underlying structures.

The mucous membranes may also be involved in dermatomyositis. Erythema of the palate and buccal mucosa, with or without ulceration, erythema of the gum margin (Fig. 20–23), and whitish patches on the tongue and buccal mucosa have been observed.

A sequel to the inflammatory phase of the disease is the occurrence of calcinosis. Cutaneous calcinosis, more characteristic of juvenile rather than adult-onset dermatomyositis, is seen in 44 to 70 per cent of children as compared with 20 per cent of adults with dermatomyositis (Fig. 20–24).[5, 37] Most commonly seen on the buttocks and about the shoulders and elbows, subcutaneous calcium deposits may produce local pain and can be extruded, leading to ulcers, sinuses, or cellulitis. Calcinosis, although often resulting in impaired function, is associated with a longer survival time and, accordingly, is viewed as a favorable prognostic sign. Sometimes patients may present with widespread calcification without apparent preceding illness. In such cases it is suspected that calcinosis may be the result of an old dermatomyositis.

The course of dermatomyositis in children differs from that in adults. Children rarely have Raynaud's phenomenon, malignancies are not present, and the mortality rate is lower; but morbidity is

higher, and functional recovery is less. Whereas in adults the disease usually begins in a healthy-appearing individual, in children respiratory illness often precedes the onset of dermatomyositis.

Diagnosis. The diagnosis of dermatomyositis is made on clinical grounds and depends on the typical cutaneous manifestations and evidence of muscle involvement and weakness. It can be confirmed by evaluation of muscle mass by magnetic resonance imaging (MRI), electromyography, measurement of serum aldolase, aspartate aminotransferase, alanine aminotransferase, lactic dehydrogenase, and serum creatine phosphokinase levels, and biopsy of a muscle of the shoulder or pelvic girdle (preferably a muscle that is tender). The muscles most commonly biopsied are the deltoid, supraspinatus, and quadriceps.

Tests for rheumatoid factor may be positive in about 10 per cent of cases of dermatomyositis, LE cells may be seen occasionally, and a positive antinuclear factor may be found in about one third of cases of dermatomyositis. In addition, in patients without clinical or muscle enzyme changes, an increase in 24-hour urinary creatine excretion may be an early indicator of myositis.[38] Since laboratories frequently test 24-hour urine creatinine excretion, ordering a 24-hour measurement of urinary creatine and creatinine concentration will avert laboratory misinterpretation of the desired study.

Five diagnostic criteria have been suggested for dermatomyositis and polymyositis. These include (1) progressive symmetrical weakness of the limb-girdle muscles and anterior neck flexors, with or without dysphagia or respiratory weakness; (2) muscle biopsy evidence of myositis and necrosis; (3) elevation of muscle-derived serum enzyme levels, particularly creatinine phosphokinase, but also the aminotransferases, lactic dehydrogenase, and aldolase; (4) electromyographic evidence of myopathy; and (5) the typical cutaneous findings of dermatomyositis. A definitive diagnosis of dermatomyositis can be made when specific skin findings and three of the above criteria (including the rash) are present; a diagnosis of polymyositis can be established with four of the criteria (without

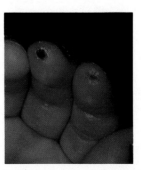

Figure 20–21. Angiitis with ulcerations on tips of the index and third fingers in a young child with acute dermatomyositis.

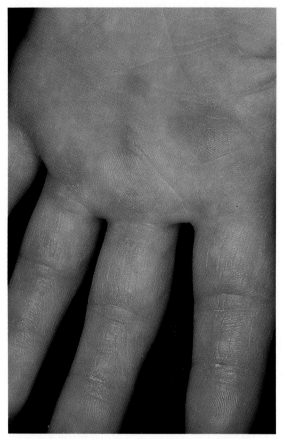

Figure 20–22. Palmar erythema in an 8-year-old with dermatomyositis.

the rash). A probable diagnosis of dermatomyositis requires two of the above criteria plus the rash.

Treatment. The course of juvenile dermatomyositis is highly variable. Its onset can be insidious with subtle weakness, anorexia, malaise, abdominal pain, and the gradual development of a rash. In other instances, the onset of the disorder can be fulminant, with fever, profound weakness, and severe multisystemic involvement. About one third of childhood cases have a relatively brief course with spontaneous or corticosteroid-induced remission within 1 or 2 years; about one third will have an intermediate course, with one or two remissions followed by relapse; in the other third the disorder may be characterized by active disease with persistent symptoms lasting well beyond 2 years.

Acetylsalicylic acid and other nonsteroidal antiinflammatory agents are of value in reducing the pain, tenderness, and inflammatory activity of this disorder. Without specific therapy, about one third of affected children recover completely, usually within 1 year of onset; with corticosteroid management, however, the death rate has been reduced from about 33 per cent to less than 10 per cent.[39] Long-term follow-up of chronically affected chil-

dren indicates that in most instances, the disease subsides after about 3 years, leaving various degrees of disability. If the child can be kept alive for 3 to 5 years, although calcinosis and mild manifestations of disease may persist, all medication can often be discontinued.

Hospitalization is advisable in the acute stages, because the disease processes may involve the muscles of respiration or deglutition and necessitate tracheotomy or the use of a mechanical respirator. A physical therapy program aimed at prevention of deformities and increasing muscle strength should be initiated early. Physical rest is extremely important during active phases of dermatomyositis. It may permit control on much lower corticosteroid dosages than otherwise would be possible. When palatorespiratory muscles are affected, great care is required to prevent aspiration and to ensure adequate respiration.

Severe dermatomyositis may be accompanied by diffuse cardiomyopathy. Although this is a rare complication, nonspecific electrocardiographic abnormalities are found in about 20 per cent of cases. In severely affected patients, respiratory insufficiency must be watched for carefully. When direct measurements of ventilation or arterial Pco_2 indicate that this is occurring, it is usually necessary to perform a tracheostomy. Tube feedings or intravenous maintenance may be required when dysphagia is present. In those instances in which prompt vigorous therapy is begun, palatal-respiratory function is monitored, adequate physical therapy is actively pursued, and meticulous long-term follow-up is maintained, successful outcome occurs in over two thirds of the cases.

Most childhood forms of dermatomyositis require high-dosage corticosteroid therapy. The initial dose of prednisone is 2 to 3 mg/kg/day, usually a dose of 60 mg of prednisone or its equivalent (up to 90 to 100 mg every day if that proves insufficient). As soon as a response is attained, as judged by muscle enzyme levels, the dosage may be reduced by decrements of about 15 per cent (at intervals of about 2 weeks) over 10 to 12 months.

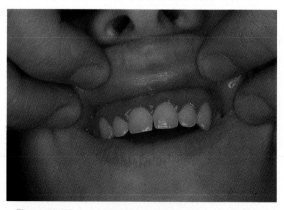

Figure 20–23. A vivid red hue on the gum line, the first clue to the diagnosis in this patient with dermatomyositis.

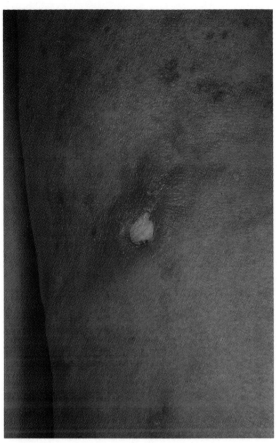

Figure 20–24. Cutaneous calcinosis in dermatomyositis.

Some patients may fail to respond even to very large doses of corticosteroids. Cytotoxic agents such as azathioprine (Imuran) in dosages of 1 to 3 mg/kg (up to 200 mg/day), methotrexate (either orally or through intramuscular or intravenous injection in a dosage of 1 mg/kg/week, with a maximum of 20 to 25 mg/week), or cyclosporine (2.5 to 5.0 mg/kg/day) may be used in severe life-threatening forms of dermatomyositis, or when the disease cannot be adequately managed with prednisone alone. When patients still fail to respond, plasmapheresis, alone or in combination with im-

munosuppresive therapy, may prove to be beneficial. Oral antimalarial agents have also been helpful in controlling the cutaneous manifestations of dermatomyositis. Although there is a risk of retinopathy in patients receiving long-term antimalarial use, experience with hydroxychloroquine (Plaquenil) suggests that this risk is minimal when appropriate dosage regimens, clinical supervision and periodic ophthalmic examinations are conducted.[40–44]

Although areas of calcinosis frequently disappear spontaneously, for patients with severe calcinosis, disodium etidronate or a diet low in phosphorus and calcium in conjunction with aluminum hydroxide gels (15 to 30 ml 4 times a day) may lower serum phosphorus and aid in the removal of cutaneous calcification.[45–47]

During the active phase of dermatomyositis, children are particularly at risk for sudden, overwhelming gram-negative sepsis secondary to aspiration due to weak palatal-respiratory function or perforation of a viscus. This risk is intensified by the masking effects of corticosteroids. A high index of suspicion, therefore, must be maintained for these complications, and early aggressive therapy must be instituted when necessary.

SCLERODERMA

Scleroderma can be classified into two categories, a variety limited to the skin (morphea, linear scleroderma) and the multisystemic disease, systemic scleroderma (progressive systemic sclerosis). Localized (cutaneous) scleroderma is discussed in Chapter 25.

Systemic scleroderma is a generalized disorder of connective tissue affecting the skin, lungs, heart, gastrointestinal tract, joints, and kidneys (Table 20–5). Seen in all age groups, although relatively uncommon in childhood, it has been reported in children as young as 15 months of age,[48–51] and, as in adults, the disorder occurs three to four times more frequently in women than in men. The pathogenesis of progressive systemic sclerosis is believed to be related to genetic factors, vascular abnormalities, abnormal collagen metabolism, and immunologic abnormalities. Of major importance are the vasospastic phenomena with endothelial

Table 20–5. CLINICAL FEATURES OF SYSTEMIC SCLEROSIS

1. Acrosclerosis (in 95%)
   a. Cutaneous sclerosis of digits (sclerodactyly)
   b. Raynaud's phenomenon
2. Subcutaneous calcification and/or ulceration
3. Telangiectatic mats, cuticular telangiectasia
4. Characteristic facies (tight skin, fixed stare, pinched nose, and perpetual grimace)
5. Variable degrees of internal organ involvement
   a. Polymyositis
   b. Esophageal and gastrointestinal disorders
   c. Cardiovascular, pulmonary, joint, or renal abnormalities
6. CRST and CREST variants generally tend to have a more benign course and more favorable prognosis

damage that precede digital, pulmonary, and renal fibrosis, cell-mediated abnormalities that facilitate the proliferation of fibroblasts and collagen synthesis, and decreased levels of collagenase resulting in the firm hidebound appearance of scleromatous tissue.[52] Although morphea and systemic scleroderma on rare ocasions occur in the same patients, the relationship between morphea and systemic scleroderma is controversial and not well understood. Most authorities, however, believe that morphea is essentially a benign disease that, particularly in children, resolves spontaneously, and if a transition from morphea to scleroderma does indeed occur, it is extremely rare. The presence of nail fold changes, Raynaud's phenomenon, or both, with or without localized areas of involvement, however, should alert the physician to further exploration.

Initially, scleroderma was divided into two forms, acrosclerosis and diffuse scleroderma. Acrosclerosis, accounting for 85 to 95 per cent of all cases, is characterized by cutaneous sclerosis of the digits (sclerodactyly) (Fig. 20–25) and Raynaud's phenomenon. It was initially thought that diffuse scleroderma was rapidly fatal and that acrosclerosis generally had a long and benign course. This concept now appears to be incorrect. The only value of this classification is that it describes the mode of onset and the distribution of lesions.

Raynaud's phenomenon, although extremely uncommon in childhood, is frequently the first sign of systemic scleroderma in this age group. Precipitated by cold or emotional stress, it is characterized by pallor, cyanosis, and hyperemia with pain, burning, numbness, tingling, swelling, and hyperhidrosis of the affected fingers or toes and, at times, the nose, lips, cheeks, ears, and chest. This disorder is present in almost all patients with systemic scleroderma, in 10 to 30 per cent of patients with systemic lupus erythematosus, in some cases of dermatomyositis and mixed connective tissue

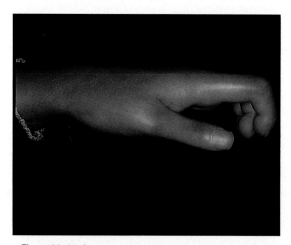

Figure 20–25. Cutaneous sclerosis (sclerodactyly) with flexion contractures in a young woman with scleroderma.

disease, and in other individuals as an idiopathic disorder of variable severity.[5]

Even in prepubertal years, systemic scleroderma has a preponderance of female patients. The appearance of the face is characteristic. The forehead is smooth and cannot be wrinkled, and atrophy and tightening of the skin give a characteristic appearance due to a fixed stare, pinched nose, prominent teeth, pursed lips, reduced oral aperture, and a perpetual grimace-like facies (Fig. 20–26). The hands become shiny, with tapered fingertips and restricted movements. Subcutaneous calcification and ulceration (Fig. 20–27) may be seen as well as telangiectases and hypopigmentation and hyperpigmentation. These pigmentary changes may be homogeneous or may have a "salt and pepper"–like appearance due to retained perifollicular hyperpigmentation in areas of hypopigmentation.

Three varieties of telangiectasia are characteristic of scleroderma. These include linear telangiectasia of the cuticles similar to that seen in other connective tissue disorders (Fig. 20–28), sharply defined telangiectatic macules of linear, oval, square, and multiangular configurations that vary from 1 to 6 mm in diameter (telangiectatic mats), and in a very small percentage of patients, telangiectasia similar to that seen in patients with Rendu-Osler-Weber disease (see Chapter 9). Capillary microscopy of the nail folds performed with an ophthalmoscope may be useful in confirming the diagnosis of scleroderma. Enlarged, dilated nail fold capillaries forming "giant" or sausage-shaped capillary loops, seen in 75 per cent of patients with systemic sclerosis, although they cannot be distinguished from those seen in dermatomyositis, can be differentiated from the capillary changes of systemic lupus erythematosus.[53] Pterygium inversum unguis–like changes (adherence of the distal portion of the nail beds to the ventral surface of the nail plate and obliteration of the space that normally separates these two structures) and replacement of the normal finger pad by hemisphere-like round finger pads have also been described in patients with systemic sclerosis.[54, 55]

Polymyositis and involvement of the esophagus probably are the most common extracutaneous sites of sclerotic change in scleroderma. Other gastrointestinal disturbances include constipation, regurgitation, weight loss, and malabsorption. Although cardiovascular, respiratory, and renal involvement have been described, these do not appear to be prominent in childhood forms of this disorder.

Patients with *limited cutaneous scleroderma*, the CREST syndrome (*c*alcinosis cutis, *R*aynaud's phenomenon, *e*sophageal dysfunction, *s*clerodactyly, and *t*elangiectasia), generally have a more slowly progressive form of the disease, may be identified by an anticentromere antibody, tend to develop clinical features later in life than in systemic sclerosis, and usually have a more favorable prognosis. Although some patients with the

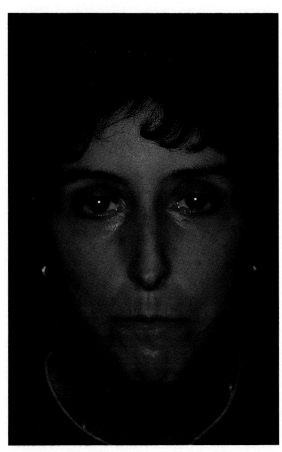

Figure 20–26. Scleroderma. Smooth atrophic skin, pinched nose, and telangiectatic mats are evident on the face of a young woman with scleroderma.

CREST syndrome may develop severe pulmonary hypertension, more extensive cutaneous lesions, and visceral involvement, the patients with this subset generally tend to have a relatively benign course. When esophageal dysfunction is absent, this variant of the disorder has been termed the *CRST syndrome.*

The diagnosis of systemic scleroderma is easily established when cutaneous sclerosis of the face and hands is present, particularly when it is associated with Raynaud's phenomenon, telangectasia, and visceral involvement. Symptoms or signs of dysphagia or gastroesophageal reflux (or radiologic demonstration of an aperistaltic dilated esophagus) help confirm the diagnosis. Although patients with visceral scleroderma without apparent cutaneous involvement have been described, it has been suggested that in such cases cutaneous features may have been present but were unappreciated at the time the diagnosis was established.[5]

The histologic appearance of the skin in systemic scleroderma is often similar to that seen in morphea (localized scleroderma), so that a histologic differentiation of the two disorders is frequently difficult. However, in early lesions of systemic scleroderma the inflammatory reaction is less pronounced, and a mild cellular infiltrate is present around the dermal vessels and eccrine coils and in the subcutaneous tissue. Lesions of systemic scleroderma show more pronounced degenerative changes in the collagen bundles and vessel walls in the later stages, and the marked inflammatory changes seen in active borders of morphea do not occur. The most common immunofluorescent staining pattern in sera of patients with systemic scleroderma is speckled, antinuclear antibodies are frequently present, and, seen in a relatively high incidence (50 per cent of patients with CREST syndrome as compared with 3 per cent of patients with progressive systemic sclerosis), the presence of anticentromere antibodies usually implies a good prognosis.[56–58]

Treatment. No specific therapy is available, and, except for extracorporeal photophoresis (currently under investigation in various research centers), management of progressive systemic sclerosis is mainly supportive. General measures include avoidance of factors producing vasospasm (tension, fatigue, stress, and cold weather) and minimizing trauma to the hands. Rest is important and, if polyarthritis is present, salicylates or other nonsteroidal anti-inflammatory agents may be beneficial. Calcium channel blockers such as nifedipine (Procardia), which reduces smooth muscle contraction by reducing the uptake of calcium, in dosages of 10 to 20 mg three times a day, and pentoxifylline (Trental), which lowers blood viscosity, thus increasing blood flow, can help control the severity of Raynaud's phenomenon and digital ulcers (nifedipine and pentoxifylline are currently not recommended for use in the treatment of Raynaud's phenomenon in the Physicians' Desk Reference and their use and dosage in children are not defined). In addition, D-penicillamine (which interferes with collagen metabolism and has a poorly understood immunosuppressive action), colchicine, and potassium *p*-aminobenzoate (Potaba) have been recommended for patients with this disorder, but none has been reported to be universally effective.[59,60] Treatment of gastrointestinal symptoms includes small frequent feedings, with elevation of the head of the bed, bland diet,

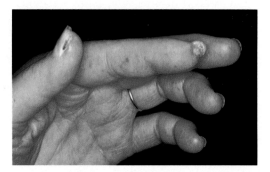

Figure 20–27. Scleroderma. Note calcinosis on the fingertips and flat mat-like telangiectatic vessels on the fingers.

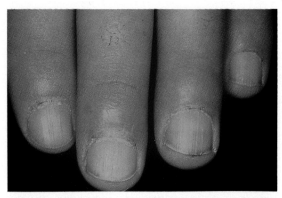

Figure 20–28. Thrombosed cuticular telangiectases without cuticular erythema. In contrast to other connective tissue diseases, cuticular hyperemia is relatively uncommon in scleroderma.

and antacids. Corticosteroids, because of complications from long-term therapy, should be reserved for those with debilitating arthritis not controlled by nonsteroidal anti-inflammatory agents, patients with extensive cutaneous edema with severe recurring digital ulcerations, and acute toxic phases of the disease. Corticosteroids do not appear to help the sclerodermatous process and, in many cases, may even be harmful. Support groups for patients with scleroderma are the United Scleroderma Foundation, Inc., P.O. Box 350, Watsonville, CA 95077 (1-800-722-HOPE) and the Scleroderma Society, Inc., 1725 York Avenue #29F, New York, NY 10128 (212-427-7040).

EOSINOPHILIC FASCIITIS

First described by Shulman in 1974, eosinophilic fasciitis (diffuse fasciitis with eosinophilia) is a scleroderma-like disease characterized by diffuse infiltration of the skin of the extremities and trunk without visceral involvement or Raynaud's phenomenon (Table 20–6). Seen in children as well as adults, the disorder bears a close resemblance to scleroderma and is thought by many authorities to be a variant of morphea or systemic sclerosis. The high male preponderance of eosinophilic fasciitis (a male-to-female ratio of 3:1), its lack of visceral involvement, a low incidence of serologic abnormalities, and prompt response to systemic corticosteroids suggest that it actually represents a separate and distinct disorder.[61, 62]

The disorder is characterized by a sudden onset following strenuous physical activity; painful swelling, induration, and scleroderma-like changes of the skin of the extremities; marked thickening of the subcutaneous fascia; absence of systemic changes; transient peripheral eosinophilia early in the disease; hypergammaglobulinemia; an elevated sedimentation rate; and a good response to systemic corticosteroids. Most patients are young to middle-aged men. In the majority of patients onset of the disorder follows trauma or excessive physical exertion and is marked by painful swelling and tenderness of the hands, forearms, feet, and legs; severe induration of the skin and subcutaneous tissues; and, at times, carpal tunnel syndrome with flexion contractures of the fingers and marked limitation of motion of the hands and feet. Primarily affecting the skin of the arms and legs, and occasionally that of the trunk, hands, and feet, the cutaneous features consist of a cobblestone or puckered appearance with a yellowish or erythematous color. The skin is indurated, taut, and bound down without pigmentary change. Although the extremities are usually the areas of initial involvement, the disease may progress to the trunk and face. Visceral involvement is rare, but there have been reports of visceral changes (similar to those seen in scleroderma) involving the esophagus, lungs, and heart and hematologic abnormalities such as pancytopenia, aplastic anemia, megakaryocytic aplasia, and antibody-mediated thrombocytopenia.[63]

Eosinophilia and hypergammaglobulinemia in the form of elevated IgG levels are commonly observed laboratory findings, but antinuclear antibody reactions remain negative. Blood eosinophilia, often the first clue to the condition, is a transient but striking feature. Histopathologic findings in early cutaneous lesions of eosinophilic fasciitis consist of edema of the lower subcutis and deep fascia with infiltration by lymphocytes, plasma cells, histiocytes, and intravascular or perivascular eosinophils in the trabeculae of the subcutaneous tissue. As the illness progresses, these structures and the dermis become collagenized, thickened, and sclerotic; and focal or diffuse eosinophilia may be observed in the fascia, lower subcutis, or both.

Although eosinophilic fasciitis frequently resolves spontaneously, or with physiotherapy alone, systemic corticosteroids seem to hasten resolution. The length of time required for improvement, however, varies for individual patients. It is not uncommon, therefore, for affected individuals

---

Table 20–6. EOSINOPHILIC FASCIITIS

1. A scleroderma-like disease without Raynaud's phenomenon or visceral involvement
2. Painful swelling and induration of skin and subcutaneous tissue (sudden onset following trauma, stress, or strenuous physical activity) with cobblestone or puckered appearance
3. Eosinophilia and hypergammaglobulinemia common, but antinuclear antibody reactions remain negative
4. Good response to sytemic corticosteroids

to be on systemic corticosteroids for years with relapses following the termination of this therapy. In such instances, a trial of cimetidine (Tagamet) may be considered.[64] Although most patients appear to have an excellent prognosis for recovery, the presence of hematologic abnormalities such as pancytopenia, aplastic anemia, leukemia, and Hodgkin's disease introduces complicating factors that may modify the prognosis.

EOSINOPHILIA-MYALGIA SYNDROME

Eosinophilia-myalgia syndrome, recognized in 1989, is a chronic multisystemic disorder characterized by blood eosinophilia and myalgias linked to the ingestion of tryptophan, a precursor of serotonin used as a popular over-the-counter remedy for various disorders such as insomnia and premenstrual syndrome, in weight loss programs, and in substance abuse centers. As of July 1990 a total of 1,531 cases, including 27 deaths, from the eosinophilia-myalgia syndrome were reported in the United States. Although the specific ingredient associated with this disorder has not been clarified, the condition appears to be associated with a contaminant in the manufacture of tryptophan similar to that observed in the toxic oil syndrome, a disorder associated with the use of illegally prepared oil used in cooking that occurred in Spain in 1981.[65-68]

Cutaneous features, seen in approximately two thirds of patients with this disorder, included a diffuse asymptomatic maculopapular eruption and small 1- to 5-mm mucinous papules on the trunk and extremities; swelling of extremities, usually in conjunction with nonpitting edema and a brawny induration of the skin suggestive of that seen in individuals with eosinophilic fasciitis; taut, bound-down thickened skin clinically identical to scleroderma; urticaria; angioedema; peripheral edema; paresthesias; livedo reticularis; ecchymoses with an absence of detectable coagulation abnormalities; alopecia; palmar fasciitis and nerve entrapment similar to that seen in the carpal tunnel syndrome; tightening of the skin of the face; and, in one patient at least, multiple subcutaneous nodules that on histopathologic examination revealed intense infiltration with eosinophils. Other features associated with this disorder include neuritis; progressive neuropathy (resulting in paralysis and, in some patients, death); trismus; the sicca syndrome without salivary gland enlargement; myalgia, and/or arthralgia; fatigue; cardiac arrhythmias; shortness of breath; cough; dyspnea; peripheral blood eosinophilia; leukocytosis; increased aldolase levels; and elevations in liver enzyme function tests.

Although the disorder subsided when the tryptophan was discontinued, oral corticosteroids (10 to 60 mg/day of prednisone, or its equivalent) were helpful in the management of severely affected individuals.

SJÖGREN'S SYNDROME

Sjögren's syndrome is a chronic autoimmune disorder of unknown etiology characterized by keratoconjunctivitis sicca (inflammation of the cornea and the conjunctiva with dryness and atrophy), xerostomia (dryness of the mouth from lack of normal secretion), enlargement of the salivary and lacrimal glands (as a result of lymphocytic and plasma cell infiltration), and a connective tissue disease (rheumatoid arthritis in at least 50 per cent of cases, systemic lupus erythematosus, dermatomyositis, or scleroderma) (Table 20-7). Other disorders associated with Sjögren's syndrome include chronic hepatobiliary disease, Hashimoto's thyroiditis, panarteritis, and interstitial pulmonary fibrosis.

Although rarely reported in childhood, as of 1989 approximately 42 cases of Sjögren's syndrome had been reported in children and adolescents.[69-72] More than 90 per cent of patients are female, and the disease generally begins after the patient has reached the age of 40 years. The most prominent dermatologic manifestations are associated with dryness of the gingiva and mucous membranes of the mouth, and, at times, the conjunctivae, nose, pharynx, larynx, vagina, and respiratory tract. The tongue may become smooth, red, and dry, and in severe cases there may be difficulty in swallowing dry food. The lips may be cracked,

---

Table 20–7. SJÖGREN'S SYNDROME

1. Major clinical features
   a. Keratoconjunctivitis sicca (dryness and atrophy of cornea and conjunctiva)
   b. Xerostomia (dryness of mouth) and fatigue are common
   c. Chronic enlargement of salivary glands
   d. Association with connective tissue disease
      (1) Usually rheumatoid arthritis
      (2) Occasionally systemic lupus erythematosus, dermatomyositis, or scleroderma
2. Cutaneous features
   a. Dryness and scaling of skin (with partial or complete loss of perspiration)
   b. Sparse, dry, brittle hair
   c. Purpura (usually lower extremities)
   d. Raynaud's phenomenon and telangiectasia of fingers and lips

fissured, or ulcerated, particularly at the corners of the mouth; the teeth frequently undergo rapid and severe decay; the eyes may be reddened and moist; and thick, tenacious secretions forming ropy mucous strands in the inner canthi may be noted (particularly when the patient first arises in the morning). Other ocular manifestations include a burning sensation, as when a foreign body is present in the eye, and inability to produce tears in response to irritants or emotion.

Fatigue is a prominent symptom. Other clinical manifestations include arthritis or other connective tissue disease; vasculitis; dryness, in about 50 per cent of affected patients, and scaling of the skin; sparse, dry, and brittle hair; purpura, especially on the lower extremities (the most common cutaneous manifestation); telangiectasias of the lips and fingers; Raynaud's phenomenon; annular erythema[73]; hoarseness; epistaxis; atrophic rhinitis; recurrent upper respiratory tract infection; and otitis media.

The diagnosis of Sjögren's syndrome can be made when any two of the three major features (keratoconjunctivitis sicca, xerostomia, and rheumatoid arthritis or other connective tissue disorder) are present. Diagnostic studies include scintigraphy (a determination of uptake, concentration, and excretion of intravenously injected radioactive material by major salivary glands); demonstration of decreased salivary flow by secretory sialography; isotope scanning and ultrasonography of the salivary glands; biopsy of the salivary glands of the lips; careful examination of the eyes, including Schirmer's test (less than 5 mm wetting of a strip of filter paper inserted under the lower eyelid); the Saxon test (an oral equivalent of the Schirmer test); conjunctival staining with rose bengal solution; filamentary keratitis on slit lamp examination; and serologic evidence of a systemic autoimmune disorder.[74] Among the hematologic and serologic changes in Sjögren's syndrome are leukopenia (with or without an accompanying splenomegaly), a relative lymphocytosis, eosinophilia, hypergam-

maglobulinemia, and positive tests for rheumatoid factor, antinuclear factor, antithyroglobulin factor, anti-Ro (SSA), and other nonspecific antibodies.

The management of Sjögren's syndrome includes treatment of the dry skin, keratoconjunctivitis, xerostomia, and associated connective tissue or lymphoproliferative disorders. Since patients with Sjögren's syndrome may also be at risk for extraglandular diseases (such as other autoimmune disease and lymphoma), long-term follow-up is indicated.[75] Although systemic corticosteroids are capable of reducing the swelling of the salivary glands, they usually do not improve the function of affected glands. Side effects frequently outweigh the benefits of this form of therapy, but if the accompanying systemic disease is severe, treatment with systemic corticosteroids, immunosuppressive drugs, or both, may be helpful.

MIXED CONNECTIVE TISSUE DISEASE

Mixed connective tissue disease (Sharp's syndrome), originally described by Sharp in 1972, is a mixed "overlap syndrome" characterized by the combination of clinical features and laboratory data similar to those of systemic lupus erythematosus, scleroderma, dermatomyositis, polymyositis, rheumatoid arthritis, and/or Sjögren's disease (Table 20–8), unusually high titers of circulating antibodies to nuclear ribonucleoprotein (RNP) antigen, and speckled antinuclear antibody (ANA) on direct immunofluorescence of normal skin.[76–79] Its features include cutaneous photosensitivity, a heliotrope rash over the eyelids, alopecia, malar telangiectasia or erythema or both, cutaneous lesions of lupus erythematosus, mucosal dryness, hyperpigmentation, hypopigmentation, mucosal dryness, sclerodactyly, puffy fingers with cutaneous sclerosis, and a tapered or sausage appearance of the fingers. The most common presenting features are joint complaints (arthritis or arthralgia), Raynaud's phenomenon, or cutaneous lupus ery-

Table 20–8. MIXED CONNECTIVE TISSUE DISEASE

1. A combination of clinical features and laboratory data of systemic lupus erythematosus, scleroderma, dermatomyositis, polymyositis, rheumatoid arthritis and/ or Sjögren's disease
2. Cutaneous features
   a. Cutaneous photosensitivity
   b. A heliotrope rash over eyelids
   c. Alopecia
   d. Malar telangiectasia and/or erythema
   e. Cutaneous lesions of lupus erythematosus
   f. Hyperpigmentation and/or hypopigmentation
   g. Periungual erythema
   h. Livedo reticularis
   i. Mucosal dryness
   j. Arthritis or arthralgia
   k. Tapered or sausage-shaped fingers
3. Laboratory features
   a. Anti-RNP titer greater than 1:1,000
   b. Speckled distribution of IgG in epidermal nuclei on direct immunofluorescence

thematosus. Although some patients with mixed connective tissue disease have deforming arthritis, the most common symptom is an evanescent nonerosive nondeforming polyarthritis similar to that seen in patients with systemic lupus erythematosus.

The most important diagnostic features are Raynaud's phenomenon, periungual telangiectasia, swelling of the hands with a tapered sausage appearance to the fingers, abnormal pulmonary function tests, myositis, disturbances of esophageal motility, joint pain, alopecia, cutaneous lesions suggestive of cutaneous lupus erythematosus, dermatomyositis, and/or scleroderma, and antibodies in high titer to ribonucleoprotein. Approximately two thirds of children with mixed connective tissue disease have cardiac involvement, including pericarditis, myocarditis, congestive heart failure, and aortic insufficiency; about 10 per cent have renal disease; and about 10 per cent of individuals have neurologic abnormalities (trigeminal sensory neuropathy, "vascular" headaches, seizures, multiple peripheral neuropathies, and cerebral infarction or hemorrhage). When mixed connective tissue disease occurs in childhood, it may mimic juvenile rheumatoid arthritis. Distinct differences, however, frequently exist between adult and childhood forms of mixed connective tissue disease. Severe thrombocytopenia appears to be limited to childhood forms, the incidence of renal and cardiac involvement is higher in children than in adults, and some children have a defect in polymorphonuclear leukocyte chemotaxis and, as a result, an increased risk for overwhelming bacterial infections.

The most distinguishing laboratory marker for this disease is the demonstration of serum antibody specific for ribonuclear protein, a ribonuclease-sensitive component of extractable nuclear antigen. In addition, most patients with mixed connective tissue disease have high (greater than 1:1,000) serum titers of antinuclear antibody in a speckled pattern, and a high titer of rheumatoid factor is present in up to 50 per cent of patients. Although LE cells may also be found in up to one third of patients with mixed connective tissue disease, indicating the close association of these two disorders, in contrast to most cases of systemic lupus erythematosus, patients with mixed connective tissue disease lack antibodies to DNA. When mixed connective tissue disease was first described, it was thought to have a better prognosis than systemic lupus erythematosus and to be readily amenable to corticosteroid therapy. Although corticosteroid therapy produces symptomatic improvement in many patients, and life-threatening disease manifestations are not as common as in systemic lupus erythematosus, mixed connective tissue disease is at times much more severe than originally suspected. Most patients, however, have a relatively benign disease; the course frequently may be one of remission and relapse similar to that observed in patients with systemic lupus erythematosus; and recent studies suggest significant morbidity and mortality from pulmonary or renal involvement and overwhelming bacterial infection. Patients should be treated according to the particular systems of involvement with high doses of corticosteroids and, when necessary, immunosuppressive agents similar to those recommended for the treatment of patients with severe systemic lupus erythematosus.

References

1. Calabro JJ, Marchesano JM: Rash associated with juvenile rheumatoid arthritis. J. Pediatr. 72:611–619, 1968.

   The clinical significance of the cutaneous eruption of Still's disease.

2. Hurwitz S: The Skin and Systemic Disease in Children. Year Book Medical Publishers, Chicago, 1985.

   An overview of the cutaneous features of systemic disorders in children with emphasis on the recognition of dermatologic signs and their significance in the diagnosis and treatment of internal disease in the pediatric age group.

3. Szer I: Rheumatic diseases in children. In Gellis SS, Kagan BM (Eds.): Current Pediatric Therapy 13. W.B. Saunders Co., Philadelphia, 1990, 337–342.

   An updated review of the management of connective tissue disorders of childhood.

4. Lehman TJA, McCurdy DK, Bernstein BH, et al.: Systemic lupus erythematosus in the first decade of life. Pediatrics 83:235–239, 1989.

   Systemic lupus erythematosus in children younger than the age of 10 years compared with children with SLE diagnosed in the second decade of life revealed no statistical difference in morbidity or mortality rates in either group.

5. Braverman IM: Skin Signs of Systemic Disease, 2nd ed. W.B. Saunders Co, Philadelphia, 1981.

   An invaluable well-written text emphasizing cutaneous features and their role in the diagnosis of systemic disease.

6. Camisa C: Vesiculobullous systemic lupus erythematosus: A report of four cases. J. Am. Acad. Dermatol. 18:93–100, 1988.

   A review of vesiculobullous SLE, a disorder that appears to share some of the morphologic, histopathologic, and immunopathologic features of dermatitis herpetiformis.

7. Rappersberger K, Tschachler E, Tani M, et al.: Bullous disease in systemic lupus erythematosus. J. Am. Acad. Dermatol. 21:745–752, 1989.

   A review of three women with systemic lupus erythematosus and vesiculobullous skin lesions.

8. Lowe L, Rapini RR, Golitz LE, et al.: Papular dermal mucinosis in lupus erythematosus. J. Am. Acad. Dermatol. 27:312–315, 1992.

   A report of two patients with lupus erythematosus in whom a truncal papulonodular eruption characterized by dermal mucin, but without the usual histologic features of lupus erythematosus, was prominent.

9. Millard LG, Rowell NR: Chilblain lupus erythematosus (Hutchinson): A clinical and laboratory study of 17 patients. Br. J. Dermatol. 98:497–506, 1978.

   Although chilblains often precedes the onset of discoid or systemic lupus erythematosus, it also may appear years after the onset of discoid lupus erythematosus.

10. Taieb A, Hehunstre J-P, Goetz J, et al.: Lupus erythematosus panniculitis with partial genetic deficiency of C2 and C4 in a child. Arch. Dermatol. 122:576–582, 1986.

A report of a 7-year-old girl with a relapsing corticosteroid-responsive panniculitis associated with hypocomplementemia in whom the disorder appeared to have been initiated by an infection with toxoplasmosis.

11. Fox JN, Klapman MH, Rowe L: Lupus profundus in children: Treatment with hydroxychloroquine. J. Am. Acad. Dermatol. 16:839–844, 1987.

A report of two young girls with discoid lupus erythematosus and lupus profundus, one with onset at 3 1/2 years of age, the other at 8 years of age, successfully treated with hydroxychloroquine.

12. Sontheimer RD, Thomas JR, Gilliam JN: Subacute cutaneous lupus erythematosus: A cutaneous marker for a distinct lupus erythematosus subset. Arch. Dermatol. 115:1409–1415, 1979.

A review of clinical and laboratory features in 27 patients with subacute lupus erythematosus, a disorder which the authors describe as a subset of lupus erythematosus intermediate in severity between that of discoid and systemic LE.

13. Callen JP, Kulick KB, Stelzer G, et al.: Subacute cutaneous lupus erythematosus. J. Am. Acad. Dermatol. 15:1227–1237, 1986.

A review of 49 patients with a specific cutaneous nonscarring form of lupus erythematosus.

14. DeSpain J, Clark DP: Subacute cutaneous lupus erythematosus presenting as erythroderma. J. Am. Acad. Dermatol. 19:388–397, 1988.

A report of a patient with subacute cutaneous lupus erythematosus presenting with exfoliative erythroderma in whom complete remission was obtained by a short course of systemic cortiosteroids and long-term hydroxychloroquine therapy.

15. Tan EM, Cohen AS, Fries J, et al.: The 1982 revised criteria for the classification of systemic lupus erythematosus. Arthritis Rheum. 25:1271–1277, 1982.

16. Provost TT, Reichlin M: Antinuclear antibody–negative systemic lupus erythematosus: I. Anti-Ro(SSA) and anti-La(SSB) antibodies. J. Am. Acad. Dermatol. 4:84–89, 1981.

Since antinuclear antibody–negative anti-Ro(SSA)–positive lupus erythematosus patients generally demonstrate a photosensitive dermatitis and accordingly are frequently seen and evaluated initially by dermatologists, the authors emphasize the value of anti-Ro and anti-La antibodies in the diagnosis of such individuals.

17. Lever WF, Schaumburg-Lever G: Connective tissue diseases. In Histopathology of the Skin, 7th ed. J. B. Lippincott Co., Philadelphia, 1990, 494–522.

A comprehensive review of the classification, pathogenesis, and histopathology of connective tissue disorders.

18. Febré VC, Lear S, Reichlin M, et al.: Twenty per cent of biopsy specimens from sun-exposed skin of normal young adults demonstrate positive immunofluorescence. Arch. Dermatol. 127:1006–1011, 1991.

The demonstration of a bright continuous band of immunofluorescence in 10 (20 per cent) of otherwise normal patients suggests that immunofluorescent study of sun-exposed skin is nonspecific and adds little information to the clinical and histopathologic findings of patients with lupus erythematosus.

19. Nordby CA, Pelachyk JM, Burnham TK: Large speckle-like thready and thready antinuclear antibody patterns as markers for different clinical presentations in lupus erythematosus. J. Am. Acad. Dermatol. 17:427–433, 1987.

A retrospective review of 51 patients with lupus erythematosus, their immunofluorescent antinuclear antibody patterns and their significance.

20. Rasmussen JE: Antimalarials—are they safe to use in children? Pediatr. Dermatol. 1:89–91, 1983.

A review of antimalarials and their use and misuse in children

concludes that, when used with proper precautions, these agents are indeed safe and can be used in children as well as adults.

21. Leads from the MMWR: Childhood chloroquine poisonings—Wisconsin and Washington. J.A.M.A. 260:1363, 1988.

When used for the prophylaxis and treatment of malaria, chloroquine has been shown to be safe if used in the recommended dosage range.

22. Madhok R: Fatal exacerbation of systemic lupus erythematosus after griseofulvin. Br. Med. J. 291:249, 1985.

A report of a 22-year-old woman with a 6-year history of systemic lupus erythematosus who died of progressive renal failure, fulminant small vessel vasculitis, generalized myositis, and respiratory distress 7 days after starting griseofulvin therapy.

23. Shornick JK, Formica N, Parke AL: Isotretinoin for refractory lupus erythematosus. J. Am. Acad. Dermatol. 24:49–52, 1991.

In a report of six patients with cutaneous lupus erythematosus resistant to conventional therapies, isotretinoin resulted in rapid clinical improvement in all cases.

24. Chamiedes L, Truex RC, Vetter V, et al.: Association of maternal lupus erythematosus with congenital complete heart block. N. Engl. J. Med. 297:1204–1207, 1977.

Six infants with complete heart block suggest immune complexes either pass from mother to fetus or are produced by the fetus as a response to maternal antigen.

25. Draznin TH, Esterly NB, Furey NL, et al.: Neonatal lupus erythematosus. J. Am. Acad. Dermatol. 1:437–442, 1979.

Report of an infant and a review of 22 previously reported infants with cutaneous lesions, congenital atrioventricular heart block, or hematologic manifestations of neonatal LE.

26. Lee LA, Weston WL: Lupus erythematosus in childhood. Dermatol. Clin. 4:151–160, 1986.

A comprehensive review of childhood and neonatal lupus erythematosus.

27. Korkij W, Soltani K: Neonatal lupus erythematosus: A review. Pediatr. Dermatol. 1:189–195, 1984.

A review of neonatal lupus erythematosus, its pathophysiology, systemic manifestations, and prognosis.

28. Olson NY, Lindsley CB: Neonatal lupus syndrome. Am. J. Dis. Child. 141:908–910, 1987.

A review of neonatal lupus erythematosus, its immunologic abnormalities and clinical manifestations.

29. Franco HL, Weston WL, Peebles C, et al.: Autoantibodies directed against sicca syndrome antigens in the neonatal lupus syndrome. J. Am. Acad. Dermatol. 4:67–72, 1981.

Clinical and serologic studies on three infants with the neonatal lupus syndrome and their mothers revealed an association with antibodies to the sicca (Sjögren) syndrome.

30. Provost TT, Watson R, Gammon WR: The neonatal lupus syndrome associated with U₁RNP (nRNP) antibodies. N. Engl. J. Med. 316:1135–1138, 1987.

A report of two infants with cutaneous lesions of neonatal lupus erythematosus syndrome who, along with their mothers, were positive for the anti-U₁RNP antibody and negative for the anti-Ro (SSA) and anti-La (SSB) antibodies.

31. Lockshin MD, Gibofski A, Peebles CL, et al.: Neonatal lupus erythematosus with heart block: Family study of a patient with anti-SS-A and SS-B antibodies. Arthritis Rheum. 26:210–213, 1983.

Studies of serologic antibodies in an infant with neonatal lupus erythematosus and congenital heart block and her mother suggest that the HLA system may not be the sole genetic factor determining susceptibility to neonatal lupus erythematosus.

32. Jordan JM, Valenstein P, Kredich DW: Systemic lupus ery-

thematosus with Libman-Sachs endocarditis in a 9-month-old infant with neonatal lupus erythematosus and congenital heart block. Pediatrics *84*:574–577, 1989.

A report of an infant with neonatal lupus erythematosus and congenital heart block with evolution, soon after birth, to systemic lupus erythematosus with Libman-Sachs endocarditis who died at the age of 12 months.

33. Laxer RM, Roberts EA, Gross KR, et al.: Liver disease in neonatal lupus erythematosus. J. Pediatr. *116*:238–242, 1990.

In a report of four infants with neonatal lupus erythematosus who had liver biopsies for significant hepatic disease, the authors speculate that maternal anti-Ro or anti-La antibodies may produce liver injury manifested as neonatal hepatitis and subsequent hepatic fibrosis.

34. Kissel JT, Mendell JR, Rammohan KW: Microvascular deposition of complement membrane attack complex in dermatomyositis. N. Engl. J. Med. *314*:329–334, 1986.

Data provide evidence that dermatomyositis, particularly in childhood forms, results from an immune-mediated vasculopathy.

35. Bowles NE, Dubowitz V, Sewry CA, et al.: Dermatomyositis, polymyositis, and Coxsackie-B virus infection. Lancet *1*:1004–1007, 1987.

Demonstration of coxsackievirus B in muscles of four of seven patients with juvenile dermatomyositis and one of two patients with adult polymyositis suggests that the chronic presence of virus in muscle may provoke a release of foreign antigens that together with abnormalities in immunoregulation may explain the pathogenesis of dermatomyositis and polymyositis.

36. Lell ME, Swerdlow ML: Dermatomyositis of childhood. Pediatr. Ann. *6*:203–211, 1977.

Childhood dermatomyositis, unlike the adult variety, is not associated with an increased incidence of malignancy.

37. Cook DC, Rosen FS, Banker BQ: Dermatomyositis and focal scleroderma. Pediatr. Clin. North Am. *10*:979–1016, 1963.

An inclusive review of dermatomyositis and focal scleroderma in childhood.

38. Rowell NR, Fairris GM: Biochemical markers of myositis in dermatomyositis and polymyositis. Clin. Exp. Dermatol. *11*:69–72, 1986.

In a study of 26 patients, 24-hour urinary creatine excretion was shown to be an excellent marker of active myositis.

39. Sullivan DB, Cassidy JT, Petty RE, et al.: Prognosis in childhood dermatomyositis. J. Pediatr. *80*:555–563, 1972.

Of 18 children treated with corticosteroids and physical therapy, all had a favorable response.

40. Jacobs JC: Methotrexate and azathioprine treatment of childhood dermatomyositis. Pediatrics *59*:212–217, 1977.

Methotrexate and azathioprine are helpful in children with dermatomyositis who do not respond to prednisone alone.

41. Heckmatt J, Hasson N, Saunders C, et al.: Cyclosporin in juvenile dermatomyositis. Lancet *1*:1063–1066, 1989.

Although the use of cyclosporine in the treatment of 14 patients with juvenile dermatomyositis was encouraging, the authors advise caution in the use of this modality because of possible side effects.

42. Dantzig P: Juvenile dermatomyositis treated with cyclosporine. J. Am. Acad. Dermatol. *22*:310–311, 1990.

A 4-year-old girl with dermatomyositis was successfully treated with oral cyclosporine (2.5 mg gradually increased to 3.5 mg/kg/day) as the initial treatment of her disorder.

43. Dau PC, Bennington JL: Plasmapharesis in childhood dermatomyositis. J. Pediatr. *98*:237–240, 1981.

Plasmapharesis can at times be beneficial for severely affected patients with dermatomyositis.

44. Woo TY, Callen JP, Voorhees JJ, et al.: Cutaneous lesions of dermatomyositis are improved by hydroxychloroquine. J. Am. Acad. Dermatol. *10*:592–600, 1984.

Although the cutaneous lesions of seven patients with cutaneous lesions of dermatomyositis showed good response to hydroxychloroquine (400 mg/day for 2 weeks followed by 200 mg/day), the treatment did not appear to have any notable effect on the myositis.

45. Rabens SF, Bethune JE: Disodium etidronate therapy for dystrophic cutaneous calcification. Arch. Dermatol. *111*:357–361, 1975.

Disodium etidronate (10 mg/kg/day orally) seemed to arrest and partially reverse the progression of the calcification process in a patient with extensive disabling dystrophic cutaneous calcifications.

46. Nassim JM, Connolly CK: Treatment of calcinosis universalis with aluminum hydroxide. Arch. Dis. Child. *45*:118–121, 1970.

A 9-year-old child with dermatomyositis and calcinosis universalis had considerable clearing of calcinosis on aluminum hydroxide gel.

47. Mazzafarin G, Lafferty FW, Pearson OH: Treatment of calcinosis with phosphorus deprivation. Ann. Intern. Med. *77*:741–745, 1972.

A 16-year-old boy with a 7-year history of calcinosis improved on aluminum hydroxide antacids and a diet low in phosphorus and calcium.

48. Goel KM, Shanks RA: Scleroderma in childhood. Arch. Dis. Child. *49*:861–865, 1974.

Five children, 2 1/2 to 10 years of age, with childhood forms of systemic sclerosis.

49. Sullivan DB, Cassidy JT: Scleroderma in the child. J. Pediatr. *85*:770–775, 1974.

Review of 12 children with systemic scleroderma.

50. Urano J, Kohno H, Watanabe T: Unusual case of progressive systemic sclerosis with onset in early childhood and following infectious mononucleosis. Eur. J. Pediatr. *136*:285, 1981.

A report of a 15-month-old girl who developed systemic sclerosis following infectious mononucleosis.

51. Larréque M, Canuel C, Bazex J, et al.: Systemic scleroderma in childhood: Report of 5 cases and review of the literature. Ann. Derm. Venereol *110*:317–326, 1983.

A report of five children with progressive systemic sclerosis and a review of the literature.

52. Krieg T, Meruer M: Systemic scleroderma: Clinical and pathophysiologic aspects. J. Am. Acad. Dermatol. *18*:457–481, 1988.

A comprehensive review of scleroderma, its clinical manifestations, pathogenesis, and treatment.

53. Statham BM, Rowell NR: Quantification of the nail fold capillary abnormalities in systemic sclerosis and Raynaud's syndromes. Acta Derm. Venereol. *66*:139–143, 1986.

A review of nail fold capillary abnormalities and their significance in patients with connective tissue disorders.

54. Patterson JW: Pterygium inversum unguis–like changes in scleroderma. Arch. Dermatol. *113*:1429–1430, 1977.

A report of six patients with scleroderma with nail findings suggestive of pterygium inversum unguis.

55. Mizutani H, Mizutani T, Okada H, et al.: Round fingerpad sign: An early sign of scleroderma. J. Am. Acad. Dermatol. *24*:67–69, 1991.

Fibrosis of the dermis results in round fingerpads in individuals with scleroderma.

56. Tuffanelli DL, McKeon F, Kleinsmith DM, et al.: Anticentromere and anticentriole antibodies in the scleroderma spectrum. Arch. Dermatol. *119*:560–566, 1983.

A study of serum samples from 106 patients (including 80 in the scleroderma spectrum) by indirect immunofluorescent microscopy and the value of anticentromere and anticentriole antibody study in patients with scleroderma.

57. Steen VD, Ziegler GL, Rodnan GP, et al.: Clinical and laboratory association of anticentromere antibody in patients with systemic sclerosis. Arthritis Rheum. 27:125–131, 1984.

The finding of anticentromere antibodies, an antibody directed against the centromere region (Kinetochore) of the chromosome, in about 50 per cent of the patients with the CREST syndrome and only 3 per cent of patients with progressive systemic sclerosis and diffuse scleroderma supports the distinctiveness of the CREST syndrome.

58. Chen Z, Fedrick JA, Pandey JP, et al.: Anticentromere antibody and immunoglobulin allotypes in scleroderma. Arch. Dermatol. 121:339–344, 1985.

A study of 55 patients with disorders in the scleroderma spectrum revealed that those who had anticentromere antibodies had fewer organs involved and a better prognosis.

59. Rodeheffer RJ, Rommer JA, Wrigley F, et al.: Controlled double-blind trial of nifedipine in the treatment of Raynaud's phenomenon. N. Engl. J. Med. 308:880–883, 1983.

The calcium channel blocker nifedipine produced symptomatic relief in 21 (66 per cent) of 32 patients with Raynaud's phenomenon.

60. Steen VD, Medsger TA Jr, Rodnan GP: D-Penicillamine therapy in progressive systemic sclerosis (scleroderma): Retrospective analysis. Ann.Intern. Med. 97:652–659, 1989.

A study of patients with progressive systemic sclerosis treated with D-penicillamine in daily dosages of 500 to 1500 mg revealed that patients thus treated had less cutaneous and visceral involvement and a better 5-year survival rate than those treated with other modalities.

61. Shulman LE: Diffuse fasciitis with eosinophilia: A new syndrome? Trans. Assoc. Am. Physicians 88:70–86, 1975.

Four patients with firm puckered skin on the extremities and sometimes the trunk with eosinophilia following severe or unusual physical exertion.

62. Patrone NA, Kredich DW: Eosinophilic fasciitis in a child. Am. J. Dis. Child. 138:363–365, 1984.

Prednisone therapy resulted in sustained subjective and objective improvement in a 13-year-old boy with a 3-year history of eosinophilic fasciitis.

63. Doyle JA: Eosinophilic fasciitis: Extracutaneous manifestations and associations. Cutis 34:259–261, 1984.

Visceral changes of the esophagus, lungs, and heart similar to those in scleroderma are described in patients with eosinophilic fasciitis.

64. Solomon G, Barland P, Rifkin H: Eosinophilic fasciitis responsive to cimetidine. Ann. Intern. Med. 97:547–549, 1982.

Induration of the skin of a 53-year-old man with eosinophilic fasciitis cleared within a few days after starting cimetidine (Tagamet), 400 mg every 6 hours, for a suspected ulcer induced by prednisone.

65. Swygert LA, Maes EF, Sewell LE, et al.: Eosinophilia-myalgia syndrome: Results of national surveillance. J.A.M.A. 264:1698–1703, 1990.

A report of a newly recognized disorder that occurred in epidemic proportions during 1989 apparently associated with the ingestion of tryptophan.

66. Slutsker L, Hoesley F, Miller DVM, et al.: Eosinophilia-myalgia syndrome associated with exposure to tryptophan from a single manufacturer. J.A.M.A. 264:213–217, 1990.

A comparison of the brand and source of tryptophan used by 58 patients with eosinophilia-myalgia syndrome suggests a contaminant or an alteration in a subset of tryptophan manufactured by a single company as a cause of the disorder.

67. Kaufman LD, Seidman RJ, Phillips ME, et al.: Cutaneous manifestations of tne L-tryptophan–associated eosinophilia-myalgia syndrome: A spectrum of sclerodermatous disease. J. Am Acad. Dermatol. 23:1063–1069, 1990.

A review of 30 patients with eosinophilia-myalgia syndrome.

68. Troy JL: Eosinophilia-myalgia syndrome. Mayo Clin. Proc. 66:535–538, 1991.

A comprehensive overview of eosinophilia-myalgia syndrome, its pathogenesis and clinical features.

69. Athreya BH, Norman ME, Myers AR, et al.: Sjögren's syndrome in children. Pediatrics 59:931–937, 1977.

A report of 2 girls with Sjögren's syndrome with onset at 7 and 12 1/2 years of age and subsequent clinical diagnoses of systemic lupus erythematosus.

70. Chudwin DS, Daniels TE, Wara DW, et al.: Spectrum of Sjögren syndrome in children. J. Pediatr. 98:213–217, 1981.

A report of eight children and 21 previously reported cases of Sjögren's syndrome in children.

71. Deprettere AJ, Van Acker KJ, De Clerck LS, et al.: Diagnosis of Sjögren's syndrome in children. Am. J. Dis. Child. 142:1185–1187, 1988.

A report of four children and a review of 23 other childhood cases of Sjögren's syndrome.

72. McCurdy FA: Primary Sjögren syndrome in adolescence: A case report and review. Int. Pediatr. 4:344–348, 1989.

A report of an 11 1/2-year-old girl with Sjögren's syndrome and a discussion of this disorder as manifested in childhood and adolescence.

73. Teramoto N, Katayama I, Arai H, et al.: Annular erythema: A possible association with primary Sjögren's syndrome. J. Am. Acad. Dermatol. 20:596–601, 1989.

A report of four patients suggests that annular erythema mimicking the erythema of Sweet's syndrome may be considered to be a cutaneous manifestation of Sjögren's syndrome.

74. Kohler PF, Winter ME: A quantitative test for xerostomia: The Saxon test, an oral equivalent of the Schirmer test. Arthritis Rheum. 28:1128–1132, 1985.

A description of a simple low-cost technique to test for xerostomia in which a folded sterile gauze pad is weighed before and after chewing for 2 minutes in order to measure the amount of saliva production in patients suspected of having Sjögren's syndrome.

75. Hansen LA, Prakash UBS, Colby TV: Pulmonary lymphoma in Sjögren's syndrome. Mayo Clin. Proc. 64:920–931, 1989.

A review of 50 patients with Sjögren's syndrome and an associated lymphoma in which 10 patients had pulmonary involvement suggested that pulmonary infiltrates in patients with Sjögren's syndrome should prompt consideration of the possibility of an associated non-Hodgkin's lymphoma.

76. Sharp GC, Irvin WS, Tan EM, et al.: Mixed connective tissue disease: An apparently distinct rheumatic disease syndrome associated with a specific antibody to extractable nuclear antigen (ENA). Am. J. Med. 52:148–159, 1972.

A description of 25 patients with arthritis or arthralgias, swollen hands, Raynaud's phenomenon, esophageal abnormalities, myositis, hypergammaglobulinemia, leukopenia, and high titers of ENA.

77. Fraga A, Gudino J, Ramos-Niembro F, et al.: Mixed connective tissue disease in childhood: Relationship with Sjögren's syndrome. Am. J. Dis. Child. 132:263–265, 1978.

Of three children with mixed connective tissue disease (MCTD), two met the criteria for systemic lupus erythematosus, two had polymyositis, and all three had cutaneous, vascular, and esophageal features of scleroderma, juvenile rheumatoid arthritis, and Sjögren's syndrome.

78. Gilliam JN, Prystkowsky SD: Mixed connective tissue disease syndrome: Cutaneous manifestations of patients with epidermal nuclear staining and high titer serum antibody to ribonuclease-sensitive extractable nuclear antigen. Arch. Dermatol. 113:583–586, 1977.

Ribonucleoprotein antibodies and epidermal nuclear staining provide readily detectable immunologic markers for mixed connective tissue disease.

79. Singsen BH: Mixed connective tissue disease in childhood. Pediatr. Rev. 7:309–314, 1986.

A comprehensive review of mixed connective tissue disease, its clinical features and management in children.

21

ENDOCRINE DISORDERS AND THE SKIN

Endocrine diseases frequently display cutaneous features that provide rewarding clues to the physician who is asked to diagnose or assist in the management of unusual dermatoses or systemic disorders of patients in the pediatric age group as well as in adults. Some of these conditions and their dermatologic features, clinical manifestations, and therapy are reviewed in this chapter.

THYROID DISORDERS

The spectrum of thyroid disease in pediatric patients is broad and may manifest as hypothyroidism (congenital or acquired), hyperthyroidism, tumors of the thyroid, and acute, subacute, or chronic thyroiditis. Of these, thyroiditis, the most common cause of thyroid disease in children and adolescents, accounts for many of the enlarged thyroid disorders formally designated as "adolescent" goiter. Also the most common cause of juvenile hypothyroidism (with or without goiter), the incidence of thyroiditis may be as high as 1 per cent in children. Most children affected with thyroiditis are clinically euthyroid and asymptomatic (some may merely present with symptoms of pressure in the neck). Those with clinical signs of hypothyroidism or hyperthyroidism will be described in the sections on the respective disorders.

Hypothyroidism

The term *hypothyroidism* refers to a group of clinical disorders that result from inadequate production of thyroid hormone. Congenital or acquired, hypothyroidism in the first 2 or 3 years of life may result in irreversible damage to the nervous system. Beyond this age, however, most effects of hypothyroidism are reversible.

Congenital hypothyroidism, a disorder of thyroid deficiency present from birth or early infancy, may develop as a result of agenesis or dysgenesis of the thyroid gland; by defective synthesis of thyroid hormone caused by an enzymatic defect; by the presence of antithyroid antibodies in a pregnant mother; by lack of maternal iodine during pregnancy (endemic goiter); or by the ingestion of antithyroid medications such as propylthiouracil or methimazole (Tapazole) by pregnant women being treated for thyrotoxicosis. Of these, thyroid dysgenesis is the most common cause of congenital hypothyroidism (Table 21–1). Although "cretinism" is often used synonymously with congenital hypothyroidism, current texts suggest the avoidance of this uncomplimentary term.

Congenital hypothyroidism is estimated to occur in 1 in 2,500 to 1 in 7,000 newborns.[1, 2] The classic clinical features include puffy myxematous facies; depressed nasal bridge; hypertelorism (broaden-

Table 21–1. ETIOLOGY OF CHILDHOOD HYPOTHYROIDISM

1. Congenital hypothyroidism
   a. Thyroid agenesis or dysgenesis (over 80%)
   b. Inborn defect of thyroid hormone synthesis
   c. Maternal causes
      1. Maternal antithyroid antibodies
      2. Endemic goiter (maternal iodine deficiency)
      3. Ingestion of goitrogenic (antithyroid agents) or radioactive iodine therapy
2. Acquired hypothyroidism
   a. Hashimoto's (chronic lymphocytic) thyroiditis
   b. Thyroid dysgenesis (with delayed failure of thyroid remnants)
   c. Inborn defect in synthesis of thyroid hormone
   d. Thyroidectomy or radioactive thyroid ablation
3. Antithyroid ingestion

Hurwitz S: The Skin and Systemic Disease in Children. Year Book Medical Publishers, Chicago, 1985.

ing of the ridge of the nose with an increased width between the eyes); a large protruding tongue; thick lips; coarse brittle hair; short neck; large fontanelles with wide cranial sutures; hoarse cry; abdominal distention; umbilical hernia; an otherwise unexplained heart murmur; goiter; hypotonia; cold, mottled or jaundiced skin; a sallow complexion; translucent "alabaster"-like ears; stunted growth; delayed and defective dentition; poor weight gain; poor peripheral circulation with subnormal body temperature and intolerance to cold; inactivity; broad hands; stubby fingers; seborrhea of the scalp; purpura; prolonged relaxation phase of tendon reflexes; mental retardation; delayed motor development with neurologic damage such as lack of coordination and ataxia; docility (affected infants are described as "good" babies); lethargy; poor feeding; constipation; myxedema; and dry skin (Table 21–2).

Although congenital hypothyroidism may present in the newborn with no clinical signs, a large goiter may cause hyperextension of the neck of the fetus resulting in malpresentation and complications in labor and delivery and most affected infants manifest a constellation of the clinical features described above. Radiologic examination in a term infant may reveal absence of the distal femoral epiphyses, and laboratory findings include a low serum thyroxine (T_4) and triiodothyronine (T_3) resin uptake and elevated levels of thyroid-stimulating hormone (TSH). A rapid radioimmunoassay measurement of serum T_4 and TSH levels on filter paper, heel-stick, or cord blood samples in the first few days of life is helpful as an early screening procedure for newborns. Ultrasound and radionuclide scanning can also help detect the presence or absence of thyroid tissue. Because of the potential risk of radiation exposure, however, radionuclide scanning must always be performed by experienced personnel with optimum equipment and the minimal recommended isotope tracer dose.[2, 3]

Acquired hypothyroidism in children younger than the age of 5 or 6 years is usually caused by a delayed failure of thyroid remnants (with thyroid dysgenesis). It can also develop as a result of inborn defects of thyroid hormone synthesis, ingestion of antithyroid agents, thyroidectomy or ablation following radiation, and chronic thyroiditis or hypothalamic-pituitary disease. After the age of 5 or 6 years, although the same etiologies may be involved, chronic lymphocytic thyroiditis (Hashimoto's disease) appears to be the most common cause of this disorder.

The clinical manifestations of acquired hypothyroidism depend on the age of the child at onset and on the extent of the dysfunction. Seen in approximately 1 in 500 to 1 in 1,000 children (with a female-to-male ratio of 6 : 1), the later in life that acquired hypothyroidism occurs the less the impairment of growth and development.

The onset of acquired hypothyroidism is often insidious. Clinical signs are frequently subtle, with a decrease in growth rate, delayed dentition, mild obesity (with myxedema), an increase in upper to lower body segment ratio, delayed puberty, developmental delay, and a decreased quality in school performance. If the hypothyroidism persists without therapy the classic features of hypothyroidism become apparent. Symptoms include generalized puffiness, with thick lips and puffiness about the eyes, nose, and cheeks producing a typical dull expressionless facies (Fig. 21–1); lethargy; poor appetite; constipation; short stature; bradycardia; decreased blood pressure with narrow pulse pressure; goiter; protuberant abdomen and buttocks; pale, thick, cool skin with sallow appearance; coarse hair; hypertrichosis (Fig. 21–2); flabby pseudohypertrophic muscles; poor wound healing; and delayed deep tendon reflexes. Although hypothyroidism usually delays the onset of

Table 21–2. CLINICAL FEATURES OF CONGENITAL HYPOTHYROIDISM

Puffy (myxedematous) facies
Sallow complexion
Wide anterior fontanelles and sutures
Macroglossia and thick lips
Hypertelorism, depressed nasal bridge
Coarse, brittle hair
Hoarse cry
Translucent ("alabaster") ears
Umbilical hernia and abdominal distention
Otherwise unexplained heart murmur
Hypotonia and slow reflexes
Short, stubby fingers, broad hands
Short lower extremities
Seborrhea of scalp, purpura
Prolonged relaxation phase of tendon reflexes
Cold, mottled, or jaundiced skin
Sluggishness and inactivity
Delayed motor development, mental retardation
Lack of coordination and ataxia
Poor weight gain, stunted growth
Subnormal body temperature, poor circulation, and intolerance to cold
Delayed/defective dentition and, in some cases, myxedema

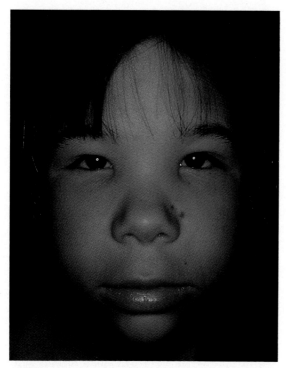

Figure 21–1. Typical expressionless facies with thick lips and puffiness of the eyes, nose, and cheeks in a 10-year-old girl with acquired hypothyroidism. (Hurwitz S: The Skin and Systemic Disease in Children. Year Book Medical Publishers, Chicago, 1985.)

long bones may reveal delayed appearance of ossification centers. Besides epiphyseal dysgenesis, a decrease in the anteroposterior diameter and breaking of the vertebral body (similar to that seen in patients with Hurler's disease) may be noted. Other laboratory features include an elevated serum cholesterol level; and, since untreated children with hypothyroidism do not grow, a low serum alkaline phosphatase level may help establish the diagnosis.

Treatment. The treatment of congenital hypothyroidism consists of thyroxine in a dosage of 10 μg/kg/day for the newborn (usually 25 to 50 μg/day during the first 6 months of life) and 2 to 5 μg/kg/day after 1 year of age, with an eventual maximal dose of 100 to 150 μg in teenagers. Weight gain in infants should be monitored daily and is probably the most sensitive indicator. Overtreatment may result in clinical signs of hyperthyroidism (diarrhea, hyperirritability, disturbed sleep patterns, excessive fluid and food intake with poor weight gain or weight loss, jitteriness, diaphoresis, hyperdefecation with or without diarrhea, and tachycardia). Since the administration of normal doses of thyroxine to infants with congenital hypothyroidism may trigger congestive heart failure owing to

puberty, some children will develop paradoxical precocious puberty with elevated serum gonadotropin concentrations (Table 21–3).

Patients with hypothyroidism complain of cold intolerance and frequently require a sweater or jacket when everyone else is comfortably warm. The hair typically disappears from the outer part of the eyebrows and becomes sparse, dry, and thin. Nails are brittle, grow slowly, and show longitudinal and transverse striations. The tongue and oral mucous membranes become thickened, and speech becomes slow and labored. As a result of deposition of mucin, the hands and feet frequently become puffy, the skin becomes rough and dry, and purpura and ecchymoses may be present.

Children with acquired hypothyroidism have a pleasant disposition but do poorly scholastically. Unfortunately, because they are usually placid, quiet, and good natured, teachers frequently fail to recognize their intellectual deficiency and think of them as ideal students. Such children, therefore, may continue to present satisfactory scholastic records despite their intellectual deficiency.

The same diagnostic tests are used in acquired as in congenital hypothyroidism. The diagnosis of primary hypothyroidism is confirmed by a low T_4 and T_3 resin uptake and an elevated serum TSH concentration. In cases of long duration, a lateral radiograph of the skull may reveal enlargement of the sella turcica, and radiologic examination of

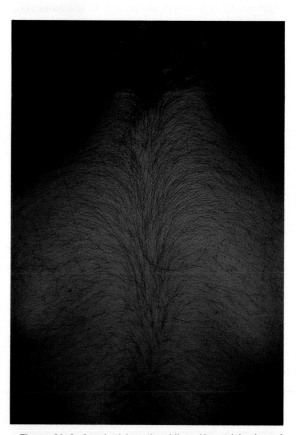

Figure 21–2. Acquired hypothyroidism. Hypertrichosis and rough dry skin are evident on the upper back of a 10-year-old girl. (Hurwitz S: The Skin and Systemic Disease in Children. Year Book Medical Publishers, Chicago, 1985.)

Table 21–3. CLINICAL FEATURES OF
ACQUIRED HYPOTHYROIDISM

Generalized puffiness (thick lips and puffiness around eyes)
  with a dull expressionless facies
Mild obesity, myxedema
Decreased growth rate and short stature (increase in upper to
  lower body segment ratio)
Delayed puberty, protuberant abdomen and buttocks
Delayed development and dentition
Poor scholastic performance
Placid disposition
Lethargy, poor appetite, and constipation
Bradycardia, decreased blood pressure with narrow pulse
  pressure
Thick, pale, cool skin (with sallow appearance)
Hypertrichosis with coarse hair
Flabby pseudohypertrophic muscles
Delayed deep tendon reflexes
Cold intolerance
Goiter
Rough dry skin, brittle nails (with longitudinal striations)
Slow labored speech
Coarse hair and hypertrichosis
Puffy hands and feet
Purpura or ecchymoses
Delayed or precocious puberty

rapid mobilization of fluid accumulated during the myxedematous state and cardiac deaths have been reported in the early phases of thyroid replacement, it is recommended that children with congenital hypothyroidism be referred to a pediatric endocrinologist and hospitalized for careful monitoring, particularly during the early phases of therapy.

The treatment of choice for children with acquired hypothyroidism is thyroxine (Synthroid) in a dosage of 3 to 5 μg/kg (to a maximum of 100 to 150 μg), with adjustments according to the individual's age and clinical and biochemical response. The dosage should be adjusted at 2- to 4-week intervals to a level that maintains the serum T_4 concentration in the mid-range of normal with normal T_3 and TSH concentrations. Fortunately, in contrast to patients with congenital hypothyroidism, irreversible brain damage is usually not a problem when the hypothyroidism is acquired after the age of 2 to 3 years.

The treatment of acquired hypothyroidism, however, may at times lead to temporary periods of personality upheaval characterized by argumentativeness and the loss of the patient's previous docile personality. School performance may accordingly deteriorate during this period as the child adjusts to a resurgence of energy and a loss of interest in scholastic achievements. In such instances, parents and teachers need to be supportive and appropriate guidance and counseling may be required. Fortunately, this period of adjustment generally lasts only a few months.

Hyperthyroidism

Hyperthyroidism, a relatively uncommon disorder of childhood, occurs most frequently in the 11- to 16-year old age group and is five or six times more common in girls than in boys. Only one-fifth as common as hypothyroidism in childhood, about 5 per cent of all patients with hyperthyroidism are younger than 15 years of age. Thyrotoxicosis can also occur in the newborn period, and in infants as young as 2 days to 2 months of age it can be life threatening. This disorder, *termed neonatal thyrotoxicosis* or *transient neonatal hyperthyroidism,* is often transient and may last for about 6 months, or it may persist indefinitely. Neonatal thyrotoxicosis is characterized by irritability, flushing, tachycardia, exophthalmos, goiter, weight loss, voracious appetite, and other features of Graves' disease. Affected infants invariably are offspring of women who have or have had thyrotoxicosis caused by long-acting thyroid stimulator (LATS) transferred from the mother to the infant during pregnancy.

Although most cases of hyperthyroidism in children are associated with autoimmune thyroid disease (diffuse toxic goiter, [Graves' disease]), it may also be associated with chronic lymphocytic thyroiditis (Hashimoto's thyroiditis), hyperfunctioning thyroid nodules, or hypersecretion of TSH. Despite the fact that a number of immunologic reactions have been demonstrated in Graves' disease, the events that precipitate these immune reactions remain obscure.

The clinical features of hyperthyroidism include nervousness, emotional lability, tachycardia and palpitation, heat intolerance, weakness, fatigue, tremors, hyperactivity, increased appetite, weight loss, increased systolic and pulse pressure, accelerated growth, sleep disturbances, school problems, vomiting, diarrhea, thyroid gland enlargement, and, at times, exophthalmos (Table 21–4). The skin is thin but not atrophic, warm, soft, moist, smooth, and velvety. Flushing of the face, increased sweating (particularly of the palms and soles), and palmar erythema are common. The nails grow rapidly, are shiny, and may have onycholysis (separation or loosening of the nail plate from the nail bed) with distal upward curvature (Plummer's nails). Chronic urticaria and general-

Table 21–4. CLINICAL FEATURES OF
HYPERTHYROIDISM (THYROTOXICOSIS)

Thyroid gland enlargement and at times exophthalmos
Nervousness, emotional lability
Tachycardia and palpitation
Increased systolic and pulse pressure
Heat intolerance, weight loss
Weakness, fatigue
Hyperactivity and tremors
Increased appetite and accelerated growth
Sleep disturbances and school problems
Vomiting and diarrhea
Warm, soft, smooth, and velvety skin
Flushing of face, increased sweating, palmar erythema
Rapidly growing shiny nails, onycholysis with upward
  curvature (Plummer's nails)
Pruritus, chronic urticaria
Addisonian pigmentation
Pretibial myxedema and thyroid acropathy

ized pruritus are uncommon manifestations of thy-rotoxicosis, and chronic active hyperthyroidism can be complicated by addisonian hyperpigmentation. The latter feature, believed to be caused by increased melanocyte-stimulating hormone (MSH) secretion from the pituitary, is probably not as common today since most patients with hyperthyroidism are now treated earlier. Patients with hyperthyroidism also have an increased incidence of alopecia areata and/or vitiligo, and about one third have a history or clinical features of atopic dermatitis.

Other cutaneous features of hyperthyroidism include pretibial myxedema and thyroid acropachy. *Pretibial myxedema*, seen in approximately 5 per cent of patients with Graves' hyperthyroidism and usually associated with exophthalmos, is a localized form of myxedema characterized by flesh-colored, pink, or purplish brown to yellow asymptomatic or pruritic plaques or nodules on the anterolateral aspect of the legs, at times extending to the dorsal aspect of the feet.[4] The overlying epidermis is thin with a waxy and sometimes translucent quality with prominent hair follicles. The hypertrichosis with dilated hair follicles and accentuation of coarse hairs may be responsible for the orange peel (peau d'orange) or pigskin-like appearance of lesions in these areas.

TSH, LATS, and 7S γ-globulin have been implicated as the cause of acid mucopolysaccharides in the skin of patients with pretibial myxedema, and current studies suggest that the serum of patients with this disorder contains a nonimmunoglobulin protein that stimulates the skin fibroblasts to produce mucin and proteins.[5] The pathogenesis of the skin lesions in pretibial myxedema appears to be distinct and unrelated to the mechanisms proposed for the other clinical and biochemical features of Graves' disease, Hashimoto's thyroiditis, and hypothyroidism, and the disorder may be treated with topical, intralesional, or systemic corticosteroids.[6]

The clinical features of *thyroid acropachy* are clubbing of digits, diaphyseal periosteal proliferation of distal bones, and thickening of the soft tissues over the distal extremities. Reported to occur in up to 1 per cent of patients with Graves' disease, and rarely seen in children, it is usually found in patients with a combination of exophthalmos, pretibial or localized myxedema, and past or present hyperthyroidism, and appears to be related to LATS in the serum of affected patients. Diagnostic signs include reduced temperature without obvious abnormality over areas of localized myxedema and increased width of the diaphyses of distal short bones (especially the mid-diaphyseal areas of the metacarpals, metatarsals, and phalanges and, in severe cases, the distal long bones [radius, ulna, tibia, and fibula]). Typical physical findings include drumstick-like clubbing, enlargement of the hands and feet, and radiographic changes (fluffy, spiculated, or homogeneous subperiosteal thickening with new bone formation and spicules perpendicular to the long axis of the bone).[7]

In patients with clinical signs and symptoms suggestive of hyperthyroidism, careful physical examination will usually demonstrate the presence of enlargement of the thyroid gland. To confirm the clinical suspicion, increased serum levels of T_4 and T_3 can be determined by radioimmunoassay, and TSH measured by radioimmunoassay will identify those few cases caused by TSH hypersecretion. If there is a question of pretibial myxedema, the demonstration of edema and large bluish deposits of mucin, with splitting up of collagen bundles extending down to the subcutaneous tissue, on histopathologic examination of cutaneous biopsy specimens will help confirm this clinical feature of thyrotoxicosis.

Treatment. Treatment of hyperthyroidism in children may be accomplished by the use of antithyroid drugs such as propylthiouracil (5 to 7 mg/kg/day, generally 150 to 450 mg/day), or methimazole (Tapazole), 0.4 to 0.7 mg/kg/day, generally 15 to 50 mg/day, in three divided doses; by thyroidectomy; or by radioiodine ablation. In patients with severe disease or distressing cardiovascular symptoms such as thyroid storm (high fever, tachycardia, sweating, and reduced mental state ranging from confusion to coma), propranolol (1 to 2 mg/kg/day) is a useful adjunctive form of therapy. Potassium iodide (2 to 4 mg/kg/day), administered as Lugol's solution or saturated solution of potassium iodide, potentiates the action of thionamide drugs and inhibits thyroid hormone secretion. The effect of potassium iodide, however, is transient. This drug, therefore, is seldom used except for short-term treatment of severe disease or preoperative preparation of patients for surgery.[8–10]

In patients in whom the goiter is three or more times greater than normal size, once euthyroidism has been produced by appropriate antithyroid therapy, subtotal thyroidectomy has been recommended. In patients in whom the goiter appears to be larger than 60 g at surgery, however, near-total thyroidectomy is suggested.[8]

MULTIPLE ENDOCRINE NEOPLASIA SYNDROMES

The multiple endocrine adenomatosis (MEA) syndromes, also termed the *multiple endocrine neoplasia (MEN) syndromes*, are familial disorders characterized by hyperplasia or tumors involving more than one endocrine gland. The clinical manifestations are inconsistent and reflect the variable involvement of hormone-producing tissues. Although the pathogenesis of the multiple syndromes is unknown, they are all inherited in an autosomal dominant pattern with variable expressivity and high penetrance (Table 21–5).[1]

The *mucosal neuroma syndrome*, the prototype of these syndromes, is a term used to describe a group of disorders characterized by multiple mu-

Table 21–5. MULTIPLE ENDOCRINE ADENOMATOSIS SYNDROMES

1. Multiple endocrine adenomatosis type I (MEA I, MEN I, Wermer's syndrome, multiple endocrine neoplasia type 1)
   a. Tumors of the anterior pituitary, pancreatic islet cells, parathyroids, and adenomas of the thyroid and adrenal cortex
   b. Lipomas, bronchial and intestinal carcinoid tumors, and schwannomas and thymomas (less common)
2. Multiple endocrine adenomatosis type II (MEA II, MEN II or 2A, Sipple syndrome, multiple endocrine neoplasia type 2a)
   a. Medullary carcinoma of the thyroid, pheochromocytoma and parathyroid tumor or hyperplasia
   b. Medullary carcinoma of the thyroid is inherited as an autosomal dominant trait (pheochromocytoma and parathyroid disease have lower degree of penetrance)
3. Multiple endocrine adenomatosis III type (MEA III, MEN III, or IIB, mucosal neuroma syndrome, multiple endocrine neoplasia type 2b or 3)
   a. Major components include multiple neuromas, medullary thyroid carcinoma, and pheochromocytoma
   b. Other features include characteristic facies, skeletal abnormalities, and ganglioneuromatosis of lips and gastrointestinal tract

cosal neuromas, intestinal ganglioneuromatosis, medullary thyroid carcinoma, parathyroid adenoma, and/or hyperplasia and pheochromocytoma. Other terms used to denote variations of this combination include multiple mucosal neuroma syndrome, medullary thyroid carcinoma syndrome, oral mucosal neuroma–medullary thyroid carcinoma syndrome, multiple endocrine adenomatosis III (MEA III), and multiple endocrine neoplasia (MEN) type 2b or 3. Although variations of the above features may occur sporadically (perhaps as the result of new mutations), most cases of the mucosal neuroma syndrome are transmitted as an autosomal dominant trait.

A relationship between carcinoma of the thyroid and pheochromocytoma was first described by Eisenberg in 1932, but it was not until almost 30 years later (1961) that Sipple reported a patient with this combination of findings.[11] Since then, reports of this association with other findings such as parathyroid hyperplasia and multiple mucosal neuromas have frequently been known as the Sipple syndrome (MEA II and MEN 2a). Endocrine neoplasias may occur singly or in various clinical patterns. *MEA type I* (multiple endocrine adenomatosis, multiple endocrine neoplasia type I) is characterized by tumors of the pituitary gland, tumors of the pancreatic islets, and adenomas of the thyroid, adrenal cortex, and parathyroid glands; *MEA type II* (multiple endocrine neoplasia type 2a) is characterized by neoplasia of the C cells of the thyroid (medullary carcinoma), adrenal medulla (pheochromocytoma), and parathyroid glands (chief cell hyperplasia or adenoma); and *MEA type III* (sometimes termed multiple endocrine neoplasia *type 2b* or *the mucosal neuroma syndrome*) is characterized by the association of multiple mucosal neuromas, medullary thyroid carcinoma, and pheochromocytoma (Table 21–5).

Mucosal neuromas (seen in 80 per cent of patients with the mucosal neuroma syndrome) may present at multiple sites (the lips, tongue, eyes, and gastrointestinal tract) and represent the hallmark of this disorder. Labial involvement results in diffusely enlarged lips with a characteristic fleshy, blubbery, or negroid appearance, the upper lip being more affected than the lower (Figs. 21–3 and 21–4). Lingual neuromas, generally limited to the anterior third of the tongue, appear as pink, sessile, or pedunculated nodules. These may be congenital or may be noted in the first few years of life and often represent the first markers heralding this syndrome (See Fig. 21–3). Nasal, laryngeal, and gingival neuromas may be present, and cutaneous involvement has also been seen on rare occasions. Neuromas may also be seen at the limbus of the conjunctivae and at the margins of the eyelids, with thickening of the eyelid margins and displacement of the cilia (Fig. 21–5).

Intestinal ganglioneuromatosis may commonly be seen as another form of mucosal neuroma in this disorder. Here, failure to thrive, constipation, or diarrhea may lead to further evaluation and eventual demonstration of the full abnormality.[12]

Physical features of patients with MEA type III (the mucosal neuroma syndrome, MEN syndrome type 2b) include a marfanoid appearance with long slender limbs and fingers, poor muscular development with very little subcutaneous fat, and skeletal defects such as kyphoscoliosis, pectus excavatum (funnel chest), and pectus carinatum (pigeon breast). Other abnormalities, such as a high-arched palate and pes cavus, may also be seen.

Medullary carcinoma of the thyroid, a malignancy seen in only 5 to 10 per cent of all thyroid cancers, is the major endocrine tumor of this syndrome. Here the perifollicular cells of the thyroid (termed *"C" cells* because of their secretion of calcitonin, the calcium-lowering polypeptide hormone) may be the source of other humoral substances such as prostaglandin and serotonin in

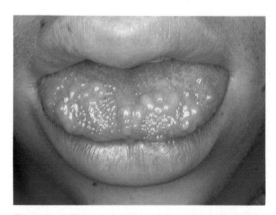

Figure 21–3. Characteristic lingual neuromas and protuberant fleshy lips in a 16-year-old boy with multiple mucosal neuroma syndrome.

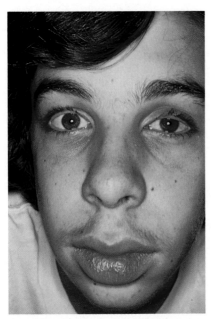

Figure 21–4. Characteristic facies with diffusely enlarged lips in multiple mucosal neuroma syndrome. (Hurwitz S: The Sipple syndrome. Society Transactions. Arch. Dermatol. *110:*139, 1974 copyright © 1974, American Medical Association).

some patients. Histopathologic examination of medullary carcinoma of the thyroid reveals sheets of rather uniform, round to spindle-shaped cells, often binucleated, with eosinophilic cytoplasm. The increased calcitonin released by these cells lowers serum calcium, thus stimulating a compensatory parathyroid response resulting in hyperparathyroidism or parathyroid adenoma. Parathyroid abnormalities, therefore, seen in 10 to 20 per cent of patients with multiple mucosal neuroma syndrome, represent a secondary response and are not the direct result of genetic aberration.

Pheochromocytoma may be present in 38 per cent of patients with the Sipple syndrome (MEA type II, MEN type 2a). In two thirds of those affected, the tumors are bilateral. Here the chromaffin cells of the adrenal medulla and sympathetic nerves and ganglia, also derived from primitive neural crest ectoderm, synthesize catecholamines, norepinephrine, and epinephrine, with resultant hypertension, tachycardia, anxiety, hyperhidrosis, weight loss, and/or fatigue.

Treatment. Since medullary thyroid carcinoma and pheochromocytoma will develop in a high percentage of patients with the mucosal neuroma syndrome, early recognition and removal of medullary carcinoma of the thyroid gives the best chance for survival. Unfortunately, most patients with medullary carcinoma die in their early 20s or 30s. Adequate therapy, therefore, includes thyroidectomy and a search for parathyroid hyperplasia, hypercalcinosis, and nephrocalcinosis. Calcitonin levels should be followed, pheochromocytomas and eye lesions should be sought, and since this syndrome

appears to be genetic in origin, all relatives should be examined and appropriately counseled.[13]

PARATHYROID DISORDERS

Disorders of the parathyroid glands (hyperparathyroidism and hypoparathyroidism) affect the skin in various ways and often present significant cutaneous features that can assist the primary or consulting physician in the diagnosis and management of affected individuals. Although primary parathyroid disease is uncommon in children, the parathyroids play a major role in the regulation of calcium and phosphorus metabolism, and associated abnormalities manifest distinctive clinical patterns.

Hyperparathyroidism

Primary hyperparathyroidism, one of the least common endocrine disorders of infancy and childhood, is rarely diagnosed in children younger than 16 years of age. When seen, it is usually due to a familial, genetically determined hyperplasia of the parathyroid, a malignant neoplasm of the parathyroid, a secondary reaction to some other disease such as is seen in patients with multiple endocrine adenomatosis (multiple endocrine neoplasia), or chronic renal insufficiency.[14, 15]

The clinical features of hyperparathyroidism include systemic effects of hypercalcemia: failure to thrive, muscular weakness, lethargy, anorexia, vomiting, fever, headache, constipation, weight loss, polydipsia, polyuria, mental retardation, metastatic calcification, and, with marked hypercalcemia, stupor, or death. Of these, metastatic calcification is the most common cutaneous manifestation. Hypercalcemia may also produce an ophthalmologic finding known as *band kera-*

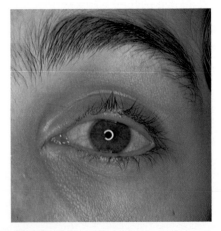

Figure 21–5. Multiple mucosal neuroma syndrome. Neuromas of the eyelid margins cause thickening of the margins and displacement of the cilia.

topathy. A result of calcium and phosphate deposition beneath Bowman's capsule, band keratopathy appears as a superficial corneal opacity resembling frosted or ground glass in a band-like configuration with white flecks or "holes" in the band resulting in a "Swiss cheese"-like appearance. Concentric with the limbus of the cornea but separated from it by a margin of uninvolved cornea, this finding is not specific for hyperparathyroidism; it may also be seen as a manifestation of hypercalcemia secondary to vitamin D intoxication, uremia, or sarcoidosis and is not commonly found in patients with hyperparathyroidism when serum phosphorus levels are low and glomerular function is maintained.

Hyperparathyroidism secondary to chronic renal failure may also produce cutaneous manifestations. The skin of the uremic patient may be pruritic, dry, scaly, sallow, and hyperpigmented; the sallow appearance is partially due to anemia, and the hyperpigmentation appears to be the result of decreased renal clearance of melanocyte-stimulating hormone (MSH). Hyperphosphatemia caused by decreased renal clearance may also produce a secondary calcification of the arteries, skin, subcutaneous fat, and, at times, muscle. This may be manifested as infarcted and ecchymotic areas or as plaques of calcinosis with periodic extrusion of calcium.

The diagnosis of hyperparathyroidism is established by consistent elevations of total serum calcium above 12 mg/dl, the reduction of serum phosphorus concentrations below 4 mg/dl, and elevated levels of parathyroid hormone. High alkaline phosphatase levels usually indicate bone disease. This complication of hyperparathyroidism may be demonstrated radiographically by generalized demineralization of bones, destructive changes at the growing ends of long bones, subperiosteal erosions (particularly in the phalanges, metacarpals and lateral portions of the clavicles), and, in more advanced disease, generalized rarefaction, cysts, tumors, fractures, and deformities. Radiographs of the abdomen may reveal renal calculi or nephrocalcinosis, and ultrasonography and radioisotope scanning can confirm the diagnosis of primary hyperparathyroidism associated with an isolated parathyroid adenoma.[14] In infants with parathyroid hyperplasia, cupping and fraying at the ends of long bones and ribs may suggest rickets, and severe demineralization and pathologic fractures are common.

The treatment of hyperparathyroidism requires subtotal or complete parathyroidectomy with careful postoperative management of calcium levels. A compromise procedure is the removal of all of the parathyroids with autotransplantation of the parathyroid tissue into the muscles of the patient's forearm. The treatment of hypercalcemia requires maintenance of hydration and production of calciuresis and natriuresis by sodium-losing diuretics such as furosemide (1 mg/kg three to four times daily) or by ethacrynic acid, with replacement of the sodium and potassium lost in the urine. The diet should be low in calcium, sources of vitamin D should be eliminated, and patients should not be exposed to sunshine during the period of hypercalcemia.

Intravenous isotonic saline (at two to four times the normal maintenance rate) combined with thiazide diuretics or furosemide should be given to increase urinary calcium losses and, in patients resistant to therapy, calcitonin is available as Calcimar (salmon calcitonin), 4 to 10 MRC units/kg every 3 to 4 hours intramuscularly with a maximum initial dose of 100 units.[16] Uremic pruritus may respond to phototherapy with ultraviolet light in the UVB (290–320 mm) range, given cautiously, so as not to stimulate excessive vitamin D production of calcium.[17, 18]

Hypoparathyroidism

Hypoparathyroidism in childhood may develop as a congenital idiopathic disorder that may occur in adults as late as the third or fourth decade of life, but usually appears in the neonatal period or in later infancy or childhood, or as an acute condition following inadvertent removal or damage of the parathyroid glands during thyroid surgery. Congenital hypoparathyroidism may occur alone, may be seen as an autoimmune disorder where it may occur alone or with other endocrine disorders, or may be a hereditary condition associated with an increased familial incidence of other endocrinologic disorders (Addison's disease, pernicious anemia, and Hashimoto's thyroiditis), candidiasis, and/or vitiligo.[4] When associated with hypoplasia of the thymus and immunologic defects, the condition is known as the DiGeorge syndrome.

Idiopathic or congenital hypoparathyroidism usually is first manifested by tetany or seizures and, in 25 to 50 per cent of patients, ectodermal defects. The skin of affected individuals is rough, dry, thick, and scaly; the hair and eyebrows are sparse; and the nails are short and thin with brittleness and crumbling of the distal half or, in less severe cases, longitudinal grooves in the proximal nail plate or irregular longitudinal cracking along the distal nail edge.[4] When hypoparathyroidism occurs while the teeth are developing, pitting, ridging, absence of dental enamel, and absence or hypoplasia of the permanent teeth may result. Other clinical manifestations include tetany, convulsions, carpopedal spasm, muscle cramps and twitching, numbness or tingling of the extremities, laryngeal stridor, exfoliative dermatitis, mental retardation, chronic diarrhea (especially in infants), photophobia, keratoconjunctivitis, blepharospasm, and, in 50 per cent of affected patients, cataracts.

Mucocutaneous candidiasis is also seen as a complication in 15 per cent of patients with idiopathic hypoparathyroidism (but not in those with postsurgical hypoparathyroidism). In addition, one third to one half of infants and young children who manifest mucocutaneous candidiasis have an associated endocrinopathy. The candidal infection occurs most frequently on the lips, in the mouth, on the perineum, in the vagina, and, less frequently, on the nails. Although reasons for this predisposition to candidiasis are unknown, the hair, nail, and skin abnormalities appear to be related to a defect in cell-mediated immunity and an ectodermal defect seen in patients with this disorder.[4]

The clinical manifestations of hypoparathyroidism associated with surgical removal or injury of the parathyroid glands differ from those seen in patients with idiopathic or congenital hypoparathyroidism. These include thinning or loss of hair, the development of horizontal grooves (Beau's lines) in the nails, or a complete loss of nails following episodes of tetany (these abnormalities revert to normal when hypocalcemia is controlled). Hyperpigmentation (predominantly on the face and distal extremities resembling chloasma, pellagra, or addisonian pigmentation) may also occur in cases of post-thyroidectomy hypoparathyroidism. Although cutaneous calcification has been noted, this complication is relatively uncommon.

Pseudohypoparathyroidism

Pseudohypoparathyroidism is a hereditary disorder in which there is an abnormal response in the receptor tissues, particularly the kidneys and skeletal system, to parathyroid hormone (rather than a deficiency of parathyroid hormone). This causes a hypocalcemia, tetany, and hyperphosphatemia that mimics idiopathic hypoparathyroidism in every way except for the presence of candidiasis.[4] Children with pseudohypoparathyroidism are short and stocky and have a round face, plethoric cheeks, short pudgy hands and feet, and stunted growth (probably a result of premature closure of the epiphyses). The most striking abnormality is growth failure of the fourth and fifth metacarpals and metatarsals and, at times, proximal phalanges, causing the fourth and fifth fingers and toes to be strikingly short. The index finger is longer than the middle finger, and when patients with this disorder make a fist a depression is present where the knuckles should be. Most patients with pseudohypoparathyroidism have some degree of mental retardation and intracranial calcification, and ectopic subcutaneous and periarticular calcification and ectopic bone formation are frequently present. The diagnosis of pseudohypoparathyroidism is established in short individuals with round facies and short metacarpal and/or metatarsal bones when plasma calcium levels are decreased, plasma phosphate levels are increased, and parathyroid hormone levels are elevated. Individuals with this disorder do not respond appropriately to the administration of exogenous parathyroid hormone. Calcification of the basal ganglia is seen on radiologic examination, and approximately 60 per cent

of patients with this disorder have subcutaneous osteomas, first seen as nontender nodules on the extremities in the vicinity of large joints.[6]

Pseudopseudohypoparathyroidism is a congenital variant or incomplete form of pseudohypoparathyroidism in which serum calcium, phosphate, and parathyroid hormone levels are normal. Although patients with pseudopseudohypoparathyroidism are physically indistinguishable from individuals with pseudohypoparathyroidism, those with pseudopseudohypoparathyroidism do not develop hypocalcemia and tetany.[4]

The treatment of hypoparathyroidism is dependent on the restoration of normal serum levels of calcium and phosphate, while avoiding the deleterious effects of hypercalcemia. Although large doses of vitamin D were the mainstay of therapy for many years, dihydrotachysterol (DHT) and 1,25-dihydroxyvitamin D_3 (calcitriol) appear to be safer. The usual daily dose of calcitriol is 0.25 to 1.0 μg (approximately 0.015 to 0.025 μg/kg/24 hr); that for dihydrotachysterol (DHT) is 0.1 to 0.5 mg for infants and young children; for older children and adults it is 0.5 to 1.0 mg (0.01 to 0.02 mg/kg/24 hr). Patients who do not respond to treatment with DHT or 1,25-dihydroxyvitamin D_3 may benefit from additional calcium, either as calcium lactate or gluconate, in dosages of 5 to 10 g/day.[16] The treatment of pseudohypoparathyroidism requires restriction of dietary phosphate and, in some cases, administration of vitamin D or its derivatives similar to that of patients with idiopathic hypoparathyroidism.

The DiGeorge Syndrome

The DiGeorge syndrome is a classic example of isolated T-cell deficiency that develops as a result of faulty embryologic development of the thymus and the parathyroid glands (a congenital malformation of the third and fourth pharyngeal pouches). Oral candidiasis is an almost constant finding in patients with this disorder, and overwhelming fungal, viral, or bacterial infection usually leads to death early in infancy (in these patients the thymus is absent or hypoplastic). Affected individuals demonstrate parathyroid deficiency (with lack of parathyroid hormone), T-cell dysfunction, and, in 90 per cent of patients, congenital defects of the heart and great vessels (truncus arteriosus, interrupted aortic arch, double aortic arch or aberrant subclavian artery). Features of this disorder include hypocalcemia and tetany at an early age, chronic diarrhea, interstitial pneumonia, failure to thrive, micrognathia, hypertelorism, low-set ears, bifid uvula, shortened lip philtrum, bowed mouth, chronic purulent rhinitis, maculopapular eruptions, mental retardation, calcification of the central nervous system, nephrocalcinosis, and cardiac malformations.[19, 20]

The management of the DiGeorge syndrome is directed toward control of the hypoparathyroidism, treatment of recurrent infection, and, whenever possible, surgical correction of the congenital cardiac or great vessel defects. If a cellular immune defect is documented, fetal thymic transplantation has been successful; an alternate to thymic transplantation is the injection of the thymic humoral factors contained in thymosin fraction V.

DISORDERS OF THE ADRENAL GLANDS

Adrenal gland dysfunction may result in a variety of systemic disorders with significant cutaneous manifestations. Those of particular interest to the pediatrician, dermatologist, and pediatric dermatologist are Addison's disease, Cushing's syndrome, and the adrenogenital syndrome.

Addison's Disease

Deficient production of cortisol and/or aldosterone may result from a wide variety of congenital or acquired lesions of the hypothalamus, pituitary, or adrenal cortex. Addison's disease, a metabolic disorder caused by a deficient production of adrenocortical hormones, is characterized by weakness, anorexia, hypotension, loss of body hair, low values of serum sodium and chloride, high levels of serum potassium, and melanin hyperpigmentation of the skin (Fig. 21–6) and mucous membranes (Fig. 21–7). Relatively uncommon in children, most cases occur during the third through fifth decades. Until recently, tuberculosis of the adrenal glands was the most frequent etiologic factor, but histoplasmosis, coccidioidomycosis, cryptococcosis, amyloidosis, metastatic malignancies, and cutaneous T-cell lymphoma (mycosis fungoides) have been identified as frequent causative agents in adults. In children, most instances of Addison's disease appear to be idiopathic, congenital, or the result of hemorrhage or an acute infection involving the adrenal cortex. About half

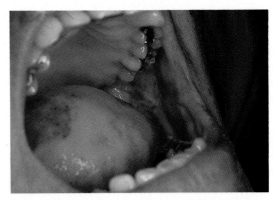

Figure 21–7. Addison's disease. Note hyperpigmentation of the mucous membranes of the mouth. (Hurwitz S: The Skin and Systemic Disease in Children. Year Book Medical Publishers, Chicago, 1985.)

of the patients with idiopathic Addison's disease demonstrate antibodies against adrenal tissue, suggesting autoimmunity as a basis for the disorder. This form of Addison's disease (particularly when seen in association with other autoimmunities) often occurs in siblings, suggesting an autosomal recessive cause in some children with this disorder.

Hyperpigmentation, the most prominent cutaneous feature of Addison's disease (see Fig. 21–6), appears to be the result of increased production of melanocyte-stimulating hormone by the pituitary gland (a compensatory phenomenon associated with decreased cortisol production by the adrenals). Seen in 92 per cent of patients, the hyperpigmentation is most intense in the flexures, at sites of pressure and friction, in creases of the palms and soles, in sun-exposed areas, and in normally pigmented areas such as the genitalia and areolae. Pigmentation of the conjunctivae and vaginal mucous membranes is common, and pigmentary changes of the oral mucosae include spotty or streaked blue-black to brown hyperpigmentation of the gingivae, tongue, hard palate, and buccal mucosa (see Fig. 21–7).

Vitiligo also occurs in up to 15 per cent of patients with Addison's disease. When seen together with hyperpigmentation, this combination produces a striking picture of hypopigmentation and hyperpigmentation. In addition to the pigmentary changes, calcification and fibrosis of the pinna of the ear may also occur. Since calcinosis of the cartilage of the ear may also be seen in patients with acromegaly, hypopituitarism, hyperthyroidism, diabetes, sarcoidosis, ochronosis, trauma, frostbite, and bacterial chondritis, it cannot be considered to be diagnostic of Addison's disease.[4]

The diagnosis of Addison's disease is suggested by its clinical features (hyperpigmentation, salt craving, postural hypotension, fasting hypoglycemia, and episodes of shock during severe illness) and may be confirmed by serum electrolyte studies and ACTH-stimulated cortisol level determinations. Treatment requires replacement with gluco-

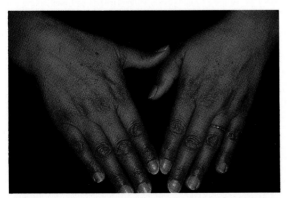

Figure 21–6. Hyperpigmentation of the skin of the hands (Addison's disease). (Hurwitz S: The Skin and Systemic Disease in Children. Year Book Medical Publishers, Chicago, 1985.)

corticoid and mineralocorticoid hormones, 12 to 20 mg/m²/day of hydrocortisone administered in two or three divided doses (with supplementation during stress at three times the maintenance dose) and fludrocortisone (Florinef) 0.05 to 0.1 mg/day.

Cushing's Syndrome

Cushing's syndrome is a term used to describe a disorder characterized by truncal obesity ad hypertension caused by increased blood levels of glucocorticoid hormones. It may be exogenous, caused by administration of systemic corticosteroids and sometimes cutaneous absorption following long-term use of topical corticosteroids, or endogenous, caused by tumors of the adrenal cortex or hypersecretion of pituitary adrenocorticotropic hormone (ACTH). The term *Cushing's disease* refers to patients with cushingism resulting from endogenous sources, such as bilateral adrenal hyperplasia resulting from ACTH secretion by the pituitary gland or by a primary adenoma or carcinoma of the adrenal gland. In infants and early childhood the disorder is caused by adrenocortical tumors (benign adenoma, primary adrenocortical hyperplasia, or malignant carcinoma). In children older than the age of 7, the etiology is usually caused by bilateral adrenal hyperplasia (Cushing's disease); and in older children, as in adults, Cushing's syndrome is often caused by exogenous corticosteroid administration.

Cushing's syndrome is relatively rare in childhood but may occur at any age, even in early infancy. The cutaneous manifestations include a characteristic plethoric "moon" facies (Fig. 21–8) with telangiectasia over the cheeks; patchy cyanosis over the upper arms, breasts, abdomen, buttocks, thighs, and legs; an increased amount of fine lanugo hair on the face and extremities; fatty deposits over the back of the neck ("buffalo hump"); increased fat deposits on the torso with a contrasting thinning of the arms and legs; purplish atrophic striae at points of tension such as the lower abdomen, thighs, buttocks, upper arms, and breasts; fragility of dermal blood vessels with increased tendency to bruisability and ecchymoses at sites of trauma; poor wound healing; frequent fungal infection (predominantly *Trichophyton rubrum* and *Pityrosporon orbiculare*); frequent and recurrent pyoderma; and corticosteroid acne, a disorder usually manifested in older children and adults characterized by red, smooth, dome-shaped papules or small pustules seen primarily on the upper trunk, arms, neck, and, to a lesser degree, the face. Addisonian hyperpigmentation, although unusual in Cushing's syndrome, may occur in Cushing's disease when production of ACTH and related peptides is increased.

The diagnosis of Cushing's syndrome is suggested by the presence of weakness and muscle wasting, truncal obesity, osteoporosis, diabetes

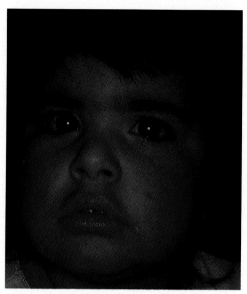

Figure 21–8. Cushing's syndrome. A characteristic "moon" facies with plethora and telangiectasia of the cheeks in a 3-year-old girl on long-term systemic corticosteroid therapy. (Hurwitz S: The Skin and Systemic Disease in Children. Year Book Medical Publishers, Chicago, 1985.)

mellitus and/or hypertension, and the previously described cutaneous manifestations. The clinical impression may be confirmed by elevated plasma 17-hydroxycorticoid levels with absence of the normal diurnal variation, by increased 24-hour urinary 17-hydroxycorticoid and 17-ketosteroid excretion, by the dexamethasone suppression test, and, when anterior pituitary abnormality is present, by visual field examination and radiologic, ultrasonic, or computed tomographic examination of the sella turcica.

The treatment of Cushing's syndrome depends on the etiology. When the disorder is endogenous, treatment should be directed at the pituitary (through surgery, irradiation, or isotope ablation) or adrenal glands (by total or subtotal adrenalectomy). When the disorder is caused by an ectopic source of ACTH, treatment should be directed at the underlying disease. In patients in whom bilateral adrenal tumors are present and bilateral adrenalectomy is indicated, lifelong glucocorticoid and mineralocorticoid therapy must be maintained. About 16 per cent of patients with Cushing's syndrome eventually develop pituitary tumors or addisonian hyperpigmentation, or both, following treatment by adrenalectomy (despite adequate adrenocortical replacement therapy). This phenomenon is called Nelson's syndrome. Treatment with metapyrone and/or aminoglutethimide prior to adrenalectomy seems to diminish the incidence of complications in these patients, and cyproheptadine (Periactin) appears to reduce ACTH levels and ameliorate clinical symptoms in some patients with Nelson's syndrome.

The Adrenogenital Syndrome

The adrenogenital syndrome is a condition in which there is excessive secretion of androgenic steroids by the adrenal cortex. It may result in adrenocortical insufficiency and salt wasting and may produce sudden death in newborns and virilization effects in patients who survive infancy (masculinization of the female [pseudohermaphroditism] and pseudoprecocious puberty in the male). Caused by adrenocortical hyperplasia, the adrenogenital syndrome is a genetic disorder resulting from a deficiency of one of several enzymes required for the formation of cortisol and, at times, aldosterone.

Virilizing adrenal tumors, although rare, are the most common type of adrenal tumor in the young. The apparent increased frequency of this disorder in females (by a 2:1 ratio) is probably related to the fact that clinical manifestations are more obvious in females than in males. In girls and adolescent females, the predominant clinical manifestations are hirsutism, features of Cushing's syndrome mixed with virilism in a masculine distribution, early appearance of pubic hair, clitoral enlargement, suppression of breast development, and delay in menarche. Clinical features of virilization in women include amenorrhea, clitoral enlargement, hirsutism in a masculine distribution, acne vulgaris manifested by comedones and deep cystic and pustular lesions, deep voice, increased muscle mass, and a male habitus. A similar tumor in prepubertal boys produces macrogenitosomia paecox and hirsutism without testicular maturation. In both girls and boys, muscles are well developed and there is rapid statural growth with marked advance in osseous maturation resulting in early epiphyseal closure and an inability to achieve full growth.

The *congenital adrenogenital syndrome* results in masculinization of girls in the form of pseudohermaphroditism with clitoral hypertrophy or labioscrotal fusion and the formation of a phallic urethra. Other clinical features include the premature development of pubic and axillary hair; deepening of the voice; and melanocyte-stimulating hormone hyperpigmentation of the skin, areolae, genitalia, palmar creases, and buccal mucosa. These patients are taller than normal during early childhood but are abnormally short during adolescence and adulthood because of premature closure of the epiphyses.

Obvious hirsutism in young children with virilism in girls or premature sexual development in boys is strongly suggestive of congenital adrenal hyperplasia or the adrenogenital syndrome, with elevation of total neutral urinary 17-ketosteroids serving as the laboratory key to diagnosis. When 17-ketosteroid levels are extremely high, the diagnosis of a neoplasm of the adrenal cortex should be suspected. As a means of differentiating the disorders, virilizing adrenal tumors do not demonstrate supression of plasma androgens or urinary 17-ketosteroids during a dexamethasone suppression test. Furthermore, since tumoral secretion is not ACTH dependent, the administration of ACTH has no effect on steroid production of patients with adrenal tumors.

The management of patients with the adrenogenital syndrome depends on the cause and course of the disorder. Physiologic amounts of cortisone acetate administered intramuscularly and oral hydrocortisone suppress the production of adrenal androgens and improve the virilization in affected individuals, but are contraindicated in the treatment of patients with adrenocortical tumors. For patients with adrenal tumors, the treatment is surgical. Since most of these tumors are malignant in the pediatric age group, surgical removal with postoperative irradiation is frequently recommended as the treatment of choice.

PITUITARY DISORDERS

Hyperpituitarism

The excessive secretion of growth hormone by pituitary tumors (usually an eosinophilic adenoma) produces gigantism in children whose epiphyses have not yet closed and acromegaly in adults. Although acromegaly is rare in chidren, it has been reported in infancy and childhood and transitional acromegalic features may also be seen in adolescents.[21] Clinical features of excessive secretion of growth hormone include coarsening of the features with overgrowth of soft tissues; cutis verticis gyrata; thick edematous eyelids; a large triangular-shaped nose; lantern jaw; macroglossia with, occasionally, a deeply furrowed tongue; a thick protruding lower lip; broad spade-like hands with short squat fingers; prominent pores; short, flat, wide, thickened, hardened, and rapidly growing nails, at times with absence of the lunula, longitudinal striations, and splitting; hirsutism; hyperpigmentation similar to that seen in patients with Addison's disease and, sometimes, acanthosis nigricans (see Chapter 25). Although the cause of hirsutism is not well understood, the hyperpigmentation appears to be related to increased secretion of melanocyte-stimulating hormone.

Cutis verticis gyrata, manifested by coarse furrowing of the skin of the vertex of the scalp and posterior aspect of the scalp and neck (Fig. 21–9), is caused by an increase in dermal collagen; and, as a result, excessive skin may buckle and form furrows and ridges that resemble gyri of the cerebral cortex. In addition to its being an occasional manifestation of hyperpituitarism, cutis verticis gyrata may occasionally occur as a primary disorder without other associated abnormalities. It may also be seen as part of a sex-linked dominant disorder (pachydermoperiostosis, a disorder manifested by thickening of the skin, accentuation of the skin of

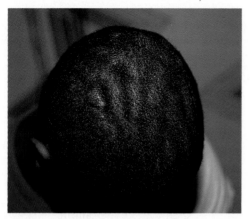

Figure 21–9. Cutis verticis gyrata. Coarse furrowing of the skin is seen on the vertex of the scalp of a 17-year-old boy. (Courtesy of Barry Goldberg, M.D.)

the face and scalp, clubbing of the fingers and periostosis of the long bones); with Apert's syndrome (acrocephalosyndactyly), a rare autosomal dominant disorder characterized by craniostenosis, broadened tower-skull deformity, syndactyly, ankyloses and progressive synostoses of the hands, feet, and spine, and, in most patients, some degree of mental redardation; as a result of inflammatory disorders of the scalp; and in patients with cerebriform intradermal nevi, myxedema, leukemia, syphilis, acanthosis nigricans, tuberous sclerosis, Ehlers-Danlos syndrome, amyloidosis, and diabetes mellitus.[22–24].

Hypopituitarism

Pituitary insufficiency (hypopituitarism) is a disorder or group of disorders resulting from a deficiency in secretion of one or more hormones derived from the pituitary gland. These include idiopathic hypopituitarism (panhypopituitarism, Simmond's disease), the least common variety; Sheehan's syndrome (pituitary deficiency usually arising as a result of hemorrhage or infarct); pituitary tumors; congenital abnormalities; or ablation of the pituitary gland by surgery or x-irradiation used for the treatment of local tumors.

The most obvious cutaneous manifestations of pituitary insufficiency are pallor, secondary to anemia and decreased cutaneous blood flow, and a tendency to severe sunburn and decreased ability to tan (due to a decrease in melanin pigmentation secondary to diminished or absent secretion of a melanocyte-stimulating factor from the pituitary).[4] Other features include a smooth, waxy, or myxedematous, coarse, dry, and scaly skin (resulting from hypothyroidism). The face may be slightly puffy, and pale or yellowish (secondary to carotenemia); the skin and subcutaneous tissue are thin, and when coupled with wrinkling around the eyes and

mouth may lead to an aged appearance; and gonadal hypofunction produces a loss of axillary, pubic, and body hair. Other manifestations of hypopituitarism include retardation of skeletal growth and thin opaque fragile slow-growing nails (often with a loss of the lunula). In addition, brown spots may be seen beneath the nail and onycholysis or longitudinal ridging may be present.

DISORDERS ASSOCIATED WITH DIABETES

At least 30 per cent of diabetics have some type of cutaneous involvement during the course of their illness. The disorders arise in a variety of ways. Some are caused by infectious agents; some result from vascular, metabolic, or nutritional disturbances; some arise as a result of medications; and some are idiopathic.[4] Cutaneous disorders associated with diabetes mellitus discussed in this section include necrobiosis lipoidica diabeticorum, diabetic dermopathy, bullosis diabeticorum, granuloma annulare (believed in some instances, perhaps, to be related to diabetes mellitus), and thick skin, stiff joints, and finger pebbling. Scleredema diabeticorum (scleredema of Buschke) is discussed in Chapter 25.

Necrobiosis Lipoidica Diabeticorum

Necrobiosis lipoidica diabeticorum (NLD) is a degenerative disorder of the dermal connective tissue often seen in patients with diabetes mellitus characterized by atrophic plaques on the anterior surface of the lower legs. Although the etiology of this disorder is unknown, it appears to be related to an alteration of dermal connective tissue owing to angiopathy of small vessels with inflammation and occlusion of dermal vessels (possibly a diabetes-related endarteritic obliterative vascular occlusion).[25–27]

Necrobiosis lipoidica diabeticorum precedes the onset of diabetes in 20 per cent of patients. More than half the patients have active diabetes mellitus, and an abnormal glucose tolerance test is demonstrable in 50 to 87 per cent of patients with this disorder.[4] Although statistics vary, necrobiosis lipoidica diabeticorum occurs in 0.1 to 0.3 per cent of diabetics. It appears to be approximately 10 times more common in juvenile diabetics than in adult-onset disease and occurs three times more often in women than in men. In 90 per cent of patients it is localized to one or both pretibial areas; in the remaining individuals it may occur on the trunk, face, scalp, arms, palms, or soles. The disorder may occur at any age. It was noted at birth in one patient but usually develops in the third or fourth decade of life and has a peak incidence in persons between 50 and 60 years of age.[4]

A typical lesion begins as an erythematous pap-

ule or nodule with a sharply circumscribed border.
It enlarges and slowly develops into an oval yellowish red sclerotic plaque with an irregular outline and a violaceous margin. The center of the
plaque is often depressed or atrophic and shows a
waxy translucent surface coursed by telangiectatic
vessels (Fig. 21–10). Lesions are usually asymptomatic. Trauma to the atrophic skin is poorly tolerated, and ulceration, although rare in childhood,
may occur in up to 30 per cent of patients with this
disorder.[28]

The diagnosis of necrobiosis lipoidica diabeticorum is suggested by the presence of sharply demarcated waxy plaques with violaceous borders on
the lower portion of the legs. In atypical locations, especially in patients who do not have
clinical diabetes, the disorder may be confused
with granuloma annulare, rheumatoid nodules,
and sarcoidosis. Characteristic of the histopathology are degeneration of collagen surrounded by
lymphocytes, histiocytes, and epithelioid cells;
thickening of vessel walls; proliferation of vessels
in the mid and lower dermis; and the presence of
lipid-filled giant cells.

The treatment of necrobiosis lipoidica diabeticorum is, in general, not very satisfactory. Since
trauma may produce stubborn painful ulcerations,
protection of the legs, elastic stockings, and bed
rest may be useful. Although patients may be seen
without evidence of diabetes, the presence of lesions should alert one to the possibility of this diagnosis, and an appropriate search for frank diabetes,
latent diabetes, or a prediabetic state should be
initiated.

Lesions of necrobiosis lipoidica diabeticorum

are usually symptom free and are often only of
diagnostic or cosmetic importance. Cosmetic
makeup or dark hose may help hide lesions. Topical corticosteroids (alone or under occlusion) or
intralesional corticosteroid injection may improve
and clear some lesions. Since patches of necrobiosis are ordinarily atrophic, however, caution must
be exercised to prevent further atrophy or ulceration. Ulcerative lesions are best treated conservatively with compresses, topical antibiotics, or
topical benzoyl peroxide in 10 to 20 per cent concentrations.[29] Extensive ulcerations may require
excision and full-thickness skin grafts. Poor healing owing to vascular damage and recurrences in
and around grafts, however, is not uncommon.
Aspirin and dipyridamole (Persantine), alone or in
combination, and pentoxifylline (Trental), although safety and effectiveness of pentoxifylline in
children below the age of 18 years have not been
established, have been reported to have a beneficial effect in some patients with this disorder.[30, 31]

Diabetic Dermopathy

Diabetic dermopathy is a characteristic dermatosis seen in 50 per cent of male patients and approximately 30 per cent of female patients with diabetes
mellitus, and, on rare occasions, in children. The
lesions are round or oval, red or reddish brown
flat-topped papules that slowly evolve into discrete, sharply circumscribed, atrophic, hyperpigmented, or scaly patches; sometimes only depressed areas with normal skin color are seen.
Lesions generally measure 1 or 2 cm or less in
diameter, and although they may occur on the
scalp, forearms, or trunk, they usually appear on
the anterior aspect of the thighs and shins of affected individuals. Although the precise pathogenesis of diabetic dermopathy is still undetermined, the presence of these characteristic lesions
can serve as a helpful clue to the diagnosis of diabetic individuals.[28]

The histopathologic features of lesions consist of
a combination of vascular disease and minor collagen changes. Vessel walls thickened with periodic acid–Schiff-positive material are seen in the
upper dermis, and slight collagen change and mi-
croangiopathy are seen in the dermis and subcutis.

Lesions of diabetic dermopathy are in large part
uninfluenced by treatment. Individual lesions
tend to disappear spontaneously after 1 1/2 to 2
years leaving annular, hyperpigmented, or normal
colored, slightly depressed or atrophic areas, but
the development of new lesions often creates an
impression that individual lesions persist for
longer periods of time. Treatment should emphasize protection of the shins from trauma, and bed
rest, open wet compresses, and topical antibiotics
should be used to assist healing of inflammatory
and crusted lesions.

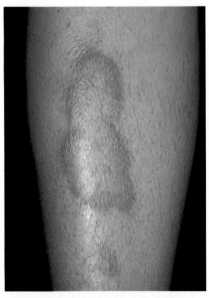

Figure 21–10. Necrobiosis lipoidica diabeticorum. A yellowish
red oval atrophic plaque has a waxy translucent surface, telangiectatic vessels, and a characteristic violaceous margin.

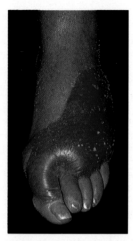

Figure 21–11. Bullous dermatosis in diabetes mellitus (bullosis diabeticorum). Painless bullae appeared on the dorsal aspect of the foot of a patient with diabetes mellitus. (Courtesy of Department of Dermatology, Yale University School of Medicine.)

Bullous Dermatosis in Diabetes Mellitus

Bullosis diabeticorum is a rare disorder that consists of large asymptomatic bullous lesions that develop rapidly on the distal extremities, especially the hands and feet (Fig. 21–11).[32, 33] Although many of the patients have peripheral neuropathy, this complication of diabetes is not present in all. The bullae are painless, clear, and noninflammatory. They develop rapidly, without evidence of trauma, ultraviolet exposure, or vascular insufficiency, and heal slowly and spontaneously.[33]

The etiology of bullosis diabeticorum is not known. Treatment consists of aseptic aspiration or incision and drainage and the use of topical antibiotics to prevent infection.

Granuloma Annulare

Granuloma annulare is a relatively common cutaneous disorder characterized clinically by papules or nodules that are grouped in a ring-like or circinate distribution. Although granuloma annulare may occur on any part of the body, it usually begins on the lateral or dorsal surfaces of the hands or feet. Females are affected twice as frequently as males. Granuloma annulare may occur at any age. Children and young adults, however, are most commonly affected, with over 40 per cent of cases appearing in children younger than 15 years of age.[34]

The cause of granuloma annulare is unknown. Various studies have shown latent diabetes to be present in a third of patients with this disorder.[35] Although still open to controversy, this finding (demonstrated in some adults but not in children) suggests that the underlying defect may be related to diabetes and to vascular changes associated with

the diabetic state. Other hypotheses suggest a humoral or delayed-type cell-mediated hypersensitivity reaction to some unidentified antigen. In some individuals granuloma annulare has been noted following trauma, sun exposure, and insect bites. The above theories, although attractive, still remain unsubstantiated and require further confirmation.[36–38]

The range of clinical lesions of granuloma annulare is broad, but the classic ringed eruption is characteristic. Early lesions begin as smooth, flesh-colored or pale red papules that slowly undergo central involution and peripheral extension to form rings with clear centers and elevated borders of continuous papules or nodules (Fig. 21–12). The rings are oval or irregular and vary from 1 to 5 cm in diameter. Lesions may be single or multiple; multiple lesions are more common in young children than in older patients; but numerous widely disseminated lesions can occur at any age (Fig. 21–13). Variants of granuloma annulare include a generalized form *(generalized granuloma annulare)*, characterized by a diffuse papular eruption on sun-exposed areas, especially on the nape of the neck and "V" area of the upper chest[39]; *perforating granuloma annulare,*[40] a disorder usually seen as asymptomatic grouped papules (some of which have a central umbilicated scale or crust) found mainly on the extremities of children as well as adults; familial forms[38]; a linear form[41]; and subcutaneous forms, most often seen on the legs, scalp, palms, and buttocks, and often confused with rheumatoid nodules (rheumatoid nodules, however, are usually larger and subcutaneous rather than intradermal). Localized granuloma annulare, the most common type, develops in two thirds of patients before the age of 30 years, and generalized granuloma annulare occurs in about 15 per cent of patients.

The histologic features of granuloma annulare

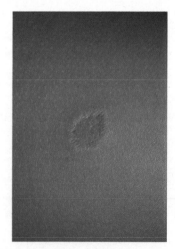

Figure 21–12. Granuloma annulare. Flesh-colored papulonodular lesions appear in an annular configuration.

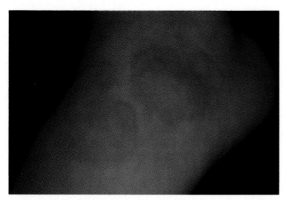

Figure 21–13. Granuloma annulare. Multiple papulonodular lesions occur in an annular configuration on the dorsal aspect of the foot of a 4-year-old child.

are characterized by well-demarcated oval foci of collagenous degeneration surrounded by lymphocytes, histiocytes, and fibroblasts, often in a palisading pattern; giant cells are uncommon. In perforating granuloma annulare, serial sections disclose extrusion of necrobiotic material through the epidermis (similar to that seen in patients with elastosis perforans serpiginosa).

Lesions of granuloma annulare usually disappear spontaneously, often within several months to several years. Although 50 to 73 per cent of lesions disappear within 2 years (with no residual scarring), recurrences are common and may be seen, usually at the original site, in up to 40 per cent of patients. At times, as simple a procedure as an injection of intralesional saline or a small biopsy may be followed by complete involution.

Although topical corticosteroids, corticosteroids under occlusion, and intralesional corticosteroids hasten resolution of lesions, because of the potential risk of dermal atrophy associated with such therapy, reassurance of eventual spontaneous resolution may be all that is necessary for treatment of the cosmetic aspect of this disorder. In individuals with generalized or cosmetically disfiguring granuloma annulare, potassium iodide, corticosteroid therapy, chloroquine, niacinamide (niacin), dapsone, alkylating agents, and photochemotherapy have been recommended.[42] Since it has been suggested that patients with granuloma annulare may be candidates for diabetes mellitus, it is often recommended that patients (particularly adults with the generalized form) be investigated for this possibility.[28]

Stiff Joints, Thick Skin, and Finger Pebbling

Stiff joints (limited joint mobility), most commonly affecting the proximal interphalangeal joints, have been described in up to one third of young insulin-dependent diabetics and in up to

one third of patients with both type I (juvenile-onset, insulin dependent) and type II (adult-onset, non-insulin-dependent) diabetics. Although hardness and thickening of the skin commonly occurs as the result of trauma or manual labor, type II diabetics can also manifest tight waxy skin, limited joint mobility, multiple grouped papules on the extensor surface on the fingers and knuckles (this has been termed *finger pebbling*), and pad-like hyperkeratoses over the distal knuckles and proximal nail folds identical to that produced in response to manual labor or repeated trauma (Fig. 21–14).[43, 44] Although the pathogenesis of joint stiffness and skin pebbling is unknown, it has been suggested that increased glycosylation and altered cross-linking of collagen in the dermis may lead to the cutaneous abnormalities seen in individuals with this disorder. It should be noted, however, that finger pebbling and knuckle pads may occur as normal variants or as a result of trauma or manual labor and thus do not necessarily indicate the presence of a diabetic state.[43, 44]

THE GLUCAGONOMA SYNDROME

Patients with glucagon-secreting pancreatic tumors may have a distinctive pruritic dermatosis characterized by configurate areas of erythema, followed by erosions, crusting, flaccid vesiculopustules, and eventual shedding of the skin, because of superficial necrosis, in cycles of 7 to 14 days.[45] Termed *necrolytic migratory erythema*, the cutaneous lesions generally arise on the face, lower abdomen, perineum, buttocks, or distal extremities. Seen most commonly in postmenopausal women, with a female-to-male ratio of 4:1, and extremely rare in the pediatric age group, the disorder may also be seen in women as young as 19 years of age.[46]

Other manifestations of the glucagonoma syndrome, possibly associated with nutritional deficiencies, include a xerotic eczema-like eruption with a faint papular component; beefy red tongue;

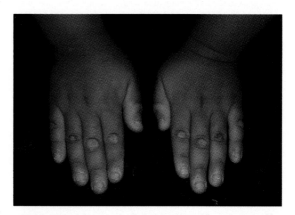

Figure 21–14. Traumatically induced knuckle pads caused by a knuckle-biting habit.

periorificial and intertriginous lesions resembling those seen in patients with chronic candidiasis, acrodermatitis enteropathica, or niacin deficiency; glossitis; stomatitis; angular cheilitis; nail hypertrophy; brittle or crumbling nails; weight loss; a normochromic anemia unresponsive to iron therapy; glucose intolerance or mild-onset diabetes; and hypoaminoacidemia. Elevated glucagon levels occur in virtually all patients in whom determinations are made. The histology of the cutaneous lesions is characterized by irregular acanthosis with spongiosis, subcorneal and midepidermal clefts, fusiform keratinocytes with pyknotic nuclei, and absence of acantholysis. Biopsies, when performed, should be taken from the edge of early lesions where the characteristic epidermal changes are most evident.

The cutaneous lesions respond to amino acid infusions, intravenous and topically administered zinc, and somatostatin or somatostatin analogues (currently available only on an experimental basis). In patients in whom metastases have occurred or complete removal of the tumor is impossible, treatment with chemotherapeutic agents such as streptozotocin (a methylnitrosurea analogue available for the treatment of unresectable or metastatic islet cell tumors), 5-fluorouracil, chlorozotocin, doxorubicin, dacarbazine, or a long-acting stomatostatin analogue can be beneficial.[47]

References

1. Hurwitz S: The Skin and Systemic Disease in Children. Year Book Medical Publishers, Chicago, 1985.

   The cutaneous features of systemic disorders in childhood.

2. Muir A, Daneman D, Daneman A, et al.: Thyroid scanning, ultrasound, and serum thyroglobulin in determining the origin of congenital hypothyroidism. Am. J. Dis. Child. 142:214–216, 1989.

   In a review of screening techniques for congenital hypothyroidism, thyroid scanning appears to be the most accurate.

3. American Academy of Pediatrics Committee on Genetics: Newborn screening for congenital hypothyroidism: Recommended guidelines. Pediatrics 80:745–749, 1987.

   The American Academy of Pediatrics guidelines for the diagnosis of congenital hypothyroidism.

4. Braverman IM: Skin Signs of Systemic Disease. W. B. Saunders Co., Philadelphia, 1981.

   A comprehensive review of the cutaneous manifestations of systemic disease.

5. Cheung HS, Nicoloff JJ, Kamiel MB, et al.: Stimulation of fibroblast activity of serum of patients with pretibial myxedema. J. Invest. Dermatol. 71:12–27, 1978.

   Studies on fibroblast activity and their role in the possible pathogenesis of pretibial myxedema.

6. Feingold KR, Elias PM: Endocrine-skin interactions: Cutaneous manifestations of pituitary disease, thyroid disease, calcium disorders and diabetes. J. Am. Acad. Dermatol. 17:921–940, 1987.

   A review of endocrine disorders and pathophysiologic mechanisms that account for their cutaneous changes.

7. Goette DK: Thyroid acropachy. Arch. Dermatol. 116:205–206, 1980.

   A report of thyroid acropachy in a 48-year-old man without exophthalmos.

8. Buckingham BA, Costin G, Roe T, et al.: Hyperthyroidism in children: A re-evaluation of treatment. Am. J. Dis. Child. 135:112–117, 1981.

   A comprehensive review of hyperthyroidism and its treatment in childhood.

9. Gorton C, Sadeghi-Nejad A, Senior B: Remission in children with hyperthyroidism treated with propylthiouracil: Long-term results. Am. J. Dis. Child. 141:1084–1086, 1987.

   In a review of 69 hyperthyroid children treated with propylthiouracil, although 64 per cent experienced a remission with therapy, 47 per cent relapsed.

10. Lippe BM, Landaw EM, Kaplan SA: Hyperthyroidism in children treated with long-term medical therapy: Twenty-five per cent remission every two years. J. Clin. Endocrinol. Metab. 64;1241–1245, 1987.

    A study of 60 children with hyperthyroidism treated with methimazole or propylthiouracil.

11. Sipple JH: Association of pheochromocytoma with carcinoma of the thyroid gland. Am. J. Med. 31:163–166, 1961.

    Case report and recognition of the association of pheochromocytoma with medullary carcinoma of the thyroid.

12. Anderson TE, Spackman TJ, Schwartz SS: Roentgen findings in intestinal ganglioneuromatosis: Its association with medullary thyroid carcinoma and pheochromocytoma. Radiology 101:93–96, 1971.

    Radiographic findings suggest a diagnosis of intestinal ganglioneuromatosis and multiple mucosal neuroma syndrome.

13. Gagel RF, Tashjian AH, Cummings T, et al.: The clinical outcome of prospective screening for multiple endocrine neoplasia 2a. An 8-year experience. N. Engl. J. Med. 318:478–484, 1988.

    A study of a large family comprising 117 members with multiple endocrine neoplasia 2a followed over a period of 18 years reaffirms the value of regular prospective screening and early treatment in reducing the morbidity and mortality of medullary thyroid carcinoma and pheochromocytoma in individuals with this disorder.

14. Allen DB, Friedman AL, Hendricks A: Asymptomatic primary hyperparathyroidism in children: Newer methods of preoperative diagnosis. Am. J. Dis. Child. 140:819–821, 1986.

    A report of an 11-year-old boy with asymptomatic primary hyperparathyroidism related to a parathyroid adenoma and a review of the diagnosis and management of this uncommon disorder of childhood.

15. Lang PJ Jr: The clinical spectrum of parathyroid disease. J. Am. Acad. Dermatol. 5:733–749, 1981.

    A comprehensive review of parathyroid disease, its clinical and cutaneous manifestations.

16. Wolfsdorf JI: Parathyroid disease. In Gellis SS, Kagan BM (Eds.): Current Pediatric Therapy 11. W. B. Saunders Co., Philadelphia 1984, 293–295.

    An authoritative review of the management of parathyroid disorders in childhood.

17. Gilchrest BA, Rowe JW, Brown RS, et al.: Ultraviolet phototherapy of uremic pruritus: Long-term results and possible mechanism of action. Ann. Intern. Med. 91:17–21, 1979.

    Uremic pruritus improved in 32 of 38 patients after a course of six to eight ultraviolet B exposures.

18. Taylor R, Taylor AEM, Diffey BL, et al.: A placebo-controlled trial of UV-A phototherapy for the treatment of uraemic pruritus. Nephron 33:14–16, 1983.

    A significant reduction of pruritus occurred in both the visible blue-light and UVA-treated groups of patients receiving phototherapy three times a week for 6 weeks.

19. Conley ME, Beckwith JB, Mancer JFK, et al.: Spectrum of the DiGeorge syndrome. J. Pediatr. 94:888–890, 1979.

A review of 25 patients with the DiGeorge syndrome in whom the diagnosis was established on the basis of autopsy reports and clinical records.

20. DiGeorge AM: The endocrine system. In Behrman RE, Vaughn VC III (Eds.): Nelson's Textbook of Pediatrics, 12th ed. W. B. Saunders Co., Philadelphia, 1983, 1432–1514.

An authoritative review of endocrine disorders, their diagnosis and management in children.

21. Blumberg DL, Sklar CA, David R, et al.: Acromegaly in an infant. Pediatrics 83:998–1002, 1989.

A report of a 21-month-old girl with acromegaly (the youngest verified case to date) in whom macrocephaly was the initial clinical feature of the disorder.

22. Garden JM, Robinson JK: Essential primary cutis verticis gyrata: Treatment with the scalp reduction procedure. Arch. Dermatol. 120:1480–1483, 1987.

A report of a patient with cutis verticis gyrata successfully treated with a scalp reduction procedure using a Y-shaped incision.

23. Orkin M, Frichot MC, Zelickson FS: Cerebriform intradermal nevus: A cause of cutis verticis gyrata. Arch. Dermatol. 110:575–582, 1974.

24. Lasser AE: Cerebriform intradermal nevus. Pediatr. Dermatol. 1:42–44, 1983.

A report of two patients with cerebriform intradermal nevi with an emphasis on the importance of early diagnosis and aggressive surgical excision and plastic reconstruction.

25. Bauer MF, Hirsch P, Bullock WK, et al.: Necrobiosis lipoidica diabeticorum. Arch. Dermatol. 90:558–566, 1964.

The relationship between necrobiosis and diabetic angiopathy.

26. Engel MF, Smith JG: The pathogenesis of necrobiosis lipoidica, a forme fruste of diabetes mellitus. Arch. Dermatol. 93:272–281, 1966.

The relationship between necrobiosis lipoidica and diabetes mellitus.

27. Quimby SR, Muller SA, Schroeter Al: The cutaneous immunopathology of necrobiosis lipoidica diabeticorum. Arch. Dermatol. 124:1364–1371, 1988.

Vascular deposits of immunoreactants in cutaneous vessels of involved and uninvolved skin in patients with necrobiosis lipoidica diabeticorum correlated with vascular changes demonstrated on histopathologic examination suggest the importance of vascular alterations as primary events in the pathogenesis of this disorder.

28. Huntley AC: The cutaneous manifestations of diabetes mellitus. J. Am. Acad. Dermatol. 7:427–455, 1982.

A comprehensive review of the dermatologic signs and symptoms of diabetes mellitus.

29. Hanke CW, Bergfeld WF: Treatment with benzoyl peroxide of ulcers on legs within lesions of necrobiosis lipoidica diabeticorum. J. Dermatol. Surg. Oncol. 4:701–704, 1978.

Terry cloth dressings impregnated with 20 per cent benzoyl peroxide lotion applied three times a day under Saran wrap occlusion resulted in complete healing of ulcers of necrobiosis lipoidica diabeticorum.

30. Eldor A, Diaz EG, Naparstek E: Treatment of diabetic necrobiosis with aspirin and dipyridamole. N. Engl. J. Med. 298:1033, 1978.

A report of a patient with necrobiosis lipoidica diabeticorum in whom treatment with aspirin (1 g/day) and dipyridamole (225 mg/day) resulted in complete healing within 6 weeks.

31. Littler CM, Tschen EH: Pentoxifylline for necrobiosis lipoidica diabeticorum. J. Am. Acad. Dermatol. 17:314–315, 1987.

Pentoxifylline, 400 mg orally three times a day, resulted in significant fading of lesions and healing of ulcers after 1 month of treatment in a 72-year-old diabetic woman with necrobiosis lipoidica diabeticorum.

32. Cantwell AR, Martz W: Idiopathic bullae in diabetics— bullosis diabeticorum. Arch. Dermatol. 96:42–44, 1967.

A review of the problem of bullous dermatosis in diabetes.

33. Bernstein JE, Medenica M, Soltani K, et al.: Bullous eruption of diabetes mellitus. Arch. Dermatol. 115;:324–325, 1979.

A 24-year-old man with severe diabetes experienced two episodes of bullae associated with intense ultraviolet exposure (perhaps associated with nephropathy rather than neuropathy).

34. Wells RS, Smith MA: The natural history of granuloma annulare. Br. J. Dermatol. 75:199–205, 1963.

Of 208 patients, 73 per cent cleared spontaneously within 2 years.

35. Romaine R, Rudner E, Altman J: Papular granuloma annulare and diabetes mellitus: Report of cases. Arch. Dermatol. 98:152–154, 1968.

Three patients with papular granuloma annulare and previously unrecognized diabetes mellitus.

36. Muhlbauer JA: Granuloma annulare. J. Am. Acad. Dermatol. 3:217–230, 1980.

A review of granuloma annulare, its pathogenesis, clinical presentation and therapy.

37. Muhlemann, MF, Williams DRR: Localized granuloma annulare is associated with insulin-dependent diabetes mellitus. Br. J. Dermatol. 110:325–329, 1984.

A prospective study of 577 patients with granuloma annulare, in contrast to an anticipated incidence of 0.9 per cent, revealed a 2.8 per cent incidence of insulin-dependent diabetes mellitus.

38. Friedman SJ, Winkelmann RK: Familial granuloma annulare: Report of two cases and review of the literature. J. Am. Acad. Dermatol. 16:600–605, 1987.

Two sisters with identical histocompatibility antigens and granuloma annulare suggests that the development of granuloma annulare among family members may represent a genetically infuenced cell-mediated immune response to an unknown antigen.

39. Dabski K, Winkelmann RK: Generalized granuloma annulare: Clinical and laboratory findings in 100 patients. J. Am. Acad. Dermatol. 20:39–47, 1989.

In a review of 100 biopsy-proved cases of generalized granuloma annulare, diabetes mellitus was diagnosed in 21% of patients in contrast to an incidence of 9.7 per cent in 1,350 patients with localized granuloma annulare and a 10.3 per cent incidence in 1,383 patients with all forms of granuloma annulare.

40. Izumi A: Generalized perforating granuloma annulare. Arch. Dermatol. 108:708–709, 1973.

In a report of a case of generalized perforating granuloma annulare in a 6-year-old girl the author suggests that children may be more prone to this variant of granuloma annulare.

41. Harpster EF, Mauro T, Barr R: Linear granuloma annulare. J. Am. Acad. Dermatol. 21:1138–1141, 1989.

A report of a patient with an unusual linear lesion with histologic features consistent with a diagnosis of granuloma annulare.

42. Ma A: Response of generalized granuloma annulare to high-dose niacinamide. Arch. Dermatol. 119:836–839, 1983.

A patient with generalized granuloma annulare experienced

resolution of her lesions after 6 months of treatment with niacinamide (1,500 mg/day).

43. Buckingham B, Perejda AJ, Sandborg C, et al.: Skin, joint and pulmonary changes in type I diabetes mellitus. Am. J. Dis. Child. *140*:420–423, 1986.

   Thickening, tightening, or a waxy quality of the skin were found in 190 (51 per cent) of 375 diabetic patients attending a summar camp.

44. Huntley AC: Finger pebbles: A common finding in diabetes mellitus. J. Am. Acad. Dermatol. *14*:612–617, 1986.

   In a survey of 60 patients with diabetes, 45 (75 per cent) were found to have a pebbly appearance of the knuckles and distal finger skin.

45. Vandersteen PR, Scheithauer BW: Glucagonoma syndrome: A clinicopathologic, immunocytochemical and ultrastructural study. J. Am. Acad. Dermatol. *12*:1032–1039, 1985.

   An excellent review of the glucagonoma syndrome and its clinical characteristics.

46. Riddle MC, et al.: Glucagonoma syndrome in a 19-year-old woman. West J. Med. *129*:68–72, 1978.

   A report of glucagonoma syndrome in a 19-year-old woman, the youngest case of this disorder apparently recorded to date.

47. Schwartz RA, Chorzelski TP: Glucagonoma syndrome. In Demis DJ (Ed): Clinical Dermatology, 18th ed., J.B. Lipincott, Co., Philadelphia, 1991, Unit 4-12A.

   A comprehensive review of the glucagonoma syndrome, its pathogenesis, clinical manifestations, and management.

22

INBORN ERRORS OF METABOLISM

The inborn disorders of metabolism are a group of hereditary diseases that are transmitted by mutant genes and result in various metabolic and clinical defects. Most of the severe errors of metabolism are transmitted by autosomal recessive genes requiring two heterozygous mates to produce a homozygous child manifesting the clinical disorder. The number of known inborn errors of metabolism is continually increasing, and many of them once thought to result from a simple enzymatic defect can now be subdivided into several distinct entities, each with different enzymatic deficiencies and varying clinical features.

PHENYLKETONURIA

Phenylketonuria (phenylpyruvic oligophrenia) is an autosomal recessive disorder of amino acid metabolism characterized by mental retardation, diffuse hypopigmentation, seizures, an eczematoid dermatitis, and photosensitivity (Table 22–1). Caused by a defect in the hydroxylation of phenylalanine to form tyrosine, the incidence of phenylketonuria has been estimated to be approximately 1 in 10,000 to 1 in 20,000 births, and it affects males and females with equal frequency.

Most commonly seen in individuals of northern European ancestry, 90 per cent of affected individuals are blond, blue eyed, and fair skinned. A peculiar musty odor, attributable to decomposition products (phenylacetic acid or phenylacetaldehyde) in the urine and sweat, is characteristic and by itself often suggests the diagnosis. Infants appear to be normal at birth and develop manifes-

tations of delayed intellectual development sometime between 4 and 24 months of age. Early symptoms may include severe vomiting to such a degree that pyloromyotomy has been carried out because of a misdiagnosis of pyloric stenosis. Skeletal changes include microcephaly, short stature, pes planus, and syndactyly. Eczematous dermatitis appears in 10 to 50 per cent of patients, and affected individuals may have indurated scleroderma-like skin changes. Although many patients have a typical flexural distribution of atopic dermatitis, others have an ill-defined, poorly described eczematous dermatitis that follows no specific pattern (Fig. 22–1).

The diagnosis of phenylketonuria depends on the demonstration of elevated serum levels of phenylalanine (20 mg/dl or higher, 10 to 50 times that of normal), normal or elevated levels of plasma tyrosine (normal is approximately 1 mg/dl), or elevated urinary levels of phenylpyruvic acid. The latter can be detected by a characteristic green or blue color that results when a few drops of urine are added to a 10 per cent solution of ferric chloride. Since diagnosis and initiation of dietary treatment of classic phenylketonuria must be completed before the child is 30 days of age if developmental retardation is to be prevented, most newborns in North America and Europe are screened by the Guthrie test (a bacterial inhibition assay method in which several drops of capillary blood obtained by heel stick may indicate an elevated level of phenylalanine).

Management consists of a diet low in phenylalanine content starting at as early an age as possible. This can be initiated by the use of products such as

Table 22–1. ERRORS OF METABOLISM

Disorder	Inheritance	Defect	Clinical Features	Diagnosis	Treatment
Phenylketonuria	Autosomal recessive (1 in 10,000 to 20,000 births)	Phenylalanine hydroxylase	90% are blond, blue-eyed and fair skinned; musty odor; eczematous dermatitis; photosensitivity; mental retardation; microcephaly; short stature	Guthrie test, Ferric chloride test, Phenistix	Low phenylalanine diet
Homocystinuria	Autosomal recessive (1 in 200,000 live births)	Cystathionine synthetase	Ectopia lentis, myopia, arachnodactyly in 50%, seizures, mental retardation, cerebrovascular accidents, sparse light or blond easily friable hair, malar flush, widepored facies, "Charlie Chaplin–like" gait and "rocker-bottom" feet	Cyanide nitroprusside test	Low methionine diet with pyridoxine (vitamin B_6)
Alkaptonuria (ochronosis)	Autosomal recessive (1 in 3 to 5 million individuals)	Homogentisic acid oxidase	Dark urine; blue to brownish black pigment on nose, malar region, sclerae, ears, axillae, genitalia; staining of clothing (beads of ink-like perspiration); arthritis; contractures; rupture of Achilles tendon; mitral and aortic valvulitis and/or calcific aortic stenosis	Ferric cyanide reduction	Low protein (low phenylalanine low tyrosine) diet with added ascorbic acid
Wilson's disease (hepatolenticular degeneration)	Autosomal recessive	Abnormal ceruloplasmin metabolism	Kayser-Fleischer rings, hyperpigmentation of legs, azure lunulae, neurologic and hepatic dysfunction	Aminoaciduria, decreased or absent ceruloplasmin	Chelating agents (BAL, versenate, or D-penicillamine)

Hurwitz S: The Skin and Systemic Disease in Children. Year Book Medical Publishers, Chicago, 1985.

Lofenalac (Mead Johnson), a casein hydrolysate formula from which most of the phenylalanine has been removed, or a synthetic amino acid preparation devoid of phenylalanine such as Phenyl-Free (Mead Johnson). When kept on appropriate restriction of phenylalanine, the patient becomes free of seizures, the electroencephalogram reverts to normal, the eczema clears, and the skin and hair regain their normal color. The effect of treatment on intellectual function, however, depends on the age at which therapy is initiated. With initiation of appropriate therapy within the first several weeks of life, preferably prior to 6 weeks to 2 months of age, normal mental development can usually be achieved. With delay in therapy beyond this period, the beneficial effect is lessened, and when therapy is started after 2 ½ years of age, little benefit can be achieved. However the diagnosis of phenylketonuria must be firmly established before treatment is initiated since phenylalanine restriction in infants without phenylpyruvic oligophrenia frequently produces dire results. As yet there is no agreement as to how long the low phenylalanine diet should be continued. In recent years many physicians have discontinued the diet when the patient reached 5 to 6 years of age. Others, however, believe that the diet should be maintained at least until adolescence and perhaps longer.[1, 2]

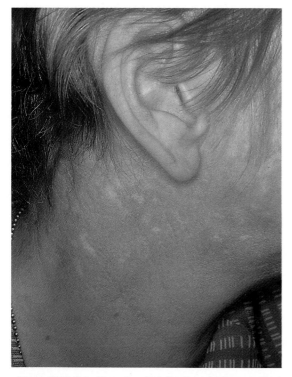

Figure 22–1. Fair skin and an ill-defined poorly circumscribed eczematous eruption in a patient with phenylketonuria.

HOMOCYSTINURIA

Homocystinuria is an autosomal recessive disorder of methionine metabolism associated with an absence or deficiency of cystathionine synthetase, the hepatic enzyme that catalyzes the formation of cystathionine from homocystine and serine. Common in Ireland (1 in 40,000 births) but rare elsewhere, with an overall incidence of less than 1 in 200,000 births, the disorder is characterized by ectopia lentis, arachnodactyly, chest and spinal deformities similar to those seen in Marfan's syndrome, seizures, developmental retardation, generalized osteoporosis, life-threatening vascular complications (occlusion of coronary, renal, and cerebral arteries), and increased urinary excretion of homocystine (see Table 22–1). The hallmark feature of this disorder, subluxation of the ocular lenses, occurs in most patients by the age of 10 years.

The typical appearance of affected individuals usually develops during the first or second year of life. It consists of sparse, light or blond, easily friable hair; malar flush; a coarse, wide-pore appearance of the facial skin; and erythematous blotches (cutis reticulata) on the skin of the face and extremities suggestive of livedo reticularis. The skin has been described as thin, and children may become quite flushed with exertion. Patients are usually tall and thin, resembling individuals with Marfan's syndrome. Bowed extremities are common, and arachnodactyly is reported to occur in about 50 per cent of cases. In addition, platyspondylia (congenital flattening of the vertebral bodies) and hollowing out of the vertebral bodies by pressure of the vertebral disks are seen on radiography; kyphoscoliosis, pectus carinatum; and genu valgum are common; some patients have rocker-bottom feet; and most have a shuffling toe-out "Charlie Chaplin–like" gait.

Central nervous system involvement is manifested by developmental retardation, which becomes evident within months to years after birth; and, although average intelligence has been reported in patients with homocystinuria, mental retardation may be severe by adolescence. Disturbances of gait are common, many electroencephalographic abnormalities may be noted, and severe focal or generalized seizures may occur. Other abnormalities include hepatomegaly, hyperinsulinemia with deranged carbohydrate metabolism, and inguinal hernia. Focal neurologic signs may develop as the result of cerebrovascular accidents, and life-threatening vascular complications, probably initiated by damage to vascular endothelium, may occur at any age, presenting a persisting mortal threat; nearly one fourth of patients die of vascular disease before the age of 30.

The presence of homocystinuria is suggested by the clinical features and can be confirmed by a urinary cyanide-nitroprusside test and by amino acid chromatography of the serum and urine. Unfortunately, there are no neonatal manifestations of homocystinuria and not all newborns with this disorder have increased blood methionine levels. The cyanide-nitroprusside test, when positive, consists of a beet red color indicating the presence of a compound containing a sulfhydryl group. A positive test result should be followed by a quantitative analysis of the amino acids of the urine, and the presence of homocystine in the urine establishes the diagnosis.

The treatment of homocystinuria consists of a low methionine diet, supplemented with cystine and folate, and approximately half of the patients with this disorder will respond to oral supplements of pyridoxine, a cofactor for cystathionine synthetase, in dosages of 50 to 1,000 mg/day. As with phenylketonuria, effective treatment depends on early diagnosis and early institution of therapy.[3–5]

ALKAPTONURIA (OCHRONOSIS)

Alkaptonuria (ochronosis) is a rare inborn error of tyrosine metabolism in which homogentisic acid, an intermediate product in the metabolic pathway of phenylalanine and tyrosine degradation, accumulates in the tissues and is excreted in the urine because of a lack of homogentisic acid oxidase, an enzyme normally found in the liver and kidney. A rare autosomal recessive disorder with an incidence of 1 in 200,000 live births, the disorder is characterized by homogentisic aciduria, dark urine, blue to bluish brown or black-brown cartilaginous pigmentary changes, and, to some extent, dermal deposition of pigment (ochronosis), degenerative joint disease, and vascular abnormalities (see Table 22–1).

Although alkaptonuria can be detected in infancy by the presence of dark brown stains on urine-moistened diapers, the disorder is often inapparent until adulthood when degenerative joint disease develops. Homogentisic acid has an affinity for connective tissue and is polymerized to a blue to brownish black cutaneous pigmentation that becomes most apparent on the nose, the malar region of the face, the ears, axillae, genitalia, sclerae, eyelashes, and nail beds (this is termed *ochronosis*). The ears, besides appearing blue to blue-brown, also become tender and stiff from staining of the underlying cartilage.[6] Dusky pigmentation of the hands is associated with underlying discoloration of the tendons; the fingernails may appear blue to gray, and subcutaneous leg calcifications have been described. Perspiration, especially in the axillary, inguinal, and malar regions, may contain appreciable amounts of pigment that appear as beads of ink on the skin, with staining of the clothes as a presenting complaint.

Dark urine, a classic finding of this disorder, may not occur in every alkaptonuria patient. Oxidation of homogentisic acid in the urine to a melanin-like pigment is responsible for the brown-black color

change; alkalinization of the urine or diaper will hasten this phenomenon. This can be done simply by the addition of a 10 per cent sodium hydroxide solution to a wet diaper or by washing the diapers with an alkaline soap. Other causes of black or dark urine such as porphyria, bilirubinemia, myoglobinuria, and hematuria, however, should not be confused with alkaptonuria.

Spondylitis and osteoarthritis of the major weight-bearing joints, arthritic complications of alkaptonuria, are believed to be a direct result of the deposition of the black pigment in cartilage. Most debilitating is the progressive arthritis that begins in the fourth decade and is seen in about 50 per cent of older patients with alkaptonuria. Other complications include synovial effusions, contractures, calcification of intervertebral disks and large joints, and, at times, rupture of the Achilles tendon. Valvular changes secondary to pigment deposition and subsequent calcification may result in mitral and aortic valvulitis and/or calcific aortic stenosis,[6] and renal lesions leading to renal insufficiency and degenerative cardiovascular disease, seen as myocardial infarction, often lead to death in affected patients.

The treatment of alkaptonuria and ochronosis is best achieved by a low protein diet with dietary control of phenylalanine and tyrosine intake. Long-term application of this diet, however, is frequently impractical. Since vitamin C protects homogentisic acid against oxidation and thus may prevent deposition of the black polymer of homogentisic acid to tendons and cartilage, early institution of ascorbic acid therapy has been suggested as a possible means of decreasing pigment formation and deposition. The efficacy of this form of therapy, however, has not been established.

TRIMETHYLAMINURIA

Trimethylaminuria (the fish odor syndrome) is a metabolic disorder in which accumulation of trimethylamine in the sweat and urine gives rise to an unpleasant fishy odor to the skin, sweat, and urine. Associated with an inability of the liver to metabolize the normal amount of trimethylamine generated in the intestinal tract by bacterial degradation of choline and lecithin-containing foods such as fish, egg yolk, liver, kidney, soy beans, meat, wheat germ, milk, and yeast, since the excessive production of trimethylamine in patients with this disorder exceeds the capacity of the normal liver to demethylate or oxidize it to the nonodorous oxide, the trimethylamine excreted through the skin, lungs, and urine results in an unpleasant body odor similar to that of rotting fish.

Although relatively rare, when present, trimethylaminuria produces a very difficult situation for the patient, the patient's associates, and family. The diagnosis of trimethylaminuria can be confirmed by gas chromatography of aseptically collected urine, acidified to a pH of 2.0 with hydrochloric acid and kept frozen until the test is done; and treatment is best accomplished by avoidance and limitation of choline-containing foods such as milk, egg yolk, liver, kidney, soy beans, and·saltwater fish.[7-9]

HEPATOLENTICULAR DEGENERATION (WILSON'S DISEASE)

Hepatolenticular degeneration, an autosomal recessive abnormality in the hepatic excretion of copper that results in toxic accumulations of the metal in the liver, brain, and other organs, is characterized by a triad of progressive neurologic dysfunction, hepatic cirrhosis, and pathognomonic pigmentation of the corneal margins (the Kayser-Fleischer ring) (see Table 22–1). The disorder, caused by an inability of the body to synthesize normal amounts of ceruloplasmin, can be detected as early as 4 years of age but usually manifests during adolescence. Although initial signs of the disorder are generally neurologic (intention tremors, dysarthria, ataxia, incoordination, personality changes, and worsening school performance and handwriting), signs of liver insufficiency (jaundice, ascites, hepatomegaly, hematemesis, and spider angiomas) are frequently the first clinical features of this condition.[10]

Kayser-Fleischer rings are seen as dense golden brown or greenish brown pigmentation localized near the limbus of the cornea. Occurring in about 95 per cent of patients with this disorder and best visualized by side lighting and slit lamp examination, this discoloration is produced by the deposition of copper in Descemet's membrane at the periphery of the cornea. Once believed to be pathognomonic of Wilson's disease, Kayser-Fleischer rings may also be seen in other copper overload states such as primary cirrhosis, intrahepatic cholestasis of childhood (Byler's syndrome), and chronic active hepatitis. Blue or azure lunulae of the nails have been reported in individuals with this disorder, but also have been observed in normal individuals and as a complication of phenolphthalein or quinacrine ingestion and argyria. In addition, patients may manifest a vague greenish discoloration on the skin of the face, neck, and genitalia, and hyperpigmentation, due to increased melanin deposition, may also be seen on the anterior aspects of the lower legs with no increase in copper or iron in biopsy specimens of the skin.

Hepatolenticular degeneration is a progressive disease and, if untreated, is inevitably fatal, with death resulting from a complication of infection, hepatic disease, or liver failure. Treatment depends on removal of accumulated copper depositions in the body. Chelating agents such as D-penicillamine and zinc acetate (25 to 50 mg three times a day) are helpful, and trientine (triethylene tetramine dihydrochloride), another copper chelating agent, also appears to be effective in selected patients.[11] The dosage of penicillamine for children younger than 10 years of age is 0.5 to 0.75 g/day (in adults the dosage is 1.0 to 1.15 g/day) and, since discontinuation of therapy can result in rapid deterioration, treatment is lifelong. Penicillamine, however, can produce allergic or toxic reactions, fever, cutaneous rashes, leukopenia, thrombocytopenia, and elastosis perforans serpiginosa; and since penicillamine inhibits pyridoxine-dependent enzymes, patients should also be given daily supplements of vitamin B_6 (12.5 to 25.0 mg/day). In an effort to minimize copper deposition, patients should be encouraged to limit their ingestion of copper-rich foods such as liver, nuts, chocolate, cocoa, mushrooms, brain, shellfish, dried foods, and broccoli. Occasional dietary indiscretion, however, is of little significance if effective chelation is maintained.

LESCH-NYHAN SYNDROME

Lesch-Nyhan syndrome, an inherited disorder of purine metabolism affecting males, is characterized by mental retardation, choreoathetoid movements, self-mutilation, and gout-like manifestations of hyperuricemia.[12] A sex-linked (X-linked) disorder, Lesch-Nyhan syndrome is caused by a deficiency of hypoxanthine-guanine phosphoribosyl transferase (HG-PRTase) which leads to an overproduction of uric acid and the clinical features associated with this disorder (Table 22–2). Patients appear normal at birth and may develop normally for 6 to 8 months, the first recognizable sign of the disease often manifesting as a result of orange uric acid crystals (resembling grains of sand) in the diaper, as renal stones, or as hematuria during the early months of life.

The onset of cerebral manifestations may be subtle, with difficulty in sitting or standing without help, involuntary movements, dystonia, spasticity, and increased deep tendon reflexes. Although mental retardation may vary in degree it usually is severe, and abnormal behavior remains a striking characteristic of the disease. The main clinical feature of this disorder is a loss of tissue about the mouth or fingers that occurs, not because of an inability to feel pain, but as a result of the child's habit of compulsive self-destructive biting of these areas. In time, without adequate restraints, all of the lower lip that is accessible to the teeth may be chewed away. The face, fingers, and wrists may also be mutilated, and since young children frequently bite others (such as parents or nurses) particular caution should be exercised when handling children with this disorder.

Not to be confused with Riga-Fede disease, a benign disorder characterized by small sublingual ulcerations and at times ulcerations or amputation of the tip of the tongue by repetitive trauma induced by raking the underside of the tongue over the lower incisors, the Lesch-Nyhan syndrome can

Table 22–2. LESCH-NYHAN SYNDROME

1. X-linked
2. Hypoxanthine-guanine phosphoribosyl transferase (HG-PRTase) deficiency
3. Hyperuricemia, mental retardation, spastic cerebral palsy, choreoathetosis, and aggressive self-mutilating behavior
4. Orange uric acid crystals (resembling grains of sand) in diaper often first sign
5. Diagnosis: increased levels of uric acid in blood and urine
6. Allopurinol (100–300 mg/day) helpful

Hurwitz S: The Skin and Systemic Disease in Children. Year Book Medical Publishers, Chicago, 1985.

be confirmed by the clinical presentation and laboratory demonstration of increased levels of uric acid in the blood and urine. Heterozygous females may be detected by the presence of two populations of fibroblasts in tissue culture of fibroblasts grown from a skin biopsy, with only one cell-line showing the key enzyme. Management includes the use of allopurinol (in dosages of 100 to 300 mg/day in divided doses) in an effort to control uric acid levels, tophaceous deposits, nephropathy, and gouty arthritis. Physical restraints (hand bandages and elbow splints) may be used to help control the self-mutilating behavior of patients. Lip biting may require extraction of deciduous teeth, but permanent teeth should be spared, since lip biting usually diminishes with age.

BIOTIN DEFICIENCY

Biotin, part of the vitamin B complex, is required for the function of three carboxylase enzymes: (1) 3-methyl crotonyl-CoA carboxylase, essential for the catabolism of leucine; (2) propionyl CoA carboxylase, essential for the catabolism of isoleucine, threonine, valine, and methionine; and (3) pyruvic acid carboxylase, required for the gluconeogenesis and regulation of carbohydrate metabolism.[13] Biotin deficiency may be induced by a biotin-deficient diet: a diet in which patients ingest large quantities of raw egg white (which contains the protein avidin that binds to biotin, thus preventing its absorption in the intestine) and/or prolonged parenteral nutrition to which biotin has not been added (Table 22–3). The resulting deficiency is manifested by anorexia, lassitude, a pale tongue, grayish pallor of the skin, atrophy of the lingual papillae, anemia, muscle pains, dryness of the skin, and a scaly dermatitis, all of which disappear following biotin administration or by cooking, boiling, or steaming of egg white (which causes avidin to lose its biotin-binding capacity).

Besides nutritionally induced biotin deficiency, there are two metabolic biotin-responsive carboxylase deficiency disorders: an acute neonatal form and a juvenile form. The neonatal form appears in the first few weeks of life with metabolic acidosis,

ketosis, alopecia totalis, and a bright scaly erythematous rash. A result of deficient holocarboxylase synthetase activity, patients with this form of the disorder do not survive without the benefit of early diagnosis and treatment. The juvenile form of the disorder, which develops 2 or 3 months after birth, is the result of biotinidase deficiency, an autosomal recessive disorder in which patients have low levels of biotin in the blood and urine and impaired biotin absorption and/or transport. It is characterized by seizures, intermittent acidosis, recurrent infections, dermatitis (often periorificial, resembling acrodermatitis enteropathica) (Fig. 22–2), sparse hair (alopecia), keratoconjunctivitis, ataxia, hypotonia, and glossitis. Both disorders are complicated by life-threatening acidosis and massive ketosis.[14]

The diagnosis of biotin deficiency can be established by a decreased concentration of plasma biotin and an increase in the urinary metabolites 3-hydroxyisovaleric acid, 3-methylcrotonylglycine, 3-hydroxypropionic acid, methylcitric acid, and lactic acid. The neonatal form of biotin deficiency is fatal, but biotin deficiency associated with the ingestion of raw eggs, biotin-deficient parenteral therapy, and the juvenile form of the disorder can be treated by intravenous multivitamins containing 60 μg of biotin or by the oral administration of 10 mg of biotin daily.[13]

DISORDERS OF TYROSINE METABOLISM

Although the relationship of tyrosine to the synthesis of melanin has been well known since the early and mid-20th century, the effect of dietary tyrosine on the skin was not cited in the dermatologic literature until ophthalmologic and cutaneous involvement became recognzied as clinical features of tyrosinemia.[15] Clinical disorders of tyrosine metabolism include neonatal tyrosinemia, tyrosinemia I, and tyrosinemia II (the Richner-

Table 22–3. BIOTIN DEFICIENCY

1. Dietary (biotin deficient diet or ingestion of raw eggs)
2. Biotin-deficient parenteral therapy
3. Metabolic forms
   a. Neonatal (multiple carboxylase deficiency)
      1. Metabolic acidosis, ketosis, and erythematous rash
      2. Patients do not survive without early treatment
   b. Juvenile form (impaired biotin absorption and/or transport)
      1. Ataxia, hypotonia, seizures, intermittent acidosis, recurrent infections
      2. Periorificial dermatitis and alopecia
4. Diagnosis confirmed by low plasma biotin and an increase in urinary metabolites
5. Avoidance of raw eggs (for avidin-type) and intravenous or oral biotin supplementation

Hurwitz S: The Skin and Systemic Disease in Children. Year Book Medical Publishers, Chicago, 1985.

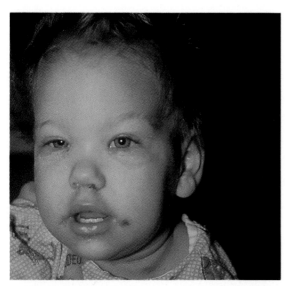

Figure 22–2. Scaly periorificial dermatitis in a child with biotin-responsive carboxylase deficiency. (Williams ML, Packman S, Cowan MJ: Alopecia and periorificial dermatitis in biotin-responsive multiple carboxylase deficiency. J. Am. Acad. Dermatol. 9:97–103, 1983.)

Hanhart syndrome) (Table 22–4). Of these, only the Richner-Hanhart syndrome exhibits cutaneous manifestations.

Neonatal Tyrosinemia. Infants (particularly those who have birth weights below 2500 g) exposed to high-protein diets may develop a syndrome of tyrosinemia, lethargy, and motor impairment termed *transient neonatal tyrosinemia*. A relative deficiency of p-hydroxyphenyl-pyruvate oxidase in premature infants has been hypothesized as the basis of this disorder. Data on the levels of this enzyme and tyrosine aminotransferase, however, are lacking since neonatal tyrosinemia is a self-limiting disorder and investigative studies would require liver biopsies, which would create a potential risk to this group of otherwise healthy infants. Affected infants can be treated by a low protein diet with, perhaps, ascorbic acid supplementation. Although urinary excretion of tyrosine and p-hydroxyphenylpyruvic acid may be aided by the administration of ascorbic acid, the efficacy of vitamin C supplementation for patients with this disorder remains questionable.

Tyrosinosis (Tyrosinemia I). Tyrosinosis is an autosomal recessive disorder characterized by failure to thrive, vomiting, diarrhea, and hepatomegaly. A deficiency in fumarylacetoacetate hydrolase, resulting in an increase in succinylacetone (a metabolite that interferes with cell growth and inhibits δ-aminolevulinic acid dehydratase), appears to be associated with the cause of this disorder. The acute form of tyrosinosis is caused by a severe enzyme deficiency and is associated with liver failure, a cabbage-like odor, and often death during the first year of life. In the milder chronic form,

patients have chronic liver disease with cirrhosis, renal tubular dysfunction with the de Toni-Fanconi syndrome, vitamin D–resistant rickets, acute intermittent porphyria-like symptoms, pancreatic islet cell hyperplasia, and hypoglycemia; and in more than one third of patients hepatomas may be present. The treatment of tyrosinemia I consists of a low-tyrosine, low phenylalanine, low methionine diet and liver transplantation for severe cirrhosis or hepatoma. Supplemental dietary cysteine has also been recommended, but its value remains questionable.[15]

Tyrosinemia II (Richner-Hanhart Syndrome). The Richner-Hanhart syndrome (tyrosinemia II, oculocutaneous tyrosinosis) is an autosomal recessive disorder that affects both sexes equally and is manifested by tyrosinemia, bilateral keratitis, photophobia, increased lacrimation, redness and inflammation of the eyes, dendritic ulcers, palmar and plantar hyperkeratosis and erosions, and, at times, profound mental retardation. A result of a deficiency of hepatic tyrosine aminotransferase, the disease is characterized by ocular, neurologic, and cutaneous features. Ophthalmic abnormalities, usually appearing during the first few months of life, often present as the first sign of this condition. They consist of photophobia, increased lacrimation, redness and inflammation of the eyes, dendritic ulcers, bilateral keratitis often leading to corneal opacities, and thick corneal and conjunctival plaques with increased vascularity.

Cutaneous changes appear shortly after the ocular lesions and, limited to the palms and soles (especially the distal phalanges and thenar and hypothenar eminences), they are manifested by

---

Table 22–4. DISORDERS OF TYROSINE METABOLISM

1. Neonatal tyrosinemia
   a. A relative deficiency of p-hydroxyphenyl-pyruvate oxidase in prematures
   b. Tyrosinemia, lethargy, and motor impairment
   c. May be treated by a low protein diet with ascorbic acid supplementation
2. Tyrosinosis (tyrosinemia I)
   a. Autosomal recessive inheritance
   b. A deficiency in fumarylacetoacetate hydrolase
   c. Failure to thrive, vomiting, diarrhea, cabbage-like odor, hepatomegaly, and often death in first year of life
   d. A milder form with chronic liver disease, renal tubular dysfunction (with the de Toni-Fanconi syndrome), vitamin D–resistant rickets, pancreatic islet cell hyperplasia, and (in one third of cases) hepatomas
   e. Treatment: a low tyrosine, low phenylalanine, and low methionine diet
3. Tyrosinemia II (Richner-Hanhart syndrome)
   a. Autosomal recessive
   b. Tyrosinemia, keratitis, palmar and plantar hyperkeratosis with erosions, and, at times, mental retardation
   c. Diagnosis confirmed by elevated levels of tyrosine in blood and urine and increased urinary tyrosine metabolites
   d. Treatment: low tyrosine, low phenylalanine diet (Low PHE-TYR Diet Powder, Mead Johnson Product 3200 AB)

Hurwitz S: The Skin and Systemic Disease in Children. Year Book Medical Publishers, Chicago, 1985.

tender annular erosions and blisters, often with crusting and hyperkeratosis (Fig. 22–3). Believed to be related to intracytoplasmic needle-shaped tyrosine crystalline inclusions,[16] the keratoses may vary from crusting and hyperkeratotic lesions 1 to 2 mm in diameter, sometimes in a linear configuration, to diffuse hyperkeratosis of the palms and soles. With pain a common feature, young children frequently prefer crawling rather than walking during the first few years of life.

Neurologic features vary from mild to moderate degrees of mental retardation. Since they can be prevented or modified by appropriate therapy, early diagnosis and treatment of this disorder is suggested. The diagnosis of tyrosinemia II is established by the clinical features and increased levels of tyrosine in the blood and urine of affected patients. Other laboratory abnormalities include elevated levels of urinary tyrosine metabolites (*p*-hydroxyphenylacetic acid, *p*-hydroxyphenylpyruvic acid, and *N*-acetyl tyrosine).

The lowering of plasma tyrosine levels can be initiated with a low-tyrosine, low-phenylalanine diet commercially available as Mead Johnson Low PHE-TYR Diet Powder (Product 3200 AB). With appropriate therapy, the ophthalmic and cutaneous manifestations clear over a few days to weeks. However, dietary management must not be termi-

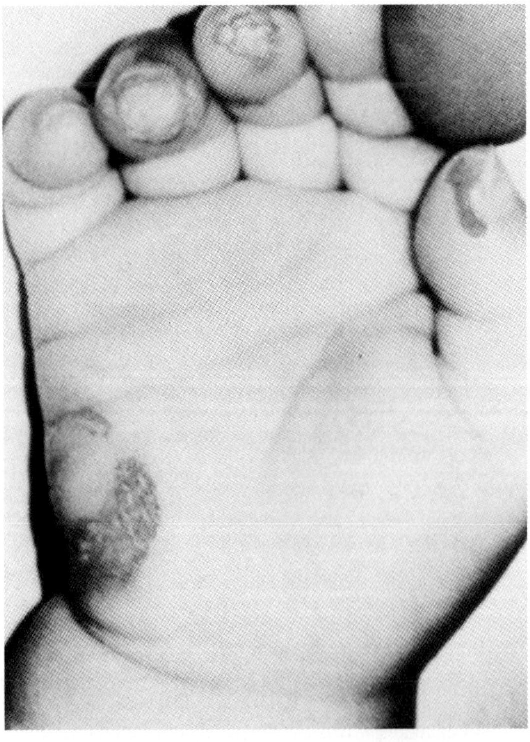

Figure 22–3. Erosions on the palm and fingertips in a child with tyrosinemia II (Richner-Hanhart syndrome). (Goldsmith LA: Tyrosinemia II. Lessons in molecular pathophysiology. Pediatr. Dermatol. 1:25–34, 1983.)

nated since discontinuation of therapy results in recurrence of exacerbations of the disorder.

ACRODERMATITIS ENTEROPATHICA

Acrodermatitis enteropathica is a hereditary disorder that generally appears in early infancy and is characterized by acral and periorificial vesiculobullous, pustular, and eczematoid skin lesions; alopecia; nail dystrophy; diarrhea; glossitis; stomatitis; behavior changes; and frequent secondary infection to bacterial or candidal organisms. Although the clinical characteristics of this disease were originally described by Danbolt and Closs in 1930, it was not until 1942 that they defined the disorder as a specific entity and, because of the acral distribution of skin lesions and associated gastrointestinal abnormalities, designated it by its present name.[17]

The inheritance pattern of acrodermatitis enteropathica is believed to be autosomal recessive with nearly equal incidence in male and female patients. Involvement in siblings, but not in parents, and a history of familial occurrence in 65 per cent of patients conforms to this suggested mode of transmission.[18]

The etiology of acrodermatitis enteropathica remained controversial until 1973 when Moynahan first demonstrated low serum zinc levels and a rapid response to the administration of zinc sulfate in patients with this disorder.[19, 20] Although many questions regarding the precise pathogenesis remain unanswered, the basic defect appears to be related to a gastrointestinal malabsorption of zinc. Three hypotheses have been proposed to explain reduced absorption of zinc in acrodermatitis enteropathica, but so far none has been satisfactorily documented. Moynahan has suggested that the malabsorption is caused by formation of an unabsorbable peptide–zinc complex in the intestinal lumen. Others suggest that the malabsorption is caused by a lack of zinc-binding ligands in the small intestine (the absorption of zinc in the intestine is believed to be assisted by a ligand that binds zinc and facilitates the transport of the trace element across the mucosa), or by trapping of zinc in the wall of the intestinal lumen[3] (it appears that the zinc-binding ligands absent from the child's intestine are supplied by the mother's breast milk). This best explains the frequency in which acrodermatitis enteropathica develops in breast-fed infants when breast-feeding is discontinued and cow's milk is introduced into the infant's diet.[21]

In addition to the classic inherited disease, syndromes of zinc deficiency mimicking acrodermatitis enteropathica may also occur in individuals receiving long-term parenteral nutrition with inadequate zinc supplementation,[22] patients who have had intestinal bypass procedures,[23] premature infants wtih low zinc storage (particularly those fed exclusively with human milk),[24, 25] as a complication of regional enteritis (Crohn's disease),[26] in infants with acquired immunodeficiency syndrome (AIDS) as a result of diarrhea (causing inadequate absorption of zinc),[27] in patients with cystic fibrosis with poor zinc absorption,[28] in chronic alcoholics with poor nutrition and individuals on zinc-deficient vegetarian diets,[29] and in patients with low pancreatic enzyme levels resulting in poor intestinal absorption of zinc.[30] Essential fatty acid deficiencies (manifested by periorificial dermatitis and a generalized xerotic or eczematous dermatitis) and biotin-carboxylase deficiency syndromes, as described earlier, can also produce a similar clinical picture.[31]

Clinical Manifestations. The triad of dermatitis, diarrhea, and alopecia classically appears at the time of weaning from breast to cow's milk. Although some patients are never diagnosed until adulthood, it appears that these individuals actually had their disease in a mild form during childhood. The onset of symptoms, therefore, usually begins early in life, generally between the age of 1 or 2 weeks to 20 months, with an average age of onset at 9 months.

Typically, infants with acrodermatitis enteropathica are listless, anoretic, and apathetic. Tissue wasting is present with an associated failure to thrive. During periods of exacerbation, frothy, bulky, foul-smelling diarrheal stools, typical of those in patients with celiac syndrome, are present. Other findings include conjunctivitis, photophobia, stomatitis, perlèche, recurring candidal or bacterial infection, and alopecia of the scalp, eyelashes and/or eyebrows. Children suffering from this disorder exhibit a striking uniformity of appearance, mainly because of the alopecia and periorificial lesions.

The syndrome usually begins with small moist erythematous lesions localized around the body orifices (mouth, nose, ears, eyes, and perineum) and symmetrically located on the buttocks and extensor surface of major joints (elbows, knees, hands, and feet), the scalp, and the fingers and toes (the acral aspect of this disorder) (Figs. 22–4 through 22–6). The cutaneous lesions are similar to those of severe candidiasis or pustular psoriasis, depending on the areas that are affected.

Drooling and change of hair color to red are additional findings seen during the active phase of the disease. Other features include growth retardation in 80 per cent and mental changes in the form of schizoid features, with frequent crying, irritability, and restlessness during periods of exacerbation in 40 per cent of patients.[17–19]

The basic cutaneous lesion of acrodermatitis enteropathica is a vesiculobullous eruption that arises from an erythematous base. The blisters quickly collapse and begin to dry and crust, and sharply marginated lichenified or psoriasiform plaques develop at these sites. On the face, the eroded and crusted peribuccal plaques may appear impetiginized, and secondary infection with *Candida albicans* is common. When the fingers and

toes are involved there is marked erythema and swelling of the paronychial tissues, often with subsequent nail deformity. If unrecognized or untreated, acrodermatitis enteropathica follows an intermittent but relentlessly progressive course and, as a consequence of general disability, infection, or both, frequently ends in death. Since patients suffer from frequent and persistent bacterial and candidal infection, it has been theorized that a zinc-dependent defect in chemotaxis may contribute to this susceptibility. These findings suggest an important role for zinc in neutrophil and monocyte chemotaxis and a correctable immune defect in patients with this disorder.[32]

The diagnosis of acrodermatitis enteropathica is based on the clinical features of a dermatitis localized around the body orifices, buttocks, extensor surfaces of the major joints, scalp, fingers, and toes; recurrent or persistent paronychias with nail dystrophy in association with the dermatitic features; recurrent infections; diarrhea; photophobia; irritability; failure to thrive; and low serum zinc levels. In addition, low serum alkaline phosphatase levels *(even when the serum zinc level is normal)*, low serum lipid levels, and defective chemotaxis may be found. Skin biopsy is not diagnostic and shows a variable picture dependent on the age and clinical appearance of the lesions. There may be hyperkeratosis, parakeratosis, intraepidermal pustules, spongiosis, acanthosis with downward projection of the rete pegs, and a mild polymorphic infiltrate in the upper region of the dermis. Although acrodermatitis may at times be seen in patients without

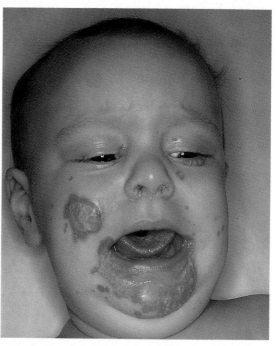

Figure 22–4. Moist erythematous plaques on the cheek and chin of a 7-month-old infant with acrodermatitis enteropathica.

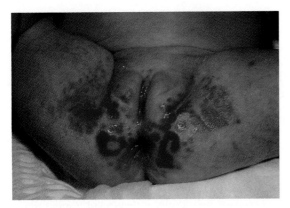

Figure 22–5. Characteristic reddish brown eczematoid plaques on the upper medial thighs and perianal areas of a 6-week-old infant with acrodermatitis enteropathica.

hypozincemia,[33] a decrease in zinc levels in plasma, erythrocytes, hair, and urine may be considered diagnostic (serum zinc levels of 70 to 110 μg/dl are considered normal and levels of 50 μg/dl or lower, the hallmark of acrodermatitis enteropathica, are diagnostic).[34] Blood zinc determinations should always be done prior to treatment to determine whether the patient truly has acrodermatitis enteropathica. It should be noted, however, that there may be sources of error caused by zinc contamination of glass tubes and rubber stoppers. Blood samples, therefore, should be collected in acid-washed sterile plastic tubes with the use of acid-washed plastic syringes.

Until the recognition of the role of zinc in the etiology of this disorder, diiodohydroxyquinoline, with or without breast milk, was the mainstay of therapy.[31, 33a, 35, 36] It now appears that the beneficial effects of diiodohydroxyquinoline, however, may have been a result of zinc contamination during the manufacturing of this preparation. Currently, zinc gluconate, acetate, or sulfate in dosages of 5 mg/kg/day, given in divided doses two or three times a day, is highly effective in the management of this disorder. With adequate therapy (usually 50 mg/day for infants and 150 to 200 mg/day for older children), improvement in temperament and decrease in irritability can generally be noted within 1 or 2 days, the appetite improves in a few days, and diarrhea and skin lesions begin to respond within 2 or 3 days after the initiation of therapy.[35] Hair growth begins after 2 to 3 weeks of therapy, and increase in the growth of the infant generally occurs within approximately 2 weeks. Available in tablets containing 15 mg of elemental zinc (the amount of elemental zinc is usually listed on the product label as the zinc equivalent), zinc sulfate or gluconate tablets may be crushed and mixed in syrup by the pharmacist or given in fruit juice and, generally well tolerated by patients, provide a safe and highly effective form of therapy for this severe and at times fatal disorder of infancy and childhood. Since dietary

sources of zinc include meat, fish, poultry, eggs, and dairy products, variations in intake of these foods may account for variations in zinc levels and the amount of supplemental zinc required to control the disorder and maintain appropriate serum zinc levels. After the patient's condition appears to be stabilized, therefore, zinc levels should be monitored at periodic (6- to 12-month) intervals, followed by the adjustment of supplemental zinc to the lowest effective dosage schedule, and since foods have a major although variable effect on the absorption of zinc, it appears to be prudent that zinc be administered 1 or 2 hours before meals.

THE HYPERLIPIDEMIAS

The hyperlipidemias (hyperlipoproteinemias) represent a group of metabolic diseases characterized by persistent elevation of plasma cholesterol levels, triglyceride levels, or both. Since plasma lipids circulate in the form of high-molecular-weight complexes bound to protein, the term *hyperlipidemia* also indicates an elevation of lipoproteins, hence justification for introduction of the term *hyperlipoproteinemia* for this group of disorders.

Plasma lipoproteins differ significantly in electrostatic charges, thus permitting their separation by electrophoretic techniques into four major fractions (chylomicrons and β-, pre-β-, and α-lipoproteins). By means of ultracentrifugation it is also possible to separate the plasma lipoproteins into four major groups (chylomicrons and very low density, low density, and high density lipoproteins), which correlate well with those separated by electrophoresis. These techniques allow classification of the familial hyperlipidemias into five groups, designated as hyperlipoproteinemias I through V, each with its own specific clinicopathologic, prognostic, and therapeutic features (Table 22–5).[37–39]

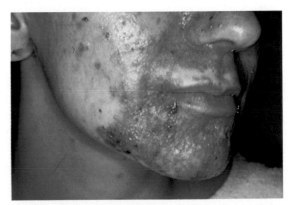

Figure 22–6. Periorificial eruption of acrodermatitis enteropathica. (Braverman IM: Skin Signs of Systemic Disease. W.B. Saunders Co., Philadelphia, 1970.)

Clinical Manifestations. Xanthomas are lipid-containing papules, nodules, or tumors that may be found anywhere on the skin and mucous membranes. Although the mechanism of their formation is not completely understood, it appears that serum lipids infiltrate the tissues where they are phagocytized by macrophages (histiocytes) and deposited, particularly in areas subjected to stress and pressure. Although they may suggest the presence of hyperlipidemia and can provide clues to the underlying disorder, when seen alone they are not diagnostic. Complete clinical and biochemical evaluations, therefore, are required before the true nature of the underlying disorder can be determined. Depending on their gross appearance, anatomic location, and mode of development, xanthomas can be categorized as *plane, eruptive* or *papuloeruptive, tendinous,* or *tuberous.* Recognition of these lesions is important inasmuch as they present visible cutaneous clues to possible metabolic abnormalities and frequently assist in diagnosis of specific metabolic disease entities.

Plane (Planar) Xanthomas. Soft, flat, macular, or slightly elevated, yellow to orange or brownish yellow, intracutaneous, macular, or slightly elevated plaques, plane xanthomas are generally seen on the face, sides of the neck, upper trunk, elbows, and knees, but may occur anywhere on the body and have a marked predilection for surgical or acne scars and the palmar creases. The most frequently seen xanthomas are those that occur on or near the eyelids during middle age. Termed *xanthelasmas* or *xanthoma palpebrarum,* they rarely occur in children or adolescents. When present, however, they require studies for diabetes mellitus, Hand-Schüller-Christian disease, myeloma, and hepatic or liver disorders; a search for xanthomas elsewhere on the body; and an investigation of plasma lipids for evidence of familial hyperlipidemia. Although approximately two thirds of individuals with xanthelasma may have normal lipid levels, these cutaneous lesions may prove to be the first clues to the presence of hyperlipoproteinemia type II disease. If the physician is to prevent the vascular consequences of type II disease, it is helpful if the disorder is detected early. Lesions that develop in palmar creases and flexural surfaces of the fingers, termed *xanthoma striatum planum,* generally portend the presence of hepatic disease or familial hyperlipidemia (types II and III).

Eruptive (Papuloeruptive) Xanthomas. These lipoidal lesions appear in crops and consist of multiple 1-mm to 4-mm red to yellow-orange papules sometimes surrounded by an erythematous base. Although they may involve the trunk and oral mucosa, they have a predilection for sites subjected to pressure or trauma, particularly the extensor surfaces of the arms, legs, and buttocks.[40] Papuloeruptive xanthomas are almost always associated with hypertriglyceridemia and are generally seen in patients with uncontrolled diabetes mellitus, in mild diabetics who are asymptomatic yet have high triglyceride levels, in patients with nephrotic syndrome,[41] or in patients with hyperlipoproteinemia I, III, IV, and V (Fig. 22–7).

Tendinous Xanthomas. Multiple skin-colored or yellowish, smooth, freely movable subcutaneous nodules and tumors, tendinous xanthomas have a predilection for the extensor tendons of the elbows, knees, heels, hands, and feet. These nontender, firm nodules measure 1 cm or more in diameter and are best seen or palpated on the Achilles tendon and the tendons on the dorsal aspect of the hands. They frequently occur in association with xanthelasma, tuberous lesions, and coronary atherosclerosis, usually occur in patients with hypertriglyceridemia, generally indicate the presence of hypercholesterolemia, and appear almost exclusively in patients with familial liproproteinemia type II and III.[3, 42]

Tuberous (Tuberoeruptive) Xanthomas. Large, firm, nodular or tumorous, sessile or pedunculated, flesh-colored or yellowish to red, tuberous xanthomas are lipid deposits that occur on the palms and extensor surfaces subject to stress or trauma, particularly the elbows, knees, hands, and buttocks. Located in the dermis and subcutaneous layers, they can enlarge to 5 cm or more in diameter and, in contrast to tendon xanthomas, are not attached to underlying structures. Generally associated with increased serum triglycerides (either on an acquired or familial basis), tuberous xanthomas are most frequently seen in association with types II, III, and IV lipoproteinemia.[43]

Other xanthomas, not part of the hyperlipoproteinemia spectrum, include *xanthoma dissemina-*

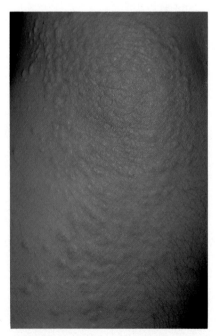

Figure 22–7. Eruptive xanthomas on the knee in a 13-year-old child with type III lipoproteinemia. (Courtesy of Department of Dermatology, Yale University School of Medicine.)

tum, an uncommon clinical entity characterized by red-yellow or mahogany-colored papular and nodular lesions with a predilection for the flexural creases (see Chapter 24), and *verruciform xanthomas,* a rare disorder manifested by solitary 0.2- to 2.0-cm verrucous papillary or flat to lichenoid, gray to reddish pink, sessile, occasionally pedunculated lesions most commonly seen on the oral mucosa and lips and occasionally on the penis, scrotum, vulva, groin, digits, nostrils, and areas of epidermal hyperplasia such as epidermal nevi (Fig. 22–8). Although the cause is unknown, current evidence suggests that verruciform xanthomas represent a reaction pattern initiated by an irritating or traumatic event.[44–47] Histologic examination of verruciform xanthomas reveals a uniform hyperkeratosis with a slightly papillated surface, acanthosis, marked elongation of the rete ridges extending to a uniform level in the dermis, and large foam cells identical to the foamy histiocytes that characterize xanthomas. Verruciform xanthomas are not associated with any underlying metabolic disorder and tend to persist indefinitely; although therapy is generally unnecessary and recurrences are common, local surgical excision is almost always curative.

Classification. The classification of the hyperlipidemic disorders is based on the classification by Fredrickson and Lees. Based on electrophoretic and ultracentrifugal analyses of serum lipoproteins, they are designated as type I, hyperchylomicronemia; type II, increased betalipoprotein; type III, increased beta- and prebetalipoprotein; type IV, increased prebetalipoprotein; and type V, combined hyperchylomicronemia and hyperprebetalipoproteinemia (of these, types I and II are the most common in childhood) (see Table 22–5).

Type I Hyperlipoproteinemia (Bürger-Grütz Disease). A rare autosomal recessive disorder, type I hyperproteinemia is characterized by an elevation of fasting serum triglycerides carried in the form of chylomicrons. The defect in type I disease, expressed as soon as the infant takes fat, probably lies in the faulty removal of normal chylomicrons from the serum because of a deficiency of lipoprotein lipase activity. Hyperlipemia is usually discovered accidentally because of lactescence (manifested by a creamy or chocolate appearance of whole blood), or because of the appearance of xanthomas, bouts of abdominal pain, or hepatic and splenic enlargements. Occasionally the disease may be noted for the first time during examination of a patient presenting with severe abdominal pain and signs of peritoneal irritation.

Episodic abdominal pain, seen in approximately one half of affected children, is very common and frequently manifested by clinical signs of acute abdominal distress. General malaise and anorexia are common, and abdominal spasm, rigidity, rebound tenderness, leukocytosis, and fever may be present. Sometimes, particularly in patients younger than the age of 6 years, the pain is caused by lipid accumulations in the liver and spleen. In others it may be due to splenic infarct or pancreatitis associated with this disorder.

About two thirds of children with type I disease are seen with xanthomas that, in almost all cases, are of the eruptive type. They may appear at any site, including the mucous membranes, and are most commonly seen on the buttocks, thighs, arms, forearms, chest, back, and face. Xanthelasmas and tendinous xanthomas account for less than 2 per cent of the lesions seen in such patients. Eruptive xanthomas usually occur suddenly when the hyperlipemia is severe and resolve rapidly when the chylomicrons decrease after institution of a low-fat diet.

Type II Hyperlipoproteinemia (Familial Hypercholesterolemia). Best understood and most important from a pediatric point of view, type II hyperlipoproteinemia is an autosomal dominant disorder characterized by cutaneous xanthomas, increased concentrations of plasma cholesterol, and a high incidence of coronary artery disease.

Seen in approximatly 1 in 250 to 500 persons in the general population, there are two groups of patients with type II disease. In patients homozygous for this disorder plasma cholesterol levels are extremely high (often reaching 700 to 1000 mg/dl). Cutaneous xanthomas usually develop during childhood, often in the first years of life, and affected individuals frequently die of ischemic heart disease in their 20s and 30s. In a second group, affected persons are presumably heterozygous for this disorder. They develop tendon xanthomas (usually after age 30), and even though serum cholesterol levels are markedly elevated, patients have a normal longevity without a significant increase in atherosclerosis and coronary heart disease.

Although the exact defect in type II disease is as yet not completely understood, it appears to be related to a derangement of cholesterol metabolism. Studies suggest deficiency of hydroxymethylglutaryl coenzyme A reductase (HMG-CoA reduc-

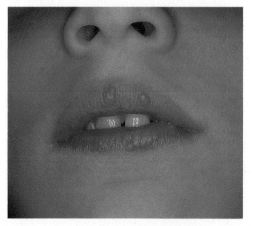

Figure 22–8. Xanthoma verruciformis on the lips of a 5-year-old girl.

Table 22–5. THE HYPERLIPOPROTEINEMIAS

Type	Clinical Features	Biochemical Features	Inheritance
I (Bürger-Grütz)	Common in infancy and early teens Episodic abdominal pain Eruptive xanthomas Lipemic plasma Lipemia retinalis	Exogenous fat-induced hyperlipemia	Autosomal recessive
II (Familial hypercholesterolemia)	Onset in childhood or adulthood Crops of eruptive xanthomas, tendinous and tuberous xanthomas Xanthelasma Atherosclerosis and coronary disease	High cholesterol levels	Autosomal dominant
III (Broad-beta disease)	Onset in adulthood (uncommon in childhood) Plane xanthomas in palmar creases A high incidence of cardiovascular disease	Endogenous hyperlipemia Abnormal glucose tolerance Increased cholesterol, β-lipoproteins, and triglycerides	Autosomal recessive
IV (Familial hyperbetalipoproteinemia)	Unusual before age 20 Eruptive tuberous xanthomas on elbows, knees, heels, and wrists Obesity Hepatosplenomegaly Abdominal pain Lipemia retinalis Premature cardiovascular disease	Endogenous carbohydrate-induced hyperlipidemia Laboratory findings similar to those in type III	Autosomal recessive
V (Familial hyperchylomicronemia with hyperbetalipoproteinemia)	Combination of types I and IV Rare in childhood Eruptive and tuberous xanthomas Obesity Hepatosplenomegaly Lipemia retinalis	Exogenous and endogenous Increase in both chylomicrons and pre-β-lipoproteins	(?) Recessive inheritance

tase) with an associated defect in fibroblast cell receptors that bind β-lipoproteins, with a resulting elevation of plasma β-lipoprotein and cholesterol.

Cutaneous xanthomas reportedly occur in 40 to 50 per cent of patients with type II disease. These include tendinous xanthomas in 40 to 50 per cent of cases, xanthelasmas in 23 per cent, and tuberous lesions in 10 to 15 per cent of affected individuals. Large pendulous tuberous xanthomas may occur in children with this disorder; eruptive xanthomas, however, are unusual.

Arcus cornea (also termed *arcus lipoides* or *arcus juvenilis*), consisting of lipid deposits of cholesterol, triglycerides, and phospholipids around the edge of the cornea, is commonly seen in association with this disease. The significance of arcus cornea depends on the age of the patient. When seen in childhood, it is almost always a sign of hyperlipoproteinemia.

Type III Hyperlipoproteinemia (Familial Hyperbeta- and Prebetalipoproteinemia). Often referred to as broad-beta disease, type III hyperlipoproteinemia is an autosomal recessive disorder characterized by xanthomas, a high incidence of cardiovascular disease, frequent abnormal tolerance to glucose, and an increase in serum levels of both cholesterol and triglycerides. The precise na-

ture of type III disease is unknown, but it appears to be associated with a disturbance in the clearance of remnant lipoproteins, with accumulations of both cholesterol and triglycerides. It is uncommon in childhood and nearly always first diagnosed in adulthood (usually around middle age) (see Fig. 22–7).

Electrophoresis of plasma proteins shows a broad beta band. Seventy-five to 80 per cent of patients with this disorder have xanthomas. They may include the full range of xanthomatous lesions from eruptive xanthomas to tendinous nodules. Soft planar xanthomas (striatum palmare) in the palmar creases are a very common feature of familial type III hyperlipoproteinemia. However, since they may also be seen in individuals with the type II disorder and in patients with liver disease, they are not an exclusive feature of type III hyperlipoproteinemia. Atherosclerotic vascular complications are common in patients with type III disease. Although both coronary and peripheral artery diseases may occur, the latter are relatively more common in patients with type III as compared with type II forms of this disorder.

Type IV Disease (Familial Hyperbetalipoproteinemia). The most common form of familial hyperlipoproteinemia, type IV, is an endogenous carbohydrate-induced disorder (in contrast to type I, which is fat-induced). Characterized by obesity and elevation of serum prebetalipoproteins, type IV disease may be familial or acquired. The familial type appears to be inherited as an autosomal dominant disease. Usually not seen before the age of 20 years, type IV hyperlipoproteinemia may appear in children with renal disease or in diabetics who have become ketotic. The cutaneous lesions seen with this disorder are eruptive, tuberous, and palmar. Cardiovascular disease is extremely common and hepatosplenomegaly, abdominal pain, and lipemia retinalis may occur.[39]

Type V Disease (Familial Hyperchylomicronemia with Hyperprebetalipoproteinemia). A combination of type I and type IV disease, type V is a complex abnormality of both endogenous and exogenous origin characterized by increased concentrations of both chylomicrons and prebetalipoproteins. Although the exact mode of inheritance is still unclear, it appears to be a recessive disorder. Patients are usually obese, and their lipemia is often discovered in late adolescence or early adulthood because of the eruptive xanthomas, hepatosplenomegaly, and acute abdominal crises similar to those seen in individuals with type I disease. Although type V hyperlipoproteinemia may have its onset in adolescence, it has only rarely been reported in childhood.[48]

TANGIER DISEASE

Tangier disease (familial high density lipoprotein deficiency) is a unique rare heritable disorder characterized by hypocholesterolemia, an almost complete absence of plasma high density lipoprotein, and storage of cholesterol esters in many tissues of the body. Seen in children as well as adults, it derives its name from the Chesapeake Bay island home of the first two patients described with this disorder.

The biochemical defect of Tangier disease is uncertain but appears to be related to a defect in the synthesis of high-density lipoprotein associated with a double dose of a rare mutant gene. The clinical manifestations include hypocholesterolemia (50 to 125 mg/dl) and low phospholipid levels in association with normal or slightly elevated triglyceride levels (150 to 250 mg/dl) and enlarged tonsils with distinctive alternating bands of red, orange, or yellowish white striations overlying the normal red mucosa. Lipid deposits may be accompanied by a persistent maculopapular eruption over the trunk and abdomen, hepatosplenomegaly, lymph node enlargement, infiltration of the cornea in adults, and alterations in the intestinal and rectal mucosa. Several patients have had recurrent peripheral neuropathy.

The prognosis in Tangier disease is unknown. Children may have no detectable abnormality except in the tonsils and plasma. Adults, however, have shown more extensive cholesterol ester deposition in the rectal mucosa, skin, and cornea.[39]

THE ALAGILLE SYNDROME

The Alagille syndrome (arteriohepatic dysplasia, Watson-Alagille syndrome) is a disorder in which affected infants have congenital intrahepatic biliary hypoplasia, cholestasis, hyperlipidemia, hypercholesterolemia, xanthomatosis, ocular defects, vertebral anomalies (butterfly vertebrae), cardiac and renal abnormalities, often with a characteristic facies, and, at times, physical and mental retardation. Although its inheritance is uncertain, familial transmission has been reported. Clinical features include an atypical facies (prominent forehead, hypertelorism, eyes deeply set in orbits, atrophy of the iris, a pointed, bulbous or saddle-shaped nose, and a sharply pointed chin), occasional porphyria cutanea tarda–like photosensitivity, cardiovascular disease (generally pulmonic stenosis), vertebral abnormalities, hypogonadism, biliary hypoplasia, hypercholesterolemia, jaundice, and pruritus. Although the overall syndrome is distinctive, none of the features (except the hepatic anomaly) is invariably present. Death prior to 5 years of age due to cardiac failure, renal failure, or both, has occurred, but the prognosis of children with the Alagille syndrome is generally better than that of patients with congenital biliary atresia (in whom survival to 2 years of age is unusual).[49, 50]

THE MUCOPOLYSACCHARIDOSES

The mucopolysaccharidoses are inherited disorders of mucopolysaccharide metabolism characterized by widespread accumulation of mucopolysaccharide (the major component in the ground substance of connective tissue) in tissues and cultured skin fibroblasts, with excessive excretion in the urine. First described by Hunter in 1917 (and labeled "gargoylism" in 1936), these disorders can now be divided into at least six somewhat related clinical entities on the basis of their clinical features, their mode of inheritance, and the nature of the accumulated mucopolysaccharide.[51–53]

Although the precise biochemical defect is still not well understood, current evidence suggests a deficiency of β-galactosidase, leading to abnormal accumulation of mucopolysaccharides in cells of the connective tissue and many organs.[53] The usual distinguishing features of the various syndromes of mucopolysaccharidosis (MPS), therefore, are based on the presence or degree of somatic and skeletal involvement, mental retardation, corneal clouding, cardiopulmonary changes, hepatosplenomegaly, and hearing loss, and on the mode of inheritance and the nature of their accumulated polysaccharides (Table 22–6). Hunter's syndrome (MPS II) is an X-linked recessive disorder; all others are autosomal recessive. They can be differentiated from the mucolipidoses, a group of disorders characterized by an accumulation of sphingolipids or glycolipids in the visceral and mesenchymal cells, which exhibit clinical and skeletal signs of the mucopolysaccharidoses but differ from them by the normal urinary excretion of uronic acid containing acid mucopolysaccharides (with the exception of mucosulfatidosis), and by the presence of clinical features usually seen in the sphingolipidoses (Niemann-Pick disease and Gaucher's disease).

The cutaneous changes of all six forms of mucopolysaccharidosis consist of pale, coarse, and dry skin with hirsutism, especially over the back and extremities, and thickened, roughened, taut inelastic skin, especially over the fingers.

Hurler's Syndrome. The most common of the mucopolysaccharidoses, Hurler's syndrome (mucopolysaccharidosis I-H, MPS I in McKusick's original classification), is the classic prototype of this group of disorders. Seen in approximately 1 in 100,000 births, it appears in the first year of life and is a particularly grave disorder, with death occurring in almost all cases before the age of 10 years usually from cardiac failure or respiratory infection.

Cardinal features of the Hurler syndrome include coarsening of facial features; macrocephaly with frontal bulging; premature closure of the sutures, with hyperostosis frequently leading to a scaphocephalic skull; flattened nasal bridge with a saddle-shaped appearance; hypertelorism; pro-tuberant tongue; short neck; protuberant abdomen due to hepatic and splenic enlargement; deformity of the chest; shortness of the spine; laxity of the abdominal wall with inguinal and umbilical hernias; broad hands with stubby fingers; a claw hand due to stiffening of the phalangeal joints; limitation of extensibility of the joints; severe, progressive mental retardation; and marked retardation of growth. Although the majority of infants are normal or above normal in length during the first year of life, growth rate decreases by 2 years of age. By age 3 almost all patients are below the third percentile for stature. Clouding of the cornea develops in all patients with Hurler's syndrome. On inspection this feature is most apparent if light is shone on the cornea from the side (slit lamp examination confirms the finding).

Diagnosis is based on the clinical picture and identification of excessive mucopolysaccharides in the urine by the toluidine blue test and the gross albumin turbidity test. Routine histopathologic examination of the skin shows vacuolization of the cytoplasm in some of the epidermal cells (due to mucopolysaccharide), with displacement of the nucleus to one side, and occasional solitary swollen cells at all levels of the epidermis. Large vacuolated mononuclear cells ("gargoyle cells") are present beneath the basement membrane as well as in the periappendageal and perivascular areas.

As yet there is no effective definitive treatment of mucopolysaccharidosis. Although initial reports

Table 22–6. THE MUCOPOLYSACCHARIDOSES

Syndrome	Clinical Features	Biochemical Features	Inheritance
Hurler (MPS I–H)	Severe retardation Corneal clouding Hepatosplenomegaly Chondrodystrophy Dwarfism Grave manifestations and early death	Chondroitin sulfate B, heparan monosulfate Excessive urinary excretion of dermatan sulfate and heparan sulfate	Autosomal recessive
Scheie (MPS I–S; formerly MSP V)	Corneal clouding Severe osteochondro-dystrophy Aortic incompetence Retinitis pigmentosa	Keratosulfate Excessive urinary excretion of dermatan sulfate and heparan sulfate	Autosomal recessive
Hunter (MPS II)	Less severe than Hurler Longer survival Lack of corneal involvement Cutaneous markers over scapula, posterior axilla, or thigh Atypical retinitis pigmentosa	Chondroitin sulfate B, heparan monosulfate	X-linked recessive
Sanfilippo (MPS III)	Aggressive behavior Severe neurologic involvement Mild somatic changes	Heparitin monosulfate Excessive urinary excretion of heparan sulfate	Autosomal recessive
Morquio (MPS IV)	Normal intelligence Striking dwarfism Corneal opacity Severe osteoporosis and atlantoaxial dislocation	Chondroitin sulfate B Marked urinary excretion of keratin sulfate and chondroitin sulfate	Autosomal recessive
Maroteaux-Lamy (MPS VI)	Normal intelligence Dwarfism Severe corneal and bony lesions	Chondroitin sulfate B Increased urinary excretion of dermatan sulfate	Autosomal recessive

of beneficial effects from plasma infusions were exciting and promising, subsequent studies indicate no clinical or biochemical results from this technique.[54, 55] Prenatal diagnosis of the mucopolysaccharidoses is now possible through the study of cultured amniotic fluid cells and the amniotic fluid itself. The clinical course of patients is usually progressively downhill, with death in those with the fully expressed syndrome from either respiratory tract infection or cardiac failure, generally before the age of 10 years.

Scheie's Syndrome. Originally considered to be a distinctive form of mucopolysaccharidosis, Scheie's syndrome (mucopolysacharidosis I-S, formerly MPSV) now appears to represent a variant of Hurler's syndrome (MPS 1-H). It is characterized by stiff joints, coarse facies, corneal clouding, excessive body hair, retinitis pigmentosa, aortic regurgitation, few other somatic effects, and normal intellect. Patients with Scheie's syndrome excrete excessive amounts of dermatan sulfate and heparan sulfate. Hurler's and Scheie's syndromes, despite their striking clinical differences, are similar by fibroblast culture. They are both corrected by the Hurler factor and both show deficiency of the same enzyme, α-L-iduronidase.

Hunter's Syndrome. Hunter's syndrome (mucopolysaccharidosis II, MPS II) is distinguished from Hurler's syndrome by an X-linked recessive inheritance, longer survival, lack of corneal clouding, characteristic cutaneous markers, and a different pattern of mucopolysaccharide excretion (chondroitin sulfate B and heparitin sulfate). The clinical picture in all respects is generally less severe than that seen in Hurler's syndrome (Fig. 22–9). Mental retardation progresses at a slower rate, humping of the lumbar area (gibbus) does not occur, and progressive deafness is a frequent feature. Hearing loss is present in about 50 per cent of patients with Hunter's syndrome, and children are often brought to a physician at about 3 years of age because of lack of speech. Although deafness also occurs in Hurler's syndrome (MPS I), severe mental retardation and death at an early age cause it to be a relatively inconspicuous feature of this disorder.

Distinctive cutaneous changes are highly chracteristic of MPS II (Hunter's syndrome) and probably represent a marker of this disorder. These pathognomonic lesions consist of firm flesh-colored to ivory-white papules and nodules that often coalesce to form ridges or a reticular pattern in symmetrical areas between the angles of the scapulae and posterior axillary lines, the pectoral ridges, the nape of the neck, and/or the lateral aspects of the upper arms and thighs (Fig. 22–10). They appear before age 10 and can spontaneously disappear. Although a reliable marker when present, the majority of cases reported with this syndrome fail to mention this finding, so the precise incidence of this cutaneous feature is unknown.[56]

Sanfilippo's Syndrome. Sanfilippo's syndrome (MPS III) is an autosomal recessive disorder char-

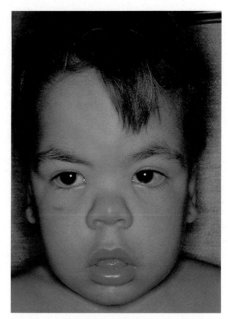

Figure 22–9. Coarse facial features in a child with Hunter's syndrome (mucopolysaccharidosis II).

acterized by aggressive behavior, severe mental retardation, coarse hair, coarse immobile facies, and relatively less severe somatic changes than those seen in MPS I and MPS II. Thickening of the skin and subcutaneous tissues produces coarse features with prominent eyebrows, thickened nares, thick lips, and a lack of expressive facial movement.[57-59] The hair is coarse, and loss of extension

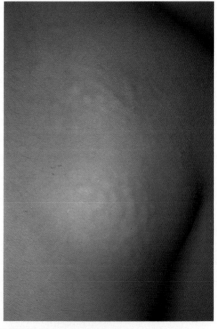

Figure 22–10. Distinctive, firm, flesh-colored papules and nodules in a reticular pattern on the shoulder and scapular area (a cutaneous marker of Hunter's syndrome, MPS II).

of the interphalangeal joints of the hands develops, but not to a degree sufficient to cause the typical claw hand deformities seen in patients with Hurler's and Hunter's syndromes. When the diagnosis is indeterminate, examination of urinary mucopolysaccharides reveals excessive excretion of heparan sulfate (the only mucopolysaccharide excreted in excessive amounts in this disorder).

Morquio's Syndrome. Morquio's syndrome (MPS IV) is an autosomal recessive disorder characterized by normal intelligence, striking dwarfism (usually not apparent until the child reaches 2 or 3 years of age), and distinctive skeletal findings with marked osteoporosis of all bones. Usually the joints are not stiff. A barrel chest with pigeon breast (pectus carinatum) deformity, relatively short trunks and neck, an appearance of disproportionately long extremities, and looseness of some joints are characteristic features. Marked excretion of keratan sulfate and chondroitin sulfate A (about two or three times greater than normal) in the urine is a characteristic feature during childhood in patients with the Morquio syndrome. These findings, however, slowly decrease, reaching normal levels during adulthood.

Maroteaux-Lamy Syndrome. Mucopolysaccharidosis VI (Maroteaux-Lamy syndrome) is an autosomal recessive disorder characterized by dwarfism, coarse facies, clouding of the corneas (frequently with severe impairment of vision), severe osseous changes, flexion contractures of the hands, normal intellect, and increased urinary excretion of dermatan sulfate. No estimates as to its incidence exist. Most authorities, however, consider this disorder to be extremely rare.[60]

THE MUCOLIPIDOSES

The mucolipidoses are a group of disorders that exhibit clinical and skeletal signs of the mucopolysaccharidoses and clinical features seen in patients with sphingolipidoses. This group includes three disorders specifically termed *mucolipidosis I, II,* and *III, gangliosidosis, juvenile sulfatidosis, fucosidosis, mannosidosis,* and perhaps, *lipogranulomatosis.*

Mucolipidosis I. Mucolipidosis I (lipomucopolysaccharidosis) is an autosomal recessive disorder characterized by mild Hurler's syndrome–like clinical manifestations, moderate progressive mental retardation, skeletal changes of dysostosis multiplex, normal urinary mucopolysaccharide excretion, and coarse refringent inclusions in cultured fibroblasts similar to but without the clear perinuclear halo of those seen in mucolipidosis II. Previously called lipomucopolysaccharidosis, mucolipidosis I is a lysosomal storage disease that results from a deficiency of acid neuraminidase with accumulation of sialic acid–rich macromolecular compounds. This disorder should be differentiated from the cherry-red spot–myo-

clonus syndrome (characterized by bilateral macular cherry-red spots, progressive myoclonus beginning in adolescence without mental retardation and progressive visual deterioration), which also demonstrates a deficiency of acid neuraminidase.

Mucolipidosis I should be included in the differential diagnosis of disorders that display a Hurler's syndrome–like phenotype in infancy. The measurement of urinary levels of bound sialic acid represents a simple screening procedure, and confirmation of the diagnosis can be accomplished by the demonstration of isolated acid neuraminidase deficiency in cultures of skin fibroblasts.

Mucolipidosis II. Mucolipidosis II (ML II, I-cell disease) is an autosomal recessive Hurler's syndrome–like disorder characterized by small orbits and prominent eyes, puffy and swollen eyelids, a pattern of tortuous veins around the orbits, fullness of the lower part of the face, full rounded cheeks that appear flushed because of many fine telangiectases, a prominent maxilla (which produces a fish mouth appearance), gingival hypertrophy, a severe type of dysostosis multiplex, short neck, thick and rigid skin (particularly on the ears and neck), stiffness of all joints with considerable reduction in range of motion, and death, usually due to severe respiratory tract infection and cardiac failure, at about 4 years of age.

Mucolipidosis II can be distinguished from Hurler's syndrome by the presence of hypertrophic gums, vacuolated lymphocytes in the peripheral blood, striking inclusions ("I-cell disease" refers to these) in fibroblast cultures from cutaneous biopsy, normal urinary mucopolysaccharide excretion, and a 10- to 100-fold increase in the specific activity of several plasma acid hydrolases.[61, 62] Prenatal diagnosis of this disorder can be confirmed by enzyme assays of amniotic fluid.[63]

Mucolipidosis III. Mucolipidosis III (pseudo-Hurler's polydystrophy) is an autosomal recessive disorder characterized by mental retardation, early restriction of joint mobility, and normal mucopolysacchariduria. Children with this disorder usually present at or about the age of 3 years, with stiffness of the joints as the main complaint. Most patients have coarse facies, short stature, fine ground-glass corneal clouding, and a moderate degree of mental retardation with IQs of 65 to 85. Aortic valve disease is present in most patients with this disorder.

GM₁ Gangliosidosis. GM_1 gangliosidosis, caused by generalized accumulation of GM_1 ganglioside due to a β-galactosidase deficiency, is characterized by coarse facies with depressed nasal bridge, full cheeks and puffy eyelids, corneal clouding, cherry-red spots in the macular region, kyphoscoliosis, radiographic changes of dysostosis multiplex, hepatosplenomegaly, marked psychomotor retardation, progressive cerebral deterioration, and death usually before the age of 2 years. Features resembling the mucopolysaccharidoses include bone changes, hepatosplenomegaly, and corneal clouding. Those suggesting a sphingolipidosis include large head, cherry-red spot of the macula, and progressive neurologic deterioration.

Juvenile Sulfatidosis. Juvenile sulfatidosis with mucopolysacchariduria (also called the Austin type of leukodystrophy) is a very rare Hurler's syndrome–like disorder characterized by mild Hurler's syndrome–like features, slowly progressive neurologic deterioration that begins in the second year of life, and death, generally in the early teens.

"STIFF SKIN" SYNDROME

A unique combination of skin and joint defects, presumably a form of focal mucopolysaccharidosis, the "stiff skin" syndrome is characterized by localized areas of stony-hard skin, mild hirsutism, limited mobility of various joints, and normal urinary mucopolysaccharide excretion.[64, 65] In one patient the areas of the skin with less severe involvement had a cobblestone appearance suggestive of that occurring in patients with the Hunter's syndrome–type of mucopolysaccharidosis.

Although the exact nature of this disorder is unknown, the presence of abnormal amounts of hyaluronidase-digestible acid mucopolysaccharide in the dermis, as well as an increase in cytoplasmic metachromatic material in cultured fibroblasts, suggests a focal abnormality of mucopolysaccharide metabolism. The presence of this constellation of findings in a mother and her two children suggests a heritable disorder of the autosomal dominant type. The fact that the siblings were the progeny of a consanguineous marriage between cousins, however, cannot exclude an autosomal recessive pattern of inheritance.

References

1. Holtzman NA, Kronmal RA, van Doorninck W, et al.: Effect of age at loss of dietary control on intellectual performance and behavior of children with phenylketonuria. N. Engl. J. Med. *314:*593–598, 1986.

   A study of 119 ten-year-olds with phenylketonuria suggests that phenylalanine restriction in children with PKU should be continued beyond the age of 8 years.

2. Azen CG, Koch R, Friedman EG, et al.: Intellectual development in 12-year-old children treated for phenylketonuria. Am. J. Dis. Child. *145:*35–39, 1991.

   Intelligence and achievement test scores of 95 twelve-year-old children with phenylketonuria support a recommendation that dietary restriction of phenylalanine be maintained throughout adolescence.

3. Hurwitz S: The Skin and Systemic Disease in Children. Year Book Medical Publishers, Chicago, 1985.

   A review of the clinical and cutaneous manifestations of systemic disorders of childhood.

4. Schimke RN: Low-methionine diet of homocystinuria. Ann. Intern. Med. *70:*642–643, 1969.

   A low methionine diet supplemented with pyridoxine appears to be beneficial for patients with homocystinuria.

5. Carson NAJ, Carré IJ: Treatment of homocystinuria with pyridoxine. Arch. Dis. Child. *44:*387–392, 1969.

   Response of 6 of 11 patients to high dosages of oral pyridoxine suggests two basic defects in cystathionine synthetase: (1) a pyridoxine-dependent syndrome and (2) a pyridoxine-resistant disorder associated with deficiency of apoenzyme.

6. Wyre D: Alkaptonuria with extensive ochronosis. Arch. Dermatol. *115:*461–463, 1979.

   A report of a 59-year-old woman with extensive ochronosis suggests that evaluation of a patient's renal status should be performed whenever alkaptonuria and ochronosis are extensive or have a rapid onset.

7. Lee CWG, Yu JS, Turner BB, et al.: Medical intelligence: Trimethylaminuria: Fishy odors in children. N. Engl. J. Med. *295:*937–938, 1976.

   A report of three children with trimethylaminuria.

8. Shelley ED, Shelley WB: The fish odor syndrome: Trimethylaminuria. J.A.M.A. *251:*253–255, 1984.

   Elimination of fish, eggs, liver, and kidneys from the diet of a 31-year-old man with trimethylaminuria helped control the disorder.

9. Rothschild JG, Hansen RC: Fish odor syndrome: Trimethylaminuria with milk as chief dietary factor. Pediatr. Dermatol. *3:*38–39, 1985.

   In a 10-year-old boy with a high milk intake (2 to 3 liters/day) and a 2-year history of rotting fish odor, restriction of milk and foods containing choline and trimethylamine oxide eliminated the offensive odor.

10. Reilly CA: Wilson's disease. Pediatr. Rev. *5:*217–222, 1989.

    A comprehensive review of Wilson's disease, its clinical manifestations and management.

11. Scheinberg IH, Jaffe ME, Sterleib I: The use of trientine in preventing the effects of interrupting penicillamine therapy in Wilson's disease. N. Engl. J. Med. *317:*209–213, 1987.

    In 13 patients in whom penicillamine had to be discontinued because of serious adverse reactions, trientine was successfully introduced with good results.

12. Lesch M, Nyhan WL: Familial disorder of uric acid metabolism and central nervous system function. Am. J. Med. *36:*561–570, 1964.

    A report of two brothers with hyperuricemia, choreoathetosis, and mental retardation suggests the presence of a rare inherited disorder in which an excess of uric acid or one of its products or precursors could produce unusual neural and behavioral characteristics.

13. Williams ML, Packman S, Cowan MJ: Alopecia and periorificial dermatitis in biotin-responsive multiple carboxylase deficiency. J. Am. Acad. Dermatol. *9:*97–103, 1983.

    A report of three patients with infantile-onset biotin-responsive multiple carboxylase deficiency.

14. Nyhan WL: Inborn errors of metabolism. Arch. Dermatol. *123:*1696–1698a, 1987.

    A comprehensive review of biotin and biotin-deficiency disorders.

15. Goldsmith LA: Tyrosinemia II: Lessons in molecular pathophysiology. Pediatr. Dermatol. *1:*25–34, 1983.

    A comprehensive review of tyrosinemia II with emphasis on its biochemistry and clinical features.

16. Shimizu N, Masaaki I, Ito K, et al.: Richner-Hanhart's syndrome: Electron microscopic study of skin lesions. Arch. Dermatol. *126:*1342–1346, 1990.

    Abnormal needle-shaped inclusions, considered to be "crystalline ghosts" presumably of tyrosine seen on ultrastructural examination, are suggested to be an important factor in the pathogenesis of cutaneous lesions in patients with the Richner-Hanhart syndrome.

17. Danbolt N, Closs K: Acrodermatitis enteropathica. Acta Derm. Venereol. *23:*127–169, 1942.

    A study of two children with acrodermatitis enteropathica.

18. Wells BT, Winkelmann RK: Acrodermatitis enteropathica: Report of 6 cases. Arch. Dermatol. *84*:90–102, 1961.

Review of acrodermatitis enteropathica based on a compilation of 58 cases in the world literature and six additional cases that had previously been labeled with other diagnoses.

19. Moynahan EJ, Barnes PM: Zinc deficiency and a synthetic diet for lactose intolerance. Lancet *1*:676–677, 1973.

A patient with lactose intolerance and acrodermatitis enteropathica who improved only after the addition of zinc to his diet led to the discovery of zinc deficiency and its role in the etiology of acrodermatitis enteropathica.

20. Moynahan EJ: Acrodermatitis enteropathica: A lethal inherited human zinc-deficiency disorder. Lancet *2*:399–400, 1974.

Nine children and one infant wth acrodermatitis enteropathica became completely symptom free and could eat a normal diet after they started receiving zinc supplements.

21. Casey CE, Walravens PA, Hambidge KM: Availability of zinc: Loading tests with human milk, cow's milk, and infant formulas. Pediatrics 68:394–396, 1981.

The difference between the bioavailability of zinc from human milk, as compared with cow's milk and infant formulas, appears to be related to the presence of zinc-binding ligands (molecules which bind to other molecules and enhance zinc uptake across the intestinal mucosa).

22. Arlette JP, Johnston MM: Zinc deficiency dermatitis in premature infants receiving prolonged parenteral alimentation. J. Am. Acad. Dermatol. 5:37–42, 1981.

A report of 10 patients with acrodermatitis enteropathica as a result of hypozincemia associated with long-term zinc-deficient parenteral nutrition.

23. Herson VC, Phillips AF, Zimmerman A: Acute zinc deficiency in a premature infant after bowel resection and intravenous alimentation. Am. J. Dis. Child. *135*:968–969, 1981.

A report of a premature infant who developed clinical features of acrodermatitis enteropathica as a result of low zinc levels following bowel resection and zinc-deficient intravenous fluid therapy.

24. Parker PH, Helinek JL, Meneely PH: Zinc deficiency in a premature infant fed exclusively human milk. Am. J. Dis. Child. *136*:77–78, 1982.

A report of zinc deficiency in a breast-fed premature infant and a discussion of potential factors contributing to its occurrence.

25. Zimmerman AW, Hambidge M, Lepow ML, et al.: Acrodermatitis in breast-fed premature infants: Evidence for a defect of mammary zinc secretion. Pediatrics *69*:176–183, 1982.

A report of two breast-fed premature infants with low zinc content in their mothers' breast milk resulting in hypozincemia and acrodermatitis enteropathica.

26. McClain C, Soutor C, Zieve L; Zinc deficiency: A complication of Crohn's disease. Gastroenterology 78:272–279, 1980.

A report of four patients with regional ileitis who had low mean zinc levels; two developed cutaneous lesions of acrodermatitis enteropathica.

27. Tong TK, Andrew LR, Mickell JJ: Childhood AIDS manifesting as acrodermatitis enteropathica. J. Pediatr. *108*:424–428, 1986.

A 14-month-old premature infant with poor weight gain, pneumonia, orofacial rash, hepatosplenomegaly, chronic diarrhea, candidal infection, pancytopenia, and low zinc levels suggesting a diagnosis of acrodermatitis enteropathica was subsequently found to have AIDS (the low zinc levels apparently resulted from severe diarrhea associated with the patient's disorder).

28. Hansen RC, Lerner R, Revsin B: Cystic fibrosis manifesting with acrodermatitis enteropathica–like eruption: Associa-

tion with essential fatty acid and zinc deficiencies. Arch. Dermatol. *119*:51–55, 1983.

A refractory dermatitis resembling acrodermatitis enteropathica in a 5-month-old infant with cystic fibrosis.

29. Freeland-Graves JH, Bodzy PW, Eppright MA: Zinc status of vegetarians. J. Am. Dietet. Assoc. 77:655–661, 1980.

Studies of 79 vegetarians and 41 nonvegetarians revealed that a number of patients on strict vegetarian diets develop low zinc serum levels as a result of inadequate dietary zinc intake.

30. Krieger I, Evans GW: Acrodermatitis enteropathica without hypozincemia: Therapeutic effect of pancreatic enzyme preparation due to a zinc-binding ligand. J. Pediatr. 96:32–36, 1980.

Picolinic acid, a chelating ligand present in pancreatic Viokase, was presumed to be responsible for increased zinc absorption in a 12-month-old girl with acrodermatitis enteropathica.

31. Miller SJ: Nutritional deficiency and the skin. J. Am. Acad. Dermatol. *21*:1–30, 1989.

A comprehensive review of cutaneous changes manifested in patients with dietary deficiency states and inherited disorders of metabolism.

32. Weston WL, Huff JC, Humbert JR, et al.: Zinc correction of defective chemotaxis in acrodermatitis enteropathica. Arch. Dermatol. *113*:422–425, 1977.

Investigation of the monocyte system in three patients with acrodermatitis enteropathica revealed a zinc-correctable suppressed cellular chemotaxis of monocytes during zinc deficiency.

33. Garrets M, Molokhia M: Acrodermatitis enteropathica without hypozincemia. J. Pediatr. 91:492–494, 1977.

An 8-year-old child who had acrodermatitis enteropathica and higher than normal serum zinc levels.

33a. Dillaha CH, Lorincz AL, Aavik OR: Acrodermatitis enteropathica—review of the literature and a report on a case successfully treated with Diodoquin. J.A.M.A. *152*:509–512, 1953.

The serendipitous use of diiodohydroxyquin (Diodoquin) resulted in the use of this agent in the therapy of acrodermatitis enteropathica for many years.

34. Neldner KH, Hambidge KM: Zinc therapy of acrodermatitis enteropathica. N. Engl. J. Med. *292*:879–882, 1975.

Oral zinc sulfate (200 mg/day) results in rapid resolution of acrodermatitis enteropathica in a 23-year-old woman with a history of this disorder present since the age of 6 months.

35. Michaelssohn G: Zinc therapy in acrodermatitis enteropathica. Acta Derm. Venereol. *54*:377–381, 1974.

An 18-year-old male with widespread skin changes of acrodermatitis enteropathica and incipient optic atrophy probably due to chlorquinaldol therapy improved on oral zinc in dosages of 45 mg three times a day.

36. Fleischer DI, Hepler RS, Landau JW: Blindness during diiodohydroxyquin (Diodoquin) therapy: A case report. Pediatrics 54:106–108, 1974.

The third report of optic neuritis: a 2-year-old boy who developed major loss of visual acuity and degenerative changes in his optic nerves and retinas during long-term high dosages of Diodoquin therapy.

37. Fleischmajer R, Dowlati Y, Reeves JRT: Familial hyperlipidemias—diagnosis and treatment. Arch. Dermatol. *110*:43–50, 1974.

A practical review of the clinical, biochemical, and therapeutic features of the hyperlipidemias.

38. Fredrickson DS, Levy RJ, Lees RS: Fat transport in lipoproteins: An integrated approach to mechanisms and disorders. N. Engl. J. Med. 276:32–44; 94–103; 148–156; 215–225; 273–281, 1967.

Analysis and classification of the hyperlipoproteinemic disorders.

39. Polano MK, Baes H, Hulsmans AM, et al.: Xanthomata in primary hyperlipoproteinemia—a classification based on the lipoprotein pattern of the blood. Arch. Dermatol. *100*:387–400, 1969.

A review of the classification of hyperlipoproteinemia based on analyses of the lipid and lipoprotein levels and cutaneous xanthomata of 23 patients.

40. Parker F: Xanthomas and hyperlipidemias. J. Am. Acad. Dermatol. *13*:1–30, 1985.

A comprehensive review of xanthomas, their pathogenesis, significance, and management.

41. Teltscher J, Silverman RA, Stork J: Eruptive xanthomas in a child with nephrotic syndrome. J. Am. Acad. Dermatol. *21*:1147–1149, 1989.

A 4-year-old boy with steroid-resistant nephrotic syndrome, extreme hyperlipidemia, and eruptive xanthomas was treated successfully with gemfibrozil (Lopid), a low fat diet and antihistamines.

42. Cruz PD, East C, Bergstresser PR: Dermal, subcutaneous, and tendon xanthomas: Diagnostic markers for specific lipoprotein disorders. J. Am. Acad. Dermatol. *19*:95–111, 1988.

A comprehensive review of lipoprotein metabolism xanthomas, their significance, and differential diagnosis.

43. Roederer G, Xhignesse M, Davignon J: Eruptive and tuberoeruptive xanthomas of the skin arising on sites of prior injury: Two case reports. J.A.M.A. *260*:1282–1283, 1988.

Eruptive and tuberoeruptive xanthomas arising at sites of minor skin injury are described in two patients with type IV and type III hyperlipidemia; in one patient lesions appeared following a cat scratch, in the other massive bee stinging preceded the appearance of a constellation of xanthomas.

44. Mountcastle EA, Lupton GP: Verruciform xanthomas of the digits. J. Am. Acad. Dermatol. *20*:313–317, 1989.

A report of a patient with multiple verruciform xanthomas on a hand and foot and a review of the literature.

45. Buchner A, Hansen LS, Merrill PW: Verrucous xanthoma of the oral mucosa: Report of five cases and review of the literature. Arch. Dermatol. *117*:563–565, 1981.

An analysis of five patients with verruciform xanthomas and a review of an additional 29 cases gleaned from the literature.

46. George WM, Azadeh B: Verruciform xanthoma of the penis. Cutis *44*:167–170, 1987.

A report of a 33-year-old man with a 25-year history of a verruciform xanthoma on the prepuce of the penis.

47. Palestine RJ, Winkelmann RK: Verruciform xanthoma in an epithelial nevus. Arch. Dermatol. *118*:686–691, 1982.

A report of a verrucous xanthoma that developed on an epithelial nevoid-type eruption on a phocomelic extremity of an 11-year-old girl.

48. Yeshuron D, Chung H, Gotto AM Jr, et al.: Primary type V hyperlipoproteinemia in childhood. J.A.M.A. *236*:2518–2520, 1977.

A 9-year-old girl with type V disease.

49. Weston CFM, Burton JL: Xanthomas in the Watson-Alagille syndrome. J. Am. Acad. Dermatol *16*:1117–1121, 1987.

A report of a 26-year-old woman with the Alagille syndrome, a form of intraductular hypoplasia that contrary to biliary atresia bears a relatively good prognosis.

50. Camacho-Martinez F, Moreno-Gimenez JC, Sanchez-Pedreno P: Correspondence: Xanthomatous biliary cirrhosis in Alagille's syndrome. J. Am. Acad. Dermatol. *18*:746–748, 1988.

A commentary on the Alagille syndrome, its significance and clinical features.

51. McKusick VA, Kaplan D, Wise D, et al.: Genetic mucopolysaccharidoses. Medicine *44*:445–483, 1965.

A critical review of the mucopolysaccharidoses.

52. Hunter G: A rare disease in two brothers. Proc. R. Soc. Med. *10*:104–116, 1917.

A detailed report of two brothers with typical features of mucopolysaccharidosis I (the Hunter syndrome).

53. Gerich JE: Hunter's syndrome: Beta-galactosidase deficiency in the skin. N. Engl. J. Med. *280*:799–802, 1969.

Deficient activity of β-galactosidase in the skin of two siblings with Hunter's syndrome and their mother, a carrier of the sex-linked disorder.

54. DiFerrante N, Nichols BL, Donnelly PV, et al.: Induced degradation of glycosaminoglycans in Hurler's and Hunter's syndromes by plasma infusion. Proc. Natl. Acad. Sci., U.S.A. *68*:303–307, 1971.

Treatment of seven patients (two with the Hurler and five with the Hunter syndrome) with plasma infusions followed by decreased excretion of urinary acid mucopolysaccharides and an associated clinical improvement.

55. Dekaban AS, Holden KR, Constantopoulos G: Effects of fresh plasma or whole blood transfusions on patients with various types of mucopolysaccharidosis. Pediatrics *50*:688–692, 1972.

Failure of fresh plasma and whole blood transfusions in the treatment of five children with mucopolysaccharidosis.

56. Prystkowsky SD, Maumanee IH, Freeman RG, et al.: A cutaneous marker in the Hunter syndrome: A report of four cases. Arch. Dermatol. *113*:602–605, 1977.

Distinctive flesh-colored to ivory-white papules and nodules, characteristic of the Hunter syndrome, serve to separate this disorder from the other mucopolysaccharidoses.

57. Leroy JC, Crocker AC: Clinical definition of Hurler-Hunter phenotypes: Review of 50 patients. Am J. Dis. Child. *112*:518–530, 1966.

A review of children with Hurler's disease, Hunter's syndrome, the Sanfilippo disorder, and the Scheie type of mucopolysaccharidosis.

58. Danks DM, Campbell PE, Cartwright E, et al.: Sanfilippo syndrome; clinical, biochemical, radiologic, hematologic, and pathologic features of nine cases. Aust. Paediatr. J. *8*:174–186, 1972.

A large series of cases of the Sanfilippo form of mucopolysaccharidosis.

59. Kaplan P, Wolfe LS: Sanfillippo syndrome type D: J. Pediatr. *110*:267–271, 1987.

Sanfillipo's syndrome type D is described as a syndrome with at least three or possibly four enzymatic defects.

60. Spranger IW, Koch F, McKusick VA, et al.: Mucopolysaccharidosis VI (Maroteaux-Lamy disease). Helv. Peadiatr. Acta *25*:337–362, 1970.

Review of 19 patients with MPS VI.

61. Terashima Y, Katsuya T, Isomura S, et al.: I-cell disease, report of three cases. Am. J. Dis. Child. *129*:1083–1090, 1975.

I-cell disease can be differentiated from the Hurler syndrome (MPS I) by the presence of hypertrophied gums, vacuolated lymphocytes in the peripheral blood, and a normal level of urinary mucopolysaccharides.

62. Gellis S, Feingold M: Picture of the Month, I-cell disease (mucolipidosis II). Am. J. Dis. Child. *131*:1137–1138, 1977.

Manifestations of a patient with I-cell disease.

63. Aula P, Rapola J, Antio S, et al.: Prenatal diagnosis and fetal pathology of I-cell disease (mucolipidosis II). J. Pediatr. *87*:221–226, 1975.

Early prenatal diagnosis of I-cell disease can be confirmed by enzyme assays of lysosomal hydrolases in cell cultures of amniotic fluid and ultrastructural studies of fetal skin.

64. Esterly NB, McKusick VA: The stiff skin syndrome. Pediatrics 47:360–369, 1971.

Four patients with localized areas of stony-hard skin, mild hirsutism, and limitation of joint mobility—a connective tissue disorder possibly resulting from an abnormality of mucopolysaccharide metabolism.

65. Jablonska S, Schubert H, Kikuchi I: Congenital fascial dystrophy: Stiff skin syndrome: A human counterpart of the tight-skin mouse. J. Am. Acad. Dermatol. 21:943–950, 1990.

A report of four patients with the stiff skin syndrome.

23

NEUROCUTANEOUS DISORDERS

Neurofibromatosis
Tuberous Sclerosis
Incontinentia Pigmenti
Hypomelanosis of Ito (Incontinentia Pigmenti Achromians)

The neurocutaneous disorders consist of a group of hereditary conditions with cutaneous, nervous system, and internal manifestations. Since the skin and nervous system share a common embryologic origin, it is not surprising that there are a large number of neurologic conditions associated with cutaneous manifestations. Of these, neurofibromatosis, tuberous sclerosis, incontinentia pigmenti, and hypomelanosis of Ito (incontinentia pigmenti achromians) have striking cutaneous markers.

NEUROFIBROMATOSIS

Neurofibromatosis (von Recklinghausen's disease) is an autosomal dominant disorder characterized by cutaneous pigmentation (café au lait spots) and tumors of the nervous system, which present as changes in the skin, bones, endocrine system, and muscle. It is estimated to occur approximately once in 2,500 to 3,000 births, with no significant difference in respect to sex, race, or color.[1] About 50 per cent of cases probably represent new mutations (Table 23–1).

Neurofibromatosis has been classified into eight distinct types, each with prognostic significance and implications for genetic counseling. The gene for neurofibromatosis I (NF I) is localized to the proximal long arm of chromosome 17, and the gene for neurofibromatosis II (NF II) is localized to the long arm of chromosome 22.[2, 3] The eight currently described subtypes of neurofibromatosis are as follows:

1. *Neurofibromatosis I* (NF I), an autosomal dominant disorder, accounts for at least 85 per cent of cases with an incidence of 1:4000, and is the classic or peripheral form of neurofibromatosis, encompassing the more classic features of this syndrome (multiple café au lait spots, axillary freckling, cutaneous neurofibromas, and Lisch

nodules). The café au lait spots are numerous and widespread, and the central nervous system lesions are primarily tumors of the optic nerve. Although optic gliomas, the most commonly encountered central nervous system tumor, seen in 15 per cent of patients with NF I, may present at a young age and one third of individuals with optic gliomas will be at risk for glioma-related dysfunctions, only 20 per cent of patients with this complication develop visual impairment.[4, 5]

2. *Neurofibromatosis II* (NF II), the acoustic or central form of neurofibromatosis, also autosomal dominant with an incidence of 1:50,000, is characterized by a 90 per cent incidence of bilateral acoustic neuromas. Café au lait spots tend to be few, large, and relatively light in color, neurofibromas are few, Lisch nodules are absent, and the skin tumors are likely to be schwannomas rather than neurofibromas. Although NF II is generally thought of as an adult disease, symptoms, the first of which is usually unilateral hearing loss, generally begin in the teens or shortly after puberty.[6, 7]

3. *Neurofibromatosis III* (NF III), "mixed" neurofibromatosis, is a disorder of undefined inheritance combining features of NF I and NF II. Patients generally have few large lightly colored café au lait lesions, more numerous cutaneous neurofibromas, and a higher frequency of central nervous system tumors (optic gliomas, neurilemmomas, and meningiomas) than individuals with NF I. Multiple central nervous system (brain and spinal cord) tumors are the hallmark of NF III.

4. *Neurofibromatosis IV* (NF IV) is a variant form, with variable inheritance and many café au lait macules and neurofibromas that, although cutaneous, acoustic, and other central nervous system lesions may be present, does not fit well into other subsets of neurofibromatosis. The cutaneous characteristics are intermediate between those of NF I and NF II.

5. *Neurofibromatosis V* (NF V), segmental neurofibromatosis, is a rare disorder characterized by

Table 23–1. NEUROFIBROMATOSIS

1. Autosomal dominant
   a. 1 in 2,500 to 3,000 births
   b. 50% represent new mutations
   c. NF-I comprises over 85% of cases; NF-II encompasses approximately 10%
2. Cutaneous and ophthalmic manifestations
   a. Café au lait spots
   b. Axillary freckling (Crowe's sign)
   c. Neurofibromas
   d. Blue-red and pseudoatrophic macules
   e. Lisch nodules (seen in only 5% of children younger than 3 years of age and 97 to 100% of postpubertal patients)
3. Systemic manifestations
   a. Neurologic, osseous, endocrine
   b. 7% are at risk for severe disease and another 5% are at risk for moderate disease

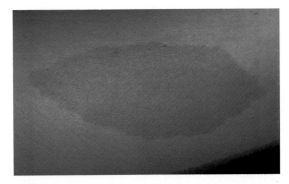

Figure 23–1. Café au lait spot. Six café au lait spots larger than 1.5 cm in diameter suggest a diagnosis of multiple neurofibromatosis (von Recklinghausen's disease). In children 5 years of age or younger, six or more café au lait spots 0.5 cm or greater probably indicate the presence of this disorder.

café au lait macules and neurofibromas limited to a single dermatome, and perhaps multiple dermatomes; unlike other forms of neurofibromatosis that are autosomal dominant, this disorder is considered to be the result of postzygotic mutation. Genetic transmission has not been documented.[8–11]

6. *Neurofibromatosis VI* (NF VI) is characterized by café au lait spots indistinguishable from those of NF I and an absence of neurofibromas, Lisch nodules, and neural crest tumors.

7. *Neurofibromatosis VII* (NF VII), "late-onset" neurofibromatosis, is a disorder in which cutaneous or deep tumors appear later in life, after the age of 20 years; pseudoarthrosis, learning disabilities, and heritability have not been reported.

8. *Neurofibromatosis VIII* (NF VIII), neurofibromatosis of unspecified type, encompasses patients who display neurofibromas and do not fit neatly into any of the other categories but, because of their clinical characteristics, the diagnosis of neurofibromatosis may be appropriate.[10]

Of note is the fact that Joseph Merrick, the famed "Elephant Man" of the 1800s, did not have neurofibromatosis. Mr. Merrick, who had no family history of neurofibromatosis, no café au lait spots, nor histologic evidence of neurofibromas, probably had the *Proteus syndrome* (a condition frequently misdiagnosed as neurofibromatosis), a disorder characterized by partial gigantism of the hands or feet, asymmetry of the arms, varicosities, linear verrucous epidermal nevi, macrocephaly, cranial hyperostosis, and hypertrophy of the long bones.[12]

Cutaneous Manifestations.

Café au Lait Spots. Café au lait spots (Fig. 23–1), a hallmark of neurofibromatosis, may occur anywhere on the body. Although usually present at birth, they may make their appearance during the first few months (or even up to 1 year of age) and often continue to increase in size and number during the first decade, especially the first 2 years of life; most patients with neurofibromatosis demonstrate their café au lait spots by the age of 9 years.[13] Although giant café au lait spots as large as 15 cm in

diameter may be seen in otherwise normal individuals, as well as patients with neurofibromatosis, the lesions characteristically average 2 to 5 cm in diameter.

Crowe and associates have postulated that the existence of six or more café au lait spots greater than 1.5 cm (15 mm) in diameter probably indicates the presence of neurofibromatosis (Fig. 23–2.) Although 10 to 20 per cent of normal individuals have one or more café au lait spots, these characteristic macules are seen in 95 per cent of patients with neurofibromatosis, and 78 per cent of patients with von Recklinhausen disease demonstrate six or more such lesions.[14] This "six spot" criterion, while not a hard and fast rule, is valuable, particularly in young children and adolescents before the cutaneous neurofibromas make their appearance. In prepubertal children, six or more café au lait spots 5 mm or more in diameter can help establish the diagnosis (Table 23–2).[15, 16]

Another form of café au lait pigmentation, termed *axillary freckling* (Crowe's sign), also serves as a valuable diagnostic aid in the early recognition of neurofibromatosis (Fig. 23–3).[17] Seen in 20 to 50 per cent of patients with the disease, axillary freckling appears as multiple 1- to 4-mm café au lait spots in the axillary vault. Lack of sun exposure in this area prevents confusion with true freckles. Although highly characteristic, axillary freckling is not necessarily pathognomonic. It may also be seen in Watson's syndrome, an autosomal disorder characterized by café au lait spots, pulmonary stenosis, and low intelligence.

Microscopic examination of café au lait spots reveals increased pigment in the basal layer of the epidermis. Giant melanin granules measuring up to 5 mm in diameter in both melanocytes and basal cells have been observed in the melanocytes and keratinocytes of the epidermis, particularly in the café au lait spots, of patients with neurofibromatosis.[18–20] Giant pigment granules, however, are not specific for the café au lait spots of neurofi-

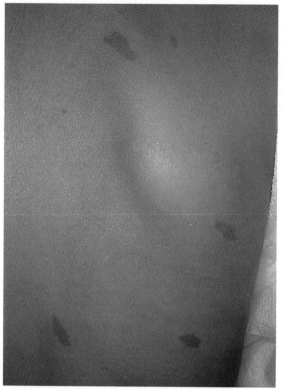

Figure 23–2. Multiple café au lait spots on the upper back of a 12-year-old girl with neurofibromatosis (von Recklinghausen's disease).

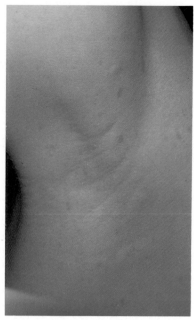

Figure 23–3. Axillary freckling (Crowe's sign). Multiple 1- to 4-mm café au lait spots in the axilla also serve as a valuable aid to the early diagnosis of multiple neurofibromatosis.

Table 23–2. DIAGNOSTIC CRITERIA FOR NEUROFIBROMATOSIS I AND II

A. Criteria for the diagnosis of neurofibromatosis I (NF I, von Recklinghausen neurofibromatosis) are met in an individual if two or more of the following are found:
1. Six or more café au lait macules over 5 mm in greatest diameter in prepubertal and over 1.5 cm in postpubertal individuals.
2. Two or more neurofibromas of any type, or one plexiform neurofibroma.
3. Multiple freckles (Crowe's sign) in the axillary or inguinal regions.
4. A distinctive osseous lesion such as sphenoid dysplasia or thinning of long bone cortex, with or without pseudoarthrosis.
5. Optic glioma.
6. Two or more iris hamartomas (Lisch nodules) on slit lamp examination or biomicroscopy.
7. A first-degree relative (parent, sibling, or offspring) with NF I by the above criteria.

B. Criteria for neurofibromatosis II include:
1. Computed tomographic or magnetic resonance imaging evidence of bilateral internal auditory canal masses consistent with acoustic neuromas

or
2. A first-degree relative with NF II and either:
  a. Unilateral eighth nerve mass
  or
  b. Two of the following: neurofibroma, meningioma, glioma, schwannoma, juvenile posterior subcapsular lenticular opacity

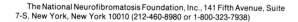

The National Neurofibromatosis Foundation, Inc., 141 Fifth Avenue, Suite 7-S, New York, New York 10010 (212-460-8980 or 1-800-323-7938)

bromatosis. They are also found occasionally in café au lait spots of persons without neurofibromatosis, are occasionally absent in café au lait spots of adults with neurofibromatosis, appear to be regularly absent in the café au lait spots of children with this disorder, and have been noted in normal epidermis and in other pigmentary conditions such as the melanocytic macules of patients with the multiple lentigines syndrome, Albright's syndrome, and the speckled lentiginous nevus (nevus spilus).[21] The diagnosis, however, may be helped by the fact that the café au lait spots of patients with neurofibromatosis contain more dopa-positive melanocytes per square centimeter than the surrounding normal skin, and in individuals without neurofibromatosis there are fewer dopa-positive melanocytes per square centimeter in the café au lait spots than the normal surrounding skin.[21, 22] Recent studies have also disclosed that the so-called macromelanosome is not a large melanosome but an autophagosome merged with a secondary lysosome (this has been termed a *melanin macroglobule*),[22] and café au lait macules with more than 10 melanin macroglobules per five high-power fields are only present in patients with von Recklinghausen's neurofibromatosis. Unfortunately, the value of this finding in patients younger than the age of 15 years is yet to be determined.[23]

Café au lait spots also occur in Albright's syndrome (McCune-Albright syndrome, polyostotic fibrous dysplasia with endocrine dysfunction, sexual precocity, and precocious somatic development, especially in girls) and other disorders (see Chapter 8). In this disorder the pigmented lesions are few, light to dark brown, usually large and unilateral, frequently have a jagged irregular border (resembling the coast of Maine), and generally stop abruptly at the midline. This is in contrast to the smooth outline (resembling the coast of California) and light brown color of the spots seen in von Recklinghausen's disease.

Other cutaneous pigmentary changes have been noted in patients with neurofibromatosis but lack the diagnostic significance attributed to axillary freckling and multiple café au lait spots. These include minute, freckle-like café au lait spots distributed in other regions of the body, areas of leukoderma, and diffuse graying or bronzing of the skin suggestive of the color seen in patients with argyria.

Neurofibromas. Von Recklinghausen's disease is also characterized by dermal fibromas and dermal or subcutaneous neurofibromas of Schwann cell origin derived from peripheral nerve sheaths. Solitary neurofibromas without other cutaneous findings are not diagnostic of neurofibromatosis and may be seen in individuals without evidence of this disorder. Whereas neurofibromas occurring as solitary lesions without café au lait spots or family history of neurofibromatosis may arise at any age, the cutaneous tumors of neurofibromatosis generally appear in late childhood or adolescence. Their appearance is frequently associated with puberty. They vary in number from a few to hundreds, with a progressive increase in size and number as the patient becomes older. Neurofibromas may occur anywhere on the body, with no specific site of predilection other than the fact that they usually avoid the palms and soles. They may appear as superficial tumors varying from 1 to 2 mm to several centimeters in diameter, or as discrete beaded, nodular, elongated masses seen along the course of nerves, usually the trigeminal or upper cervical nerves. *Plexiform neuromas* (plexiform neurofibromas) involve deeply located large nerves and show irregular nerve fascicles as a result of an increase in endoneural matrix and perineurium. They may reach enormous proportions; have a "bag-of-worms" consistency; can be present at birth; usually involve the limbs; are often associated with hypertrophy of the underlying soft tissues and bones; may at times cause pain, muscle weakness, atrophy, or slight sensory loss; have a predisposition to neurofibrosarcoma; and are not necessarily confined to patients with neurofibromatosis.

Generally flesh colored, neurofibromas tend to have a distinctive violaceous hue when small. As they enlarge they become pink, blue, or pigmented. Small tumors may be deep seated, sessile, or dome shaped; and as they become larger they become globular, pear shaped, pedunculated, or pendulous (Fig. 23–4). With moderate digital pressure the smaller lesions may be invaginated into an

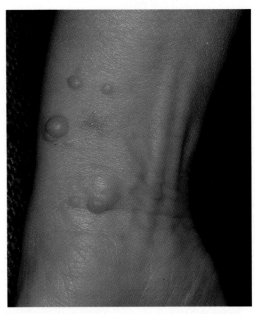

Figure 23–4. Neurofibromas. Skin-colored globular and dome-shaped nodules in a patient with neurofibromatosis (von Recklinghausen's disease). With moderate pressure neurofibromas may be invaginated into an underlying dermal defect, an almost pathognomonic maneuver termed *buttonholing* (Hurwitz S: The Skin and Systemic Disease in Children. Year Book Medical Publishers, Chicago, 1985.)

underlying dermal defect, an almost pathognomonic maneuver termed *buttonholing*.[24]

Although a benign course for neurofibromas is usual, some of the tumors may undergo malignant change. Neurofibrosarcomas, also referred to as malignant schwannomas, may develop in patients with neurofibromatosis, but this is not common.[21] Because of a tendency to report unusual cases, the literature reflects a high incidence of malignant transformation, with a range between 2 and 16 per cent (a more accurate figure for this complication appears to be 2 to 3 per cent). Although fibrosarcomatous malignant degeneration has occurred in early childhood, it is rare before the age of 40. Malignant degeneration may be heralded by rapid enlargement or pain, but malignant growth, once it develops, is often slow, with few metastases. In addition, large plexiform neuromas appear to have a higher incidence of malignant change, and excision of such lesions should be performed prophylactically when feasible. The prognosis for neurofibrosarcomas is poor. Extensive spread along the involved nerve requires aggressive surgical treatment, and local recurrences are common.

Blue-Red Macules and Pseudoatrophic Macules. Blue-red macules and pseudoatrophic macules (involuted neurofibromas) have also been described as characteristic lesions of neurofibromatosis. They arise before or after puberty and become slightly elevated and dome shaped; and new lesions may continue to appear. The blue-red lesions may have small blood vessels leading to a conglomerate appearance of telangiectasia and a reddish or bluish discoloration (due to stasis of blood) on exposure to cold.[25]

Lisch Nodules. Asymptomatic yellowish brown melanocytic hamartomas on the iris (Lisch nodules) have also been described in patients with the classic form of neurofibromatosis (NF I). The most common clinical feature of NF I, these lesions are seen in only 5 per cent of children younger than 3 years of age, 55 per cent of children 5 or 6 years of age, 94 per cent of children older than the age of 6 years, and 97 to 100 per cent of postpubertal patients with neurofibromatosis. Although not seen in normal persons or, except in one case, patients with the central (acoustic) form of neurofibromatosis, they may be seen in patients with mixed neurofibromatosis (NF III). Lisch nodules may at times be detected without magnification, but they are usually best visualized by an experienced ophthalmologist using a slit lamp microscope or binocular biomicroscopy. Since many children with neurofibromatosis 5 years of age or younger, and up to 3 per cent of postpubertal patients do not have Lisch nodules, their absence does not discount the diagnosis. All unaffected parents and children whose status is in question, therefore, should have a thorough ophthalmologic examination as a part of their evaluation so that appropriate genetic counseling can be provided.[26, 27]

Systemic Manifestations. In almost all patients neurofibromatosis can be diagnosed in the first year of life, and some form of systemic problem or compromise generally develops before the age of 20 years.[26] There is marked variability, however, in the overall severity and progression of classic neurofibromatosis. It can cause serious problems, and even death in the newborn, or may produce only mild or insignificant problems during the lifetime of the affected individual.

The severity of cutaneous involvement is not indicative of the extent of disease in other organs. Neurologic manifestations have been reported in as high as 40 per cent of patients and may involve any part of the central nervous system. Acoustic neuroma, rare and unilateral in NF I but more common and often bilateral in NF II, and optic glioma (most common in patients with NF I), are the most common lesions of the cranial nerves. Deafness therefore is common in patients with NF II, and glioma of the optic nerve, the most common central nervous system tumor and the one primarily seen in patients with NF I, may occasionally produce exophthalmos, decreased visual acuity, or restricted ocular movements.[5]

Neurologic disease occurs in more than half the cases of neurofibromatosis and includes retardation, seizure disorders, and tumors. Seizures are reported to occur in 8 to 13 per cent of patients (of these about half are associated with intracranial tumors); and intellectual compromise in the form of hyperactivity, learning disability, or mild to moderate mental retardation, found in up to 10 to 20 per cent of patients, may vary from a mild learning disability to severe retardation. The degree of mental deficiency, although occasionally severe, fortunately is usually mild to moderate and not progressive.

As many as 50 per cent of patients with neurofibromatosis may have osseous defects associated with this disorder. All bony changes may be explained by the development of neurofibromas lying within or in close proximity to bone. Of these, spinal deformity, particularly scoliosis or kyphosis, is the most common and may occur in over 10 per cent of patients.

The autonomic nervous system may also be affected and the gastrointestinal tract is involved in about 10 per cent of patients with neurofibromatosis. Intestinal neurofibromas with bleeding of the overlying mucosa have been reported. Complications, therefore, include vague abdominal discomfort, melena, hematemesis, bowel obstruction, and even intestinal perforation. Endocrine disorders include acromegaly, menstrual abnormalities, delayed or incomplete sexual development, gynecomastia, hyperthyroidism or hypothyroidism, infertility, Addison's disease, hyperparathyroidism, and diabetes. In children the most common endocrine abnormality is sexual precocity. Between 5 and 20 per cent of patients with pheochromocytoma also have neurofibromatosis; only 1 of every 223 patients with neurofibromatosis, however, is found to have a pheochromocytoma.[1, 24]

Since it has been noted that an increased incidence of juvenile chronic myelogenous leukemia has been found among patients with NF I, and that patients with a combination of juvenile xanthogranuloma and neurofibromatosis have an increased risk of chronic myelogenous leukemia or acute monomyelocytic leukemia, it is suggested that patients with neurofibromas or neurofibromatosis and juvenile xanthogranulomas be evaluated periodically for this possibility.[28–31]

Diagnosis. The diagnosis of neurofibromatosis depends on the number and size of café au lait spots (the earliest manifestation of this disorder), axillary freckling, Lisch nodules when present, and cutaneous neurofibromas. In individuals with inconclusive cutaneous changes, giant pigment granules (melanin macroglobules), or an increased number of melanocytes in the café au lait macules compared with the surrounding skin, although not diagnostic, may help establish the diagnosis. If there are at least six café au lait spots, larger than 1.5 cm in postpubertal children or adults or 5 mm or more in prepubertal children, the diagnosis of NF I is suggested, but not definitive. If axillary freckling is also present, the diagnosis is more likely. A careful search of the skin for neurofibromas, ocular examination for Lisch nodules, and determination of whether other family members are known or suspected to have neurofibromatosis is helpful (see Table 23–2). If the diagnosis of neurofibromatosis is in doubt, or at least not confirmed, this point should be made clear and referrals should be made for appropriate evaluation. If the diagnosis is certain or likely and the child's family history is negative, both parents should be examined for cutaneous or systemic manifestations, and slit lamp or binocular biomicroscopic examination should be performed in an effort to establish the presence or absence of Lisch nodules.

Treatment. Since many patients have minor or incomplete forms of this disorder, reassurance for parents of children affected with mild forms of neurofibromatosis is helpful. Treatment consists of surgical excision or dermabrasion of tumors that are disfiguring, interfere with function, or are subject to irritation, trauma, or infection. Periodic complete physical examinations are necessary, with particular attention to possible hypertension, skeletal deformities, endocrine disorders, gastrointestinal complications, and involvement of cranial nerves II and VIII. Plexiform neurofibromas and vertebral dysplasia may be signaled by an abnormal hair whorl or hairy nevus overlying the spinal column, and, although malignant degeneration of cutaneous tumors before age 40 is rare, complete surgical excision with histopathologic examination is mandatory if cutaneous neurofibromas become painful or show signs of rapid enlargement.

Genetic counseling is another important aspect of treatment, since there is a 50 per cent chance of transmitting neurofibromatosis with each pregnancy. In addition, an affected adult has about a 40 per cent chance of having a mildly affected child and a 12.5 per cent chance of having a moderately to severely affected child. In most affected families, 75 per cent of patients afflicted with the disorder will have minimal to mild disease; of these, there is a 25 per cent lifetime risk of moderate to severe involvement. A correlation has been made between the presence of hypertelorism (increased breadth of the nasal bridge with corresponding increased width between the eyes) and midline or orbital plexiform neuromas and central nervous system abnormalities in patients with neurofibromatosis.[32] Because of the high incidence of central nervous system abnormalities with this combination, a computed tomographic (CT) scan, or resonance imaging (MRI) and electroencephalography are recommended as part of the workup for such patients; and because of the possibility of other associated anomalies, CT scan of the orbits and auditory canals, developmental mental testing, audiometry, ophthalmologic examination, electroencephalograms, spinal radiographs, and blood pressure and urinary evaluations for the possibility of pheochromocytoma are suggested for all patients with neurofibromatosis. Children with neurofibromatosis should have an intelligence test and psychological testing before they enter school, and their hearing should be tested (because of the possibility of acoustic neuromas). Since patients who manifest both juvenile xanthogranulomas and neurofibromas or neurofibromatosis may have a predisposition to leukemia,

patients with this combination should be checked periodically for this possibility.

TUBEROUS SCLEROSIS

Tuberous sclerosis is a relatively uncommon disorder of irregular but dominant autosomal inheritance of variable penetrance occurring with an incidence of about 5 to 7 per 100,000 individuals. Of these, 50 to 70 per cent appear to arise from new mutations. It is classified as a neurocutaneous syndrome in which the brain, eyes, skin, heart, kidneys, lungs, and bones may be affected. The full entity is defined by a triad of seizures, mental deficiency, and a variety of pathognomonic skin lesions (Table 23–3). The latter include adenoma sebaceum, shagreen patches, periungual and gingival fibromas, and hypopigmented macules. Although café au lait spots have an increased incidence (26 per cent) in this disorder, they are not a diagnostic sign of tuberous sclerosis.[33]

Primarily a defect in the organization of connective tissue in which hyperplasia of ectodermal and mesodermal tissue leads to a variety of hamartomas in the nervous system, skin, heart, kidneys, and other organs in which the gene is linked to the distal long arm of chromosome 9, the exact pathogenesis is unclear.[34]

Clinical Manifestations. Adenoma sebaceum, present in 80 to 90 per cent of cases, is the most common skin manifestation associated with this disorder. The term *adenoma sebaceum* is a misnomer; these lesions represent angiofibromas, hamartomas composed of fibrous and vascular tissue. The lesions usually appear as 1 to 4 mm dome-shaped nodules with a smooth surface (see Figs. 8–39, 8–40, and 23–5). They range from pink to red and often are accompanied by fine telangiectasia. Lesions of adenoma sebaceum are usually located in a bilaterally symmetrical distribution in the nasolabial folds, cheeks, and chin and sometimes on the forehead and scalp. They are rarely found on the upper lip except for the central area immediately below the nose. The lesions, rarely present at birth, usually appear at some time between the second and fifth birthdays, often not until puberty. Since only 13 per cent of children with tuberous

Table 23–3. TUBEROUS SCLEROSIS

1. Autosomal dominant
   a. 5 to 7 per 100,000 individuals
   b. 50% to 70% represent new mutations
2. Cutaneous manifestations
   a. Hypopigmented macules (in 70% to 90% of cases)
   b. Adenoma sebaceum (angiofibromas)
   c. Shagreen patches
   d. Periungual and gingival fibromas
   e. Tooth pits
3. Systemic manifestations (in 80% to 90% of patients): central nervous system involvement; cardiac rhabdomyomas; retinal gliomas; renal hamartomas or carcinomas, or enlarged cystic kidneys; cystic lesions in lungs, osseous lesions

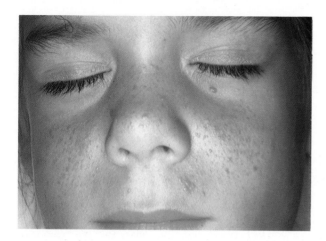

Figure 23–5. Adenoma sebaceum. Small, discrete, reddish pink, dome-shaped angiofibromas are evident in a bilaterally symmetrical distribution on the cheeks, nose, and upper lip of a 5-year-old girl with tuberous sclerosis.

sclerosis develop the facial lesions of adenoma sebaceum during the first year of life, it appears that this is not the best early marker of this condition.

Fibromas also develop around and under the nails of the fingers and toes (periungual and subungual fibromas) (Fig. 23–6) and on the gums (gingival fibromas). The periungual and subungual fibromas, seen in about 50 per cent of patients, appear at puberty as firm, flesh colored growths. Because of their relatively late appearance they too are of little value in the early diagnosis of this disorder.

Shagreen patches are seen in 21 to 83 per cent of patients with tuberous sclerosis (Figs. 8–41 and 23–7). They develop during early childhood, usually between the patient's second and fifth birthdays. They generally develop on the trunk (most frequently the lumbosacral area) and appear as flesh-colored to yellowish or yellowish orange, slightly elevated plaques of dermal connective tissue. Seen as single or multiple lesions measuring 2 to 10 cm or more in diameter, they frequently have an orange-peel or pigskin appearance resembling shagreen leather.

White macules, seen in 70 to 90 per cent of patients with tuberous sclerosis, are a particularly valuable early marker of this disorder. Although

delayed appearance of hypopigmented macules in patients with tuberous sclerosis has been reported,[35] reports of their late appearance is questionable since these hypopigmented lesions can often be overlooked during infancy unless careful examination (including the use of a Wood's lamp in a completely darkened room) has been undertaken. Hypopigmented macules, therefore, are generally present at birth or appear shortly thereafter, may enlarge as the infant grows, and persist throughout life, but otherwise do not change in size or shape (see Figs. 16–13, 23–8, and 23–9). In addition to the characteristic hypopigmented macules, there is also an increased incidence of tuberous sclerosis in patients with poliosis and partial albinism (see Fig. 16–12) and individuals with tuberous sclerosis have an increased number of café au lait spots.[33, 36, 37] Although the etiologies of hyperpigmentation and hypopigmentation are unknown, since melanocytes are derived from the neural crest, it is not surprising that these changes are found in patients with disorders involving the central nervous system.

A striking feature of the white spots of tuberous sclerosis is the marked variability in size and shape of lesions. They range from 0.4 to 7 cm or more, with the majority of lesions measuring between

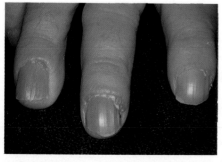

Figure 23–6. Periungual fibromas. Firm, flesh-colored growths are present in the periungual region of a patient with tuberous sclerosis.

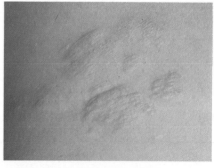

Figure 23–7. Shagreen patches. Slightly elevated flesh-colored plaques of connective tissue with an orange-peel (peau d'orange) surface on the lumbosacral area of a girl with tuberous sclerosis.

Figure 23–8. Lance-ovate ash-leaf-shaped hypopigmented macule of tuberous sclerosis.

1 and 3 cm in diameter. They are usually oval or semioval and have highly irregular margins (Fig. 23–9). Although ash-leaf-shaped lance-ovate hypopigmented macules (see Fig. 23–8) have been described as the characteristic lesions of tuberous sclerosis,[38] in Braverman and my series only 18 per cent of the white spots of tuberous sclerosis were found to be truly ash-leaf shaped.[33]

The white spots of tuberous sclerosis have often been termed *vitiliginous* by nondermatologists, but these partially depigmented lesions are unrelated to vitiligo and can be differentiated by many characteristics. Vitiligo represents an acquired form of hypopigmentation characterized by sharply demarcated "ivory white" macules surrounded by hyperpigmented skin. The completely depigmented ivory white macules of vitiligo may

Figure 23–9. An irregular hypopigmented macule on the thigh of an 18-year-old young woman with tuberous sclerosis. Only 18 per cent of leukodermatous lesions of tuberous sclerosis are lance-ovate in shape.

occur at any age but are rare in infants. Although lesions of vitiligo may appear on any part of the body, they frequently have a bilateral or symmetrical distribution, with involvement of the skin of the face and neck, of the backs of hands and forearms, over bony prominences, and in body folds and periorificial areas. They often change in size and shape, frequently spread, and occasionally may show partial to complete repigmentation. Conversely, the leukoderma of tuberous sclerosis is usually present at birth and is located over the abdomen, back, and anterior and lateral surfaces of the arms and legs. It is a dull white, with incomplete depigmentation (in comparison to the ivory white color of vitiligo), does not alter in shape or size with age, and appears to be related to a defect of melanosome melanization. The basic cause of this pigmentary disturbance remains obscure.

The difference between hypopigmented lesions of tuberous sclerosis and vitiligo can be demonstrated by electron microscopy. Whereas the completely depigmented lesions of vitiligo reveal an absence or decrease in the number of melanocytes, the partially depigmented macules of tuberous sclerosis have a normal number of melanocytes with a decrease in the size, synthesis, and melanization of melanosomes.[38]

Another peculiar form of speckled leukoderma may be seen as small 1 to 3 mm hypopigmented lesions (white freckles) in a confetti-like pattern over the pretibial area in some patients with tuberous sclerosis (Fig. 23–10). Although occasionally seen in normal individuals, they, too, can serve as helpful markers in the diagnosis of patients with this disorder.[33] Of further significance, in addition to the increased incidence of tuberous sclerosis in patients with partial albinism,[36, 37] the presence of one or more tufts of white hair in an infant with seizures should suggest the possibility of a diagnosis of tuberous sclerosis.[39]

In view of the high frequency of white macules present at birth in patients with tuberous sclerosis, infants and children, particularly those with seizure disorders, should be screened for the characteristic but easily overlooked dull-white macules that are now recognized as the earliest cutaneous markers of tuberous sclerosis. In individuals with light pigmentation, however, these macules can be extremely faint. Illumination of the skin with a Wood's light in a darkened room can be helpful in detecting hypopigmented spots that contrast poorly with surrounding normal skin.

Tooth pits (seen as punctate, round or oval, 1 to 2 mm randomly arranged enamel defects), particularly in the permanent teeth, appear to be another marker of tuberous sclerosis. Recent studies suggest that when tooth pits are seen in numbers of five or more, they may prove to be pathognomonic of this disorder. (Fig. 23–11).[40, 40a, 40b]

The systemic lesions of tuberous sclerosis may produce severe symptoms and possibly death. Central nervous system involvement may lead to convulsions and mental retardation. Seizures, seen

Figure 23–10. White freckles. Multiple 1- to 3-mm hypopigmented lesions in a confetti-like pattern on the leg of a patient with tuberous sclerosis.

in 80 to 90 per cent of patients with tuberous sclerosis, may begin as infantile spasms, in which sudden repetitive myoclonic contractions of most of the body musculature are combined with flexion, extension, opisthotonos, and tremors. By 2 or 3 years of age, focal or generalized seizures and mental retardation may become evident. Extensive CNS involvement leads to hypsarrhythmia (salaam seizures), with electroencephalographic findings of multifocal high-voltage spikes and slow chaotic waves. Later in life the seizure pattern may change

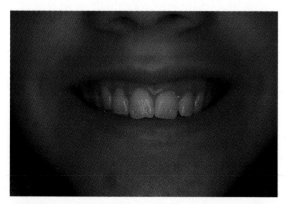

Figure 23–11. Tooth pits. Tooth pits are said to be pathognomonic of tuberous sclerosis when present in numbers of five or more; this patient was a healthy 15-year-old girl with no evidence of this disorder.

to a petit mal variety, and in less severe cases generalized or focal motor seizures may develop.

Retardation may be mild or severe and appears in 62 per cent of affected individuals. Sclerotic calcification in the brain is visible as "tubers" on radiographs in 50 to 75 per cent of individuals. In young children, when skull radiographs are not diagnostic, findings of small calcifications and ventricular dilatation on magnetic resonance imaging (MRI) or computed tomographic (CT) scan are helpful in the diagnosis of this disorder.[41] Forty to 80 per cent of patients with tuberous sclerosis have renal hamartomas (angiomyolipomas), renal cell carcinomas, or enlarged cystic kidneys resembling those of polycystic kidney disease.[42] Rhabdomyomas in the heart may be associated with congestive heart failure, murmurs, cyanosis, or sudden death, and the association of Wolff-Parkinson-White syndrome with supraventricular tachycardia has been reported. The eyes may have characteristic retinal lesions (gliomas) referred to as phakomas. Fundoscopy may show multiple, raised, mulberry-like lesions on or adjacent to the optic nerve head or flat, disk-like lesions in the periphery of the retina. Ophthalmologic examination may reveal flat, partially transparent noncalcified tumors, nodular calcified tumors, or tumors containing features of both. Cystic lesions in the lungs may rupture and produce spontaneous pneumothorax, often with a radiographic honeycombed appearance, and about 85 per cent of patients with tuberous sclerosis have osseous manifestations with the bones, particularly those of the hands and feet, demonstrating cysts and periosteal thickenings.

Diagnosis. Although formes frustes of tuberous sclerosis are common, the appearance of characteristic skin lesions in children with epilepsy, mental retardation, or both, should establish a diagnosis of tuberous sclerosis. The diagnosis is readily apparent when the classic triad of adenoma sebaceum, epilepsy, and mental retardation is present. In the absence of all features of the syndrome, however, diagnosis depends on the cutaneous manifestations, family history (with examination of family members), ophthalmologic examination, bone survey for cortical thickening and phalangeal cysts, skull radiographs, magnetic resonance imaging or computed tomography, intravenous pyelography or ultrasonic examination of the kidney for renal hamartomas, and chest radiography for honeycombing of the lungs.

Management. Seizure disorders associated with tuberous sclerosis often respond to anticonvulsant therapy. Death, when it occurs, may result from status epilepticus, pulmonary or renal insufficiency, or cardiac failure. Adenoma sebaceum requires no treatment except for cosmetic reasons. Best results are seen following cryosurgery, electrodesiccation and curettage, dermabrasion, or laser beam therapy; of these the latter currently appears to be the easiest and least traumatic. Although surgery may be required for relief of symptoms from internal tumors of tuberous sclerosis, surgical removal is often unsatisfactory. Genetic counseling against childbearing is recommended for patients with the disorder (even those with mild forms of tuberous sclerosis), since their children may be more severely affected than they are. However, 50 to 70 per cent of patients with tuberous sclerosis may be mutations and, unless there is evidence of tuberous sclerosis in other members of the family, genetic counseling (although of primary importance in the management of individuals with this disorder) is not completely effective in the prevention of new cases. Recognition of cutaneous markers, however, is useful and often leads to the identification of unrecognized or mildly affected individuals with formes frustes of the disorder. It is suggested, therefore, that all family members at risk for tuberous sclerosis have skin examination, funduscopic examination, skull, hand, and foot radiographs, cranial computed tomography, and ultrasound examination, which can be utilized as a noninvasive technique instead of excretory urography.[43]

Although it has been stated that most patients with tuberous sclerosis die before the age of 25, with death usually caused by malignant central nervous system neoplasm or status epilepticus, that 30 per cent of affected children die before age 5, and that 5 to 15 per cent of patients die before adulthood and only 5 per cent live beyond the age of 30, it should be noted that there is wide variability in the expression of the disease. All patients with skin lesions do not develop seizures or mental deficiency, and many patients with mild or abortive forms of the disorder, unrecognized, live out a normal life span. These high morbidity figures, therefore, appear to be overly pessimistic and require further evaluation.

INCONTINENTIA PIGMENTI

Incontinentia pigmenti (Bloch-Sulzberger syndrome) is a hereditary disorder that affects the skin, central nervous system, eyes, and skeletal system. Although the genetics of this disorder have not been delineated, the familial tendency with almost exclusive involvement of females (97 per cent) suggests that transmission is X-linked dominant and that the disorder is prenatally lethal to hemizygous males.[44, 45] This explains the predominance of female patients with this disorder. The fact that males with incontinentia pigmenti are no more severely affected than their female counterparts suggests that the disease in living male patients may be the result of spontaneous mutation.

Clinical Manifestations. The disorder generally appears at birth or shortly thereafter (90 per cent of patients have cutaneous lesions within the first 2 weeks of life; 96 per cent have their onset before the age of 6 weeks). Although the cutaneous lesions have four distinct phases, their sequence is

irregular and overlapping of stages is common. (Table 23–4).[46]

Phase 1. The first phase of incontinentia pigmenti begins with inflammatory vesicles (Fig. 23–12) or bullae that develop in crops over the trunk and extremities, often persisting for weeks to months. An interesting and unexplained feature of this phase of the disorder is the high degree of eosinophilia (from 18 to 50 per cent) that is present in 74 per cent of patients during the first 2 weeks of life. Biopsy of a small blister during this vesicular stage reveals an inflammatory dermatitis with epidermal vesicles filled with eosinophils.

Phase 2. The vesicular stage is followed by an intermediate phase characterized by irregular linear warty or verrucous lesions (Fig. 23–13) on one or more extremities, usually the backs of the hands and feet. This stage, seen in 70 per cent of patients with incontinentia pigmenti, resolves spontaneously, usually within a period of several months.

Phase 3. During or shortly following this intermediate verrucous stage, the highly characteristic pigmentary state begins. The pigmentation, the hallmark of the disease, seen in almost 100 per cent of patients, is characterized by bands of slate-brown to blue-gray splattered Chinese-figure–like patches arranged in swirl-like formations on the extremities and trunk (Figs. 23–14 through 23–16). This stage tends to increase in intensity until the patient's second year of life. It persists for many years and gradually fades and, in many cases, completely disappears by adolescence or early adulthood. It is from this pigmentary stage that the disease derives its name (because histologically melanin appears to drop down from the melanocytes into the dermis).

Although the pigmentary changes were originally considered to be a postinflammatory phenomenon secondary to the vesiculobullous or verrucous stages, the pigment fails to follow the pattern, shape, or location of the bullous and verrucous lesions. Electron microscopic studies, however, conclude that all three stages are related to each other and that pigmentary incontinence may represent a phagocytic phenomenon.[47]

Phase 4. A fourth phase consisting of depigmented lesions may also be detected in individuals with incontinentia pigmenti.[48] Seen as isolated streaked hypopigmented lesions or in

Table 23–4. INCONTINENTIA PIGMENTI

1. X-linked dominant, prenatally lethal to males (97% are females; living males probably represent mutations)
2. Four cutaneous phases (inflammatory vesicles or bullae, verrucous lesions, whorled hyperpigmentation, and hypopigmented patches)
3. Eosinophilia in over 70% of patients (often until 20th week of life)
4. Systemic manifestations in 79% (20% at birth) (dental, 68%; ocular, 35%; central nervous system, 30%; cardiac, occasionally, and skeletal, 13%)

Hurwitz S: The Skin and Systemic Disease in Children. Year Book Medical Publishers, Chicago, 1985.

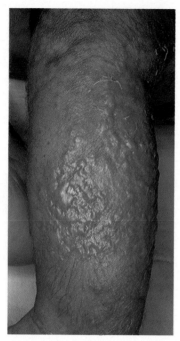

Figure 23–12. Incontinentia pigmenti (vesicular stage). Multiple vesicles and bullae, many in a linear distribution (the first phase of incontinentia pigmenti) are seen on the leg of a 2-week-old infant.

conjunction with other manifestations, they have been noted on the arms, thighs, trunk, and particularly the calves of children as well as adults (Fig. 23–17), and studies have shown a diminution of hair, sweat pores, sweat coils, and sweating in these areas.[49] The presence of these lesions, although frequently overlooked, may serve as a clue to the hereditary pattern and may play a role in the genetic counseling of families of individuals with this disorder.

Systemic Manifestations. Systemic manifestations occur in a high percentage of patients with incontinentia pigmenti. Almost 80 per cent of patients have one or more abnormalities of the hair

(Fig. 23–18), eyes, central nervous system, and/or structural development. Thirty per cent of patients have central nervous system involvement. Of these, 3.3 per cent have seizures, and although many individuals are bright or have normal intellect, 16 per cent have low mentality and 13 per cent have spastic abnormalities. Ophthalmic changes are present in 35 per cent of patients; 18 per cent have strabismus; and an equal number demonstrate more serious eye involvement (cataracts, optic atrophy, or retinal damage). Alopecia is seen in 38 per cent of patients; nail dystrophy is present in 7 per cent of individuals; painful grayish white verrucous or keratotic subungual tumors may be seen (usually during the second or third decades of life); and, at times, lytic defects may be noted on roentgenographic examination of the distal phalanges of affected as well as unaffected fingers.[50, 51] In addition, 64 per cent of patients have dental anomalies (delayed dentition, partial anodontia, pegged or conical teeth) (Fig. 23–19).[44] Occasionally, cardiac anomalies and skeletal malformations (such as microcephaly, syndactyly, supernumerary ribs, hemiatrophy, or shortening of the arms or legs) may occur. In a four-generation study of a family with incontinentia pigmenti, several members also had woolly hair nevus syndrome and six of seven patients had alopecia and agenesis or hypoplasia of eyebrows and eyelashes.[45]

Diagnosis. The combination of vesicular and linear, nodular, or warty lesions in a female infant is pathognomonic of this disorder, and the characteristic Chinese-figure–like pigmentation is a hallmark of the disease. Because of the risk of involvement of other children and a potential for ocular, dental, osseous, and neurologic changes, it is important that physicians, particularly pediatricians and family practitioners, usually the first to see the patient, be familiar with this entity and be able to diagnose and counsel patients seen with this disorder.

Histopathologic examination of vesicular lesions in the first stage of incontinentia pigmenti reveals a dermal infiltrate composed of lymphocytes, polymorphonuclear leukocytes, and numerous eo-

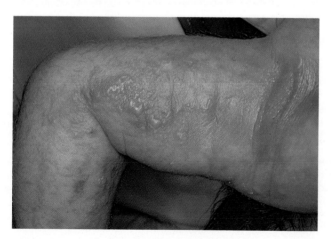

Figure 23–13. Vesicular and verrucous lesions on the thigh of the 2-week-old infant with incontinentia pigmenti in Figure 23–12. Although incontinentia pigmenti has four distinct cutaneous phases, their sequence is irregular and overlapping is common.

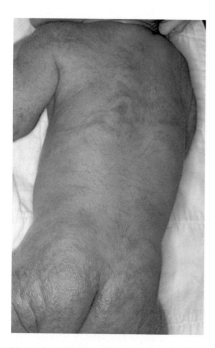

Figure 23–14. Swirl-like bands of slate-brown to blue-gray hyperpigmentation in a child with incontinentia pigmenti.

sinophils and mononuclear cells in the vesicles as well as the epidermis and dermis. Features of the second stage consist of acanthosis, irregular papillomatosis, and hyperkeratosis. The basal cells show vacuolization and a decrease in their melanin content. The dermis shows a mild chronic inflammatory infiltrate intermingled with melanophages. The third stage is characterized by extensive deposits of melanin within melanophages located in the upper dermis. Usually this dermal hyperpigmentation is found in association with diminution of pigment in the basal layer and the cells of the basal layer show vacuolization and degeneration.

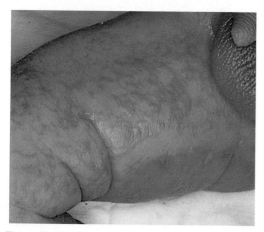

Figure 23–15. Chinese figure–like hyperpigmentation in a male newborn with incontinentia pigmenti.

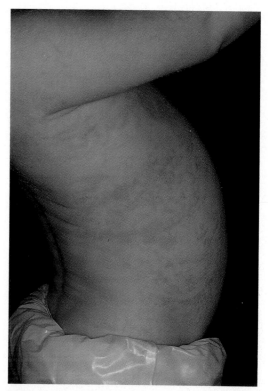

Figure 23–16. Chinese figure–like pigmentation in a linear, swirled pattern on the trunk of a 2-year-old girl with incontinentia pigmenti.

Treatment. No special therapy is required for the skin lesions of incontinentia pigmenti. Genetic counseling for carrier females is advisable, however, since up to 80 per cent of affected children have associated congenital defects. Seizures in the first week of life associated with incontinentia pigmenti seem to indicate a poor prognosis with subsequent developmental delay. Absence of seizures early in life, however, especially in conjunction with normal developmental milestones, appears to predict normal development, and generally tends to offer a good prognosis.[52]

HYPOMELANOSIS OF ITO (INCONTINENTIA PIGMENTI ACHROMIANS)

Hypomelanosis of Ito, initially called incontinentia pigmenti achromians, is a condition of hypopigmentation first described by Ito in 1952. The name incontinenti pigmenti achromians was coined because hypopigmenation of the skin appeared in a linear swirled pattern that resembled a negative image of the hyperpigmentation see in patients with incontinentia pigmentia (Fig. 23–20).[53, 54] Histologic examination of the hypopigmented areas reveals a decrease in the number of melanin granules in the basal area and a complete

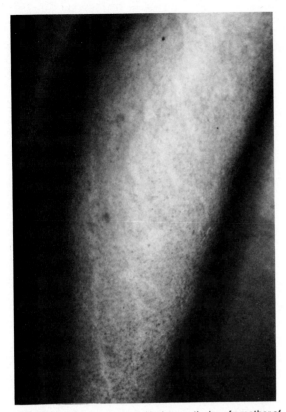

Figure 23–17. Hypopigmented lesions on the leg of a mother of an infant with incontinentia pigmenti, the fourth stage of the disorder. (Courtesy of Robert Hartmann, M.D.)

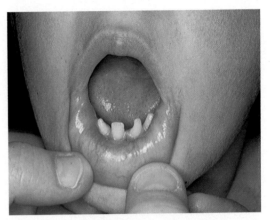

Figure 23–19. Pegged (conical) teeth. Approximately two thirds of patients with incontinentia pigmenti have dental anomalies (anodontia, pegged or conical teeth, or delayed dentition).

Although multiple cases of hypomelanosis of Ito have been described in several families and it may represent an autosomal dominant disorder, its genetic pattern remains unclear.[55–57] The disorder is often seen at birth, or early in infancy or childhood, and persists for many years. In a few patients the lesions may be patchy and confined to relatively limited areas of the body (see nevus achromicus); in most patients, however, the hypopigmented areas are more extensive, are often bilateral, appear to be more pronounced on the ventral surface of the trunk and the flexor surfaces of the limbs, and tend to run parallel to one another following

absence of melanin in other areas. With the dopa reaction, the hypopigmented areas contain fewer and smaller melanocytes than normal and sparse, short dendrites. Since there is no histologic evidence of pigment incontinence and the disorder is distinct from and unrelated to incontinentia pigmenti, these two disorders should not be confused with one another (Table 23–5). Thus, most authorities currently favor the term *hypomelanosis of Ito* rather than incontinentia pigmenti achromians.

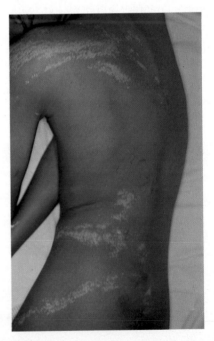

Figure 23–20. Incontinentia pigmenti achromians (hypomelanosis of Ito). Macular, linear, or swirl pattern of hypopigmentation are present. Approximately 50 per cent of patients with incontinentia pigmenti achromians have internal manifestations.

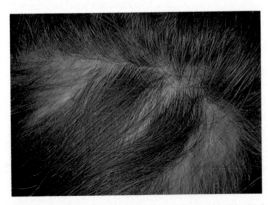

Figure 23–18. Cicatricial alopecia in a 7-year-old girl with incontinentia pigmenti. Alopecia is seen in 25 to 38 per cent of patients with this disorder.

Table 23–5. HYPOMELANOSIS OF ITO
(INCONTINENTIA PIGMENTI ACHROMIANS)

1. Genetic pattern unclear (perhaps autosomal dominant)
2. Hypopigmentation often in a linear swirled pattern
3. 50% have systemic manifestations (central nervous system dysfunction; ocular disturbances; musculoskeletal anomalies; hair, nail and dental anomalies)

Hurwitz S: The Skin and Systemic Disease in Children. Year Book Medical Publishers, Chicago, 1985.

the lines of Blaschko. To date, involvement of the scalp, palms, and soles has not been noted.[58]

Approximately 50 per cent of patients with hypomelanosis of Ito have internal manifestations. These include central nervous system dysfunction (seizure disorders and delayed development), ocular disturbances (strabismus, heterochromia iridis, microphthalmia, and nystagmus), musculoskeletal anomalies (i.e., macrocephaly, scoliosis, asymmetry of the limbs, weakness, hypotonicity, asymmetry of the head, dwarfism, small stature, hemiatrophy, delayed fontanelle closure, spina bifida occulta, genu valgum, dislocation of the hips, polydactyly, syndactyly, irreducible flexion of one or more fingers [camptodactyly], lordosis, and bifid thumbs). In addition, affected patients may have hair anomalies (i.e. diffuse alopecia, generalized hirsutism, facial hypertrichosis, coarse, curly, or slow growing hair), cleft lip and palate, malformed auricles, hypertelorism, cataracts, chorioretinal atrophy, skin anomalies (i.e., decreased sweat response, decreased capillary resistance, morphea, and ichthyosis), dental anomalies (i.e., anodontia and dental dysplasia), transverse ridging of the nails, hepatomegaly, diaphragmatic hernia, and diastasis recti.[54–60]

The report of familial cases of hypomelanosis of Ito and incontinentia pigmenti, and the fact that at least one mother and child had skin lesions of incontinentia pigmenti before the onset of hypomelanosis of Ito suggests a possible relationship between the two disorders.[60]

Since hypopigmented lesions appear infrequently in early infancy and young children, the appearance of such lesions, particularly in the absence of previous inflammatory skin disease, should alert the physician to possible association with systemic disease. All patients with systematized hypopigmented lesions, therefore, should be evaluated for anomalies; a careful developmental evaluation should be obtained; and if scoliosis or asymmetry is present, since the likelihood of seizures with this combination is high, an electroencephalogram and neurologic assessment are indicated.[60, 61]

References

1. Crowe FW, Schull WJ, Neel JV: A Clinical, Pathologic Genetic Study of Multiple Neurofibromatosis. Charles C Thomas, Springfield, Illinois, 1956.

A classic monographic survey of von Recklinghausen's disease.

2. Riccardi VM: von Recklinghausen neurofibromatosis. N. Engl. J. Med. 30:1617–1627, 1981.

A comprehensive authoritative review of neurofibromatosis.

3. Sloan JB, Fretzin DF, Bovenmyer DA: Genetic counseling in segmental neurofibromatosis. J. Am. Acad. Dermatol. 22:461–467, 1990.

A report of two children with segmental neurofibromatosis and a review of the literature with regard to possible hereditary transmission of this disorder.

4. Eldrige R, Denckla MB, Bien E, et al.: Neurofibromatosis type 1 (Recklinghausen's disease): Neurologic and cognitive assessment with sibling controls. Am. J. Dis. Child. 143:833–837, 1989.

In a controlled study of 13 pairs of siblings (in which one of each pair was affected with NF I), although the patients affected with NF 1 had no increase in mental retardation, attention deficit, or specific learning disorders, they had a higher incidence of subtle neurologic abnormalities and IQ scores lower than those of their unaffected siblings.

5. Listernick R, Charrow J, Greenwald MJ, et al.: Optic gliomas in children with neurofibromatosis type 1. J. Pediatr. 114:788–792, 1989.

In a review of 85 children with NF-1, none of whom had ophthalmic symptoms, 10 (15 per cent) were found to have gliomas of one or both optic nerves.

6. Wertelecki W, Rouleau GA, Superneau DW, et al.: Neurofibromatosis 2: Clinical and DNA linkage studies of a large kindred. N. Engl. J. Med. 319:278–283, 1989.

Clinical and DNA studies of 15 males and 8 females of a large kindred with neurofibromatosis 2.

7. Richards SS, Bachysnki BN: Ophthalmic manifestations of neurofibromatosis type 2. Int. Pediatr. 5:270–274, 1990.

A report of a patient with neurofibromatosis type 2 with a review of the literature and a discussion of the ophthalmologic findings of individuals with this subtype of neurofibromatosis.

8. Pullara TJ, Greeson D, Stoker GL, et al.: Cutaneous segmental neurofibromatosis. J. Am. Acad. Dermatol. 13:999–1003, 1985.

A report of 2 patients with multiple cutaneous neurofibromas restricted to a dermatomal portion of the skin.

9. Stotts JS, Steinman HK: Congenital, segmental pigmented lesions. Arch. Dermatol. 123:251–253, 1987.

A report of a 64-year-old woman with multiple hyperpigmented macules and neurofibromas on the left side of her upper back, the left side of her chest, left breast, the medial aspect of her left arm and left axilla (segmental neurofibromatosis), a rare disorder with to the authors' knowledge only 13 case reports in the world literature at the time this review was written.

10. Crowe FW: Multiple neurofibromatosis (von Recklinghausen's disease). In Demis DJ (Ed.): Clinical Dermatology, 17th ed. J.B. Lippincott Co, Philadelphia, 1990, unit 24–2.

A comprehensive review of neurofibromatosis, its various types and clinical manifestations.

11. Conejo-Mir JS, Saval H, Martinez FC: Segmental neurofibromatosis. J. Am. Acad. Dermatol. 20:681–682, 1989.

A report of a 28-year-old black man with segmental neurofibromatosis on the lateral aspect of his right abdomen.

12. Tibbles J, Cohen M: The Proteus syndrome: The elephant man diagnosed. Br. Med. J. 293:683–685, 1986.

Joseph Merrick, "the elephant man," probably suffered from the Proteus syndrome, a rare disease named for the Greek god Proteus (the polymorphous one), rather than neurofibromatosis.

13. Riccardi VM: Pathophysiology of neurofibromatosis: IV. Dermatologic insights into heterogeneity and pathogenesis. J. Am. Acad. Dermatol. *3*:157–166, 1980.

A systematic evaluation of 102 patients with, or at risk for, neurofibromatosis.

14. Crowe FW, Schull WJ: Diagnostic importance of the café-au-lait spot in neurofibromatosis. Arch. Intern. Med. *91*:758–766, 1963.

Six or more café au lait spots greater than 1.5 cm in diameter probably indicate the presence of neurofibromatosis.

15. Whitehouse D: Diagnostic value of the café-au-lait spot in children. Arch. Dis. Child. *41*:316–319, 1966.

In children 5 years of age and younger, the criterion for neurofibromatosis is modifed to five café au lait spots or more, 0.5 cm or greater in diameter.

16. Obringer AO, Meadows AT, Zackai EH: The diagnosis of neurofibromatosis-1 in the child under the age of 6 years. Am. J. Dis. Child. *143*:717–719, 1989.

Using the National Institutes of Health criteria, 112 of 160 children younger than the age of 6 years were diagnosed as having NF-1.

17. Crowe FW: Axillary freckling as a diagnostic aid in neurofibromatosis. Ann. Intern. Med. *61*:1142–1143, 1962.

Twenty per cent of patients with neurofibromatosis display axillary freckling (Crowe's sign).

18. Benedict PH, Szabo G, Fitzpatrick TB, et al.: Melanotic macules in Albright's syndrome and in neurofibromatosis. J.A.M.A. *25*;618–626, 1968.

Melanocytes in café au lait spots have characteristic giant melanin granules.

19. Jimbo K, Szabo G, Fitzpatrick TB: Ultrastructural giant pigment granules (macromelanosomes) in cutaneous pigmented macules of neurofibromatosis. J. Invest. Dermatol. *61*:300–309, 1973.

Giant pigment granules are noted in melanocytes and keratinocytes in the epidermis of patients with neurofibromatosis, not in the café au lait spots of normal individuals.

20. Morris TJ, Johnson WG, Silvers DN: Giant pigment granules in biopsy specimens from café au lait spots in neurofibromatosis. Arch. Dermatol. *118*:385–388, 1982.

Giant pigment granules in 6 of 8 dopa-incubated epidermal biopsy specimens suggested that large numbers of giant pigment granules from café au lait spots, although not specific, may be helpful in the diagnosis of neurofibromatosis.

21. Lever WF, Schaumburg-Lever G: Tumors of neural tissue: Neurofibromatosis. In Histopathology of the Skin, 6th ed. J. B. Lippincott Co., Philadelphia, 1983, 667–674.

The histopathology of café au lait spots in neurofibromatosis.

22. Nakagawa H, Hori Y, Sato S, et al.: The nature and origin of the melanin macroglobule. J. Invest. Dermatol. *83*:134–139, 1984.

Studies suggest that giant melanin granules are not macromelanosomes but represent autolysosomes referred to as melanin macroglobules.

23. Martuza RL, Philippe I, Fitzpatrick TB, et al.: Melanin macroglobules as a cellular marker of neurofibromatosis: A quantitative study. J. Invest. Dermatol. *85*:347–350, 1985.

Electron microscopic studies of café au lait spots suggest that the presence of ten or more melanin macroglobules (MMG) per five high-powered microscopic fields (at least in patients older than 15 years of age) help establish the diagnosis of von Recklinghausen's neurofibromatosis.

24. Bravermann IM: Neurocutaneous disorders. In Skin Signs of Systemic Disease, 2nd ed. W. B. Saunders Co., Philadelphia, 1981, 777–800.

A comprehensive review of the cutaneous features of neurocutaneous disease.

25. Westerhof W, Konrad K: Blue-red macules and pseudoatrophic macules: Additional cutaneous signs of neurofibromatosis. Arch. Dermatol. *118*:577–581, 1982.

A report of two patients with pseudoatrophic blue-red macules and review of four additional patients exhibiting blue-red macules as early cutaneous features of neurofibromatosis.

26. Riccardi VM: The multiple forms of neurofibromatosis. Pediatr. Rev. *3*:293–298, 1982.

An authoritative review of neurofibromatosis and its various forms as manifested in childhood.

27. Lubs M-LE, Bauer MS, Formas ME, et al.: Lisch nodules in neurofibromatosis type-I. N. Engl. J. Med. *324*:1264–1283. 1991.

In a study of 167 patients with neurofibromatosis, the authors conclude that Lisch nodules are specifically diagnostic for neurofibromatosis-I.

28. Hurwitz S: The Skin and Systemic Disease in Children. Year Book Medical Publishers, Chicago, 1985.

An overview of cutaneous features and their relationship to systemic disorders in childhood.

29. Bertak M: Juvenile chronic myelogenous leukemia and dermal histiocytosis in vonRecklinghausen's disease. Am. J. Dis. Child. *133*:831–833, 1979.

A review of chronic myelogenous leukemia and dermal histiocytosis in patients with von Recklinghausen's disease.

30. Cooper PH, Frierson HF, Kayne AL, et al.: Association of juvenile xanthogranuloma with juvenile myeloid leukemia. Arch Dermatol *120*:371–375, 1984.

In a report of a child with multiple juvenile xanthogranulomas who developed juvenile chronic myeloid leukemia at the age of 30 months, the authors comment on the possible relationship of multiple café au lait spots, juvenile xanthogranulomas, juvenile chronic myeloid leukemia, and neurofibromatosis.

31. Morier P, Mérot Y, Paccaud D, et al.: Juvenile chronic granulocytic leukemia, juvenile xanthogranulomas, and neurofibromatosis. J. A. Acad. Dermatol. *22*:962–965, 1990.

A report of a 22-month-old boy with juvenile xanthogranulomas, neurofibromatosis, and chronic granulocytic leukemia and a review of 23 previously published cases.

32. Westerhof W, Delleman J, Walters E, et al.: Neurofibromatosis and hypertelorism. Arch. Dermatol. *120*:1579–1581, 1984.

A report of eight patients with hypertelorism and neurofibromatosis in which all were shown to have central nervous systemic involvement.

33. Hurwitz S, Braverman IM: White spots in tuberous sclerosis. J. Pediatr. *77*:587–594, 1970.

Hypopigmented macules, the earliest sign of tuberous sclerosis, present in 18 of 23 children with this disorder.

34. Fryer AE, Connor JM, Povey S, et al.: Evidence that the gene for tuberous sclerosis is on chromosome 9. Lancet *1*:659–660, 1987.

Linkage analysis of 19 families with tuberous sclerosis support the assignment of the gene for tuberous sclerosis to the distal long arm of chromosome 9.

35. Oppenheimer EY, Rosman NP, Dooling EC: The late presence of hypopigmented macules in tuberous sclerosis. Am. J. Dis. Child. *139*:408–409, 1985.

Report of children with tuberous sclerosis in whom the white macules did not become apparent until later in childhood.

36. Nickel WR, Reed WB: Tuberous sclerosis. Arch. Dermatol. *85*:209–216, 1962.

Tuberous sclerosis, a hereditary disease with protean manifestations, reported as being present in every organ and almost every structure of the body.

37. Hurwitz S: Society Transactions: Discussion on tuberous sclerosis. Arch. Dermatol. *104*:336–337, 1971.

A patient with partial albinism, hypopigmented macules, and tuberous sclerosis, and a discussion of various forms of leukoderma in tuberous sclerosis.

38. Fitzpatrick TB, Szabó G, Hori Y, et al.: White leaf-shaped macules: Earliest visible sign of tuberous sclerosis. Arch. Dermatol. *98*:1–6, 1968.

All patients with seizures, regardless of age, should be examined for white macules, which may be the only early visible sign of tuberous sclerosis.

39. McWilliam RP, Stephenson JBP: Depigmented hairs, the earliest sign of tuberous sclerosis. Arch. Dis. Child. *53*:961, 1978.

The presence of one or more tufts of white hair in an infant with seizures suggests a diagnosis of tuberous sclerosis.

40. Hoff M, van Gransven MF, Jongeblood WL, et al.: Enamel defects associated with tuberous sclerosis. Oral Surg. Oral Med. Oral Pathol. *40*:261–269, 1975.

Tooth pits—a new sign of tuberous sclerosis?

40a. Milnarczyk G: Oral Surg. Oral Med. Oral Pathol. *71*:63–67, 1991.

Enamel pitting was present in the adult dentition of 100 per cent of 50 patients with tuberous sclerosis (of the tuberous sclerosis patients who were younger than 11 years of age, 76 per cent had pitting).

40b. Robertson DM: Dental enamel pits in tuberous sclerosis. Arch. Ophthalmol. *110*:319, 1992.

Rose bengal ophthalmic strips provide a good means of identification for dental enamel pits in patients with tuberous sclerosis when dental plaque-disclosing solution is not available.

41. Richardson EP J: Tuberous sclerosis—another success for magnetic resonance imaging. Mayo Clin. Proc. *64*;371–373, 1989.

Magnetic resonance imaging (MRI), although it may miss calcifications, can also be helpful for the early diagnosis of tuberous sclerosis.

42. Weinblatt ME, Kahn E, Kochen J: Renal cell carcinoma in patients with tuberous sclerosis. Pediatrics *80*:898–903, 1987.

A report of an adolescent with renal carcinoma and tuberous sclerosis, a reminder that in addition to its well-described association with brain tumors, renal cell carcinoma may also be seen in patients with tuberous sclerosis.

43. Cassidy SB, Pagan RA, Pepin M, et al.: Family studies in tuberous sclerosis: Evaluation of apparently unaffected parents. J.A.M.A. *249*:02–1304, 1983.

Criteria for the evaluation of family members of patients with tuberous sclerosis.

44. Carney RG: Incontinentia pigmenti: A world statistical analysis. Arch. Dermatol. *112*:535–542, 1976.

Analysis of 653 patients (593 females, 16 males) with incontinentia pigmenti (sex not reported in 44 cases).

45. Wiklund DA, Weston WL: Incontinentia pigmenti: A four generation study. Arch. Dermatol. *116*:701–703, 1980.

A review of seven members of a family spanning four generations with incontinentia pigmentia.

46. El-Benhawi MO, George WM: Incontinentia pigmenti: A review. Cutis *41*:259–262, 1988.

A report of a 6-week-old girl with incontinentia pigmenti in whom several stages of cutaneous lesions (vesiculobullae, lichenoid papules and verrucous lesions) presented simultaneously.

47. Schaumburg-Lever G, Lever WF: Electron microscopy of incontinentia pigmenti. J. Invest. Dermatol. *61*:151–158, 1973.

Electron microscopic studies revealing common features in the first three stages of incontinentia pigmenti suggest that all three are related to each other.

48. Wiley HE III, Frias JL: Depigmented lesions in incontinentia pigmenti: A useful sign. Am. J. Dis. Child. *128*:546–547, 1974.

Streaked hypopigmented lesions on the calves or other areas of individuals with incontinentia pigmenti.

49. Moss C, Ince P: Anhidrotic and achromian lesions in incontinentia pigmenti. Br. J. Dermatol. *116*:839–849, 1987.

Three women with incontinentia pigmenti with hairless anhidrotic hypopigmented streaks on the limbs as their predominent cutaneous abnormality: Seven other patients diagnosed in infancy were found to have similar lesions.

50. Mascaró J, Palou J, Vives P: Painful subungual keroatotic tumors in incontinentia pigmenti. J. Am. Acad. Dermatol. *13*:913–918, 1985.

In a report of a 23-year-old woman with incontinentia pigmenti, subungual tumors on several fingers had a histology almost indistinguishable from that seen in patients with keratoacanthomas.

51. Simmons DA, Kegel MF, Scher RK, et al.: Subungual tumors in incontinentia pigmenti. Arch Dermatol. *122*:1431–1434, 1986.

In a 22-year-old woman with incontinentia pigmenti, painful subungual tumors and lytic defects (demonstrated by radiographic evaluation) were found in the distal phalanges of affected as well as unaffected fingers.

52. O'Brien JE, Feingold M: Incontinentia pigmenti: A longitudinal study. Am. J. Dis. Child. *139*:711–712, 1985.

This review of the long-term course of 15 patients with incontinentia pigmenti offers helpful prognostic information for families of patients with this disorder.

53. Ito M: Studies on melanin I: Incontinentia pigmenti achromians: A singular case of nevus depigmentosus systematicus bilateralis. Tohoku J. Exp. Med. 55(Suppl 1): 57–59, 1952.

A disorder with systematized depigmented macules.

54. Hamado T, Saito T, et al.: Incontinentia pigmenti (Ito). Arch. Dermatol. *96*:673–676, 1967.

A syndrome in which cutaneous markers resemble a negative image of incontinentia pigmenti.

55. Schwartz MF, Esterly NB, Fretzin DF: Hypomelanosis of Ito (incontinentia pigmenti achromians): A neurocutaneous syndrome. J. Pediatr. *90*:236–240, 1977.

Ten patients ranging in age from 1 1/2 to 21 years of age with developmental or neurologic abnormalities and hypomelanosis of Ito (a cutaneous sign of possible defects in other organ systems).

56. Rubin NG: Incontinentia pigmenti achromians. Arch. Dermatol. *105*:424–425, 1972.

Multiple cases of incontinentia pigmenti achromians in a family suggest an autosomal dominant basis to this disorder.

57. Sybert VP: Hypomelanosis of Ito. Pediatr. Dermatol. 7:74–76, 1990.

An overview of hypomelanosis of Ito and its inherited aspects.

58. Pinto FJ, Bolognia JL: Disorders of hypopigmentation in children. Pediatr. Clin. North Am. 38:991–1017, 1991.

An overview of hypopigmented lesions, their significance, diagnosis, and management in children.

59. Jelinek JE, Bart RS, Schiff GM: Hypomelanosis of Ito ("incontinentia pigmenti achromians"). Arch. Dermatol. *117*:596–601, 1973.

A report of three cases and review of the literature.

60. Takematsu H, Sato S, Igarashi M, et al.: Incontinentia pigmenti achromians (Ito). Arch. Dermatol. *119*:391–395, 1983.

In a study of 3 children and a review of 70 previously documented cases of hypomelanosis of Ito, at least one mother and child had skin lesions of incontinentia pigmenti before the onset of the cutaneous lesions of hypomelanosis of Ito, suggesting a possible relationship between the two disorders.

61. Ruiz-Maldonado R, Toussaint S, Tamayo L, et al.: Hypomelanosis of Ito: Diagnostic criteria and report of 41 cases. Pediatr. Dermatol. *9*:1–10, 1992.

Proposed diagnostic criteria and a 20-year study of 41 patients with hypomelanosis of Ito.

THE MONONUCLEAR PHAGOCYTE (RETICULO-ENDOTHELIAL) AND LYMPHORETICULAR SYSTEM

The mononuclear phagocyte system, previously referred to as the reticuloendothelial system, represents a group of diseases derived from cells of the monophagocytic system that participate in a variety of immunologic and inflammatory processes. A description of these clinical disorders is presented in this chapter with emphasis on their pathogenesis, clinical features, and management in childhood.

HISTIOCYTOSIS IN CHILDREN

Histiocytosis X

Histiocytosis X is a term originated by Lichtenstein in 1953 to identify three related clinical entities of unknown etiology characterized by histiocyte proliferation.[1] This classification includes the triad of Letterer-Siwe disease, Hand-Schüller-Christian disease, and eosinophilic granuloma. Each of these disorders presents a distinct clinical picture with overlapping transitional stages suggesting that they are all variants of the same basic disease process. The X in the title only serves to remind us of the lack of a specific etiology for this group of disorders. Although numerous etiologies have been proposed, their pathogenesis remains obscure. These include a disturbance of intracellular lipid metabolism, a reactive histiocytic response to an infectious process, and a neoplastic disorder of histiocytes. Proof of unity of these three syndromes is recognized by their histologic similarity, the presence of Langerhans cells with positive S-100 stains, and electron microscopic demonstration of Langerhans granules (Birbeck's granules) in the cytoplasm of histiocytes in all three syndromes.

LETTERER-SIWE DISEASE

Letterer-Siwe disease is seen at the severe fulminating end of the histiocytosis spectrum, as the acute disseminated form of the disease. Studies of Letterer-Siwe disease in monozygotic twins, reports of familial incidence, and cases of consanguinity suggest a hereditary influence, perhaps an autosomal recessive gene with reduced penetrance. It usually occurs during the first year of life and, although described in adults,[2] is almost exclusively limited to children up to 3 years of age. In virtually all patients with Letterer-Siwe disease, skin markers may represent the first recognizable sign of the disorder. The infant may appear healthy for many months before fever, anemia, thrombocytopenia, adenopathy, hepatosplenomeg-

Table 24–1. LETTERER-SIWE DISEASE

1. Usually in first year of life (almost exclusively in children up to age 3)
2. Not necessarily uniformly fatal
3. Cutaneous features (seen in 80% of patients)
   a. Scaly erythematous seborrhea-like rash
   b. Petechiae, purpuric papules and nodules
   c. Vesicles and crusted papules may predominate in infants.
4. Other features: fever, anemia, thrombocytopenia, adenopathy, hepatosplenomegaly, skeletal tumors
5. Buccal and gingival ulcerations, chronic otitis media, and ulcerations of the postauricular, inguinal, or perineal lesions may represent important diagnostic clues.

Modified from Hurwitz S: The reticuloendothelial disorders. *In* The Skin and Systemic Disease in Children. Year Book Medical Publishers, Chicago, 1985.

aly, or skeletal tumors become apparent (Table 24–1).[3, 4]

Cutaneous involvement, which occurs in 80 per cent of patients, is usually part of the initial presentation of the disease. It frequently begins with a scaly, erythematous seborrhea-like eruption on the scalp, behind the ears, and in the axillary, inguinal, or perineal areas. On close inspection, the presence of basic lesions of histiocytosis (reddish brown or purpuric papules) may identify the disorder (Figs. 24–1 through 24–5). In infants, vesicular or crusted papules may predominate (Fig. 24–6). Purpuric nodules on the palms and soles of infants appear to be a particularly bad prognostic sign of this disorder (Figs. 24–7 and 24–8). Buccal and gingival ulcerations, chronic otitis media, and ulceration of the postauricular, inguinal, or perineal regions also represent important diagnostic clues. When the diagnosis is indeterminant, the character and distribution of lesions should suggest the true nature of the eruption. Diagnosis, then, can be confirmed easily by skin biopsy.

This disease was considered to be an invariably fatal disorder until 1951 when Aronson reported the first incidence of recovery.[5] Since then, addi-

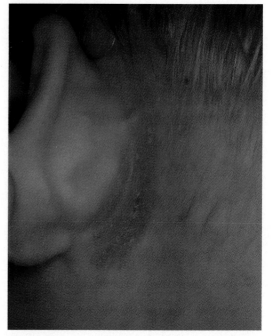

Figure 24–2. A persistent seborrhea-like erythematous eruption with purpuric papules in the postauricular area of a 14-month-child with Letterer-Siwe disease. (Hurwitz S: The reticuloendothelial disorders. *In* The Skin and Systemic Disease in Children. Year Book Medical Publishers, Chicago, 1985.)

tional long-term survivals have been reported. Careful clinical reviews have shown that prognosis is related to age at onset, duration of symptoms, and the degree of systemic involvement. Benign and purely cutaneous forms, although rare, have been reported.[6–9] The absence of thrombocytopenia and a lack of extensive visceral involvement favor a good prognosis.

The highest mortality is seen in patients younger than the age of 6 months, particularly those with widespread systemic involvement. Purpura of the palms, a finding seldom seen in other skin disease,

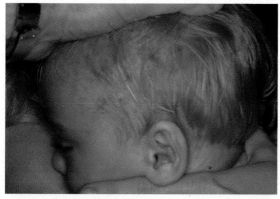

Figure 24–1. Histiocytosis X. A scaly, erythematous seborrhea-like eruption is present on the scalp of a 14-month-old infant with Letterer-Siwe disease. (Hurwitz S: The reticuloendothelial disorders. *In* The Skin and Systemic Disease in Children. Year Book Medical Publishers, Chicago, 1985.)

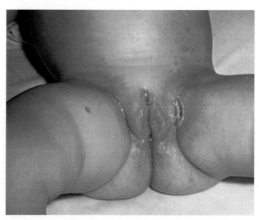

Figure 24–3. Histiocytosis X (Letterer-Siwe disease) in the diaper area. (Braverman IM: Skin Signs of Systemic Disease. W.B. Saunders Co., Philadelphia, 1970.)

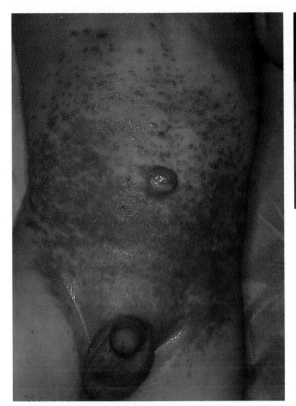

Figure 24–4. A persistent reddish brown pruritic papular eruption on the abdomen, groin, and genital region of a 14-month-old infant with Letterer-Siwe disease.

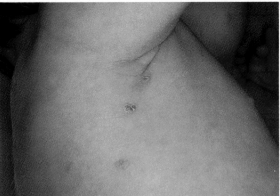

Figure 24–6. Crusted and vesicular lesions in a 1-month-old infant with congenital Letterer-Siwe disease.

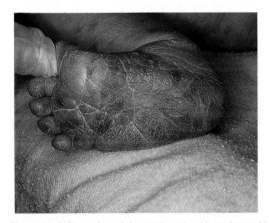

Figure 24–7. Purpuric nodules on the sole of a newborn with congenital Letterer-Siwe disease (a particularly bad prognostic sign of Letterer-Siwe disease).

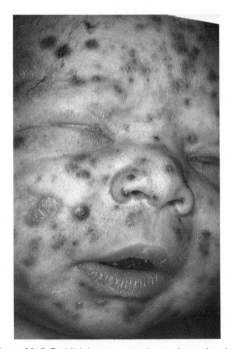

Figure 24–5. Reddish brown purpuric papules and nodules in a newborn with congenital histiocytosis (Letterer-Siwe disease).

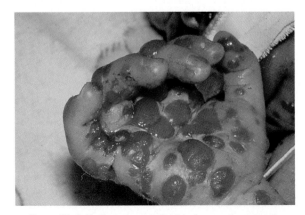

Figure 24–8. Erythematous nodular lesions on the palm of an infant with congenital Letterer-Siwe disease. (Courtesy of Marilyn Jones, M.D.)

early age at onset, and lung involvement appear to be signs of a particularly poor prognosis. Death may be caused by pulmonary, hepatic, or splenic involvement and is frequently attributed to hemorrhage, anemia, or infection. Although in general Letterer-Siwe disease often implies a fatal outcome, the disease course varies, therapy is often beneficial, spontaneous remissions have occurred, and at times the illness may evolve into a more chronic phase of histiocytosis X such as Hand-Schüller-Christian disease.[10]

HAND-SCHÜLLER-CHRISTIAN DISEASE

This is the variant of histiocytosis X generally seen in patients between 2 and 6 years of age (Table 24–2). Classically, this syndrome consists of a triad of osteolytic defects, diabetes insipidus, and exophthalmos. The bony lesions are invariably present; only 50 per cent of patients, however, have diabetes insipidus, and a mere 10 per cent demonstrate exophthalmos. Chronic otitis media secondary to histiocytic infiltration of the mastoid is common. Histiocytic proliferation may also cause necrosis, ulcerations, and small tumors of the gums and oral mucous membranes. Radiographs of the skull often reveal sharply defined areas of osseous rarefaction, termed *geographic skull,* or erosions of the tooth-bearing portion of the mandible, with loosening or extrusion of the teeth. The lungs and pleura represent a major cause of disability and are affected in 30 per cent of patients, with death resulting from pulmonary fibrosis, associated ventricular hypertrophy, and right-sided heart failure.

Skin lesions, seen in 30 to 50 per cent of patients, are similar to those of the Letterer-Siwe syndrome, except that in Hand-Schüller-Christian disease purpura is less common and the skin lesions are neither as vivid nor as destructive. The skin lesions consist of coalescing, scaling or crusted, brown to flesh-colored papules. Occasionally, lesions of long duration develop a shiny yellowish hue. As in Letterer-Siwe disease, granulomatous infiltrates with ulceration are also found in the axillary or anogenital areas.

EOSINOPHILIC GRANULOMA

Eosinophilic granuloma represents the third and most benign form of histiocytosis X. Usually seen in young adults and children older than the age of 6 years, the onset is insidious (Table 24–3). The patient is generally free of symptoms until headaches, localized pain, tenderness, or swelling of soft tissues suggests the diagnosis. In children, eosinophilic granuloma often represents an early or transitional form of Letterer-Siwe or Hand-Schüller-Christian disease. In adults it is usually a benign, although chronic, illness. The disorder may present as single or multiple skeletal lesions and often goes undetected until a spontaneous fracture or an incidental radiographic examination suggests the diagnosis. Although the course is usually benign, 10 per cent of patients manifest multifocal disease within 6 months.[11]

Skin lesions are relatively rare but may be identical to those seen in Letterer-Siwe or Hand-Schüller-Christian disease. Again they may consist of crusting of the scalp (suggesting seborrheic dermatitis); reddish brown papules or nodules in the retroauricular and perineal areas; or ulcerated granulomatous lesions of the buccal mucous membranes or inguinal, perineal, or vulvar regions. The course is characteristically chronic, with a strong tendency to spontaneous remission. Diabetes insipidus, pulmonary lesions, and Langerhans granules have been reported, adding to the evidence that all three forms of histiocytosis are caused by a common disease process.

MANAGEMENT OF HISTIOCYTOSIS X

Therapeutic regimens for histiocytosis X vary widely, and since the disease is of variable activity, evaluation of therapy is often difficult. In general, patients with diffuse systemic disease of the reticulohistiocytic system suffer impaired immunity, and, subsequently, diminished resistance to infection. Blood transfusions and antibiotics may improve the long-term outlook for such patients, in

---

Table 24–2. HAND SCHÜLLER-CHRISTIAN DISEASE

1. Generally in children 2 to 6 years of age
2. A triad of osteolytic defects, diabetes mellitus, and exophthalmos
3. Other features: chronic otitis media, necrosis, ulcerations and small tumors of gums and oral mucous membranes, and pulmonary involvement (30%)
4. Cutaneous lesion (in 30 to 50%)
   a. Similar to Letterer-Siwe disease (coalescing scaling or crusted brown to flesh-colored papules)
   b. Purpura less common and lesions less vivid and less destructive than those in patients with Letterer-Siwe disease
5. The lungs and pleura represent a major cause of disability.

Modified from Hurwitz S: The reticuloendothelial disorders. *In* The Skin and Systemic Disease in Children. Year Book Medical Publishers, Chicago, 1985.

Table 24–3. EOSINOPHILIC GRANULOMA

1. Least severe form of histiocytosis X
2. Usually in children older than 6 years and adults
3. Clinical features
   a. Headaches, localized pain, tenderness or swelling of soft tissues suggest the diagnosis
   b. Single or multiple skeletal lesions
   c. Cutaneous lesions (relatively rare, but identical to those of Letterer-Siwe and Hand-Schüller-Christian disease)
      (1) Reddish brown papules or nodules in retroauricular and perineal areas
      (2) Ulcerated granulomatous lesions of buccal mucous membranes and inguinal, perineal, or vulvar areas
   d. Course characteristically chronic with a strong tendency to spontaneous remission

Modified from Hurwitz S: The reticuloendothelial disorders. *In* The Skin and Systemic Disease in Children. Year Book Medical Publishers, Chicago, 1985.

particular for those with anemia, leukopenia, or thrombocytopenia.

Immunosuppressive drugs currently appear to offer the greatest hope for survival. Simultaneous combination of drugs has been most effective. This suggests that aggressive combination regimens with good symptomatic care may achieve further long-term remissions, and possibly eventual cure. Prednisone, in dosages averaging 2 to 4 mg/kg/day, may result in complete clearing of lesions or remissions lasting from 12 to 30 months. Alkylating agents such as nitrogen mustard, chlorambucil (Leukeran), and cyclophosphamide (Cytoxan) appear to be highly effective. Procarbazine offers a very limited response and a high incidence of toxicity.

Nitrogen mustard (mechlorethamine) gives a rapid effect and may be administered intravenously in dosages of 0.2 to 0.5 mg/kg. For long-term therapy, chlorambucil may be given orally in dosages of 0.1 to 0.3 mg/kg/day, for several months, depending on the course of the disease. A year or more of therapy is frequently required to control histiocytosis.

The plant alkaloids vinblastine and vincristine have produced some notable successes. Vinblastine may be given in weekly or semiweekly intravenous injections of 0.1 to 0.3 mg/kg for many weeks. This drug, however, causes bone marrow suppression, neuritis, alopecia, and gastrointestinal side effects. Therapy, therefore, should be initiated in low dosages with gradual increments, as tolerated, in an effort to minimize side effects.

Methotrexate, 1.25 mg/day, alone or in combination with corticosteroids, although potentially toxic, is also an effective mode of therapy. Intermittent dosages (once or twice a week as opposed to daily doses) may prove to be less toxic. Cyclophosphamide, 3 mg/kg/day, appears to be less toxic and is especially beneficial when combined with corticosteroids or when combined with corticosteroids and vinblastine.

In general, patients with Hand-Schüller-Christian disease and eosinophilic granuloma are more responsive to therapy than patients with Letterer-Siwe disease. Radiation therapy, particularly when initiated early in the course of the disease, is very effective for localized skeletal lesions. Diabetes insipidus is controllable with vasopressin (Pitressin) by injection or nasal insufflation. X-irradiation or curettage is effective for bone lesions of eosinophilic granuloma.

Histiocytosis X, although still a potentially fatal disorder, particularly in young children, can be diagnosed early by characteristic cutaneous manifestations. The skin signs may appear alone or in combination with systemic symptoms. Although the disease reputedly has a poor prognostic outlook, it often presents in much less severe form, so that prognosis is often more optimistic than the literature suggests. Vigorous therapeutic approaches, with a combination of corticosteroids, immunosuppressive drugs, and general supportive measures, appear to offer the greatest hope for survival. With accumulation of data, the fatalistic approach to the disease must be reassessed. Aggressive chemotherapy and good supportive care may allow children not only hope for long-term remission but even complete cure.

Non-X Histiocytic Disorders

In addition to the previously described triad of disorders characterized by proliferation of histiocytes and Langerhans cells in the skin, bones, liver, spleen, lungs, and/or lymph nodes, a number of histiocytoses characterized by dermal accumulation of histiocytes, but lacking Langerhans granules, have been described under the designation of non-X histiocytoses. Some of these are described in the following sections.

XANTHOMA DISSEMINATUM

Xanthoma disseminatum is a rare, benign, mucocutaneous xanthomatosis of unknown cause affecting the skin, oral mucosa, and, at times, the pharynx and larynx. Although in the past some authors assumed a relationship between this disorder and histiocytosis-X, its predominance in adults, common involvement of the oral mucosa, larynx, and pharynx, rarity of osseous lesions, and prevalence of foam cells, uncommon in lesions of histiocytosis X, suggest that xanthoma disseminatum warrants separate consideration. Predominantly a disorder of young adult males, in 30 per cent of patients the disorder begins before the age of 15 (Table 24–4). Cutaneous lesions, which may number in the hundreds, consist of closely set, round to oval, yellowish orange or yellowish to mahogany brown or purple papules, nodules, and plaques that are present mainly on the face, flexor surfaces of the neck, antecubital fossae, periumbilical area, perineum, and genitalia. The lips, eyelids, and conjunctivae

Table 24–4. XANTHOMA DISSEMINATUM

1. Usually a disorder of young men (30% start before the age of 15 years)
2. A rare benign proliferative xanthomatous disorder (possibly a variant of Hand-Schüller-Christian disease?)
3. Cutaneous lesions
   a. Closely set round to oval, yellowish orange or yellowish brown to mahogany-brown or purple papules, nodules, and plaques
   b. Usually on face, flexor surface of neck, antecubital fossae, periumbilical area, perineum, and genitalia
4. Other features
   a. Xanthomatous deposits in mouth, pharynx, larynx, and trachea (in one third to 40% of cases) may lead to respiratory difficulty
   b. Diabetes insipidus in 40% and, at times, meningeal involvement (seizures, growth retardation, and increase in cerebrospinal fluid protein level)

Modified from Hurwitz S: The reticuloendothelial disorders. *In* The Skin and Systemic Disease in Children. Year Book Medical Publishers, Chicago, 1985.

may be involved, and xanthomatous deposits have been observed in the mouth and upper respiratory tract (epiglottis, larynx, and trachea in one third to 40 per cent of cases), occasionally leading to respiratory difficulty.[12, 13]

The distribution of lesions, their histologic features, and the usual lack of disturbed lipid metabolism help establish the diagnosis. Histologic examination of lesions shows xanthoma cells, eosinophilic histiocytes, numerous Touton giant cells, and an inflammatory infiltrate. In early lesions large histiocytes dominate the histologic picture; with time, lipidization of histiocytes increases with formation of foam cells and the more typical histologic features of the disorder become apparent.

Meningeal involvement, especially at the base of the skull, resulting in diabetes insipidus, occurs in 40 per cent of patients; other manifestations of meningeal involvement include seizures, growth retardation, and an increase in cerebrospinal fluid protein level.

Except for severe laryngeal involvement occasionally necessitating tracheostomy, the disease tends to run a chronic but benign course and the disorder generally tends to regress spontaneously. If diabetes insipidus occurs, it usually is mild and may be transient, so that continued therapy with vasopressin injections (Pitressin) becomes unnecessary. Ocular or respiratory tract pathologic problems, however, may justify a more aggressive approach with localized radiation therapy or alkylating agents such as chlorambucil.

JUVENILE XANTHOGRANULOMA

Juvenile xanthogranuloma, a designation that is replacing the term *nevoxanthoendothelioma*, represents a benign, self-limiting disease of infants, children, and occasionally adults, characterized by one or several and occasionally numerous red to yellow nodules located on the skin and other organs. The lesions have no relationship to nevi, and endothelial cells are not responsible for the histogenesis of this disorder. Accordingly, the earlier term, *nevoxanthoendothelioma* (a misnomer), has been replaced by the name *juvenile xanthogranuloma* (Table 24–5). Since histiocytes represent the basic cell, and internal organs similar to those seen in Hand-Schüller-Christian disease occasionally occur, many authors consider juvenile xanthogranuloma to be a reactive granuloma of unknown cause or an abortive cutaneous form of histiocytosis. The absence of Langerhans cells and Birbeck's granules on electron microscopy represents a strong argument differentiating juvenile xanthogranuloma from the group of disorders classified under the designation of histiocytosis X.

The condition is characterized by solitary or multiple yellow to reddish brown papules and nodules of the face (Fig. 24–9), scalp, neck, and sometimes the subungual areas[14] and the proximal

Table 24–5. JUVENILE XANTHOGRANULOMA (NEVOXANTHOENDOTHELIOMA)

1. 0.5 to 1 cm yellow to reddish brown papules and nodules (solitary or multiple); giant 4 to 10 cm in diameter lesions may at times be seen
    a. Usually on face, scalp, neck or proximal extremities
    b. Occasionally in mouth, vaginal orifice, or perineal area
2. Ninety per cent are self-limiting purely cutaneous lesions
3. Occasionally may affect the lungs, pericardium, meninges, spleen, liver, testes, or eyes
4. Possible association of leukemia in patients with a combination of neurofibromatosis and juvenile xanthogranuloma

Modified from Hurwitz S: The reticuloendothelial disorders. *In* The Skin and Systemic Disease in Children. Year Book Medical Publishers, Chicago, 1985.

portions of the extremities or trunk. Lesions also occur on mucous membranes or at mucocutaneous junctions (the mouth, vaginal orifice, and perineal area). Typically the lesions are present at birth (20 per cent) or during the first 6 to 9 months of life, and may persist or continue to erupt for years.[15] They run a benign course, often increasing in number until about 1 to 1½ years of age, and then involute spontaneously. There may be as few as one or two lesions or as many as several hundred. They may range from several millimeters to 1 cm or more in diameter, and frequently they have a discrete, firm, or rubbery consistency. On occasion, large juvenile xanthogranulomas, measuring 4 to 10 cm in diameter (giant juvenile xanthogranulomas), have been reported.[16, 17] Although such lesions also tend to resolve spontaneously, they may at times (because of their large size) break down in the center and at times suppurate (Fig. 24–10). When this occurs, bacterial cultures, appropriate antibiotics, and surgical excision may be required.

The histology of juvenile xanthogranulomas varies with the stage of the lesion. Early lesions may show large accumulations of histiocytes without lipid infiltration intermingled with only a few lymphoid cells and eosinophils. S-100 (an acidic protein classically associated with neuroepithe-

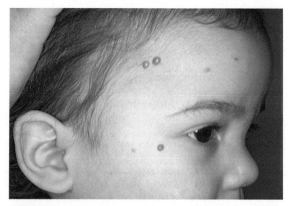

Figure 24–9. Yellow to reddish brown papular and nodular lesions on the face of an infant with juvenile xanthogranulomas (nevoxanthoendotheliomas).

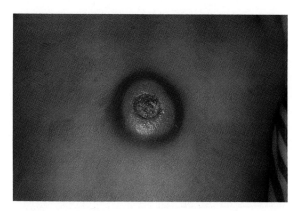

Figure 24–10. A large (2.5 × 3-cm) juvenile xantho-granuloma with central necrosis, infection, and crusting on the back of an 8-month-old infant. (Courtesy of Barry Richter, M.D.)

lium but also found in melanocytes, nevus cells, eccrine glands, and Langerhans cells) stains are negative. In mature lesions a granulomatous infiltrate containing foam cells, foreign body giant cells, and Touton giant cells as well as histiocytes, lymphocytes, and eosinophils is usually present. The presence of giant cells, mostly Touton giant cells, showing a "wreath" of nuclei surrounded by foamy cytoplasm is typical.[15]

The vast majority (90 per cent or more) of patients with juvenile xanthogranuloma have a self-limiting cutaneous disease. Although rare cases lasting until adulthood have been reported, generally those that have their onset after the first year of life manifest complete healing, usually within 1 to 5 years. Regarded as a disorder limited to the skin until 1949, when Blank and co-workers reported a lesion on the iris in a 4-month-old infant,[18] lesions may also occur in the lung, pericardium, central nervous system,[19] liver, spleen, and testes. Patients with pulmonary involvement often show spontaneous regression of lesions. Ocular tumors of the iris or epibulbar area, however, the most frequent internal complication, often require therapy if extensive glaucoma, hemorrhage, or blindness is to be avoided. Once the proper diagnosis has been established, therapy for ocular lesions includes radiation and topical or systemic corticosteroids; skin lesions, however, involute spontaneously and generally require no treatment.

As stated in the discussion of neurofibromatosis, there have been patients with a combination of juvenile xanthogranulomas and café au lait spots or neurofibromatosis who developed chronic myelogenous leukemia or acute monomyelocytic leukemia. Patients with this combination, therefore, should be checked periodically for the possibility of an associated leukemia.[20]

NECROBIOTIC XANTHOGRANULOMA

Necrobiotic xanthogranuloma, a rare disorder usually reported in adults, is characterized by sharply demarcated indurated plaques and nod-

ules that are usually yellow to reddish brown or violaceous and have a predilection for periorbital areas, trunk, and proximal extremities. Lesions vary in size, may at times be as large as 10 cm or more in diameter, and often ulcerate and heal with areas of atrophy and telangiectasia. Visceral necrobiotic xanthogranulomatous lesions may be noted in the heart, skeletal muscles, larynx, spleen, and ovary; patients with this disorder tend to have an accompanying IgG monoclonal gammopathy; and bone marrow examination reveals atypical plasma cells and multiple myeloma.[21] Histopathologic examination of cutaneous lesions is characterized by granulomatous masses presenting as focal aggregates or large intersecting bands occupying the dermis or subcutis, extensive hyaline necrobiosis, and numerous large giant cells of the Touton and foreign body type, foam cells, and lympyhocytes. The course of the disorder is chronic and progressive and may be associated with proliferation of plasma cells in the bone marrow, paraproteinemia, multiple myeloma, and sometimes Hodgkin's disease. Treatment options include systemic corticosteroids, cytotoxic drugs, and plasmapheresis, with varying degrees of success.[21, 22]

CONGENITAL SELF-HEALING RETICULOHISTIOCYTOSIS

Congenital self-healing reticulohistiocytosis, first described by Hashimoto and Pritzker in 1973, is a rare disorder, usually present at birth or within the first several days or weeks of life. It is characterized by solitary or multiple, reddish brown, pink, or purplish papules, nodules, or papulo-vesicular lesions mainly on the face, scalp, trunk and extremities (Fig. 24–11) that tend to break down in the center, form ulcerated craters, and involute spontaneously within 1 year (usually within 2 or 3 months) leaving white atrophic scars. On histopathologic examination the lesions show densely aggregated histiocytes with abundant eo-

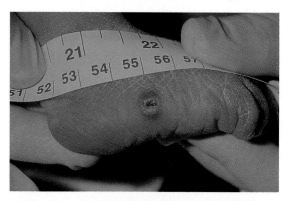

Figure 24–11. Self-healing reticulohistiocytosis. (Courtesy of Jane Grant-Kels, M.D.; reprinted from Kapila PK, Grant-Kels JM, Allred C, et al.: Congenital spontaneously regressing histiocytosis. Case report and review of the literature. Pediatr. Dermatol. 2:312–317, 1985.)

sinophilic cytoplasm with a ground-glass appearance and a mixture of lymphocytes, neutrophils, and eosinophils (Table 24–6).[23–27] Although its nosology remains unclear, it is believed by some to represent a predominantly cutaneous form of eosinophilic granuloma.[24] Since its course is benign and self-limiting, it is important to distinguish this disorder from histiocytosis X and other histiocytic conditions.

BENIGN CEPHALIC HISTIOCYTOSIS

Benign cephalic histiocytosis is a self-healing form of histiocytosis that, although at times generalized, is usually seen on the upper face, scalp, or neck, and occasionally the shoulders during the first 3 years of life. It is characterized by multiple red to yellow 2- to 5-mm papulonodular lesions that do not increase in size and eventually resolve over months to years (generally 2 to 5 years) leaving atrophic pigmented scars. Viewed by some authorities to be a variant of generalized eruptive histiocytoma, histopathologic examination of lesions reveals a thinned epidermis overlying a well-circumscribed upper dermal infiltrate composed primarily of histiocytes with irregularly shaped nuclei and sparse cytoplasm intermingled with a few lymphocytes and eosinophils. Foam cells, Touton giant cells, Langerhans cells, and Birbeck's granules are absent, and electron microscopic examination reveals clustered intracytoplasmic comma-shaped or worm-like bodies. The absence of Langerhans cells distinguishes this entity from lesions of histiocytosis X, and the absence of Touton giant cells distinguishes it from juvenile xanthogranuloma. Since lesions generally tend to heal, therapy is unnecessary (Table 24–7).[28–31]

GENERALIZED ERUPTIVE HISTIOCYTOMA

Generalized eruptive histiocytoma is a rare benign self-healing dermatosis characterized by recurrent crops of small, yellow to reddish, generally symmetrical 1- to 2-mm papules that appear on the lower trunk, on the extensor aspect of the extremi-

Table 24–6. CONGENITAL SELF-HEALING RETICULOHISTIOCYTOSIS

1. Solitary or multiple, small, pink, red, purplish or reddish brown papules, nodules, or papulovesicular lesions mainly on the face, scalp, trunk, and extremities
2. Lesions tend to occur during the first few days of life, grow in size and number during the first few weeks, and regress over a period of several weeks to months.
3. Histopathology:
   a. A dermal infiltrate of pleomorphic histiocytic cells with abundant eosinophilic cytoplasm, with or without epidermal involvement, often with an admixture of lymphocytes, neutrophils, and eosinophils
   b. Langerhans granules, concentrically laminated and nonlaminated dense bodies, octopus-like bodies, worm-like bodies, comma-like bodies, myeloid figures, and positive S-100 protein uptake

Table 24–7. BENIGN CEPHALIC HISTIOCYTOSIS

1. A self-limiting cutaneous eruption that generally begins in the first 2 or more years
2. Slightly raised hemispheric yellowish red, 2- to 5-mm papulonodular lesions on the face, scalp, neck, arms, shoulders, and, at times, the buttocks, thighs, and perineal areas
3. Lesions tend to fade over a period of years, leaving hyperpigmented atrophic scars.
4. Histopathologic features: histiocytes with irregularly shaped nuclei and sparse cytoplasm; a few intermingled lymphocytes and eosinophils; absence of Touton giant cells; and worm-like or comma-shaped intracytoplasmic bodies on electron microscopy

ties, and, rarely, on the mucous membranes. Although generally regarded as a disorder of adults, childhood forms have been reported, and it has been seen in infants as young as 3 and 8 months of age.[31–33] The lesions regress after a few months, leaving macular hyperpigmentation. As a result of the continuous development of new lesions, however, the disorder may persist indefinitely.

The histologic picture is one of a monomorphous infiltrate of histiocytes with large pale nuclei and abundant pale cytoplasm; S-100 staining is negative, and multinucleated giant cells are generally but not always absent. Since the disorder is self-limiting and asymptomatic, treatment is unnecessary.

PROGRESSIVE NODULAR HISTIOCYTOMA

Progressive nodular histiocytoma is an extremely rare disorder characterized by a widespread eruption of hundreds of yellowish brown papules 2 to 10 mm in diameter and raised 1- to 3-cm nodules. Conjunctival, oral, and laryngeal lesions may occur. Typically the face is heavily involved with merging lesions, imparting a leonine appearance; new lesions progressively occur, and ulceration, without spontaneous resolution, is common. The histopathologic examination of lesions reveals a massive infiltrate of histiocytic-appearing cells admixed with masses of lymphocytes; occasional Touton giant cells may be seen, and, in the fibrous areas, fibroblasts and collagen predominate with the collagen bundles occasionally arranged in a stariform or matted pattern. Chemotherapy with vinblastine and electron beam therapy and surgical excision of lesions currently appear to be treatments of choice for this disorder.[3, 34]

MULTICENTRIC RETICULOHISTIOCYTOSIS

Primarily a disorder of adults during the fifth decade of life and at times seen in adolescents, multicentric reticulohistiocytosis is a systemic granulomatous disorder characterized by polyarthritis and cutaneous lesions consisting of firm, reddish brown to yellow lesions that vary from a few millimeters in diameter to conglomerate nodules measuring several centimeters in diameter. Occurring most frequently on the fingers and hands, often with a "coral bead" arrangement along the nail folds, the face (particularly the nose and paranasal areas), scalp (particularly behind the ears), neck, and trunk are also common sites of involvement. Nodular lesions on the arms, elbows, and knees may resemble rheumatoid nodules or juxta-articular nodes of syphilis. Mucous membrane lesions, which are seen in one half of the patients, most frequently present on the lips, buccal mucosa, nasal septum, tongue, palate, and gingiva; and in one half to two thirds of patients polyarthritis and arthralgia are the initial manifestations. In many cases there is rapid progression to a destructive form of arthritis (arthritis mutilans), with often the distal interphalangeal joint being most severely affected.

Histologically, there are numerous large eosinophilic histiocytes with abundant eosinophilic fine granular cytoplasm with a ground-glass appearance and foreign body–type multinucleated giant cells.[31] In some instances (about one fourth of the reported cases) the disorder regresses within 6 to 8 years; in others, however, the disease remains stationary or progresses to persistent joint disease with severe articular deformities and disfigurement of the hands, face, and scalp. Alkylating agents such as cyclophosphamide or nitrogen mustard may help prevent disfiguring arthritis in skin lesions, but the course of the disorder is capricious, cutaneous lesions are often resistant to therapy, and about one half of the patients eventually suffer from destructive arthritis.

MALIGNANT HISTIOCYTOSIS

Malignant histiocytosis, originally described in 1939 as histiocytic medullary reticulosis, is an uncommon malignant histiocytic disorder that often has an acute onset and used to progress to a fatal course within a few months (Table 24–8). Clinical features include fever, wasting, generalized lymphadenopathy, hepatosplenomegaly, jaundice, and pancytopenia; and extensive erythrophagocytosis by histiocytes in marrow, liver, spleen, and lymph nodes is classically seen. Although involvement of the skin or subcutaneous tissues has been estimated to occur in about 10 per cent of cases, in children the incidence appears to be somewhat higher.

Cutaneous lesions consist of petechiae, purpura, eczematous lesions, and erythematous papules, nodules, or plaques that often undergo ulceration. Anemia, leukopenia, and thrombocytopenia are major laboratory abnormalities, and the cutaneous infiltrate, which is usually located in the middle to lower portion of the dermis and subcutaneous fat, is characterized by masses of normal and atypical histiocytes with focal areas of necrosis and acute and chronic inflammation. The atypical histiocytes display large, pleomorphic, vesicular nuclei, and

Table 24–8. MALIGNANT HISTIOCYTOSIS

1. Acute onset, malaise, fever, wasting, generalized lymphadenopathy, hepatosplenomegaly, pancytopenia
2. Affects children as well as adults
3. Cutaneous features (in 10%): papules, nodules, or plaques that undergo ulceration
4. Previously invariably fatal within weeks or months, but survivals up to 6 years or more with chemotherapy have occurred.

Hurwitz S: The reticuloendothelial disorders. *In* The Skin and Systemic Disease in Children. Year Book Medical Publishers, Chicago, 1985.

some contain phagocytized erythrocytes, nuclear debris, and fragments of leukocytes in their cytoplasm. Although generally considered to be an almost uniformly fatal disorder, with death occurring within weeks or months, occasional remissions and responses to chemotherapy with 6-year or more survivals have been reported.[35, 36]

Sarcoidosis

Sarcoidosis is a systemic granulomatous disorder of unkown etiology with widespread manifestations predominantly affecting the lungs, eyes, skin, and reticuloendothelial system. Rarely seen in children, the greatest incidence of this disorder is in patients between 20 and 40 years of age. Although the youngest reported patient was a 2-month-old infant, of the relatively few childhood cases in the literature, most have occurred in the preadolescent or adolescent age group (between 9 and 15 years of age) (Table 24–9).[37]

The disease occurs in blacks, Asians, and whites and appears to be most common among Scandinavians, American blacks, and whites of the southeastern United States. Although there have been case reports involving white children of Northern European ancestry, and rarely seen in African blacks, most children with sarcoidosis in the United States have been black and from the "sarcoid belt" of the southeastern states.[11, 37, 38]

Table 24–9. SARCOIDOSIS

1. A systemic granulomatous disorder of unknown etiology (an abnormal host response with delayed hypersensitivity and abnormal immunoregulation?)
2. Relatively uncommon in children (most cases in the United States are in blacks from the southeastern United States)
3. Skin lesions (in up to 50%), lungs (50%), ocular lesions (25%), splenomegaly (17%), osseous lesions (12%), cranial nerve paresis (5%), hilar lymphadenopathy (70%), peripheral lymphadenopathy (30%), hepatomegaly (20%)
4. Cutaneous lesions
   a. Soft red to yellowish brown or violaceous flat-topped papules
   b. Nodules or infiltrated plaques
   c. Subcutaneous tumors
   d. Scaly erythematous patches
5. Serum angiotensin-converting enzyme levels (often of diagnostic value in adults but less significant in children)

Hurwitz S: The reticuloendothelial disorders. *In* The Skin and Systemic Disease in Children. Year Book Medical Publishers, Chicago, 1985.

The etiology of sarcoidosis is unknown. Although many agents (mycobacteria, fungi, viruses, and bacteria) have been postulated to be involved in its pathogenesis, the cause appears to be the end result of multiple factors, with an abnormal host response, delayed hypersensitivity, and abnormal immunoregulation contributing to its clinical features.

Clinical Manifestations. The signs and symptoms of sarcoidosis are due primarily to local tissue infiltration and injury from pressure and displacement by sarcoidal lesions. The skin, lungs, eyes, liver, spleen, lymph nodes, bones, muscles, nervous system, and exocrine glands may be involved, with clinical manifestations of the disorder dependent on the organ or system affected and its degree of involvement.

Rare in children, when the disease occurs before the age of 6 years it characteristically involves the skin, as well as the eyes and synovial tissues, in a chronic progressive course. In older children and adolescents it resembles adult disease, with fever, cough, weight loss, abdominal pain, adenopathy, parenchymal lung disease, hypergammaglobulinemia, and hypercalcemia. Preschool-aged children, however, differ in that they tend to have polyarthritis and severe uveitis (frequently suggesting a diagnosis of juvenile rheumatoid arthritis), cutaneous manifestations, and a conspicuous absence of pulmonary abnormalities.[39–42] The majority of cutaneous lesions in this age group consist of asymptomatic eczematous or infiltrated plaques and papules, and children frequently have ichthyosiform cutaneous manifestations.[40]

Arthralgias, low-grade fever, and abdominal pain are the most frequent symptoms in children with sarcoidosis. Pulmonary involvement, the earliest and most frequently seen symptom in adults, although less common, also occurs in childhood forms of this disorder. Symptoms referable to the lungs are usually mild and often consist of a dry hacking cough, with or without mild to moderate dyspnea. The most common radiographic finding in children is that of bilateral hilar lymph node enlargement, with or without detectable lung changes. Ocular involvement, too, is extremely common in children. Uveitis and iritis constitute the most frequently observed lesions, but keratitis, retinitis, glaucoma, and involvement of the eyelids and lacrimal glands may also occur (Figs. 24–12 and 24–13). Although the world literature suggests that eye lesions in children are not usually severe, involvement of the eye, with resultant partial or total blindness, occurs in a relatively high percentage of children with sarcoidosis.[37]

Facial nerve paralysis and central nervous system involvement, although common in adults, are rare in children. Ossesous involvement is also rarely noted in children. When present, however, the metacarpals, metatarsals, and phalanges are the bones most frequently affected. Uveoparotid fever (a combination of uveitis, parotitis, and Bell's palsy) and Sjögren's syndrome without arthritis,

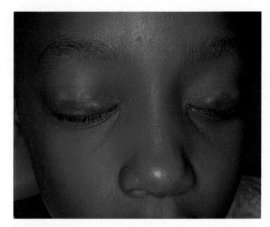

Figure 24–12. Granuloma annulare of upper eyelid resembling sarcoidosis.

although often seen in adults, are quite rare in children. Parotid gland enlargement and peripheral adenopathy are common in children, and hepatic and splenic involvement, although clinically uncommon, are frequently seen at autopsy. A recently described entity, Blau's syndrome (familial granulomatous arteritis of juvenile onset, familial granulomatous arthritis), characterized by generalized erythematous papules and plaques, iritis, arthritis, and synovial cysts overlying the ankle and wrist joints, with an absence of pulmonary involvement, skeletal abnormalities and lymphadenopathy, although similar in many respects to childhood sarcoidosis, appears to represent a unique autosomal dominant familial disorder rather than a variant of sarcoidosis.[43, 44]

Cutaneous Manifestations. Cutaneous lesions of sarcoidosis include papules, nodules, infiltrated plaques, subcutaneous tumors, ichthyosis (ich-

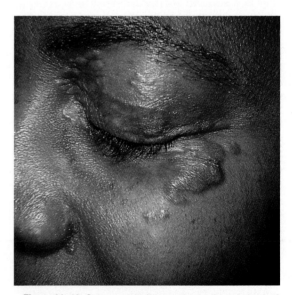

Figure 24–13. Cutaneous lesions on the eyelid and cheek of a patient with sarcoidosis. (Courtesy of Eugene Mirrer, M.D.)

thyotic sarcoid), hypopigmentation, and scaly erythematous patches with little or no palpable infiltration, with the latter often leaving pitted scars in children younger than 6 years of age.[39] Less commonly there may be follicular and palmar lesions, and fusiform changes of the fingers and slight contracture of the hands (pseudoclawing) may, at times, be seen. The most common lesions are soft, red to yellowish brown or violaceous flat-topped papules, with a predilection for the face; and the lesions often tend to occur in areas of trauma or scarification.[45, 46] Although the extremities, neck, and trunk may be affected, an annular configuration of these lesions around the nares, lips, and eyelids is highly characteristic of this disorder. Frequently these lesions will present a waxy or translucent appearance. Occasionally the mucous membranes may be involved as well. If the cutaneous lesions are pressed out with a glass slide (diascopy), a characteristic yellowish brown or "apple-jelly" color may be demonstrated.

Other forms of sarcoidosis in the skin have received special designations. One of these is *lupus pernio* (Fig. 24–14), a variant in which soft infiltrated violaceous plaques are located on the nose, cheeks, ears, forehead, dorsa of the hands, fingers, and toes. *Angiolupoid* is a term used to describe purplish infiltrated plaques or nodules, particularly on or around the nose, with a characteristic telangiectatic vascular component. Since lesions along the nasal rim are often associated with upper respiratory tract involvement, direct and indirect laryngoscopic examination of such patients has been suggested.[47] *Erythrodermic sarcoidosis* is a term used to describe a relatively rare variant of sarcoidosis. Characterized by extensive, sharply demarcated, brownish red, scaly patches with little or no palpable infiltration, these lesions (generally seen on the legs, buttocks, and trunk, and occasionally simulating a generalized exfoliative dermatitis) often involute spontaneously. Another form of skin involvement is a nodular vasculitis with a granulomatous infiltrate largely confined to the subcutaneous tissue. This variant, termed the *Darier-Roussy* type of sarcoidosis, is characterized by skin-colored or violaceous, round or oval, deep-seated nodules and appears primarily on the trunk and legs, usually without subjective symptoms.

Erythema nodosum, occasionally seen in association with sarcoidosis, is a striking but not diagnostic finding; it represents a hypersensitivity phenomenon and is not specific for this disorder.

Diagnosis. There is no single fully reliable test for sarcoidosis. Since the clinical picture may be mimicked by other diseases, histologic proof is advisable. In typical lesions, the characteristic histopathologic finding consists of islands of large, pale-staining epithelioid cells containing few if any giant cells intermingled with histiocytes and lymphocytes. Because of the sparse rim of lymphoid cells in typical cases, they are often referred to as "naked" tubercles. Occasionally asteroid bodies or Schaumann bodies are found in the giant cells. Schaumann bodies (round or oval, laminated, and calcified, especially at their periphery) stain dark blue because of the presence of calcium. The star-shaped asteroid bodies stain best with phosphotungstic acid–hematoxylin, which stains the center brown-red and the spikes blue. Schaumann and asteroid bodies, however, have been observed in other granulomas, such as tuberculosis, leprosy, and berylliosis, and therefore are not specific for this disorder.[48] The Kveim test consists of intradermal injection of a 10 per cent suspension of human sarcoidal tissue (usually from the spleen or lymph nodes) in normal saline. Following the injection a small papule may develop 4 to 6 weeks later, and biopsy reveals distinctive sarcoidal granulomas. Although useful and found to have prognostic as well as diagnostic value, because of variability of the test suspension, the Kveim test is not always reliable and therefore now rarely used. Tuberculin, histoplasmin, and coccidioidin tests and evaluation for cat-scratch disease should be performed, however, since these conditions may closely resemble sarcoidosis in children. The diagnosis, unfortunately, is often hindered by a lack of the classic laboratory findings of hyperglobulinemia, hypercalcemia, leukopenia, and eosinophilia, and although occasionally found, they rarely prove to be reliable diagnostic features of sarcoidosis in childhood.

In addition, 50 to 60 per cent of patients (and up to 80 per cent of children) with active sarcoidosis have elevated serum levels of angiotensin-converting enzyme. Although serum angiotensin-converting enzyme levels can be used as an indicator of disease activity, especially in individuals with pulmonary sarcoidosis, they are often elevated in other granulomatous diseases and normal individuals younger than the age of 20, and are

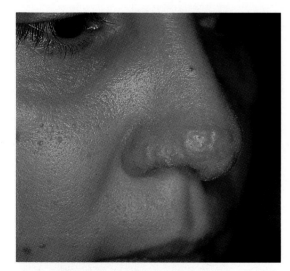

Figure 24–14. Cutaneous sarcoidosis on the nose (lupus pernio). (Courtesy of Department of Dermatology, Yale University School of Medicine.)

frequently normal when sarcoidosis is limited to the skin. Thus, although not a specific test for the differentiation of different forms of hypercalcemia, it may indicate progressive disease with a relatively poor prognosis and thus may serve as a chemical marker of successful treatment of patients with sarcoidosis.[48–50]

Treatment. The natural course of sarcoidosis in childhood is insidious and smoldering and often regresses completely after many years. Mortality is reported to be about 5 per cent, and tuberculosis has been estimated to occur in 10 per cent of children with sarcoidosis. Since the etiology is unknown, although specific therapy is not available, corticosteroids can suppress the acute manifestations of the disorder. Because of the well-known hazards of prolonged systemic corticosteroid therapy, the indications for treatment are determined by the specific organ system involved and the severity of the involvement. Corticosteroids should be used in patients with persistent hypercalcemia; joint involvement; lesions of the nasal, laryngeal, and bronchial mucosa; severe, debilitating, or rapidly progressing lung disease; central nervous system lesions; disfiguring skin and lymph node lesions; persistent facial palsy; myocardial involvement; hypersplenism; and ocular sarcoidosis. In ocular sarcoidosis, corticosteroid ophthalmic preparations may be used in conjunction with the systemic therapy. In children the dose of prednisone is 1 mg/kg/day, with gradual reduction to the lowest dosage that will suppress the symptoms and signs of the disorder. Although the course of treatment is usually about 6 months, the duration is determined by the response to therapy and the type or severity of involvement. Other drugs occasionally used in the treatment of adult sarcoidosis, such as oxyphenbutazone, chloroquine, potassium *p*-aminobenzoate, azathioprine, chlorambucil, and transfer factor, are generally not used for the treatment of childhood forms of sarcoidosis and require further evaluation.[51]

LYMPHOCYTOMA CUTIS

Lymphocytoma cutis (lymphadenosis benigna cutis, pseudolymphoma of Spiegler-Fendt) is a benign inflammatory disorder characterized by increased hyperplasia of the reticuloendothelial tissue of the skin. It can occur at any age and seems to affect women two to three times as frequently as men. Although the etiology remains unknown, some cases appear to follow insect bites, actinic injury, or other trauma.[52] Transfer from person to person by serial passage[53] and a spirochetal infection (a borreliosis) transmitted by an arthropod (see Chapter 10) also suggest an infectious etiology, at least in some patients with this disorder.[54]

Clinical Manifestations. From a clinical point of view there are two forms of lymphocytoma cutis. The first presents as a localized or circumscribed form. Seen in infants and children as well as adults, the localized form rapidly increases in incidence from infancy through adolescence to early adulthood, and then gradually declines.

The localized form generally is confined to one region. As a rule, it begins as a discrete firm purple or yellowish brown solitary nodule or as a number of regionally limited swellings. Lesions may begin as pea-sized nodules and enlarge slowly, frequently reaching a size measuring 4 or 5 cm in diameter. In over 60 per cent of cases the localized lesions make their appearance on the face, ears, or scalp (usually the cheek, forehead, or tip of the nose). Occasionally other regions of the body may be involved, particularly the forearms, genitalia, or areolae of the breasts (Fig. 24–15). Prognosis in the localized form is good. The chances for complete recovery are favorable, often with spontaneous healing after months or years, or following treatment.

The disseminated form of lymphocytoma cutis is less common in all age groups. It is rarely seen in infancy and young children. Generally occurring in middle-aged adults, it appears as firm bluish red papules or nodules, usually on the face, but sometimes on the trunk and extremities. Lesions tend to grow rapidly, spread, and often persist throughout life. Although lymphocytoma cutis can be confused clinically and histologically with lymphoma, long-term studies indicate that the disseminated form is benign and identical to the localized form of the disorder.

Histopathologic examination must differentiate lesions of lymphocytoma cutis from malignant lymphoma. Lymphocytoma cutis is characterized by a dense proliferation of mature nonneoplastic-appearing lymphoid and reticulum cells in the der-

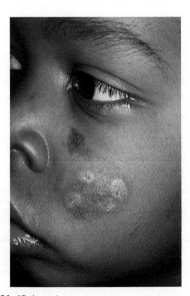

Figure 24–15. Lymphocytoma cutis on the left cheek of a 4-year-old black child.

mis. The arrangement often resembles a well-delineated germinal center surrounded by small mature lymphocytes. The lymphocytic infiltrate is separated from the epidermis by a clear grenz zone of connective tissue and can be differentiated from malignancy by the presence of plasma cells or eosinophils, lack of extension into the deep dermis and subcutaneous fat, and the absence of abnormal reticulum cells and mitoses (Fig. 24–16).

Treatment. The prognosis, particularly for the localized form of lymphocytoma cutis, is good, and the chances of complete recovery are favorable. The circumscribed lesions heal spontaneously after months or years, or after treatment. Good results have been achieved with the use of penicillin. Bäfverstedt has found that disseminated lesions may at times also be penicillin sensitive.[54] The effect of penicillin, however, is inconsistent, and radiation, particularly in adults, still seems to be the most widely used method of therapy. Cryosurgery with liquid nitrogen and argon laser therapy have also been recommended, and although the argon laser beam can reduce and help camouflage resistant lesions, complete resolution is generally not obtained with this modality.[54a, 55]

In the treatment of children I prefer to avoid radiation therapy whenever possible. If lesions do not disappear spontaneously, penicillin should be tried and topical, intralesional, or systemic corticosteroid therapy, cryosurgery or argon laser therapy may give a favorable response. In the event of failure, although recurrences are possible, lesions in the circumscribed form usually respond rapidly to radiation therapy. The disseminated form does not respond as readily to radiation therapy and shows a greater tendency to recur. Lesions may frequently tend to spread and persist throughout life, but maintain a benign course. Cases of lymphocytoma cutis reported to have changed from a benign to malignant lymphoma were probably misdiagnosed, representing malignant lymphoma from the outset.

LEUKEMIA

Leukemia, the most common form of childhood cancer, accounts for about one third (2,000 to 2,500) of an estimated 7,000 new cases of childhood neoplastic disorders in the United States each year. Patients usually present with constitutional or toxic symptoms of infection or systemic disease, but cutaneous lesions present as the initial manifestation in 50 per cent of infants with congenital leukemia, 10 to 50 per cent of patients with monocytic leukemia, and 6 to 10 per cent of those with lymphocytic and granulocytic leukemias. Although the cutaneous features of various leukemias and lymphomas often tend to resemble one another, each will frequently have its own characteristic appearance and distribution. In acute and chronic lymphocytic leukemia, the face and extremities are the primary areas of involvement; in granulocytic leukemia the trunk is primarily affected; in monocytic leukemia the entire cutaneous surface may display skin lesions; and in patients with acute monocytic leukemia, florid oral and cutaneous lesions are characteristic.[10]

Leukemia can be quite varied in its presentation and often mimics other diseases. Systemic manifestations of leukemia include fever, anemia, pallor, lethargy, anorexia, irritability, lymphadenopathy, hepatosplenomegaly, overt signs of bleeding such as petechiae or ecchymoses, bone pain and arthralgia associated with periosteal or bony involvement, and, particularly in individuals with central nervous system involvement, headache and vomiting. Cutaneous manifestations may be grouped into various categories. These include cutaneous lesions resulting from leukemic infiltration of the skin and subcutaneous tissues (leukemia cutis, granulocytic sarcoma, and extramedullary tumor masses); nonspecific lesions such as ichthyosis, hyperpigmentation, hyperkeratosis of the palms and soles, severe eczematous eruptions, Sweet's syndrome, pyoderma gangrenosum, erythema multiforme, and hypereosinophilic syn-

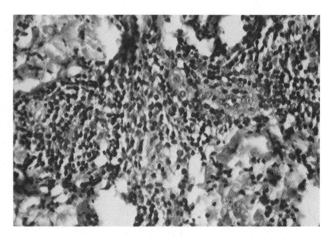

Figure 24–16. Lymphocytoma cutis. Microscopic features consist of a dense proliferation of mature benign-appearing lymphoid and reticulum cells in the dermis.

drome; toxic or immunologic responses to tumor antigens ("leukemids"); opportunistic infections; cutaneous lesions associated with bone marrow dysfunction (petechiae, purpura, ecchymoses, or cutaneous erythropoiesis in infants manifesting as blueberry muffin lesions); lesions in cutaneous scars; and cutaneous manifestations resulting from radiation therapy and chemotherapy.[56–62]

Leukemia Cutis

The specific cutaneous lesions of leukemia are usually seen as discrete pink, red-brown or purple macules, papules, or tumors (Figs. 24–17 through 24–19). The solid masses are firm but not stony hard, and tumors of monocytic leukemia tend to be large and purplish or "plum-colored."[10] Although acute lymphocytic leukemia, the most common childhood form of this disorder, accounts for 60 per cent of childhood leukemias, primary cutaneous lesions are seen in only 0.5 to 1 per cent of affected children and, although helpful, usually do not present as reliable early markers of acute lymphocytic leukemia in childhood.

Leukemic infiltrates may arise in scars from recent surgery, burns, trauma, intramuscular injections, and lesions of herpes simplex or herpes zoster infections.[58] In addition, leukemic plaques can cause thickening of the scalp, eyebrows, and cheeks producing a typical leonine facies. Especially common in acute monocytic and acute myelomonocytic leukemia, patients with oral involvement may present with painful teeth, hyperplasia of the intradental papillae, gingival involvement (friable bleeding gums and a swollen reddish appearance often completely covering the teeth), and sore throat and ulcerations of the buccal or gingival mucosae suggesting a diagnosis of Vincent's angina. Nonspecific lesions ("leukemids"), presumed to result from toxic effects of the underlying disorder, such as prurigo-like papules, maculo-

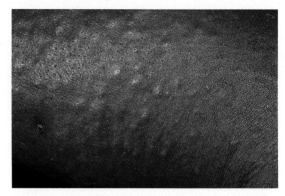

Figure 24–18. Leukemia cutis. (Courtesy of Neal S. Penneys, M.D.)

papular eruptions (see Fig. 24–18), vesiculobullous lesions, urticaria, generalized erythroderma, exfoliative hyperpigmentation, chloroma, erythema multiforme, Sweet's syndrome (see chapter 18, Fig. 18–18), and erythema nodosum may also be seen.

Green tumors, granulocytic sarcomas (formally called chloromas), the sole pathognomonic lesions of leukemia, can arise at the same time as acute granulocytic leukemia or may precede the disease by 1 or more years before the underlying disorder becomes apparent. Seen primarily in children younger than the age of 18 years, granulocytic sarcomas, which result from infiltration of immature granulocytic cells, may also arise at sites other than the skin, such as the bones (the periosteum of the orbital and cranial bones and, at times, the sinuses, sternum, vertebrae, pelvis, and long bones), lacrimal glands, lymph nodes, and breast. Seen in 2.9 per cent of all patients with acute myelogenous leukemia, lesions vary from 1 to 3 cm in diameter and the green color, caused by the enzyme myeloperoxidase (veroperoxidase), fades on exposure to air.

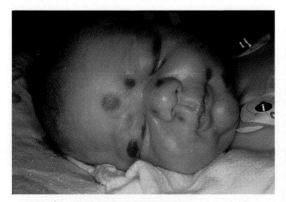

Figure 24–17. Acute lymphocytic leukemia with cutaneous lesions on the face of a newborn. (Courtesy of Ann Lucky, M.D.)

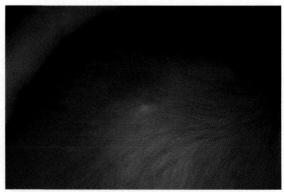

Figure 24–19. A nodular lesion on the scalp of a 4-month-old infant with congenital leukemia.

Congenital Leukemia

Congenital leukemia, characterized by the proliferation of cells of the myelomonocytic, lymphoid, or erythroid series, is an extremely rare disorder. With fewer than 150 cases reported in the world literature, cutaneous lesions are seen in 50 per cent of cases as its initial manifestation. Lesions may vary from a few millimeters to several centimeters in diameter and may be skin colored or reddish brown to blue-gray. Nodular lesions have a firm "woody" texture and are freely movable over the underlying subcutaneous tissue (see Figs. 24–17 and 24–19).

The diagnosis of leukemia requires correlation of the history and physical findings, morphologic interpretation of peripheral blood smears and bone marrow, and evaluation of relevant laboratory data. Although cutaneous biopsies of lesions of leukemia cutis may suggest the diagnosis, they often mimic a variety of inflammatory and neoplastic diseases, and touch smears, peripheral blood smears, and bone marrow evaluation are generally required in an effort to make a definitive diagnosis. Except for granulocytic sarcoma, in which lesions show a massive infiltrate of immature granulocytic cells with abundant cytoplasm and large oval nuclei, histologic examination of cutaneous lesions of leukemia cutis reveals a dermal infiltrate with a variable appearance depending on the specific leukemic cell type.

The cure rate of leukemia depends not only on its type but also on therapy. For this reason, children should be treated by a skilled pediatric oncologist or at a pediatric hematology/oncology research and treatment center. If death occurs, it is usually attributed to hematologic abnormalities such as hemorrhage, disseminated intravascular coagulation, septicemia, other severe infection, or complications of therapy. With currently available treatment, approximately 50 per cent of children with acute lymphoblastic leukemia are cured, and an even higher cure rate is expected in the future. Chemotherapy, currently the mainstay of treatment, varies with the type of leukemia, with combinations of prednisone, asparaginase, vincristine, and other agents (e.g., methotrexate, mercaptopurine, daunorubicin, cyclophosphamide, and cytarabine) in addition to the supportive measures necessary to prevent drug- or disease-related complications.

NEUROBLASTOMA

Neuroblastoma, a tumor that arises from the primitive neurocrest cells that form the adrenal medulla and sympathetic nervous system, is the most common malignant tumor in infancy, and, in childhood ranks fourth in frequency to leukemia, lymphoma, and central nervous system tumors. Although neuroblastoma represents less than 8 per cent of childhood cancer, it is responsible for 15 per cent of cancer deaths in childhood. This malignancy usually appears in the newborn or young child (more than 50 per cent of cases are diagnosed in children younger than 2 years of age). The most common presentation is an abdominal mass that is hard, smooth, nontender, and most often palpated in the flank. Cutaneous features, seen in 2.6 per cent of all patients and 32 per cent of newborns with this disorder, may at times be seen as the initial sign of the disease. These include "raccoon eyes" (periorbital ecchymoses resulting from orbital metastases), heterochromia irides (the result of involvement of the sympathetic innervation of the iris that controls eye color), and highly characteristic firm, nontender, blue or bluish gray metastatic nodules (Fig. 24–20) that, due to release of catecholamines, tend to blanch and develop a surrounding halo of erythema within 2 or 3 minutes after being palpated, stroked, or rubbed. Although blueberry muffin lesions, vascular tumors, cutaneous lesions of leukemia, and cysts may sometimes be confused with cutaneous lesions of neuroblastoma, their characteristic blanching following palpation or rubbing, careful physical examination with blood pressure evaluation, cutaneous biopsy, ultrasonograms, abdominal and chest radiographs, computed tomography, and careful search for products of catecholamine metabolism (vanillylmandelic acid and homovanillic acid) generally lead to the appropriate diagnosis.[63, 64]

HODGKIN'S DISEASE

Lymphomas, a group of malignant neoplasias derived from B or T lymphocytes, and rarely from histiocytes, are subdivided into Hodgkin's disease, possibly derived from activated or transformed T-helper cells, non-Hodgkin's lymphomas, largely derived from B lymphocytes, and mycosis fungoides (cutaneous T-cell lymphoma), derived from T lymphocytes.[48]

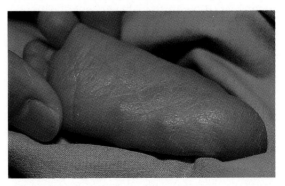

Figure 24–20. Bluish gray nodules on the foot of an infant with neuroblastoma. (Courtesy of Kenneth Greer, M.D.; reprinted from Nguyen TQ, Fisher GB Jr., Tabbarah SO, et al.: Stage IV-S metastatic neuroblastoma presenting as skin nodules at birth. J. Int. Dermatol. 27:712–713, 1988.)

Hodgkin's disease, a malignant lymphoma in which the Reed-Sternberg giant cell (a large typically multinucleated cell with abundant cytoplasm) is the central histologic feature, occurs primarily in two age groups. This tumor causes approximately 4 per cent of childhood malignancies, rarely occurs before the age of 5 years, and increases to a peak level in teenagers and young adults between 15 and 34 years of age; a second peak occurs in adults older than the age of 40. Although its etiology remains unknown, a virus of low virulence and infectivity has been suggested as a cause, and some suspect a genetic predisposition to the disorder. In 90 per cent of cases, Hodgkin's lymphoma is initially limited to the lymph nodes, with superficial lymph nodes more commonly the first site of involvement than visceral lymph nodes. It presents as a painless enlargement of the cervical lymph nodes, and occasionally of the supraclavicular, axillary, or inguinal lymph nodes. Usually first noted by the patient or parents, the enlargement is firm, nontender, and often discrete, involving single or multiple lymph nodes. The patient's condition, otherwise, may initially be normal, but with progressive involvement fever, anemia, and weight loss are common. Cutaneous manifestations are found in 13 to 40 per cent of patients and, as with leukemia and other carcinomas, both specific and nonspecific lesions are found.[10] Specific cutaneous lesions (those with histologic features of Hodgkin's disease) occur in 0.5 to 7.5 per cent of patients and probably less frequently in children. Although such lesions are generally seen as late rather than early manifestations, they generally present as pink, reddish brown, violaceous, plum-colored or dark purple papules or nodules and often coalesce to form large tumors or plaques. Varying from a few millimeters to several centimeters in diameter, lesions are usually localized to the upper trunk, neck and scalp, and ulcerations may sometimes occur.

Nonspecific skin signs include pruritus (which occurs in up to 50 per cent of patients and frequently appears as the first cutaneous feature of the disorder), pallor, purpura, papules, pyoderma, hyperpigmentation (in 10 to 30 per cent of patients), hyperpigmented scars, exfoliative erythroderma, acquired ichthyosis, nonspecific eczematous or psoriasiform plaques, prurigo nodularis, hyperkeratosis of the palms and soles, urticaria, loss of body hair, nail dystrophy, follicular mucinosis, erythema nodosum, erythema multiforme, herpes simplex virus infection, and herpes zoster virus infection. Vesicular and bullous lesions, although rare, when seen usually appear as a terminal manifestation.[65-69]

The prognosis of Hodgkin's lymphoma has improved substantially over the past several decades. In early (stage I) disease, over 90 per cent of patients can be cured by radiation therapy alone or in conjunction with chemotherapy such as nitrogen mustard, vincristine, procarbazine, prednisone, doxorubicin, bleomycin, vinblastine, or dacarbazine. In advanced stages, a combined approach (radiation therapy, total nodal irradiation, and various combinations of chemotherapeutic agents) is generally required. Although many therapeutic and management problems remain, Hodgkin's disease may now be approached with considerable more optimism, and up to 80 to 90 per cent of children with stage III and up to 80 per cent of those with stage IV disease can now be expected to survive for periods of 5 years or more.

NON-HODGKIN'S LYMPHOMAS

The non-Hodgkin's lymphomas are a group of lymphocytic malignancies with different histopathologic features and clinical behaviors. They account for approximately 6 per cent of malignancies in children younger than 15 years of age and are most commonly seen in children between 7 and 11 years of age. Cutaneous manifestations occur in up to 26 per cent of patients and in about 5 per cent of patients they appear as the initial manifestation of the disease. Nonspecific cutaneous manifestations include pruritus, a papular dermatitis resembling dermatitis herpetiformis, erythema multiforme, herpes zoster, purpura, exfoliative dermatitis, poikiloderma, and perhaps scleromyxedema (papular mucinosis, lichen myxedematosis), a disorder characterized by mucin deposition and fibroblast proliferation in the upper dermis producing lichenoid waxy papules, plaques, nodules, and diffuse thickening of the skin of the face, forearms, and trunk.[70] Specific lesions consist of cutaneous nodules that vary from 3 to 10 mm in diameter. They are typically dusky red to plum-colored or brown and are often grouped or arranged in annular or arciform configurations; ulcerations are common.

The diagnosis of non-Hodgkin's lymphoma depends on a careful history, physical examination, complete blood cell count and differential, chest radiograph, and biopsy of lymph nodes, bone marrow, or other involved tissues. Histopathologic examination of specific lesions is characterized by a dense dermal lymphocytic infiltrate composed of a monomorphic population of cells with atypical nuclei, frequently extending to the subcutaneous tissue. Differentiation from pseudolymphoma, however, is often difficult and frequently requires clinical correlation, careful histologic evaluation, and, at times, immunotyping and electron microscopic evaluation.

With appropriate surgery, radiation and chemotherapy, more than half the children affected with early-stage non-Hodgkin's lymphoma can be cured; and although the prognosis for children with advanced disease is less favorable, 60 to 80 per cent of children with advanced-stage disease may be treated successfully with intensive therapy.

CUTANEOUS T-CELL LYMPHOMA

Cutaneous T-cell lymphoma (mycosis fungoides) is a chronic, frequently fatal neoplasm of helper T cells whose initial clinical manifestations appear in the skin, often remaining there for years before terminating as a malignant lymphoma with lymph node and visceral involvement. Generally seen in patients in the fifth to seventh decades of life, it may also be seen in children, adolescents, and young adults (Table 24–10).[71, 72] Although its etiology remains unknown, current hypotheses suggest a viral origin, chronic antigenic stimulation in which epidermally located antigens act as stimulants for blast formation of T cells, or a malignant lymphoma in which the mycosis cell (a T lymphocyte) represents the neoplastic cell. In some patients, a phenytoin hypersensitivity syndrome (the Dilantin hypersensitivity syndrome), characterized by fever, rash, lymphadenopathy, and hepatitis associated with leukocytosis and eosinophilia, with clinical, pathologic, and immunologic features of cutaneous T-cell lymphoma, has been noted.[73]

Clinically as well as histologically cutaneous T-cell lymphoma can be divided into erythematous, plaque, and tumor stages. The disorder may begin with any of the stages, only one or two phases may be noted, or lesions of all three stages may be present at the same time.

The erythematous (premycotic) stage is characterized by pruritus and flat erythematous, eczematous, psoriasiform, or poikilodermatous lesions; and in some patients the disorder may begin with a pigmented purpura-like eruption simulating Schamberg's capillaritis.[74]

In the plaque (mycotic) phase the premycotic lesions become infiltrated and well demarcated and appear as red or reddish brown to purple slightly indurated plaques. Central clearing often develops, and the lesions may assume serpiginous, arciform, horseshoe, or other bizarre shapes. In many instances, the entire integument may become infiltrated, producing thickened red skin with or without scaling, with islands of normal skin often remaining for a time before the universal erythroderma becomes complete.[10] Although extensive exfoliative erythroderma may occur in atopic, contact, or seborrheic dermatitis, psoriasis,

or pityriasis rubra pilaris, patients with de novo onset of persistent generalized erythroderma and no evidence for drug eruption should be evaluated for the possibility of cutaneous T-cell lymphoma.

In the third (tumor) stage, multiple, round, dome-shaped or irregular raised tumors may appear (Figs. 24–21 and 24–22). These are flesh colored or smooth brown to bluish red lesions covered with a thin, stretched, atrophic-appearing epidermis, with or without telangiectasia. Lesions often undergo necrosis or ulceration and at times may disappear spontaneously. Once tumors, lymphadenopathy, or cutaneous ulceration occurs, the prognosis is extremely poor, and up to 50 per cent of patients may die within 2½ to 4 years.[11]

Other Clinical Features and Variants. A disorder termed *parapsoriasis en plaque* has been defined as both a benign and a premalignant disorder. Lesions of the premalignant variety are characterized by round or oval, yellowish to red, smooth or slightly scaly plaques 2 to 4 cm in diameter that occur chiefly on the trunk and thighs. In patients in whom parapsoriasis en plaque progresses to cutaneous T-cell lymphoma, the skin assumes a dusky reddish brown hue on which numerous telangiec-

Table 24–10. MYCOSIS FUNGOIDES (CUTANEOUS T-CELL LYMPHOMA)

1. Generally seen in fifth to seventh decades of life, occasionally in childhood and early adulthood
2. Etiology unknown (?chronic antigenic stimulation in skin)
3. Cutaneous lesions
   a. Erythematous (premycotic) stage
   b. Plaque (mycotic) stage
   c. Tumor stage
4. Poor prognosis (50% mortality within 2 to 4 years of onset) of tumor stage

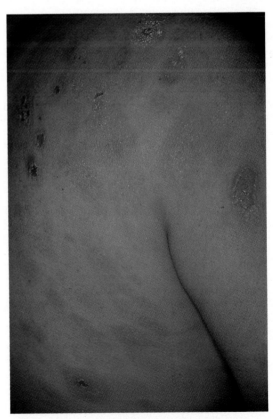

Figure 24–21. Mycosis fungoides (cutaneous T-cell lymphoma). Erythematous plaque-like lesions show crusting and ulceration. (Courtesy of Department of Dermatology, Yale University School of Medicine.)

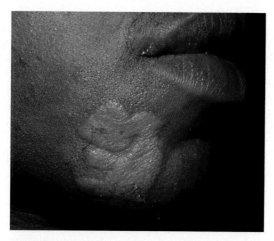

Figure 24–22. A nodular tumor on the chin of a 10-year-old black boy with mycosis fungoides (cutaneous T-cell lymphoma). (Courtesy of Emily Omura, M.D.; reprinted from Hurwitz S: The reticuloendothelial disorders. *In* The Skin and Systemic Disease in Children. Year Book Medical Publishers, Chicago, 1985.)

tatic vessels involve the entire skin. Poikilodermatous lesions become atrophic with a folded wrinkled telangiectatic surface, mild scaling, and hyperpigmentation and hypopigmentation; and eventually plaque-like infiltration and ulcerations develop. *Alopecia mucinosa* (follicular mucinosis) has also been shown to be a feature of mycosis fungoides and, on occasion, malignant lymphoma in adults. Although it can at times be seen as a manifestation of the disorder in children, in the majority of cases (children and adults younger than the age of 40), it is generally regarded as a benign condition not associated with mycosis fungoides. Although most cases of follicular mucinosis in childhood represent a benign self-limiting process, with persistence of lesions the disorder, even in children, may on rare occasions also be associated with a lymphoma.[68]

About 15 per cent of patients with mycosis fungoides develop generalized or universal redness and scaling of the skin with weeping, crusting, fissuring, and some degree of hyperpigmentation. Pruritus is usually severe, and excoriations are prominent. Some patients are simply red with little alteration of the epidermis (*l'homme rouge*). Thickening of the palms and soles (keratoderma palmaris et plantaris), ectropion, leonine facies, dystrophic nails, lymphadenopathy associated with leukocytosis and abnormal mononuclear cells, and alopecia of the scalp are often seen. *Sézary syndrome*, a disorder characterized by generalized erythroderma with intense itching, peripheral lymphadenopathy, and the presence of Sézary cells (atypical cells with large grooved nuclei) in the infiltrate of the skin and the peripheral blood, although at first believed to be an independent entity, with infrequent exceptions appears to represent one of many manifestations of mycosis fungoides.[10]

Diagnosis. In the premycotic stage cutaneous T-cell lymphoma may be extremely difficult to diagnose. Pruritus with or without skin lesions may be the only finding. Skin lesions are usually nondescript and eczematous, frequently suggesting a diagnosis of psoriasis, parapsoriasis, eczema, seborrheic dermatitis, or neurodermatitis. The histology of the lesion is usually not helpful at this stage. When clinical infiltration is noted, however, histopathologic examination of lesions usually exhibits changes consistent with this disorder. Although the histopathology varies with the stage of the disease, a multiplicity of cell types with pleomorphism of the histiocytes, immature and atypical reticulum cells, scattered mycotic figures, a patchy infiltrate in the lower dermis, and the presence of Pautrier microabscesses in the epidermis help establish the diagnosis.

Treatment. Since most patients live for many years before cutaneous T-cell lymphoma becomes life threatening, early stages of the disease may be treated conservatively with topical and systemic antipruritics and topical corticosteroids. For those with more advanced disease, localized radiation therapy, PUVA therapy, electron beam therapy, topical use of nitrogen mustard (Mustargen), systemic chemotherapy, interferon therapy, and extracorporeal photochemotherapy are currently recommended.[75, 76]

References

1. Lichtenstein L: Histiocytosis X: An integration of eosinophilic granuloma of bone, Letterer-Siwe disease, and Schüller-Christian disease as related manifestations of a single nosological entity. Arch. Pathol. *84:*102, 1953.

   The three disorders are grouped into one entity termed *histiocytosis X.*

2. Kuttner BJ, Friedman KJ, Burton CS III, et al.: Letterer-Siwe disease in an adult. Cutis *39:*142–146, 1987.

   A 67-year-old woman with adult Letterer-Siwe disease, one of 31 cases reported in adults 16 years of age or older.

3. Gianotti F, Caputo R: Histiocytic syndromes: A review. J. Am. Acad. Dermatol. *13:*383–404, 1985.

   An authoritative review of the clinical, histologic, and ultrastructural features of the histiocytic syndromes.

4. Esterly NB, Maurer HS, Gonzalez-Crussi F: Histiocytosis X: A seven-year experience at a children's hospital. J. Am. Acad. Dermatol. *13:*481–496, 1985.

   A review of the clinical features and therapeutic regimens of 32 children with histiocytosis.

5. Aronson RP: Streptomycin in Letterer-Siwe disease. Am. J. Dis. Child. *117:*236–238, 1969.

   The first reported case of recovery of a patient with Letterer-Siwe disease.

6. Esterly NB, Swick HM: Cutaneous Letterer-Siwe disease. Am. J. Dis. Child. *117:*236–238, 1969.

   A 2½-year-old girl with purely cutaneous manifestations of Letterer-Siwe disease had a striking remission due to vincristine sulfate (Velban) and was subsequently controlled on oral cyclophosphamide (Cytoxan).

7. Freeman S: A benign form of Letterer-Siwe disease. Aust. J. Dermatol. *12:*165–171, 1971.

A 3-month-old infant with histiocytosis improved (on topical corticosteroids alone) by 10 months of age.

8. Bierman HR: Apparent cure of Letterer-Siwe disease. J.A.M.A. *196:*368–370, 1966.

Seventeen-year survival of identical twins with histologically proven Letterer-Siwe disease.

9. Wolfson SL, Botero F, Hurwitz S, et al.: "Pure" cutaneous histiocystosis X. Cancer *48:*2236–2238, 1981.

A report of two children with cutaneous lesions of histiocytosis X successfully treated with oral corticosteroids.

10. Braverman IM: Skin Signs of Systemic Disease, 2nd ed. W. B. Saunders Co., Philadelphia, 1981.

An invaluable well-written text emphasizing the cutaneous features and their role in the diagnosis of systemic disease.

11. Hurwitz S: The reticuloendothelial disorders. In The Skin and Systemic Disease in Children. Year Book Medical Publishers, Chicago, 1985.

An overview of the reticuloenthelial system and its cutaneous manifestations in systemic disorders of childhood.

12. Mishkel MA, Cockshott WP, Nazir DJ, et al.: Xanthoma disseminatum: Clinical, metabolic, pathologic and radiologic aspects. Arch. Dermatol. *113:*1094–1100, 1977

Report of a case of xanthoma disseminatum with a review of the clinical, metabolic, and pathologic features.

13. Kumakari M, Sudoh M, Miura Y: Xanthoma disseminatum. J. Am. Acad. Dermatol. *4:*291–299, 1981.

A report of a 40-year-old Japanese woman with xanthoma disseminatum and diabetes insipidus with histologic and ultrastructural studies of the cutaneous features of the disorder.

14. Frumkin A, Roytman M, Johnson SF: Juvenile xanthogranuloma underneath a toenail. Cutis *40:*244–245, 1987.

A report of a 3-year-old boy with a subungual juvenile xanthogranuloma.

15. Cohen BA, Hood A: Xanthogranuloma: Report on clinical and histologic findings in 64 patients. Pediatr. Dermatol. *6:*262–266, 1989.

A report of 64 patients with juvenile xanthogranuloma supports the concept that lesions of this disorder are benign, generally limited to the skin, and although they generally are self-limiting (particularly in individuals who develop them after the age of 20 years), they may at times persist and occasionally continue to erupt for years.

16. Campbell L, McTigue MK, Esterly NB, et al.: Giant juvenile xanthogranuloma. Arch. Dermatol. *124:*1723–1728, 1988.

A report of a 5½-month-old infant with an 8×5-cm juvenile xanthogranuloma: since the lesion began to regress spontaneously, therapy was not required.

17. Resnick SD, Woosley J, Azizkhan RG: Giant juvenile xanthogranuloma: Exophytic and endophytic variants. Pediatr. Dermatol. *7:*185–188, 1990.

A report of two children with xanthogranulomas larger than 2 cm in diameter.

18. Blank H, Eglick PG, Beerman H: Nevoxanthoendothelioma with ocular involvement. Pediatrics *4:*349–354, 1949.

Nevoxanthoendothelioma in the eye of a 4-month old.

19. Flach DB, Winkelmann RK: Juvenile xanthogranuloma with central nervous system lesions. J. Am. Acad. Dermatol. *14:*405–411, 1986.

A report of two boys with extensive cutaneous lesions of juvenile xanthogranuloma who subsequently developed disabling central nervous system involvement.

20. Cooper PH, Frierson HF, Kayne AL, et al.: Association of juvenile xanthogranuloma with juvenile myeloid leukemia. Arch. Dermatol. *120:*371–375, 1984.

A review of reported cases of juvenile chronic myelogenous leukemia associated with juvenile xanthogranulomas. Although cutaneous lesions in such cases may have histopathologic similarities like those of sporadic juvenile xanthogranulomas, they are more often likely to be multiple, papular, and confluent.

21. Kossard S, Winkelmann RK: Necrobiotic xanthogranuloma with paraproteinemia. J. Am. Acad. Dermatol. *3:*257–270, 1980.

A report of eight patients with inflammatory, ulcerative, atrophic nodules, xanthomatous plaques, subcutaneous nodules, and paraproteinemia.

22. Finelli LG, Ratz JL: Plasmapharesis, a treatment modality for necrobiotic xanthogranuloma. J. Am. Acad. Dermatol. *17:*351–354, 1987.

A report of a 55-year-old woman with a 9-year history of lower extremity ulcerations, pancytopenia, hepatosplenomegaly and IgG monoclonal paraproteinemia in whom successful healing of the ulcerated lesions and lowering of the paraproteinemia were achieved by plasmapharesis when cytotoxic therapy failed.

23. Hashimoto K, Bale GF, Hawkins HK, et al.: Congenital self-healing reticulohistiocytosis (Hashimoto-Pritzker type). Int. J. Dermatol. *25:*516–522, 1986.

A review of 16 cases of congenital self-healing reticulohistiocystosis.

24. Kapila PK, Grant-Kels JM, Allred C, et al.: Congenital, spontaneously regressing histiocytosis: Case report and review of the literature. Pediatr. Dermatol. *2:*312–317, 1985.

A report of a 1-day-old girl with congenital self-healing reticulohistiocytosis whose lesions resolved spontaneously within several weeks.

25. Jordaan HF, Drusinsky SF: Congenital self-healing reticulohistiocytosis: A report of a case. Pediatr. Dermatol. *3:*473–475, 1986.

A report of a newborn male with a solitary lesion of congenital self-healing reticulohistiocytosis.

26. Timpatanapong P, Rochanawutanon M, Siripoonya P, et al.: Congenital self-healing reticulohistiocytosis: Report of a patient with a strikingly large tumor mass. Pediatr. Dermatol. *6:*28–32, 1989.

A report of a male infant with multiple brownish red to bluish red firm papulonodular lesions, the largest of which measured about 8 cm in diameter with clinical, histopathologic, and ultrastructural findings of congenital self-healing reticulohistiocytosis.

27. Herman LE, Rothman KF, Harawi S, et al.: Congenital self-healing reticulohistiocytosis: A new entity in the differential diagnosis of neonatal papulovesicular eruptions. Arch. Dermatol. *126:*210–212, 1990.

An infant with congenital self-healing reticulohistiocytosis with papulovesicles, superficial erosions and hemorrhagic crusted lesions as predominant cutaneous manifestations of the disorder.

28. Gianotti F, Caputo R, Ermacore E, et al: Benign cephalic histiocytosis. Arch. Dermatol. *122:*1038–1043, 1986.

A report of 13 patients with benign cephalic histiocytosis and a comprehensive review of their clinical and histopathologic features.

29. Eisenberg EL, Bronson DM, Barsky S: Benign cephalic histiocytosis. J. Am. Acad. Dermatol. *12:*328–331, 1985.

A report of a 4-year-old boy with benign cephalic histiocytosis and a review of the clinical and histologic features of this disorder.

30. De Luna ML, Glikin I, Golberg J, et al.: Benign cephalic histiocytosis: Report of four cases. Pediatr. Dermatol. *6:*198–201, 1989.

A report of four patients with benign cephalic histiocytosis with a review of the differential diagnosis, clinical and histologic features of this disorder.

31. Roper SS, Spraker MK: Cutaneous histiocytosis syndromes. Pediatr. Dermatol. *3*:19–30, 1985.

The histiocytic syndromes of childhood and guidelines for their evaluation.

32. Winkelmann RK, Kossard S, Fraga S: Eruptive histiocytoma of childhood. Arch. Dermatol. *116*:565–570, 1980.

A report of a 9-year-old girl with generalized eruptive histiocytomas.

33. Caputo R, Ermacora E, Gelmetti C, et al.: Generalized eruptive histiocytoma in children. J. Am. Acad. Dermatol. *17*:449–454, 1987.

A report of four children with generalized eruptive histiocytomas.

34. Burgdorf WHC, Kusch SL, Nix TE, et al.: Progressive nodular histiocytoma. Arch. Dermatol. *117*:644–649, 1981.

A report of a patient with lesions characteristic of progressive nodular histiocytoma and a review of the clinical, histologic, and ultrastructural features of the disorder.

35. Morgan NE, Fretzin D, Variakojis D, et al.: Clinical and pathologic cutaneous features of malignant histiocytosis. Arch. Dermatol. *119*:367–372, 1983.

A review of the clinical and pathologic features of the skin in five patients with malignant histiocytosis.

36. Wick MR, Sanchez NP, Crotty CP, et al.: Cutaneous malignant histiocytosis: A clinical and histopathologic study of eight cases, with immunohistochemical analysis. J. Am. Acad. Dermatol. *8*:50–62, 1983.

A report of eight patients with malignant histiocytosis in whom cutaneous involvement was a prominent feature at the initial presentation of the disorder.

37. Kendig EL: Medical progress: Sarcoidosis among children—a review. J. Pediatr. *61*:229–278. 1962.

A review of sarcoidosis demonstrates the value of corticosteroids in children with severe involvement.

38. Beier RF, Lahey MD: Sarcoidosis among children in Utah and Idaho. J. Pediatr. *65*:350–359, 1964.

Eight Caucasian children with sarcoidosis (mostly of northern European ancestry) in Utah and Idaho.

39. Rasmussen JE: Sarcoidosis in young children. J. Am. Acad. Dermatol. *5*:560–570, 1981.

A report of a 1-year-old child with sarcoidosis and a review of its diagnosis and management in childhood.

40. Mallory SB, Paller AS, Ginsburg BC, et al.: Sarcoidosis in children: Differentiation from juvenile rheumatoid arthritis. Pediatr. Dermatol. *4*:313–319, 1987.

In a report of four young children with sarcoidosis with severe joint manifestations, three of the four had ichthyosiform manifestations suggesting a possible association between severe joint disease and ichthyosiform changes in children with this disorder.

41. Lindsley CB, Godfrey WA: Childhood sarcoidosis manifesting as juvenile rheumatoid arthritis. Pediatrics *76*:765–768, 1985.

A report of two children with sarcoidosis originally misdiagnosed as having juvenile rheumatoid arthritis.

42. Pattishal EN, Strope GL, Spinola SM, et al.: Childhood sarcoidosis. J. Pediatr. *108*:169–177, 1986.

A retrospective review of 60 patients, 2 to 21 years of age, with sarcoidosis.

43. Rotenstein D, Gibbas DL, Majmudar B, et al.: Familial granulomatous arteritis with polyarthritis of juvenile onset. N. Engl. J. Med. *306*:86–90, 1982.

A review of an entity consisting of familial forms of granulomatous arteritis and juvenile polyarthritis.

44. Blau EB: Familial granulomatous arthritis, iritis and rash. J. Pediatr. *107*:689–693, 1985.

A report of a 6½-year-old girl with an autosomal dominant disorder that affected 10 family members in three generations.

45. Olumide YM, Bandele EO, Elesha SO, et al.: Cutaneous sarcoidosis in Nigeria. J. Am. Acad. Dermatol. *21*:1222–1224, 1989.

In a review of 43 patients with sarcoidosis in which 30 per cent had cutaneous lesions, sarcoidal infiltration of scarification marks was the most common cutaneous feature.

46. Alabi GO, George AO: Cutaneous sarcoidosis and tribal scarifications in West Africa. Int. J. Dermatol. *28*:29–31, 1989.

In a report of seven patients with cutaneous lesions of sarcoidosis, the most common presentation consisted of sarcoidal lesions on tribal scarification marks.

47. Jorizzo JL, Koufman JA, Thompson JN, et al.: Sarcoidosis of the upper respiratory tract in patients with nasal rim lesions: a pilot study. J. Am. Acad. Dermatol. *22*:439–444, 1990.

Three of four patients with nasal rim lesions of sarcoidosis in whom laryngoscopy revealed sarcoidosis of the respiratory tract suggests that patients with this variant of sarcoidosis should be referred for otolaryngological examination, regardless of the presence or absence of symptoms.

48. Lever WF, Schaumburg-Lever G: Histopathology of the Skin, 7th ed. W.B. Saunders Co., Philadelphia, 1990.

An authoritative review of the histopathology of cutaneous lesions.

49. Rodriguez G, Shin BC, Abernathy RS: Serum angiotension-converting enzyme activity in normal children and in those with sarcoidosis. J. Pediatr. *99*:69–72, 1981.

A review of serum angiotensin-converting enzyme activity and its significance in children with sarcoidosis.

50. Lufkin EG, DeRemee RA, Rohrbach MS: The predictive value of serum angiotensin-converting enzyme activity in the differential diagnosis of hypercalcemia. Mayo Clin. Proc. *58*:447–451, 1983.

In a review of serum angiotensin-converting enzyme measurements in a large number of patients with various granulomatous, metabolic, and hypercalcemic disorders the authors suggest that activity of the enzyme, although not a specific test for the differential diagnosis of various forms of hypercalcemia, can be used as a chemical marker of successful treatment of patients with sarcoidosis.

51. Kendig EL Jr: Sarcoidosis. In Gellis SS, Kagan BM (Eds.): Current Pediatric Therapy 13. W.B. Saunders Co., Philadelphia, 1990, 687–688.

An authoritative review of the management of sarcoidosis in childhood.

52. Bäfverstedt B: Lymphadenosis benigna cutis (LABC): Its nature, course and progress. Acta Derm. Venereol. *40*:10–18, 1960.

Clinical and histopathologic studies of lymphadenosis benigna cutis (lymphocytoma cutis).

53. Paschoud JM: Die Lumphadenosis benigna cutis als übertragbare Infektions-krankheit. Hautarzt *8*:197, 1957; *9*:153, 263, and 311, 1958.

Demonstration that lymphadenosis benigna cutis (lymphocytoma cutis) can be transferred from person to person and by serial passage suggests an infective etiology, at least in some patients with this disorder.

54. Bäfverstedt B: Lymphadenosis benigna cutis. Acta Derm. Venereol. *48*:1–6, 1968.

Differentiation of two distinct forms of lymphadenosis benigna cutis (lymphocytoma cutis).

54a. Kuflik AS, Schwartz RA: Lymphocytoma cutis: A series of five patients successfully treated with cryosurgery. J. Am. Acad. Dermatol. 26:449–452, 1992.

A report of five patients with lymphocytoma cutis, all of whom responded to treatment with 15 to 20 second liquid nitrogen open spray cryosurgery; four of the five patients cleared with one treatment (one required a second).

55. Wheeland RG, Kantor GR, Bailin PL, et al.: Role of the argon laser in treatment of lymphocytoma cutis. J. Am. Acad. Dermatol. 14:267–272, 1986.

Although the argon laser can be used as a means of improving the cosmetic appearance and alleviating symptoms of lymphocytoma cutis, it fails to provide complete histologic clearing of the disorder.

56. Stawiski MA: Skin manifestations of leukemias and lymphomas. Cutis 21:814–818, 1978.

A review of cutaneous manifestations and their value in the diagnosis of leukemias and lymphomas.

57. Peterson AO Jr, Jarratt M: Pruritus and nonspecific nodules preceding myelomonocytic leukemia. J. Am. Acad. Dermatol. 2:496–498, 1980.

A report of a patient with myelomonocytic leukemia in whom generalized persistent pruritus and the intermittent appearance of nonspecific necrotic nodules preceded other manifestations of leukemia by 4 years.

58. Baden TJ, Gammon WR: Leukemia cutis in acute myelomyonocytic leukemia: Preferential localization in a recent Hickman catheter scar. Arch. Dermatol. 123:88–90, 1987.

A report of a patient with acute myelomyonocytic leukemia in whom cutaneous leukemic infiltration demonstrated a predilection for a scar at the site of a catheter placement suggests that careful cutaneous examination of recent scars may provide an early clue of leukemic relapse.

59. Heskel NS, White CR, Fryberger S, et al.: Aleukemic leukemia cutis: Juvenile chronic granulocytic leukemia presenting with figurate cutaneous lesions. J. Am. Acad. Dermatol. 9:423–427, 1983.

A report of a 3½-year-old girl who had a figurate cutaneous eruption that led to the diagnosis of leukemia.

60. Gottesfeld E, Silverman RA, Coccia PF, et al.: Transient blueberry muffin appearance of a newborn with congenital myeloblastic leukemia. J. Am. Acad. Dermatol. 21:347–351, 1989.

A report of an infant with congenital leukemia and blueberry muffin-like lesions.

61. Su WPD, Buechner SA, Li C-Y: Clinicopathologic correlations in leukemia cutis. J. Am. Acad. Dermatol. 11:121–128, 1984.

A comprehensive review of the clinical and histopathologic features of leukemia cutis.

62. Gilman AL, Cohen BA, Urbach AH, et al.: Pyoderma gangrenosum as a manifestation of leukemia in childhood. Pediatrics 81:846–848, 1988.

A report of two children in whom pyoderma gangrenosum was the initial manifestation of their leukemic disorder.

63. Lucky AW, McGuire J, Komp DM: Infantile neuroblastoma presenting with cutaneous blanching nodules. J. Am. Acad. Dermatol. 6:389–391, 1982.

A report of an 8-week-old girl in whom blanching cutaneous metastatic nodules led to the diagnosis of neuroblastoma.

64. Nguyen TQ, Fisher GB Jr, Tabbarah SO, et al.: Stage IV-S metastatic neuroblastoma presenting as skin nodules at birth. J. Int. Dermatol. 27:712–713, 1988.

An infant with congenital neuroblastomas was noted to have bluish gray cutaneous lesions and an abdominal mass at birth.

65. Silverman CL, Strayer DS, Wasserman TH: Cutaneous Hodgkin's disease. Arch. Dermatol. 118:918–928, 1982.

A report of a patient with Hodgkin's disease initially seen for a cutaneous lesion on a buttock.

66. White RM, Patterson JW: Cutaneous involvement in Hodgkin's disease. Cancer 55:1136–1145, 1985.

A review of 16 patients with histologically specific cutaneous involvement by Hodgkin's disease.

67. Simon S, Azevedo SJ, Byrnes JJ: Erythema nodosum heralding recurrent Hodgkin's disease. Cancer 56:1470–1472, 1985.

A report of two young men in whom recurrence of Hodgkin's disease was heralded by the appearance of cutaneous lesions of erythema nodosum.

68. Gibson LE, Muller SA, Peters MS: Follicular mucinosis of childhood and adolescence. Pediatr. Dermatol. 5:231–235, 1988.

Although most reports suggest that follicular mucinosis in childhood is a benign self-limiting process, this study of 59 patients with persistence of their cutaneous lesions demonstrated that follicular mucinosis, even in childhood, may be persistent and associated with lymphoma.

69. Shelnitz LS, Paller AS: Hodgkin's disease manifesting as prurigo nodularis. Pediatr. Dermatol. 7:136–139, 1990.

A report of a 13-year-old girl with prurigo nodularis as the presenting sign of stage IIA Hodgkin's disease.

70. Garcia RG, Garcia SG, Vilela DS, et al.: Scleromyxedema associated with non-Hodgkin lymphoma. Int. J. Dermatol. 28:670–671, 1989.

This, the second reported case of scleromyxedema in a patient with non-Hodgkin lymphoma, suggests the possibility of a more than casual relationship between the two disorders.

71. Koch SE, Zackheim HS, Williams ML, et al.: Mycosis fungoides beginning in childhood and adolescence. J. Am. Acad. Dermatol. 17:563–570, 1987.

A report of 12 patients with mycosis fungoides (including one patient who had histologic documentation of the disorder at 5 years of age) whose lesions began before the age of 20 years.

72. Peters MS, Thibodeau SN, White JW Jr, et al.: Mycosis fungoides in children and adolescents. J. Am. Acad. Dermatol. 22:1011–1018, 1990.

A review of mycosis fungoides in five children who developed the disorder prior to the age of 20 years suggests that physicians often hesitate to perform or delay skin biopsies in children. Thus, the incidence of mycosis fungoides in patients younger than 20 years of age may be higher than reported.

73. D'Incan M, Souteyrand P, Bignon YJ, et al: Hydantoin-induced cutaneous pseudolymphoma with clinical, pathologic, and immunologic aspects of Sézary syndrome. Arch. Dermatol. 128:1371–1374, 1992.

What is believed to be the first case report of a patient with a Sézary-like syndrome associated with phenytoin therapy.

74. Barnhill RL, Braverman IM: Progression of pigmented purpura-like eruptions to mycosis fungoides. J. Am. Acad. Dermatol. 19:25–31, 1988.

A report of three males with pigmented purpuric eruptions, with onset ranging from the ages of 14 to 30 years, in whom the dermatosis eventually progressed into mycosis fungoides.

75. Olsen EA, Rosen ST, Vollmer RT, et al.: Interferon alfa-2a in the treatment of cutaneous T cell lymphoma. J. Am. Acad. Dermatol. 20:395–407, 1989.

Findings in fourteen (64 per cent) of 22 patients with stages Ia to IVa cutaneous T cell lymphoma suggest that recombinant human leukocyte interferon alfa-2a is an effective and well-tolerated single-agent therapy for early and advanced cutaneous T cell lymphoma.

76. Edelson R, Berger C, Gasparro F, et al.: Treatment of cutaneous T-cell lymphoma by extracorporeal photochemotherapy: Preliminary results. N. Engl. J. Med. *316*:297–303, 1987.

In a study of 41 patients with cutaneous T-cell lymphoma, extracorporeal photochemotherapy (orally administered methoxsalen followed by extracorporeal ultraviolet A exposure) appeared to offer a safe, effective approach for treatment of many patients with widespread cutaneous T-cell lymphoma.

UNCLASSIFIED DISORDERS

MASTOCYTOSIS

Mastocytosis is a term used to describe a group of clinical disorders characterized by the accumulation of mast cells in the skin and at times, generally in adults, other organs of the body. It may appear at any time from birth to middle age; approximately three fourths of all cases develop during infancy or early childhood (generally before the age of 2), and most of the remaining 25 per cent begin at or after puberty (usually between the ages of 15 and 40).[1, 2] The etiology is unknown. Although reports of mastocytosis in twins, siblings, and families suggest an inherited basis for this disorder, the overwhelming majority of patients have no familial association.[3–6]

The clinical spectrum of mastocytosis includes (1) single or multiple small cutaneous nodules (solitary mastocytoma) (Fig. 25–1); (2) multiple hyperpigmented macules or papules (urticaria pigmentosa) (Figs. 25–2 through 25–4); (3) a diffuse form in which virtually all of the skin is infiltrated with mast cells (diffuse cutaneous mastocytosis) (Fig. 25–5); (4) unusual telangiectases of the trunk and extremities usually seen in adults and rarely in children (telangiectasia macularis eruptiva perstans); (5) systemic mastocytosis, a condition in which mast cell proliferation occurs in various or-gan systems (the skin, liver, spleen, lymph nodes, lungs, bones, and gastrointestinal tract); and (6) a rare malignant form of mast cell leukemia seen primarily in adults and rarely in children (Table 25–1).

The classification of the forms of mastocytosis, often confusing because of their varied manifestations, can be simplified by separation into childhood and adult varieties. In children the disorder appears in three forms: (1) individual lesions (solitary mastocytosis); (2) a generalized form termed *urticaria pigmentosa;* and (3) a relatively rare variant (diffuse cutaneous mastocytosis). All three of these childhood forms may display vesicular or bullous variants. Seen primarily in children younger than 2 years of age, they may be termed *bullous mastocytoma* (Fig. 25–6), bullous urticaria pigmentosa (Fig. 25–4 and 25–7), or bullous mastocytosis (Figs. 25–5 and 25–8). Although the cause of vesiculation in this age group remains unknown, it presumably is related to histamine- or other chemical mediator-induced transudate in a group susceptible to vesicle formation by insecure attachments of the epidermis to the underlying dermis.[7]

Clinical Manifestations. The prognosis and course of mastocytosis depends on the clinical presentation and its age at onset. In general, chil-

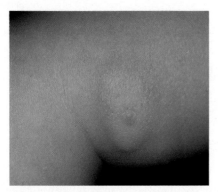

Figure 25–1. Solitary mastocytoma. A 1.5- to 2-cm flesh-colored to reddish brown nodular aggregation of mast cells is evident on the upper arm of a young infant. Stroking or gentle rubbing of such lesions causes localized erythema and urticarial wheals (Darier's sign) due to mast cell liberation of histamine and perhaps other chemical mediators.

dren who develop the disorder before the age of 10 years have a better prognosis than adults (in childhood it is almost always a purely cutaneous disease that resolves spontaneously). In adults, however, the skin lesions seldom disappear, and 30 to 55 per cent of patients have evidence of systemic involvement (Fig. 25–9).[1, 2]

The diagnosis of cutaneous mastocytosis is aided by a phenomenon known as Darier's sign. This finding, a hallmark of the disorder, is seen in 90 per cent of patients with cutaneous mastocytosis and consists of localized erythema and urticarial wheals that develop after gentle mechanical irritation, such as might be induced by a tongue blade or

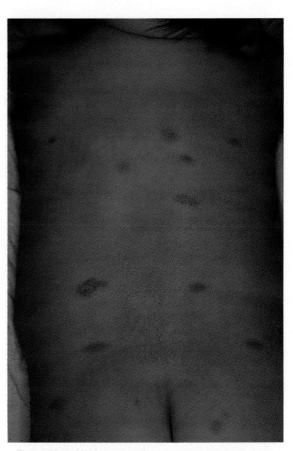

Figure 25–3. Multiple, reddish brown, hyperpigmented macules and papules on the back of a 5-month-old infant with urticaria pigmentosa.

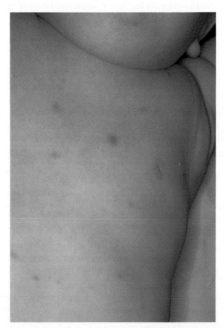

Figure 25–2. Urticaria pigmentosa. Multiple hyperpigmented macules and nodules appear on the chest and abdomen of a young infant. Note positive Darier's sign on the upper aspect of the chest.

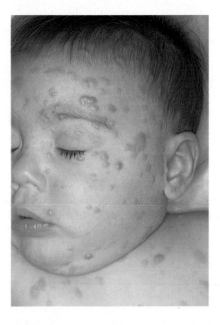

Figure 25–4. Bullous urticaria pigmentosa. Vesicles and bullae are prominent features of this form of mast cell disease.

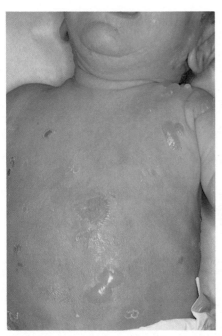

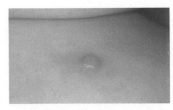

Figure 25–6. Bullous mastocytoma. A blister and Darier's sign (erythema and urtication following gentle rubbing) are seen in a solitary mastocytoma on the chest of a young infant.

Figure 25–5. Bullous mastocytosis. Diffuse cutaneous erythrodermic mastocytosis with extensive bulla formation.

the blunt end of a pen or pencil (see Figure 25–2). Erythema and urtication, apparently the result of liberation of histamine by mast cells, usually develop within a few minutes and may persist as long as 30 minutes to several hours. The degranulation of mast cells seems to be correlated with an increased production of cyclic adenosine monophosphate and prostaglandin D_2, with histamine, heparin, and prostaglandin D_2 being responsible for many of the systemic features noted in patients with this disorder.[8]

Solitary Mastocytosis. The terms *solitary mastocytosis* and *solitary mastocytoma* are used when there are one or more isolated or individual lesions, a variant estimated to occur in 10 to 15 per cent of all cases of mastocytosis. Lesions usually

Table 25–1. CLINICAL SPECTRUM OF MASTOCYTOSIS[*]

1. Solitary mastocytoma
2. Urticaria pigmentosa
3. Diffuse cutaneous mastocytosis
4. Telangiectasia macularis eruptiva perstans (usually in adults, rare in children)
5. Systemic mastocytosis
   a. Primarily seen in adults and in infants with diffuse cutaneous mastocytosis
   b. Asymptomatic systemic involvement of a limited degree may occur in urticaria pigmentosa of childhood, but it is uncommon
   c. Mast cell leukemia or lymphoma, at times (in adults)

* Childhood forms of mastocytosis include solitary mastocytoma, urticaria pigmentosa, and diffuse cutaneous mastocytosis. All three may display vesicular or bullous variations.
Modified from Hurwitz S: The Skin and Systemic Disease in Children. Year Book Medical Publishers, Chicago, 1985.

appear at birth or early in infancy, increase somewhat in size for several months, and eventually regress spontaneously, usually within a period of several years. (see Figure 25–1). In most patients with this form of mastocytosis, lesions are indeed solitary. Many children, however, may develop as many as three or four individual lesions (in one instance, a 4-month-old infant had nine solitary mastocytomas),[9] and a few patients with solitary mastocytosis have been reported to progress to a generalized form of urticaria pigmentosa.[10]

Solitary mastocytomas may occur on any part of the body but are noted most frequently on the arms (especially near the wrists), the neck, and trunk. Clinically they are seen as slightly elevated flesh-colored to light-brown or tan plaques or nodules. Occasionally they may display a yellowish or pink hue. Lesions are usually round or oval and generally measure 1 to 5 cm in diameter. They may have a thick or rubbery quality with a smooth or pebbly peau d'orange (orange peel–like) consistency. Darier's sign is positive, and stroking or rubbing of lesions may at times produce symptoms of flushing or colic.

Infant skin is more likely to respond to various noxious stimuli by forming blisters. Accordingly, bullous lesions are seen as common variants of this disorder. When present in association with solitary lesions of mastocytosis, this disorder (frequently misdiagnosed as bullous impetigo) is termed *bullous mastocytoma* (see Figure 25–6). This tendency toward vesiculation and bulla formation usually disappears within 1 to 3 years.

Solitary mastocytomas have the most favorable prognosis of all cutaneous forms of mastocytosis. Symptoms, when present, are usually mild, and spontaneous resolution within a period of several years is the rule (almost always before the age of 10). Parents should be advised that symptoms, if present, usually abate after 1 or 2 years (even before the lesions disappear) and that surgical excision, except in cases that are symptomatic and troublesome, is generally unnecessary.

Urticaria Pigmentosa. Urticaria pigmentosa, seen in about two thirds of patients with cutaneous mastocytosis, is the most common manifestation of the mastocytosis syndrome.[1] Primarily a disease of children, the disorder may be present at birth, with the majority of cases originating during the first 3 to 9 months of life. In a study of 139 patients with urticaria pigmentosa, 86 per cent had the onset of

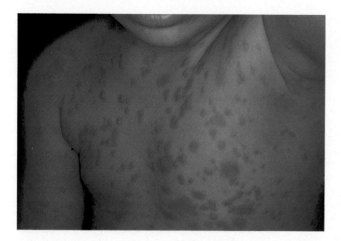

Figure 25–7. Bullous urticaria pigmentosa. Vesicles and bullae are prominent features of this form of mast cell disease.

their disorder before 15 years of age; the remaining had their onset between ages 15 and 40.[3]

Cutaneous Manifestations. The cutaneous lesions of urticaria pigmentosa generally appear as multiple, reddish brown (occasionally yellowish brown) hyperpigmented macules, papules, or nodular lesions that urticate in a characteristic manner when traumatized (Darier's sign) (see Figure 25–2). When the normal-appearing skin also urticates it usually does so to a lesser extent. Dermographism of apparently uninvolved skin occurs in one third to one half of all patients with urticaria pigmentosa. This finding, when present, appears to be due to an increase in mast cells throughout the dermis of otherwise apparently normal skin. Dermographism by itself, however, is not diagnostic of this disorder. It may also be seen in approximately 5 per cent of the general population; in up to 25 to 50 per cent of normal individuals when extraordinarily firm stroking is performed; in patients with thyroid disorders, diabetes, and phenylketonuria; during infectious bacterial disease, pregnancy, and menopause; after the ingestion of certain medications such as penicillin; following wasp or bee stings; and during arthropod infestations.[8]

Lesions of urticaria pigmentosa may occur anywhere on the body but generally tend to involve the trunk, often in a symmetrical fashion. In later stages lesions may spread to the extremities and

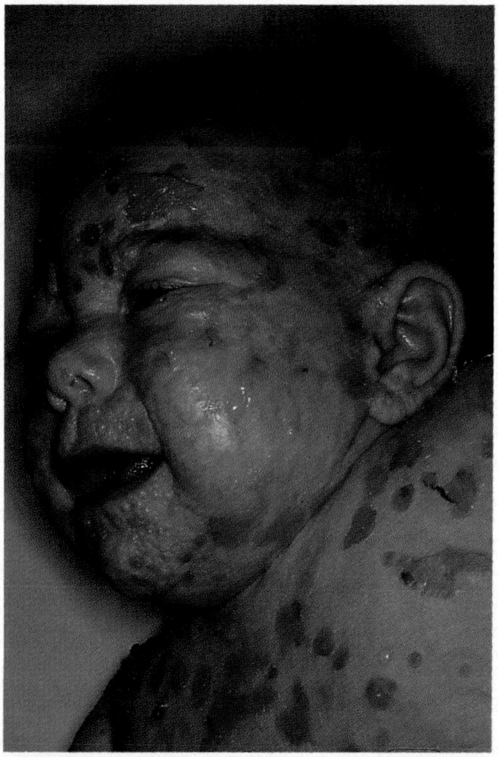

Figure 25–8. Diffuse cutaneous and erythrodermic mastocytosis in a 3-month-old infant. The skin is diffusely thickened with a boggy or doughy appearance, and extensive bullous eruptions are present. This variant is termed bullous mastocytosis; with time the boggy, doughy appearance tends to improve.

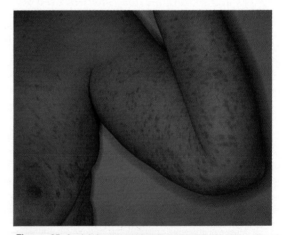

Figure 25–9. Adult-type urticaria pigmentosa. Generalized reddish brown, freckle-like lesions are characteristic of the adult form of urticaria pigmentosa. These cutaneous lesions tend to persist indefinitely, and 30 to 55 per cent of adult patients with urticaria pigmentosa have some evidence of systemic involvement.

the neck. Involvement of the scalp, face, palms, and soles, although occasionally present, is infrequent and relatively uncommon; a few cases have been reported in which lesions were present on the buccal, palatal, or pharyngeal mucosa or on the anal mucous membrane.

Individual lesions are usually round or oval, vary from 1 mm to several centimeters in diameter, and generally are larger in children than in adults. Pigmentation, particularly in older lesions, is common. The reason for increased pigmentation of lesions is unknown. Increased levels of tyrosinase due to reduction of tyrosine inhibitor by the release of mucopolysaccharides from the mast cells have been suggested as the cause of this phenomenon. This hypothesis, however, remains unsubstantiated and requires further investigation and corroboration.[1]

Vesicles or bullae occasionally occur as prominent features of urticaria pigmentosa of childhood (see Figures 25–4 and 25–7). Although the mechanism of vesiculation is unknown, this appears to be related to the release of histamine and perhaps other chemical mediators and the well-known fact that infantile skin blisters more easily than adult skin. When bullae are present in addition to pigmented skin lesions, the disease is termed *bullous urticaria pigmentosa.*[7]

Telangiectasia macularis eruptiva perstans is a variant generally seen in patients with the adult form of urticaria pigmentosa. This variant, although relatively uncommon in childhood, has been reported in children with this disorder.[1] Patients with telangiectasia macularis eruptiva perstans have an extensive eruption of small persistent brownish red hyperpigmented telangiectatic macules on the trunk and extremities with little or no tendency toward urtication. This relatively uncommon disorder is thought by some to be related to frequent dilatation of blood vessels by repeated release of histamine; and although this concept remains unsubstantiated, it has been suggested that patients with this variant may have an increased incidence of peptic ulcer.[2]

Prognosis. The prognosis and course of urticaria pigmentosa depends on the clinical presentation and age at onset. When seen in children younger than age 10, it has an excellent prognosis and is almost always a cutaneous disorder that tends toward spontaneous remission; in about one half of the cases in which the condition has its onset in infancy or early childhood the lesions disappear spontaneously by adolescence and another 25 per cent will have partial resolution of lesions by adulthood.[11] Although systemic involvement has been reported in up to 5 per cent of children with onset of urticaria pigmentosa before 10 years of age, as compared with 10 to 30 per cent of older children, in a review of childhood cases having widespread and occasionally fatal extracutaneous mast cell infiltrates (liver, spleen, lymph nodes, and bone marrow), it was found that these patients had diffuse cutaneous or erythrodermic forms of

mastocytosis rather than true urticaria pigmentosa. In adults the skin lesions seldom disappear and 30 to 55 per cent of adults with mastocytosis have evidence of systemic involvement.[12]

Although generalized flushing in urticaria pigmentosa may occur when large amounts of histamine, vasodilating prostaglandin (PGD_2) and perhaps other biologically active metabolites of arachidonic acid are liberated, the pruritus associated with this disorder is usually rather mild and intermittent. Urticaria and pruritus may be induced by inadvertent or deliberate rubbing of lesions or by exercise, hot baths, spicy foods, or the ingestion of histamine-releasing drugs.

Systemic involvement. When systemic mastocytosis occurs almost any organ or tissue of the body may be affected. The most frequently involved tissues and organs are the bones, liver, spleen, lymph nodes, and peripheral blood. Mast cell accumulations, however, have also been found in the lung, kidney, gastrointestinal tract, skeletal muscle, myocardium, pericardium, omentum, and other tissues. Hepatomegaly, present in 10 to 15 per cent of patients, and splenomegaly (usually seen in association with hepatic enlargement) seem to occur in an equal percentage of patients. Although an incidence as high as 30 per cent has been reported for bone involvement (either localized or diffuse areas of osteoporosis or osteosclerosis) in patients with systemic disease, 10 or 15 per cent appears to be a more realistic figure for this association.[1]

Since systemic involvment occurs in 10 to 30 per cent of children with urticaria pigmentosa whose skin lesions appear after the age of 10 years and in 30 to 55 per cent of adults with mastocytosis, all patients with late-onset or adult forms of mastocytosis should be evaluated for this possibility.[13] Although the measurement of urinary histamine excretion may be of indirect help in the diagnosis of systemic mastocytosis, increased serum histamine levels have been detected in individuals without histaminuria. Patients with chronic myelocytic leukemia, polycythemia vera, drug reactions, urticaria, and severe insect bite reactions may also have increased urinary excretion of histamine metabolites. Thus, although urinary histamine evaluation may sometimes be helpful, further experience and correlation with the clinical and histologic picture are required to substantiate the validity of this laboratory study for the diagnosis of systemic disease.[14] Symptoms of the mastocytosis syndrome may include intense pruritus, urticaria, headache, flushing, tachycardia, gastrointestinal symptoms, nonspecific abnormalities of blood clotting, hypotension, and syncope. Patients with bone involvement may have bone pain. Hemorrhagic diatheses, although rare, may be related to hepatosplenic involvement, heparin liberation, or the infrequent association of mastocytosis with mast cell leukemia or lymphoma.

The development of leukemia or a related malignant condition affecting tissues of the reticuloendothelial system is the main hazard in adult patients with mastocytosis. The presence of mast cells in the peripheral blood of patients with mastocytosis accordingly is a grave prognostic sign. A 5-year-old child with urticaria pigmentosa and acute lymphoblastic leukemia was reported on by Fromer and associates in 1973. Although perhaps coincidental, this report raises the question as to whether this association may have been more than a chance occurrence.[15]

Diffuse Cutaneous and Erythrodermic Mastocytosis. Diffuse cutaneous mastocytosis is a relatively rare form of childhood mastocytosis that bears little clinical resemblance to urticaria pigmentosa. In this disorder large areas of the dermis are infiltrated with mast cells, and the skin develops a thickened boggy, doughy, and at times lichenified appearance. The cutaneous surface may be smooth, or it may contain numerous minute papules that give it a Scotch-grained leather-like appearance, frequently with a yellow carotenemia-like tint or a diffusely reddened appearance (diffuse erythrodermic mastocytosis) (see Figure 25–5). In some cases diffuse cutaneous mastocytosis may be accompanied by multiple cutaneous lesions and extensive bullous eruptions. In this variant, termed *bullous mastocytosis* (see Figure 25–8), the prognosis seems to be related to the age at onset of bullous lesions. When bullae develop early in the neonatal period, the prognosis is more guarded and systemic involvement frequently occurs. With delayed onset of blisters, however, extracutaneous manifestations appear to bear less significance and the prognosis is more favorable.[7]

The diffuse cutaneous forms of mastocytosis may present symptoms of intense generalized pruritus, flushing, temperature elevation, vomiting, diarrhea, abdominal pain, gastrointestinal ulceration, and acute respiratory distress, with wheezing, cyanosis, apnea, and, at times, severe shock-like states. In a review of eight infants with this variant, two died; five of the remaining six had mast cell infiltration of the reticuloendothelial system; and one had gastrointestinal involvement, an increased number of mast cells in the bone marrow, and mast cells in the peripheral blood. Although this disorder has a less favorable prognosis, the blistering and boggy Scotch-grained appearance of the skin generally tend to improve with time.[16]

Diagnosis. Although cutaneous mastocytosis without clinically obvious skin lesions has been described,[17] typical cases generally present little diagnostic problem to physicians familiar with this disorder. Urtication following the mechanical irritation of lesions (Darier's sign) is highly diagnostic and will frequently help to confirm the true nature of the disease. Atypical and more unusual forms of cutaneous mastocytosis, however, are more difficult to diagnose and require a high index of suspicion on the part of the clinician.

When the diagnosis is indeterminate, cutaneous biopsy can help confirm the true nature of the disorder. Since loss of granules may occur owing to handling of lesions during biopsy, the injection of local anesthetic too close to lesions or biopsy of a lesion that had previously been urticated tends to make histopathologic identification of mast cells difficult. Specimens accordingly should be handled gently and removed whenever possible without previous urtication, and avoidance of local anesthetic infiltration directly into the area of the biopsy site may be necessary to establish the proper histopathologic diagnosis.

All forms of mastocytosis are characterized by abnormal accumulation of mast cells. In the macular and papular types of lesions, there generally is a sparse mast cell infiltrate in the upper dermis, usually with a perivascular and periappendageal distribution. A relative scarcity of mast cells in some sections may make histologic confirmation difficult, and at times the true nature of the disorder may be established only after repeated biopsies have been performed.

Cutaneous biopsy specimens of juvenile forms of urticaria pigmentosa are characterized by dense aggregates of mast cells in the subpapillary layers and midcutis. The cells may have a peculiar arrangement, being packed into tumor-like clumps or arranged in strands or columns of varying width. The dense packing of mast cells may cause them to appear cuboidal, polyhedric, or flattened, thus resembling fibroblasts with spindle-shaped nuclei. Nodular lesions and isolated mastocytomas tend to have massive mast cell infiltrates throughout the entire corium, and the skin of patients with diffuse cutaneous mastocytosis has a band-like infiltrate of mast cells close to the epidermis. Mast cells are characterized by the presence of metachromatic granules in their cytoplasm. Although these granules frequently are not visible on routine stains, they generally can be visualized after staining with Giemsa, azure A, methylene-blue or toluidine-blue stains (Fig. 25–10); the histopathologic finding of 12 to 15 mast cells per blood vessel or 10 or more mast cells per high-power field can help confirm the diagnosis.[18] Brownstein and Rabinowitz have further suggested that 6 or more mast cells per high-power field should make one suspicious; and in a patient with clinical features, 3 to 4 mast cells per high-power field can help confirm the diagnosis.[19]

Treatment. There is no satisfactory treatment for mastocytosis. Children with diffuse cutaneous mastocytosis and those with onset after the age of 5 to 10 years should be closely observed and screened for possible involvement of other organs. Proper screening in such cases includes frequent examination of blood smears, thrombocyte, bleeding, and coagulation time studies, and, if indicated by history, gastrointestinal survey and bone scans. Patients with all forms of this disorder should try to avoid potential mast cell degranulators such as aspirin, codeine, opiates, procaine, spicy foods, cheese, excessive ingestion of alcohol, and polymyxin B, and should be aware that radiographic dyes, medications used in surgical patients (e.g., scopolamine, *d*-tubocurarine, gallamine, decamethonium, and pancuronium [Pavulon]), hot

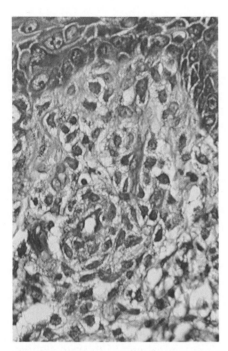

Figure 25–10. Mastocytosis. Cuboidal, polyhedric, or flattened mast cells are characterized by metachromatic granules in their cytoplasm (frequently not visible on routine stains, the metachromatic granules generally can be visualized after special staining).

baths, and vigorous rubbing after showering or bathing should be avoided in patients with mastocytosis.[20] Hydroxyzine (Atarax or Vistaril), 2 to 3 mg/kg/day in divided doses, and various antihistamines are helpful for the relief of pruritus and may modify flushing or other symptoms associated with the mastocytosis syndrome. Cyproheptadine (Periactin) has the advantage of both antihistamine and antiserotonin activity and for some patients it is the drug of choice for the management of symptoms associated with this disorder. Since H_1 and H_2 receptors are present on many cells, concomitant use of an H_1 and H_2 antagonist such as cimetidine (Tagamet) or ranitidine (Zantac) may also be considered.[18, 21, 22] Since clinical experience in children is limited, however, cimetidine and ranitidine are generally not recommended for children unless anticipated benefits outweigh their theoretical or potential risks.

Oral cromolyn sodium (disodium cromoglycate), available as Gastrocrom, in dosages of 20 to 40 mg/kg/day in four divided doses for infants and children up to the age of 2 years, 100 mg four times a day for children 2 to 12 years of age, and 800 mg a day for adults, has been helpful in the management of patients with gastrointestinal involvement, urticaria, and blistering associated with bullous and diffuse cutaneous forms of mastocytosis and in adults with systemic involvement. The full benefit of this medication, however, should not be anticipated for up to 2 to 3 weeks after the initiation of therapy.[23, 24]

Because mast cell degranulation is a calcium-dependent process, oral calcium-channel blockers such as nifedipine and ketotifen have been used for this purpose.[25, 26] In addition, although potent topical and intralesional corticosteroids can help clear cosmetically objectionable or symptomatic lesions,[27, 28] this approach is not recommended for general use. Alfa-2b interferon, oral psoralen, and long-wave ultraviolet light (PUVA) therapy have also been used, even in infancy, for some individuals with mastocytosis. Unfortunately, however, since relapses may at times occur after PUVA treatment is discontinued and at least one patient was reported to have a severe anaphylactic reaction after a single injection of interferon, these approaches are generally not recommended at this time for children with cutaneous mastocytosis.[29–30]

MORPHEA

Morphea (also termed *localized* or *circumscribed scleroderma*) is a disorder of unknown etiology manifested by localized atrophy, hardening (sclerosis), and depigmentation of the skin. Seen primarily in children and young adults, with a 3:1 female-to-male ratio, the average age at onset is about 5 years. The condition is characterized by discrete circumscribed nontender sclerotic patches with an ivory-colored center and a surrounding violaceous halo. The relationship between morphea and systemic scleroderma (progressive systemic sclerosis) is controversial and not well understood. If a transition from morphea to scleroderma does occur, it is, in all probability, extremely rare.

Although the etiology of morphea is unknown and remains speculative, it is suggested that the disorder may represent a cutaneous injury pattern or immunologic event stimulating collagen production, induration, or hardening. An infectious agent, such as *Borrelia*, the etiologic agent of erythema migrans and Lyme disease, has been suggested (at least in some patients in western Europe); and the occasional coexistence of lesions of morphea and lichen sclerosus et atrophicus suggests that these two disorders may be the result of similar etiologic events or closely related pathologic processes.[31–33]

Clinical Manifestations. The onset of morphea is insidious and begins with flesh-colored, erythematous, or purplish plaques that evolve into firm, waxy, ivory to yellow-white shiny lesions, with or without a surrounding lilac or violaceous inflammatory zone (Figs. 25–11 and 25–12). Affected areas, in order of decreasing frequency, are the thorax, trunk, neck, extremities, and face.

The disorder can be divided into four basic patterns, which may be termed *guttate, plaque, generalized,* and *linear.* Guttate morphea is a relatively uncommon variant. In the guttate form lesions are chalk white and oval, measure only a few millimeters in diameter, and are distributed on the anterior chest, shoulders, neck, and other areas

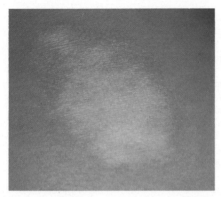

Figure 25–11. Morphea. A circumscribed ivory to yellow-white atrophic plaque is surrounded by a violaceous or lilac-colored inflammatory border.

of the body. Considerable confusion frequently exists between guttate morphea and lichen sclerosus et atrophicus, and patients have been seen in which typical lesions of both disorders occur.

Plaque-like lesions occur as indurated areas of skin, which at first are purplish. After a period of weeks to months they lose their color, especially in the central part of the lesions, and appear as scle-

rotic ivory-colored waxy areas with a lilac or violaceous edge. In this form, lesions vary from a few centimeters to several inches in diameter and, at times, fusion of many plaque-like lesions may result in a more generalized form of morphea.

Linear lesions of morphea occur primarily in children. Generally affecting the limbs (occasionally the head or trunk), their clinical appearance is similar to that of plaque-like forms but the violaceous peripheral ring is inconspicuous or only present at the advancing border. Lesions present as linear band-like areas of induration with hyperpigmentation, hypopigmentation, and atrophy of the skin, underlying subcutaneous tissue, muscles, fascia, and even bones. When there is deep involvement and fixation to underlying structures, this disorder has been termed *disabling pansclerotic morphea* (Fig. 25–13). This variant, usually affecting girls from 1 to 14 years, tends to have a relentless disabling course and may produce marked disability in the form of flexion contractures and musculoskeletal atrophy of the extremities.[34] Although the finding of antinuclear antibodies, DNA, and rheumatoid factor in some patients with linear scleroderma and reports of linear scleroderma in patients with systemic lupus erythematosus help support the role of immunologic mechanisms in the pathogenesis and a possible relationship between cutaneous morphea and sys-

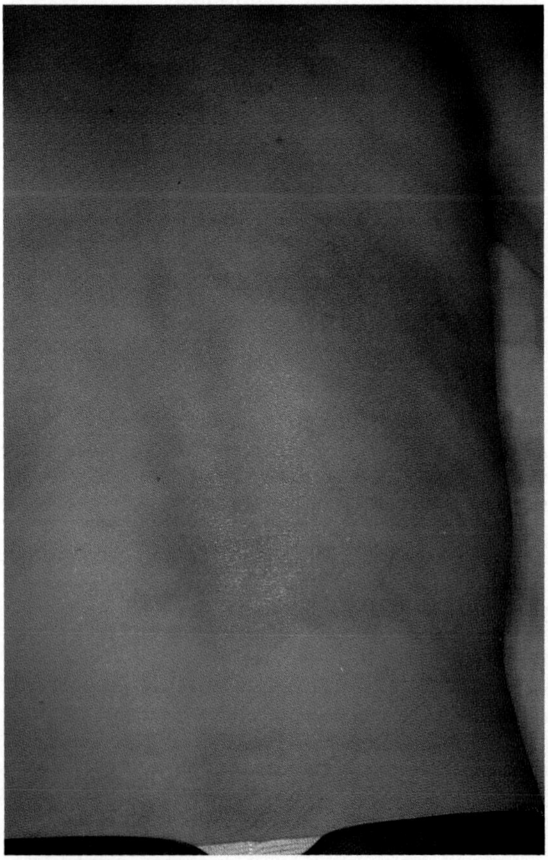

Figure 25–12. Plaque-like morphea. A hyperpigmented indurated sclerotic plaque on the lumbar area of a child with morphea.

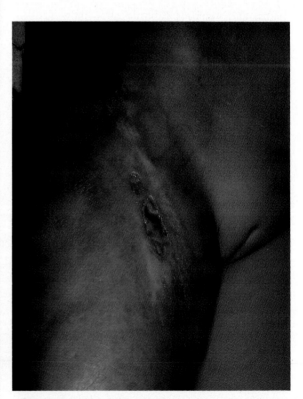

Figure 25–13. Pansclerotic morphea on the hip and thigh of a 7-year-old girl who in addition to her cutaneous lesions had flexion contractures and disability.

temic sclerosis, their significance to date remains unclear.[35–37]

Coup de sabre is a form that appears specifically on the face and frontoparietal scalp. In this variant a linear depressed groove, often with an associated zone of alopecia, resembles a saber wound or cut on the frontoparietal scalp. The groove may extend downward into the cheek, nose, and upper lip, and, at times, may involve the mouth, gum, chin, or neck (Fig. 25–14). The coupe de sabre variety probably represents a mild form of progressive facial hemiatrophy (the Parry-Romberg syndrome), a condition of slowly progressive atrophy of the soft tissue of the corresponding half of the face, accompanied at times by contralateral jacksonian epilepsy, trigeminal neuralgia, alopecia, enophthalmos, or atrophy of the ipsilateral half of the upper lip, gum, and tongue.

Occasionally, roughening of one surface of the long bones underlying a linear area of morphea may be noted. This disorder, termed *melorheostosis,* is characterized radiographically by a picture suggesting that of wax flowing down the side of a candle.[38]

Localized morphea may at times resemble vitiligo, other forms of macular atrophy, or lesions of lichen sclerosus et atrophicus. The histopathologic features of morphea consist of increased thickening and condensation of the connective tissue, with edema, homogenization, fibrosis, and sclerosis of collagen. Blood vessels are reduced in size

and are surrounded by round cell infiltration. As the disorder progresses, hair and glandular structures become atrophic, and the dermis is converted into a dense mass of connective tissue containing many dilated lymphatic spaces and but few blood vessels.

In cases of linear scleroderma there may be sclerosis of fat and fascia, calcinosis may be present, and the underlying muscle may show an interstitial myositis. Although the histologic picture of morphea frequently may resemble that of systemic scleroderma, lesions of systemic scleroderma show more pronounced degenerative changes in the collagen bundles and vessel walls in the later stages, the epidermis may show epidermal atrophy with a disappearance of rete ridges in areas of involvement, and the marked inflammatory changes seen in the active border of plaques of morphea do not occur in active lesions of systemic scleroderma.

Treatment. Although the treatment of morphea remains unsatisfactory, spontaneous recovery, particularly in children, is common. Guttate and plaque-like lesions of morphea generally tend to improve within 3 to 5 years. Residual hypopigmentation, hyperpigmentation, and occasionally atrophy, however, may persist for long periods of time. Lesions of linear morphea tend to last longer, but they, too, have a tendency to improve over a period of years. Linear lesions of the coup de sabre variant and facial hemiatrophy, conversely, generally tend to persist. Occasionally, calcinosis requiring surgical removal may develop in linear lesions, contractures may limit movement of joints, and sometimes clawing of the hand may be a sequela of this variant of localized scleroderma.

Topical or intralesional corticosteroid therapy has been reported to hasten resolution of lesions, but this form of therapy is generally unrewarding, can result in localized atrophy, and is not recommended. Physiotherapy, massage, warm baths, and exercise, however, are frequently helpful for patients with linear morphea in whom strictures may result. In addition, corticosteroids, antimalarials, phenytoin, methotrexate, penicillamine, salazopyrine, cyclosporine, and colchicine have been recommended for treatment of patients with this disorder.[39–41] Considering the variable course of morphea and the side effects associated with penicillamine (bone marrow depression, allergic reactions, nephrotic syndrome, dermatomyositis, a lupus erythematosus–like illness, Sjögren's syndrome, thyroiditis, pemphigus, anetoderma, myasthenia gravis, chronic bronchoalveolitis, and Goodpasture-like syndrome), its use should be limited to the most severe and disfiguring forms of the disorder.[42, 43]

LICHEN SCLEROSUS ET ATROPHICUS

Lichen sclerosus et atrophicus (LSA) is a distinctive benign cutaneous disorder of unknown etiology. Seen in children as well as adults, the disorder

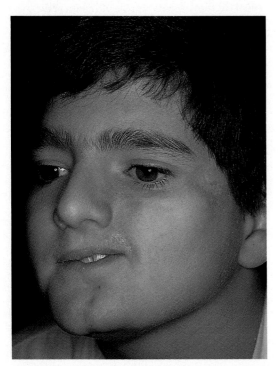

Figure 25–14. Coup de sabre. A localized groove-like form of scleroderma (resembling a sabre cut) is present on the face of a 12-year-old boy.

may occur at any age, in any race, and in both sexes. The youngest case reported was that of an infant only a few weeks of age; 85 to 90 per cent of cases appear in females; 10 to 15 per cent of affected individuals have the onset of their disorder before the age of 13; and the majority of cases in childhood (70 per cent) had the onset of the disorder prior to 7 years of age.[44, 45]

Clinical Manifestations. The eruption of lichen sclerosus et atrophicus is characterized by sharply defined, small, pink to ivory white, slightly raised, flat-topped papules a few millimeters in diameter that aggregate and coalesce into plaques of various sizes. As the condition progresses, atrophy and delling (fine follicular plugs on the surface of macules) may become highly diagnostic features of the disorder. The anogenital region is involved in the majority of cases (75 per cent of affected children have anogenital involvement). Of those who have involvement elsewhere on the body, up to 42 per cent are reputed to have an associated anogenital involvement.[44] Extragenital lesions are asymptomatic and may begin asymmetrically but eventually generally become distributed in a symmetrical manner over the clavicles, on the chest and back, around the umbilicus, and on the flexor surfaces of the extremities, neck, and axillae (Fig. 25–15).

The Koebner phenomenon has been documented in cases of lichen sclerosus et atrophicus in childhood; lesions may develop in surgical scars or sites of vaccination, and exacerbations of quiescent lesions may occur following local trauma or irritation.[44] As previously stated in the discussion of localized or circumscribed scleroderma, lesions of lichen sclerosus et atrophicus occasionally occur in association with morphea, and it has been suggested that guttate morphea actually may represent a variant of lichen sclerosus et atrophicus.

In females the anogenital lesions frequently tend to surround both the vulva and perianal regions in an hour-glass or figure-eight pattern (Fig. 25–16). When seen on the dorsum of the glans penis in males, the disorder has been termed *ba-*

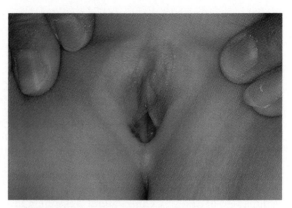

Figure 25–16. Hypopigmentation, hemorrhagic erosions, and ulcerations of the genital region of a 6-year-old girl with lichen sclerosus et atrophicus (familiarity with this disorder will help avoid a misdiagnosis of sexual abuse).

lanitis xerotica obliterans. A vaginal discharge may precede the vulval lesions in about 20 per cent of affected girls, and pruritus vulvae appears in about 50 per cent of girls affected with this disorder. Anogenital lesions may at times extend to include the skin on the inner aspect of the thighs; in many girls the white coloring may be replaced by reddening and blistering, and tiny hemorrhages and excoriations may be present, especially on the labia minora and clitoris.

Except for anogenital lesions in which the cutaneous features may be complicated by excoriation, maceration, infection, or contact dermatitis due to topical therapy, the diagnosis of lichen sclerosus et atrophicus is usually not difficult. Differential diagnosis should include the possibility of vitiligo, morphea, lichen planus, and, when anogenital lesions are present, the possibility of child abuse or a dermatitis such as might be seen in association with pinworm infestation, candidiasis, or bacterial vulvovaginitis.

The microscopic features of lichen sclerosus et atrophicus consist of marked hyperkeratosis with plugging of the hair follicles, thinning of the stratum malpighii (sometimes with loss of rete ridges), hydropic degeneration of the basal layer, marked edema with homogenization of the collagen in the upper dermis, and a band-like, predominantly lymphocytic infiltrate in the mid-dermis.

Prognosis. The prognosis of lichen sclerosus et atrophicus with onset in childhood is somewhat better than that of adult forms of this disorder. Involution in adults is uncommon and is usually accompanied by residual atrophy, and there is a distinct relationship between adult lichen sclerosus et atrophicus, leukoplakia, and squamous cell carcinoma. The possibility of malignancy as a sequela of lichen sclerosus et atrophicus in childhood, however, is extremely rare.

In half of the childhood cases, most lesions clear within 1 to 10 years (with an average of 5 years), and approximately two thirds of cases improve or undergo involution before or at about the time of

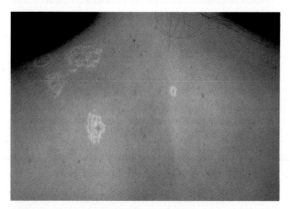

Figure 25–15. Multiple, white, atrophic lesions of lichen sclerosus et atrophicus on the upper back.

puberty, without atrophy.[44, 45] In the remaining one third, the condition tends to persist; and, in females, atrophy of the clitoris and labia minora, with fusion of the latter, and stricture of the introitus may occur.[45] In patients in whom improvement has taken place, however, the disorder may be reactivated years later by trauma, pregnancy, or the administration of anovulatory drugs.[46, 47]

Treatment. The course of lichen sclerosus et atrophicus is generally not influenced by topical therapy. Topical corticosteroids (hydrocortisone), emollient creams, and topical antipruritic agents such as those containing pramoxine (Prax) or pramoxine and hydrocortisone (Pramasone) offer symptomatic relief to the vulva and perianal lesions. If secondary infection is present, topical anticandidal or antibacterial agents may be added. Although 2 per cent testosterone propionate in soft paraffin or petrolatum has been shown to be beneficial, side effects such as clitoral hypertrophy, hypertrichosis, or increased libido suggest caution in its use, particularly in children.[47] As an alternative, a 1 per cent topical formulation of progesterone (100 mg/30 g in Aquaphor or petrolatum) may be considered; and, although further studies are required, p-aminobenzoate (Potaba) and topical cyclosporine have also been suggested as adjuncts for the management of patients with this disorder.[48] Although vulvar lichen sclerosus et atrophicus in childhood does not predispose to neoplasia, the incidence of squamous cell carcinoma in adult cases has been estimated as 4.4 per cent.[46] Patients with cases persisting beyond puberty, or having onset after puberty, accordingly should be observed at intervals of 6 to 12 months for the possibility of leukoplakia or carcinoma. If carcinoma is suspected, cutaneous biopsy is recommended in adults; and newly arising nodules, erosions, or ulcers in lesions of lichen sclerosus et atrophicus that persist for more than a few weeks require histologic examination.

SCLEREDEMA

Scleredema (also termed *scleredema adultorum of Buschke*) is a rare condition of unkown etiology characterized by a diffuse brawny induration of large areas of the skin. Since at least 50 per cent of cases occur in childhood, the term *adultorum* is a misnomer. Appearing twice as frequently in females as in males, 22 per cent of cases begin between 10 and 20 years of age and an additional 29 per cent of cases appear before the age of 10; the disorder has also been described in a 3-month-old infant.[49, 50]

Although scleredema may begin spontaneously, 65 to 95 per cent of patients have the onset of their disorder within a few days to 6 weeks following an acute febrile illness. Of these, 58 per cent of the infections are streptococcal, and recent studies suggest an association with severe long-standing diabetes mellitus.[51–54] Whether the disorder represents a toxic disturbance in ground substance resulting from bacterial toxins, an autoimmune process, or a manifestation of allergic sensitization remains obscure.

The onset of scleredema is usually sudden, and the disorder generally begins on the posterior aspect of the neck and shoulders, with gradual extension to the face, anterior aspect of the neck, scalp, chest, upper back, and arms (Fig. 25–17). The abdomen, genitalia, buttocks, thighs, legs, hands, and feet are less frequently involved. Although the disorder is usually restricted to the skin, involvement of the tongue, pharynx, and esophagus may result in dysarthria and dysphagia. Ocular manifestations consist of induration of the eyelid and conjunctiva and trophic corneal changes. There may be pleural, pericardial, or peritoneal effusion, cardiac disease, skeletal muscle dysfunction, paraproteinemia, and, as a result of induration of the skin overlying the joints, restriction of motion in association with hydroarthrosis.[55]

The diagnosis of scleredema is usually suggested by the sudden onset of symmetrical cutaneous induration, particularly if there is a preceding history of infection or long-term diabetes and obesity. Although the histologic changes are nondiagnostic, the clinical diagnosis may be supported by a mild inflammatory infiltrate and separation of the collagen bundles (particularly those in the lower two thirds of the dermis) by empty spaces created by the swelling and splitting of collagen bundles. The demonstration of greatly increased amounts of mucopolysaccharide may be done more easily when a special fixative such as cetylpyridinium chloride is used.

The disease usually reaches its maximum development within 2 to 6 weeks; in most cases, the prognosis is good, with spontaneous resolution usually occurring within 6 months to 2 years. About one fourth of patients, however, may exhibit only partial improvement, with persistent areas of

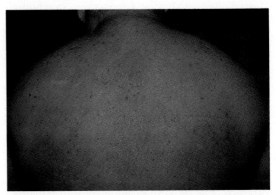

Figure 25–17. Scleredema (scleredema of Buschke). Diffuse, symmetrical, nonpitting induration of the skin of the upper back. (Courtesy of Department of Dermatology, Yale University School of Medicine.)

residual induration.[56] In patients in whom the disorder is associated with obesity and diabetes, the cutaneous induration may persist for many years, and on rare occasions patients have manifestations of their disorder for as long as 20 to 40 years.

There is no effective treatment of scleredema. Owing to the high incidence of streptococcal infection (particularly in children), bacterial cultures are recommended, and appropriate antibiotics should be initiated when indicated. Other suggested forms of therapy include warm baths, massage, systemic corticosteroids, thyroid and pituitary extracts, and the subcutaneous injection of hyaluronidase and fibrinolysin. None of these, however, has proved beneficial in the management of this disorder.

MACULAR ATROPHY (ANETODERMA)

Macular atrophy, frequently termed *macular anetoderma* (Gk, meaning "relaxed skin"), describes an idiopathic atrophy of the skin characterized by oval lesions of thin, soft, loosely wrinkled, depigmented outpouchings of skin that result from weakening of the connective tissue of the dermis. The disorder may be classified as primary macular anetoderma, which arises from apparently normal skin, or as secondary macular anetoderma, which follows previous inflammatory and infiltrative dermatoses such as secondary syphilis, sarcoidosis, leprosy, lupus erythematosus, tuberculosis, urticarial lesions, purpura, lichen planus, acne vulgaris, urticaria pigmentosa, and varicella, or penicillamine treatment in patients with Wilson's disease.[57] A peculiar laxity of the eyelid (blepharochalasis) may also follow chronic or recurrent dermatitis of the eyelids. When eyelid changes are seen in association with adenoma of the thyroid and progressive enlargement of the lips due to inflammation of the labial salivary glands, the disorder is termed *Ascher's syndrome.*

Based on whether an inflammatory reaction occurred before the appearance of the atrophy, two types of primary macular anetoderma have been described: anetoderma of Jadassohn, in which the atrophic lesions are preceded by inflammation, and anetoderma of Schweninger-Buzzi, in which there is no evidence of inflammation. Although the underlying etiopathogenesis of primary anetoderma has not been established, serologic and direct immunofluorescent findings suggest that immunologically mediated mechanisms play a role in the elastolytic process seen in individuals with this disorder.

Anetoderma of Jadassohn is characterized by crops of round or oval pink macules 0.5 to 1 cm in diameter that develop on the trunk, shoulders, upper arms, thighs, sacral area, and occasionally face or scalp (Fig. 25–18). Usually seen in females in their teens to 30s, and occasionally in children, the anetoderma begins with a sharply defined red spot,

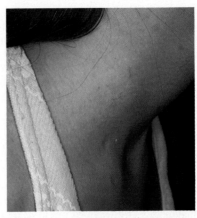

Figure 25–18. Macular anetoderma of the Jadassohn type. White, shiny, oval or round atrophic herniations yield to gentle pressure (atrophic herniation or outpouching reappears when the pressure is released).

which grows peripherally and becomes round or oval and slightly depressed. As the redness disappears the atrophic stage begins. The lesion then becomes distinctly white and shiny, develops an atrophic hernia-like outpouching, and assumes a livid red or yellowish color. The lesions then develop a characteristic atrophic, wrinkled, and pale herniation, which yields on pressure, admitting the finger through the surrounding ring of normal skin. Much like an umbilical hernia, the bulge reappears when the finger is released and at times, fatty tissue may infiltrate the lesions, giving them a more firm, soft tumor-like appearance.

Anetoderma of Schweninger-Buzzi is manifested by the sudden appearance of large numbers of bluish white macules, some of which are protuberant, without any preceding inflammatory eruption. Women are affected more commonly than men. Lesions are generally seen on the trunk, neck, face, shoulders, extremities, and back and range from 10 to 20 mm in diameter. Seen during childhood or adult life, the disease is slowly progressive and new lesions appear one by one or in groups, a few at a time, over a period of years. The essential difference in this form of anetoderma is a lack of inflammation and the relative absence of coalescence of lesions.

In all forms of macular anetoderma the primary histopathologic feature is the destruction and loss of elastic fibers. In the Jadassohn type, early lesions show a perivascular infiltrate consisting of polymorphonuclear leukocytes, eosinophils, and "nuclear dust" (a histologic picture of vasculitis). In the later atrophic stage of the Jadassohn form and in the Schweninger-Buzzi type, little or no inflammatory infiltration is present, elastic fibers are absent, and the collagen bundles appear more or less swollen and homogenized. In all forms of macular anetoderma, fragmentation, contractions, and loss of elastic tissue is highly characteristic. This change is a constant and diagnostic feature, and unless sections are stained for elastic tissue, the diagnosis frequently can be overlooked.

There is no known etiology for this group of disorders, and except perhaps for surgical excision of cosmetically objectionable lesions, no form of therapy appears to be effective.

ATROPHODERMA OF PASINI AND PIERINI

Atrophoderma of Pasini and Pierini is a relatively uncommon atrophic disorder of the skin. Of unknown etiology, it is seen more commonly in females, may appear at any age (including infancy), and usually begins on the trunk during the late teens or early 20s. A chronic condition that tends to persist indefinitely, this disorder is characterized by asymptomatic bluish brown to violaceous, oval, round, or irregular, smooth well-circumscribed patches with a depressed center and a "cliff-drop" border.

The atrophy begins as an asymptomatic, slightly erythematous macular lesion on the trunk (particularly the back). Initially there may be a singular lesion, but more often there are multiple lesions, varying from 1 to 12 cm in diameter. Within 1 or 2 weeks the lesions develop a slate gray to brown pigmentation. The atrophic patches extend very slowly, increase in number for 10 years or more, and then generally persist without apparent change. During this period new lesions may occur and old ones slowly enlarge. At times lesions are indistinguishable from those of morphea. Indeed, typical lesions of morphea and atrophoderma may occur in different areas in the same patient; and although opinions differ, it has been suggested that this disorder may represent an atrophic variant of morphea.[58–60] Against this hypothesis is the fact that lesions of atrophoderma lack induration and sclerosis and the lilac ring characteristic of morphea.

Because histologic changes are often minimal, cutaneous biopsy should include an area of surrounding normal skin for comparison. The histopathologic features of early lesions consist of mild homogenization of the collagen bundles and a scattered lymphocytic infiltrate. Melanin is increased in the basal layer, and there may be thinning of the connective tissue, with a slight perivascular infiltration in the upper dermis. Older lesions demonstrate slight atrophy of the epidermis, a decrease in the size of the dermal papillae, flattening of the rete pegs, and, in the deeper dermal layers, thickening of the collagen bundles with an increase in their eosinophilia.[58]

The course of atrophoderma is benign, and there is no known effective treatment. The disorder remains active for months to years and lesions persist indefinitely, but there are no reports of systemic involvement or complications.

STRIAE (STRIAE DISTENSAE)

Striae (striae distensae, "stretch marks") are linear depressions of the skin that are initially pink or purple and later become white, shiny, and atrophic. Seen primarily in areas subject to stretching such as the lower back, buttocks, thighs, breasts, abdomen, inguinal areas, and shoulders, they may develop physiologically in up to 35 per cent of girls and 15 per cent of boys between the ages of 9 and 16 years and with other conditions associated with an increased production of glucocorticoids by the adrenal glands.[61] The most frequent causes of this disorder appear to be stretching exercises, rapid growth, obesity, adolescence, pregnancy, Cushing's disease, and prolonged use of systemic and potent topical corticosteroids (see Figures 13–18 and 3–20).[62, 63] Although the precise etiology is not clearly understood, formation of striae appears to be related to stress-induced rupture of connective tissue, destruction of collagen and elastin, and dermal scarring in which glucocorticoids suppress fibroblastic activity and newly synthesized collagen fills the gaps between ruptured collagen fibers.[64] Although therapy for this disorder is generally unsatisfactory, most striae that occur during adolescence tend to become less noticeable with time. It has been suggested that topical tretinoin (0.1 per cent Retin-A cream), applied once daily for 6 to 12 weeks, may be helpful for some patients, and avoidance of extreme stretching of the skin may be beneficial.[65]

ACANTHOSIS NIGRICANS

Acanthosis nigricans is a cutaneous disorder characterized by light brown to black verrucous or papillomatous hypertrophic lesions, which may occur on any part of the body but characteristically appear on the nape and sides of the neck, in the axillae, and in the groin (Fig. 25–19). In addition to the characteristic areas there may be verrucous hyperkeratosis of the knuckles, genitalia, perineum, face, thighs, breasts, and flexural regions of the elbows and knees. Acanthosis nigricans may begin during childhood, at puberty, or during later adult life. Hyperpigmentation, the first cutaneous change, is followed by an increase in skin markings and varying degrees of localized hypertrophy of the epidermis in the affected areas. The disorder probably represents a reaction of the skin to different stimuli. In some patients it appears before, after, or concomitantly with the onset of an endocrine disorder or internal malignancy.

Some individuals have a familial tendency to this disorder, and, in obese individuals, an undiscovered endocrinopathy may be responsible for the characteristic cutaneous changes. Acanthosis nigricans also has been reported in association with excessive doses of niacin, corticosteroids, di-

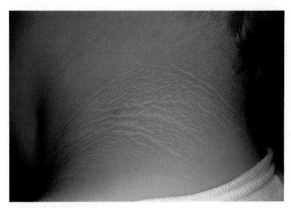

Figure 25–19. Acanthosis nigricans on the posterior aspect of the neck of an 8-year-old girl.

ethylstilbestrol, oral contraceptives, and various insulin-resistance states.[66–68] The suggestion that acanthosis nigricans is caused by release of a pituitary or ectopically produced peptide hormone is consistent with clinical observations of individuals with this disorder.[69]

Although four types of this disorder have been described in the past, many authorities currently include pseudoacanthosis nigricans, previously used to describe acanthosis nigricans in obese individuals, under the classification of benign acanthosis nigricans.[70]

Acanthosis Nigricans Associated With Malignancy. In middle-aged and older adults, acanthosis nigricans is frequently associated with adenocarcinoma, generally of the stomach (but it may appear elsewhere in the gastrointestinal tract, the lung, breast, gallbladder, pancreas, testes, uterus, ovaries), and, in rare instances, with lymphoma or squamous cell carcinoma. Most cases of acanthosis nigricans associated with malignancy begin after puberty or in adulthood. A few cases, however, have been observed in childhood.[71] Because of the high association of malignancy in middle-aged and older adults, patients who develop acanthosis nigricans after 30 years of age without evidence of endocrine disease or obesity should be investigated for possible malignancy, particularly adenocarcinoma of an abdominal or thoracic organ. If benign, genetic or "syndromal" acanthosis nigricans, obesity, and endocrinopathy are excluded, patients who manifest acanthosis in childhood should also be investigated for this rare possibility.[70]

Benign Acanthosis Nigricans. True benign acanthosis nigricans may represent an obesity-dependent disorder or a rare genetic dermatosis that greatly resembles ichthyosis hystrix and follows an irregular autosomal dominance. It can be present at birth or may develop in childhood or, more commonly, at puberty; when associated with obesity, it is usually obesity-dependent and regresses with weight loss. In cases that begin before puberty, it frequently becomes intensified at that

time, possibly as the result of hormonal stimulation. After this increase in intensity, the dermatosis frequently becomes stationary or may tend to subside.

"Syndromal" Acanthosis Nigricans. "Syndromal" acanthosis nigricans occasionally may appear as a feature of several specific syndromes. Included among these are Bloom's syndrome (in which acanthosis nigricans may appear in the axillae during childhood or puberty), Crouzon's syndrome (craniofacial dysostosis), Lawrence-Seip syndrome (lipodystrophy, muscular hypertrophy, and accelerated osseous maturation), insulin-resistant diabetes,[66, 68] Prader-Willi syndrome, pituitary hypogonadism, polycystic ovary disease, lupus erythematosus, lupoid nephritis, dermatomyositis, scleroderma, and Rud's syndrome (ichthyosis, hypogonadism, mental deficiency, epilepsy, and infantilism).

Epidermal and pigmented nevi, erythrasma, and endocrine disorders with hyperpigmentation (Addison's disease) may at times simulate acanthosis nigricans. The histologic features of acanthosis nigricans include marked acanthosis, hyperkeratosis, papillomatosis, and an increase in pigment cells in the basal layer and upper dermis where melanophores containing pigment are found.

Treatment. Treatment of acanthosis nigricans depends primarily on careful exclusion of endocrine disease or internal malignancy as a cause of this disorder. When acanthosis nigricans develops in teenagers and young adults, with or without obesity, it is necessary to determine whether the patient has endocrine disease. In children, acanthosis nigricans is generally not considered to be a manifestation of internal malignancy. Between the ages of 12 and 30 the most common abnormalities associated with this disorder are obesity of Cushing's syndrome; in patients older than 30, obesity and malignancy are most commonly seen. Relative to the cosmetic appearance of the cutaneous lesions, correction of known precipitating factors (obesity, endocrinologic disease, and internal malignancy) is necessary, and topical retinoic acid (tretinoin, Retin-A), 10 to 20 per cent urea, lactic acid formulations (Lacticare, Epilyt, or 12% Lac-Hydrin), 5 to 20 per cent salicylic acid in an emollient cream (such as Ureacin creme), or Keralyt gel, followed by gentle periodic abrasion with a polycellulose pad such as a Buf-Puf or loofah sponge provide some degree of improvement.

CONFLUENT AND RETICULATED PAPILLOMATOSIS

First described by Gougerot and Carteaud, confluent and reticulated papillomatosis is a rare cutaneous papillomatous disorder characterized by persistent verrucous papules that are confluent in the center and reticulated at the periphery. Believed by some authorities to be a variant of acanthosis nigricans, the disorder, seen primarily in adolescents (particularly girls at or near puberty) and young adults, appears initially on the upper chest, usually in the sternal area, with extension to the breasts, neck, axillae, superior portion of the shoulders, and spinal, intrascapular, sacral and pubic areas, and occasionally to the face. Although the cause of the disorder is unknown, its clinical resemblance to tinea versicolor, occasional reports identifying *Malassezia* (*Pityrosporum orbiculare*) in lesions of some patients, and a response, at least in some patients, to topical 2.5 per cent selenium sulfide shampoo, sodium hyposulfite, topical antifungal agents, or topical keratolytic compounds suggest that the dermatosis may perhaps represent a host response to the yeast phase of *Malassezia furfur* or a genetically determined disorder of keratinization colonized with *Pityrosporum orbiculare* as a secondary phenomenon.[72, 73]

POROKERATOSIS

Porokeratosis is an uncommon chronic progressive disorder of keratinization and may appear in several forms: (1) classic porokeratosis of Mibelli, an autosomal dominant disorder generally seen in children or young adults; (2) a disorder that appears on sun-exposed surfaces (disseminated superficial actinic porokeratosis), generally seen in adults during the third of fourth decades of life; and (3) a superficial form that begins on the palms and soles and subsequently involves other areas of the body.

Porokeratosis of Mibelli may appear as one, a few, or many lesions that persist indefinitely (Figs. 25–20 through 25–22). Linear and zosteriform types resembling linear epidermal nevi have also

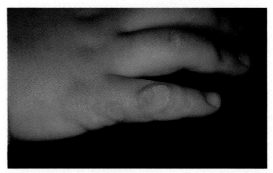

Figure 25–21. Porokeratosis of Mibelli. A circinate plaque with a characteristic raised peripheral ridge surmounted by a furrow on a finger of a 2½-year-old girl.

been described. A hypothesis that the linear form of porokeratosis is the result of a Koebner response in a genetically predisposed individual has been proposed but requires verification.[74]

The skin lesions of porokeratosis of Mibelli may appear at any age, but usually first appear during childhood. Affecting males two or three times more frequently than females, the disorder has a predilection for the face, neck, forearms, and hands, but also may affect the feet, ankles, scalp (where it may produce areas of alopecia), the buccal mucosa, and glans penis. The initial lesion begins as a crateriform hyperkeratotic papule that gradually eventuates in an atrophic plaque of circinate or irregular contour measuring from a few millimeters to several centimeters in diameter. The diagnostic feature of this disorder is the raised hyperkeratotic peripheral ridge surmounted by a furrow. This pathognomonic finding is often referred to as the "great wall of China."

Porokeratosis of Chernosky, the second form of porokeratosis (disseminated superficial actinic porokeratosis, DSAP) usually appears during the third or fourth decade of life. Occasionally seen in adolescents 16 years of age or older, the disorder appears on sun-exposed areas of the skin. Lesions

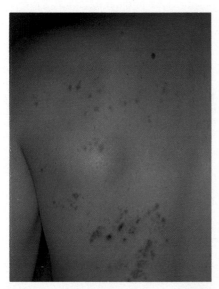

Figure 25–20. Porokeratosis of Mibelli. Circinate plaques with raised hyperkeratotic borders are surmounted by a furrow (the so-called great wall of China).

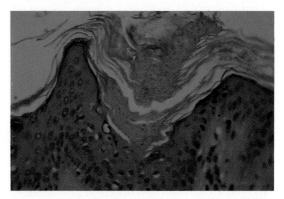

Figure 25–22. Porokeratosis of Mibelli. A photomicrograph of the peripheral raised edge of a lesion of porokeratosis of Mibelli shows a keratin-filled invagination and its central parakeratotic "cornoid lamella." (Courtesy of Department of Dermatology, Yale University School of Medicine.)

are usually multiple, with most patients having over 50 lesions; are primarily limited to the extremities; and measure 0.1 to 4.5 cm in diameter, with most lesions measuring 0.5 to 1.0 cm. In contrast to lesions of porokeratosis of Mibelli the ridges are only slightly elevated above the cutaneous surface.[75]

Porokeratosis plantaris, palmaris, et disseminata (porokeratosis punctata palmaris et plantaris) has been recognized as a third variant of porokeratosis that does not appear to fit into either of the previously defined forms of this disorder.[76] An autosomal dominant genodermatosis, the disorder begins in the late teens or early 20s, and lesions appear on the palms and soles, with subsequent involvement of other areas of the body, including parts not exposed to sunlight. The disorder is bilateral and fairly symmetrical, and males appear to be affected twice as frequently as females.

Lesions of porokeratosis have been likened to epidermal nevi and are believed to arise from a mutant clone of faulty keratinization. They should be differentiated from epidermal nevi, lesions of granuloma annulare and tinea corporis, warts, and lesions of elastosis perforans serpiginosa. The pathognomonic microscopic feature is the cornoid lamella, which corresponds to the sharply defined margin of the lesion and is seen as a narrow column of lighter-staining keratin containing parakeratotic cells that begin in the malpighian layer and extend upward through the granular and keratin layers (See Figure 25–22). The granular layer is absent beneath the cornoid lamella; and within the center of the ring formed by the cornoid lamella, most lesions present a thin atrophic malpighian layer, with effacement of rete ridges, varying amounts of atrophy of the dermis, and chronic inflammatory infiltrate.

Treatment. Lesions of porokeratosis are primarily cosmetic, slowly progressive, and relatively asymptomatic. However, since development of squamous cell carcinoma or Bowen's disease within lesions has been reported, lesions that are not or cannot be removed should be carefully observed for possible neoplastic change.[77] Small circumscribed lesions may be excised or destroyed by cryotherapy, electrodesiccation and curettage, dermabrasion, or carbon dioxide laser beam surgery, but recurrences are common; and although topical 5-fluorouracil cream and etretinate have been reported to be effective for the treatment of disseminated superficial porokeratosis, further evaluation will be required to determine their long-term effectiveness.

MELKERSSON-ROSENTHAL SYNDROME

In 1928 Melkersson described the association of recurrent swelling of the lips and recurrent facial paralysis. In 1931 Rosenthal noted the association of fissured tongue in patients with this disorder. This disorder, termed the *Melkersson-Rosenthal*

syndrome, although widely reported in the European literature (with an incidence of 1 in 2,000 cases in one dermatology clinic), is relatively uncommon in the United States, perhaps owing to a low incidence of suspicion in this country. This syndrome is characterized by a triad of recurrent facial paralysis, facial edema, and a furrowed or "scrotal" tongue (sometimes accompanied by macrocheilitis). Furrowing of the tongue, seen in 0.5 per cent of the general population, occurs in 30 per cent of patients with this disorder, and facial palsy appears in 30 per cent. The attacks usually disappear within days or weeks but frequently tend to persist after several recurrences. When the disorder is limited to the lips, the term *cheilitis granulomatosa* or *Meischer's granulomatous cheilitis* may be applied (Fig. 25–23).

The presumed etiology is attributed to a lability of the autonomic nervous system with a resultant vasomotor edema. The paralysis is attributed to granulomatous involvement of nerves, compression of the nerve in its bony canal by edema, or primary vasomotor injury due to temporary insufficiency of the supplying blood vessels.[78–80] Attacks usually start during adolescence with paralysis of a facial nerve, repeated attacks of migraine, and edema of the circumoral tissue of the upper lip or cheeks and occasionally the gingivae, sublingual area, and lower lip. Usually the edema is asymmetrical, but sometimes the whole face may be involved. The histopathology reveals a tuberculoid type of granuloma with lymphedema and perivascular lymphocytic infiltrate. With time, the infiltrate becomes more dense and pleomorphic and focal granulomas indistinguishable from sarcoidal granulomatosis can be seen.[81]

Although there is no completely satisfactory

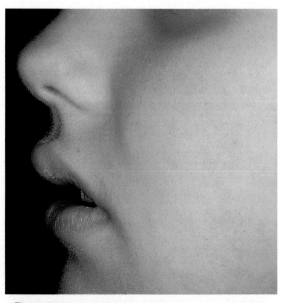

Figure 25–23. Cheilitis granulomatosa (Meischer's granulomatous cheilitis) on the upper lip of an 11-year-old girl.

treatment for this disorder, the removal of odontogenic or sinus foci of infection, intralesional corticosteroid injections, metronidazole (Flagyl), possibly because of its antiinflammatory properties, and, in long-standing cases with chronically enlarged tissues (once the disorder is quiescent), debulking of tissue and cheiloplasty may at times be helpful.[81a, 82]

GRAFT-VERSUS-HOST DISEASE

The *host-versus-graft reaction* is a condition that tends to occur when a leukocyte-poor or leukocyte-free graft or transplant (skin, heart, or kidney) is placed in a normal individual. In this disorder the host's circulating leukocytes react against the foreign tissue and, usually within 1 or 2 weeks, cause destruction of the grafted tissue.

In *graft-versus-host disease* the reverse happens. Immunoincompetent recipients of foreign immunocompetent cells in exchange transfusions or organ transplants are unable to react immunologically and the grafted donor cells mount an attack against the host tissues. In many cases, this may prove to be fatal. Examples of graft-versus-host reaction include the reactions that occur in patients with leukemia treated by a combination of irradiation or chemotherapy with bone marrow grafts, patients with certain severe immunodeficiencies treated with bone marrow transplants, immunodeficient infants through maternal-fetal transfer of leukocytes, and occasionally infants with hemolytic disease treated with intrauterine or exchange transfusions.

The *graft-versus-host disease syndrome* is characterized by anorexia, severe diarrhea, colitis, hepatosplenomegaly, liver dysfunction, marked wasting, pleural effusions, bone marrow aplasia, an erythematous maculopapular rubella-like eruption, extensive exfoliation, and marked susceptibility to infection. The cutaneous features include an eruption that generally begins on the face and head 5 to 12 days after the transplant has been performed. The rash rapidly spreads to the trunk and arms, becomes confluent, and leads to a generalized erythema and edema. The reaction may then regress and disappear, generally in about 6 weeks, or may develop into a generalized, dry, scaling scarlatiniform or toxic epidermal necrolysis–like rash accompanied by bullae, alopecia, and/or nail dystrophy.[83]

In some cases the eruption may progress to a generalized exfoliative erythroderma within a period of several weeks after the grafting. This erythroderma may progress to dermal sclerosis, epidermal atrophy, hyperkeratosis, ulceration, and reticular hyperpigmentation. After several weeks or months the eruption enters a quiescent stage and the skin appears thin, atrophic, or parchment-like, frequently with a bronze hue.

The differential diagnosis of the cutaneous manifestations of graft-versus-host disease includes seborrheic dermatitis, Leiner's disease, acrodermatitis enteropathica, histiocytosis X, drug eruption, lichen planus, viral exanthems, exfoliative erythroderma, poikiloderma vasculare atrophicans, and toxic epidermal necrolysis. In such instances, cutaneous biopsy can frequently be an aid to early diagnosis. The histopathologic features of graft-versus-host disease consist of epidermal atrophy, exocytosis, acantholysis, liquefactive degeneration of basal cells, and individual cell dyskeratosis or necrosis. "Mummified" bodies surrounded by satellite lymphocytes, which appear within discrete epidermal spaces of the stratum spongiosum ("satellite cell necrosis"), are characteristic and can facilitate early histopathologic diagnosis of this disorder.[84]

Individuals with graft-versus-host disease are acutely and potentially fatally ill. Accordingly, systemic antibiotic therapy, systemic corticosteroids, antileukocytic serum, thalidomide, or immunosuppressive therapy have been utilized in an attempt to eliminate complicating infection and reduction of the severity of the reaction. PUVA therapy may at times be beneficial for patients with cutaneous manifestations of lichenoid chronic graft-versus-host disease.[85, 85a]

CUTANEOUS REACTIONS TO COLD

Cutaneous reactions to cold include a varied group of clinical and pathologic disorders. When exposure is extreme, the condition produces the picture of immersion foot or frostbite; when the exposure is less severe and associated with dampness, perniosis (chilblains) may result. Frostbite is caused by exposure to freezing cold. Trench foot and immersion foot are caused by a combination of cold and wetness, but perniosis represents an exaggerated response to cold and dampness in a predisposed or susceptible individual.

Frostbite

Frostbite is a disorder caused by the actual freezing of tissue at temperatures of extreme cold (−2°C to −10°C). At these temperatures the duration of exposure, wind velocity, dependency of an extremity, and factors such as fatigue, injury, immobility, general health, and racial predisposition potentiate the effects of the cold.

Although the mechanism of frostbite is not clearly understood, it appears to be related to direct cold injury to the cell, indirect injury due to ice crystal formation, and impaired circulation to the area of involvement. Frostbite generally affects exposed areas, such as the toes, feet, fingers, nose, cheeks, and ears. The frozen area becomes cold, and waxy, the skin becomes white or slightly yellow, and, except for the initial feeling of cold and discomfort, there is little to no pain. It is only on rewarming that the extent of tissue damage becomes apparent.

In mild cases there is redness and discomfort with return to normal within a period of a few hours. In more severe cases cyanosis or mottling appears. This is followed by erythema and swelling; the numbness is replaced by burning pain, and in a period of 24 to 48 hours, vesicles and bullae appear. Eventually crusts form and the adjacent skin that is thin, tender, and red (Fig. 25–24). More severe forms tend to develop gangrene, and in extreme cases necrosis of the skin and loss of the affected parts (nerves, muscles, tendons, and periosteum) may occur.

The early treatment of frostbite consists of covering of the affected areas with other body surfaces and warm clothing. The use of local dry heat is hazardous and should be avoided. Current studies reveal that rapid rewarming produces more pain, hyperemia, and large blebs and bullae but will result in an increased rate of healing and reduction of tissue loss and sequelae. This is best accomplished by immersion of the involved parts in a warm water bath at temperatures of 40°C to 44°C until all frozen tissues are thawed. Pain during the thawing and immediately after thawing should be treated with potent analgesics and sedatives. Treatment should include the administration of tetanus toxoid, gentle cleanisng with a germicidal preparation, open methods of treatment with reverse isolation, avoidance of pressure and even light contact, bed rest until the period of

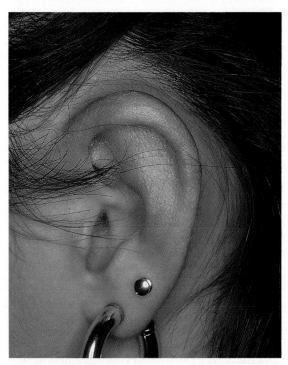

Figure 25–24. Frostbite on the ear of a 16-year-old girl.

acute inflammation has subsided, and vigorous treatment of infection when present. If surgical measures are required, they should be delayed as long as possible. Since the prediction of tissue loss is difficult, amputation of necrotic tissue is best deferred for a period of at least 60 to 90 days to allow time for contracture, shrinkage, and the formation of a definitive line of demarcation between necrotic and viable tissue.

Trench Foot (Immersion Foot)

Trench foot or its equivalent, immersion foot, is a cold-induced nonfreezing injury of the extremities that occurs in individuals constantly exposed to a wet and cold environment. Generally seen in polar explorers, soldiers, and seamen, the disorder resembles a mild to moderate frostbite and is uncommon in children.

During exposure there is usually an initial uncomfortable feeling of coldness followed by virtually no discomfort and, at times, a feeling of warmth as the nerves become sensitive. The limb becomes cold, numb, blue, swollen, and pulseless. The pain is aggravated by heat and relieved by cold, and the ischemic tissue is prone to infection. In severe cases there is muscle weakness, joint stiffness, and gangrene. The gangrene, however, is superficial and nearly always heals without tissue loss.

In addition, immersion of the feet in relatively warm water for long periods of time may produce a syndrome characterized by a wrinkling, blanching, and maceration of the skin on the plantar and lateral aspects of the feet known as tropical immersion foot, "swamp foot," or "jungle rot." The disorder tends to occur in military personnel during military operations in flooded terrain or rice paddies in tropical areas and in individuals who wear insulated boots for long periods of time. Although itching and burning may persist for several days, the disorder differs from that of cold-wet immersion foot in that it is nondestructive and, in most cases, entirely reversible, leaving no residual disability.[86]

The application of a silicone grease prior to water immersion, changing to dry socks, wearing of porous shoes or boots whenever possible, and allowing the feet to be open to the air and dry out for several hours each day can help prevent or delay the development of tropical immersion foot.

The treatment of classic immersion foot is similar to that recommended for frostbite and consists of bed rest in a warm bed to promote reflex vasodilatation of the peripheral blood vessels. Trauma and direct warmth to the skin should be avoided, and the affected limb should be kept slightly elevated outside the bed clothing and cooled by fans or by lower room temperature. Although any of the sequelae of frostbite may occur, early signs of demarcation may be misleading and extensive gangrene is rare.

Perniosis

Perniosis (chilblains) is an exaggerated response to cold in individuals with a constitutional predisposition to the disorder. Characterized by the occurrence of localized cyanosis, nodules, or ulcerations on exposed extremities in cold and damp weather, the disorder, although common in Great Britain, Ireland, and Northern Europe, is relatively uncommon, often unrecognized, or commonly misdiagnosed in the United States.

In affected individuals, cold exposure appears to lower skin temperature and increase vasoconstriction, ultimately resulting in tissue anoxemia and the skin lesions seen in association with this disorder. Perniosis may occur at any age but seems to affect children and young women in particular, and shoe boots made of a waterproof outer covering and insulated lining may be responsible for cases in girls when the linings become cold and wet (Fig. 25–25).[87] Perniotic lesions may also be seen in patients with lupus erythematosus (see Figure 20–10), and a possible association has been described in patients with chronic myelomonocytic leukemia.[88]

Mild cases are manifested by an initial blanching, and then by ill-defined erythematous macules that become infiltrated and vary from a dark pink to a violaceous hue. In most cases the disorder is characterized by edematous patches of erythema or cyanosis that appear 12 to 24 hours after exposure to cold. Initially patients are usually unaware of the disorder. With time the areas become edematous and bluish red and eventually develop numbness, tingling, pruritus, burning, or pain.

Individual lesions tend to appear in a symmetrical distribution principally on the dorsal aspect of the phalanges of the fingers and toes and on the heels, lower legs, thighs, nose, and ears. The course is usually a self-limiting over 2 or 3 weeks. In young girls and adolescent women who wear skirts rather than slacks, the calves and shins are common sites of involvement. Chronic perniosis occurs repeatedly during cold weather and disappears during warm weather. Blistering and ulceration occasionally occur, and at times, lesions may heal with residual areas of pigmentation.

Treatment consists of proper clothing to prevent undue exposure to cold, antipruritics, and soothing lotions or ointments; in severe cases, elevation of the affected areas, vasodilating agents (nicotinic acid, priscoline, and nifedipine) and antibiotics for patients with associated secondary infection should be used.[89]

CUTANEOUS REACTIONS TO HEAT

Erythema ab Igne

Erythema ab igne is an acquired persistent reticulated erythematous and pigmented condition of the skin produced by prolonged or repeated exposure to moderately intense heat from fireplaces, heating appliances, or radiators. Although relatively uncommon in North America and Continental Europe where central heating of the home is predominant, the disorder is common in Great Britain and may be seen in young girls or older women who expose their legs to heating systems for warmth and on the abdomens and lower backs of individuals who use hot water bottles or heating pads for excessively prolonged periods of time.

The disorder is characterized by a mottled appearance of the skin exposed to the heat and eventually is manifested by a reticulated, annular, or gyrated erythema that progresses to a pale-pink to purplish dark-brown color with superficial venular telangiectasia and hyperpigmentation (Fig. 25–26). As in burn scars, squamous cell carcinomas have been reported in plaques of erythema ab igne. When present, they tend to be aggressive, with metastases occurring in over 30 per cent of cases, and have a poor prognosis.

Treatment of erythema ab igne consists of protection from further exposure to the offending heat source. Once exposure to heat is discon-

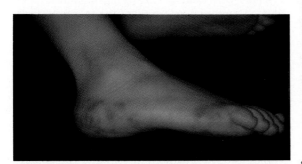

Figure 25–25. Perniosis (chilblains) on the heel and lateral aspect of the foot of a 7½-year-old girl.

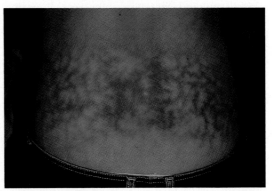

Figure 25–26. Erythema ab igne. Reticular brown pigmentation on the lower back following prolonged exposure to a heating appliance. (Courtesy of Department of Dermatology, Yale University School of Medicine.)

tinued the color may fade to some degree. In general, however, the discoloration will persist indefinitely and pigmentation is frequently permanent.

PANNICULITIS

Panniculitis is a term applied to describe a group of disorders in which the major focus of inflammation is in the subcutaneous fat. Although it is difficult to develop a firm classification of acute panniculitis, since the lesions may appear in a sporadic fashion as a result of many conditions, it can be classified as panniculitis without systemic disease, such as may be seen secondary to trauma or cold (cold panniculitis), and as poststeroidal panniculitis, drug-induced panniculitis, panniculitis of infancy, and panniculitides associated with systemic disorders. The latter include connective tissue disease (such as lupus erythematosus or scleroderma), Behçet's syndrome, lymphoproliferative disease (lymphoma, histiocytosis), nutritional deficiency, diabetes, thyroid disease, α_1-antitrypsin deficiency, generalized lipodystrophy, and pancreatic disease. In most instances, the histopathologic picture is characterized by an early stage of nonspecific inflammation with varying degrees of vascular change followed by phagocytosis of fat, a granulomatous reaction, and a final stage of fibrosis. Because of the difficulty in assigning every case of panniculitis to one of the recognized entities, some cases become classified as nondefinite or nonspecific forms of panniculitis.[90]

Panniculitis in childhood, as in adults, may be an isolated and localized disease process or a manifestation of a systemic disorder. Although the reason for the inflammatory process is unknown, an immune mechanism may be involved and in infants an underlying biochemical defect in the metabolism of fat may lead to the cause of the disorder.

Lesions appear singly or in crops, tend to be flat or raised, discrete and well circumscribed, or irregular and diffuse, erythematous, purple, bluish, or hyperpigmented; they persist for variable periods of time ranging from 1 week or less to several months. Thus, panniculitis of the newborn period or childhood, just as with any other form of panniculitis, must be evaluated on an individual basis with careful clinical and laboratory investigation to rule out the possibility of severe or systemic disease.[91]

Cold panniculitis, which is more common in infants than adults, is characterized by painful erythematous plaques or subcutaneous nodules that develop in exposed areas within hours after exposure to the cold (Fig. 25–27). Lesions appear 1 to 3 days after exposure and subside spontaneously, generally after a few weeks to a few months, leaving a temporary residual pigmentation that may at times persist for 1 month or more. The development of cold panniculitis in children appears to

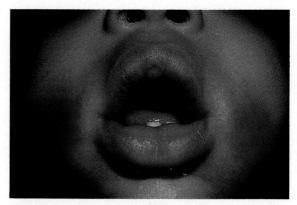

Figure 25–27. Cold panniculitis (popsicle panniculitis). (Courtesy of Douglas H. MacGilpin, M.D.)

be related to the fact that subcutaneous fat solidifies more readily at lower temperatures in infants and young children than it does in adults.

Factitial panniculitis, a disorder in which red or purple-red nodules result from the injection of various foreign substances into the subcutaneous tissue, can result in a bizarre clinical and histologic picture that frequently defies diagnosis until the true cause of disorder (self-inoculation) is suspected. In such instances the diagnosis can be assisted by the finding of birefringent particles by polarized light or, in the case of injected oily substances such as silicone, a characteristic histologic Swiss cheese–like picture in which oil cysts surrounded by fibrosis and inflammation can help to establish the true nature of the disorder.

Poststeroidal panniculitis, a rare entity of childhood, is characterized by small, sometimes pruritic or painful, subcutaneous nodules on the cheeks, arms, trunk, and buttocks of young children, shortly (generally within 2 to 4 weeks) after the sudden discontinuation of systemic corticosteroid therapy. Histologic features, a patchy lobular panniculitis with cleft-containing fat cells surrounded by histiocytic giant cells, resemble those of subcutaneous fat necrosis of the newborn. Although the lesions tend to improve if corticosteroid therapy is reinstituted, they tend to regress spontaneously, thus reinstitution of corticosteroid therapy is unnecessary.[92]

Weber-Christian disease (relapsing febrile nodular nonsuppurative panniculitis) is a rare disorder. Primarily seen in women between the ages of 20 and 60 years, and occasionally in children, including those in the neonatal period, it is characterized by the appearance of crops of tender nodules and plaques in the subcutaneous fat, usually in association with mild fever, malaise, and, at times, myalgia and arthralgia. Although the lesions may be symmetrically distributed on the trunk, the upper extremities, and rarely the face, the thighs and legs are the primary areas of involvement. Lesions tend to last for 15 to 25 days and, as they involute, may leave a central depression in the skin. Nodules lasting for longer periods have also been described; and sometimes the lesions, usually those on the thigh and lower abdomen, undergo liquefaction and discharge an oily, yellowish to yellowish brown liquid through the necrotic overlying skin. The etiology of Weber-Christian syndrome is unknown, and in general the prognosis is good, with attacks becoming less severe and ultimately ceasing. Its association with systemic disease suggests that multiple pathophysiologic and perhaps immunologic mechanisms may lead to the fat necrosis seen in individuals with this disorder.[93] Although in general the prognosis is good and the disorder frequently resolves after a few months, recurrences are common and patients frequently continue to suffer recurrent attacks for up to 10 or more years. Possible underlying causes such as pancreatic disease must be considered in adulthood, and corticosteroids are usually effective if given in relatively high doses during acute attacks.

Lipogranulomatosis subcutanea (the Rothmann-Makai syndrome) appears to represent a rare variant of Weber-Christian disease and occurs most often in children. Although the disease is often pictured as beginning in infancy with a few slightly tender large subcutaneous plaques, the disease is perhaps best regarded as a spontaneously resolving localized form of lobular panniculitis, with no fever, systemic symptoms, or visceral manifestations. Although corticosteroids, sulfonamides, and antibiotics have been used, there appears to be no effective treatment and in most instances the condition regresses spontaneously within a year.

Other forms of panniculitis include erythema nodosum (see Chapter 18); pancreatic panniculitis, a disorder that probably results from breakdown of subcutaneous fat caused by enzymes released into the circulation from a nodular or neoplastic pancreatic disease; cytophagic panniculitis (a rare proliferative disorder of histiocytes characterized by fever, subcutaneous nodules, and abnormal hepatic function); erythema induratum, believed by many to be a manifestation of tuberculosis (a deep-seated subcutaneous infiltration of the lower legs, especially the calves, that often ulcerates before healing and results in atrophic scars); traumatic panniculitis, a disorder consisting of hard, indurated, inflamed nodules following a blunt injury; subacute nodular migratory panniculitis (Vilanova's disease), a disorder of unknown etiology believed by some to be a variant of erythema nodosum in which individual lesions instead of remaining fixed in size and position extend peripherally to form large plaques with central clearing; aspartame-induced granulomatous panniculitis (an idiosyncratic reaction to the ingestion of saccharin)[94]; and, as noted earlier, panniculitis associated with α_1-antitrypsin deficiency, a relatively uncommon subset characterized by recurrent nodules that break down to discharge an oily yellow fluid or undergo ulceration. It is likely that cases reported in the past as liquefying Weber-Christian panniculitis may have represented cases of panniculitis caused by α_1-antitrypsin deficiency.[95]

FAMILIAL MEDITERRANEAN FEVER

Familial Mediterranean fever (benign paroxysmal peritonitis, familial paroxysmal polyserositis, familial recurrent polyserositis, Armenian disease) is an autosomal recessive disorder of unknown etiology seen almost exclusively in individuals of Armenian or Arabic origin and individuals of Jewish descent from central and eastern Europe (Table 25–2). Characterized by acute febrile attacks with peritonitis, pleuritis, synovitis, abdominal, chest, and articular pain, and an insidious development of amyloidosis, it occurs one to one and one-half times more frequently in men than in women.[96]

There appear to be two phenotypes of familial Mediterranean fever. Type I (the common variant) is characterized by recurrent attacks of fever and short, self-limiting episodes of peritonitis, pleuritis, arthritis, and erysipelas-like cutaneous lesions, with renal amyloidosis manifesting as the nephrotic syndrome eventually developing in at least one fourth of affected patients. Type II (a more rare variant) is characterized by amyloidosis as the initial or sole manifestation of the disorder. Principally involving the kidneys, this complication is particularly common in non-Ashkenazic (Sephardic) Jews and Arabs.

Attacks of familial Mediterranean fever usually begin in early childhood (during the first decade in 67 per cent of cases and by the second decade in 90 per cent) and continue throughout life. Most are self-limiting and may be followed by prolonged asymptomatic intervals, sometimes lasting several years. Attacks of peritonitis (often suggestive of acute appendicitis) and pleuritis begin suddenly and subside spontaneously within 72 hours. Although symptoms of joint inflammation persist longer, sometimes for several months, they rarely leave residual damage.

Cutaneous lesions, seen in approximately 10

Table 25–2. FAMILIAL MEDITERRANEAN FEVER

1. An autosomal recessive disorder
2. Generally seen in Armenians, Arabs, and Ashkenazic Jews
3. Acute febrile attacks with peritonitis, pleuritis, synovitis, and abdominal, chest, and articular pain often begin in childhood (during the first decade in 67% and by the second decade in 90%)
4. Cutaneous lesions in 10% of cases (urticaria, erythematous papules, vesicles, subcutaneous nodules, and erysipelas- or cellulitis-like lesions)
5. Amyloidosis in 25% (with eventual death in 90% of patients with renal amyloidosis), primarily in Sephardic Jews and Arabs
6. Fat-free diet, aspirin, and bed rest, with colchicine for those unresponsive to dietary management

Modified from Hurwitz S: The Skin and Systemic Disease in Children. Year Book Medical Publishers, Chicago, 1985.

per cent of patients, may include urticaria, erythematous papules, vesicles, bullae, subcutaneous nodules histologically resembling periarteritis nodosa, and painful tender erythematous lesions usually appearing on the calves, around the ankles, and on the dorsal aspects of the feet (Fig. 25–28). These erysipelas-like or cellulitis-like lesions, the most frequent cutaneous manifestations, may occur as the only manifestation of an attack or may accompany the arthritic symptoms and, like the arthritis, may be precipitated by trauma.

Amyloidosis occurs in about 25 per cent of patients and causes death in 90 per cent of individuals affected with this complication before the age of 40. There appears to be no relationship between the age at onset and the type, frequency, or severity of attacks, but renal amyloidosis appears to be more common in Sephardic Jews. Ashkenazic Jews and individuals of Armenian descent, therefore, have a better prognosis.

The diagnosis of familial Mediterranean fever is dependent on the above constellation of clinical features in individuals of certain ethnic backgrounds. Rectal biopsy appears to be the diagnostic procedure of choice. Histopathologic examination reveals acute inflammation of the involved serosa (and amyloidosis in those individuals affected with this complication).

Familial Mediterranean fever is a severe, chronic, incurable disorder with an unpredictable and often fatal course in a significant number of patients (those with renal amyloidosis). Although there is no completely effective therapy, a fat-free diet, aspirin, and bed rest are beneficial; colchicine (0.6 mg two or three times daily) has been reported to be effective in preventing attacks in approximately 70 per cent of adult patients in high-risk populations and seems to minimize deterioration of renal function in patients with amyloidosis with proteinuria who do not have the nephrotic syndrome. Colchicine, however, is not listed in the manufacturer's official directive, and it is currently suggested that this form of therapy be reserved for those children who are incapacitated by frequent and severe attacks and do not respond to dietary fat restriction.[97]

PYODERMA GANGRENOSUM

Pyoderma gangrenosum is a severe, chronic, inflammatory disorder of the skin characterized by a painful sloughing ulceration with purulent base and an elevated dusky blue or reddish purple undermined border surrounded by a red areola (Fig. 25–29).[98, 99] Most often found on the lower extremities (especially the anterior tibial surface), but also elsewhere on the body, and usually seen in adults, the disorder has also been reported in infants and children (particularly adolescents). Pathergy (the development of lesions at sites of minor trauma), which occurs in 20 per cent of patients with this disorder, may be more common in childhood cases.[100, 101] Although the disorder may occur without associated disease, it frequently develops in patients with a variety of systemic disorders, namely, ulcerative colitis, regional enteritis, a rheumatoid arthritis–like disorder, chronic hepatic disease, hematologic disorders (myelogenous leukemia, acute lymphoblastic leukemia, myeloid metaplasia, and polycythemia vera), and

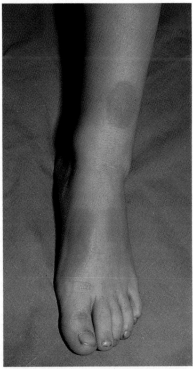

Figure 25–28. Erythematous nodules on the dorsal aspect of the foot and pretibial area of a child with familial Mediterranean fever. (Courtesy of James E. Rasmussen, M.D.; reprinted from Hurwitz S: The Skin and Systemic Disease in Children. Year Book Medical Publishers, Chicago, 1985.)

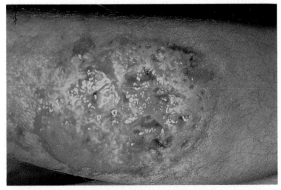

Figure 25–29. Pyoderma gangrenosum. This painful ulceration has a purulent base and an undermined elevated border. (Courtesy of Department of Dermatology, Yale University School of Medicine.)

various paraproteinemias, including multiple myeloma. Although the cause of pyoderma gangrenosum remains unknown, it appears to have an immunogenic etiology, perhaps a cell-mediated hypersensitivity or a vasculitis triggered by a variety of predisposing factors (Table 25–3).[98, 99]

The diagnosis of pyoderma gangrenosum is based on clinical features and the elimination of other causes of cutaneous ulceration simulating this condition. The histologic appearance of lesions is not diagnostic. Early lesions show areas of necrosis with edema and infiltration of polymorphonuclear leukocytes and lymphocytes; older lesions show epidermal proliferation, acanthosis, fibroblastic activity, and, on occasion, multinucleated giant cells.

Since the pathogenesis of pyoderma gangrenosum remains unknown, treatment is empirical and relies on various systemic and topical approaches in conjunction with a vigorous attempt to control the underlying disease. Topical therapy is directed toward debridement of the underlying base of lesions, 0.25 per cent acetic acid soaks, wet dressings with potassium permanganate, whirlpool baths, silver sulfadiazine cream, benzoyl peroxide, pigskin dressings, hyperbaric oxygen, topical corticosteroid creams, and intralesional corticosteroids. Systemic corticosteroids are usually the drug of choice for patients resistant to topical therapy. If pathogenic organisms can be cultured from lesions, specific antibiotic therapy may be instituted. Other therapeutic modalities include 2 per cent topical sodium cromoglycate solution, dapsone, sulfapyridine, minocycline, clofazimine, rifampin, thalidomide, and immunosuppressive agents such as cyclophosphamide or cyclosporine, but their efficacy requires further investigation and evaluation.

WELLS' SYNDROME (EOSINOPHILIC CELLULITIS)

Eosinophilic cellulitis (Wells' syndrome), a rare disorder first described by Wells in 1971, is an acute inflammatory cutaneous disorder characterized by recurrent sudden outbreaks of erythema-tous, often painful or pruritic, edematous urticaria-like or infiltrated eruptions, often with sharp rosy or violaceous borders (Fig. 25–30). Seen in children as well as adults, the disorder usually starts with a prodromal burning sensation or itching, spreads rapidly over 2 or 3 days, and gradually subsides to be replaced by a blue or slate-colored induration that persists for several weeks and then slowly fades, often leaving a temporary area of atrophy similar to that seen in patients with morphea. Although its etiology and pathogenesis are unknown, a number of triggering mechanisms such as insect bites, fungal infections, drug eruptions (particularly penicillin), or underlying hematologic disease suggest a hypersensitivity reaction as the cause of the disorder.[102, 103]

The clinical picture is striking, and the affected areas frequently resemble acute bacterial cellulitis, urticaria, insect bites, or a vesiculobullous contact dermatitis and may cover large areas of the limb, the face, or trunk. Histopathologic features, although not pathognomonic, evolve through several stages and are generally helpful in establishing the appropriate diagnosis. The acute stage is characterized by a dense cellular infiltrate composed predominantly of eosinophils and marked dermal edema. In the subacute stage, masses of histiocytes, eosinophils, and palisading

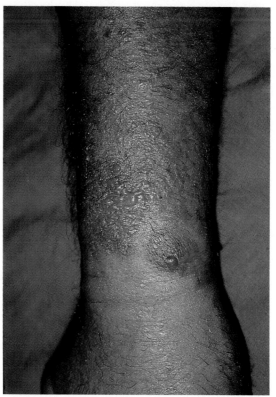

Figure 25–30. Wells' syndrome (eosinophilic cellulitis). Erythematous urticaria-like infiltrative lesions are shown on the forearm. (Courtesy of Kenneth E. Greer, M.D.)

Table 25–3. PYODERMA GANGRENOSUM

1. A severe, chronic, inflammatory disorder with a painful sloughing ulceration with a purulent base, an undermined elevated border, and a surrounding red areola
2. An immunologic abnormality (cell-mediated hypersensitivity or vasculitis?)
3. May be seen in association with ulcerative colitis, regional enteritis, chronic hepatitis, arthritis, and various paraproteinemias and hematologic disorders
4. *Treatment:* topical therapy, intralesional corticosteroids, systemic corticosteroids, dapsone, sulfapyridine, and perhaps rifampin, thalidomide, clofazimine, topical sodium cromoglycate or immunosuppressive therapy

Modified from Hurwitz S: The Skin and Systemic Disease in Children. Year Book Medical Publishers, Chicago, 1985.

giant cells may be seen around the fibrinoid collagen (these elongated areas of collagen with their bright red granular deposits of fibrin are referred to as "flame figures").

Although the prognosis of Wells' syndrome is generally excellent, and most lesions tend to fade spontaneously over a period of weeks to years, systemic corticosteroids hasten resolution and dapsone, griseofulvin, and colchicine have sometimes been found to be effective.

ANOREXIA NERVOSA AND BULIMIA

Anorexia nervosa and bulimia are severe disorders associated with potentially serious medical complications, psychiatric morbidity, and, at times, debilitating or deadly complications.[104, 105] In both disorders, patients have an intense preoccupation with food and attempt to lose weight by vomiting, abusing laxatives, diuretics, diet pills, or emetics. Cutaneous features include increased lanugo-like body hair, excessive loss of subcutaneous fat, pretibial or pedal pitting edema without hypoproteinemia, dry skin, brittle hair and nails, hypercarotenemia, and petechiae and purpura in association with hypoplastic bone marrow and thrombocytopenia. Emesis-associated complications include recurrent sore throats, hoarse voice, dental erosions, and characteristic hand lesions (elongated superficial ulcerations and hyperpigmented calluses or scars on the dorsal aspect of the hands, particularly the second and third fingers of one hand), the result of repeated abrasion of the skin against the maxillary incisors during self-induced emesis. Because of the potential severity of these disorders, it is important that physicians, particularly in view of the fact that patients tend to deny their illness or minimize the severity of their symptoms, recognize the early signs and symptoms of these potentially life-threatening conditions.

THE BATTERED CHILD

Although its true incidence is unknown, child abuse is an increasingly common cause of morbidity and mortality in childhood and has been termed the *battered child syndrome* by Kempe and his associates. It has been shown that 10 per cent of young children seen in emergency departments for injuries have findings that suggest physical abuse and an additional 10 per cent have injuries judged to be the result of gross neglect.[106, 107]

Child abuse may occur at any age but generally is reported in children younger than the age of 6, with the highest incidence in those younger than 3 years of age.

Affecting more than 2 million children a year, 2,000 to 5,000 children in the United States die annually of some form of physical abuse, and 90 to 95 per cent of all children suffering from child abuse have skin manifestations. The possibility of child neglect or abuse, therefore, should be considered in any child with unusual injuries. Particularly suspect are those with multiple abrasions, bruises, ecchymoses, lacerations, soft tissue hematomas, and multiple scars or fractures. Instances in which there is a delay in reporting the injury, in which the degree and type of injury are at variance with the history of trauma, or in which the parents are evasive or vague as to the cause of injury also are suspicious and should be investigated for the possibility of abuse.

Clinical Manifestations. The following characteristics help to distinguish skin lesions on the battered child from those of other cutaneous disorders. Ecchymoses and bruises on the hands and face, adult human bites, and bruises or scratches on the cheeks, mouth, lips, lower back, buttocks, or inner thighs are particularly suspect; and clustering of lesions on the face, head, trunk, buttocks, hands, or proximal extremities should alert the examiner to the possibility of child abuse. The configurations of lesions in battered children are morphologically similar to the implements used to inflict the trauma. Multiple evenly spaced marks, curvilinear loops, and arcuate lesions, as may be induced by lashing with a doubled-over belt, clothesline, or electric cord, are pathognomonic of traumatically induced lesions. They are usually ecchymotic, but they may also present as abrasions or lacerations.[108, 109] Shackles on the wrists, ankles, or neck leave easily identifiable rings, which are red if fresh and brown and hyperpigmented if of long standing. Ligature marks on the neck or extremities, bruises on the fingers, face, trunk, hand, or shoulders, and grab marks (fingertip bruises) on the shoulders, hands, or legs are particularly suspicious and should suggest the possibility of deliberate trauma. Other clues include the fact that the child does not look to its parent for comfort, poor medical compliance by the parents, and a general lack of warmth between mother and child.

Burns and traumatic bruises are the two most common injuries seen in child abuse. Burns induced by cigarettes, matches, or other heated objects are frequently mistaken for lesions of impetigo. Cigarette burns leave "dug-out" craters, and linear contact burns involving the buttocks, hands, and feet require careful investigation. It should be noted that children will not stay in contact with a hot surface or scalding hot water. They normally test the heat of the water and step into the bath with one foot at a time. Accordingly, symmetrical burns on the feet (particularly the dorsal aspect), the buttocks, or hands require careful investigation and evaluation. Other forms of contact burn include those induced by holding the child against a hot radiator, hot comb, or hair dryer. These burns follow the contour of the heated object, and, in many cases, failure to thrive, malnutrition, dehydration, and poor skin hygiene may complete the picture.

Bite marks are another pathognomonic sign of nonaccidental trauma. The human bite is differentiated easily from the dog bite by its contusing and crushing characteristics; dog bites rip and tear the flesh. Traumatic alopecia may occur when the parent pulls the child's hair, since the hair often provides a handle that can be used to grab or jerk at the child. This type of injury is analogous to dislocated joints or other physical injuries that occur as a result of twisting or wrenching an extremity.[108]

Treatment. Management of child abuse or neglect requires a high index of suspicion on the part of the examining physician. Although there is frequently great reluctance to believe that injuries are deliberately inflicted, traumatic lesions of a suspicious nature require consultation with child abuse experts and full investigation as soon as possible. The patient's chart should be tagged with some distinctive coding so that future injury will not be overlooked, all siblings should be examined as soon as possible, the incident should be reported to a protective agency, and psychiatric evaluation should be obtained as soon as possible.

If the child is considered to be at risk, hospitalization may be vital for protection as well as diagnostic assessment. Management of cutaneous lesions is generally symptomatic, with careful attention to prevention of infection and, when indicated, to improved nutrition and hygiene. History or physical evidence of ecchymoses, contusions, or easy bruisability requires complete skeletal survey for the possibility of old or new fractures and a complete workup for bleeding disorders, including platelet counts and bleeding, clotting, prothrombin, and thromboplastin times.

Once a diagnosis of child abuse or neglect has been established, treatment requires intensive cooperation between the physician, family, and social agency. Although battered children generally do better when they are able to remain with their parents and siblings while the family receives intensive psychiatric and social assistance, permanent removal of the child from the parents' care must be considered when the likelihood of parental response to treatment seems remote. On the other hand, one must also be attuned to the fact that public opinion and social awareness, having increased considerably in recent years, may occasionally precipitate overzealous action with little regard to the parents' claims and feelings. It is imperative, therefore, that disorders such as phytophotodermatitis, mongolian spots, cupping or coin rubbing (Cao-Gio), osteogenesis imperfecta, Ehlers-Danlos syndrome (Fig. 25–31), lichen sclerosus et atrophicus (see Figure 25–16), localized vulvar pemphigoid (an uncommon form of childhood bullous pemphigoid),[110] and other benign perianal or genital disorders not be mis-

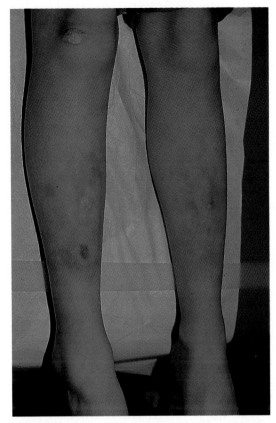

Figure 25–31. Ehlers-Danlos disease in a young girl. The parents were accused of child abuse for 2 years before the true nature of the dermatosis was discovered. (Courtesy of Marilyn Jones, M.D.)

diagnosed, confused with, or misinterpreted as child abuse.[111, 112]

References

1. Sagher R, Even-Paz Z: Mastocytosis and the Mast Cell. Year Book Medical Publishers, Chicago, 1967.

   An encyclopedic appraisal of mastocytosis, the mast cell, and its physiologic and pathologic processes.

2. Demis DJ: The mastocytosis syndrome: Clinical and biological studies. Ann. Intern. Med. 59:194–206, 1963.

   Symptoms of the mastocytosis syndrome can be correlated with increased excretion of histamine.

3. Selmanowitz VJ, Orentreich NO, Tiagco CC, et al.: Uniovular twins discordant for cutaneous mastocytosis. Arch. Dermatol. 102:34–41, 1970.

   A report of uniovular twins discordant for cutaneous mastocytosis, with discussion of the genetic patterns of this disorder.

4. Selmanowitz VJ, Orentreich NO: Mastocytosis: A clinical genetic evaluation. J. Hered. 61:91–94, 1970.

   Of the more than 600 cases of mastocytosis that have been reported, 40 known familial cases suggest a possible genetic etiology to this disorder.

5. Boyano T, Carrascosa T, Val J, et al.: Urticaria pigmentosa

in monozygotic twins. Arch. Dermatol. *126*:1375–1376, 1990.

A report of monozygotic twins who presented simultaneously with urticaria pigmentosa.

6. Oku T, Hashizume H, Yokote R, et al.: The familial occurrence of bullous mastocytosis (diffuse cutaneous mastocytosis). Arch. Dermatol. *126*:1478–1484, 1990.

A report of three children and their mother with diffuse cutaneous mastocytosis suggests the presence of an autosomal dominant trait of genetic inheritance in some patients with this disorder.

7. Orkin M, Good RA, Clawson CC, et al.: Bullous mastocytosis. Arch. Dermatol. *101*:547–564, 1970.

A review of bullous mastocytosis, its differential diagnosis, clinical course, and prognosis.

8. Keahy TM: The pathogenesis of urticaria. Dermatol. Clin. *3*:13–28, 1985.

A comprehensive review of the pathogenesis of urticaria and physiologic compounds known to be capable of inducing mast cell degranulation.

9. Burkhardt GG: Letters to the editor: Benign mastocytomas. Arch. Dermatol. *118*:449–450, 1982.

A 4-month-old male infant with nine "solitary" mastocytomas.

10. Lantis SH, Koblenzer PH: Solitary mast cell tumor: Progression to disseminated urticaria pigmentosa in a Negro infant. Arch. Dermatol. *99*:60–63, 1969.

Although solitary mastocytosis is considered to be the most benign form of mastocytosis, an unusual progression to widespread urticaria pigmentosa is reported.

11. Klaus SN, Winkelman RK: Course of urticaria pigmentosa in children. Arch. Dermatol. *86*:116–119, 1962.

Twenty-six patients with mastocytosis with onset in the first decade of life support the supposition that urticaria pigmentosa in children is almost always a cutaneous disorder that resolves spontaneously.

12. Hurwitz S: The Skin and Systemic Disease in Children. Year Book Medical Publishers, Chicago, 1985.

An overview of the cutaneous manifestations of systemic disorders of childhood.

13. Caplan RM: Urticaria pigmentosa and systemic mastocytosis. J.A.M.A. *194*:1077–1080, 1965.

A review of urticaria pigmentosa, its clinical manifestations, and its prognosis.

14. Keyzer JJ, de Monchy JGR, von Doormal JJ, et al.: Improved diagnosis of mastocytosis by measurement of urinary histamine metabolites. N. Engl. J. Med. *309*:1603–1605, 1983.

In a study of eight patients with mastocytosis, although urinary histamine metabolites were found to be increased in patients with systemic involvement, except for one patient with widespread deeply infiltrated lesions, skin involvement alone was usually not associated with elevated histamine metabolite levels.

15. Fromer JL, Jaffe N, Paed D: Urticaria pigmentosa and acute lymphoblastic leukemia. Arch. Dermatol. *107*:283–284, 1973.

The coexistence of acute lymphoblastic leukemia in a child with urticaria pigmentosa.

16. Burgoon CF, Graham JH, McCafree DL: Mast cell disease: A cutaneous variant with multisystem involvement. Arch. Dermatol. *98*:590–605, 1968.

A review of eight patients with evidence of diffuse cutaneous mastocytosis and widespread systemic disease suggests a more guarded prognosis for patients with this variant of childhood mastocytosis.

17. Kendall ME, Fields JP, King LE Jr: Cutaneous mastocytosis without clinically obvious skin lesions. J. Am. Acad. Dermatol. *10*:903–905, 1984.

A report of a woman with intractable pruritus who, despite an absence of cutaneous lesions, was found to have a proliferation of mast cells in her skin and increased urinary histamine and prostaglandin metabolite excretion, thus broadening the spectrum of mast cell disease and generalized pruritus.

18. Barklow SL, Marney SR: Mastocytosis: One year's experience. South. Med. J. *80*:51–54, 1987.

A review of 10 adult patients with systemic mastocytosis treated by a combination of H_1 and H_2 histamine antagonists. In the absence of skin lesions in all 10 patients, the diagnosis was made by cutaneous punch biopsy (the criterion for diagnosis was the presence of more than 10 mast cells per high power field).

19. Brownstein MH, Rabinowitz AD: The invisible dermatoses. J. Am. Acad. Dermatol. *8*:579–588, 1983.

An overview of the histopathologic approach to the diagnosis of a variety of dermatoses.

20. DiBacco RS, DeLee VA: Mastocytosis and the mast cells. J. Am. Acad. Dermatol. *7*:709–722, 1982.

An authoritative review of mastocytosis and mast cell disease.

21. Gerard JW, Ko C: Urticaria pigmentosa: Treatment with cimetidine and chlorpheniramine. J. Pediatr. *94*:843–844, 1979.

Chlorpheniramine (2.5 mg every 8 hours) and cimetidine (60 mg every 6 hours) were helpful in the management of a 3-year-old boy with bullous mastocytosis (when used in combination the results appeared to be better than either drug used alone).

22. Fenske NA, Lober CW, Pautler SE: Congenital bullous urticaria pigmentosa. Treatment with concomitant use of H_1- and H_2-receptor antagonists. Arch. Dermatol. *121*:115–118, 1985.

An infant with recurrent episodes of fever, irritability, decreased feeding, recurrent bullous formation, erosions with secondary infection, and septicemia was successfully managed by the concomitant use of cyproheptadine (0.25 mg/kg/day) and cimetidine (30 mg/kg/day).

23. Welch EA, Alper JC, Bogaars H, et al.: Treatment of bullous mastocytosis with disodium cromoglycate. J. Am. Acad. Dermatol. *9*:349–353, 1983.

A report of the use of oral cromolyn sodium (100 to 200 mg/day) for the control of pruritus, dermatographism, and bulla formation in two infants with bullous mastocytosis.

24. Frieri M, Alling DW, Metcalfe DD: Comparison of the therapeutic efficacy of cromolyn sodium with that of combined chlorphenamine and cimetidine in systemic mastocytosis: Results of a double-blind clinical trial. Am. J. Med. *78*:9–14, 1985.

In a double-blind study, although the cutaneous manifestations of systemic mastocytosis were well controlled by a combination of H_1 and H_2 antagonists, oral cromolyn sodium appeared to be more effective for the gastrointestinal symptoms in individuals with this disorder.

25. Fairley JA, Pentland AP, Voorhees JJ: Urticaria pigmentosa responsive to nifedipine. J. Am. Acad. Dermatol. *11*:740–743, 1984.

The successful use of nifedipine (10 mg three times a day) in the suppression of cold-induced urtication and flushing in a 20-year-old college student with urticaria pigmentosa suggests that calcium-channel blockers may represent a useful class of therapeutic agents for the management of mast cell release.

26. Czarnetzki BM: A double-blind cross-over study of the ef-

fect of ketotifen in urticaria pigmentosa. Dermatologica *166*:44–47, 1983.

Ketotifen (2 mg/day) was shown to be effective in the treatment of 10 adults with urticaria pigmentosa.

27. Barton J, Lavker RM, Schechter NM, et al.: Treatment of urticaria pigmentosa lesions with corticosteroids. Arch. Dermatol. *121*:1516–1523, 1984.

A report of successful treatment of individual lesions of urticaria pigmentosa by intralesional corticosteroids, 10 mg (0.25 ml) of triamcinolone acetonide (40 mg/ml) into individual lesions, 30 mg (0.75 ml) into a 5 × 1-cm linear band of confluent lesions, and topical 0.05 per cent betamethasone dipropionate (Diprolene) ointment under occlusion to areas of urticaria pigmentosa (8 hours daily for 6 weeks).

28. Guzzo C, Lavker R, Roberts LJ II, et al.: Urticaria pigmentosa: Systemic evaluation and successful treatment with topical steroids. Arch. Dermatol. *127*:191–196, 1991.

Seventeen patients with adult-onset urticaria pigmentosa treated with 0.05 per cent betamethasone dipropionate ointment over half the body under occlusion nightly for 6 weeks had almost complete resolution of their lesions; although slow return of lesions may occur after 6 months following the completion of therapy, the therapeutic response could be extended by topical corticosteroid application once a week.

29. Christophers E, Honigsmann H, Wolff K, et al.: PUVA-treatment of urticaria pigmentosa. Br. J. Dermatol. *98*:701–702, 1978.

Although nine adults and one child with urticaria pigmentosa responded to PUVA therapy, relapses occurred within 3 to 6 months after treatment was discontinued.

30. Kolde G, Frosch PJ, Czarnetzki BM: Response of cutaneous mast cells to PUVA in patients with urticaria pigmentosa: Histomorphic, ultrastructural, and biochemical investigations. J. Invest. Dermatol. *83*:175–178, 1984.

A comprehensive overview of PUVA therapy in the management of patients with urticaria pigmentosa.

30a. Kluin-Nelemans HC, Hanneke C: Response to interferon alfa-2b in a patient with systemic mastocytosis. N. Engl. J. Med. *326*:619, 1992.

A combination of alfa-2b interferon and prednisone may be helpful for the treatment of systemic mast cell disease.

31. Aberer E, Kollegger H, Kristoferitch W, et al.: Neuroborreliosis in morphea and lichen sclerosus et atrophicus. J. Am. Acad. Dermatol. *19*:820–825, 1988.

Although there is no general agreement about the spirochetal origin of morphea and lichen sclerosus et atrophicus, the isolation of *Borrelia* organisms (from one patient) and the detection of spirochetes on histologic sections and significant antibodies to *B. burgdorferi* (in 50 per cent of patients with morphea and 45 per cent of patients with lichen sclerosus et atrophicus) suggests that *Borrelia* infection may indeed be the cause, at least in some patients, of both disorders.

32. Hoesly J, Mertz LW, Winkelmann RK: Localized scleroderma (morphea) and antibody to *Borrelia burgdorferi*. J. Am. Acad. Dermatol. *17*:455–458, 1987.

ELISA and IFA studies in patients with morphea suggests that although there may not be a specific association with *B. burgdorferi* infection and morphea, patients with morphea who have cross-reacting circulating antibodies may eventually provide insight into the cause and pathogenesis of this disorder.

33. Uitto J, Santa Cruz DJ, Bauer EA, et al.: Morphea and lichen sclerosus et atrophicus. J. Am. Acad. Dermatol. *3*:271–279, 1980.

The coexistence of lesions of morphea and lichen sclerosus et atrophicus in 10 patients suggests that these two disorders may represent closely related pathologic processes.

34. Diaz-Perez JL, Connolly SM, Winkelmann RK: Disabling pansclerotic morphea of children. Arch. Dermatol. *116*:169–173, 1980.

A report of 14 children with a unique disabling syndrome of generalized morphea involving all levels of the skin (the dermis, panniculus, fascia) and at times even muscle and bone.

35. Woo TY, Rasmussen JE: Juvenile linear scleroderma associated with serologic abnormalities. Arch. Dermatol. *121*:1403–1405, 1985.

The finding of antinuclear antibody titers of 1:40 or greater in 13 of 24 patients with juvenile linear scleroderma (3 of whom had significant internal involvement), dermatomyositis, nephritis consistent with systemic lupus erythematosus, or Raynaud's phenomenon; rheumatoid factor titers of 1:20 or greater in 7 of 17 patients (5 of whom also had elevated antinuclear antibody titers); and 5 patients with antinuclear antibody and rheumatoid factor titers (2 of whom had systemic diseases such as nephritis and Raynaud's phenomenon) suggest long-term observation with periodic evaluation for patients with this disorder.

36. Falanga V, Medsger TA, Reichlin M: High titers of antibodies to single-stranded DNA in linear scleroderma. Arch. Dermatol. *121*:345–347, 1985.

Report of seven patients with severe linear scleroderma and high antibody titers to double-stranded DNA suggests that these antibodies may define a subgroup of patients with linear scleroderma who have more severe and extensive involvement of skin and underlying tissues.

37. Falanga V, Medsger TA Jr, Reichlin M, et al.: Linear scleroderma: Clinical spectrum, prognosis, and laboratory abnormalities. Ann. Intern. Med. *104*:849–857, 1986.

In a study of 53 patients with linear scleroderma, the presence of eosinophilia, antinuclear antibody and single-stranded DNA binding was correlated with active disease.

38. Soffa DJ, Sire DJ, Dodson JH: Melorheostosis with linear sclerodermatous skin changes. Radiology *114*:577–578, 1975.

A 5-year-old girl with linear morphea and radiologic evidence of melorheostosis, the 12th reported patient with overlying cutaneous changes of fewer than 200 reported cases of patients with melorheostosis.

39. Neldner KH: Treatment of localized scleroderma with phenytoin. Cutis *22*:569–572, 1978.

Phenytoin sodium (Dilantin) in dosages of 100 mg two or three times a day produced significant reversal of linear scleroderma in five patients, including one with the coup de sabre form of the disorder.

40. Czarnecki DB, Taft EH: Generalized morphea successfully treated with salazopyrine. Acta. Dermatol. Venereol. *62*:81–82, 1982.

Salazopyrine (Azulfidine) in a dosage of 1 g twice daily for 10 months induced remission of generalized morphea in a 60-year-old woman.

41. Falanga V, Medsger TA Jr: D-Penicillamine in the treatment of localized scleroderma. Arch. Dermatol. *126*:609–612, 1990.

Results in seven (64 per cent) of 11 patients with extensive localized scleroderma after long-term use of D-penicillamine suggests that this modality, although it has many side effects, may be used (if carefully monitored) for the treatment of patients with severe forms of localized scleroderma.

42. Wojnarowska F: Dermatomyositis induced by penicillamine. J. R. Soc. Med. *73*:884–886, 1980.

A 50-year-old woman with rheumatoid arthritis developed clinical evidence of dermatomyositis after 6 months of penicillamine therapy; the dermatomyositis slowly abated once the penicillamine was discontinued.

43. Uitto J, Jimenez S: Editorial: Fibrotic skin diseases: Clinical presentations, etiologic considerations, and treatment options. Arch. Dermatol. *126*:661–664, 1990.

A comprehensive review of the etiologic considerations and treatment options of various forms of fibrotic skin disease.

44. Chernosky ME, Derbes VJ, Burks JW Jr: Lichen sclerosis et atrophicus in children. Arch. Dermatol. *75*:647–652, 1957.

A survey of the literature with review of 35 cases and a report of four patients with childhood lichen sclerosus et atrophicus.

45. Clark JA, Muller SA: Lichen sclerosus et atrophicus in children: A report of 24 cases. Arch. Dermatol. *95*:476–482, 1967.

Of 24 children with lichen sclerosus et atrophicus, 70 per cent had the onset of the disorder prior to 7 years of age; of these 11 of 22 had spontaneous involution of lesions.

46. Wallace HJ: Lichen sclerosus et atrophicus. Trans. St. John's Hosp. Derm. Soc. *57*:9–30, 1971.

An extensive 20-year study of 395 patients with lichen sclerosus et atrophicus.

47. Tremaine RDL, Miller RAW: Lichen sclerosus et atrophicus. Int. J. Dermatol. *28*:10–16, 1989.

A comprehensive overview of the pathogenesis, clinical features, and therapy of lichen sclerosus et atrophicus.

48. Penneys NS: Treatment of lichen sclerosus with potassium para-aminobenzoate. J. Am. Acad. Dermatol. *10*:1039–1042, 1984.

A report of 5 patients in whom significant clinical improvement appeared after the administration of Potaba (2 to 4 g/day) suggests that potassium p-aminobenzoate may be a useful adjunct for the management of patients with symptomatic lichen sclerosus et atrophicus.

49. Greenberg LM, Geppert C, Worthen HG, et al.: Scleredema "adultorum" in children: Report of three cases with histochemical study and review of world literature. Pediatrics *32*:1044–1054, 1963.

A review of scleredema in childhood and its differentiation from scleroderma and dermatomyositis.

50. Heilbron B, Saxe N: Scleredema in an infant. Arch. Dermatol. *122*:1417–1419, 1986.

In a report of a biopsy-proven case of scleredema in a 3-month-old infant with fatal cytomegalovirus pneumonia it was speculated that the cause of death was related to decreased chest excursion caused by the scleredematous encasement of the skin.

51. Bradford WD, Cook CD, Vawter GF, et al.: Scleredema of childhood: Report of five cases. J. Pediatr. *68*:391–399, 1966.

In a review of 31 children and adults and a report of 5 children with scleredema most cases were preceded by an acute upper respiratory (particularly streptococcal) tract infection.

52. Fleischmajer R, Faludi G, Krol S: Scleredema and diabetes mellitus. Arch. Dermatol. *101*:21–26, 1970.

Of eight patients with scleredema, two had glucose tolerance and insulin assays typical of chemical or latent diabetes, six had overt maturity-onset diabetes, and five were known to have long-term diabetes (15 to 25 years in duration).

53. Cohn B, Whaler CE Jr, Briggaman RA: Scleredema adultorum of Buschke and diabetes mellitus. Arch. Dermatol. *101*:27–35, 1970.

Three patients with scleredema and diabetes mellitus of 15 to 20 years' duration suggests an association between these two disorders.

54. Venencie PY, Powell FC, Su WPD, et al.: Scleredema: A review of thirty-three cases. J. Am. Acad. Dermatol. *11*:128–134, 1984.

A comprehensive overview of scleredema, its clinical features, pathogenesis and management.

55. Ohta A, Uitto J, Oikarinen AI, et al.: Paraproteinemia in patients with scleredema: Clinical findings and serum effects on skin fibroblasts in vitro. J. Am. Acad. Dermatol. *16*:96–107, 1987.

A review of four patients with scleredema and paraproteinemia suggests that a variety of circulating factors in the serum, perhaps paraprotein, may enhance the synthesis of extracellular macromolecules by dermal fibroblasts, thus providing a mechanism for fibrosis.

56. Curtis AC, Shulak BM: Scleredema adultorum, not always a benign disease. Arch. Dermatol. *92*:526–541, 1965.

Contrary to previous concepts, 25 per cent of patients with scleredema adultorum showed either no improvement or only partial improvement 2 or more years after the onset of the disease.

57. Davis W: Wilson's disease and penicillamine-induced anetoderma. Arch. Dermatol. *113*:976, 1977.

A report of 2 brothers (3 and 15 years of age) with Wilson's disease who developed anetoderma, presumably as a complication of penicillamine (Cuprimine) therapy.

58. Canizares O, Sacks PM, Jaimovich L, et al.: Idiopathic atrophoderma of Pasini and Pierini. Arch. Dermatol. *77*:42–60, 1968.

A description of five cases of atrophoderma with separation of this disorder from morphea.

59. Jablonska S, Szczepanski A: Atrophoderma of Pasini and Pierini: Is it an entity? Dermatologica *125*:226–241, 1962.

A hypothesis that atrophoderma may be an abortive form of scleroderma in which the typical features of scleroderma fail to develop, perhaps because of a lack of autonomic nervous system involvement.

60. Berman A, Berman GD, Winkelmann RK; Atrophoderma (Pasini-Pierini): Findings on direct immunofluorescent, monoclonal antibody, and ultrastructural studies. Int. J. Dermatol. *27*:487–490, 1988.

Studies suggest that the pathogenesis of atrophoderma may be related to the presence of T lymphocytes and macrophages around dermal blood vessels and that this disorder may represent a form of morphea without sclerosis.

61. Sisson WR: Colored striae in adolescent children. J. Pediatr. *45*:520–540, 1954.

The occurrence of striae in nonobese adolescents (35 per cent of the girls and 15 per cent of the boys examined) appeared to be associated with an increase in 17-ketosteroids.

62. Stroud JD, Van Dersal JV: Striae. Arch. Dermatol. *103*:103–104, 1971.

A report of two patients with ulcerated striae believed to be related to high-dose systemic corticosteroids used for the treatment of dermatomyositis in one and, in the second, a topical formulation containing triamcinolone and an anticandidal agent (Mycolog) for the treatment of candidiasis in the inguinal area.

63. Barkey WF: Striae and persistent tinea corporis related to prolonged use of betamethasone dipropionate 0.05% cream/clotrimazole 1% cream (Lotrisone cream). J. Am. Acad. Dermatol. *17*:518–519, 1987.

The development of striae following prolonged use of a betamethasone dipropionate-clotrimazole formulation (Lotrisone) twice a day for a period of 8 months reaffirms the need for appropriate precautions in the use of high-dose corticosteroids.

64. Shuster S: The cause of striae distensae. Acta. Derm. Venereol. *59*:161–169, 1979.

Stretch and intradermal rupture and changes of interfibrillary materials such as glycosaminoglycans are hypothesized as important factors in the production of striae.

65. Elson ML: Treatment of striae distensae with topical tretinoin. J. Dermatol. Surg. Oncol. 16:267–270, 1990.

Daily application of 0.1 per cent Retin-A cream over a period of 12 weeks appeared to improve the appearance of striae in all but 1 of 16 patients.

66. Richards GE, Cavallo A, Meyers WJ III, et al.: Obesity, acanthosis nigricans, insulin resistance, and hyperandrogenemia: Pediatric perspective and natural history. J. Pediatr. 107:893–897, 1985.

A review of acanthosis nigricans, obesity, insulin resistance, and increased plasma testoserone levels in young women with female postmenarchal hyperandrogenemia.

67. Dix JH, Levy WJ, Fuenning C: Remission of acanthosis nigricans, hypertrichosis, and Hashimoto's thyroiditis with thyroxin replacement. Pediatr. Dermatol. 3:323–326, 1986.

A report of a 13-year-old girl with acanthosis nigricans, hypertrichosis, and Hashimoto's thyroiditis in whom the cutaneous lesions improved with thyroid hormone therapy suggests that hypothyroidism, in some patients at least, may be directly involved in the pathogenesis of acanthosis nigricans.

68. Barth JH, Ng LL, Wajnarowska F, et al.: Acanthosis nigricans, insulin resistance, and cutaneous virilism. Br. Dermatol. 118:613–619, 1988.

A study of 13 patients with hypoandrogenism, insulin resistance, and acanthosis nigricans.

69. Lerner AB: On the cause of acanthosis nigricans. N. Engl. J. Med. 281:106–107, 1969.

Peptide hormones from the pituitary gland or ectopically produced by a neoplasm as a possible cause of acanthosis nigricans.

70. Curth HO: The necessity of distinguishing four types of acanthosis nigricans. Proceedings, XIII Congress Internationalis Dermatologiae–München, Berlin, Springer-Verlag, 1967, 557–558.

Addition of a fourth benign type to the previously described forms of acanthosis nigricans.

71. Curth HO, Hilberg AW, Machacek GF: The site and histology of the cancer associated with malignant acanthosis nigricans. Cancer 15:364–382, 1962.

Acanthosis nigricans as a clue to internal adenocarcinoma.

72. Hamilton D, Tavafoghi V, Shafer JC, et al.: Confluent and reticulated papillomatosis of Gougerot and Carteaud: Its relation to other papillomatoses. J. Am. Acad. Dermatol. 2:401–410, 1980.

A report of four patients (two adolescents and two young adults) with confluent and reticulated papillomatosis and a comprehensive review of the literature.

73. Nordby CA, Mitchell AJ: Confluent and reticulated papillomatosis responsive to selenium sulfide. Int. J. Dermatol. 25:194–199, 1986.

A report of a 15-year-old black male adolescent with a 2½ year history of confluent and reticulated papillomatosis successfully treated with selenium sulfide.

74. Eyre WG, Carson WE: Linear porokeratosis of Mibelli. Arch. Dermatol. 105:426–429, 1972.

Two patients with porokeratosis of Mibelli in a linear distribution suggest a Koebner-type response in individuals genetically predisposed to this disorder.

75. Chernosky ME, Freeman RG: Disseminated superficial actinic porokeratosis (DSAP). Arch. Dermatol. 96:611–624, 1967.

Clinical and investigative studies in 31 patients with ultraviolet light–induced porokeratosis.

76. Guss SB, Osbourn RA, Lutzner MA: Porokeratosis plantaris, palmaris et disseminata. Arch. Dermatol. 104:366–373, 1971.

Eight patients in four generations of one family present a third variant of porokeratosis that could not be classified as either the Mibelli or Chernosky type.

77. James WD, Rodman OG: Squamous cell carcinoma arising in porokeratosis of Mibelli. Int. J. Dermatol. 25:389–391, 1986.

A review of 29 cases of malignant degeneration in lesions of porokeratosis of Mibelli (squamous cell carcinoma, Bowen's disease, and basal cell carcinoma) reaffirms the need for careful evaluation and removal, when possible, of lesions of porokeratosis.

78. Wadlington WB, Riley HD Jr, Lowbeer L: The Melkersson-Rosenthal syndrome. Pediatrics 73:502–506, 1984.

A report of four patients with the Melkersson-Rosenthal syndrome and the review of the pathology, clinical features, and management of this disorder.

79. Swerlick RA, Cooper PH: Cheilitis glandularis: Reevaluation. J. Am. Acad. Dermatol. 10:466–472, 1984.

A report of two adults and three children with actinic, atopic, or factitious cheilitis as an unusual reaction pattern to chronic irritation of the lips.

80. Yuzuk S, Trau H, Levy A, et al.: Melkersson-Rosenthal syndrome. Int. J. Dermatol. 24:456–457, 1985.

A report of a 13-year-old girl with progressive edema of the upper lips and a fissured tongue who, prior to the onset of the edema, suffered recurrent infections of the nose and sinuses.

81. Greene RM, Rogers RS III: Melkersson-Rosenthal syndrome: A review of 36 patients. J. Am. Acad. Dermatol. 21:1263–1270, 1990.

In a review of 36 patients with the Melkersson-Rosenthal syndrome, 8 of 14 biopsy specimens revealed histopathologic features of granulomatous cheilitis.

81a. Kano Y, Shiohara T, Yagita A, et al.: Treatment of recalcitrant cheilitis granulomatosa with metronidazole. J. Am. Acad. Dermatol. 27:629–630, 1992.

A report of a patient in whom oral metronidazole (Flagyl), 500 mg twice daily for three months, cleared not only the Crohn's disease but the cheilitis granulomatosa as well.

82. Allen CM, Camisa C, Hamzeh S, et al.: Cheilitis granulomatosa: Report of six cases and review of the literature. J. Am. Acad. Dermatol. 23:444–450, 1990.

A comprehensive review of cheilitis granulomatosa, its clinical and histologic features, and approach to therapy of this disorder.

83. Peck GL, Herzig GP, Elias PM: Toxic epidermal necrolysis in a patient with graft-vs-host reaction. Arch. Dermatol. 105:561–571, 1972.

Graft-versus-host reaction in a 22-year-old man with acute lymphocytic leukemia treated with allogeneic bone marrow transplantation results in toxic epidermal necrolysis.

84. Grogan TM, Odom RB, Burgess JH: Graft-vs-host reaction. Arch. Dermatol. 113:806–812, 1977.

Cutaneous biopsy as an aid to early diagnosis of graft-versus-host reaction.

85. Jampel RM, Farmer ER, Vogelsang GB, et al.: PUVA therapy for chronic cutaneous graft-vs-host disease. J. Am. Acad. Dermatol. 127:1673–1678, 1991.

Studies on six patients confirm PUVA as an effective and safe therapy for patients with cutaneous changes of lichenoid chronic graft-versus-host disease.

85a. Crawford CL: Thalidomide neuropathy. N. Engl. J. Med. 327:735, 1992.

The use of thalidomide for the treatment of graft-versus-host disease may result in neuropathy, a complication (seen in 25 per cent of patients) that may at times be severe and often is persistent.

86. Taplin D, Zaias N: Tropical immersion foot syndrome. Milit. Med. *131*:814, 1966.

A review of immersion foot in tropical climates and its differentiation from classic cold immersion foot.

87. Coskey RJ, Mehregan AH: Shoe boot pernio. Arch. Dermatol. *109*:56–57, 1974.

Pernio (chilblain) in young women due to cold and the wet lining of shoe boots.

88. Kelly JW, Dowling JP: Pernio: A possible association with chronic myelomonocytic leukemia. Arch. Dermatol. *121*:1048–1052, 1985.

A report of pernio in a man with chronic myelomonocytic leukemia and four retrospective cases suggests the possibility of a distinct relationship between the two disorders.

89. Dowd PM, Rustin MHA, Lanigan S: Nifedipine in the treatment of chilblains. Br. Med. J. *293*:923–924, 1986.

Nifedipine (20 mg three times a day) was found to be effective in the treatment of severe recurrent perniosis.

90. Thiers BH: Panniculitis. Dermatol. Clin. *1*:537–551, 1983.

A comprehensive overview of the panniculitides, their pathogenesis, classification, and therapy.

91. Aronson IK, Zeitz HJ, Variakojis D: Panniculitis in children. Pediatr. Dermatol. *5*:216–230, 1988.

A report of 4 new cases and a review of 23 additional cases of childhood panniculitis.

92. Silverman RA, Newman AJ, LeVine MJ, et al.: Poststeroid panniculitis: A case report. Pediatr. Dermatol. *5*:92–93, 1988.

A report of firm, red, subcutaneous plaques that developed on the cheeks of a 19-month-old girl during a 1-month period of rapid corticosteroid withdrawal.

93. Sorenson RU, Abramowsky CR, Stern RC: Ten-year course of early-onset Weber-Christian syndrome with recurrent pneumonia: A suggestion for pathogenesis. Pediatrics *78*:115–120, 1986.

A 10-year-old boy with infant-onset systemic Weber-Christian disease.

94. Novick NL: Aspartame-induced granulomatous panniculitis. Ann. Intern. Med. *102*:206–207, 1985.

A report of bilateral granulomatous nontender nodules on the legs of a 22-year-old woman with a history of daily consumption of 36 to 44 ounces of a saccharine-containing diet soft drink.

95. Smith KC, Su WPD, Pittelkow MR, et al.: Clinical and pathologic correlations in 96 patients with panniculitis, including 15 patients with deficient levels of alpha$_1$-antitrypsin. J. Am. Acad. Dermatol. *21*:1192–1196, 1989.

α_1-Antitrypsin levels in 96 patients with various forms of biopsy-proved panniculitis suggest that the clinical finding of panniculitis with ulceration and the histologic findings of acute inflammation, necrosis, hemorrhage, and elastic tissue degeneration justify evaluation for possible α_1-antitrypsin deficiency syndrome.

96. Braverman IM: Connective tissue (rheumatic) diseases. In Braverman, IM: Skin Signs of Systemic Disease. W.B. Saunders Co., Philadelphia, 1981, 255–377.

An overview of the cutaneous features seen in disorders of the connective tissue.

97. Zemer D, Pras M, Sohar E, et al.: Colchicine in the prevention and treatment of amyloidosis of familial Mediterranean fever. N. Engl. J. Med. *314*:1001–1005, 1986.

In a study of 1070 patients with familial Mediterranean fever, colchicine appeared to be effective in the prevention

of amyloidosis and additional deterioration of renal function in patients who had proteinuria without the nephrotic syndrome.

98. Shwaegerle SM, Bergfeld WF, Senitzer D, et al.: Pyoderma gangrenosum: A review. J. Am. Acad. Dermatol. *18*:559–568, 1988.

A comprehensive review of pyoderma gangrenosum, its pathophysiology, and currently available therapeutic approaches to the management of individuals with this disorder.

99. Prystkowsky JH, Kahn SN, Lazarus GS: Present status of pyoderma gangrenosum: Review of 21 cases. Arch. Dermatol. *125*:57–64, 1989.

A review of 22 patients with pyoderma gangrenosum emphasizes the importance of using optimal laboratory techniques for the detection of IgA monoclonal gammopathies in patients with this disorder and aggressive therapeutic approaches, particularly when vital structures are threatened.

100. Powell FC, Perry HO: Pyoderma gangrenosum in childhood. Arch. Dermatol. *120*:757–761, 1984.

In a review of eight children with pyoderma gangrenosum, removal of the affected bowel in three patients with inflammatory bowel disease was followed by complete remission of all cutaneous lesions.

101. Glass AT, Bancila E, Milgraum S: Pyoderma gangrenosum in infancy: The youngest reported patient. J. Am. Acad. Dermatol. *25*:109–110, 1991.

A report of a 7-month-old infant believed to be the youngest patient with pyoderma gangrenosum recorded in the English-language medical literature.

102. Nielsen T, Schmidt H, Søgaard H: Eosinophilic cellulitis (Wells' syndrome) in a child. Arch. Dermatol. *117*:427–429, 1981.

A report of an 11-year-old boy with eosinophilic cellulitis of the scalp who developed persistent atrophic alopecia during the regressive phase of the disorder.

103. Aberer W, Konrad K, Wolff K: Wells' syndrome is a distinctive disease entity and not a histologic diagnosis. J. Am. Acad. Dermatol. *18*:105–114, 1988.

A comprehensive review of Well's disease, its pathogenesis, clinical diagnosis, and therapy.

104. Gupta MA, Gupta AK, Haberman HF: Dermatologic signs in anorexia and bulimia nervosa. Arch. Dermatol. *123*:1386–1390, 1987.

Dermatologic changes in patients with anorexia nervosa and bulimia nervosa can serve as early signs of these severe and potentially dangerous eating disorders.

105. Williams JF, Friedman IM, Steiner H: Hand lesions characteristic of bulimia. Am. J. Dis. Child. *140*:28–29, 1986.

Characteristic cutaneous lesions on the hands can lead physicians to the diagnosis or exacerbation of symptoms in patients with bulimia.

106. Kempe CH, Silverman FN, Steele BF, et al.: The battered-child syndrome. J.A.M.A. *181*:17–24, 1962.

In a survey of 302 cases of physically abused children reported in 1 year, 85 resulted in permanent brain injury and 33 resulted in death.

107. Friedman SB, Morse CW: Child abuse: A five-year follow-up of early case findings in the emergency department. Pediatrics *54*:404–410, 1974.

A follow-up study of 156 children younger than 6 years of age with injuries believed to represent cases of suspected abuse, gross neglect, or possible accidental injury.

108. Ellerstein NE: The cutaneous manifestations of child abuse and neglect. Am. J. Dis. Child. *133*:906–909, 1979.

Cutaneous findings, the most easily recognizable physical manifestations of child abuse and neglect.

109. Schachner L, Hanken DE: Assessing child abuse in childhood condyloma acuminata. J. Am. Acad. Dermatol. *12*:157–160, 1985.

A check list of subjective and objective criteria for the evaluation of individuals suspected of suffering child abuse.

110. Levine V, Sanchez M, Nestor M: Localized vulvar pemphigoid in a child misdiagnosed as sexual abuse. Arch. Dermatol. *128*:804–806, 1992.

A 3-year-old girl with vulvar erosions misdiagnosed as a case of child abuse was inappropriately removed from her parent's care until the correct diagnosis of localized vulvar pemphigoid was made approximately 11 months later.

111. De Jong AR, Rose M: Frequency and significance of physical evidence in legally proven cases of child sexual abuse. Pediatrics *84*:1022–1026, 1989.

In a retrospective review of sexual abuse court records the authors conclude that physical evaluation in conjunction with the quality of the history obtained and the ability of the child to tell his or her story effectively will frequently determine the outcome of litigation.

112. Bays J, Jenny C: Genital and anal conditions confused with child sexual abuse trauma. Am. J. Dis. Child. *144*:1319–1322, 1990.

A review of seven children in whom dermatologic, traumatic, infectious, and congenital disorders were confused with sexual abuse.

INDEX

Note: Page numbers in *italics* refer to illustrations; page numbers followed by t refer to tables.